PRECLINICAL DEVELOPMENT HANDBOOK

Toxicology

PRECLINICAL DEVELOPMENT HANDBOOK

Toxicology

SHAYNE COX GAD, PH.D., D.A.B.T.
Gad Consulting Services
Cary, North Carolina

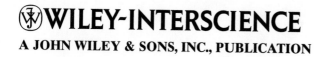

WILEY-INTERSCIENCE
A JOHN WILEY & SONS, INC., PUBLICATION

Published by John Wiley & Sons, Inc., Hoboken, New Jersey
Published simultaneously in Canada

For general information on our other products and services or for technical support, please contact
our Customer Care Department within the United States at (800) 762-2974, outside the United States
at (317) 572-3993 or fax (317) 572-4002.

Wiley also publishes its books in a variety of electronic formats. Some content that appears in print
may not be available in electronic formats. For more information about Wiley products, visit our web
site at www.wiley.com.

Library of Congress Cataloging-in-Publication Data is available.

ISBN: 978-0-470-24846-1

Printed in the United States of America

10 9 8 7 6 5 4 3 2 1

CONTRIBUTORS

Duncan Armstrong, AstraZeneca R & D, Alderley Park, Macclesfield, Cheshire, United Kingdom, *Secondary Pharmacodynamic Studies and* In Vitro *Pharmacological Profiling*

Michael Balls, FRAME, Nottingham, United Kingdom, *Preclinical Drug Development Planning*

Alan S. Bass, Schering-Plough Research Institute, Kenilworth, New Jersey, *Current Practices in Safety Pharmacology*

Nirmala Bhogal, FRAME, Nottingham, United Kingdom, *Preclinical Drug Development Planning*

C. Anita Bigger, U.S. Food and Drug Administration, Center for Drug Evaluation and Research, Silver Spring, Maryland, In Vitro *Mammalian Cell Mutation Assays*

Eric A. G. Blomme, Global Pharmaceutical Research and Development, Abbott Laboratories, Abbott Park, Illinois, *Genomics; Toxicogenomics in Preclinical Development*

Joanne M. Bowen, Royal Adelaide Hospital Cancer Centre, and University of Adelaide, Adelaide, South Australia, *Use of Project Teams in Preclinical Development; Relationship between Animal Models and Clinical Research: Using Mucositis as a Practical Example*

Joanne Bowes, AstraZeneca R & D, Alderley Park, Macclesfield, Cheshire, United Kingdom, *Secondary Pharmacodynamic Studies and* In Vitro *Pharmacological Profiling*

William J. Brock, Brock Scientific Consulting, LLC, Montgomery Village, Maryland, *Regulatory Issues in Preclinical Safety Studies (U.S. FDA)*

Arie Bruinink, Materials–Biology Interactions, Materials Science & Technology (EMPA), St. Gallen, Switzerland, In Vitro *Toxicokinetics and Dynamics: Modeling and Interpretation of Toxicity Data*

Maribel E. Bruno, National Center for Toxicogenomics, National Institute of Environmental Health Sciences, Research Triangle Park, North Carolina, *Toxicoproteomics: Preclinical Studies*

Juan Casado, Spanish National Cancer Center (CNIO), Madrid, Spain, *Proteomics*

J. Ignacio Casal, Spanish National Cancer Center (CNIO), Madrid, Spain, *Proteomics*

José A. Centeno, Armed Forces Institute of Pathology, Washington, DC, *Toxicologic Pathology*

Robert Combes, FRAME, Nottingham, United Kingdom, *Preclinical Drug Development Planning*

Mary Ellen Cosenza, Amgen Inc., Thousand Oaks, California, *Safety Assessment of Biotechnology-Derived Therapeutics*

Mark Crawford, Cerep, Redmond, Washington, *Secondary Pharmacodynamic Studies and* In Vitro *Pharmacological Profiling*

Dipankar Das, University of Alberta, Edmonton, Alberta, Canada, *Preclinical Development of Protein Pharmaceuticals: An Overview*

N.J. Dent, Country Consultancy Ltd., Copper Beeches, Milton Malsor, United Kingdom, *Auditing and Inspecting Preclinical Research and Compliance with Good Laboratory Practice (GLP)*

Jacques Descotes, Poison Center and Claude Bernard University, Lyon, France, *Safety Assessment Studies: Immunotoxicity*

Krista L. Dobo, Pfizer Global R&D, Groton, Connecticut, In Vivo *Genotoxicity Assays*

Shayne Cox Gad, Gad Consulting Services, Cary, North Carolina, *Repeat Dose Toxicity Studies; Irritation and Local Tissue Tolerance Studies in Pharmaceutical Safety Assessment; Carcinogenicity Studies; Bridging Studies in Preclinical Pharmaceutical Safety Assessment*

Rachel J. Gibson, Royal Adelaide Hospital Cancer Centre, and University of Adelaide, Adelaide, South Australia, *Use of Project Teams in Preclinical Development; Relationship between Animal Models and Clinical Research: Using Mucositis as a Practical Example*

Gary A. Gintant, Abbott Laboratories, Abbott Park, Illinois, *Current Practices in Safety Pharmacology*

Robin C. Guy, Robin Guy Consulting, LLC, Lake Forest, Illinois, *Drug Impurities and Degradants and Their Safety Qualification*

Andreas Hartmann, Novartis Pharma AG, Basel, Switzerland, In Vivo *Genotoxicity Assays*

Kenneth L. Hastings, sanofi-aventis, Bethesda, Maryland, *Regulatory Issues in Preclinical Safety Studies (U.S. FDA)*

Ronald D. Hood, Ronald D. Hood & Associates, Toxicology Consultants, Tuscaloosa, Alabama; and Department of Biological Sciences, Tuscaloosa, Alabama, *Reproductive and Developmental Toxicology*

Robert H. Heflich, U.S. Food and Drug Administration, National Center for Toxicological Research, Jefferson, Arkansas, In Vitro *Mammalian Cell Mutation Assays*

Dorothy M. K. Keefe, Royal Adelaide Hospital Cancer Centre, and University of Adelaide, Adelaide, South Australia, *Use of Project Teams in Preclinical Development; Relationship between Animal Models and Clinical Research: Using Mucositis as a Practical Example*

Joanne R. Kopplin, Druquest International, Inc., Leeds, Alabama, *Selection and Utilization of CROs for Safety Assessment*

Prekumar Kumpati, University of Pittsburgh, Pittsburgh, Pennsylvania, *Bacterial Mutation Assay*

Duane B. Lakings, Drug Safety Evaluation, Inc., Elgin, Texas, *Regulatory Considerations*

Hans-Jörg Martus, Novartis Pharma AG, Basel, Switzerland, In Vivo *Genotoxicity Assays*

B. Alex Merrick, National Center for Toxicogenomics, National Institute of Environmental Health Sciences, Research Triangle Park, North Carolina, *Toxicoproteomics: Preclinical Studies*

Jacques Migeon, Cerep, Redmond, Washington, *Secondary Pharmacodynamic Studies and* In Vitro *Pharmacological Profiling*

Martha M. Moore, U.S. Food and Drug Administration, National Center for Toxicological Research, Jefferson, Arkansas, In Vitro *Mammalian Cell Mutation Assays*

Dennis J. Murphy, GlaxoSmithKline Pharmaceuticals, King of Prussia, Pennsylvania, *Current Practices in Safety Pharmacology*

Robert M. Parker, Hoffmann-LaRoche, Inc., Nutley, New Jersey, *Reproductive and Developmental Toxicology*

Hans-Gerd Pauels, Dr. Pauels—Scientific and Regulatory Consulting, Münster, Germany, *Immunotoxicity Testing: ICH Guideline S8 and Related Aspects*

Roger Porsolt, Porsolt & Partners Pharmacology, Boulogne-Billancourt, France, *Current Practices in Safety Pharmacology*

R. Julian Preston, National Health and Environmental Effects Research Laboratory, U.S. Environmental Protection Agency, Research Triangle Park, North Carolina, In Vitro *Mammalian Cytogenetic Tests*

Ronald E. Reid, University of British Columbia, Vancouver, British Columbia, Canada, *The Pharmacogenomics of Personalized Medicine*

Ward R. Richter, Druquest International, Inc., Leeds, Alabama, *Selection and Utilization of CROs for Safety Assessment*

Michael G. Rolf, AstraZeneca R & D, Alderley Park, Macclesfield, Cheshire, United Kingdom, *Secondary Pharmacodynamic Studies and* In Vitro *Pharmacological Profiling*

Dimitri Semizarov, Global Pharmaceutical Research and Development, Abbott Laboratories, Abbott Park, Illinois, *Genomics; Toxicogenomics in Preclinical Development*

Evan B. Siegel, Ground Zero Pharmaceuticals, Inc., Irvine, California, *Regulatory Considerations*

Peter K.S. Siegl, Merck Research Laboratories, West Point, Pennsylvania, *Current Practices in Safety Pharmacology*

Sonu Sundd Singh, Nektar Therapeutics India Private Limited, Secunderabad, India, *Toxicokinetics: An Integral Component of Preclinical Toxicity Studies*

Mavanur R. Suresh, University of Alberta, Edmonton, Alberta, Canada, *Preclinical Development of Protein Pharmaceuticals: An Overview*

John Taylor, ProPhase Development Ltd, Harrogate, United Kingdom, *Immunotoxicity Testing: ICH Guideline S8 and Related Aspects*

Paul B. Tchounwou, Jackson State University, Jackson, Mississippi, *Toxicologic Pathology*

Jean-Pierre Valentin, AstraZeneca R & D, Alderley Park, Macclesfield, Cheshire, United Kingdom, *Secondary Pharmacodynamic Studies and* In Vitro *Pharmacological Profiling*

Jeffrey F. Waring, Global Pharmaceutical Research and Development, Abbott Laboratories, Abbott Park, Illinois, *Toxicogenomics in Preclinical Development*

CONTENTS

PREFACE

This *Preclinical Development Handbook: Toxicology* focuses on the methods of identifying and understanding the risks that are associated with new potential drugs for both large and small therapeutic molecules. This book continues the objective behind this entire *Handbook* series: an attempt to achieve a through overview of the current and leading-edge nonclinical approaches to evaluating the nonclinical safety of potential new therapeutic entities. Thanks to the persistent efforts of Mindy Myers and Gladys Mok, the 31 chapters cover the full range of approaches to identifying the potential toxicity issues associated with the seemingly unlimited range of new molecules. These evaluations are presented with a thorough discussion of how the approaches fit into the mandated regulatory requirements for safety evaluation as mandated by the U.S. Food and Drug Administration and other regulatory authorities. They range from studies on potential genotoxicity and cardiotoxicity in cultured cells to a two-year study in rats and mice to identify potentially tumorigenic properties.

The volume differs from the others in this series in that although the methods used by the researchers are fixed by regulation at any one time, these methods are increasingly undergoing change as it is sought to become ever more effective at identifying potential safety issues before they appear in patient populations. Although we will never achieve perfection in this area, we continue to investigate new ways of trying to do so.

1

PRECLINICAL DRUG DEVELOPMENT PLANNING

Nirmala Bhogal, Robert Combes, and Michael Balls

FRAME, Nottingham, United Kingdom

Contents

1.1   INTRODUCTION

1.1.1   Overview of Objectives

It is well recognized that productivity in drug development has been disappointing over the last decade, despite the steady increase in R&D investment [1] and advances in techniques for producing potentially new candidate molecules. The principal problems appear to be a lack of efficacy and/or unexpected adverse reactions, which account for the majority of drug withdrawals and drugs undergoing clinical testing being abandoned. This high attrition rate could be dramatically reduced by improving the preclinical testing process, particularly by taking account of multidisciplinary approaches involving recent technologies, and by improving the design of preclinical projects to facilitate the collection and interpretation of relevant information from such studies, and its extrapolation to the clinical setting.

The objective of this chapter is to provide an overview of the early drug discovery and development processes. The main focus is the use of *in vitro* and *in silico* methods. This is because these techniques are generally applied during the earliest stages to identify new targets (target discovery) and lead compounds (drug discovery), as well as for subsequent drug development. They are also used to resolve equivocal findings from *in vivo* studies in laboratory animals, to guide selection of the most appropriate preclinical *in vivo* models, and to help define the mechanistic details of drug activity and toxicity. However, the use of animals in preclinical testing is also considered, since animal data form part of new medicine dossiers submitted to regulatory bodies that authorize clinical trials and the marketing of new products. The drug development process that will be considered is shown in Fig. 1.1. Definitions of the terminology and abbreviations/acronyms used in this chapter are listed in Table 1.1.

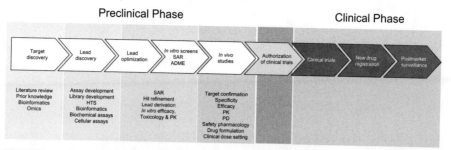

FIGURE 1.1   The key stages of drug discovery and development. A typical series of methods and strategies uses preclinical phases. Note that some of the studies may not be required and the process can be iterative. Refer also to Fig. 1.2 for a more detailed description of toxicity testing planning.

1.1.2   Drug Development Models

An essential part of drug development is the selection of the most appropriate animal, *ex vivo*, *in vitro*, or *in silico* systems, to allow the collection of information that can be interpreted in terms of the effects of a new therapeutic agent in humans or in one or more subpopulations of humans. There are several deciding factors that guide model selection. During early drug discovery screening, the main consideration is whether the chosen model can cope with large libraries of potentially bioactive molecules. It is generally accepted that, while nonanimal models generally lack the sophistication of studies on vertebrate animals and are based on nonclinical endpoints, they are a useful means of filtering out poor candidates during early drug discovery. The possibility of false hits during this stage is accepted as a trade-off, but it is also recognized that data from the use of several techniques and prior information can assist with the weeding out of false hits. The drug development process involves a more extensive evaluation using *in vitro* and *in silico* approaches and preclinical studies in vertebrate animals on a limited number of potential therapeutic agents.

The drive toward the use of systems biology approaches that take into account the roles of multiple biological and physiological body systems earlier in the drug development process has prompted a dramatic change in the way that data from cell-based studies are used. In many instances, data from several tests can be assembled and analyzed by using *in silico* models to gain a systems biology overview of drug ADMET and activity. Advances in comparative genomics have also opened up the scope for using zebra fish (*Brachydanio rerio*) and invertebrate organisms, such as nematode worms (*C. elegans*) and the fruit fly, *Drosophila melanogaster*, during the early stages of drug development. Likewise, advances in information mining, bioinformatics, data interpretation, the omics technologies, cell culture techniques, and molecular biology have the potential to greatly enhance the drug development process. Ironically, up to now, few of these methodologies has been standardized, formally validated, and accepted for regulatory use. Indeed, *in vitro* data are generally considered supplementary to animal data, rather than as an alternative source of information that is useful and applicable in its own right. Nevertheless, *in vitro* approaches provide information about the mechanisms of action

TABLE 1.1 Terminology and Abbreviations

Term	Definition
2D heteronuclear NMR	Two radionuclides are used to construct a two-dimensional map of a binding site by NMR.
Agglomeration	The process of particle attraction and adhesion.
Algorithm	A set of rules to assist with problem solving.
Allometric scaling	The process by which size, blood volume, and anatomical features of an organism are taken into account during extrapolation of information from animals to humans.
Analogue-based minimization	The process of using information about variants of the natural ligand for a target to derive a minimum number of features required of a smaller substance, so that binding affinity, efficacy, and/or specificity for the target in question are retained.
Antisense	A piece of genetic material that is the exact opposite of the natural messenger RNA that encodes a potential protein.
Bioaccumulation	The buildup of a drug or its metabolite(s) in a particular tissue or cell type.
Bioavailability	A measure of the amount of an administered drug that reaches its intended site of action.
Bioinformatics	The management and analysis of information, in order to use computer-based processes to understand biological events.
Biokinetic	Describes the key physiological processes that follow the exposure of an organism to a chemical or drug.
Biomarker	A molecular indicator of a biological event.
Biotechnology product	Replacement therapeutics or recombinant protein or DNA products isolated from or produced by using GM animals, cell cultures, plants, or microorganisms.
Biotransformation	The process by which a substance is chemically or functionally modified within the body, which usually involves the action of specific enzymes.
Combinatorial library	Large libraries of chemicals generated by a combination of acquisition and understanding of the requirements for recognition of a particular target.
Comparative genomics	The study of human genetics by reference to the genetics of other organisms as a means of deciphering human gene organization and function.
Cytotoxicity	A measure of the ability of a substance to damage or kill a cell.
Decision tree	A support tool for selection among competing choices and their possible consequences.
DNAzymes	A DNA-modifying enzyme.
Drug mimetic	A drug or drug-like molecule with a structure or modulatory activity that resembles that of a substance found within the body.
Druggable genome	The sum of the genes, their encoded disease-related proteins, or gene expression regulatory elements, which can functionally be modulated by drugs and drug-like molecules.

Druggable proteins — Proteins that bind drugs with a binding affinity below 10μM.

Drug discovery — The identification of a potential therapeutic agent.

Drug development — The progress of a lead from drug discovery toward a marketable drug.

Drug-like compound — A compound that has a molecular weight typical of a drug (around 500 daltons) and a structure that indicates it may have pharmaceutical properties.

Efficacy — The capacity of an agent to cause the desired biological effect.

Endpoint — The measurable effect of a substance on a biological system.

Epitope — The recognition site on a molecule for a particular molecule or class of molecules.

Eukaryotic — Describes organisms whose cells possess a nucleus and other membrane-bound vesicles, including fungi, plants, and animals.

Ex vivo — Literally, "out of the living"—used to refer to experiments that are conducted on tissues or cells isolated directly from a living organism.

Gene silencing — The process of preventing a gene from being expressed.

Genome — The entire genetic makeup of an organism.

Genomics — The study of the genetic makeup of an organism.

Genotoxicity — The adverse effects of a substance on the genetic makeup of a cell or organism.

Glucuridonation — The process of conjugating the uronic acid of glucose to substances, to detoxify or inactivate them.

Hapten — A substance that must combine with a carrier, in order to induce specific antibody production.

Hematotoxicity — The adverse effects of a substance on blood cells or on the cells or processes that produce specific types of blood cells.

Hit — The product of the high-throughput screening of large libraries of drug-like compounds, fragments, peptides, or proteins, identified by predominantly one-shot affinity, activity, or *in silico* methods.

Homeobox — DNA sequences found throughout the genome of most organisms that regulate gene expression, particularly during early development.

Homolog — A molecule with corresponding structures or functions in two or more species.

Humanized — The product of a process that is aimed to confer more human-like properties on a molecule, cell, or living organism.

Hydrophobicity — The tendency of a molecule to repel or exclude water molecules. (Means the same as lipophilicity.)

Immunogenicity — The ability of a substance to stimulate an immune response.

Immunohistochemistry — The testing of the ability of a tissue to be stained with an antibody.

Immunoprecipitation — The ability of an antibody–molecule complex to pull a second molecule out of solution as a result of interactions between the antibody recognizing molecule and secondary molecule.

Indels — Insertional or deletion mutations in DNA.

In silico — Using computer-based methods and virtual systems.

In vitro — Literally, "in glass"—used to refer to maintenance of tissues, cells, or cell fractions outside the body from which they were derived.

TABLE 1.1 *Continued*

Term	Definition
In vivo	Literally, "within the living"—used to refer to experiments conducted on intact living organisms.
Isozyme	Variants of enzymes that catalyze the same reaction(s) but differ from each other in primary structure and/or electrophoretic mobility.
Karyotype	The chromosomal complement of an organism.
Lead compound	A compound identified by hit generation that has suitable physicochemical and functional properties to serve as a starting point for the development of a potentially marketable drug.
Lipophilicity	The affinity of a molecule for a lipophilic environment.
Log P	The octan-1-ol/water partition coefficient—used to express lipophilicity.
Macroparticle	Particulate matter of a crystalline nature, generally exceeding a 10 nm diameter.
Margin of safety (MOS)	A ratio of the maximum amount of a substance that causes no effect in animals and the actual exposure (intended or otherwise) of the human population.
Meta-analysis	A statistical process for combining information from different sources.
Metabolic competence	The ability of a system to metabolize.
Metabonomics	The study of metabolic responses to drugs and chemicals.
Microfluidics	Small-scale systems comprised of chambers connected by a fluid matrix.
Molecular dynamics	Computer simulations of the movement of atoms, based on changes in the energy required to maintain certain conformations.
Monte Carlo simulation	A statistical method for studying systems, especially those with large numbers of coupled degrees of freedom.
Nanomedicines	Therapeutic agents based on the use of nanoparticles.
Nanoparticle	A microscopic particle with a unit size not exceeding 100 nm.
Oligonucleotide	A short stretch of synthetic DNA.
Omics	Technologies relating to the study of the genome, proteome, or metabolic responses of cells, tissues, and organisms.
Organotypic	An *in vitro* system designed to preserve or reconstitute the 3D structure of a tissue or organ, to mimic the *in vivo* situation.
Patch clamping	A process for measuring electrical activity across a living membrane by using electrodes.
Permeability	The ability to cross a living membrane.
Phage display	A system whereby a protein is displayed on the surface of a bacterial virus (a bacteriophage).
Phagocytic	Describes the engulfing of a molecule, a microorganism or part of an organism, by leukocytes (a type of white blood cell).
Pharmacokinetic	Describes the uptake, biotransformation, and distribution of a pharmaceutical agent and its metabolites in the tissues, and their subsequent elimination.
Pharmacophore	A collection of electrical and molecular features that define interactions between a molecule and its binding site on its target.

6

Plasma clearance rate	The speed at which a substance is removed from the blood.
Polymorphisms	Genetic differences within the population that occur for a given gene at a frequency of 1% or more.
Posttranslational modification	The process by which a protein is altered after it is synthesized, by the additional or removal of specific moieties.
Potency	The comparative ability of a drug to induce the desired effect.
Prokaryote	Cellular organisms that lack a distinct nuclear membrane or membrane-bound organelles (e.g., bacteria).
Proteome	The total protein complement encoded by the genome of an organism.
Proteomics	The study of protein expression patterns in specific cells, tissues, or organisms.
Quantum dot	Nanocrystals comprised of a semiconductor metal core.
Reactive oxygen species	Oxygen radicals or super-radicals that are capable of causing cellular damage.
Recombinant DNA technology	The process of DNA manipulation in an artificial environment.
Redox	The process of loss of oxygen or gain of hydrogen by one molecule accompanied by the gain of oxygen or loss of hydrogen by another molecule.
Reporter gene	A gene that is expressed in response to an upstream biochemical event, which can be used to monitor that event.
Reverse pharmacology	The screening of a library of compounds against one particular target to identify a lead for drug development.
RNA aptamers	RNA-based molecules that bind to enzymes.
RNAi	RNA interference—process of silencing or dampening protein expression.
Signal-to-noise ratio	Measure of the signal strength (change being observed) against the background within an experiment.
Therapeutic agent	A chemical, protein/peptide, DNA, stem cell, natural product, or biotechnology product that forms the active component of a finished pharmaceutical product.
Therapeutic index	The ratio between the toxic dose and the therapeutic dose of a drug, which is related to the MOS.
Three Rs	The principles of *replacement* of animal experiments, *reduction* of the number of animals used in a given study, or *refinement* of the procedures used, in order to minimize suffering and distress.
Toxicogenomics	The use of genomics and bioinformatics to identify and characterize mechanisms of action, based on changes in gene expression as monitored by the production of mRNA transcripts.
Toxicokinetic	Describes the uptake, biotransformation, distribution, and effects of a directly or indirectly toxic substance and its metabolites in the tissues, and their subsequent elimination.
Transcription	The process of messenger RNA production from a gene.
Transgene	A gene or variant of a gene that is inserted into the genetic makeup of an organism.
Vector DNA/RNA	Carrier DNA/RNA that may also facilitate the expression and/or cellular uptake of foreign genetic material by cells and tissues.
Xenobiotic	A chemical or other substance that is not a natural component of the makeup of the organism exposed to it.

TABLE 1.1 *Continued*

Abbreviation/Acronym	Full Name
ADME(T)	absorption, Distribution, Metabolism, Elimination (Toxicity)
ADR	Adverse Drug Reaction
BBB	Blood–Brain Barrier
BCS	Biopharmaceutics Classification System
BRET	Bioluminescent Resonance Energy Transfer
cAMP	Cyclic Adenosine Monophosphate
CASE	Computer Automated Structure Evaluation
CBER	Center for Biologics, Evaluation and Research
CDER	Center for Drugs, Evaluation and Research
CoMFA	Comparative Molecular Field Analysis
COMPACT	Computerized Optimized Parametric Analysis of Chemical Toxicology
CRE	Cyclic-amp Responsive Element
CYP	Cytochrome P450
CYP450-DMO	Cytochrome P450-Dependent Monooxygenase
DEREK	Deduction of Risk from Existing Knowledge
ECVAM	European Centre for the Validation of Alternative Methods
ELISA	Enzyme-linked Absorbance Assay
EMEA	European Medicines Agency
EPA	Environmental Protection Agency
ERE	Estrogen Responsive Element
FACS	Fluorescence-Activated Cell Sorting
FDA	Food and Drug Administration
FRET	Fluorescent Resonance Energy Transfer
GFP	Green Fluorescent Protein
GPCR	G-Protein-Coupled Receptor
HESC	Human Embryonic Stem Cell
HTS	High-Throughput Screening
IAM	Immobilized Artificial Membrane
ICCVAM	Interagency Coordinating Committee on the Validation of Alternative Methods
ICH	International Conference for Harmonization
IND	Investigational New Drug
LC-MS/MS	Liquid Chromatography and Tandem Mass Spectrometry

LD$_{50}$	Lethal Dose that kills 50% of a test group (of animals)
Log P	Octan-1-ol/water partition coefficient
MAP kinase	Mitogen-Activated Protein Kinase
MCASE	Multi-CASE
MDCK	Madin–Darby Canine Kidney
MOS	Margin of Safety
MS	Mass Spectrometry
MTD	Maximum Tolerated Dose
NCE	New Chemical Entity
NCTR	FDA National Center for Toxicological Research
NMR	Nuclear Magnetic Resonance
OECD	Organization for Economic Co-operation and Development
PAMPA	Parallel Artificial Membrane Permeation Assay
PBPK	Physiologically Based Pharmacokinetic
PCR	Polymerase Chain Reaction
PK	Pharmacokinetic
pK_a	The acid-ionization constant
PTFE	Polytetrafluoroethylene
QSAR	Quantitative
QSAR–ES	Quantitative Structure–Activity Relationship—Expert System
QT Interval	The time between the start of the Q wave and the end of the T wave in the heart's electrical cycle
SAR	Structure–activity Relationship
SPA	Scintillation Proximity Assay
SPR	Surface Plasmon Resonance
TOPKAT	The Open Practical Knowledge Acquisition Toolkit
UFAW	Universities Federation for Animal Welfare

of a drug that is vital for the design of *in vivo* animal studies and can add substantial weight to the product dossier submitted to regulatory bodies.

Increasingly, predictions about the ways in which a particular chemical is likely to interact with its desired cellular target are made by undertaking *in silico* modeling. These results are used to filter out poor candidate molecules according to chemical class and structural or functional features during drug discovery. However, filtering of this kind is sometimes impossible, so lead identification still relies to some extent on serendipitous finds from random libraries, rather than on rational lead discovery. For instance, for new chemical entities (NCEs) for which there are no data, i.e., are first-in-class, *in silico* screenings are difficult to handle, particularly where there is also limited knowledge of the structure of the active site of the target. Also, there might be a lack of important information for other compounds. For example, predicting drug effects can be seriously compromised when ADME data on the behavior of a molecule in different tissues and species are lacking. This is confounded by the reality that this kind of information for different individuals will always be limited. Both of the above situations are most evident in the case of large molecules, such as (1) peptides and proteins with complex structures and multiple conformations, (2) humanized products that could be differentially immunogenic in different species, and (3) nanoparticle formulations.

1.1.3 Information Required Prior to Drug Authorization/Approval

Once a new therapeutic candidate has been successfully identified from preclinical studies, the next stage involves the authorization of clinical studies. The information required prior to the authorization of any clinical trial is crucial for the design and execution of preclinical studies, irrespective of whether the aim is to define drug action or provide safety information. Such information includes (1) manufacturing quality, (2) physicochemical properties, (3) efficacy, (4) proposed mechanism of action, (5) selectivity, (6) ADME, and (7) possible adverse effects in humans.

In the United States, the Food and Drug Administration (FDA) handles drug approvals. The FDA has fast tracked this process for treatments for serious diseases where no therapies currently exist [2]. Drug developers are required to submit an Investigational New Drug (IND) Application, in which evidence from preclinical studies is provided for review by the FDA. The FDA decides whether it is reasonably safe for the company to test the drug in humans. Under the FDA's jurisdiction, the Center for Drugs, Evaluation and Research (CDER) and the Center for Biologics, Evaluation and Research (CBER) are responsible for reviewing different types of therapeutic agent applications (Table 1.2). Note that these changes in jurisdiction mean that biological products, the testing of which was at one point based on limited animal tests (because of their poor predictivity), are likely to require more stringent testing under the CDER [3].

The FDA has exclusive executive control over decisions regarding drug approvals in the United States. However, in Europe, it is possible to have a drug approved by a number of different routes. This is because companies can apply either via the EMEA (European Medicines Agency) for pan-European approval or via one or more national agencies. However, since November 2005, all new drugs for the major diseases, including AIDS, cancer, diabetes, and neurodegenerative disorders, and

TABLE 1.2   CDER and CBER:[a] **Review of New Therapeutic Agent Applications**

CDER

- Traditional small molecule therapeutics
- Growth hormone, insulin, and other endocrine peptide therapeutics
- Monoclonal antibodies
- Proteins (e.g., cytokines, enzymes, and other novel proteins), except those specifically assigned to the CBER, namely, vaccines and blood products that are assigned to CBER
- Immunomodulatory agents (but not vaccines)
- Growth factors intended to modulate hematopoiesis *in vivo*
- Combination products where the primary mode of action is that of an agent assigned to the CDER

CBER

- Products composed of human, bacterial, or animal cells or fragments of cells, for use as preventative or therapeutic vaccines
- Gene therapy products
- Vaccines
- Allergenic extracts used for the diagnosis and treatment of allergic diseases
- Antitoxins, antivenins, and venoms
- Blood and blood products from humans or animals
- Combination products where the primary mode of action is that of an agent assigned to the CBER

[a]The CDER and CBER are afforded jurisdiction by the U.S. FDA.

medicinal products developed by means of biotechnological processes must be approved via the EMEA.

With the globalization of the pharmaceutical industry, the International Conference on Harmonization (ICH) guidelines have, since 1990, set out to standardize drug applications in terms of their content and format. Japan, the United States and the European Union (EU) comply with these requirements for the quality, safety, and efficacy assessment of new drugs. These guidelines operate alongside national requirements. Quality assessment guidelines are provided to standardize the assessment of drug stability (shelf-life), and the management of risks due to impurities, such as residual solvents and infectious agents, such as viruses (which can be present when a drug is isolated from plants, animals, humans, or cell lines). The guidelines also require the standardization of cell lines, test procedures, acceptance criteria, and procedures for formulation and development. Efficacy guidelines are also provided, to standardize the conduct, interpretation, and reporting of clinical trials.

There are some important practical considerations that should be borne in mind when conducting preclinical studies. The most comprehensive guidelines are those provided for drug safety testing, which cover a number of toxicological endpoints, including carcinogenicity, genotoxicity, reproductive and developmental toxicity, and immunotoxicity. Some of the guidelines apply generically to all new drugs, while others focus on specific types of therapeutic agents, such as biotechnology products. These guidelines are essential reading for researchers engaged in drug development and are considered in more detail throughout the remainder of this chapter.

Another important source of reference is the Organization for Economic Co-operation and Development (OECD). By ratifying the convention of the OECD, many European countries, Australia, Japan, New Zealand and the United States have agreed to abide by a set of test guidelines for assessing the human health effects of chemicals [4], which apply equally to the testing of therapeutic agents. Later, we refer to a number of nonanimal methods and refinements of animal procedures accepted by the member countries of the OECD.

1.2 FINDING NEW DRUG TARGETS

1.2.1 Background

Until relatively recently, drug development focused on a limited number of targets, against which NCEs with a desired effect could be selected. These "druggable" targets were once most extensively investigated by using animal models. However, greater access to recombinant DNA technology means that most early screens are now conducted primarily by using different genetically engineered cell lines expressing putative targets that can be arrayed into high density plastic plate formats suitable for interactions between the targets and potential lead chemicals (for methods, see later discussion).

Overington et al. [5] derived a consensus figure for the number of therapeutic drug targets for the FDA-approved drugs that were available in 2005. They identified 324 drug targets for all classes of approved therapeutic agents, which were targeted by in excess of 1357 drugs, of which 1204 were small molecules and 166 were biologicals. Cell surface receptors and channels represented the targets for >50% of all the FDA-approved drugs. A further 10% of the drugs, including monoclonal antibodies, also target other cell surface proteins. Most of the remaining targets were enzymes, nuclear receptors, DNA, or ribosomes. These targets represent a minute fraction of the genome, and a mere 3% (266 proteins) of the predicted proteome.

According to this survey, on average 5.3 new druggable targets are discovered each year. This means that many more potential drug targets remain to be discovered. Whether a potential drug target will be a good therapeutic target, however, depends on whether (1) it plays a key role in gene regulation, (2) it is selectively expressed in certain disease states or tissues, and (3) it has a definable and unique binding site.

Often, a further important piece of information is the nature or identity of the endogenous modulator. For example, >1000 G-protein-coupled receptors (GPCRs) have been cloned from various species, including 160 distinct human subtypes with known ligands, although these represent only a limited set of targets for current therapeutic agents. A further 100 or so are orphan receptors, for which there is currently no known natural ligand. In such cases, the starting point is the gene, from which the protein receptor can be expressed and used to screen large combinatorial libraries of chemicals in the search for a modulator. Such a reverse pharmacology strategy uses the orphan receptor as a "hook" for screening libraries and hit generation, where little is known about the natural ligand. In many cases, receptor models use the crystal structure of rhodopsin as a template, as this is the only GPCR whose structure has been resolved. The importance of GPCRs is emphasized by the fact that, although >20% of the top 200 current best-selling drugs interact with these cell surface receptors, they generate worldwide sales of drugs such as cimetidine, losartan, and ropinerole of over $20 billion (U.S.) [6].

1.2.2 Impact of New Technologies on Target Discovery

Comparative genetics can provide much relevant information, particularly with regard to the role of human-specific genes and the suitability of animal models for drug development. The application of microarray techniques, standards, and resources that permit the comparison of gene expression patterns across species and between cell types and tissues has started to provide some insight into the metabolic and biochemical differences between health and disease states. A good example of this is the Cancer Genome Anatomy Project (www.ncbi.nlm.nih.gov/CGAP) [7], in which mutational sites in cancer cells have been identified.

A cursory examination of the 373 completed genome sequences for archeal, prokaryote, and eukaryote [8] species suggests that, although genome size increases from archea through prokaryotes to eukaryotes, genome size is not directly linked to the number of genes within the functional genomes, nor with evolutionary status. It is, however, clear that, as the complexity of organisms increases, so does the complexity of gene regulation and the level of genetic redundancy—the ability of several genes to rescue loss-of-function of another gene. Nevertheless, for highly conserved genes, such as those that are involved in early development, and homeobox genes, studies on early life stages of species such as zebra fish and invertebrate models can indicate the roles of genes. However, in general, such studies are more relevant to safety pharmacology than to mechanistic and efficacy studies. It is worth bearing in mind that computational predictions and statistical analyses have suggested that the bacterial *Escherichia coli* and human genomes account for 35 common metabolic pathways, namely, those that are important in biosynthesis and in degradation and respiratory processes [9], and that, possibly as a result of bacterial infection, a number of bacterial genes have become permanently integrated in the human genome [9, 10]. This opens up the possibility of using bacterial studies to decipher a limited number of biochemical pathways affected by drugs, as well as for genotoxicity testing.

Unicellular eukaryotes, such as yeast, share remarkable genetic and functional similarities with multicellular eukaryotes. The most useful yeast strain in terms of dissecting protein and gene interactions is *Saccharomyces cerevisiae*. At 12,100 kilobases, the *S. cerevisiae* genome is much smaller than the human genome. However, because its gene density is 50 times greater than that of the human genome, genes found in the *S. cerevisiae* genome resemble around 30% of the genes associated with diseases in humans [11]. Since the entire genome of *S. cerevisiae* encodes no more than 6000 proteins, it is relatively straightforward to investigate gene function in yeast and make genome-wide microarray measurements. Such data, together with information from other sources, have made it possible to identify a number of putative drug targets [12] and protein–protein interactions [13], thereby facilitating the development of extensive maps of protein and gene interactions. Such studies in *S. cerevisiae* have been particularly useful in neurodegenerative and ageing research and in studies on diseases that arise as a consequence of mitochondrial DNA damage. One example is the observation that yeast mutants for α-synuclein result in a large change in yeast sexual reproduction, as well as causing cytotoxicity, both endpoints of which are suited to high-throughput screening assays for new treatments for Parkinson disease [14].

Subsequent studies on yeast-based models of Parkinson disease have suggested that there is substantial scope for using yeast for the high-throughput screening of chemicals for drug discovery [15]. For example, *S. cerevisiae* possesses three distinct G-protein-coupled receptors (GPCRs), which are involved in pheromone (Ste2 and Ste3 receptors) and glucose sensing (Gpr1) [16]. These receptors are related, albeit to a limited extent, to the vastly expanded human GPCR repertoire. By coupling heterologously expressed human GPCRs to the yeast MAP kinase pathway (associated with yeast mating and growth arrest), in yeasts where the MAP kinase pathway is linked to reporter gene expression [17], it is possible to monitor receptor recognition and activation by simple growth or colorimetric reporter assays.

Caenorhabditis elegans is another organism that can be used in early drug discovery. This nematode worm is transparent, has a short life span, is a mere 1 mm in length and 80 µM in diameter, reproduces every 3 days by self-fertilization to produce over 300 offspring, and is a multicellular organism composed of exactly 959 somatic cells. It displays many of the basic features of higher eukaryotes, including the possession of muscle, excretory cells, and neural cells, and has been extensively used to increase understanding of the mechanisms of gene regulation and gene function. Antisense knock-out or knock-down of gene expression can be achieved simply by feeding the worm with *E. coli* bacteria transformed with plasmid DNA containing antisense DNA. More recently, RNA interference (RNAi) has been used to manipulate the genomes of organisms such as *C. elegans*, although the possibility of transmission of RNA silencing to subsequent generations can occur [18]. Like all multicellular organisms, *C. elegans* exhibits programmed cell death (apoptosis) [19], in a way that is very similar to that seen in higher organisms as part of ageing and disease processes. Similarities between the signaling pathways involved in the regulation of cell proliferation in *C. elegans* and humans suggest that this organism might provide information on the regulation of cell proliferation, which will be of relevance to cancer therapeutics. The entire 302-cell nervous system of this worm has been mapped by electron microscopy, and although the average human possesses somewhere in the order of 100 billion neurons, it seems that neurotransmission is similar in the two species. Thus, *C. elegans* possesses the major classes of ion channels, receptors, transporters, and neurotransmitters that make it a suitable candidate for some forms of drug screening, such as the discovery of new dopaminergic drugs. Similarly, *D. melanogaster* shares much of its basic neurobiology with higher organisms, including humans. It possesses the same neurodegenerative states, neurotransmission mechanisms, and receptor homolog that are found in humans as key targets for neurally active therapeutic agents, making studies with these organisms useful for the development of treatments for conditions such as Parkinson's disease [20].

1.2.3 Data Mining

Novel drug targets can also be found in other ways, including data mining. This involves analyzing the literature, to determine the biochemistry underlying particular human diseases, and human physiology. In addition, human population genetics studies can be undertaken, to determine the roles of human genes, how they interact, the consequences of population differences at the gene level, and, ultimately, the complete physiology of the human body. In the last-named case, since the possibilities for human studies are limited, most of the information gathered comes from fundamental research that examines modes of interaction of specific substances with any given novel targets, and the modulation of their physiological roles, by combining several approaches, including *in vivo* studies.

The next step is to define whether a newly discovered potential drug target is a feasible target, by identifying the binding site of the proposed molecular target. In this respect, the potential for data mining has been greatly enhanced by the recent development of a druggable-protein database. This can provide information that is useful for deriving rules for the computational identification of drug binding sites. Indeed, there are now algorithms designed specifically for this purpose [21]. Some analyses relate to the identification of pockets within the binding site that serve as potential specific drug targets. However, this approach can be complicated, since the binding pocket that is targeted by an endogenous or natural modulator of target function might include only part of the binding site, or might lack it altogether. A recently described approach to this problem, in which 2D heteronuclear NMR is used to screen drug-like and fragment libraries for interactions with proteins, generates additional reliable data than is obtainable from conventional high-throughput screens. While such information can be used for computational application, including the refinement of protein models, it is limited by the number of protein structures that are currently available. An exception to this are quantitative structure–activity relationships (QSARs) generated by computational techniques such as CoMFA, which rely on molecular descriptors for molecules that are specific for a target, in order to generate a set of conformers that can be used to predict the ability to bind to a protein.

1.3 TRADITIONAL APPROACHES TO DRUG DISCOVERY AND DEVELOPMENT

1.3.1 Hit to Lead

The current attrition rate for NCEs can be gauged from the fact that, on average, for every 7 million molecules screened, only one product is marketed [22]. These odds have resulted in the concentration by pharmaceutical companies on refining, rather than expanding, their chemical libraries and methods. A further important factor that determines the success of early drug screening is the choice of methodologies used to identify hits and to screen potential leads and their derivatives. In this section, we describe the key stages and methodologies used for hit generation, hit confirmation, lead, identification and lead characterization (Table 1.3).

Before 1980, nearly all drugs were small molecules of around 50 to 1000 times smaller than the size of a typical protein at around 500 daltons, or smaller. Extensive combinatorial libraries of small molecules are generated in-house by all large pharmaceutical companies, often by diversity-oriented synthesis, in which small molecular building blocks are randomly combined in all possible spatial orientations. Screening libraries can consist of thousands of chemicals and rely on an appropriate hit generation and lead characterization strategy. The chemicals concerned must meet certain purity, molecular weight, lipophilicity (log P), and functional conformer criteria.

Schreiber [23] first used diversity-oriented synthesis to generate bead-attached libraries of target-oriented and diversity-oriented chemicals. This approach involves

TABLE 1.3   Key Methods Used During Hit Generation and Lead Optimization[a]

Methods	Assay Principles	Advantages	Limitations
Affinity-based biophysical methods			
Mass spectrometry	Relies on the affinity of a compound for a protein to cause mass/charge shifts.	Can handle large drug-like/ fragment mixtures.	Not truly an HTS platform; poor at resolving mixtures; false hits.
NMR	Monitors the location of radionuclides in the target–ligand complex and is used to probe the active site of folded/*in situ* proteins/DNA. A number of new higher resolution techniques (e.g., magic angle spinning NMR) do not require high purity target proteins.	Provides structural information for *in silico* platforms; suited to screening large fragment libraries.	Does not provide SAR data; false hits; weakly potent fragment hits are poorly detected.
X-ray crystallography	X-ray diffraction by crystallized protein/ protein–ligand complexes.	Provides structural information; HTS platform.	Weakly potent fragment hits are poorly detected; erroneous assumption about structural similarity can lead to some compounds being discarded; there are not crystal structures available for all target proteins.
Biochemical screens			
Scintillation proximity assay	Monitors energy transfer changes as an indicator of binding interactions.	Provides kinetic data	High background; limited plate format; not easily correlated to physiological effect.
Radiometric binding assays	Uses radioactive tracing of target– tracer/molecule interactions.	Direct measurement of binding interactions; adaptable for a wide range of possible target-based screens.	Relatively expensive to generate suitable tracer; health and safety considerations; not real-time measurements.

TABLE 1.3 *Continued*

Methods	Assay Principles	Advantages	Limitations
SPR	Commonly based on the target being immobilized on a chip and the compound mixture being passed over it. Interactions are monitored as an electrical readout.	Permits kinetic measurements; can be used to identify hits from complex mixtures.	Chip preparation and availability; requires relatively large amounts of materials; more suited to detailed mechanistic studies than HTS.
Nonradioactive assays	Includes colorimetric/ absorbance-based assays (such as ELISA), luminescence-based assays, and fluorescence-based assays (e.g., FRET, real-time fluorimetry, fluorescence correlation spectroscopy), as generally used in conjunction with cell-based assays (see below).	Generate quantitative data suited to SAR; can give real-time data; can provide mechanistic information; suitable to HTS formats.	Often more suited to later stages of lead discovery.
Cell-based assays			
Reporter gene assays	Involves the use of genes such as those encoding GFP, luciferase, and β-galactosidase coupled to a biochemical pathway modulated by a substance to monitor the extent or modulation.	Generates quantitative data suited to SAR; minimum resources needed.	Not truly HTS; can give equivocal data; false hits; not well suited for fragment screens.
FRET	Monitors energy transfer between a fluorescent energy donor and acceptor as a measure of the proximity between the two groups, commonly found on the target and a tracer.	Suitable for high density formats; provides mechanistic information; broad range of applications; real-time monitoring of interactions.	High incidence of false hits; prone to fluorescence quenching.

TABLE 1.3   *Continued*

Methods	Assay Principles	Advantages	Limitations
BRET	Similar principles to FRET.	Suitable for medium density formats; provides mechanistic information; suitable for monitoring protein–protein interactions; real-time monitoring of interactions.	Some limitations on application; involves protein engineering of the target.
Reporter gene	Based on recombinant protein engineering and expression technology to couple an endogenous pathway to the expression and/or activity of a protein from a transgene in response to drug modulation of a target.	Several commercially available plasmids (e.g., with cAMP, calcium, and estrogen responsive elements); sensitive high throughput assay formats.	High incidence of false hits; long incubation times; indirect correlation with target modulation.
Electrical readout	Includes biosensor-based methods and patch clamping.	Suitable for monitoring channel activity.	Not truly suited to HTS; limited utility
Second messenger assays	Based on a direct measurement of one of more downstream changes in signal mediators in response to drug modulation of a target. Includes assays such as those that measure changes in intracellular calcium (FLIPR/Aequroscreen), cAMP, and many more.	Direct measurement of the effects of a substance.	Only suited to some types of targets (e.g., receptor, channels, enzymes); time consuming.

TABLE 1.3 *Continued*

Methods	Assay Principles	Advantages	Limitations
Fluorophore and chromophore-based methods	Rely on the use of an ion-sensitive dye to detect intracellular changes in ion content.	Suitable for monitoring increases in intracellular calcium, potassium, and sodium ions.	Sensitivity dependent on dye chemistry.
Cell proliferation assays	Includes methods such as dye or radioisotope uptake, protein estimations, cell counting, and oxygen sensor measurements to monitor the competence, viability, and growth rate of cells.	Minimum resources needed; generic application; quantitative data can be obtained.	Difficulty equating to physiological endpoint.
In silico methods			
Protein modeling	*Ab initio* or homology-based protein structure modeling based on amino acid sequence analysis and biophysical/biochemical data.	Binding site identification and pharmacophore modeling.	Need experimental confirmation of findings.
Molecular docking/SAR/ combinatorial chemistry	Molecular dynamics simulations and energetic calculations.	Virtual screening prior to chemical synthesis.	Need experimental confirmation of findings.
PBPK modeling	Mathematical prediction of the fate of a drug.	Can be used to identify the sites of action of a drug and to estimate likely internal dose.	Reliant on large amounts of data; can involve considerable mathematical expertise.

[a]A number of different approaches are used during drug discovery and development. Here, a list of methods applicable to hit generation and lead development are listed alongside the main advantages and limitations of each method or group of methods. HTS, high-throughput screen.

the use of fragments—small chemicals—of around 120–250 kDa. Generally, these fragments display lower (10 μM to millimolar) affinities for a target than do more complex, drug-sized chemicals (affinities within the nanomolar range). It is therefore necessary to complement fragment screens by using sensitive analytical techniques, such as protein-detected or ligand-detected NMR [24], MS [25], X-ray crystallography [26], and SPR [27] (although the last named is generally more applicable for hit confirmation; see later discussion). These techniques are preferable to bioassays, such as cell-based binding or functional assays, or to the step-wise combination of hit fragments either by chemical synthesis or by combining pharmacophores [28]. Despite the fact that the method used to screen fragments affects the success of such screens, the hit rate for fragment-based lead discovery is substantially higher than that for drug-like screens, there being an apparent inverse relationship between chemical complexity and target complementarity. Indeed, a screen of <1000 fragments might identify several useful hits for lead development.

A "library in tube" method is being developed for large mixtures of chemicals, which has been adapted from a concept put forward by Brenner and Lerner in 1992 [29]. This technique involves coding each chemical with a DNA tag, in order to identify the attached chemical by PCR, such that mixtures of chemicals can be panned against a target. This approach has much potential for diversity-oriented hit generation (see Ref. 30 for a review).

Biochemical screening can be performed by using several types of readout, including those reviewed in Ref. 31. Whatever the assay used, it should display good signal-to-noise ratios and should also be reproducible. The two most commonly used screening formats are radiometric and nonradiometric assays, both of which are suitable for intact cell or tissue-based studies. Radiometric assays include filtration-based methods, where the unbound radioactive probe (generally the radioligand specific for the target) competes for ligand binding with the unlabeled screen compound, after which it is removed in readiness for scintillation counting, or for scintillation proximity assays (SPAs), where β-particle emissions from isotopes with short β-particle path lengths (namely, ^{3}H and ^{125}I) are measured *in situ* by using scintillant-impregnated microspheres. The amount of reduction of the radiolabel signal intensity due to competition is measured. The use of the former isotope renders the method amenable to a 384-plate format, while the latter is generally more suited to a 96-well format.

Nonradiometric assays include those based on colorimetric, fluorescent, luminescent, or electrical changes. Commonly used methods include proximity-based fluorescent resonance energy transfer (FRET), which can be used to monitor interactions between a fluorescent donor and an acceptor on the target, and to screen chemicals. This technique is suited for both monitoring a wide range of molecular interactions and to 1536-well formats. One example of how FRET may be useful is in the screening of enzyme inhibitors [32]. The drawbacks of this method are the high incidence of false positives and problems with fluorescent quenching. Bioluminescent resonance energy transfer (BRET) is another proximity-based screen. This method, while being prone to quenching, requires the use of proteins such as *renilla reinformis* luciferase donor and green fluorescent protein (GFP) acceptor, in the presence of coelenterazine a (luciferase substrate). BRET is generally more useful for screening interactions between large molecules, such as proteins, due to the bulky nature of acceptor and donor groups, luciferase, and GFP. Nevertheless, it can also be used to screen for chemicals that perturb such interactions, and indeed, BRET has been proposed as a screen for HIV-1 protease inhibitors [33]. The sensitivity of both FRET and BRET is dramatically improved when there is a large difference between the emission spectra prior to and following energy transfer from the donor to the acceptor group.

Other commonly used screens rely on the expression of a reporter gene (e.g., β-galactosidase or luciferase) in response to the activation of a specific pathway.

However, many more screening techniques are specific for the targets in question, as is the case for GPCRs [34] and HIV-1 [35]. An example of the usefulness of electrical readouts is the examination of the interaction between DNA and metal-locompounds. In this case, the DNA is immobilized on electrodes, and interactions with the drug can alter the electrical output [36]. Generally, these functional assays (with the notable exception of SPA) can provide a mechanistic overview of drug action. However, further insight can be gained by using surface plasmon resonance (SPR). SPR is a real-time monitoring system based on change in mass, in which microgram amounts of the target are immobilized on a chip and exposed to the test chemical. The flow rate and wash rate can be varied, such that not only can the individual chemicals in a mixture be resolved according to rank order of affinity, but also the on–off rates of binding can be monitored. Membrane protein targets, however, are difficult to isolate and refold into the chip matrix, so SPR is far more useful for the screening of drugs that target soluble proteins and DNA [37].

As a typical screen of 1 million chemicals can take 6 months to complete, there is interest in expediting hit generation by using higher density plate formats or by chemical pooling. Increasing the assay density by increasing the well density is feasible, but is highly dependent on the nature of the screen. Chemical pooling involves placing multiple chemicals into each well of a plate, with a single chemical overlap between two wells. This can reduce the screening time to a matter of weeks. However, factors such as the possibility that two of the compounds in the same well will cancel the effects of each other or will act synergistically, can result in false negatives and positives, respectively. It is also general practice to include pairs of structurally related chemicals in each screen.

A new drug can also be developed as a result of rational drug design, particularly when there is extensive knowledge of the structure and function of the target protein, as well as available computer models and the capability to dock virtual compounds into the active site. In many cases, however, the original first-in-class compound was designed by modification of the endogenous ligand for the target. The classical example of this is the design of small nonpeptide antagonists that target neuropeptide receptors (e.g., neurokinin receptors) by gradual structural minimization and constraint of the natural endogenous receptor ligands [28]. In general, the design of these smaller nonpeptide ligands, based on knowledge of the natural ligand, requires extensive peptide analogue generation and screening for efficacy and activity, so as to identify the key interactions and functional groups on the peptide that determine specificity and activity. In the above example of neurokinin receptor binding, the key interactions were identified as being with the terminal Phe-X-Gly-Leu-Met-NH_2 motif. Indeed, all ligands that retain neurokinin receptor affinity contain aromatic rings and amine groups that fit into the receptor pocket.

The latter analogue-based minimization of the natural ligand for a target protein is particularly relevant, given that larger molecules such as peptides and proteins are increasingly being investigated as clinical agents. Currently, more than 40 peptides are marketed worldwide, with some 700 more at various stages of development as drug leads. Similarly, there are some 120 antibody-, hormone-, and enzyme-based therapeutics currently on the global market. Many of these therapeutics are more specific and more active than their small molecule counterparts, and they accumulate less readily in tissues, with generally lower oral bioavailability and less stability.

They are all potentially immunogenic and are relatively expensive to manufacture. These molecules are also not generally amenable to rational design strategies and are often developed by *de novo* routes with limited *in silico* approaches, in view of the difficulties associated with docking flexible peptides and proteins into the target protein.

Screening for peptide, polypeptide, and protein therapeutic leads presents a problem, in that large libraries are generally not amenable to chemical synthesis. One solution to this problem is to use systems in which the peptide is linked to the DNA that encodes it. Phage display, for instance, is a technique that allows one or more genes encoding any number of protein variants to be expressed in an anchored form amenable to affinity probing. The genes of interest are inserted into the genome of a nonlytic phage, which is introduced into bacteria. The proteins encoded by the genes are expressed (displayed) on a defined coat protein of the respective phage. Phage display libraries of over a billion different peptide or protein sequences can be prepared, the only limitation being the efficiency with which the bacteria are infected. By using the molecular target as a probe to isolate hits from this library, it is possible to undertake successive rounds of optimization until the most specific hits are identified. Phage display, and the similar, more recent ribosomal display systems [38], can be used to screen for protein and hapten hits for drug development and have proved particularly useful with respect to the development of specific antibodies [39]. However, the need for folded proteins has led to the development of a yeast-display technology, whereby proteins are presented in their folded form on the yeast cell wall. These anchored systems all facilitate miniaturized screening and, in the case of the yeast-display libraries, FACS [40].

The techniques used for developing genetically based therapeutics share some similarities with more traditional drug discovery approaches. Genetically based therapeutics include plasmids containing transgenes for gene therapy, oligonucleotides for antisense applications, DNAzymes, RNA aptamers, and small interfering RNAs for RNAi [41]. So far, two such products have been approved for clinical use and many more are in the course of development, so this important group of therapeutics requires specific consideration in the context of preclinical planning. Very little is currently understood about the suitability of many genetically-based therapeutics. It is known, however, that the design of the vector crucially determines delivery and nuclear uptake, and also that the promoter used will determine the expression levels of the transgene and the efficiency of gene silencing (reviewed in Ref. 41). Since uptake is a key determinant of efficacy, the development of these therapeutic agents must be used together with an evaluation of DNA delivery techniques, such as microinjection, electroporation, viral delivery systems, and carrier molecules that either promote cellular endocytosis (e.g., cationic lipids or amines) or facilitate uptake (e.g., carbon nanotubes) (see Ref. 42 for a review and Section 1.4.4). Equally, the expression of the encoded DNA is reliant on the precise nucleotide sequence, with codon use often resulting in changes in the expression of the encoded protein product and, in some cases, to its cellular fate.

Whatever the discovery route for a lead compound from drug-like libraries or fragment libraries, it is clear that most of the drugs that are currently marketed are highly similar to the leads from which they were derived [43]. This makes lead discovery a crucial step in the drug discovery process. The most widely used approach to confirming leads is affinity-based screening [44], where qualitative (e.g., rank order) or quantitative (K_d, IC_{50}) measurements are used to monitor interactions between compound libraries and protein, RNA, or DNA targets, by using approaches such as standard binding assays, NMR, SPR, or X-ray crystallography. Other approaches involve the use of changes in biochemical events that have been identified from target modulation or predicted by *in silico* screening. A combination of all three approaches has the advantage over using biochemical techniques alone, of reducing the number of false hits while allowing higher screening throughputs. For instance, experimentally based screening may result in false hits, because of (1) nonspecific interactions (predominantly hydrophobic in nature), (2) aggregation or poor solubility of the drug, and (3) purities, reactive groups, or chemical stability that are not readily discernible from *in silico* predictions. MS-based methods result in fewer false positives because of nonspecific hydrophobic interactions, poor solubility, impurities, and reactive functional groups. In practice, however, the method used for hit generation is dependent on the resources available.

In the case of *in vitro* biochemical and cellular assays, miniaturized formats can be used to screen around 1 million drug-like molecules, by using 1–50 μM concentrations and a 30–50% activity cutoff between potential hits and failures [45]. Where fragment libraries are used, activity might only be detectable at substantially higher concentrations, and by using more-sensitive techniques. As a result of these selection criteria, the rate of false hits (and failures) is also relatively high.

Hit confirmation generally involves biochemical assays to confirm that the observed activity is linked to the desired mechanism of action. The choice of methodologies is important, since it is at this stage that eliminating false-positive hits becomes most important and depends on the necessary properties of the final drug. It is also at this stage that hits begin to be ranked according to specificity, activity, and suitability to be used for lead development. Indeed, data from hit confirmation studies are often amenable to structure–function analysis by using *in silico* methods that may ultimately guide decisions as to the most favorable leads.

This process is developed further during the hit-to-lead stage, in which potency is no longer considered to be the deciding factor, but selectivity, the feasibility of chemical synthesis and modification, the mechanisms of target interaction and modulation, pharmacokinetics, and patentability of the final drug have become increasingly important. Many of these issues are considered later. It is important to note, however, that determining whether individual fragment hits fulfill these criteria is much more problematical. The ability to chemically modify a hit lends itself to the three main ways of generating a lead compound from initial promising hits and subsequently derivatizing and modifying the lead to give the final drug, namely, by using biophysical or biochemical methods, cell-based screens, or *in silico* predictions.

It is at the above stage of development that the possible risks associated with a new drug candidate begin to be addressed. The affinity and specificity of the drug candidate for the desired target can often dictate whether it will be discarded at an early stage. For instance, if there is a difference of several orders of magnitude in affinities for selected targets and off-targets, the drug is less likely to have predictable side effects. That is, it is possible that a drug may have a desirable effect within one concentration range, above which it causes toxicity. The relationship between the desired therapeutic effects of a drug and its adverse effects is expressed as a margin of safety (MOS; also referred to as therapeutic index)—being the difference between the effective dose and that which gives rise to toxicity.

Two important sources of information can contribute to a widening of the MOS during lead optimization. The first is a fundamental understanding of the mechanisms of interaction with the desired target and off-targets. The second is information from combinatorial chemistry and rapid *in vitro* screens to determine the relationship between structure and activity, which can then be applied to developing computational analysis techniques. This is a fundamental principle of rational drug design, where the original lead is often structurally related to the endogenous substance that modulates target activity. On a final note, however, rational drug design is not applicable in all circumstances, and a great deal of drug discovery still relies heavily on the serendipitous discovery of new drugs by empirical screening of various chemical classes.

1.3.2 Pharmacokinetics

Introduction Lead derivation and optimization are guided by three predominant factors: efficacy, specificity, and pharmacokinetics. Pharmacokinetics is the study of the time course of drug absorption, distribution, metabolism, and excretion (ADME), and how ADME relates to the therapeutic and toxic effects of a drug. The key parameters and methods used in ADME studies are listed in Table 1.4. During the 1990s, it was noticed that many drug candidates were abandoned during clinical trials due to poor pharmacokinetics [46]. This, in part, reflects problems with

TABLE 1.4   Key ADME Parameters and Methodologies[a] for Early Studies

Physicochemical properties
   Chemical stability and degradation
   Solubility
   pK_a
   Lipophilicity ($\log P$)
Binding target screens
   Plasma protein binding
   Nonspecific interactions/binding studies
Absorption and distribution
   Passive transport into the systemic circulation system—Caco-2 MDCK cells
   P-gp substrate/transporter assays
   Absorption screening—models of the blood–brain, placental/reproductive, epithelial,
     and, corneal barriers
   PBPK modeling
Metabolism and excretion
   CYP metabolism
   CYP inhibition/induction
   Glucuronidation
   Nuclear receptor activation
   Regulation of lipid and cholesterol metabolism
   Aromatase inhibition
   Metabolite stability
   Kidney cells and tissue preparations

[a]These approaches are increasingly being used by pharmaceutical companies in an attempt to reduce drug attrition rates.

species extrapolation, allometric scaling, and the selection of suitable preclinical models.

Absorption and Distribution   For ease of administration, oral delivery is the most favored route of administration. Orally delivered drugs need to possess good gut absorption and clearance, as well as good metabolic stability; this is to ensure adequate systemic exposure. This is expressed as oral bioavailability, which is the fraction of the ingested drug that is available systemically, depends on both absorption and elimination, and which can be estimated from the equation:

$$\text{Oral bioavailability} = \text{Fraction absorbed across the intestinal wall} \times \text{Fraction}$$
$$\text{that is not cleared by the gut} \times \text{Fraction not cleared by}$$
$$\text{the liver} \times \text{Fraction not cleared by the lungs}$$

The fraction absorbed from the gut is dependent on lipophilicity ($\log P$), namely, the hydrophobicity, molecular size, and hydrogen bonding potential of the drug, and its permeability, which is dictated by van der Waals forces that are due to nitrogen and oxygen atoms, which influence the polar surface area of a drug molecule. Highly lipophilic drugs are likely to be absorbed directly from the gut into the lacteals and enter the lymphatic system before the general circulation, thus avoiding first-pass metabolism in the liver. On the other hand, small, moderately lipophilic drugs are likely to be passively or actively transported (depending on electrical charge, structure, and intermolecular interactions) across the intestinal barrier into the hepatic portal vein and are destined for the hepatobiliary system. Lipinski's rule-of-five [47] is commonly used to predict the permeability of a compound according to the rule that >5 hydrogen bonds, coupled with a molecular mass of >500 Da, a $c \log P > 5$, and >10 nitrogen and oxygen atoms are indicators of poor absorption. The full list of criteria for passive absorption through biological membranes is given in Table 1.5.

The biopharmaceutics classification system (BCS) [48] is a scientific framework for classifying drug substances based on their aqueous solubility and intestinal permeability. It takes into account three major determinants of the rate and extent of absorption following the administration of a solid oral dosage—(1) dissolution, (2) solubility, and (3) intestinal permeability—and can be used to avoid some animal studies. According to the BCS, drug substances are classified as follows:

TABLE 1.5   Criteria[a] for Absorption from the Gut for Drug-like Compounds

Rule-of-five:
- MW $\leq$ 500
- $c \log P \leq 5$
- H-bond donors $\leq$ 5
- H-bond acceptors (N and O atoms) $\leq$ 10

Additional criteria
- Polar surface area $\leq 140\,\text{Å}^2$ or Σ H-bond donors and acceptors ≤ 12
- Rotatable bonds ≤ 10

[a]These include Lipinski's criteria and experimentally determined criteria for the gut absorption of orally administered drugs.

Class I: High Solubility–High Permeability
Class II: Low Solubility–High Permeability
Class III: High Solubility–Low Permeability
Class IV: Low Solubility–Low Permeability

In the case of Class 2 and 4 drugs, dissolution is the predominant factor, and this can be estimated by using *in vitro* data that correlate well with *in vivo* results. The rate-limiting step for the absorption of a class 1 drug is gastric emptying, whereas permeability is the most important factor in the case of class 3 drugs. On a cautionary note, however, many drug-like compounds are exceptions to this rule, due to active transport mechanisms, the involvement of carriers, and possible biotransformation in the gut, and because the rule only applies to orally administered drugs. The rule is more likely to be applicable where the drug is a mimetic of a natural product. Furthermore, good oral bioavailability is shown by many drugs that are larger than 500 Da, but conformationally constrained, and/or that have reduced polar surfaces. This means that many potentially useful leads are discarded, if predictions are based solely on physicochemical indicators, without additional studies.

Thus, *in vitro* screens for the determination of bioavailability are indispensable during early drug development. *In vitro* systems range from relatively simple subcellular fractions, tissue slices or perfused organ preparations, through primary cultures and cell lines, grown either as mono cultures or cocultures, to three-dimensional organotypic cultures, which include reconstructed tissue models (see Ref. 49 for a review). For instance, *in vitro* approaches to determine permeability include the use of animal tissues or cell lines. Where a drug is absorbed by simple passive diffusion, rat everted intestinal rings [50], single-pass perfused intestinal preparations [51], and the human adenocarcinoma cell line Caco-2 [52] are often used to assess intestinal permeability. The common problem of accounting for differences in biotransformation can be addressed by supplementing these assays with a metabolic component. Everted tissue rings, in particular, can suffer from problems related to tissue viability, while the use of Caco-2 cells suffers from (1) the lack of mucus that coats the luminal surface of intestinal cells *in situ* and (2) the possibility that metabolic properties and other essential properties of the cells are lost during repeated passaging. The need for long culture times has been met by using Madin–Darby canine kidney (MDCK) cells, which, like Caco-2 cells, form a columnar epithelium with tight junctions, but which only require 3 days in culture. MDCK cells express fewer transporters, however, and are thus more suited to situations where there is little indication of the involvement of transporters, where the data from MDCK and Caco-2 cells are comparable [53]. However, where first-pass metabolism occurs, cells expressing CYP enzymes are more useful (see later discussion). A comparison of cell-based and tissue-based permeability data indicates that there are good correlations between data from such studies, at least in terms of their ability to rank drugs according to permeability [54]. However, both methods tend to underestimate the absorption of drugs that are actively transported, and to overestimate the absorption of drugs that are subject to efflux pump transport [55].

Two further methods for the assessment of absorption are (1) the use of immobilized membranes or artificial membrane (IAM) [56] chromatography and

(2) the parallel artificial membrane permeation assay (PAMPA) [57]. IAM and PAMPA are both relatively rapid screens, the latter also being amenable to a microtiter plate format. Hence, both are suitable for screening large libraries of drugs for passive diffusion. Again, these systems are only really suited to absorption studies where there is little indication that a drug might be subject to transporter/efflux protein binding, as determined by direct binding assays. For instance, the drug export pump, P-glycoprotein (P-gp), which protects the brain from toxic substances by transporting them back into the blood, and which is, incidentally, also found in tissues such as the kidney and the liver, has been used as the basis of a model system composed of porcine brain capillary endothelial cells. This system allows the ability of drugs to inhibit the efflux of a fluorescent P-gp substrate out of the cells to be readily monitored in a 96-well format [58]. This model may also be a useful supplement to many of the studies on more complex tissue and cell culture systems, given the key role of efflux proteins in determining internal drug concentrations. Indeed, the internal dose that reaches other tissues may have a crucial bearing on the use of the final marketed drug and the nature of the target patient group. Despite the fact that the placental transfer of drugs and other xenobiotics is known to occur, the process is poorly understood. What is known is that it involves efflux proteins, and that P-gp binding capacity may assist with decisions as to whether reproductive and developmental toxicity testing is likely to be required.

Dermal absorption can be determined by using organotypic skin models comprising stratified layers of epidermal cells, with each layer exhibiting morphological and functional differentiation. This has given rise to several commercially available organotypic and reconstructed human skin *in vitro* culture models, including EPISKIN™ (http://www.loreal.com) and EpiDerm™, and its fibroblast-supported version, Full Thickness EpiDerm™ (http://www.mattek.com). Multilayered models of the tracheobronchial tract are also available and permit squamous metaplasia [59], mucin production, and mucociliary clearance to be analyzed for making respiratory toxicity predictions of inhaled drug preparations [60]. Of particular relevance to the development of many cell-based organotypic models is the use of microporous substrates, which have led to physiologically more relevant culture conditions for studies of transcellular transport and cell–tissue interactions. Also, blood–brain barrier (BBB) function can be monitored by using coculture systems and reconstructed models in which sufficiently tight cell–cell junctions are formed (reviewed in Ref. 61), which might be more appropriate when it is envisaged that a delivery system might be used. For example, in models of the BBB, brain microcapillary endothelial cells can be cultured with astrocytes, glial cells, or neurones [62, 63] and "whole-brain" spheroid culture systems have been used to model absorption in neurotoxicology [64].

The nasal route is also widely used for topical and systemic targeting and has recently been considered as a suitable route for active peptide and protein administration, since the nasal mucosa has a higher permeability than the intestinal epithelial layer, because of its porous and neural pH endothelial basement membrane, and since first-pass hepatic and intestinal metabolism is largely avoided. However, mucociliary clearance is relatively fast, and the dose volume is smaller than that administered by other routes. These factors should be considered during the early development of therapeutics designed for nasal administration. *In vitro* models of human nasal absorption are particularly important, given that there are substantial differences in nasal structure and function between many laboratory animal species and humans, which complicates data extrapolation [65]. Human nasal epithelial tissues can be obtained noninvasively, but the resulting heterogeneous primary cell population is difficult to culture and maintain. This has prompted the development of a nasal absorption model, based on Calu-3 human lung adenocarcinoma cells, derived from the upper airway of the lung. The cells can be grown at the air–liquid interface, as confluent and polarized sheets, with tight junctions, which secrete mucin, while also possessing cytochrome P450 (CY)PA1 and CYP2B6 activities and transport functions [66].

As illustrated earlier, because whole perfused organs, tissue slices, tissue isolates, organ fragment cultures, and other organotypic preparations can have limited lifetimes in culture, a wide variety of cell lines are used instead of primary cells and tissues. However, it is important for the cell lines to be thoroughly characterized, since, although use of human tissue and cells is advantageous as it obviates the need for interspecies extrapolation, the more commonly used animal cell lines may also provide data of use during drug development.

Metabolism   Metabolism is a major determinant of drug efficacy and toxicity and has a major influence on drug pharmacokinetics. The metabolism of a drug will depend not only on its structure but also on the presence and expression levels of biotransformation enzymes. Metabolism is one of the main factors that determines not only how well a drug is absorbed into the systemic system but also how it is then transported to, and taken up by, specific tissues, as well as how it is eliminated. Susceptibility to biotransformation can dictate the effective dose of a drug at its intended site of action. Hence, predicting the likely routes and consequences of biotransformation is an essential part of early drug screening.

Phase I drug biotransforming enzymes include the CYP enzymes, flavin-containing monooxygenases, alcohol and aldehyde dehydrogenases, aldehyde oxidase, and peroxidase. Phase II pathways involve conjugation reactions, such as glucuronidation, glutathione conjugation, sulfation, methylation, coenzyme A conjugation, and phosphorylation. The enzymes involved are polymorphic and exist as a large number of isozyme forms that have wide substrate specificity and vary in nature and activity according to tissue and species. This is also the case for other metabolic enzymes and, indeed, for individual differences in drug response and metabolism. It is known, for instance, that there are at least 30 variants of the human CYP2D6 [67], which is responsible for the metabolism of almost one-third of all current therapeutic drugs. Phase I biotransformation is the main source of toxic intermediates or active drugs from innocuous parent chemicals (prodrugs). The main redox reaction, catalyzed by CYP-dependent monooxygenases (CYP-DMO), yields more polar and therefore more readily excretable metabolites. These by-products can exhibit biological effects that exceed, or differ from, those elicited by the parent molecule. Hence, a xenobiotic might appear to lack efficacy in an *in vitro* system, due to the absence of a biotransformation pathway necessary for its conversion into an active form.

Most of the systems described so far are not specifically designed with metabolic competence in mind. One way to circumvent problems with metabolic competence is by adding subcellular or cellular metabolizing systems and assessing the production of known metabolites [68]. For instance, by using rat liver microsomes, it is possible to monitor the biotransformation of small amounts of drugs by using capillary electrophoresis [69]. Metabolic cellular systems can be divided into three main categories: (1) metabolically competent indicator cells (e.g., hepatocytes), (2) coculture systems comprising noncompetent indicator cells (e.g., fibroblasts) mixed with metabolicallycompetent cells, and (3) genetically engineered cell lines that can simultaneously act as indicators of both selected metabolic pathways and toxicity.

Since the liver is the major site of drug metabolism, the use of primary hepatocytes has become well established for studying drug metabolism and drug interactions. Hepatocyte models composed of primary cells assembled into a double collagen layer sandwich provide an *in vivo*-like environment, which can retain some important liver functions long enough for useful data to be obtained [70]. More recently, a mini bioreactor scaffold has been devised for biotransformation studies, comprised of a polycarbonate scaffold in 6-, 24-, and 96-well formats, which supports a gas-permeable PTFE membrane, suitable for medium throughput screening [71]. Animal or human cells can be used, although the latter are often in short supply and rapidly lose their viability and phase I and II biotransforming capacities. However, using animal cells does not overcome potential problems with interspecies differences. HepG2 cells have been used, since they allegedly retain human phase I and II drug-metabolizing activities, as well as bile acid and albumin synthesizing capabilities that are normally lost during hepatocyte culture. In addition, these cells can be transformed with specific genes (e.g., CYP genes), in order to bolster their metabolic competence. Drug interactions with efflux proteins such as P-gp can also be monitored with HepG2 cells, to gauge the extent of drug uptake into the liver [72].

Krebsfaenger et al. [73] constructed a panel of Chinese hamster cell lines that stably expressed variants of the human CYP2D6 gene, or in the case of the genetically engineered and metabolically competent V79 Cell Battery™, tissue-specific human phase I or II metabolic enzymes, including a number of CYP variants, glutathione *S*-transferases, and *N*-acetyltransferases. Since the cell battery also contains cell lines that express equivalent enzymes from other species, there is some scope for resolving species differences in metabolism. This system may not be able to account for the consequences of the overexpression of enzymes, or account for the onslaught of long-range biochemical pathways that may regulate metabolism. Nevertheless, the use of polymorphic cell lines has clear advantages over the use of a genetically homogeneous cell line.

A major problem, particularly when trying to model chronic exposure effects, is simulating *in vivo* perfusion rates by using cell-based systems of biotransformation to (1) ensure the removal of metabolites, and of other products such as reactive oxygen species; and (2) avoid cofactor depletion [74, 75]. Systems based on cell or cell coculture models have been designed to address these problems. Canova et al. [76] have recently described a flat membrane bioreactor, in which primary rat hepatocytes were cultured as collagen sandwiched monolayers on a polycarbonate plate. Since this system permits continuous perfusion, the cells exhibited a high level of metabolic competence and extended viability, as compared to cells grown as adherent monolayers.

Drugs can also inhibit CYP activity without being themselves subject to CYP metabolism, thereby causing the accumulation of toxic substances by modeling the interactions between the drug and the enzyme. Some basic information about the chemical classes that are subject to biotransformation by these key enzymes is already known and can be used for such predictions. For example, CYP1A1 is very active in metabolizing polycyclic aromatic hydrocarbons, CYP2B1 and CYP1A2 preferentially metabolize aromatic amines, and CYP2E1 metabolizes low molecular weight chemicals. Perhaps the most important enzyme, CYP3A4, metabolizes larger molecules, and only six isoenzymes account for the metabolism of almost half of all the drugs in clinical use, namely, CYP1A2, CYP2C9, CYP2C19, CYP2D6, CYP3A3, and CYP3A4 [77, 78]. These enzymes are all polymorphic and (with the notable exception of CYP2D6) are inducibly expressed. Since there are a number of X-ray diffraction structures for CYPs, which can also serve as templates for the homology modeling of other isoenzymes, it is possible to use molecular dynamics simulations and molecule docking to determine whether a novel chemical class of drug candidate is likely to be subjected to CYP metabolism or act as an inhibitor [79]. The advantages of such approaches include the fact that these screens can be used to eliminate poor drug candidates prior to synthesis of the compounds, and undesirable metabolic labile sites can be modified to alter the effective dose and metabolically linked contraindications between medicines can be reduced. Some such *in silico* prediction methods rely on knowledge of the structure and physicochemical properties of the drug in question to serve as alerts. For instance, Singh et al. [80] developed a rapid and semiquantitative model for identifying CYP3A4-labile groups on the basis of exposure and the energetics of hydrogen bonds. This has been used to accurately predict CYP3A metabolism for a number of chemicals [80] (for a review, see also Ref. 81).

The most common technique used to identify metabolic stability, rate of drug biotransformation, and likely metabolic fate of a drug is LC-MS/MS. This technique has recently been automated for high-throughput automated metabolic and protein binding screening [82]. Established cell lines and cell batteries (such as the V79 Cell Battery described earlier) that are genetically engineered to express various phase I and phase II enzymes, either singly or in combination, are particularly important in this respect, since they permit the contributions of specific isozymes to metabolism to be investigated [73] during relatively fast metabolic screening.

1.4   SPECIAL CONSIDERATIONS FOR NOVEL THERAPEUTIC CLASSES

1.4.1   New Classes of Therapeutic Agents: A New Drug Development Strategy?

Over the last decade or so, there has been a dramatic change in the nature of targets, with new protein, nanomedicines, and gene-based and cell-based therapeutics being investigated at an unprecedented rate. These biotechnology-derived pharmaceuticals are mainly used for the diagnosis, prevention, and treatment of serious and chronic diseases and range from blood and blood components and antitoxins to monoclonal antibodies, growth factors, vaccines, gene transfer products, and, potentially, cell-based therapeutics, and they may incorporate nanoparticulate delivery systems. As discussed below, the complex pharmacokinetic behavior of these therapeutics is only just starting to be understood, and attempts to group the preclinical testing of them has been attempted on a very *ad hoc* basis. Nevertheless, there are some specific considerations for each type of therapeutic that should be borne in mind during early therapeutic development.

1.4.2 Protein-Based Therapeutics

Protein-based therapeutics can be subjected to a broad range of posttranslational modifications, including phosphorylation, glycosylation, and intermolecular and intramolecular bond formation, which can vary, depending on the cell or organism used to generate the product. In the case of replacement therapeutics, it is important to mimic the posttranslational modification seen in humans as precisely as possible. For novel therapeutics, the consequences of using recombinant techniques to produce a biological product, such as a monoclonal antibody, should be evaluated, to ensure that the finished product is sufficiently humanized, has folded correctly; and exhibits the type of posttranslation modification required for its proper function. In all cases, the primary aim is to avoid having the product elicit immunogenic responses that reduce its effectiveness or give rise to adverse effects.

The pharmaceutical industry has developed ways of scaling up the cell-based manufacture of biological products in serum-free and protein-free chemically defined media, in order to minimize the abnormal glycosylation of proteins. This is to comply with a regulatory requirement for the glycosylation profile of a protein to be maintained. This is particularly important, since products such as monoclonal antibodies can elicit antibody-dependent cell cytotoxicity, depending on their glycosylation state [83]. Indeed, protein-based therapeutics are often developed and characterized by mass (e.g., SPR, MS), activity (in cellular or biochemical assays), and immunogenicity assays (e.g., antibody-dependent cell-mediated cytotoxicity and immune cell proliferation assays), more so than in small chemical therapeutics. These measurements are generally obtained much earlier in the drug development process.

Other problems encountered during the development of protein-based therapeutics are caused by the fact that most of the products are human specific, potentially limiting the relevance of preclinical animal-based studies. In the case of the immunomodulatory monoclonal antibody TGN1412, a surrogate anti-rat CD28 antibody (JJ316), specific for the equivalent epitope to that recognized by TGN1412 in humans, was used to probe the mechanism of action of the therapeutic. However, subsequent studies on TGN1412 were conducted on macaques, on the basis that the CD28 antibody in this species possesses an identical TGN1412 recognition epitope to that found on the human protein. None of these preclinical models were able to predict the very serious contraindications that later materialized during Phase I trials [84]. This casts some doubt over the utility of testing surrogate molecules in a surrogate species with regard to the estimation of human safety when applied to humanized products. In the United States, the review of biological products, including monoclonal antibodies and other therapeutic agents with novel mechanisms of action, was until relatively recently conducted by the CBER. However, the CBER recognized that the utility of animal studies in the development of such therapeutic agents is often limited, due to species differences between the molecular targets. As a consequence, the jurisdiction for testing such products has now been transferred to the CDER, and it is almost certain that there will be a requirement that biological products conform to the two species test criteria adopted for other pharmaceuticals.

1.4.3 Gene Therapeutics

Advances in the use of viral vectors (e.g., adenoviruses, lentiviruses, and RNA viruses) and nonviral vectors (e.g., cells, liposomes, and DNA) have resulted in a growing interest in developing gene therapeutics for targeting single gene deficiencies, as well as cancers and neurodegenerative and tissue repair diseases. Nucleotide-based therapeutics will almost certainly be taken up by different cell types in the body via the same mechanisms. However, the key questions are the longevity of these treatments, whether they will result in incorporation into the genetic makeup of specific cell types, and the long-term consequences for the genetic makeup of germline and somatic cells. These products may therefore require early screening for reproductive and developmental toxicity, potentially via the use of fish larval forms and developmental assays with *D. melanogaster or C. elegans*. Genotoxicity screens that involve cell-based screens may also be relevant. Incidentally, the FETAX (frog embryo teratogenesis assay—*Xenopus*) test [85], a 4-day whole embryo developmental toxicity test, has been available for use for several years, but the apparent *status quo* with regard to its evaluation is consistent with concerns over its relevance to humans. The requirement for animal-based developmental, reproductive, or genotoxicity testing can then be assessed on a case-by-case basis, depending on the class of vector, transgene, and delivery method. In the absence of suitable long-term *in vitro* models, chronic toxicity studies in animals might also be justified, in which DNA integration is monitored by sensitive PCR-based techniques, although the two-year rodent assay may not be suitable for this purpose [86].

1.4.4 Nanomedicines

Nanomedicines (and ultrafines) consist of, or contain, organic or inorganic nanomaterials of variable dimensions, which, according to the U.S. Patent Office, are of 100 nm or less in size. The two main classes are carbon-based liposomes, dendrimers, fullerenes, nanotubes, nanowires, nanorods and metal oxide-based quantum dots and PEG-polyester systems. Nanomedicines, such as PEG-modified versions of existing drugs (e.g., PEG-granulocyte colony stimulating factor), are already on the market. Many other nanotechnology-based applications, such as carbon nanotube-based RNA, DNA, protein, and drug delivery systems, are being developed [87]. Indeed, between 2004 and 2005 there was a 60% increase in the number of such products in the development pipeline.

There is currently little regulatory guidance on how nanomedicines should be characterized, and each nanomedicine is generally assessed on an individual basis. It is also clear that information for macroparticle equivalents is often of limited relevance. According to the FDA, toxicity screening of nanomedicines [88] should involve (1) an assessment of physicochemical characteristics, including core and surface chemistry; (2) *in vitro* studies to determine absorption by the intended, and potentially additional, routes of exposure, binding studies, bioaccumulation/cellular uptake studies, and cytotoxicity screening; and (3) *in vivo* understanding of biokinetics and toxicity.

Nanomedicines display physical and chemical properties that are often distinct from their macroparticle counterparts. For instance, the small particle size corresponds with a high surface area: mass ratio means that not only are nanoparticles likely to be more reactive because of their quantum properties [89], they are also more likely to agglomerate in a way that makes absorption difficult to predict by using biokinetic modeling alone. This would require information about the extent of agglomeration and the proportion of each type of particle in heterogeneous mixtures of particles, as well as a fundamental understanding of how agglomeration affected different reactivities. Agglomeration is dependent on surface chemistry and charge, and this will also have a crucial bearing on uptake into different tissues [90].

Nanoparticles may be able to escape phagocytic activity and may not only have extended biological half-lives but may also elicit immunogenic and inflammatory responses, especially since they may be able to access lung tissues and be able to cross the BBB, the intestinal mucosa, and other physical barriers more readily than macroparticles. Indeed, the size of a nanoparticle is generally that of a typical protein. Note that BBB passage requires nanoparticle dimensions of 20–50 nm, whereas 70-nm particles are able to cross into the pulmonary system, and spherical fullerenes appear to accumulate in the liver [91]. However, at present, there is little information about how nanoparticles are able to interact with the immune system and with specific tissues.

Examining the tendency of nanomedicines to bioaccumulate is an important step in the nanomedicine development strategy, so the need for long-term toxicity testing cannot be overemphasized. There is already some indication as to how readily different types of carbon-based nanomaterials accumulate in different tissues [92], as well as about how physicochemical properties such as size, shape, tendency to agglomerate, surface fictionalization, and chemical composition relate to the absorption, distribution, and biokinetics of nanoparticles (see Ref. 93 for a review).

1.5 *IN VITRO* ASSAYS: APPLICATIONS IN SAFETY PHARMACOLOGY

1.5.1 Background

Many surrogate assays have been developed for the detection of toxicological endpoints. Many of those used specifically for lead development and early ADME characterization have already been considered. Here, we consider *in vitro* assays that are relevant to the early characterization of toxicologically relevant endpoints. A list of methods that are currently available for toxicological endpoints that may be more suited to high-throughput safety pharmacology have been developed and/ or validated, some of which have already been afforded OECD Test Guideline status (Table 1.6). These and other such tests may eventually expedite the safety testing of pharmaceutical products. At present, however, they are most commonly used to provide evidence to supplement animal test data. Their potential application to toxicology testing is illustrated in Fig. 1.2. Their validation status will have a bearing on the acceptability of specific tests as part of a medicine's dossier for different regulatory agencies, and there is generally a delay of several years between validation and regulatory acceptance. It should be noted that in the EU, under the terms of *Directive 86/609/EEC*, once an *in vitro* alternative to an animal test has been deemed to be reasonably and practicably available and has been validated for a specific purpose, it must be used instead of the equivalent animal test.

TABLE 1.6 Status of Nonanimal Methods that Are of Relevance to Drug Development[a]

Test Method	Test System	Endpoint	OECD TG Reference and Comments
In Vitro Test Methods for Which There Are OECD Health Effects Test Guidelines (Including Draft Guidelines Under Review for Acceptance) http://www.oecd.org/home/			
Transcutaneous electrical resistance test (TER)	Monitors changes in electrical resistance as a measure of loss of corneum integrity and barrier function; involves skin disks from euthanized rats	Skin corrosion (topical agents)	TG 430
Human skin models (EpiDerm™, EPISKIN™)	Reconstructed human epidermal equivalent (commercial system) used to assess cell viability, involving the MTT reduction test	Skin corrosion (topical agents)	TG 431
3T3 NRU phototoxicity test	BALB/c 3T3 (murine) cell line cytotoxicity based on Neutral Red uptake to measure cell viability; not a direct replacement alternative, as there is no *in vivo* equivalent test	Phototoxicity	TG 432
Corrositex™ membrane barrier test	An artificial barrier system coupled to a pH-based chemical detection system	Skin corrosion (topical agents)	Draft TG 435
Bacterial Reverse Mutation test (Ames)	Revertant bacteria detected by their ability to grow in the absence of the amino acid	Genotoxicity	TG 471
In vitro mammalian chromosome aberration test	Microscopic detection of chromosomal damage to cells in culture	Genotoxicity	TG 473
In vitro mammalian cell gene mutation test	Functional bioassays to monitor mutations in enzyme encoding genes	Genotoxicity	TG 476
Sister chromatid exchange assay	Cells in culture are examined after two rounds of division by metaphase arrest and chromosomal preparation; chromatid exchange is monitored by microscopy	Genotoxicity	TG 479
Gene mutation assay in yeast	*Saccharomyces cerivisiae* exposed to the test substance are grow under different culture conditions used to monitor mutagenic potential (cf. Ames test)	Genotoxicity	TG 480
Mitotic recombination assay in yeast	Crossover or gene conversion following exposure of yeast to the test substance; relies on different growth requirements of mutated and wild-type yeast strains	Genotoxicity	TG 481

Test	Description	Toxicity	Status
Unscheduled DNA synthesis in mammalian cells	Measures the DNA repair synthesis after deletions caused by the test substance; based on the incorporation of radioactive nucleotides into the newly synthesized DNA	Genotoxicity	TG 482
In vitro micronucleus test	Cell-based assay; supplement to TG 474 (in vivo micronucleus test); detection of chromosome damage and formation of micronuclei	Genotoxicity	Draft TG 487
Sex-linked recessive lethal test	Drosophila are exposed to the test substance. Germline transmission of mutations is monitored through two successive generations	Reproductive toxicity	TG 477

Validated Methods that Are Yet to Be Introduced into Regulatory Use

Test	Description	Toxicity	Status
EpiOcular™	Human keratinocyte derived model of the corneal epithelium barrier function	Eye irritation (topical application)	Retrospective (weight-of-evidence) validation (ECVAM)
In vitro micronucleus test	CHL/IU, CHO, SHE, or V79 cell lines are commonly used, with or without metabolic activation, to monitor damage and formation of micronuclei in interphase	Mutagenicity	Retrospective (weight-of-evidence) validation (ECVAM)
Embryonic stem cell test	3T3 cell cytotoxicity and differentiation of embryonic stem murine cell lines used to examine teratogenic potential	Developmental toxicity	Endorsed as screening test (EU)
Postimplantation rat whole embryo test	Morphological assessment of rat embryos	Developmental toxicity	Endorsed as screening test (EU)
Micromass test	Micromass cultures of rat limb are bud monitored for inhibition of cell proliferation and differentiation	Developmental toxicity	Endorsed as screening test (EU)

Methods Undergoing Validation

Test	Description	Toxicity	Status
EPISKIN™	Reconstructed human skin system used with MTT assay to monitor barrier function	Skin irritation	Report stage in EU
EpiDerm™	Similar to EPISKIN™	Skin irritation	Report stage in EU

TABLE 1.6 *Continued*

Test Method	Test System	Endpoint	OECD TG Reference and Comments
Prevalidated Methods			
SkinEthic eye model	Epithelial corneal cell line used for cytotoxicity testing based on the MTT reduction assay	Eye irritation	Appraisal stage in EU
Methods Undergoing Development, Prevalidation, or Evaluation			
Tissue culture models	Neutral Red release and silicon microphysiometry or fluorescein leakage bioassays with human keratinocytes and MDCK cells, respectively; red blood cell (RBC) hemolysis test	Eye irritation	Being reviewed by ECVAM for possible retrospective (weight-of-evidence) validation
Organotypic models	Bovine corneal opacity and permeability (BCOP) assay, with postmortem corneas; hen's egg test on the chorioallantoic membrane (HET-CAM assay); isolated rabbit and chicken eye tests (IRE and ICE)	Eye irritation	Being reviewed by ICCVAM for possible retrospective (weight-of-evidence) validation
Cell transformation assay	With SHE and BALB/c 3T3 cell lines	Carcinogenicity	
Modified Leydig cell line	Analysis of progesterone production as a measure of the test substance effects on steroid hormone production	One/two generation study	For use as part of test battery
Testis slices	Assessment of steroid production capacity of the Leydig cells upon exposure of *ex vivo* rat tissue to toxicants	One/two generation study	For use as part of test battery
Human adrenocortical carcinoma cell line	Assay to allow entire steroid pathway effects to be mapped	One/two generation study	For use as part of test battery
Placental microsomal aromatase assay	Monitors the ability of substances to affect steroid production; a subcellular microsomal assay is used industrially	One/two generation study	For use as part of test battery

[a]This is a comprehensive list of methods that have been validated or that are at various stages of development for toxicity testing. More information about these methods and how they can be applied is available from: http://www2.defra.gov.uk/research/project_data/more.asp?I=CB01067&M=KWS&V=reach&scope=0.

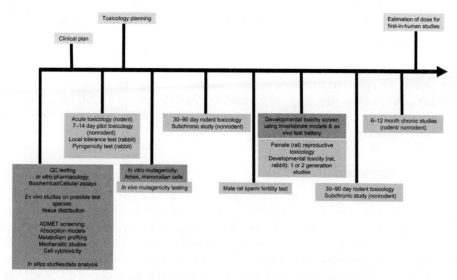

FIGURE 1.2   A typical toxicity plan from formulation of a clinical plan to first-in-human studies. The figure summarizes the general regulatory requirements and the role of *in vitro* and animal studies in preclinical safety pharmacology.

1.5.2   QT Prolongation

The recently developed ICH S7B guideline relates to the prolongation of the QT interval, the time between the start of the Q wave and the end of the T wave in the electrical cycle of the heart. Drugs that prolong the QT interval do so by blocking the activity of the human ether-a-go-go-related gene (hERG) channel found on cardiomyocytes, which plays a role in phase 3 depolarization. This can, but does not always, lead to the potentially fatal, although rare, tachyarrhythmia, Torsades des pointes. Electrophysiological recordings in cells and tissue explants can be used to screen for hERG activity. The most commonly used nonanimal assays involve studies on rabbit left ventricular wedge or perfused heart preparations [94].

Several cell-based and *in silico* prediction tools could also be used effectively for early screening. It is clear that while several classes of drugs, including antihistamines, antiemetics, antibacterials, and neuroleptics, have been associated with QT prolongation [95], not all the drugs of a particular class will cause this effect. Hence, although mutational analysis of hERG and pharmacophore modeling has helped to elucidate how several drugs block channel activity (reviewed in Ref. 96), the prediction of QT prolongation by using *in silico* methods alone is problematical. As a consequence, the first realistic step in screening for hERG-blocking activity generally depends on the use of cell-based studies. It should also be remembered that hERG activity is not the sole determinant of whether a drug is likely to cause cardiac arrhythmias, since the expression and activity of other ion channels can either mitigate or exacerbate the effects of a drug on QT interval prolongation. Metabolism and species differences in ion channel distribution and activity must also be taken into account. Species differences can be avoided by using cell lines such as Chinese hamster ovary or human embryonic kidney cells heterologously expressing hERG, since mammalian cells are the ideal system for studying potassium channel activity at physiologically relevant temperatures (see Ref. 96 for a review). This is the case even despite the fact that while patch clamping is generally more readily achievable for larger cell types, such as *Xenopus* oocytes expressing hERG, the lower temperature required for their culture can complicate data extrapolation to humans. More recently, human embryonic stem cell (HESC)-derived cell types with primary cardiomyocyte-like properties have become available [97, 98]. However, although these cells act as a suitable surrogate for cardiomyocytes, the use of HESCs raises ethical issues. Adult stem cells derived from tissues such as bone marrow have therefore also been investigated as primary cardiomyocyte surrogates [99].

1.5.3 ICH Guidelines

Pyrogenicity testing forms part of the quality control of pharmaceuticals, particularly of biotechnological products that may be contaminated with gram-negative bacteria. Five *in vitro* methods have been proposed and evaluated as possible alternatives to pyrogenicity testing in animals (usually rabbits). These are based on the use of human whole blood or blood subcellular fractions linked to interleukin-based screens. These methods have been validated under the auspices of ECVAM, and the ECVAM Scientific Advisory Committee has endorsed their use. Draft recommendations regarding the applicability of these methods were published by ICCVAM in December 2006 [100].

The ICH guidelines for the safety testing of pharmaceutical products for human use are listed in Table 1.7. In general, tests are conducted by the same route of exposure as that anticipated for clinical use. Where there is more than one route of exposure, at least two routes should be investigated. Where the intended route of human exposure is impracticable for animal studies, the route of exposure in animal studies will need to be different, although the aim is to establish whether the level of systemic exposure is similar to that via the clinical route. In the case of ocular administration, systemic exposure is not automatically assumed, so some toxicological studies, such as carcinogenicity testing, may not be required, unless there is compelling evidence to suggest otherwise. Carcinogenicity testing is not usually required for peptide and protein replacement therapeutics, unless they are significantly different from their natural counterparts. The dose used is generally derived from the MTD from 3-month toxicity studies, as well as from a consideration of toxicokinetic data and the known or predicted consequences of biotransformation of the chemical. Carcinogenicity testing may also be guided by the outcome of genotoxicity and cell transformation studies, the majority of which involve cell-based screens for gene mutation or chromosomal aberration. The ICH guidelines require three tests for genotoxicity: (1) a test for gene mutation in bacteria, (2) an *in vitro* mammalian cell or mouse lymphoma assay for chromosomal damage, and (3) an *in vivo* test for the detection of chromosomal damage in hematopoietic cells in the bone marrow of rodents.

Determination of the acute toxicity of a single dose of a pharmaceutical no longer requires an LD_{50} determination. Instead, it is most commonly derived from the maximum tolerated dose (MTD). The ICH guidelines recommend that acute toxicity is determined in a rodent and in a nonrodent species. However, in many cases, it may be possible to justify the use of a single species and/or incorporation of the MTD estimation into a dose escalation study from longer term/repeat-dose studies. The justification for conducting repeat-dose studies is partly based on the outcome of single-dose studies. This is especially the case when single-dose studies indicate

TABLE 1.7   ICH Guidelines[a] for Safety Pharmacology

ICH Guideline for Safety Pharmacology http://www.ich.org/	Description of Content
Acute Toxicity Testing	
M3(R1)—Maintenance of the ICH Guideline on Non-clinical Safety Studies for the Conduct of Human Clinical Trials for Pharmaceuticals	S4—single dose LD_{50} tests for pharmaceuticals have been abandoned; the guideline sets out the duration of acute, repeat dose, and chronic tests in animals, and the criteria for reproductive, developmental, fertility, genotoxicity, and carcinogenicity testing, as well as the times during development that each type of safety test should be performed
Carcinogenicity Testing	
S1A—Guideline on the Need for Carcinogenicity Studies of Pharmaceuticals	Long-term studies, with dosing at the MTD level or, in the United States, a dose 100-fold higher than the recommended human daily dose, are conducted in a single rodent species (the rat unless evidence suggests it is not an appropriate species), for a duration of no less than 6 months; additional rodent studies of short-term or medium-term duration may be required (generally in mice/GM mice); a weight-of-evidence approach is used to determine whether there is a likely cause for concern based on genotoxicity tests, the results of cell transformation studies, effects of same-in-class/ SAR, preoplastic lesions in repeat-dose studies, and/or long-term tissue retention of the drug or its metabolites
S1B—Testing for Carcinogenicity of Pharmaceuticals	
S1C(R1)—Dose Selection for Carcinogenicity Studies of Pharmaceuticals	
Genotoxicity Testing	
S2A—Guidance on Specific Aspects of Regulatory Genotoxicity Tests for Pharmaceuticals	Provides recommendations as to the bacterial strains and mammalian cell lines or human blood cells that could be used to detect various types of DNA damage; defines the concentrations to be used in each type of test and how to make decisions as to whether to proceed with *in vivo* animal studies
S2B—Genotoxicity: A Standard Battery for Genotoxicity Testing of Pharmaceuticals	
Toxicokinetic Studies	
S3A—Note for Guidance on Toxicokinetics: The Assessment of Systemic Exposure in Toxicity Studies	Toxicokinetic studies are normally integrated with repeat dose/3-month toxicity studies and provide multiple-dose pharmacokinetic data
S3B—Pharmacokinetics: Guidance for Repeated Dose Tissue Distribution Studies	
Chronic Toxicity Testing	
S4—Duration of Chronic Toxicity Testing in Animals (Rodent and Non Rodent Toxicity Testing)	Performed for a 6-month duration in rodents and a 9-month duration in nonrodent species

TABLE 1.7 *Continued*

ICH Guideline for Safety Pharmacology http://www.ich.org/	Description of Content
Reproductive Toxicity Testing	
S5(R2)—Detection of Toxicity to Reproduction for Medicinal Products Toxicity to Male Fertility: An Addendum to the ICH Tripartite Guideline on Detection of Toxicity to Reproduction for Medicinal Products	one- or two-generation studies (generally in rodents) may be needed, depending on the intended use, form, and route of administration of a drug; incorporates embryotoxicity studies (usually on rabbits/rodents), but also considers the merits of other test systems, such as tissue, organ, and organism cultures
Biotechnological Products	
S6—Preclinical Safety Evaluation of Biotechnology-Derived Pharmaceuticals	Pharmaceutical products from cell cultures and transgenic plants/animals, such as proteins, hormones, antibodies, and proteins extracted from human tissues, are primarily subject to these guidelines; normally, two species are used, but in some cases only a single species is relevant; if no species is relevant, the creation of a GM model is considered
Miscellaneous Safety Pharmacology	
S7A—Safety Pharmacology Studies for Human Pharmaceuticals S7B—The Non-clinical Evaluation of the Potential for Delayed Ventricular Repolarization (QT Interval Prolongation) By Human Pharmaceuticals	Defines the way in which toxicity of the major organ systems can be monitored by using animal and *in vitro* methods; one of the criteria for determining whether safety pharmacology needs to be performed is whether a drug is able to enter into the systemic system, so many topically administered drugs are excluded from full safety evaluation QT prolongation: criteria are given for *in vitro* and *in vivo* animal tests
Immunotoxicity Testing	
S8—Immunotoxicology Studies for Human Pharmaceuticals	Addresses the use of local tolerance/allergy tests at the site of injection (generally in rabbits); and the use of assays that monitor humoral and cell-mediated immunity and immunomodulation; the requirement for immunotoxicity testing is based on a weight-of-evidence approach

*The ICH website has additional information about the testing criteria and study design for each end-point. Guidelines for quality assessment are also available from this site.

that the half-life of the drug (and/or its metabolites) in organs or tissues significantly exceeds the apparent half-life of the elimination phase in plasma, and when the steady-state levels of a drug are higher in repeat-dose studies than in single-dose studies. Predicted tissue-specific retention that leads to tissue-specific toxicity is also a justification for repeat-dose studies. Pharmaceuticals developed for site-specific delivery might also require repeat-dose studies.

Determining the acute dose toxicity of biotechnology products in animals is likely to be of limited relevance to safety assessment. This is because such products (e.g., recombinant proteins) are highly human specific and are likely to give rise to immunogenicity. However, the latter effect can be investigated by using the murine local lymph node assay (LLNA). This test has been accepted in the United States and the European Union as an alternative to the guinea pig maximization test for assessing allergic contact dermatitis caused by pharmaceuticals, and is now part of the OECD Health Effects Test Guidelines (TG 429).

The possibility of using *in vitro* systems to permit the high-throughput assessment of chronic toxicity is currently very limited, predominantly due to the problems inherent in undertaking repeat exposures and maintaining long-term cultures. However, one system developed from stem cells consists of a neurosphere with an outer layer of cells surrounding a growing core [64] that can be maintained in culture for up to a year. This system might be amenable for development into a long-term assay for assessing neurotoxicological endpoints (see Section 1.3.2).

1.6 SYSTEMS BIOLOGY

Many of the screens and assays described thus far are focused on measuring a single parameter. However, although they provide information relevant to the *in vivo* assessment of new drugs, they lack some of the complexities of animal studies. Nevertheless, this can sometimes be an advantage, particularly as the effects observed during *in vivo* studies can be due to a multitude of unknown mechanisms, and this can confound data interpretation and extrapolation. As illustrated next, recent developments in the omics-based technologies and microfluidics may provide a way of addressing this caveat against the use of existing cell-based and tissue-based screens.

1.6.1 Omics-Based Technologies

Biomarkers Biomarkers discovered from, and subsequently used in, nonclinical studies can play several useful roles in drug development. During lead discovery, a biomarker can assist with the screening of chemicals, based on the ability of the candidate molecule to modulate the activity of a specific process, such as a biochemical pathway. In some cases, these biomarkers can be used to develop reporter gene screens, such as the CRE and ERE activation-linked expression of GFP or enzymes. In this way, the application of biomarkers can provide information about target interactions in support of the feasibility of a given therapeutic approach, as well as to assist in the development of high-throughput screening systems to expedite drug discovery.

Biomarkers are also relevant for selecting the most appropriate test species, since the absence of a significant marker is likely to be indicative of differences in the activities of a drug in humans and the test species. The use of biomarkers as surrogate endpoints can identify the commonality between *in vitro* and *in vivo* effects, leading to dramatic improvements in the power of meta-analysis and of other approaches, where the goal is to assemble and evaluate value of information from various sources, such as animal experiments, human studies, and *in vitro* studies. This is, of course, subject to the very careful selection of the biomarkers to be used. One consideration is a need to readily detect changes in levels of biomarkers and to be able to relate such changes to drug-related efficacy or toxicity. In the interests of animal welfare and experimental convenience, metabolites and other small molecules that can be detected noninvasively in blood, stool, hair, or urine samples are preferred. This is because such biomarkers can be continually monitored during an experiment, and large numbers of samples can be collected, thereby allowing statistically reliable data to be generated from a small number of animals. However, most importantly, such biomarkers can also be readily analyzed in body fluid and stool samples taken from participants in clinical trials and can be used in the conduct of postmarket surveillance of large cohorts of patients.

Omics Toward Biomarker Discovery   *Genomics* can be used to identify new targets, since it is now possible to analyze changes in the transcription of >20,000 genes in various cell types and tissues in multiparameter experiments. There are two key approaches: (1) the detection of cDNAs that correspond to the entire protein-encoding gene; and (2) the use of RNAi to determine the relevance of mRNA levels in terms of protein expression and gene function. Recently, these approaches have been used to assess the influence of noncoding RNAs on specific biochemical pathways in mammalian cells [101]. The application of genomics has already proved useful in fundamental research and for gaining a mechanistic understanding of drug activity. However, so far, it has made only limited contributions to drug discovery [1]. Similarly, *toxicogenomic* approaches, in which global changes in gene expression resulting from exposure of specific cells or tissues to a test substance are identified, have been of limited use up to now. Nevertheless, the microarray or serial analysis of gene expression, by using commercially derived or custom-made gene chips, such as those from Affymetrix (www.affymetrix.com/), is a technique that is already proving useful for the identification of markers of hematotoxicity and carcinogenicity [102, 103].

Proteomics is an approach that involves measuring total cellular protein and determining the posttranslational modification and fate of proteins. The most applicable techniques involve spotting cell lysates onto arrayed antibody wells to search for potential biomarkers and to profile molecular pathways. In this way, much useful information on specific protein–protein interactions has been gained by using yeast-2-hybrid systems, and coimmunoprecipitation or other affinity-based methodologies. The antibodies required for this purpose are being generated and characterized by the Human Proteome Organization (HUPO) [104]. The reason why data from proteomics can be more relevant than the information from genomic analysis is that changes in mRNA levels do not necessarily correlate with changes in protein expression. Furthermore, it is clear that a drug might alter the protein recycling/degradation/synthesis rates and/or the extent, as well as the nature, of posttranslational modification. However, proteomics is limited by the fact that some classes of proteins are difficult to resolve (e.g., membrane proteins) and it is currently not amenable to high-throughput formats.

Metabonomics is defined as "the quantitative measurement of the dynamic multi-parametric metabolic response of living systems to pathophysiological stimuli or genetic modification" [105]. It has traditionally required the use of analytical methods such as MS and NMR, in conjunction with separation techniques such as gas or liquid chromatography, which are primarily suited to the resolution of low molecular weight metabolites. Although NMR is generally less sensitive than MS-based methods, newer techniques such as magic angle spinning NMR cater for the direct metabolic profiling of as little as 20 mg of tissue or biofluids [106, 107]. Typically, drug testing by metabolic profiling involves the collection of body fluids from animals or human volunteers and is conducted alongside drug metabolism and PK studies.

In the case of animal experiments, many variables have complicated the interpretation of data from metabonomic studies in animals. Such variables include the species and strain of animal, gender, age, and the influence of diurnal variations and environmental factors and stressors. Other factors include the choice of dosing vehicle and the acclimatization period prior to the conduct of studies in metabolism cages. Nevertheless, the development of increasingly sophisticated analytical techniques (see later discussion) has permitted the use of smaller group sizes and reductions in the amounts of body fluids required, and reductions in the need for invasive studies, particularly where metabolic profiling is conducted on urine samples.

The main advantage of metabonomics over proteomics and genomics is that there is a much stronger link to a tangible physiological response to a drug, because it is not reliant on potentially delayed effects on protein expression, but rather on the measurement of biochemical changes that result from the modulation of specific pathways.

1.6.2 Microfluidics Systems

A microscale cell culture system that consists of a series of chambers each containing mammalian cells connected by a fluid network can be used to assess drug dynamics as a quasi *in vivo* surrogate system [108]. The development of robotic DNA printing systems [109] that allow cells to be transformed *in situ*, and adaptations that facilitate the growth and maintenance of such microfluidics systems, without the need for plating, can, as a result, be used for longer term as well as real-time studies [110]. The use of human cells instead of animal cells greatly increases the relevance of such systems to human safety.

1.6.3 Enabling Technologies for Multiparameter Studies

All the approaches discussed generate such a large amount of information that data analysis and interpretation can be very complicated, so complex analytical methods are needed to integrate and analyze the results. One of the most useful of these methods is pattern recognition. Pattern recognition algorithms differ widely in the ways in which data are analyzed and used to develop new hypotheses. The further development and application of these methods (reviewed in Ref. 111) could transform the ways in which systems biology approaches will facilitate the use of information from omic-based studies, data mining, pathway informatics, and other types of study, in order to gain an overview of drug action. At present, more than 150 databases, data analysis tools, and software suites are already available for this purpose [112]. These bioinformatics platforms mainly comprise commercially available clustering techniques that enable the extraction of exposure-related infor-

TABLE 1.8 Pathway Signal Databases and Generation Tools for Systems-Based Drug Development[a]

Pathway Tools

MetaCore http://metacore.com/web/index.php

A pathway modeling database

Pathway Studio www.ariadnegenomics.com

Assists with the interpretation of omics data and the generation of pathways that can be updated with information from other sources

Pathway Analyst http://path-a.cs.ualberta.ca/

Predicts pathways in which a target protein may be involved

Gepasi http://www.gepasi.org/

Software for modeling biochemical pathways; incorporates biokinetic simulation tools

Jdesigner http://sbw.kgi.edu/software/jdesigner.htm

A system that allows biochemical networks to be drawn

Whole cell biochemical pathways

Genomatica http://www.genomatica.com/index.shtml

A collection of models for whole cells and organisms that displays gene, protein, and biochemical networks

E-Cell http://www.e-cell.org/software

A simulation, modeling, and analysis tool for application to complex biological systems

Whole tissue/organ pathway tools

Human Physiome Project https://www.bioeng.auckland.ac.nz/physiome/physiome_project.php

A computational database that aims to build integrative models of biological systems, and whole organ/tissue structure and functions

Clinical data

Entelos http://www.entelos.com/

For virtual patient simulations based on normal and disease physiology, to assist in deciphering disease-related pathways

[a]The rapidly growing number of resources is impossible to list in full. However, these are some key resources that can be used during drug discovery and development.

mation on changes in proteins, in metabolites, or in gene expression, and can overlay information from different sources to find common hotspots or to identify biochemical networks. The length of the branch corresponds to the similarities between datasets. To further reduce the number of false-positive biomarkers, a common problem with all omics-based technologies, condition-specific algorithms, modeling approaches, and data-mining software packages have recently been developed (reviewed in Ref. 113; Table 1.8). There are also several tools that assist with the weighting of information from these varied approaches (Table 1.8).

1.7 COMPUTATIONAL METHODOLOGY USED IN EARLY PRECLINICAL DRUG DEVELOPMENT

1.7.1 Combinatorial Chemistry and SAR

By avoiding the incorporation of particular chemical groups into a drug, the likelihood of toxicity can be greatly reduced. Computational methods are used at the very early stages of drug development to analyze the behavior of virtual chemical libraries, in terms of target specificity and affinity, or in terms of transport across physiological barriers, metabolism, or the causation of off-target modulation [114]. These predictions can rely on either a local set of data for a limited number of structurally related chemicals or global models. The latter require a large training set for refining a computational predictive tool and are generally able to identify alerts that may result in toxicity with greater success than locally trained tools (i.e., those based on a small set of known compounds). Affinity receptor binding data are very useful for the development of predictive computational models of closely related analogues of a drug molecule, as is information on the natural ligand derived from *in vitro* target–ligand binding studies.

An ability to generate an accurate model of the target protein is also very useful. Such models can be created *ab initio* or by homology-based modeling. In fact, the protein target models themselves are generated by using several approaches, the most popular of which combines primary sequence analysis for structural signatures that indicate probable protein folding with X-ray diffraction and crystallographic studies on a protein of the same class. A variety of molecular docking programs can be used, and most algorithms are based on an assumption that the target (generally a protein) is a rigid structure, while the ligand is flexible. The notable exceptions are force-field-based methods, such as molecular dynamics and Monte Carlo simulations, which allow for flexibility in both the target and the ligand. This approach accommodates the proposed "induced fit" model for most peptide and protein ligands. Fragment-based incremental methods are similarly suitable for assembling ligands from fragments that are incrementally docked into the target.

QSAR modeling is useful when each member of the same class of chemicals (sharing key structural elements and physicochemical properties) acts by a common mechanism. It involves generating rules from a training set of molecules based on their structures and known biological activities. These rules are then used to predict the biological activity of a novel candidate molecule with structural features that fall within the applicability domain of the model. For each docking application, a scoring system to identify virtual hits and a rule base that can accommodate experimental SAR data, are essential. The reader is referred to an excellent review on this topic [115] (see also Table 1.9).

1.7.2 *In Silico* Prediction of ADME and Toxicity

Adverse drug reactions (ADRs) remain one of the major reasons why a drug that has passed through preclinical testing will eventually be dropped following clinical trials. Efforts have recently been made to develop computer-based prediction tools and other such expert systems, for use in assessing the ADR potentials of drugs. Although there are four general types of expert systems, all of them are built up from experimental toxicity data. Hence, the early prediction of whether a drug is likely to have adverse effects can be used to refine compound libraries prior to high-throughput hit generation and lead development. DEREK (Deduction of Risk from Existing Knowledge) is a knowledge-based system, which focuses on molecular substructures (or "alerts") associated with known toxicological endpoints [116, 117]. It is able to predict three different endpoints, including mutagenicity, for which it was found to be 84% correctly predictive for a set of 226 chemicals. CASE

TABLE 1.9   Examples of QSARs that Can Be Used During Lead Discovery and Optimization[a]

Database	Type of Information
ChemTree http://www.goldenhelix.com/chemtreesoftware.html	Statistical analysis QSAR for chemical library refinement
QikProp http://www.schrodinger.com	ADME prediction QSAR for lead generation and optimization
Catalyst http://www.accelrys.com/products/catalyst/	3D QSAR and query-based database management tool
CoMFA (Comparative Molecular Field Analysis) http://www.chem.ac.ru/Chemistry/Soft/COMFA.en.html	3D QSAR technique based on data from known active molecules; applicable when the structure of the target protein is unknown
VolSurf http://www.moldiscovery.com/soft_volsurf.php	Produces 2D molecular descriptors from 3D molecular interaction energy grid maps, for the optimization of *in silico* PK properties (eADME or IS-DMPK)

[a]More information about these methods and how they can be applied is available from http://www2.defra.gov.uk/research/project_data/more.asp?!=CB01067&M=KWS&V=reach&scope=0. Website links accessed 30 January 2007.

(Computer Automated Structure Evaluation) is an automated rule induction system [118]. It generates its own structural alerts by breaking down each chemical into all its possible fragments that are then classified as biophores (associated with toxicity) or biophobes (not associated with toxicity). CASE has been adapted by the FDA to provide MCASE QSAR-ES, which is able to predict carcinogenicity with an accuracy of 75% [119]. TOPKAT is an automated QSAR system [120] that uses large amounts of data for diverse compounds to build a set of descriptors. Decision tree-based methods are typified by OncoLogic [121], which, as its name suggests, is also used to predict carcinogenicity. The toxicological endpoints predicted by these and other such computer-based tools are summarized in Table 1.10. However, it should be noted that the predictivity of these tools is strictly determined by the quality of the molecular descriptors and the training set used to generate the prediction algorithm. In many cases, it may be possible to increase the predictive power of these and other such expert systems, by using more than one expert system for each endpoint. For instance, when 14 carcinogens were submitted to COMPACT and HazardExpert, used separately they predicted 10 and 8 actual carcinogens as carcinogenic, respectively, but when the two methods were used together, all 14 carcinogens were identified [122]. Tools such as INVDOCK, which combine molecular docking with structural alert profiling, may also be useful tools [123].

1.7.3   Prediction of Tissue-Specific Exposure: PBPK Modeling

A fundamental problem when using hazard data for risk assessment is the need to relate the effects detected at the dose level administered to a test system (the external dose) with the effects that would be caused by the dose that actually reaches the target in humans (the internal dose). The internal target organ dose can be predicted by undertaking toxicokinetic studies. Physiologically based biokinetic

TABLE 1.10 Examples of Computer-Based Expert Systems Available for ADME and Toxicity Predictions

Name	Type of Expert System	Website	Some of the Endpoints Predicted[a]	
CASE/ MCASE/ CASETOX	Automated rule based	www.multicase. com	• Carcinogenicity • Teratogenicity • Mutagenicity	• Acute toxicity • Chronic toxicity
DEREK	Knowledge based	www.chem.leeds. ac.uk/luk	• Teratogenicity • Mutagenicity • Respiratory sensitization	• Carcinogenicity • Skin irritation • Skin sensitization
HazardExpert	Knowledge based	www.compudrug. com	• Oncogenicity • Mutagenicity • Teratogenicity • Immunotoxicity • Neurotoxicity	• Membrane irritancy/ sensitivity • Bioavailability • Bioaccumulation
TOPKAT	Automated rule-based QSAR	www.accelrys.com	• Carcinogenicity • Mutagenicity • Developmental toxicity • Skin sensitization	• Eye irritancy • Biodegradability • Acute toxicity • Chronic toxicity
OncoLogic®	Decision tree approach	http://www.epa. gov/oppt/cahp/ actlocal/can. html	• Carcinogenicity	
COMPACT	Knowledge-based QSAR	www.surrey.ac. uk/SBMS	• Carcinogenicity via CYP1A-related and CYP2E-related metabolic activation	

[a]The endpoints that can be predicted using each expert system are based on the current status of each system. More information about these methods and how they can be applied is available from http://www2.defra.gov.uk/research/project_data/more.asp?!=CB01067&M=KWS&V=reach&scope=0. Website links accessed 30 January 2007.

(PBPK) modeling is a way of predicting ADME *in vivo* by combining results from the literature and from computational techniques [124], and by extrapolating data from *in vitro* studies between species. Some key PBPK methods are listed in Table 1.11. Plasma protein binding can have a crucial bearing on the internal dose, since it determines the free (unbound) concentration (this also has a bearing on the composition of cell culture media) [125]. Differential equations can be derived, which, when solved, provide information of relevance to humans. A better, biologically based, dose–response model of *in vivo* toxicity can then be developed from external dose data.

Significant advances are currently being made in biokinetic modeling, including the development of software programs and databases for the rapid generation of new models (http://www.hsl.gov.uk/capabilities/pbpk-jip.htm). These will improve the usefulness of this approach for evaluating large numbers of chemicals and will assist with the interpretation of *in vitro* hazard predictions for risk assessment purposes.

TABLE 1.11   Examples of Programs for the Prediction of Biokinetic Properties

Name	Supplier	Website	Properties Predicted[a]
Cloe PK®	Cyprotex	www.cyprotex.com	• Potential exposure • Absorption from GI tract • Plasma, tissue, and organ concentrations • Renal excretion • Hepatic metabolism
iDEA pkEXPRESS™	LION Bioscience	www.lionbioscience.com	• Absorption from GI tract • Systemic circulation • Bioavailability • Plasma concentration • Elimination
Megen100	Health & Safety Lab	www.hsl.gov.uk/capabilities/pbpk.htm	• Oral and intravenous absorption • Concentration–time profiles for plasma and major organs and tissues • Hepatic metabolism
PK-Sim®	Bayer Technology Services	www.bayertechnology.com	• Oral absorption • Concentration–time profiles for plasma and major organs and tissues • Bioavailability • Renal and billiary excretion

[a]More information about these methods and how they can be applied is available from http://www2.defra.gov.uk/research/project_data/more.asp?!=CB01067&M=KWS&V=reach&scope=0.

One key issue is the role of transporter proteins in the absorption and uptake of a drug or its metabolites, as this will determine the internal dose to which any particular organ is exposed. Problems with crystallizing membrane proteins have made it inherently difficult to generate 3D models of many important transporter proteins. Homology and comparative modeling can, however, be used to generate models by reference to experimental data, the structure of related proteins, and more fundamental predictions of protein folding and tertiary structure, made from the primary amino acid sequences of relevant proteins. For instance, three ATP-binding cassette (ABC) transporters of bacterial origin have been crystallized, and from these structures, comparative modeling has been used to generate models of ABC transporters that play a key role in drug efflux in humans. Another approach is to generate a pharmacophore from experimental data for known transporter binding molecules, as in the case for monoamine transporters, then to use QSAR systems to make predictions as to whether a novel drug is likely to be a transported. These approaches are discussed in more detail in Ref. 126.

1.8   ANIMAL MODELS USED IN PRECLINICAL TESTING OF PHARMACEUTICALS

1.8.1   Selection of a Suitable Test Species

Although not an absolute regulatory requirement, it is still widely accepted that drug development should involve initial studies conducted in a rodent species, followed by studies in a nonrodent species. In addition, further studies may be conducted in other species, such as the rabbit (e.g., for local tolerance and for pyrogenicity). There is often flexibility in the nature of the tests required by most regulators for a new medicine's dossier. For instance, where only a single species can be shown to be relevant, regulators may be willing to consider information from nonanimal studies to decide whether the two-species testing requirement can be waived.

The Universities Federation for Animal Welfare (UFAW) has published a handbook that lists the major characteristics of laboratory species, to which the reader is referred [127]. Perhaps of more general importance is the use of existing preclinical, clinical, and basic research data in the species selection process. Information from mechanistic and early *in vitro* studies is particularly important, as is understanding differences between species in the spatial and temporal expression of the drug target and in target modulation and activity. The starting point is understanding any significant differences between the pharmacology of the human protein and the possible test species. Sequence homology and structural homology do not guarantee the functional equivalence of species homologs. Once functional equivalence has been established by using cell expression systems, the next stage is to understand the tissue distribution of the target in the selected test species. This can involve *in vivo* studies with target-specific probes such as fluorescent or radiolabeled antibodies or ligands. In general, however, this information is more readily attainable from tissue distribution studies, including immunohistochemistry. A good illustration of how this can be important was made in a recent paper, which highlighted differences between the human and rat versus the mouse in the distribution and pharmacology of serotonin receptors, which showed that the mouse is a poor preclinical model for some classes of antipsychotic agents [128]. The rat was a more suitable rodent model, although the mouse has already been used in some preclinical studies for CNS-active serotoninergic drugs. With the greater availability of genomic information, species selection (or, indeed, the selection or generation of an appropriate GM animal model) can be made on the basis of amino acid sequence, as is the case when developing humanized antibodies. In some cases, this may obviate the need to conduct extensive studies in higher order vertebrates, such as primates.

In addition to differences in target expression, differences in plasma clearance rate and routes of excretion can also have a crucial bearing on whether a particular species or strain is used [129]. Differences between anatomical and functional properties associated with the intended route of administration (as in the case of nasal absorption, see Section 1.3.2), functional differences between species homologs of efflux and transporter proteins such as P-gp [130], and differences between the distribution and activities of key metabolic enzymes predicted to be involved in the biotransformation of a drug may limit the choice of test species.

Where more than one species is likely to be used for preclinical studies, the choice of species may also involve a consideration of the need for allometric scaling. This allows the prediction of human pharmacokinetics from the pharmacokinetics of a drug in a test species, by taking body weight into account. A recent study [131] indicates that although allometric scaling is most reliable when PK parameters are available for five species, certain three-species combinations (such as mouse/rat, monkey, and dog) are adequate, whereas other three-species combinations (such as rabbit, monkey, and dog) are significantly worse. In general, two-species combinations are poorer for making allometric predictions, and certain combinations, such as mouse and rat, rabbit and monkey, and dog and monkey, are particularly poor. However, in practice, two-species combinations are commonly used, which usually involve a rodent and a nonrodent species.

Species selection is also dependent on the feasibility of a study and on the availability and cost of acquiring and caring for the animals concerned. Developmental toxicity, for instance, could not be reasonably or ethically conducted on primates or some other vertebrate species and is generally conducted in rodents, because of their small size, shorter life spans, and the larger litter sizes produced at each generation. Preliminary studies may be conducted with fish larval forms and invertebrates.

1.8.2 Experimental Design

The ICH guidelines advocate the principles of the three Rs. That is, prior to the use of vertebrate animals, scientists are required to consider: (1) whether there are alternatives to using animals that can provide information that is as valid and acceptable to regulators as animal data; (2) where there are no replacement alternatives, how prior information and information from nonanimal experiments could be used to reduce the number of animals used; and (3) how animal experiments could be refined in order to reduce suffering (e.g., by using more humane endpoints).

The first step in designing an animal experiment is to clearly define its objectives in terms of the nature of information sought or the hypothesis to be tested. The correct grouping of animals according to their treatment (nature and frequency of intervention, etc.) and husbandry regime (light–dark cycle, handling, monitoring, etc.) reduces variation in experimental data. Standard operating procedures should be developed that take into account the scientific objectives and animal welfare issues associated with each experiment. For instance, all the animals (control, vehicle control, and test animals) should be handled with the same frequency, for the same periods of time and by the same technician, and subjected to identical procedures. Other causes of variation stem from inadvertent infections, which can be minimized by good laboratory practice, routine health surveillance, and using suitably ventilated cages. Whether food and fluid control (i.e., limiting daily supply), timed feeding and water supply, or *ad libitum* feeding and drinking are appropriate can also be an important consideration. The effects of weight, age, sex, and/or strain on the experimental outcome can have important implications for experimental design and can be accounted for in various ways, for example, by appropriate grouping of animals (some examples are given in http://oslovet.veths.no/compendia/LAS/KAP28.pdf). This is because different strains of rats can vary dramatically in their clinical responses to a drug, so selecting the most appropriate isogenic strain can be difficult and it might sometimes be appropriate to use more than one strain in each experiment. There are a number of useful resources on this topic (e.g., Ref. 132).

The number of possible variables highlights the importance of a pilot study. Pilot studies that are designed on the basis of existing information can be used to identify logistical, animal welfare, and scientific problems and to address specific scientific questions, prior to the conduct of larger animal studies [133]. Whether an experiment entails multiple endpoints, different sexes, and/or different strains, the interpretation of the data might be compromised without prior and careful statistical planning, or in the worst case scenario, be impossible, resulting in the need to repeat the experiment.

The ICH guidelines recommend carcinogenicity testing, where the weight of evidence suggests it may be required or where there is insufficient evidence to rule out the possibility of carcinogenic hazard. Such testing normally should be conducted only in rats, as there is evidence to suggest that the rat bioassay is more predictive of human risk Cancer-associated biomarkers have an enormous potential to streamline preclinical drug development and can also be used to devlop humane endpoints and facilitate temporal studies in small numbers of animals [134].

1.9 USE OF PRIOR INFORMATION

1.9.1 Sources of Prior Knowledge

Information retrieval is an important aspect of drug development, and a list of databases that provide information that can be used is given in Table 1.12. The tremendous rate at which information is increasing in volume and is diversifying requires that computational tools are developed to support the extraction and ranking of information according to its relevance and reliability. In addition, models of how different elements of a biochemical pathway interact can be derived mathematically, and such models have been used to successfully construct biochemical networks of relevance to drug discovery [135].

Some special sources of prior information include data suites that collate information about specific biochemical pathways, specific diseases, human genetics, and human sub-populations. Because most diseases have complex etiologies, particularly diseases such as cancer, heart disease, stroke, and diabetes, which arise from a combination of lifestyle, environmental, and genetic factors, several large-scale population studies are being undertaken (some examples are given in Table 1.12). These studies may contribute to a greater understanding of the complex basis of such diseases, leading to improvements in drug discovery and target selection where patterns that link genetic differences to drug effects or disease can be established.

Perhaps the most directly relevant information is that available from preclinical and clinical studies on existing therapeutic products. Usually, this information is not publicly available, but some confidential information is being incorporated into many databases. PharmaPendium™ [136] is an example of a recent public resource that includes drug safety data (preclinical and clinical) for FDA-approved drugs. Such resources are likely to prove invaluable for researchers and regulators alike.

TABLE 1.12 Information Resources[a]

Omics Databases and Resources

SRS http://srs.ebi.ac.uk/ srsbin/cgi-bin/wgetz?- page+srsq2+-noSession	A gene/protein sequence retrieval system that can be used to browse various biological sequence and literature databases
ToxExpress http://www. genelogic.com/genomics/ toxexpress/	A toxicogenomic profiling suite that can be used in biomarker discovery
MIAME http://www.mged. org/Workgroups/MIAME/ miame.html	Minimum Information About a Microarray Experiment: criteria needed to permit the interpretation of the results of the experiment unambiguously and, potentially, to reproduce the experiment
Array Track http://www.fda. gov/nctr/science/centers/ toxicoinformatics/ ArrayTrack/	Developed by FDA National Center for Toxicological Research (NCTR); an integrated suite designed to manage, analyze, and interpret microarray data
KEGG http://www.genome. jp/kegg/	Kyoto Encyclopedia of Genes and Genomes provides a complete computer representation of the cell, the organism, and the biosphere
Unigene http://www.unigene. com	Provides an organized view of the transcriptome
SNP http://www.ncbi.nlm.nih. gov/projects/SNP/	The Single Nucleotide Polymorphism database
SPAD http://www.grt. kyushu-u.ac.jp/spad/	The Signaling PAthway Database (SPAD): an integrated database for genetic information and signal transduction systems

Pharmacology, Toxicology, and Biological Systems

BIOPRINT http://www. cerep.fr/cerep/users/pages/ Collaborations/bioprint. asp	A pharmacology and ADME database that contains *in vitro* pharmacology profiles, ADR, PK and clinical data for over 2500 marketed drugs, failed drugs, and reference compounds
BioRS http://biors.gsf. de:8111/searchtool/ searchtool.cgi	A biological data retrieval system
CEBS http://www.niehs.nih. gov/cebs-df/index.cfm	Chemical Effects in Biological Systems: a knowledge base for information and resource exchange
BIND http://bond. unleashedinformatics.com	Biomolecular Interaction Network Database: designed to store full descriptions of interactions, molecular complexes and pathways
BioCarta http://www. biocarta.com/	Provides interactive graphic models of molecular and cellular pathways
BRENDA www.brenda.uni- koeln.de	A collection of enzyme functional data
CSNDB http://geo.nihs.go. jp/csndb/	Cell Signaling Networks Database: a database and knowledge base for signaling pathways of human cells
SwissProt http://expasy.org/sprot/	A protein sequence database with descriptions of the function of proteins, protein structure, posttranslational modifications, variants, etc.
TransPath http://www. biobase-international.com/ pages/index. php?id=transpath	Provides information about (mostly mammalian) signal transduction molecules and reactions, focusing on signaling cascades that change the activities of transcription factors and thus alter the gene expression profiles of a cells

TABLE 1.12   *Continued*

PathArt http://jubilantbiosys. com/ppa.htm	A database of biomolecular interactions with tools for searching, analysis and visualization of data
DSSTox http://www.epa.gov/ ncct/dsstox/index.html	The EPA's Distributed Structure-Searchable Toxicity Database for improved structure–activity and predictive toxicology capabilities
TOXNET http://toxnet.nlm. nih.gov/	A database on toxicology, hazardous chemicals, environmental health, and toxic releases
PharmGKB http://www. pharmgkb.org/	A database on relationships among drugs, diseases, and genes

Literature Database

PubMed www.pubmed.com	A database that includes over 16 million citations from MEDLINE and other life science journals for biomedical articles back to the 1950s; PubMed includes links to full text articles and other related resources
Bio-Frontier P450/CYP http://www.fqs.pl/	A database for testing CYP interactions

Human Population Genetics and Toxicity Databases and Resources

The Collaborative on Health and the Environment http://database. healthandenvironment. org/	A searchable database of links between chemical contaminants and human diseases
The Personalized Medicine Research Project (Marshfield Project) http:// www.marshfieldclinic.org/ chg/pages/default.aspx	A human population genetic database to understand the interplay of human genetics, diseases, and environmental factors
Medgene[SM] database http:// hipseq.med.harvard.edu/ MEDGENE/login.jsp	A database of disease-associated genes
CARTaGENE http://www. cartagene.qc.ca/	A source of information on the genetic variation of a large population
Latvian Genome Project http://bmc.biomed.lu.lv/gene/	Large-scale human population genetic project to discover disease linkages
Estonian Genome Project http://www.geenivaramu. ee/	A source of information on the genetic variation of a large population
The United Kingdom Biobank (UK Biobank) http://www.ukbiobank. ac.uk/	Genetic and medical information is being collected for 500,000 UK volunteers
Translational Genomic Research in the African Diaspora (TgRIAD) http://www.genomecenter. howard.edu/TGRIAD.htm	A database to understand disease, genetics, and environmental factor linkage in people of African descent
Obesity gene map database http://obesitygene. pbrc.edu/	A database of genetic markers associated with obesity
COGENE the Craniofacial and Oral Gene Expression Network http://hg.wustl. edu/cogene/	A consortium that looks at the genetics of early development, in particular, craniofacial disorders

TABLE 1.12   *Continued*

Human genome variation database http://hgvbase.cgb.ki.se/	Contains links to a number of single nucleotide polymorphism databases for particular diseases
The International HapMap Project http://www.hapmap.org/	A consortia aimed at finding genes associated with human disease and response to pharmaceuticals
GenomEUtwin http://www.genomeutwin.org/	A database of human population genetics aimed specifically at finding genetic and lifestyle linkages to disease that involves studies on twins
Public Population Project in Genomics (P3G) http://www.p3gconsortium.org/	A consortium that aims to develop a human population genetics database

*a*This is a list of resources that are applicable to understanding the output of omics-based studies and compiling a systems biology view of diseases and drug effects. Websites accessed 30 January 2007.

Other databases include the Adverse Drug Effects database [137], which stores information on approved drugs, including the severity and incidence of adverse effects, which is relevant to the discovery and design of new clinical products.

1.9.2 Standardization of Data Collection and Meta-Analysis

The quality and completeness of the available toxicological data will significantly affect the level of confidence in the preclinical data. The application of Good Laboratory Practice (GLP) should increasingly help to standardize the way in which experiments are designed, conducted, and reported, thereby improving the quality of the information available for guiding subsequent studies.

Meta-analysis is a statistical approach, which is used to combine data from different sources, but it needs to be applied with great caution. It is particularly difficult to use meta-analysis when different datasets contradict one another. Nevertheless, the use of surrogate endpoints, such as biomarkers, may dramatically improve the power of meta-analysis, since appropriate biomarkers can be used to increase the credibility of animal and human cell-based and tissue-based preclinical studies, and to facilitate extrapolation between such *in vitro* studies and preclinical *in vivo* studies, in animals and in humans.

Several potential biomarkers of exposure and toxicity can be considered. For example, such a scheme was originally proposed by Sobels [138] for the extrapolation of data on genetic damage from animals to humans, and was subsequently modified by Sutter [139] to permit *in vitro–in vivo* extrapolation. In some cases, threshold doses can be set, solely on the basis of *in vitro* tests (e.g., for some genotoxins). This parallelogram approach can then be used to extrapolate preclinical data to effects on humans, according to the paradigm:

$$\text{Human } (\textit{in vivo}) \text{ toxicity} = \frac{[\text{Rodent } (\textit{in vivo}) \text{ toxicity} \times \text{Human } (\textit{in vitro}) \text{ toxicity}]}{\text{Rodent } (\textit{in vitro}) \text{ toxicity}}$$

The concept assumes that the ratio of *in vitro* toxicity to *in vivo* toxicity for any particular endpoint is broadly comparable across species. Up to now, this approach has been used for extrapolating data on genetic damage but has proved to be less useful for extrapolating other forms of toxicity data to humans, because of the relatively complex mechanisms of toxicity that are involved. Nevertheless, in a recent paper [140], the concept was applied to a comparison of rat and human skin penetration rates *in vitro* and to predicting the *in vivo* effects of topically applied substances. As key biomarkers for drug effect and toxicological endpoints become available, the applicability of this approach is likely to expand to other areas of drug development and safety pharmacology.

1.10   CONCLUSIONS

Despite decades of research and development, the issue of adverse drug reactions that result in drug withdrawals remains a significant problem. This problem is confounded by the fact that information from clinical studies on human volunteers and patients is often kept from public scrutiny. Indeed, only a small number of pharmaceutical companies post their clinical trials information on publicly available registers. A recent study indicates that target organ toxicities in humans are not always predicted reliably by preclinical tests in animals. The predictivity of cardiovascular, hematopoietic, and gastrointestinal toxicity is around 80% but is lower for toxicity to the liver, skin, and nervous system [141]. Hence, there is an urgent need for a new approach to drug development, which involves the targeted use of new and advanced technologies that are based on defined cell systems, either as standalone alternatives to animal studies or as tools to assist with the extrapolation of animal data to humans.

Indeed, in 2004, the FDA produced a report that suggested that the fall in drug development returns was due largely to the failure to use the new technologies such as genomics, proteomics, and bioinformatics platforms to detect safety problems that cannot be identified in the more traditional animal-based methods. These newer, and often systems biology-based, approaches hold enormous potential in this respect but are very much in their infancy. One of the most significant problems is the difficulty in standardizing and validating these new technologies, in order to ensure that the quality of data and the quality of data analysis form a suitable basis for safety assessments. These systems are being developed at an unprecedented rate. For example, a consortium of global pharmaceutical giants has been assembled to put forward biomarkers and screening assays for consideration by the FDA. It remains to be seen whether this initiative will reduce the current drug attrition rate. Preclinical planning must look at both the existing regulatory requirements and the scope for cost- and time-effective studies that make the maximum use of the new and exciting technologies.

ACKNOWLEDGMENT

The authors would like to thank Dr Michelle Scrivens for her valued assistance in the preparation of this chapter.

REFERENCES

1. Challenge and Opportunity on the Critical Path to New Medical Products. US FDA March 2004. Available from http://www.fda.gov/oc/initiatives/criticalpath/whitepaper.html (accessed 29 January 2007).

2. *Guidance for Industry: Fast Track Drug Development Programs—Designation, Development, and Application Review*. Rockvill, MD: US Department of Health and Human Services Food and Drug Administration, Center for Drug Evaluation and Research (CDER), Center for Biologics Evaluation and Research (CBER); January 2006. Procedural Revision 2. Available from http://www.fda.gov/cber/gdlns/fsttrk.pdf (accessed 29 January 2007).

3. Schwieterman WD. Regulating biopharmaceuticals under CDE versus CBER: an insider's perspective. *Drug Discov Today* 2006;11(19–20):945–951.

4. Organisation for Economic Co-operation and Development. *Chemcials Testing Guidelines. Section 4: Health Effects*. Available from http://www.oecd.org/document/55/0,2340,en_2649_34377_2349687_1_1_1_1,00.html (accessed 29 January 2007).

5. Overington JP, Al-Lazikani B, Hopkins AL. How many drug targets are there? *Nat Rev Drug Discov* 2006;5(12):993–996.

6. Wilson S, Bergsma D. Orphan G-protein coupled receptors: novel drug targets for the pharmaceutical industry. *Drug Des Discov* 2000;17(2):105–114.

7. Cancer Genome Anatomy Project: National Cancer Institute. Available from www.ncbi.nlm.nih.gov/CGAP (accessed 29 January 2007).

8. Genomes on-line database version 2. Available from http://www.genomesonline.org/ (accessed 29 January 2007).

9. Romero P, Wagg J, Green ML, Kaiser D, Krummenacker M, Karp PD. Computational prediction of human metabolic pathways from the complete human genome. *Genome (Biol)* 2004;6(1): http://genomebiology.com/2004/6/1/R2 (accessed 29 January 2007).

10. Salzberg SL, White O, Peterson J, Eisen JA. Microbial genes in the human genome: lateral transfer or gene loss? *Science* 2001;292(5523):1903–1906.

11. Steinmetz LM, Scharfe C, Deutschbauer AM, Mokranjac D, Herman ZS, Jones T, Chu AM, Giaever G, Prokisch H, Oefner PJ, Davis RW. Systematic screen for human disease genes in yeast. *Nat Genet* 2002;31:400–404.

12. Hughes TR, Marton MJ, Jones AR, Roberts CJ, Stoughton R, Armour CD, Bennett HA, Coffey E, Dai H, He YD, Kidd MJ, King AM, Meyer MR, Slade D, Lum PY, Stepaniants SB, Shoemaker DD, Gachotte D, Chakraburtty K, Simon J, Bard M, Friend SH. Functional discovery via a compendium of expression profiles. *Cell* 2000;102:109–126.

13. Kumar A, Agarwal S, Heyman JA, Matson S, Heidtman M, Piccirillo S, Umansky L, Drawid A, Jansen R, Liu Y, Cheung K-H, Miller P, Gerstein M, Roeder GS, Snyder M. Subcellular localization of the yeast proteome. *Genes Dev* 2002;16(6):707–719.

14. Outeiro TF, Lindquist S. Yeast cells provide insight into alpha-synuclein biology and pathobiology. *Science* 2003;302:1772–1775.

15. Griffioen G, Duhamel H, Van Damme N, Pellens K, Zabrocki P, Pannecouque C, van Leuven F, Winderickx J, Wera S. A yeast-based model of α-synucleinopathy identifies compounds with therapeutic potential. *Biochem Biophys Acta* 2006;1762:312–318.

16. Versele M, Lemaire K, Thevelein JM. Sex and sugar in yeast: two distinct GPCR systems. *EMBO Rep* 2001;2:574–579.

17. Pausch MH, Lai M, Tseng E, Paulsen J, Bates B, Kwak S. Functional expression of human and mouse P2Y12 receptors in Saccharomyces cerevisiae. *Biochem Biophys Res Commun* 2004;324:171–177.

18. Fire A, Xu S, Montgomery MK, Kostas SA, Driver SE, Mello CC. Potent and specific genetic interference by double stranded RNA in *Caenorhabditis elegans*. *Nature* 1998;391:806–811.

19. Metzstein MM, Stanfield GM, Horvitz HR. Genetics of programmed cell death in *C. elegans*: past, present and future. *Trends Genet* 1998;14(10):410–416.

20. Nichols CD. *Drosophila melanogaster* neurobiology, neuropharmacology, and how the fly can inform central nervous system drug discovery. *Pharmacol Ther* 2006;112(3): 677–700.

21. Kellenberger E, Muller P, Schalon C, Bret G, Foata N, Rognan D. Sc-PDB: an annotated database of druggable binding sites from the protein data bank. *J Chem Inf Model* 2006;46:717–727.

22. Tapolczay D, Chorlton A, McCubbin Q. Probing drug structure improves the odds. *Curr Opin Drug Discov Dev* 2000;April:30–33.

23. Schreiber SL. Target-oriented and diversity-oriented organis synthesis in drug discovery. *Science* 2000;287(5460):1964–1969.

24. Villar HO, Yan J, Hansen MR. Using NMR for ligand discovery and optimization. *Curr Opin Chem Biol* 2004;8(4):387–391.

25. Swayze EE, Jefferson EA, Sannes-Lowery KA, Blyn LB, Risen LM, Arakawa S, Osgood SA, Hofstadler SA, Griffey RH. SAR by MS: a ligand-based technique for drug lead discovery against RNA targets. *J Med Chem* 2002;45(18):3816–3819.

26. Hartshorn MJ, Murray CW, Cleasby A, Frederickson M, Tickle IJ, Jhoti H. Fragment-based lead discovery using X-ray crystallography. *J Med Chem* 2005;48(2):403–413.

27. Lofas S. Optimizing the hit-to-lead process using SPR analysis. *Assay Drug Dev Technol* 2004;4:407–415.

28. Rees DC, Congreve M, Murray CW, Carr R. Fragment-based lead discovery. *Nat Rev Drug Discov* 2004;3:660–672.

29. Brenner S, Lerner RA. Encoded combinatorial chemistry. *Proc Natl Acad Sci USA* 1992;89:5381–5383.

30. Scheuermann J, Dumelin CE, Melkko S, Neri D. DNA-encoded chemical libraries. *J Biotechnol* 2006;126:568–581.

31. Landro JA, Taylor ICA, Stirtan WG, Osterman DG, Kristie J, Hunnicutt EJ, Rae PMM, Sweetnam PM. HTS in the new millennium. The role of pharmacology and flexibility. *J Pharmacol Toxicol Methods* 2000;44:273–289.

32. Kokko L, Johansson N, Lovgren T, Soukka T. Enzyme inihibitor screening using a homogenous proximity-based immunoassay for estradiol. *J Biomol Screen* 2005;10:348–354.

33. Kimberly H, Clement, JF, Abrahamyan L, Strebel K, Bouvier M, Kleinman L, Mouland AJ. A human immunodeficiency virus type 1 protease biosensor using bioluminescence resonance energy transfer. *J Virol Methods* 2005;128:93–103.

34. Thomsen W, Frazer J, Unett D. Functional assays for screening GPCR targets. *Curr Opin Biotechnol* 2005;16:655–665.

35. Westby M, Nakayama GR, Butler SL, Blair WS. Cell-based and biochemical screening approaches for the discovery of novel HIV-1 inihibitors. *Antiviral Res* 2005;67:121–140.

36. Mascini M, Bagni G, Di Pietro ML, Ravera M, Baracco S, Osella D. Electrochemical biosensor evaluation of the interaction between DNA and metallo-drugs. *Biometals* 2006;19:409–418.

37. Huber W. New strategy for improved secondary screening and lead optimization using high-resolution SPR characterization of compound-target interactions. *J Mol Recognition* 2005;18:273–281.

38. Hanes J, Pluckhun A. *In vitro* selection and evolution of functional proteins by using ribosomal display. *Proc Natl Acad Sci USA* 1997;94:4937–4942.

39. Silacci M, Brack S, Schirru G, Marlind J, Ettorre A, Merlo A, Viti F, Neri D. Design, construction, and characterization of a large synthetic human antibody phage display library. *Proteomics* 2005;5:2340–2350.

40. Boder ET, Wittrup KD. Yeast surface display for screening combinatorial polypeptide libraries. *Nat Biotechnol* 1997;15:553–557.

41. Patil SD, Rhodes DG, Burgess DJ. DNA-based therapeutics and DNA delivery systems: a comprehensive review. *AAPS* 2005;7(1):E61–E77.

42. Klumpp C, Kostarelos K, Prato M, Bianco A. Functionalized carbon nanotubes as emerging nanovectors for the delivery of therapeutics. *Biochim Biophys Acta* 2006;1758:404–412.

43. Proudfoot JR. Drugs, leads and drug-likeness: an analysis of some recently launched drugs. *Bioorg Med Chem Lett* 2002;12(12):1647–1650.

44. Makara GM, Athanasopoulos J. Ligand affinity binding in improving success-rates for lead generation. *Curr Opin Biotechnol* 2005;16:666–673.

45. Golebiowski A, Klopfenstein SR, Portlock DE. Lead compounds discovered from libraries: part 2. *Curr Opin Chem Biol* 2003;7:308–325.

46. Kola I, Landis J. Can the pharmaceutical industry reduce attrition rates? *Nat Rev Drug Discov* 2004;3:711–715.

47. Lipinski CA, Lambardo F, Dominy BW, Feeney PJ. Experimental and computational approaches to estimate solubility and permeability in drug discovery and development settings. *Adv Drug Deliv Rev* 1997;23:3–25.

48. Amidon GLH, Lennernäs H, Shah VP, Crison JR. A theoretical basis for a biopharmaceutic drug classification: the correlation of *in vitro* drug product dissolution and *in vivo* bioavailability. *Pharm Res* 1995;12(3):413–420.

49. Schmeichel KL, Bissell MJ. Modeling tissue-specific signaling and organ function in three dimensions. *J Cell Sci* 2003;116(12):2377–2388.

50. Leppert PS, Fix JA. Use of everted intestinal rings for *in vitro* examination of oral absorption potential. *J Pharm Sci* 1994;8:976–981.

51. Amidon GL, Sinko PJ, Fleisher D. Estimating human oral fraction dose absorbed: a correlation using rat intestinal membrane permeability for passive and carrier-mediated compounds. *Pharm Res* 1988;10:651–654.

52. Hidalgo IJ. Cultured intestinal epithelial cell models. *Pharm Biotechnol* 1996;8:35–50.

53. Irvine JD, Takahashi L, Lockhart K, Cheong J, Tolan JW, Selick HE, Grove JR. MDCK (Madin–Darby canine kidney) cells: a tool for membrane permeability screening. *J Pharm Sci* 1999;88:28–33.

54. Stewart BH, Chan OH, Lu RH, Rener EL, Schmid HL, Hamilton HW, Steinbaugh BA, Taylor MD. Comparison of intestinal permeabilities determined in multiple *in vitro* and *in situ* models: relationship to absorption in humans. *Pharm Res* 1995;12:693–699.

55. White RE. High-throughput screening in drug metabolism and pharmacokinetic support of drug discovery. *Annu Rev Pharmacol Toxicol* 2000;40:133–157.

56. Pidgeon C, Ong S, Munroe J, Hornback WJ, Kasher JS, Grunz L, Liu H, Qiu X, Pidgeon M, Dantzig A. IAM chromatography: an *in vitro* screen for predicting drug membrane permeability. *Med Chem* 1995;38:590–594.

57. Kansy M, Senner F, Gubernator K. Physicochemical high throughput screening: parallel artificial membrane permeation assay in the description of passive absorption processes. *J Med Chem* 1998;41:1007–1010.

58. Bubik M, Ott M, Mahringer A, Fricker G. Rapid assessment of P-glycoprotein–drug interactions at the blood–brain barrier. *Anal Biochem* 2006;358:51–58.

59. Gray AC, Malton J, Clothier RH. The development of a standardised protocol to measure squamous differentiation in stratified epithelia, by using the fluorescein cadaverine incorporation technique *Altern Lab Anim* 2004;32(2):91–100.

60. Gray TE, Guzman K, Davis CW, Abdullah LH, Nettesheim P. Mucociliary differentiation of serially passaged normal human tracheobronchial epithelial cells. *Am J Respir Cell Mol Biol* 1996;14(1):104–112.

61. Deli MAM, Abraham CS, Kataoka Y, Niwa M. Permeability studies on *in vitro* blood–brain barrier models: physiology, pathology and pharmacology. *Cell Mol Neurobiol* 2005;25:59–126.

62. Combes RD, Balls M, Bansil L, Barratt M, Bell D, Botham P, Broadhead C, Clothier R, George E, Fentem J, Jackson M, Indans I, Loizou G, Navaratnam V, Pentreath V, Phillips B, Stemplewski H, Stewart J. The Third FRAME Toxicity Committee: Working Toward Greater Implementation of Alternatives in Toxicity Testing. *Altern Lab Anim* 2002;32(S1):635–642.

63. Gumbleton M, Audus KL. Progress and limitations in the use of in vitro cell cultures to serve as a permeability screen for the blood–brain barrier. *J Pharm Sci* 2001;90:1681–1698.

64. Atterwill CK, Purcell WM. Brain spheroid and other organotypic culture systems in *in vitro* neurotoxicology. In Pentreath VW, Ed., *Neurotoxicology In vitro* Washington DC: Taylor and Francis; 1999, pp 213–238.

65. Harkema JR. Comparative structure, function and toxicity of the nasal airways. Predicting human effects from animal studies. In Gardner DE, Crapo JD, McCellan RO, Eds. *Toxicology of the Lung*. Washington DC: Taylor and Francis; 1999, pp 55–83.

66. Dimova S, Brewster ME, Noppe M, Jorissen M, Augustijns P. The use of human nasal *in vitro* cell systems during drug discovery and development. *Toxicol In Vitro* 2005;19:107–122.

67. Daly AK. Nomenclature for human CYP2D6 alleles. *Pharmacogenetics* 1996;6:193–201.

68. Coecke S, Rogiers V, Bayliss M, Castell JM, Doehmer J, Fabre G, Fry J, Kern A, Westmoreland C. The use of long-term hepatocyte cultures for detecting induction of drug metabolising enzymes: the current status: ECVAM Hepatocytes and Metabolically Competent Systems Task Force Report 1. *Altern Lab Anim* 1999;27(4):579–638.

69. Kim HS, Wainer IW. On-line drug metabolism in capillary electrophoresis. 1. Glucuronidation using rat liver microsomes. *Anal Chem* 2006;78:7071–7077.

70. Dunn JC, Tompkins RG, Yarmush ML. Long-term *in vitro* function of adult hepatocytes in a collagen sandwich configuration. *Biotechnol Prog* 1991;7:237–245.

71. Scmitmeier S, Langsch A, Bader A. A membrane-based small-scale bioreactor for accelerated *in vitro* drug screenings with primary hepatocytes. *Desalination* 2006;199:258–260.

72. Fearn RA, Hirst BH. Predicting oral drug absorption and hepatobiliary clearance: human intestinal and hepatic *in vitro* cell models. *Environ Toxicol Pharmacol* 2006;21:168–178.

73. Krebsfaenger N, Murdter TE, Zanger UM, Eichelbaum MF, Doehmer J. V79 Chinese hamster cells genetically engineered for polymorphic cytochrome P450 2D6 and their predictive value for humans. *ALTEX* 2003;20(3):143–154.

74. Boonstra J, Post JA. Molecular events associated with reactive oxygen species and cell cycle progression in mammalian cells. *Gene* 2004;337:1–13.

75. Prabhakaran K, Sampson DA, Hoehner JC. Neuroblastoma survival and death: an *in vitro* model of hypoxia and metabolic stress. *J Surg Res* 2004;116:288–296.

76. Canova N, Kmonickova E, Lincova D, Vitek L, Farghali H. Evaluation of a flat membrane hepatocyte bioreactor for pharmacotoxicological applications: evidence that inhibition of spontaneously produced nitric oxide improves cell functionality. *Altern Lab Anim* 2004;32:25–35.

77. Wong JM, Harper PA, Meyer UA, Bock KW, Morike K, Lagueux J, Ayotte P, Tyndale RF, Sellers EM, Manchester DK, Okey AB. Ethnic variability in the allelic distribution of human aryl hydrocarbon receptor codon 554 and assessment of variant receptor function *in vitro*. *Pharmacogenetics* 1991;1:66–67.

78. Schwarz UI. Clinical relevance of genetic polymorphisms in the human CYP2C9 gene. *Eur J Clin Invest* 2003;33:23–30.

79. Refsgaard HHF, Jensen BF, Christensen IT, Hagen N, Brockhoff PB. *In silico* prediction of cytochrome P450 inihibitors. *Drug Dev Res* 2006;67:417–429.

80. Singh SB, Shen LQ, Walker MJ, Sheridan RP. A model for predicting likely sites of CYP3A4-mediated metabolism on drug-like molecules. *J Med Chem* 2003;46:1330–1336.

81. Crivori P, Pogessi I. Computational approaches for predicting CYP-related metabolism properties in the screening of new drugs. *Eur J Med Chem* 2006;41:795–808.

82. Chovan LE, Black-Schaefer C, Dandliker PJ, Lau YY. Automatic mass spectrometry method development for drug discovery: application in metabolic stability assays. *Rapid Commun Mass Spectrom* 2004;18:3105–3112.

83. Jefferis R. Glycosylation of recombinant antibody therapeutics. *Biotechnol Prog* 2005;21:11–16.

84. Bhogal N, Combes R. TGN1412: time to change the paradigm for the testing of new pharmaceuticals. *Altern Lab Anim* 2006;34(2):225–239.

85. Fort DJ, Paul RR. Enhancing the predictive validity of Frog Embryo Teratogenesis Assay—*Xenopus* (FETAX). *J Appl Toxicol* 2002;22:185–191.

86. International Conference on Harmonisation of technical requirements for registration of pharmaceuticals for human use (25 October 2006). *ICH Considerations: General Principles to Address the Risk of Inadvertent Germline Integration of Gene Therapy Vectors.* Available from http://www.ich.org/LOB/media/MEDIA3363.pdf (accessed 29 January 2007).

87. Alonso MJ. Nanoparticles for overcoming biological barriers. *Biomed Pharmacother* 2004;58:168–172.

88. Sadrieh N. Nanaotechnology: regulatory perspective for drug development http://www.fda.gov/nanotechnology/powerpoint_conversions/regulatory_perspective_files/outline/index.html (accessed 29 January 2007).

89. Oberdörster G, Maynard A, Donaldson K, Carter J, Karn B, Kreyling W, Lai D, Olin S, Monteiro-Riviere N, Warheit S, Yang H. Principles of characterizing the potential health effects from exposure to nanomaterials: elements of a screening strategy. A report from ILSI Research Foundation/Risk Science Instate Nanomaterial Toxicity Screening Working Groups. *Particle Fibre Toxicol* 2005;2:1–36.

90. Labhesetwar V, Song C, Humphrey W, Shebucki R, Levy RJ. Arterial uptake of biodegradable nanoparticles: effects of surface modifications. *J Pharm Sci* 2000;87: 1229–1234.

91. Environmental Toxicity Council (ETC) Group: Size matters! The case for a global moratorium. 2003/04. Occasional paper series vol 7 no 1. Available from http://etcgroup. org/en/materials/publications.html?id=165 (accessed 10 September 2007).

92. Lacerda L, Bianco A, Prato M, Kostarelos K. Carbon nanotubes as nanomedicines: from toxicology to pharmacology. *Adv Drug Dev Rev* 2006;58:1460–1470.

93. Nel A, Xia T, Maedler L, Li N. Toxic potential of materials at the nanolevel. *Science* 2006;311:622–627.

94. Lawrence CL, Pollard CE, Hammond TG, Valentin JP. Nonclinical proarrhythmia models: predicting torsades des pointes. *J Pharmacol Toxicol Methods* 2005;52:46–59.

95. De Pont FI, Poluzzi E, Montanaro N. Organising evidence on QT prolongation and occurrence of torsades des pointes with non-antiarrhythmic drugs: a call for consensus. *Eur J Clin Pharmacol* 2001;57:185–209.

96. Recanatini M, Poluzzi E, Masetti M, Cavalli A, De Ponti F. QT prolongation through hERG K$^+$ channel blockade: current knowledge and strategies for the early prediction during drug development. *Med Res Rev* 2005;25:133–166.

97. Lavon N, Benvenisty N. Differentiation and genetic manipulation of human embryonic stem cells and the analysis of the cardiovascular system. *Trends Cardiovasc Med* 2003;13:47–52.

98. He JQ, Ma Y, Lee Y, Thompson JA, Kamp T. Human embryonic stem cells develop into multiple types of cardiac myocytes: action potential characterisation. *Circ Res* 2003;93:1–9.

99. Makino S, Fukuda K, Miyoshi S, Konishi F, Kodama H, Pan J, Sano M, Takahashi T, Hori S, Abe H, Hata J, Umezawa A, Ogawa S. Cardiomyocytes can be generated from marrow stromal cells in vitro. *J Bioeng Biomembr* 1999;28:379–385.

100. Draft ICCVAM test method recommendations: *In Vitro Pyrogenicity Test Methods* (December 2006). Available from http://iccvam.niehs.nih.gov/methods/pyrodocs/supp/ PWGrec12016.pdf (accessed 29 January 2007).

101. Willingham AT, Orth OP, Batalov S, Eters EC, Wen BG, Aza-Blanc P, Hogenesch JB, Sculz PG. A strategy for probing the function of noncoding RNAs finds a repressor of NFAT. *Science* 2005;309:1570–1573.

102. Yoon BI, Li GX, Kitada K, Kawasaki Y, Igarashi K, Kodama Y, Inoue T, Kobayashi K, Kanno J, Kim DY, Inoue T, Hirabayashi Y. Mechanisms of benzene-induced hematotoxicity and leukemogenicity: cDNA microarray analyses using mouse bone marrow tissue. *Environ Health Perspect* 2003;111:1411–1420.

103. Kramer JA, Curtiss SW, Kolaja KL, Alden CL, Blomme EA, Curtiss WC, Davila JC, Jackson CJ, Bunch RT. Acute molecular markers of rodent hepatic carcinogenesis identified by transcription profiling. *Chem Res Toxciol* 2004;17:463–470.

104. Nilsson P, Paavilainen L, Larsson K, Odling J, Sundberg M, Andersson AC, Kampf C, Persson A, Al-Khalili Szigyarto C, Ottosson J, Bjorling E, Hober S, Wernerus H, Wester K, Ponten F, Uhlen M. Towards a human proteome atlas: high-throughput generation of mono-specific antibodies for tissue profiling. *Proteomics* 2005;5:4327–4337.

105. Nicholson JK, Lindon JC, Holmes E. "Metabonomics": understanding the metabolic responses of living systems to pathophysiological stimuli via multivariate statistical analysis of biological NMR spectroscopic data. *Xenobiotica* 1999;29:1181–1189.

106. Bollard ME, Murray AJ, Clarke K, Nicholson JK, Griffin JL. A study of metabolic compartmentation in the rat heart and cardiac mitochondritiss using high resolution magic angle spinning ^{1}H NMR spectroscopy. *FEBS Lett* 2003;553:73–78.

107. Bollard ME, Stanley EG, Lindon JC, Nicholson JK, Holmes E. NMR-based metabonomic approaches for evaluating physiological influences on biofluid composition. *NMR Biomed* 2005;18:143–162.

108. Viravaidya K, Sin A, Shuler ML. Development of a microscale cell culture analog to probe naphthalene toxicity. *Biotechnol Prog* 2004;20:316–323.

109. Ziauddin J, Sabatini DM. Microarrays of cells expressing defined cDNAs. *Nature* 2001;411:107–110.

110. Hung PJ, Lee PJ, Sabouchi P, Lin R, Lee P. Continuous perfusion microfluidic cell culture array for high-throughput cell-based assays. *Biotechnol Bioeng* 2005;89:1–8.

111. Keun HC. Metabonomic modelling of drug toxicity. *J Pharmacol Exp Ther* 2006;109:92–106.

112. Butcher EC, Berg EL, Kunkel EJ. System biology in drug discovery. *Nat Biotechnol* 2004;22:1253–1259.

113. Ekins S, Nikolsky Y, Nikolskaya T. Techniques: application of systems biology to absorption, distribution, metabolism, excretion and toxicity. *Trends Pharm Sci* 2005;26:202–209.

114. Wilson AG, White AC, Mueller RA. Role of predictive metabolism and toxicity modelling in drug discovery—a summary of some recent advancements. *Curr Opin Drug Discov Dev* 2003;9:74–83.

115. Rester U. Dock around the clock—current status of small molecule docking and scoring. *QSAR Comb Sci* 2006;25:605–615.

116. Barratt M, Langowski J. Validation and development of the DEREK skin sensitisation rulebase by anaylsis of the BgVV list of contact allergens. In Balls M, Zeller AM, Halder M, Eds. *Progress in the Reduction Refinement and Replacement of Animal Experimentation.* New York: Elsevier; 2000, pp 493–512.

117. Zinke S, Gerner I, Schlede E. Evaluation of a rule base for identifying contact allergens by using a regulatory database: comparison of data on chemicals notified in the European Union with "structural alerts" used in the DEREK expert system. *Altern Lab Anim* 2002;30:285–298.

118. Dearden JC, Barratt MD, Benigni R, Bristol DW, Combes RD, Cronin MTD, Judson PN, Payne MP, Richard AM, Tichy N, Worth AP, Yourick JJ. The development and validation of expert systems for predicting toxicity. *Altern Lab Anim* 1997;25:223–252.

119. Matthews EJ, Contrera JF. A new highly specific method for predicting the carcinogenic potential of pharmaceuticals in rodents using enhanced MCASE QSAR-ES software. *Regul Toxicol Pharmacol* 1998;28:242.

120. Enslein K, Gombar VK, Blake BW. International Commission for Protection Against Environmental Mutagens and Carcinogens. Use of SAR in computer-assisted prediction of carcinogenicity and mutagenicity of chemicals by the TOPKAT program. *Mutat Res* 1994;305:47.

121. Woo YT, Lai D, Argus A, Arcos JC. Development of structure–activity relationship rules for predicting carcinogenic potential of chemicals. *Toxicol Lett* 1995;79:219.

122. Lewis DFV, Bird MG, Jacobs MN. Human carcinogens: an evaluation study via the COMPACT and HazardExpert procedures. *Hum Exp Toxicol* 2002;21:115.

123. Ji ZL, Wang Y, Yu L, Ha LH, Zheng CJ, Chen YZ. *In silico* search of putative adverse drug reaction related proteins as a potential tool for facilitating drug adverse effect prediction. *Toxicol Lett* 2006;164:104–112.

124. Blaauboer BJ. The integration of data on physico-chemical properties, *in vitro*-derived toxicity data and physiologically based kinetic and dynamics modelling as a tool in hazard and risk assessment: a commentary. *Toxicol Lett* 2003;138:161–171.

125. Deglmann CJ, Ebner T, Ludwig E, Happich S, Schildberg FW, Koebe HG. Protein binding capacity *in vitro* changes metabolism of substrates and influences the predictability of metabolic pathways *in vivo*. *Toxicol In Vitro* 2004;18:835–840.

126. Chang C, Ray A, Swaan P. *In silico* strategies for modelling membrane transporter function. *Drug Discov Today* 2005;10:663–671.

127. Poole TB, Ed. *The UFAW Handbook on the Care and Management of Laboratory Animals*. London: UFAW; 1999.

128. Hirst WD, Abrahamsen B, Blaney FE, Calver AR, Aloj L, Price GW, Medhurst AD. Differences in the central nervous system distribution and pharmacology of the mouse 5-hydroxytryptamine-6 receptor compared with rat and human receptors investigated by radioligand binding, site-directed mutagenesis, and molecular modelling. *Mol Pharmacol* 2003;64 (6):1295–1308.

129. Morton DM. Importance of species selection in drug toxicity testing. *Toxicol Lett* 1998;102–103:545–550.

130. Tang-Wai DF, Kajiji S, diCapua F, de Graff D, Roninson IB, Gros P. Human (MDR1) and mouse (mdr1, mdr3) P-glycoproteins can be distinguished by their respective drug resistance profiles and sensitivity to modulators. *Biochemistry* 1995;34:32–39.

131. Tang H, Mayersohn M. Accuracy of allometrically predicted pharmacokinetic parameters in humans: role of species selection. *Drug Metab Dispos* 2005;33:1288–1295.

132. Festing M, Ed. *The Design of Animal Experiments: Reducing the Use of Animals in Research Through Better Experimental Design*. London: Royal Society of Medicine Press Ltd, 2002.

133. Morris T, Goulet S, Morton D. The International Symposium on Regulatory Testing and Animal Welfare: recommendations on best scientific practices for animal care in regulatory toxicology. *ILAR J* 2002;43(Suppl):S123–S125.

134. Gold LS, Bernstein L, Magaw R, Slone TH. Inter-species extrapolation in carcinogenesis: prediction between rats and mice. *Environ Health Perspect* 1989;81:211–219.

135. Krauthammer M, Kaufmann CA, Gilliam TC, Rzhietsky A. Molecular triangulation: bridging linkage and molecular-network information for identifying candidate genes in Azheimer's disease. *Proc Natl Acad Sci USA* 2004;101:15148–15153.

136. PharmaPendium™. Elsevier MDL. Available from http://www.mdl.com/products/knowledge/pharmapendium/index.jsp (accessed 29 January 2007).

137. Adverse Drug Effects Database™. Wolters-Kluwer Health. Medi-Span Available from http://www.medispan.com/Products/index.aspx?id=18 (accessed 29 January 2007).

138. Sobels FH. Evaluating the mutagenic potential of chemicals: the minimal battery and extrapolation problems. *Arch Toxicol* 1980;46:21–30.

139. Sutter TR. Molecular and cellular approaches to extrapolation for risk assessment. *Environ Health Perspect* 1995;103:386.

140. Van Ravenzwaay B, Leibold E. The significance of *in vitro* rat skin absorption studies to human risk assessment. *Toxicol In Vitro* 2004;18:219–225.

141. Greaves P, Williams A, Eve M. First dose of potential new medicines to humans: how animals help. *Nat Rev Drug Discov* 2004;3:226–236.

2

USE OF PROJECT TEAMS IN PRECLINICAL DEVELOPMENT

Dorothy M. K. Keefe, Joanne M. Bowen, and Rachel J. Gibson
Royal Adelaide Hospital Cancer Centre and University of Adelaide, Adelaide, South Australia

Contents

Preclinical Development Handbook: Toxicology, edited by Shayne Cox Gad
Copyright © 2008 John Wiley & Sons, Inc.

2.1 GENERAL HISTORY OF PRECLINICAL DEVELOPMENT

2.1.1 What Is Preclinical Development?

As the name suggests, preclinical development of a drug is that part of drug development occurring before the drug enters human trials. During this time, safety, activity, and mechanism of action studies can occur. In fact, even once clinical trials have begun, further preclinical studies can be performed to answer developing questions. Any new therapeutic agent that has shown activity in *in vitro* and *in vivo* models still needs to be thoroughly investigated in order for it to move successfully from the laboratory to the clinic. Commonly, these are referred to as translational activities and may involve a number of different studies including scale-up synthesis of the therapeutic agent, development of analytical assays, development and manufacture of dosage formulations, and animal research studies including pharmacology and toxicology. Regulatory authorities around the world have requirements for new drugs before they can begin human studies, and companies need to comply with these. (http://www3.niaid.nih.gov/research/topics/HIV/therapeutics/intro/preclinical_drug_dev). In order for this to happen effectively, there needs to be a project team in place to manage the overall development.

2.1.2 Why Is It Important?

There are many new drugs investigated every year that are found to be active in various ways in either cell culture or animal model systems. However, few of these translate successfully to human use. This may be due to unacceptable toxicity, species variation in effect, cost–benefit ratio in production, inability to scale production sufficiently to produce quantities required in human use, and financial limitations. Having a standard set of procedures that need to be followed makes the process easier, although practical experience contributes a great deal of value.

2.1.3 Elements Associated with Preclinical Development

This includes *in vitro* and *in vivo* studies of efficacy, safety, pharmacokinetics, and pharmacodynamics, in order to produce pharmaceutical grade materials, and to make effective submission for investigational new drug status with the U.S. Food and Drug Administration (FDA) and other regulatory authorities. By the end of preclinical development there needs to be the ability to produce sufficient quantities of drug for human use, analytical assays to measure the drug and its metabolites, appropriate dosage formulations, and animal toxicology and pharmacology. All of this needs to comply with FDA and other regulatory requirements. The vast majority of drugs that enter preclinical development do not end up as marketable items. However, those that do are often able to radically improve patients' quality of life.

2.2 WHAT IS A PROJECT TEAM?

A project team in this setting is the group of people charged with taking the drug through the preclinical phase, from the time of decision regarding its potential for human use, up to the time of clinical trial. It is made up of all the key people who can organize the studies that need to be conducted and needs to include adequate administrative support, record keeping, time-line planning, and recording of milestones. A project team is vital for the success of any drug/compound undergoing preclinical development. It is able to successfully implement all aspects of drug development projects, including planning, conducting, regulatory aspects, clinical aspects, administration, ethics approval, administrative support, and reporting of results. More generically, however, a project team is a group of people brought together with a common purpose (in this case to prepare a drug for clinical development).

2.2.1 Differing Models for Project Teams

In the pharmaceutical industry, project teams can be aligned in different ways. For example, it may be appropriate to have one team that looks after the entire development of a drug, set up along lines historically used by the company. There may be standard operating procedures (SOPs) for a given company that will be applied to all new teams that are required. This team may then oversee the bringing of a new drug from basic research right through animal trials to human study. Or, there may be SOPs for preclinical study teams that are completely separate from Clinical Teams, with a hand-over of responsibility between teams once human studies are commenced. Or a new team for a new drug may be allowed (or in the case of new companies, may need) to set up a project team from scratch for a new drug. In this case, a clear idea of the aims of the project is vital. Alternatively, development of a drug may come under the responsibility of several different teams, each responsible for a certain part of the overall project; for example, there could be different project teams along department lines, doing all of the pharmacology, molecular pharmacology, bioanalysis, medicinal chemistry, business development, or marketing for all drugs under development by that particular company. There would then be a requirement for higher level liaison between groups regarding each single drug.

2.2.2 Leadership of a Project Team

Each project team is assigned a project leader who has the responsibility to run the project forward—that is, maintain an updated project plan, meet milestones, ensure personnel resources are sufficient by communicating with departmental heads, and keep management and the company updated.

This is like leadership in any situation: it contributes enormously to the success of a team, and if not present is sorely missed. There are many theories about leadership, but Griffiths [1] lists eleven competencies that are required: establishing focus, influencing others, drive to achieve, focus on customers, building relationships, fostering teamwork, attention to information, interpersonal awareness, improving performance, developing others, and empowering others. And these are all important in any project team, whatever the goal of that team. It should be noted, however, that a project team never works in isolation but needs to be aware (to a certain degree) of its position within its institution, organizational unit, and program, before it reaches the project or individual level. There also needs to be trust between a team leader and the team members for optimum success [1].

There is an increasing literature on building high performance teams and on project teams that is outside the scope of this chapter.

2.3 BENEFITS OF PROJECT TEAMS IN PRECLINICAL DEVELOPMENT

The major benefit of project teams in preclinical development is the ability to coordinate the activities of all investigators/staff in order to get the drug to clinical trial, or make a decision that it will not work, in the shortest possible time. The team acts as a repository for all information regarding the drug and ensures that all regulatory requirements are met in a timely manner so that nothing is omitted that will delay application for an investigational new drug (IND) approval.

Members of the preclinical project team include the team leader, laboratory head, scientists, students, and administrative support staff. All of these people bring together the skills that are required for the effective management of the team. These skills include budgeting, legal issues, protocol writing, report writing, publication writing, presentation of results, and building of the IND file. Mostly, the project team will be run out of a pharmaceutical company, but many academic institutions will have their own project teams working on specific issues and liaising with industry as appropriate. All members of the project team play a crucial role in any preclinical development.

There are a number of different terminologies that are often used by project teams. We have listed below some of the more common ones.

Investigational Product. A pharmaceutical form of an active ingredient or placebo being tested or used as a reference in a clinical trial, including a product with a marketing authorization used or assembled (formulated or packaged) in a way different from the approved form, or when used for an unapproved indication, or when used to gain further information about an approved use.

Investigator. Any person responsible for the conduct of the clinical trial at a trial site. If a trial is conducted by a team or individuals at a trial site, the investigator is the responsible leader of the team and may be called the principal investigator.

Sponsor–Investigatory. An individual who both initiates and conducts, alone or with others, a clinical trial, and under whose immediate direction the investigational product is administered to, dispersed to, or used by a subject. The term does not include any person other than an individual (e.g., it does not include a corporation or an agency).

Subinvestigator/Coinvestigator. Any individual member of the clinical trial team designated and supervised by the investigator at a trial site to perform critical trial-related procedures and/or to make important trial-related decisions (e.g., associates, residents, research fellows).

Animal Research Ethics Committee. An independent body constituted of veterinary, scientific, and nonscientific members, whose responsibility is to ensure the protection of the rights, safety, and well-being of animals involved in research by, among other things, reviewing, approving, and providing continuing review of trial protocol and amendments and of the methods and materials to be used in each research project.

2.3.1   Individual Responsibilities Within the Project Team

Principal Investigator   The principal investigator has a number of specific roles to play in a project team. First, the he/she is responsible for the signing of appropriate forms including regulatory forms and, if applicable, disclosing of financial interests and arrangements. The principal investigator is also responsible for signing contracts with sponsors and third parties as applicable. Other key responsibilities include supervision of each member of the project team, documentation of the delegation of responsibilities, ensuring the safety and welfare of animals (where an animal trial is being undertaken), hiring and training of members of the project team, meeting sponsor requirements, meeting with sponsors to discuss planned and ongoing studies, and finally meeting with auditors (internal, sponsor, and regulatory authorities) at the conclusion of their audits to review findings.

Providing Investigator Qualifications and Agreements   This is one of the key roles that a principal investigator has in a project team. It is essential that he/she continues to keep an up-to-date curriculum vitae, detailing experience including the proper education and training to undertake the research project or clinical trial. Furthermore, the principal investigator is responsible for signing the protocols and external contracts and documenting the financial aspects of the trial.

Assuring Protocol Compliance   By having a detailed understanding of the requirements of each research trial and clinical trial, the principal investigator can ensure that all other staff on the project team are aware of and undertaking their roles and responsibilities accurately. The principal investigator can also ensure that staff are not deviating from the protocol without prior agreements from the sponsor and/or the human and/or animal research ethics committees.

Liaisons with Human and/or Animal Research Ethics Committees   It is the role of the principal investigator of any project team to prepare animal research ethics committee applications. This involves the initial written application to conduct animal research, notifying the committee if there are any changes that need to be made to the protocols, providing the committees with results (either positive or negative), and providing the committees with annual reports and end-of-project reports.

Support Staff   All support staff of the project teams are required to fulfill those job responsibilities specific to that job title according to regulations and guidelines as well as to the appropriate standard operating procedures (SOPs) and maintain study files and archives.

Administrative Responsibilities   The administrative responsibilities of the project team lie with the principal investigator. Briefly, he/she is responsible for the hiring and training of other members of the project team, management of the business aspects of the studies (including the development and negotiation of study budgets and contracts), and overseeing the management of documents (including the filing and archiving).

2.3.2   General Responsibilities of the Project Team

Principal Investigator, Coinvestigator, Data Manager, Study Pharmacist, and Support Staff   All members of the project team are required to conduct all studies according to applicable regulations and guidelines and SOPs of the site, and according to the policies and procedures of the institution as appropriate. They are required to ensure that the principal investigator is informed in a timely manner of all study-related activities through appropriate mechanisms, to ensure the safety and welfare of animals by thoroughly understanding ongoing study protocols and to be knowledgeable about investigational products. For studies that are conducted under U.S. IND, all investigators and research personnel must comply with regulations governing disclosure of personal, professional, or financial interest in a research study that may impact upon its conduct, evaluation, or outcome. Finally, all project team members are required to comply with study protocol and procedures. (See Table 2.1.)

2.4   SPECIAL CONSIDERATIONS OF ACADEMIC PROJECT TEAMS

The project team required to complete a preclinical study varies considerably depending on the research avenue and outcomes sought. However, a reasonable model is illustrated in Fig. 2.1. The principal investigator instigates the preclinical project. He/she will then liaise with the senior research staff to adequately design a research plan to address the gaps in knowledge and questions to be answered. This is often quite a time-consuming exercise, as ideas are bounced back and forth and an appropriate course of action is decided upon. Will the study involve humans or animals? Will the study be observational or require intervention? Will the study be using novel treatments? These are just a few of the questions that need to be addressed before the study commences. The project team has a crucial role to play in this initial development of the project. More importantly, the project team will also decide whether other expertise will be required for the study. For example, will

TABLE 2.1   Major Components of Project Team Activity

Administration	Project Management	Investigator-Sponsored Trials (If Applicable)
Contract negotiations, sign contracts	Ethics committee submissions and communications	Quality assurance/quality control
Fiscal management	Regulatory files creation and maintenance	Data handling
Facilities management/availability	Data management	Record keeping
Strategic planning	Adverse event reports	Financing
Database development	Protocol implementation and management	Notification to regulatory authorities
Performance tracking	Organizational tools	Information on investigational product(s)
Quality control and assurance (including SOPs)	Office staff training	Supply and handling of investigational product(s)
Insurance and indemnity	Storing study documents	Safety information Monitoring
		Audit and noncompliance
		Premature termination or suspension of a trial
		Study reports

pharmacists, nurses, technical officers, and students be required? In many cases of preclinical development, biotechnology and pharmaceutical industries are involved, not only in aiding in funding but also in providing technology and reagents. Ethical relations need to be maintained, to ensure that there is no bias/pressure from industry. This guarantees that there is independence and transparency, which ultimately benefits everyone.

Once the research project has commenced, the tiers of the project team contribute to the daily running of the project under direct supervision from the principal investigator of the project team. Constant communication with the principal investigator is essential. Students can be involved in the studies and often play a critical role in any project team.

2.5   USING THE DARK AGOUTI (DA) RAT MODEL OF MUCOSITIS TO ILLUSTRATE

In academic preclinical research, the drivers may be slightly different from those in industry, although the structure and activity of a project team still follows the same ideals. Using our laboratory as an example, we have developed an animal model of chemotherapy- and radiotherapy-induced gastrointestinal mucositis. This is not a model used for developing a single drug for registration, rather a model we have developed to study the pathobiology and treatment of mucositis. However, we do

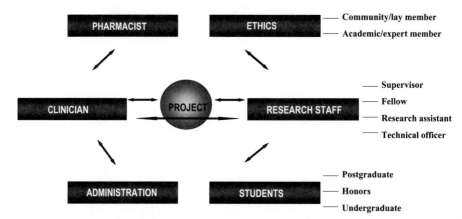

FIGURE 2.1   A diagrammatic representation of a project team in the research setting. The project team required to complete a preclinical study varies depending on research avenue and outcomes sought, however, a reasonable model includes those shown. The clinician is often the first to recognize a need for research into a particular area and instigates the preclinical project. He/She then liases with research staff to adequately design a research plan to address the gaps in knowledge and questions to be answered. The combination of clinician and senior research staff allows for multiple principal investigators to be named on any grant application. The research plan must be submitted to an ethics committee for scrutiny. Each committee is comprised of both lay and expert community members to provide a broad view of the project, allowing comments on its significance as well any potential improvements required. In many cases, the biotechnology and pharmaceutical industries are to be used in the project, by providing technology and agents, and the clinician is primarily responsible for opening dialogue with these professions. The administration department within the hospital in the form of record keeping and patient control is involved in supplying background information readily as needed. Once the project is under way, the tiers of laboratory staff contribute to the daily running of the research under supervision from the head of the lab. Constant communication with the clinician as well as data management, tissue collection, and manuscript preparation are all the responsibility of the research staff. Students are also involved through placement in certain parts of the experiment following training by technical staff.

have our own project team to run the studies, and the principles are similar so it will serve as an illustration.

An appropriate animal model was required to investigate further the mechanisms underlying alimentary mucositis. The model had few requirements: it had to have value commercially, it had to be able to be used in true translational research (i.e., research that goes from the laboratory to the clinic and from the clinic to the laboratory), and the overriding goal for the model had to be (and still is today) to improve patient outcomes. It needed to be able to be interrogated in various ways and using various different potential drugs in a standard fashion.

A model was therefore developed using subcutaneously implanted isogeneic rat breast cancer in the female dark Agouti (DA) rat. The mammary adenocarcinoma arose spontaneously in the 1970s and has been propagated ever since by passage through female rats. Female rats are used because the tumor passages more effectively through females than males. The tumor is injected (as a cell suspension) subcutaneously into both flanks and is harvested between 10 and 14 days and processed for further passage or experimental use. This model had previously been used for studies of malnutrition following chemotherapy [2, 3] and for studies of neuroprotection by glutamate [4], but had not been previously used to assess the alimentary tract following chemotherapy. The model has allowed an attempt at ameliorating intestinal toxicities following chemotherapy [5] and more recently fractionated radiotherapy, while guarding against tumor growth. More recently, the model has been refined to using tumor-naive rats [6]. The advantage of the nontumor model is a time and cost saving, whereas the advantage of the tumor model is the interaction between tumor and host.

2.5.1   Choice of Cytotoxic Agent

Initially, the detailed time course of intestinal damage and repair in the DA rat model needed to be established. In order to commence studies, an appropriate chemotherapeutic agent was required. The cytotoxic agent had to be commonly used and known to cause mucositis in the clinic. Methotrexate (MTX) is a commonly used cytotoxic agent; the mode of action is in the inhibition of dihydrofolate reductase (DHFR) [7–9]. MTX is also known to cause diarrhea and anorexia, accompanied with malabsorption, malnutrition, and dehydration in patients. Furthermore, MTX is known to inhibit epithelial proliferation and enterocyte function as well as increase the risk of gut-associated sepsis due to disruption of the mucosal barrier. This has led to gastrointestinal toxicity being the major dose-limiting factor for the use of MTX [9–11]. Therefore, MTX was deemed an appropriate choice of cytotoxic agent to begin our studies.

2.5.2   Time Course of Small Intestinal Mucositis in the DA Rat Model

Rats were assigned to experimental or control groups; experimental animals received 1.5 mg/kg MTX on days designated 0 and 1, while control animals received saline only [12]. The dose of MTX was chosen from pilot experiments, which indicated that it caused significant, nonlethal small intestinal mucositis [5]. Experimental rats were killed on days 1 (6 h following the second dose of MTX) through 5, with control rats being killed on days 1 and 5 only. This small study detailed the time course of MTX-induced small intestinal mucositis and found that the small intestine is indeed the predominant site of damage. Apoptosis increased 28-fold in the small intestinal crypts 6 h after the second dose and indicated that crypt hypoplasia and villus atrophy occurred between days 2 and 4 following treatment. Following this initial injury, the epithelium enters a rapidly proliferating state, repairing and regenerating the intestine [9, 12–14]. This small animal experiment confirmed that the time course of small intestinal mucositis in the DA rat model [12] was similar to that observed in our initial human studies [5, 15], indicating that the animal model was an appropriate model to continue developing. Furthermore, these results allowed us to continue to understand the mechanisms underlying mucositis.

2.5.3   Tumor Bearing Versus Tumor Naive?

The DA rat model was initially developed using subcutaneously implanted isogeneic rat breast cancers in the female dark Agouti rat. However, it has been well documented that patients with malignancies will have alterations in their immune function [16], including impaired delayed-type hypersensitivity, decreased lymphocytic function, and decreased lymphocyte proliferation response [16, 17]. In addition to this, tumors are known to be responsible for the secretion of different mediators, which decrease the efficiency of immunological integrals [18]. Until recently, there was no evidence on whether the presence of a tumor burden will affect the gastrointestinal response (i.e., mucositis) to chemotherapy. However, a study conducted by our laboratory found that response to chemotherapy was worse in tumor-bearing rats than tumor-naive rats, indicating that the presence of a tumor load adds to the comorbidity following chemotherapy [6].

2.5.4 Advantages of Our Rat Model of Mucositis

The DA rat model of mucositis has a number of key advantages over other animal models. First, the rats have a rapid growth and development phase. Second, there is homogeneity among all animals, meaning that we can accurately assess what damage is occurring and when. Finally, we are able to examine the entire gastrointestinal tract from mouth to anus and from epithelium to muscle. This has enabled us to develop a three-dimensional model of mucositis.

How Do We Generate Questions/Avenues to Investigate in the DA Rat Model? Many of the questions and avenues that have been investigated in the DA rat model of mucositis have stemmed from questions that need to be answered in the clinic. Our first studies in mucositis were done in humans, but it is very hard to take biopsies in real patients throughout the GIT and throughout the course of cytotoxic treatment.

2.6 OUR DA RAT MODEL OF MUCOSITIS AND PRECLINICAL DEVELOPMENT

How Do We Use the Model for Preclinical Development? The DA rat model has been used to assess the pathobiology of mucositis following various chemotherapeutic agents. Using a standard trial protocol and measuring at different levels of the GIT at different time points, we have built up a clear picture of the damage caused by various agents. We can then add any potential antimucotoxic drug of interest and assess, in the same way, whether it reduces mucosal toxicity. We have previously done this with IL-11, glutamine, Palifermin, Velafermin, and VSL#3.

How Do We Design an Appropriate Trial? Having set up the model to measure damage throughout the GIT at various time points, it is possible to decide which time points and areas of the gut are of particular interest for a given study. In small pilot studies, mortality and diarrhea can be used as endpoints. If the drug of interest shows promise in the pilot setting, then we can examine more specific time points and different areas of the GIT and make measurements including histology and apoptosis in larger, more detailed studies.

How Do We Determine Variables to Change? As with any experiment, the number of variables to be changed at each given time should be as close to one as possible.

Which one to change depends on the question being asked. For example, do we wish to compare three different doses? Or perhaps three different administration schedules? This is done by discussion with the team and the company and depends on pilot results as well as other information from earlier studies.

What Happens When Things Don't Go According to Plan?   This is a frequent occurrence in a laboratory. First, it is important not to panic! Every step of the protocol needs to be rechecked (this is one of the reasons that good record keeping is vital). Decisions need to be made with respect to altering the experiment midway, abandoning it, or restarting. No hasty decisions should be made, as they are often wrong.

2.7   HOW DO WE GENERATE QUESTIONS/AVENUES TO INVESTIGATE FOR PRECLINICAL DEVELOPMENT?

2.7.1   Questions Are Formulated by What We Need/Want to Know

There are several ways in which questions can be generated for our model. First, a pharmaceutical company may approach us to ask us to try its agent in our DA rat model. Alternatively, through careful reading of the current literature, or through scientific research discussions, we come across a question that we cannot currently answer and that we feel it would be useful to investigate. Other ways in which we can generate questions are that we learn about a new drug and seek it out for testing in our model or we seek to expand what the model can do. For example, we can try and test new chemotherapeutic agents, or test the development of the radiotherapy model. A research avenue to investigate these questions is then formulated in the rat model, using the principles of changing as few variables as possible, using minimal numbers of animals, and using adequate controls.

Following on from this, an appropriate trial is designed (in consultation with the project team) in the rat model of mucositis to answer our questions. Our questions are answered by a variety of techniques: the rat's response to treatment, histology, histopathology, intestinal morphometry, apoptosis, Western blotting, RT-PCR, and microarrays (with diarrhea and mortality in pilots).

From these experiments, we are then able to generate results that lead to potential mechanisms and invariably more questions. All of these lead to an attempt to understand mechanisms in the rat model and translation into the clinic.

With proper planning for storage of samples, further questions can be answered as and when they become important. The development of new technologies allows for this, as with the development of tissue microarray technology. Properly stored tissues can have RNA extracted for assessment.

2.7.2   Structure of Our Preclinical Team

The Mucositis Research Group head is a clinician scientist, allowing for understanding of both basic and clinical issues to ensure that the research carried out by our group is clinically relevant. There is then a laboratory manager who is responsible for day-to-day running of the laboratory, occupational health and safety, task allocation, record keeping, stock ordering, and routine finances, as well as playing a lead role in manuscript planning, mentoring of junior staff, and medium-term planning. We have a technical officer who works under supervision of the laboratory manager on the above tasks, and the rest of the staff are postgraduate students whose projects all fit into the overall goal of the group, which is to understand and then minimize gastrointestinal toxicity from anticancer treatments.

2.7.3   Team Meetings

There is an annual direction planning meeting, which looks at overall strategy: funding from partners and grant applications, priorities of research projects, student numbers and progress, manuscript planning, abstract submission plans, and conferences to be attended. A fortnightly team meeting looks at individual progress but in the group setting with reports of activity against targets, checking of laboratory record books, and updates on tasks (writing, abstracts). On alternate fortnights the laboratory head and laboratory manager meet each other person separately to assess progress in a more confidential setting. An open-door policy with regard to communication is maintained, and the overall effect is a happy, hard-working, and high-achieving workforce. The environment is supportive and optimistic, with all members of the team recognized and valued for their contributions and their differences. Turnover of staff is low, and this is a reflection of the atmosphere. In addition, *ad hoc* meetings with visiting experts are conducted as required. Team building exercises, such as the occasional lunch, the annual trip to the Multinational Association of Supportive Care Symposium, and afternoon tea for special celebrations, help to keep the team functioning well.

This is the model that has developed over the years in the Mucositis Research Group, but it is not the only possibility. There are many different organizational models, and different ones may suit different companies. This can be a problem during company mergers, as the "personality" of one group of workers may not fit with that of another! This is due to organizations having their own definite structural, humanistic, political, and cultural models. Of critical importance, however, is periodic review of goals, orientation, and general direction. This can be particularly important in a research laboratory, where the temptation can be to head off in any direction that seems interesting at the time, without stopping to think how that fits in with the overall aims of the research group.

2.8   HOW DO WE PRESENT THE RESULTS AND HOW DO WE DETERMINE WHAT THEY MEAN?

It is a principle of good science that all results should be presented and published, whether positive or negative, and it is our duty to ensure that this happens with our studies. However, it is harder in the commercial world to do this due to problems with commercial confidentiality. The importance of being transparent is essential for good science and this cannot be overstated. However, again it is somewhat easier in academia than in industry.

Different Scenarios Can Lead to Different Outcomes   Sometimes it can be the protocol that leads to a drug not working rather than the drug itself: the dose or schedule can be wrong, or an ineffective batch of drug can be used. These problems need to be checked. A timely reminder is that a single experiment always needs repeating before it can be said to be valid.

The Importance of Being Transparent   While improving company profits is obviously one of the major aims of any industry, the overriding issue in drug research and development is to produce drugs that really work, and that will improve quality and quantity of life, with minimal adverse effects. This may sound like unnecessarily stating the obvious, but it is an important component to a project team's work: getting the right answer is the goal, not getting an answer that will drive up profits, especially if it is wrong. Putting an unsafe or ineffective drug onto the market will get found out and will result in much more trouble down the track.

What Happens If the Drug Doesn't Work?   We need to check the experiment, look at potential confounders, consider changes to dose, route, or scheduling, and if possible try these. Sometimes a drug can be removed from development because the company determines not to try altering the protocol due to cost blow-outs. It is the responsibility of the project team to try to ensure the protocol chosen for the "do or die" study is the one most likely to work. However, if the drug doesn't work, then it should *not* be marketed.

Interface with Clinical Development   During the progression of preclinical research into the clinical setting, a number of questions need to be answered. Can we find the answers by studying humans? If yes, then we begin research in humans. If not, further animal or cell model studies are required to be designed so that this can be achieved. Ultimately, any research in humans will lead to further questions. Then we must again consider if these questions can be answered by looking at humans. If not, then we must go back to preclinical models of research before we can continue (Fig. 2.2).

2.9   THE FUTURE FOR PRECLINICAL PROJECT TEAMS

Potential Improvements   With the ongoing development of teams and companies, SOPs are revised, improved, and developed with the experience of the organization. This should lead to a continued refinement of project team theory as well as practical implementation within a company/academic institution. The increasing crossover between business and research should enable constant improvement, as long as the differences between science and business are respected.

New Difficulties   The same crossover can also have negative impacts, with business decisions interfering in the practice of research. Obviously, there has to be a balance, as financial imperatives have to be heeded to a certain degree. The size of a team can become unwieldy and the structure of an organization can impose dysfunction on a team. Poor leadership and management of a team can lead to failure, and it can be hard to distinguish between failure of the drug and failure of the team on some occasions.

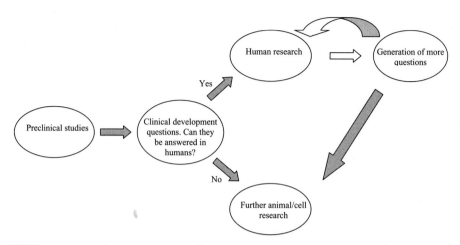

FIGURE 2.2   Development from preclinical to clinical investigations. During the progression of preclinical research into the clinical setting a number of questions need to be answered. Can we find the answers by studying humans? If yes, then we begin research in humans. If not, further animal or cell model studies are required to be designed so that this can be achieved. Ultimately, any research in humans will lead to further questions. Then we must again consider if these can be answered by looking at humans. If not, then we must go back to preclinical models of research before we can continue.

Summary   A good preclinical project team is compact, goal-oriented, well-resourced both financially and with skilled personnel, and has clear time-lines for meeting its objectives. It undergoes regular assessment against its tasks and is able to adapt to results in a positive, timely manner.

REFERENCES

1. Griffiths X. *The Art of Leading a Team*. Adelaide, Australia: KRG Consultants; 2002.
2. Rofe AM, Bourgeois CS, Washington JM, Philcox JC, Coyle P. Metabolic consequences of methotrexate therapy in tumour-bearing rats. *Immunol Cell Biol* 1994;72:43–48.
3. Rofe AM, Bais R, Conyers RA. Ketone-body metabolism in tumour-bearing rats. *Biochem J* 1986;233:485–491.
4. Boyle FM, Wheeler HR, Shenfield GM. Glutamate ameliorates experimental vincristine neuropathy. *J Pharmacol Exp Ther* 1996;279:410–415.
5. Keefe DMK. *The Effect of Cytotoxic Chemotherapy on the Mucosa of the Small Intestine*. Adelaide: Department of Medicine, University of Adelaide; 1998.
6. Gibson RJ, Bowen JM, Alvarez E, Finnie JW, Keefe DMK. Establishment of a single dose irinotecan model of gastrointestinal mucositis. *Chemotherapy* 2007;53:360–369.
7. Huennekens FM. The methotrexate story: a paradigm for development of cancer chemotherapeutic agents. *Adv Enzyme Regul* 1994;34:397–419.
8. Tenenbaum L. *Cancer Chemotherapy and Biotherapy*. Philadelphia: WB Saunders; 1994, pp 7–8.
9. Bowen JM, Gibson RJ, Cummins AG, Keefe DMK. Intestinal mucositis: the role of the Bcl-2 family, p53 and caspases in chemotherapy-induced damage. *Support Care Cancer* 2006;17:713–731.

10. Papaconstantinou HT, Xie C, Zhang W, Ansari NH, Hellmich MR, Townsend CM, Ko TC. The role of caspases in methotrexate-induced gastrointestinal toxicity. *Surgery* 2001;859–865.

11. Verburg M, Renes IB, Meijer HP, Taminiau JAJM, Buller HA, Einerhand AWC, Dekker J. Selective sparing of goblet cells and Paneth cells in the intestine of methotrexate-treated rats. *Am J Physiol* 2000;279:G1037–G1047.

12. Gibson RJ, Keefe DMK, Thompson FM, Clarke JM, Goland GJ, Cummins AG. Effect of interleukin-11 on ameliorating intestinal damage after methotrexate treatment of breast cancer in rats. *Dig Dis Sci* 2002;47:2751–2757.

13. Howarth GS, Francis GL, Cool JC, Xu X, Byard RW, Read LC. Milk growth factors enriched from cheese whey ameliorate intestinal damage by methotrexate when administered orally to rats. *J Nutr* 1996;126:2519–2530.

14. Taminiau JAJM, Gall DG, Hamilton JR. Response of the rat small-intestine epithelium to methotrexate. *Gut* 1980;21:486–492.

15. Keefe DM, Brealey J, Goland GJ, Cummins AG. Chemotherapy for cancer causes apoptosis that precedes hypoplasia in crypts of the small intestine in humans. *Gut* 2000;47:632–637.

16. Fittkau M, Voigt W, Holzhausen HJ, Schmoll HJ. Saccharic acid 1.4-lactone protects against CPT-11-induced mucosa damage in rats. *J Cancer Res Clin Oncol* 2004;130(7):388–394.

17. Evans TRJ. Vaccine therapy for cancer—fact or fiction? *Proc R Coll Physicians Edinburgh* 2001;31:9–16.

18. Broder S, Waldmann TA. The suppressor-cell network in cancer (first of two parts). *N Engl J Med* 1978;299:1281–1284.

3

RELATIONSHIP BETWEEN ANIMAL MODELS AND CLINICAL RESEARCH: USING MUCOSITIS AS A PRACTICAL EXAMPLE

RACHEL J. GIBSON, JOANNE M. BOWEN, AND DOROTHY M. K. KEEFE
Royal Adelaide Hospital Cancer Centre, and University of Adelaide, Adelaide, South Australia

Contents

Preclinical Development Handbook: Toxicology, edited by Shayne Cox Gad
Copyright © 2008 John Wiley & Sons, Inc.

3.1   GENERAL HISTORY OF THE USE OF ANIMAL MODELS

Animals have been used in "research" by humans for hundreds of years with the first recorded use of animals for research purposes by Erasistratus in Alexandria in the third century BC [1]. In the second century AD, Galen of Pergamum used animals to further understand anatomy; however, it was not until the beginning of the 19th century that "true" animal research began [2]. With the lack of appropriate anesthesia, some scientists proposed principles for animal research: experiments needed to be necessary, needed to have a clearly defined and attainable objective, should not be repeated unnecessarily, and needed to be conducted with the least possible infliction of pain on the animals [2]. This formed the basis of animal research for the next century [2].

By the late 1800s, basic anesthesia had been developed, leading to major advances in medical research. This necessitated developments in animal research [2]. Following World War II, animal research grew at a rapid rate as research into cancer, cardiovascular diseases, digestive diseases, and ageing began in earnest [2]. The development of appropriate animal models has allowed for major advances to be made for human benefit. We have improved our knowledge and understanding of many diseases including but not exclusive to AIDS, cholera, diabetes, and spinal cord injuries [3, 4]. Furthermore, animal models have allowed us to understand biology, including the physiology of reproductive biology, which has led to the development of the oral contraceptive pill [3, 4].

Today, animal research is tightly regulated, with researchers adhering to Codes of Practice [5]. The purposes of these codes are to ensure the ethical and humane care and use of animals used for scientific purposes [5]. Animal models continue to lead the way with advances in medical research.

3.2   BENEFITS OF ANIMAL MODELS IN MUCOSITIS RESEARCH

Mucositis is a major clinical problem in oncology, caused by the cytotoxic effects of cancer chemotherapy and radiotherapy. It can affect the mucosa of the oral cavity and gastrointestinal tract, causing mouth pain, ulceration, abdominal pain, bloating, vomiting, and diarrhea, depending on the target tissue [6, 7]. For many years, mucositis received little attention. However, the development of animal models has allowed considerable work to be undertaken on mucositis in the oral cavity [8–15] and in the gastrointestinal tract (GIT) [16–20]. Despite the advances, however, these investigations have separated the GIT into the oral and esophageal mucosa and the remainder of the tract, with no investigations to date having investigated the entire GIT from mouth to anus [7, 21]. There are at least two major reasons for this approach to past studies of mucositis. First, while both the upper and lower GIT are lined with mucosa, the tissue types are different. The upper GIT consists of a renewing stratified squamous mucosa, whereas the lower GIT is primarily columnar epithelium. As a consequence, the kinetics of mucositis in the two areas are vastly different, as are the clinical endpoints. Second, the ease with which the oral mucosa can be inspected and studied in *in vivo* models has been an asset compared to the remainder of the tract [7, 21]. However, it is now recognized that the entire GIT has the same embryological route of development with the differences seen being due to cellular differentiation at various sites in order to conduct specialized functions [7, 21]. With the development of appropriate animal models, we can investigate this hypothesis.

3.2.1 Oral Mucositis Animal Models

While there are a number of different animal models in oral mucositis research, two in particular have been studied extensively. Wolfgang Dorr and colleagues [8–12] have developed a radiation model in mice, which involves irradiating the tongue and snout. This model has also been able to extensively investigate the effects of combined chemotherapy and radiotherapy [22]. In addition, it has enabled detailed studies to be conducted on the effects of single dose and fractionated radiotherapy on the head. The second model, which has advanced the understanding of the mechanisms of oral mucositis, is the hamster model, which has been used extensively by Stephen Sonis and colleagues [15]. Briefly, this model of mucositis uses male golden Syrian hamsters, as unlike other rodents, they have a buccal cheek pouch that is susceptible to chemotherapy. Mucositis is able to be induced by the administration of 5-fluorouracil (5-FU) at 60 mg/kg on three days (days 0, 5, and 10). The buccal pouch mucosa is superficially irritated (mechanically scratched) on days 1, 2, and 3, resulting in mucositis in most of the animals [15].

3.2.2 Gastrointestinal Animal Models

Few animal models exist for investigating the remainder of the GIT. Howarth and colleagues [23] have developed an animal model for utilizing the sucrose breath test and also for investigating potential antimucotoxics [24, 25]. However, very few other models exist that are able to investigate the underlying mechanisms of gastrointestinal mucositis. The dark Agouti (DA) rat model of mucositis (see Section 3.4) fills this need.

The development of appropriate animal models allows us to ask specific questions about any region of the GIT, develop an appropriate line of questioning, and then investigate it. We can also measure our response to these questions by changing only one variable at a time. Other advantages of animal models include the ability to work with a homogeneous population, where all of the animals are inbred. This reduces the variability between each animal and ensures that we are getting an accurate reflection of what is occurring. Standard questions are able to be investigated in each experiment, which generate standard answers. All of these combine to reduce the time of drug development, meaning that drugs move from the research laboratory to the clinic in a more timely fashion.

3.3   DIFFICULTIES OF ANIMAL MODELS IN MUCOSITIS RESEARCH

While animal models undoubtedly have benefits, they also have difficulties and limitations. One of the first animal models for investigating mucositis was established by Sonis and colleagues [15]. While this model has enabled hypotheses to be developed for mucositis mechanisms, there is the confounding issue of wound healing. Hamsters have cheek pouches and mucositis is able to be induced by either chemotherapy (5-FU) [15, 26, 27] or radiotherapy [28]. However, following administration of the chemotherapy, the cheek pouch needs to be "mechanically" scratched or irritated in order to induce ulcerated lesions. In humans, however, the oral mucosa does not need to be superficially irritated in order to induce mucositis, and so this model cannot be compared with the clinical setting. Additionally, superficial irritation may also result in wound healing mechanisms being initiated. This highlights the fact that, despite similarities, animal models are never identical to humans, and there will always be issues with translation from animal to human research. This does not, however, devalue animal research; it just adds an appropriate note of caution. With the hamster cheek-pouch model, some agents that have appeared promising in the animals have not translated to success in humans with mucositis. One factor here may be the component of wound healing. With the need for mechanical scratching of the mucosa to allow chemotherapy to cause an ulcer, the insult to the mucosa is composed of both the scratch and the chemotherapy, and this may alter both the development of the ulcer and the recovery. In humans, no scratch is necessary. If a given agent is acting to heal the component induced by the scratch, but has no effect on the development of a chemotherapy-induced ulcer, then it would not be expected to work for chemotherapy-induced mucositis in humans. However, dose and scheduling issues are also important and cannot be overlooked. The doses used in rats do not automatically translate to humans: there may be species differences in susceptibility to different agents, and the traditional mg/kg dosing of rodents is not often used in humans, where we tend to use (for reasons that are not always logical) body surface area dosing.

An added difficulty with animal models has been introduced with the development of monoclonal antibodies for treatment of human disease. Fully humanized monoclonal antibodies may not be active in animal models and toxicities may not develop until translation occurs to the human situation.

Difficulties also arise in the DA rat model of mucositis. Unlike the hamster, in the rat, we are unable to successfully induce visible oral mucositis due to the highly keratinized nature of the epithelium (D. Wilson and D. Keefe, personal communication). This makes it difficult to successfully investigate oral mucositis. Furthermore, higher doses of chemotherapy are required to induce mucosal injury in animal models, due to the resilience of the rat GIT. Another difference is the presence of squamous epithelium in the rat stomach, which can lead to reduction in oral intake when keratinocyte growth factor, a stimulator of epithelial growth, is used. We also know that rats do not vomit, and since some vomiting is a manifestation of mucosal injury, this is a disadvantage.

The route of administration of chemotherapy has important implications for drug metabolism. In the DA rat model of mucositis, intravenous administration of chemotherapeutic drugs is extremely difficult, with administration into the tail vein being made especially difficult due to the skin pigmentation. This means that investigation into mucositis induced by drugs administered via this route is not routinely performed. Although all chemotherapeutic drugs cause damage [29, 30], the mechanisms of how they do this may be different.

Other contributing factors also cause difficulties in animal research. These include stresses in the animals from isolation due to experimental procedures, the need to anesthetize animals on a regular basis, and the effect that this has on mucosal homeostasis, and the efficacy of any investigative drugs on tumor load.

3.4 THE DARK AGOUTI (DA) RAT MAMMARY ADENOCARCINOMA MODEL OF MUCOSITIS

An appropriate animal model was required to investigate further the mechanisms underlying alimentary mucositis. The model had few requirements: it had to be capable of modeling the changes that occur in the human GIT following insult with chemotherapy; it had to have commercial value; it had to be able to be used in true translational research (research that goes from the laboratory to the clinic and from the clinic to the laboratory); and the overriding goal for the model had to be (and still is today) to improve patient outcomes. It had additional advantages of being able to be used either with or without tumor and to allow study of any organ of choice. It has subsequently also been used for a radiotherapy-induced mucositis study, and in the future combination studies could be performed.

A model was therefore developed using subcutaneously implanted isogeneic rat breast cancer in the female dark Agouti (DA) rat. The mammary adenocarcinoma arose spontaneously in the 1970s and has been propagated ever since by passage through female rats. Female rats are used because the tumor passages more effectively through females than males. It is worth noting that the tumor does not grow in culture; otherwise it would be preferential to study it using these methods. The tumor is injected (as a cell suspension) subcutaneously into both flanks and is harvested between 10 and 14 days and processed for further passage or experimental use. This model had previously been used for studies of malnutrition following chemotherapy [31, 32] and for studies of neuroprotection by glutamate [33], but had not been used to assess the alimentary tract following chemotherapy. The model has allowed attempts at ameliorating intestinal toxicities following chemotherapy [34] and more recently fractionated radiotherapy [35], while guarding paradoxically against tumor growth. More recently, the model has been refined to using tumor-naive rats [36].

3.4.1 Choice of Cytotoxic Agent

Initially, the detailed time course of intestinal damage and repair in the DA rat model needed to be established. In order to commence studies, an appropriate chemotherapeutic agent was required. The cytotoxic agent had to be commonly used and known to cause mucositis in the clinic. Methotrexate (MTX) is a commonly used cytotoxic agent; the mode of action is in the inhibition of dihydrofolate reductase (DHFR) [6, 37, 38]. MTX is also known to cause diarrhea and anorexia, accompanied with malabsorption, malnutrition, and dehydration in patients. Furthermore, MTX is known to inhibit epithelial proliferation and enterocyte function as well as increase the risk of gut-associated sepsis due to disruption of the mucosal barrier. This has led to gastrointestinal toxicity being the major dose-limiting factor for the use of MTX [6, 39, 40]. Therefore, MTX was deemed an appropriate choice of cytotoxic for our initial studies.

3.4.2 Time Course of Small Intestinal Mucositis in the DA Rat Model

Rats were assigned to experimental or control groups; experimental animals received 1.5 mg/kg MTX on days designated 0 and 1, while control animals received saline only [20]. The dose of MTX was chosen from pilot experiments, which indicated that it caused significant, nonlethal small intestinal mucositis [34]. Experimental rats were killed on days 1 (6 h following the second dose of MTX) through 5, with control rats being killed on days 1 and 5 only. This small study detailed the time course of MTX-induced small intestinal mucositis and found that the small intestine is indeed the predominant site of damage. Apoptosis increased 28-fold in the small intestinal crypts 6 h after the second dose and indicated that crypt hypoplasia and villus atrophy occurred between days 2 and 4 following treatment. Following this initial injury, the epithelium enters a rapidly proliferating state, repairing and regenerating the intestine [6, 20, 25, 41]. This small animal experiment confirmed that the time course of small intestinal mucositis in the DA rat model [20] was similar to that observed in our initial human studies [34, 42], indicating that the animal model was an appropriate model to continue developing. Furthermore, these results allowed us to continue to understand the mechanisms underlying mucositis.

3.4.3 Tumor Bearing Versus Tumor Naive

The DA rat model was initially developed using subcutaneously implanted isogeneic rat breast cancers in the female dark agouti (DA) rat. However, it has been well documented that patients with malignancies will have alterations in their immune function [43], including impaired delayed-type hypersensitivity, decreased lymphocytic function, and decreased lymphocyte proliferation response [43, 44]. In addition to this, tumors are known to be responsible for the secretion of different mediators, which decrease the efficiency of immunological integrals [45]. Until recently, there was no evidence regarding whether the presence of a tumor burden will affect the gastrointestinal response (i.e., mucositis) to chemotherapy. A study conducted by our laboratory found that the response to chemotherapy was worse in tumor-bearing rats than tumor-naive rats, indicating that the presence of a tumor load adds to the comorbidity following chemotherapy [36].

3.4.4 Advantages of Our Rat Model of Mucositis

The DA rat model of mucositis has a number of key advantages over other animal models. First, the rats have a rapid growth and development phase. Second, there is homogeneity between all animals, allowing accurate assessments of what damage is occurring and when it is occurring, in relation to chemotherapy administration and healing times. Finally, we are able to examine the entire GIT from mouth to anus and from epithelium to muscle. This has enabled us to develop a three-dimensional model of mucositis. The relative simplicity of the DA rat model of mucositis, combined with the homogeneity of the tumor, ease of interrogation of the model, investigation of other organs in the body, the reproducibility of the model, and its ability to be translated to other laboratories makes it a highly effective animal model. Furthermore, there is the ability to develop simple study protocols that allow investigation of mucosal damage as well as looking at different interventions of drugs at varying time points throughout the study, including prechemotherapy, postchemotherapy, or a combination of both. This similarity of protocols strengthens the model. A wide variety of tests are also able to be performed, from relatively simple mortality and diarrhea assessments through to the more complex gene expression studies.

3.5   GENERATION OF RESEARCH QUESTIONS/AVENUES FOR INVESTIGATION IN THE DA RAT MODEL

Many of the questions and avenues that have been investigated in the DA rat model of mucositis have stemmed from questions that need to be answered in the clinic; but with mucositis there are a vast number of questions that have never been asked, leading to an almost infinite list of potential future studies. The use of the model for mucositis occurred as a direct result of preliminary human studies into chemotherapy-induced injury to the small intestine in humans. Although the original model had been used for the study of immunology [31, 32] and to study neurotoxicity of chemotherapy, this was not carried out in tumor-bearing animals due to time constraints with respect to tumor growth and lead time to neurotoxicity [33].

3.6   HISTORY OF MUCOSITIS IN HUMANS

Mucositis is a major oncological problem caused by the cytotoxic effects of cancer chemotherapy and radiotherapy. By definition, mucositis suggests that inflammation is present; however, recent studies have shown that this is not necessarily the case [34, 42]. Rather, the name simply refers to the damage that occurs to the mucous membranes of the body [34, 42]. Mucositis affects the entire alimentary tract (AT) from mouth to anus and causes pain and ulceration in the mouth and small and large intestines. In addition, it causes abdominal bloating, vomiting, and diarrhea [6, 7, 46, 47]. The potentially severe nature of mucositis can have some further devastating effects, including a reduction or cessation of treatment (which may decrease the chance for remission) and increased stays in hospitals, leading to increased costs of treatment and use of opioids for pain management [46, 48]. Mucositis occurs in approximately 40% of patients after standard doses of chemotherapy and in 100% of patients undergoing high dose chemotherapy and stem cell or bone marrow transplantation [6, 7, 46, 47]. The frequency and severity of mucositis varies depending on the type of cancer (and therefore the treatment regimen) and on the patient's age, with the very young and the very elderly being the most affected [49].

One of the major problems with mucositis is that the mechanisms behind the development of mucositis are not fully understood, making it hard to target treatment. Recent work has shown that the entire GIT has the same embryological route of development, with the differences seen being due to cellular differentiation at various sites in order to conduct specialized functions [7]. Based on this theory, it is likely that mucositis is the same throughout the GIT, with the local differences in manifestations being due to localized specialized differentiation necessary for specific function [7]. It may be that these specialized differences in function explain why different regions of the tract, such as the small intestine, are more susceptible to "early" mucositis than other regions, such as the oral mucosa. To date, there are no investigations that have examined the entire GIT response to chemotherapy; this is most likely due to the difficulties in appropriate models.

Mucositis is a field that has rapidly evolved over the last decade. We have seen advances leading from basic clinical science questions able to be investigated in humans, to conducting detailed microarray experiments in animal models. The first step in the mucositis matrix started with relatively simple investigations of the severity and time course of changes in intestinal permeability following high dose chemotherapy and autologous blood stem cell transplantation [50]. This study involved 35 patients and found that maximum sugar permeability occurred in the small intestine 14 days after the start of chemotherapy, returning to normal 35 days after chemotherapy. Furthermore, this abnormality was found to correlate with the time frame that the patients suffered from other gastrointestinal symptoms, including anorexia and nausea [50]. This first insight into damage after chemotherapy led to further questions being asked about exactly how chemotherapy damages the small intestine.

Our second study into understanding mucositis assessed the frequency, duration, and severity of both oral and gastrointestinal symptoms after chemotherapy and also involved a clinical study. Sixty patients in total were assessed, including those with a newly diagnosed malignancy and those undergoing high dose chemotherapy and autologous peripheral blood stem cell transplantation. Patients were assessed nutritionally, completed a symptom questionnaire, performed an intestinal sugar permeability test, and underwent blood testing for serum endotoxin. A small number of patients also underwent a series of breath tests before and after chemotherapy [34]. Results from this study indicated that patients experienced gastrointestinal symptoms 3–10 days after chemotherapy, and these returned to normal by day 28. In contrast to this, patients did not experience oral symptoms until day 7 after chemotherapy, remaining until day 14 before returning to normal by day 28 [34].

These results were the first to show that chemotherapy does alter the small intestine. A third patient-based study was conducted to assess small intestinal mucosal histology. Twenty-three patients were recruited for the study and underwent an endoscopy with duodenal biopsy before and at varying time points after chemotherapy. Biopsies were assessed using a variety of techniques, including the apoptosis specific assay (TUNEL), enterocyte height, and electron microscopy [42]. We found from this study that there was a sevenfold increase in apoptosis in intestinal crypts 1 day after chemotherapy (Fig. 3.1), followed by a reduction in intestinal morphometry 3 days after chemotherapy. Values had returned to normal by 16 days

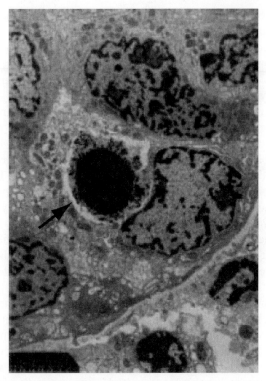

FIGURE 3.1 Electron micrograph of an apoptotic cell in the epithelial layer of the small intestinal crypt at 1 day after chemotherapy. The arrow indicates an apoptotic cell with a pyknotic nucleus (original magnification 12,000×). (Used with permission from Ref. 42.)

after chemotherapy [42]. All of these findings from the three clinical studies indicated that cancer chemotherapy does indeed damage the small intestine. Each study answered a question, but also led to more questions that needed answering. However, in order to fully understand the mechanisms of how this damage occurs, an appropriate animal model needed to be developed. While it was possible to perform upper GI endoscopy and biopsy in a small number of patients, additional more detailed investigations would have been extremely difficult and time-consuming for patients, who are heterogeneous in so many ways.

3.7 USE OF POTENTIAL ANTIMUCOTOXICS

3.7.1 Interleukin-11

One of the first potential antimucotoxics to be investigated in great detail was interleukin-11 (IL-11). IL-11 was first cloned as a stromal-cell derived multifunctional cytokine [51], and over the last decade has been the subject of much research, including early clinical trials for patients with varying malignancies [52–54]. IL-11 has also been the focus of much research into the protection and recovery of stem cells found within the hematopoietic system [55–57]. IL-11 stimulates proliferation of hematopoietic stem cells [55] as well as stimulating hematopoietic recovery following high dose chemotherapy treatment [56]. Additionally, IL-11 has been shown to have nonhematological effects and is produced in varying locations throughout the body, including the alveolar cells of the lung, chondrocytes, synoviocytes, and thyroid carcinoma cells. Thus, IL-11 may have a role in the stem cells found in the small intestinal crypts.

IL-11 and its receptor IL-11Rα are expressed within the gastrointestinal epithelium [57–59]. Animal studies have highlighted the pleiotrophic nature of IL-11 in numerous small intestinal pathologies, including those induced by cytotoxic treatment. Keith and colleagues [60] used two different models of gastrointestinal pathology and concluded that there was a strong beneficial effect of IL-11, which often led to the reduction or resolution of the pathology, although they made no attempt to elucidate the mechanisms behind this. Further studies conducted by Du and colleagues [57, 61, 62] examined the functional significance of IL-11 in mice treated with combined chemotherapy/radiotherapy. The results from these studies clearly demonstrated that mice receiving IL-11 had an increased survival rate compared with their control counterparts, as well as an elevated mitotic index within the crypt epithelial cells, indicating a more rapid recovery time [57, 61, 62]. In another study, IL-11 increased the survival of mice treated with combined chemotherapy/radiotherapy, aided the recovery of small intestinal villi, and increased cell proliferation in crypts [63]. This was a comprehensive study and analyzed different administration schedules of IL-11 including pre, pre and during, and postcytotoxic exposure. However, this study did not evaluate escalating doses of IL-11 and was unable to ascertain whether increasing the dose resulted in corresponding increases in protection [63]. Furthermore, none of the above studies used tumor-bearing animals and were therefore unable to evaluate the effect of IL-11 on the tumor, nor the confounding effect of IL-11 and chemotherapy/radiotherapy on the tumor.

In the DA rat model of mucositis, the time course of mucositis and the effect of IL-11 on preventing intestinal damage were investigated. The effect of IL-11 on untreated animals was firstly ascertained prior to investigating the effect of IL-11 on improving mucositis following treatment with the cytotoxic MTX [20]. Biological efficacy was confirmed by an increased peripheral platelet count. Small intestinal mucositis was assessed using apoptosis and intestinal morphometry and it was found that IL-11 did not reduce apoptosis following chemotherapy, but instead increased it [20]. Surprisingly, this increased level of apoptosis did not lead to increased intestinal damage, and observed intestinal morphometry levels were less severe. These findings suggest that small intestinal apoptosis itself does not inevitably lead to mucositis [20]. IL-11 has now been approved by the Food and Drug Administration for treatment of adults with solid tumors and lymphomas with severe thrombocytopenia induced by chemotherapy [64].

3.7.2 Palifermin

Palifermin (keratinocyte growth factor, KGF or Kepivance®) is a member of the heparin-binding growth factor family [65, 66] and is different from other family members in that it has a specific trophic action for epithelial cells [65, 66]. Palifermin mediates its function in a paracrine–epitheliomesechymal manner by binding to its receptor located in the epithelial region of the GIT and other tissues after synthesis by mesenchymal cells located in adjacent epithelium [67–70].

Over recent years it has been the subject of many animal and clinical studies, with particular emphasis on its interactions within the GIT. Farrell and colleagues [71] have demonstrated that palifermin is able to protect against intestinal mucositis in some animal models by improving weight loss and crypt survival. Palifermin has also been shown to be effective in protecting the oral mucosa of mice following radiation therapy [10, 11, 72–74]. These studies have clearly demonstrated that palifermin is an effective antimucotoxic.

Further evidence for the antimucotoxic effect displayed by palifermin came from a recent study in our laboratory. Using the DA rat model of mucositis, we aimed to determine whether palifermin was effective in ameliorating intestinal mucositis following chemotherapy. Our results demonstrated that palifermin pretreatment significantly reduces diarrhea and mortality after chemotherapy. This indicates that palifermin is an effective antimucotoxic for gastrointestinal mucositis [75]. These findings have led to palifermin being the first approved antimucotoxic drug used clinically in Australia, Europe, and North America from December 2004 onwards, for patients receiving stem cells transplantation, hyperfractionated radiation, and high dosage chemotherapy. However, palifermin has yet to be approved for standard cycles of chemotherapy.

3.7.3   Velafermin

Velafermin (FGF-20) is also a member of the fibroblast growth factor family [76–78], and members of this family have been implicated in the normal growth and development of the GIT [76–78]. Receptors for FGFs have been located in the epithelial region of the GIT [79, 80]. Velafermin has previously been shown to have activity in models of ulcerative colitis [77] and oral mucosal damage following cytotoxic insult [81]. Recent results from a Phase I clinical trial investigating velafermin have indicated that it is well tolerated following intravenous administration [82] and these results have led to Phase II clinical trials, which are now under way.

Further evidence for the role of velafermin has come in recent months. Using the DA rat model of mucositis, multiple doses and schedules of administration of velafermin to determine its efficacy as an antimucotoxic in gastrointestinal mucositis were assessed. While some of the investigated doses of velafermin were found to be less effective in reducing the severity of diarrhea and mortality, others appeared to increase the diarrhea and mortality. However, evidence of importance of both the dose scheduling and duration of the dosing had previously been reported by Alvarez and colleagues [81]. In their study, they reported that administration of velafermin on varying days and for varying durations led to different efficacies of the antimucotoxic, and they hypothesized that this was due to the multifactorial elements in mucositis progression. However, in our study, we identified that 16 mg/kg velafermin was a potentially effective dose. This dose of velafermin delayed the onset and reduced the duration of severe diarrhea and improved survival rates. These encouraging results indicate that velafermin has the potential to be an effective antimucotoxic, and further animal studies are now warranted in order to understand the mechanisms of action.

3.7.4   VSL#3

The probiotic compound VSL#3 (VSL Pharmaceuticals, Italy) is a new high potency preparation of highly concentrated freeze-dried living bacteria. Each sachet contains *Streptococcus thermophilus* and several species of *Lactobacillus* and *Bifidobacteria*. The compound has been examined previously in models of inflammatory bowel disease (IBD) and has level 1 evidence of effectiveness in ameliorating pouchitis and Crohn disease [83]. Being a "probiotic" means that VSL#3 is capable of exerting good effects on the host organism by improving the balance of intestinal flora and by ameliorating the growth of possible pathogenic microbes [84]. The mechanism of action appears to be through protective, trophic, and anti-inflammatory effects on bowel mucosa [85]. As such, it seems sensible that VSL#3 would also be effective in ameliorating mucositis, specifically chemotherapy-induced diarrhea (CID), which has a number of overlapping pathologies with inflammatory bowel disease (IBD), including upregulation of inflammatory mediators [86–88]. Recently, VSL#3 has been investigated within our laboratory using the DA rat mucositis model in a study comparing schedules for effectiveness of diarrhea prevention following chemotherapy. Promising results have come from the initial series of experiments indicating its potential antimucotoxic ability.

3.7.5   Other Potential Antimucotoxics

There are numerous other antimucotoxics that have been tested in animal models. These include transforming growth factor-β [89], insulin-like growth factor-1 [24, 90], whey growth factor [25], glutamine [34, 91], and epidermal growth factor [92], to name a few. It is important to continue to study these potential antimucotoxics in animal models prior to use in humans.

3.8   IRINOTECAN: A SPECIAL CASE?

Irinotecan hydrochloride (CPT-11) is a relatively new cytotoxic agent used primarily to treat colorectal carcinoma [6, 17, 75]. The mode of action is to inhibit DNA topoisomerase I [93–96]. One of the biggest problems with using this cytotoxic agent is the severe and frequent gastrointestinal toxicities, particularly diarrhea [6, 17, 75, 93–96]. The severe nature of the diarrhea, coupled with the fact that the underlying mechanisms of its development remain unknown, means that the use of irinotecan is limited. This makes an otherwise very effective drug very difficult to use clinically [75]. Although chemotherapy-induced diarrhea (CID) is well recognized [97–99], the underlying mechanisms have received very little attention. Much of the information in the published literature is based on clinical observations with very little basic science. It is therefore important that we gain a better understanding of the mechanisms behind irinotecan-induced diarrhea, as its continued use will be questionable if the dose-limiting and often life-threatening diarrhea associated with administration cannot be prevented [100].

Utilizing a number of different animal models, including the DA rat model of mucositis, the way in which the GIT responds to irinotecan has been somewhat elucidated; however, the exact mechanism of induction remains unclear [6, 17, 75, 93–96].

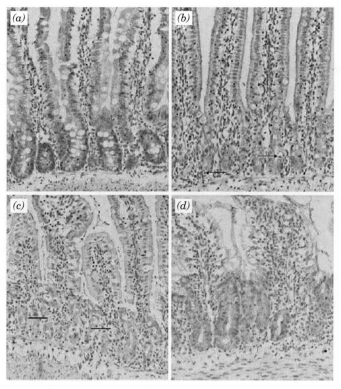

FIGURE 3.2   Photomicrographs of rat jejunum stained with hematoxylin and eosin: (A) Untreated control, (B) 6h, (C) 24h, and (D) 48h. Irinotecan treatment caused changes in morphometry, which included apoptosis (arrows) and crypt degeneration (bars) at early time points. Crypt hyperplasia and villus atrophy occurred at 48h. Original magnfication 100×. (Used with permission from Ref. 114.)

Using the DA rat model of mucositis, our laboratory has, for the first time, been able to establish the changes that occur in the GIT. We first demonstrated a clear time course of gastrointestinal mucositis, caused by irinotecan (Fig. 3.2). Furthermore, we demonstrated that irinotecan causes severe colonic damage (with apoptosis) (Figs. 3.3 and 3.4) and accompanying excessive mucus secretion, suggesting that this increased level of apoptosis, histopathological changes, and goblet cell changes may cause changes in absorption rates leading to diarrhea [17, 47]. Further animal models have investigated the effect of irinotecan on the mouse ileum and cecum. These studies have suggested that the diarrhea induced by irinotecan is the result of the malabsorption of water and electrolytes and mucin hypersecretion [95].

More recently, evidence has arisen that suggests irinotecan-induced diarrhea is a result of interactions between drug metabolism and bacterial microflora [95, 96, 101–103]. One such series of animal experiments has suggested that irinotecan-induced diarrhea is in fact due to changes in bacterial microflora [104, 105]. These studies concluded that irinotecan treatment causes changes in the microflora of the stomach, jejunum, colon, and feces of rats, and that these changes are associated with the development of diarrhea. Furthermore, these changes in microflora may

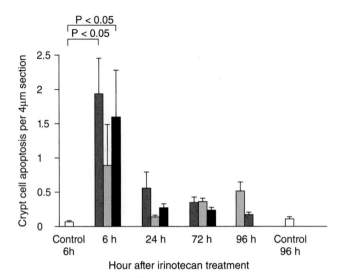

FIGURE 3.3   Effect of 100 mg/kg, 150 mg/kg and 200 mg/kg irinotecan given intraperitoneally (IP) over 2 days on jejunal crypt cell apoptosis in rats with breast cancer. Apoptosis was maximal in all doses 6 h following treatment (100 mg/kg and 200 mg/kg $P < 0.05$). White bar, control; diagonal stripes, 100 mg/kg irinotecan; dots, 150 mg/kg irinotecan; black bar 200 mg/kg irinotecan. Results are shown as mean ± SEM. (Used with permission from Ref. 17.)

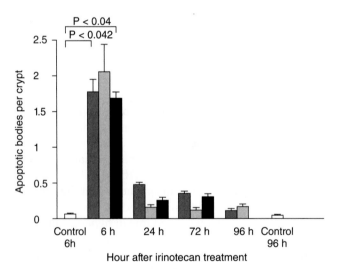

FIGURE 3.4   Effect of 100 mg/kg, 150 mg/kg, and 200 mg/kg irinotecan given IP over 2 days on colon crypt cell apoptosis in rats with breast cancer. Apoptosis was maximal in all doses 6 h following treatment (100 mg $P < 0.042$; 200 mg/kg $P < 0.04$). White bar, control; diagonal stripes, 100 mg/kg irinotecan; dots, 150 mg/kg irinotecan; black bar, 200 mg/kg irinotecan. Results are shown as mean ± SEM. (Used with permission from Ref. 17.)

have systemic effects and, in particular, may contribute to the development of chemotherapy-induced mucositis [104, 105]. These results from recent animal studies
have been able to be translated back to the clinical setting. We are currently investigating if microflora change in patients following chemotherapy. This highlights the
true translational research capacity of an appropriate animal model.

3.9   RADIOTHERAPY: A NEW APPLICATION FOR THE DA RAT MODEL OF MUCOSITIS

Radiation therapy for head and neck cancers results in 30% and 60% of patients
developing oral mucositis, while pelvic radiotherapy can lead to acute radiation
damage to the anorectal region in up to 75% of patients [106]. These symptoms can
be severe enough to interrupt the planned course of treatment in around 10% of
patients [107]. Intestinal epithelial injury is one of the major dose-limiting factors
in radiation oncology, as acute radiation mucositis severely negates the ability of
patients to tolerate higher doses of radiation, which produce greater antitumor
effects than lower doses [108]. Despite this, there is currently no appropriate animal
model for determining fractionated radiation damage to the GIT, and we have been
unable to assess how multiple fractions/doses of radiation therapy cause damage,
not only to the epithelium but to all layers of the GIT. It is important to develop
such a model as fractionated radiation therapy is a common treatment option in the
clinic, leading to severe side effects.

The DA rat model of mucositis has been used extensively in the study of chemotherapy-induced mucositis and results have clearly indicated that mucositis induced
by this model is similar to that seen in humans. Currently, there is no animal model
for fractionated radiotherapy to study damage to the GIT, with the majority of
animal models involving irradiation utilizing a single dose of whole body irradiation
[22, 109] or fractionated doses to the head and neck (snout) regions only [72]. The
research conducted by Dorr and colleagues have shown that palifermin is effective
in reducing the acute oral mucositis induced by radiation therapy [10, 22, 72–74,
109], with the positive effects seeming to be based on changes occurring to the epithelial proliferation and differentiation processes [10]. It is now of vital importance
to translate this research from a head and neck (snout) only radiation model to an
animal model that is able to study damage to the entire GIT. Many patients receive
this modality of treatment and in order to understand how fractionated doses of
radiation therapy cause mucositis in the clinic, we need an appropriate animal
model. There are differences between chemotherapy, single-dose radiation therapy,
and fractionated radiation therapy that relate to the continued, cumulative damage
of daily radiation.

3.10   NEW ADVANCES

3.10.1   Introduction

Clinical research has documented the occurrence of mucositis in cancer patients,
highlighting its prevalence and importance; however, animal research has primarily

been responsible for elucidating the mechanisms underpinning its development. The overall goal of preclinical or basic mucositis research is to reduce the burden of disease in cancer patients. Effective realization of this goal will be achieved through an enhanced focus on identifying patients who are at a greater risk of toxic effects and those who are less likely to respond to treatment with potentially life-threatening agents [110]. Increased understanding of complex disease pathways and application of a number of new technologies in preclinical models have created a renewed ability to move forward in this area.

3.10.2   Continuum of Mucosal Injury Research

The most significant advance in mucositis research in the past five years has been the development and characterization of the five-phase model of mucositis to explain its unique pathobiology [13, 86, 88]. The model includes the sequential, but not necessarily discrete, five biological stages of damage induced by cancer treatment.

1. *Initiation.* This stage occurs rapidly following administration of cancer treatment and is activated by the simultaneous effects of both DNA and non-DNA damage within epithelial and submucosal cells and generation of reactive oxygen species (ROSs).
2. *Upregulation and Message Generation.* Here DNA strand breaks and ROSs activate multiple transcription factors, including p53 and NFκB, which regulate a great number of downstream genes involved in mucosal toxicity. At the same time, non-DNA damage-associated events occurring include production of ceramide and matrix metalloproteinases, which lead to apoptosis and tissue breakdown.
3. *Signaling and Amplification.* Due to the activation of transcription factors, proinflammatory cytokines accumulate and target the tissues of the submucosa, with this damage also acting as a positive feedback signal to amplify the reaction. Furthermore, certain cytokines are capable of activating the initial transcription factors further and enhancing upregulation of metalloproteinases and ceramide.
4. *Ulceration.* This phase is considered the most significant in mucositis and is characterized by a loss of mucosal integrity with superficial bacterial colonization of the subsequent lesions. The consequences of this include activation of infiltrating mononuclear cells to release additional proinflammatory cytokines and the upregulation of proapoptotic genes, potentiating tissue injury.
5. *Healing.* Generally, mucositis resolves once cancer treatment has ceased and is likely carried out in a similar fashion to other types of mucosal healing, with epithelial cell migration, proliferation, and differentiation of healing tissue.

This model was discovered gradually, with the questions answered from a preclinical animal model of oral mucositis [15, 27, 28, 111, 112], which was further evidenced in other animal models [16, 17, 20, 104, 113–115] and confirmed in human biopsy samples [18, 116, 117]. It changed the historical thinking of mucositis as a solely epithelial-driven injury to one involving the entire mucosa and all cell types contained within. This new model of mucositis has allowed opportunities to target steps in development of injury. A definitive pathway for the disease is critical for designing experiments for testing interventions in the few mucositis-specific animal models that exist. A particular example of this is anti-inflammatory agents. Since it is now recognized as an important mechanism involved in mucosal injury, currently used agents in the treatment of other inflammatory disorders may prove useful in prevention and treatment of mucositis and should be tested in preclinical models [118].

Toxicities associated with cancer treatment include those that are localized or regional (ulcers, xerostomia, abdominal pain, malabsorption) and those that are more generalized or systemic (fatigue, lack of appetite, nausea) [119]. The recent realization of concurrent tissue-based and systemic toxicities has resulted in the new paradigm of toxicity clustering [120]. New research initiatives are now under way to further investigate the common aspects of pathogenesis in all cancer treatment-related toxicities (D. Keefe and S. Sonis, personal communication), a significant advance in the approach to this oncological problem. Interestingly, the proof of principle testing for this new way of thinking was carried out in cancer patients [120]. Translational research in the laboratory using animal testing is now occurring to examine in greater details some of the initial findings.

3.10.3 Emerging Tools in Cancer Treatment and Diagnosis Improvement Requiring Mucositis Research

Biological Response Modifiers   Although biological response modifiers (BRMs) were initially studied in the 1960s for their potential use in cancer therapy, poor trial results caused a loss in momentum in research [121, 122]. Now refreshed with renewed interest, it has become a rapidly advancing area in cancer treatment. BRMs modify the relationship between the tumor and the patient and can be divided into three main categories: (1) agents that restore, augment, or modulate the patients' normal immunological mechanisms; (2) agents that have direct antitumor effects; and (3) agents that have other biologic effects including interference with a tumor cell's ability to metastasize, promotion of cell differentiation, or interference with transformation of cells (Oncolink website). BRM agents currently being evaluated include monoclonal antibodies, interferons, interleukin 2, and tumor necrosis factor. Collectively, this form of treatment has been named immunotherapy due to its immune system regulatory properties. Side effects associated this these treatments include fever, chills, rash, vomiting, hypotension, and allergic reactions and can be severe [123, 124]. As such, patients need to be carefully monitored following administration of drugs. Although initially developed through animal-based research, it is obvious that to improve the therapeutic use of these agents, further preclinical research needs to be conducted to elucidate mechanisms for averting toxicity. The rat mucositis model is an appropriate animal model for this.

A special case is the targeted anticancer therapies, including monoclonal antibodies and small molecules [125]. Both of these are gaining a significant and expanding role in the therapy of cancer, but the use of targeted therapy remains in combination with conventional cancer treatments (chemotherapy and radiotherapy) for optimal response. A recent review of the literature surrounding the targeted anticancer therapies identified mucosal toxicities as a significant component of the treatments that was not well studied [125]. These toxicities included diarrhea and mouth ulcers [125]. Furthermore, economic considerations of these toxicities need to be addressed. The combination treatment of monoclonal antibodies with other therapeutic agents, including other antibodies, can cost upwards of $10,000–$25,000 (U.S.) a month. This has staggering financial implications for patients and challenges the healthcare system. Considering that not all patients are responsive (most likely due to differences in targeted receptors), molecular testing to assign drugs on an individual patient basis needs to quickly become part of the paradigm of biological therapy [126]. Thus, there is an obvious need to examine the mucosal toxicities as well as other systemic toxicities in order to understand the mechanism(s) of damage as well as to target appropriate prevention or treatments. Animal models may provide the most appropriate way of investigating this.

Gene Therapy   The emerging field of gene therapy is quite broad and promises a number of innovative treatments in the cancer treatment setting as well as the prevention of disease. In animal models of lung cancer, survival benefits have been demonstrated using gene therapy to create cancer vaccines, target viruses to cancer cells for lysis, decrease the blood supply to the tumor, and introduce genes into the cancer cells that either cause death or restore a normal phenotype [127, 128]. This is the next generation in cancer therapeutics thanks to the introduction of genetic engineering. However, caution must be used when applying the therapy. Current gene therapy vaccines rely on modulation of the immune system and stimulation of proinflammatory cytokines to destroy tumor cells. This could lead to perturbation of mucositis, where activation of the inflammatory cascade results in mucosal tissue damage. Continued development of gene therapy approaches in animal models will provide the necessary platform to address this and many other concerns relating to its future use in the clinic.

Pharmacogenetics   Expanding knowledge of the molecular basis of cancer and its associated diseases, such as mucositis, has shown that differences in gene expression patterns can guide therapy. The field of research concerning genetic variability in response to drugs is termed pharmacogenetics. Technologies involved in this type of research include DNA sequencing, single nucleotide polymorphism (SNP) discovery, and genotyping [129]. Clinical research dominates in this area, with the observation of patient response heterogeneity triggering interest. However, the application of the knowledge garnered from patient results to design preclinical experiments should prove valuable in the future. Realization that certain drug metabolism pathways can be manipulated to modulate cancer therapy response should be investigated in appropriate animal models.

Pharmacogenomics   Pharmacogenomics is the study of inherited differences in interindividual drug disposition and effects. Pharmacogenomics is especially important for oncology, as severe systemic toxicity and unpredictable efficacy are hallmarks of cancer therapies [130]. The recent completion of the human genome combined with emerging genomic and proteomic technologies has advanced this field considerably in the past five years. Arguably the most important discovery platform now in use is microarrays. The types of microarray in oncology molecular diagnostics are currently cDNA, oligonucleotide, and tissue based. For effective explanation of the huge amount of measurements generated by these microarrays, significant computer-based data analysis systems have been designed. The four predominant methods of data analysis have emerged as hierarchic clustering, self-organizing maps, multidimensional scaling, and pathway associations [131]. Collectively, they can be used for tumor classification and subtyping, drug and biomarker discovery, and the powerful tool of transcription profiling of whole genome mRNA expression to establish profiles of gene expression and biological pathway activation [129]. This is possible for multiple species, so application of this technology will allow a great number of questions to be answered, and of course generated, using animal models of disease. Mucositis research using the DA rat model has recently introduced microarray experiments into routine laboratory tests and generated a wealth of new directives for elucidating mucosal toxicity mechanisms and risk factors [6].

An extension of pharmacogenomics is molecular cartography, which is the science of identifying the interaction of genes and gene products that characterize the function and specialization of each individual cell in the context of cell–cell interaction, tissue and organ function, and system's biology [132]. Molecular cartography or "meta-genomics" will be an exciting area for research in the future. Again, animal models will provide the platform needed to investigate the intricate and multi-faceted interactions of genes, so as to elucidate pathological processes, including mucositis, and in the development of novel or improved modes of treatment intervention.

Toxicogenomics   Of particular importance in mucositis research is the developing field of toxicogenomics. This is the study of gene expression patterns using high throughput microarrays, automated real-time PCR, nuclear magnetic resonance, and proteomic strategies designed to detect up- and downregulation of genes associated with drug toxicity risk [133]. Toxicogenetic markers for adverse side effects identified in animal models will influence selection and optimization of lead compounds for human studies. An example of this is the discovery that inherited forms of the long QT syndrome can be caused by high affinity drug blockade associated with mutations in the HERG potassium channel regulator [134]. The true value of toxicogenomics is currently unrealized; however, with continued advances in data mining and expression profiling technologies, this will occur in the near future.

Nanomedicine   The National Cancer Institute has described nanotechnology as a significant research initiative that could transform cancer research and clinical approaches to cancer care (NCI website 2006). There are a growing number of examples of how nanotechnology tools and nanomachines are transforming the way we approach disease diagnosis, treatment, and prevention. Each has developed through animal models and many remain in the preclinical stages [134]. For example, nanopore sequencing is an ultrarapid method of sequencing based on pore nano-engineering and assembly used for the detection of SNPs and for gene diagnosis of pathogens; microneedles are micromachined needles and lancets engineered from single crystal silicon to be used for painless drug infusion, cellular injection, and a number of diagnostic procedures; and drug delivery microchips are microfabricated devices that incorporate micrometer-scale pumps, valves, and flow channels to allow controlled release of single or multiple drugs on command, especially useful in the long-term treatment of conditions requiring pulsatile release of drug following implantation. Each of these technologies will have particular and individual side effects of treatment.

The issue of toxicity is a particular concern with all new technologies, such as nanomedicine, but often is ignored. Therefore, to ensure efficient application of these technologies, it is essential that fundamental research is carried out to address this issue. In this respect, the use of a preclinical animal model is vital to development of the treatment. In the situation of mucositis, new drug delivery systems have the potential to be truly effective in reducing tumor burden but may induce considerable mucosal toxicity and should be examined fully in the model. In this respect, it should become a priority for the NIH and NCI in their respective nanotechnology funding programs.

3.11   FUTURE USE OF ANIMAL MODELS IN MUCOSITIS RESEARCH

With the constant application of drug screening and agent testing for potential cancer treatments and supportive agents to use in the clinic, the animal model of mucositis will continue to be a highly valuable tool. We are currently in an age where the biotechnology and pharmaceutical industries are progressing rapidly, offering exceptional new drugs into development. However, it remains that proper rigorous preclinical testing in appropriate and truly representative models needs to be carried out with each new antimucotoxic treatment to ensure that innovative treatment approaches are not introduced before the technology or its understanding has matured sufficiently to extract maximum benefit.

Over the next twenty years, due to the ageing population, the global incidence of cancer will greatly increase and with it mucositis. There will also be an increase in consumerism in medicine, with better informed and assertive patients seeking out novel therapies. For these reasons, the continued development of clinically useful therapies for mucositis is essential. However, the combination of complex factors including technological success, society's willingness to pay, and future healthcare delivery systems will undoubtedly influence how preclinical models are designed and implemented [135].

3.12   CONCLUSION

To summarize, this chapter has described the use of animal models for research of the clinical problem of mucositis. The strong relationship in this example, between animal investigation and translation to the clinical setting, has provided a unique opportunity to conduct effective research in what continues to be a significant oncological problem. With continuing dedication to research and drug development in this area, we will undoubtedly see further improvements in treatment.

ACKNOWLEDGMENTS

Dr. Rachel Gibson is supported by a research fellowship from The Cancer Council South Australia. Dr. Joanne Bowen is supported by a research fellowship from The Royal Adelaide Hospital.

REFERENCES

1. Straight W. Man's debt to laboratory animals. *Miami Univ Med School Bull* 1962;16:106.
2. Rowan AN. *Of Mice, Models, and Men: A Critical Evaluation of Animal Research.* Albany: State University of New York Press; 1984, p 323.
3. Smith JA, Boyd KM. *Lives in the Balance: The Ethics of Using Animals in Biomedical Research.* New York: Oxford University Press; 1991, p 352.
4. Paton W. *Man and Mouse: Animals in Medical Research.* New York: Oxford University Press; 1993, p 288.
5. National Health and Medical Research Council. *Australian Code of Practice for the Care and Use of Animals for Scientific Purposes*, 7th ed. Australian Government; 2004, pp 1–85.
6. Bowen JM, Gibson RJ, Cummins AG, Keefe DMK. Intestinal mucositis: the role of the Bcl-2 family, p53 and caspases in chemotherapy-induced damage. *Support Care Cancer* 2006;17:713–731.
7. Keefe DM, Gibson RJ, Hauer-Jenson M. Gastrointestinal mucositis. *Semin Oncol Nurs* 2004;20:38–47.
8. Dorr W, Brankovic K, Hartmann B. Repopulation in mouse oral mucosa: changes in the effect of dose fractionation. *Int J Radiat Biol* 2000;76:383–390.
9. Dorr W, Emmendorfer H, Weber-Frisch M. Tissue kinetics in mouse tongue mucosa during daily fractionated radiotherapy. *Cell Proliferation* 1996;29:495–504.
10. Dorr W, Spekl K, Farrell CL. Amelioration of acute oral mucositis by keratinocyte growth factor: fractionated irradiation. *Int J Radiat Oncol Biol Phys* 2002;54:245–251.
11. Dorr W, Spekl K, Farrell CL. The effect of keratinocyte growth factor on healing of manifest radiation ulcers in mouse tongue epithelium. *Cell Proliferation* 2002;35:86–92.
12. Dorr W, Spekl K, Martin M. Radiation-induced mucositis in mice: strain differences. *Cell Proliferation* 2002;35:60–67.
13. Sonis ST. The pathobiology of mucositis. *Nat Rev Cancer* 2004;4:277–284.
14. Sonis ST, Fey EG. Oral complications of cancer therapy. *Oncology* 2002;16:680–695.
15. Sonis ST, Tracey C, Shklar G, Jenson J, Florine D. An animal model for mucositis induced by cancer chemotherapy. *Oral Surg Oral Med Oral Pathol* 1990;69:437–443.
16. Gibson RJ, Bowen JM, Cummins AG, Keefe DMK. Relationship between chemotherapy and subsequent apoptosis and damage in the gastrointestinal tract of the rat with breast cancer. *Clin Exp Med* 2005;4:188–195.
17. Gibson RJ, Bowen JM, Inglis MR, Cummins AG, Keefe DMK. Irinotecan causes severe small intestinal damage as well as colonic damage in the rat with implanted breast cancer. *J Gastroenterol Hepatol* 2003;18:1095–1100.
18. Gibson RJ, Cummins AG, Bowen JM, Logan RM, Healey T, Keefe DMK. Apoptosis occurs early in the basal layer of the oral mucosa following cancer chemotherapy. *Asia Pacific J Clin Oncol* 2006;2:39–49.
19. Gibson RJ, Keefe DMK, Clarke JM, Regester GO, Thompson FM, Goland GJ, Edwards BE, Cummins AG. The effect of keratinocyte growth factor on tumour growth and small intestinal mucositis after chemotherapy in the rat with breast cancer. *Cancer Chemother Pharmacol* 2002;50:53–58.
20. Gibson RJ, Keefe DMK, Thompson FM, Clarke JM, Goland GJ, Cummins AG. Effect of interleukin-11 on ameliorating intestinal damage after methotrexate treatment of breast cancer in rats. *Digest Dis Sci* 2002;47:2751–2757.

21. Keefe DM. Gastrointestinal mucositis: a new biological model. *Support Care Cancer* 2004;12:6–9.

22. Dorr W, Bassler S, Reichel S, Spekl K. Reduction of radiochemotherapy-induced early oral mucositis by recombinant human keratinocyte growth factor (palifermin): experimental studies in mice. *Int J Radiat Oncol Biol Phys* 2005;62:881–887.

23. Howarth GS, Tooley KL, Davidson GP, Butler RN. A non-invasive method for detection of intestinal mucositis induced by different classes of chemotherapy drugs in the rat. *Cancer Biol Ther* 2006;5:1189–1195.

24. Howarth GS, Cool JC, Bourne AJ, Ballard FJ, Read LC. Insulin-like growth factor-I (IGF-I) stimulates regrowth of the damaged intestine in rats, when administered following, but not concurrent with, methotrexate. *Growth Factors* 1998;15:279–292.

25. Howarth GS, Francis GL, Cool JC, Xu X, Byard RW, Read LC. Milk growth factors enriched from cheese whey ameliorate intestinal damage by methotrexate when administered orally to rats. *J Nutr* 1996;126:2519–2530.

26. Sonis ST, Van Vugt AG, McDonald J, Dotoli E, Schwertschlag U, Szklut P, Keith J. Mitigating effects of interleukin 11 on consecutive courses of 5-fluorouracil-induced ulcerative mucositis in hamsters. *Cytokine* 1997;9:605–612.

27. Sonis ST, Van Vugt AG, Brien JP, Muska AD, Bruskin AM, Rose A, Haley JD. Transforming growth factor-beta 3 mediated modulation of cell cycling and attenuation of 5-fluorouracil induced oral mucositis. *Oral Oncol* 1997;33:47–54.

28. Sonis ST, Peterson RL, Edwards LJ, Lucey CA, Wang L, Mason L, Login G, Ymamkawa M, Moses G, Bouchard P, Hayes LL, Bedrosian C, Dorner AJ. Defining mechanisms of action of interleukin-11 on the progression of radiation-induced oral mucositis in hamsters. *Oral Oncol* 2000;36:373–381.

29. Ijiri K, Potten CS. Response of intestinal cells of differing topographical and hierarchical status to ten cytotoxic drugs and five sources of radiation. *Br J Cancer* 1983;47: 175–185.

30. Ijiri K, Potten CS. Further studies on the response of intestinal crypt cells of different hierarchical status to eighteen different cytotoxic agents. *Br J Cancer* 1987;55:113–123.

31. Rofe AM, Bourgeois CS, Washington JM, Philcox JC, Coyle P. Metabolic consequences of methotrexate therapy in tumour-bearing rats. *Immunol Cell Biol* 1994;72:43–48.

32. Rofe AM, Bais R, Conyers RA. Ketone-body metabolism in tumour-bearing rats. *Biochem J* 1986;233:485–491.

33. Boyle FM, Wheeler HR, Shenfield GM. Glutamate ameliorates experimental vincristine neuropathy. *J Pharmacol Exp Ther* 1996;279:410–415.

34. Keefe DMK. The effect of cytotoxic chemotherapy on the mucosa of the small intestine. MD Thesis, Department of Medicine, University of Adelaide.

35. Yeoh ASJ, Gibson RJ, Bowen JM, Yeoh E, Stringer AM, Giam K, Logan RM, Keefe DMK. Radiation therapy-induced mucositis: relationships between short and long-term fractionated radiation, NF-κB, Cox-1 and Cox-2. *Cancer Treatment Reviews* 32:645–651.

36. Gibson RJ, Bowen JM, Alvarez E, Finnie JW, Keefe DMK. Establishment of a single dose irinotecan model of gastrointestinal mucositis. *Chemotherapy* 2006;53:360–369.

37. Huennekens FM. The methotrexate story: a paradigm for development of cancer chemotherapeutic agents. *Adv Enzyme Regul* 1994;34:397–419.

38. Tenenbaum L. *Cancer Chemotherapy and Biotherapy*. Philadelphia: WB Saunders; 1994, pp 7–8.

39. Papaconstantinou HT, Xie C, Zhang W, Ansari NH, Hellmich MR, Townsend CM, Ko TC. The role of caspases in methotrexate-induced gastrointestinal toxicity. *Surgery* 2001;859–865.

40. Verburg M, Renes IB, Meijer HP, Taminiau JAJM, Buller HA, Einerhand AWC, Dekker J. Selective sparing of goblet cells and Paneth cells in the intestine of methotrexate-treated rats. *Am J Physiol* 2000;279:G1037–G1047.

41. Taminiau JAJM, Gall DG, Hamilton JR. Response of the rat small-intestine epithelium to methotrexate. *Gut* 1980;21:486–492.

42. Keefe DM, Brealey J, Goland GJ, Cummins AG. Chemotherapy for cancer causes apoptosis that precedes hypoplasia in crypts of the small intestine in humans. *Gut* 2000;47:632–637.

43. Fittkau M, Voigt W, Holzhausen HJ, Schmoll HJ. Saccharic acid 1.4-lactone protects against CPT-11-induced mucosa damage in rats. *J Cancer Res Clin Oncol* 2004; 130:388–394.

44. Evans TRJ. Vaccine therapy for cancer—fact or fiction? *Pro R Coll Physicians Edinburgh* 2001;31:9–16.

45. Broder S, Waldmann TA. The suppressor-cell network in cancer (first of two parts). *N Eng J Med* 1978;299:1281–1284.

46. Keefe DMK. Mucositis management in patients with cancer. *Support Cancer Ther* 2006;3:154–157.

47. Gibson RJ, Keefe DMK. Cancer chemotherapy-induced diarrhoea and constipation: mechanisms of damage and prevention strategies. *Support Care Cancer* 2006;14: 890–900.

48. Elting LS, Cooksley C, Chambers M, Cantor SB, Manzullo E, Rubenstein EB. The burdens of cancer therapy, clinical and economic outcomes of chemotherapy-induced mucositis. *Cancer* 2003;98:1531–1539.

49. Pico J-L, Avila-Garavito A, Naccache P. Mucositis: its occurrence, consequences, and treatment in the oncology setting. *Oncologist* 1998;3:446–451.

50. Keefe DM, Cummins AG, Dale BM, Kotasek D, Robb TA, Sage RE. Effect of high-dose chemotherapy on intestinal permeability in humans. *Clin Sci* 1997;92:385–389.

51. Paul SR, Bennet F, Calvetti JA, Kelleher KG, Wood CR, Leary AC, Sibley B, Clark SC, Williams DA, Yang Y-C. Molecular cloning of a cDNA encoding interleukin 11, a stromal cell-derived lymphopoietic and haematopoietic cytokine. *Proc Natl Acad Sci* 1990;87: 7512–7516.

52. Tepler I, Elias L, Smith JW 2nd, Hussein M, Rosen G, Chang AY, Moore JO, Gordon MS, Kuca B, Beach KJ, Loewy JW, Garnick MB, Kaye JA. A randomized placebo-controlled trial of recombinant human interleukin-11 in cancer patients with severe thrombocytopenia due to chemotherapy. *Blood* 1996;87:3607–3614.

53. Gordon MS. Thrombopoietic activity of recombinant human interleukin 11 in cancer patients receiving chemotherapy. *Cancer Chemother Pharmacol* 1996;38:S96–S98.

54. Gordon MS, McCaskill-Stevens WJ, Battiato LA, Loewy J, Loesch D, Breeden E, Hoffman R, Beach KJ, Kuca B, Kaye J, Sledge GW Jr. A phase I trial of recombinant human interleukin-11 (neumega rhIL-11 growth factor) in women with breast cancer receiving chemotherapy. *Blood* 1996;87:3615–3624.

55. Musashi M, Yang Y-C, Paul SR, Clark SC, Sudo T, Ogawa M. Direct and synergistic effects of interleukin-11 on murine hemopoiesis in culture. *Proc Natl Acad Sci* 1991;88:765–769.

56. Leonard JP, Quinto CM, Kozitza MK, Neben TY, Goldman SJ. Recombinant human interleukin-11 stimulates multilineage hematopoietic recovery in mice after a myelosuppressive regimen of sublethal irradiation and carboplatin. *Blood* 1994; 83:1499–1506.

57. Du XX, Doerschuk CM, Orazi A, Williams DA. A bone marrow stromal-derived growth factor, interleukin-11, stimulates recovery of small intestinal mucosal cells after cytoablative therapy. *Blood* 1994;83:33–37.

58. Du XX, Williams DA. Interleukin-11: a multifunctional growth factor derived from the hematopoietic microenvironment. *Blood* 1994;83:2023–2030.

59. Peterson RL, Trepicchio WL, Bozza MM, Wang L, Dorner AJ. G1 growth arrest and reduced proliferation of intestinal epithelial cells induced by rhIL-11 may mediate protection against mucositis. *Blood* 1994;86:311a.

60. Keith JC Jr, Albert A, Sonis ST, Pfeiffer CJ, Schaub RG. IL-11, a pleiotrophic cytokine: exciting new effects of IL-11 on gastrointestinal mucosal biology. *Stem Cells* 1994;12: 79–90.

61. Du XX, Liu Q, Yang Z, Orazi A, Rescorla FJ, Grosfield JL, Williams DA. Protective effects of interleukin-11 in a murine model of ischemic bowel necrosis. *Am J Physiol* 1997;272:G545–G552.

62. Du XX, Neben DT, Goldman S, Williams DA. Effects of recombinant human interleukin-11 on hematopoietic reconstitution in transplant mice: acceleration of recovery of peripheral blood neutrophils and platelets. *Blood* 1993;81:27–34.

63. Potten CS. Interleukin-11 protects the clonogenic stem cells in murine small-intestinal crypts from impairment of their reproductive capacity by radiation. *Int J Cancer* 1995;62:356–361.

64. Cairo MS, Davenport V, Bessmertny O, Goldman SC, Berg SL, Kreissman SG, Laver J, Shen V, Secola R, van de Ven C, Reaman GH. Phase I/II dose escalation study of recombinant human interleukin-11 following ifosfamide, carboplatin and etoposide in children, adolescents and young adults with solid tumours or lymphoma: a clinical, haematological and biological study. *Br J Haematol* 2005;128:49–58.

65. Bansal GS, Cox HC, Marsh S, Gomm JJ, Yiangou C, Luqmani Y, Coombes RC, Johnston CL. Expression of keratinocyte growth factor and its receptor in human breast cancer. *Br J Cancer* 1997;75:1567–1574.

66. Brauchle M, Madlener M, Wagner AD, Angermeyer K, Lauer U, Hofschneider PH, Gregor M, Werner S. Keratinocyte growth factor is highly overexpressed in inflammatory bowel disease. *Am J Pathol* 1996;149:521–528.

67. Chailler P, Basque JR, Corriveau L, Menard D. Functional characterization of the keratinocyte growth factor system in human fetal gastrointestinal tract. *Pediatr Res* 2000;48:504–510.

68. Meropol NJ, Somer RA, Gutheil J, Pelley RJ, Modiano MR, Rowinsky EK, Rothenberg ML, Redding SW, Serdar CM, Yao B, Heard R, Rosen LS. Randomized phase I trial of recombinant keratinocyte growth factor plus chemotherapy: potential role as a mucosal protectant. *J Clin Oncol* 2003;21:1452–1458.

69. Rubin JS, Bottaro DP, Chedid M, Miki K, Cunha GR, Finch PW. Keratinocyte growth factor as a cytokin that mediates mesenchymal–epithelial interaction. *EXS* 1995;74: 191–214.

70. Borges L, Rex KL, Chen JN, Wei P, Kaufman S, Scully S, Pretorius JK, Farrell CL. A protective role for keratinocyte growth factor in a murine model of chemotherapy and radiotherapy-induced mucositis. *Int J Radiat Oncol Biol Phys* 2006;66:254–262.

71. Farrell CL, Bready JV, Rex KL, Chen JN, DiPalma CR, Whitcomb KL, Yin S, Hill DC, Wiemann B, Starnes CO, Havill AM, Lu ZN, Aukerman SL, Pierce GF, Thomason A, Potten CS, Ulich TR, Lacey DL. Keratinocyte growth factor protects mice from chemotherapy and radiation-induced gastrointestinal injury and mortality. *Cancer Res* 1998; 58:933–939.

72. Dorr W, Noack R, Spekl K, Farrell CL. Amelioration of radiation-induced oral mucositis by keratinocyte growth factor (rhKGF): experimental studies. *Int J Radiat Oncol Biol Phys* 2000;46:729.

73. Dorr W, Noack R, Spekl K, Farrell CL. Modification of oral mucositis by keratinocyte growth factor; single radiation exposure. *Int J Radiat Biol* 2001;77:341.

74. Dorr W. Modification of acute radio (chemo) therapy effects in squamous epithelia by keratinocyte growth factor. *Radiother Oncol* 2001;60:S8.

75. Gibson RJ Bowen JM, Keefe DM. Palifermin reduces diarrhoea and increases survival following irinotecan treatment in tumour-bearing DA rats. *Int J Cancer* 2005;116: 464–470.

76. Stern J, Ippoliti C. Management of acute cancer treatment-induced diarrhea. *Semin Oncol Nurs* 2003;19:11–16.

77. Jeffers M, McDonald WF, Chillakuru RA, Yang M, Nakase H, Deegler LL, Sylander ED, Rittman B, Bendele A, Sartor RB, Lichenstein HS. A novel human fibroblast growth factor treats experimental intestinal inflammation. *Gastroenterology* 2002;123:1151–1162.

78. Jeffers M, Shimkets R, Prayaga S, Boldog F, Yang M, Burgess C, Fernandes E, Rittman B, Shimkets J, LaRochelle WJ, Lichenstein HS. Identification of a novel human fibroblast growth factor and characterization of its role in oncogenesis. *Cancer Res* 2001;61: 3131–3138.

79. Hughes SE. Differential expression of the fibroblast growth factor receptor (FGFR) multigene family in normal human adult tissues. *J Histochem Cytochem* 1997;45: 1005–1019.

80. Housley RM, Morris CF, Boyle W, Ring B, Blitz R, Tarpley JE, Aukerman SL, Devine PL, Whitehead RH, Pierce GF. Keratinocyte growth factor induces proliferation of hepatocytes and epithelial cells throughout the rat gastrointestinal tract. *J Clin Invest* 1994;94:1764–1777.

81. Alvarez E, Fey EG, Valax P, Yim Z, Peterson JD, Mesri M, Jeffers M, Dindinger M, Twomlow N, Ghatpande A, LaRochelle WJ, Sonis ST, Lichenstein HS. Preclinical characterization of CG53135 (FGF-20) in radiation and concomitant chemotherapy/radiation-induced oral mucositis. *Clin Cancer Res* 2003;9:3454–3461.

82. Schuster MW, Shore TB, Greenberg J, Jalilizeinali B, Possley S, Halvorsen Y-D, Annino V, Hahne W. Phase I trial of CG53135-05 to prevent mucositis in patients undergoing high-dose chemotherapy (HDCT) and autologous peripheral blood stem cell transplantation (PBSCT). *J Clin Oncol* 2005;23:6656.

83. Reid G, Hammond JA. Probiotics. Some evidence of their effectiveness. *Can Fam Physician* 2005;51:1487–1493.

84. Delia P, Sansotta G, Donato V, Messina G, Frosina P, Pergolizzi S, De Renzis C, Famularo G. Prevention of radiation-induced diarrhea with the use of VSL#3, a new high-potency probiotic preparation. *Am J Gastroenterol* 2002;97:2150–2152.

85. Petrof EO, Kojima K, Ropeleski MJ, Musch MW, Tao Y, De Simone C, Chang EB. Probiotics inhibit nuclear factor-kappaB and induce heat shock proteins in colonic epithelial cells through proteasome inhibition. *Gastroenterology* 2004;127:1474–1487.

86. Sonis ST. A biological approach to mucositis. *J Support Oncol* 2004;2:21–32; discussion 35–36.

87. Sonis ST. The pathobiology of mucositis. *Nat Rev Cancer* 2004;4:277–284.

88. Sonis ST. Pathobiology of mucositis. *Semin Oncol Nurs* 2004;20:11–15.

89. Sonis ST, Lindquist L, Van Vugt A, Stewart AA, Stam K, Qu GY, Iwata KK, Haley JD. Prevention of chemotherapy-induced ulcerative mucositis by transforming growth factor beta 3. *Cancer Res* 1994;54:1135–1138.

90. Howarth GS, Fraser R, Frisby CL, Schirmer MB, Yeoh EK. Effects of insulin-like growth factor-I administration on radiation enteritis in rats. *Scand J Gastroenterol* 1997; 32:1118–1124.

91. Huang E-Y, Wan Leung S, Wang C-J, Chen H-C, Sun L-M, Fang F-M, Yeh S-A, Hsu H-C, Hsuing C-Y. Oral glutamine to alleviate radiation-induced oral mucositis: a pilot randomized trial. *Int J Radiat Oncol Biol Phys* 2000;46:535–539.

92. Fehrmann A, Dorr W. Effect of EGFR-inhibition on the radiation response of oral mucosa: experimental studies in mouse tongue epithelium. *Int J Radiat Biol* 2005; 81:437–443.

93. Araki E, Ishikawa M, Iigo M, Koide T, Itabashi M, Hoshi A. Relationship between development of diarrhea and the concentration of SN-38, and active metabolite of CPT-11, in the intestine and the blood plasma of athymic mice following intraperitoneal administration of CPT-11. *Jpn J Cancer Res* 1993;84:697–702.

94. Cao S, Black JD, Troutt AB, Rustum YM. Interleukin 15 offers selective protection from irinotecan-induced intestinal toxicity in a preclinical animal model. *Cancer Res* 1998;58:3270–3274.

95. Ikuno N, Soda H, Watanabe M, Oka M. Irinotecan (CPT-11) and characteristic changes in the mouse ileum and cecum. *J Natl Cancer Inst* 1995;87:1876–1883.

96. Takasuna K, Hagiwara T, Hirohashi M, Kato M, Nomura M, Nagai E, Yokoi T, Kamataki T. Involvement of B-glucuronidase in intestinal microflora in the intestinal toxicity of the antitumor camptothecin derivative irinotecan hydrochloride (CPT-11) in rats. *Cancer Res* 1996;56:3752–3757.

97. Gwede CK. Overview of radiation- and chemoradiation-induced diarrhea. *Semin Oncol Nurs* 2003;19:6–10.

98. Engelking C, Rutledge DN, Ippoliti C, Neumann J, Hogan CM. Cancer-related diarrhea: a neglected cause of cancer-related symptom distress. *Oncol Nurs Forum* 1998;25: 859–860.

99. Viele CS. Overview of chemotherapy-induced diarrhea. *Semin Oncol Nurs* 2003;19: 2–5.

100. Govindarajan R. Irinotecan/thalidomide In metastatic colorectal cancer. *Oncology (Williston Park)* 2002;16:23–26.

101. Alimonti A, Gelibter A, Pavese I, Satta F, Cognetti F, Ferretti G, Rasio D, Vecchione A, Di Palma M. New approaches to prevent intestinal toxicity of irinotecan-based regimens. *Cancer Treat Rev* 2004;30:555–562.

102. Ma MK, McLeod HL. Lessons learned from the irinotecan metabolic pathway. *Curr Med Chem* 2003;10:41–49.

103. Takasuna K, Hagiwara T, Hirohashi M, Kato M, Nomura M, Nagai E, Yokoi T, Kamataki T. Inhibition of intestinal microflora beta-glucuronidase modifies the distribution of the active metabolite of the antitumor agent, irinotecan hydrochloride (CPT-11) in rats. *Cancer Chemother Pharmacol* 1998;42:280–286.

104. Stringer AM, Gibson RJ, Logan RM, Bowen JM, Yeoh ASJ, Burns J, Finnie JW, Keefe DMK. Chemotherapy-induced diarrhoea is associated with changes in the luminal environment in the DA rat. *Exp Biol Med* 2006;232:96–107.

105. Stringer AM, Gibson RJ, Bowen JM, Logan RM, Yeoh ASJ, Keefe DMK. Chemotherapy-induced mucositis: the role of gastrointestinal microflora and mucins in the luminal environment. *J Support Oncol* 2006;5:259–267.

106. Kushwaha RS, Hayne D, Vaizey CJ, Wrightham E, Payne H, Boulos PB. Physiologic changes of the anorectum after pelvic radiotherapy for the treatment of prostate and bladder cancer. *Dis Colon Rectum* 2003;46:1182–1188.

107. Yeoh EK, Russo A, Botten R, Fraser R, Roos D, Penniment M, Borg M, Sun WM. Acute effects of therapeutic irradiation for prostatic carcinoma on anorectal function. *Gut* 1998;43:123–127.

108. Egan LJ, Eckmann L, Greten FR, Chae S, Li ZW, Myhre GM, Robine S, Karin M, Kagnoff MF. IkappaB-kinasebeta-dependent NF-kappaB activation provides radioprotection to the intestinal epithelium. *Proc Nat Acad Sci USA* 2004;101:2452–2457.

109. Dorr W, Reichel S, Spekl K. Effects of keratinocyte growth factor (palifermin) administration protocols on oral mucositis (mouse) induced by fractionated irradiation. *Radiother Oncol* 2005;75:99–105.

110. Sharma R, Tobin P, Clarke SJ. Management of chemotherapy-induced nausea, vomiting, oral mucositis, and diarrhoea. *Lancet Oncol* 2005;6:93–102.

111. Sonis ST. The biologic role for nuclear factor-kappaB in disease and its potential involvement in mucosal injury associated with anti-neoplastic therapy. *Crit Rev Oral Biol Med* 2002;13:380–389.

112. Sonis ST. Mucositis as a biological process: a new hypothesis for the development of chemotherapy-induced stomatotoxicity. *Oral Oncol* 1998;34:39–43.

113. Gibson RJ, Bowen JM, Keefe DM. Palifermin reduces diarrhea and increases survival following irinotecan treatment in tumor-bearing DA rats. *Int J Cancer* 2005;116: 464–470.

114. Bowen JM, Gibson RJ, Tsykin A, Cummins AG, Keefe DMK. Irinotecan changes gene expression profiles in the small intestine of the rat with breast cancer. *Cancer Chemother Pharmacol* 2006;59:337–348.

115. Logan RM, Gibson RJ, Sonis ST, Keefe DM. Nuclear factor-kappaB (NF-kappaB) and cyclooxygenase-2 (COX-2) expression in the oral mucosa following cancer chemotherapy. *Oral Oncol* 2006;43:395–401.

116. Yeoh AS, Bowen JM, Gibson RJ, Keefe DM. Nuclear factor kappaB (NFkappaB) and cyclooxygenase-2 (Cox-2) expression in the irradiated colorectum is associated with subsequent histopathological changes. *Int J Radiat Oncol Biol Phys* 2005;63: 1295–1303.

117. Lalla RV, Schubert MM, Bensadoun RJ, Keefe D. Anti-inflammatory agents in the management of alimentary mucositis. *Support Care Cancer* 2006;14:558–565.

118. Hickok JT, Morrow GR, Roscoe JA, Mustian K, Okunieff P. Occurrence, severity, and longitudinal course of twelve common symptoms in 1129 consecutive patients during radiotherapy for cancer. *J Pain Symptom Manage* 2005;30:433–442.

119. Sonis S, Haddad R, Posner M, Watkins B, Fey E, Morgan TV, Mookanamparambil L, Ramoni M. Gene expression changes in peripheral blood cells provide insight into the biological mechanisms associated with regimen-related toxicities in patients being treated for head and neck cancers. *Oral Oncol* 2006;43:289–300.

120. Nadler LM, Stashenko P, Hardy R, Kaplan WD, Button LN, Kufe DW, Antman KH, Schlossman SF. Serotherapy of a patient with a monoclonal antibody directed against a human lymphoma-associated antigen. *Cancer Res* 1980;40:3147–3154.

121. Miller RA, Maloney DG, Warnke R, Levy R. Treatment of B-cell lymphoma with monoclonal anti-idiotype antibody. *N Eng J Med* 1982;306:517–522.

122. Bonner JA, Harari PM, Giralt J, Azarnia N, Shin DM, Cohen RB, Jones CU, Sur R, Raben D, Jassem J, Ove R, Kies MS, Baselga J, Youssoufian H, Amellal N, Rowinsky EK, Ang KK. Radiotherapy plus cetuximab for squamous-cell carcinoma of the head and neck. *N Eng J Med* 2006;354:567–578.

123. Kiewe P, Hasmuller S, Kahlert S, Heinrigs M, Rack B, Marme A, Korfel A, Jager M, Lindhofer H, Sommer H, Thiel E, Untch, M. Phase I trial of the trifunctional anti-HER2

× anti-CD3 antibody ertumaxomab in metastatic breast cancer. *Clin Cancer Res* 2006;12:3085–3091.

124. Keefe DMK, Gibson RJ. Mucosal injury from targeted anti-cancer therapy. *Support Care Cancer* 2006;15:483–490.

125. Sharkey RM, Goldenberg DM. Targeted therapy of cancer: new prospects for antibodies and immunoconjugates. *CA Cancer J Clin* 2006;56:226–243.

126. Cross D, Burmester JK. Gene therapy for cancer treatment: past, present and future. *Clin Med Res* 2006;4:218–227.

127. Vattemi E, Claudio PP. Gene therapy for lung cancer: practice and promise. *Ann Ital Chir* 2004;75:279–289.

128. Ross JS, Schenkein DP, Kashala O, Linette GP, Stec J, Symmans WF, Pusztai L, Hortobagyi GN. Pharmacogenomics. *Adv Anat Pathol* 2004;11:211–220.

129. Watters JW, McLeod HL. Cancer pharmacogenomics: current and future applications. *Biochim Biophys Acta* 2003;1603:99–111.

130. Zhang MQ. Large-scale gene expression data analysis: a new challenge to computational biologists. *Genome Res* 1999;9:681–688.

131. Chiappelli F. The molecular immunology of mucositis: implications for evidence-based research in alternative and complementary palliative treatments. *Evidence Based Complementary Alternative Med* 2005;2:489–494.

132. Hamadeh H, Amin P, Paules R, Afshari C. An overview of toxicogenomics. *Curr Issues Mol Biol* 2002;4:45–56.

133. Mitcheson JS, Chen J, Lin M, Culberson C, Sanguinetti MC. A structural basis for drug-induced long QT syndrome. *Proc Nat Acad Sci USA* 2000;97:12329–12333.

134. Moghimi SM, Hunter AC, Murray JC. Nanomedicine: current status and future prospects. *FASEB J* 2005;19:311–330.

135. Shikora K. The impact of future technology on cancer care. *Clin Med* 2002:2:560–568.

4

BACTERIAL MUTATION ASSAY

PREMKUMAR KUMPATI

University of Pittsburgh, Pittsburgh, Pennsylvania

Contents

Preclinical Development Handbook: Toxicology, edited by Shayne Cox Gad
Copyright © 2008 John Wiley & Sons, Inc.

4.1   INTRODUCTION

The population at large has been exposed to a variety of existing/new chemicals and drugs that have subsequently been shown to trigger mutations (genetic damage) and cancers, in addition to other genetic diseases. Hence, genetic toxicity testing has been an important aspect and essential component for assessing the mutagenic/carcinogenic potential of such agents and is indispensable for product development and registration. It is no wonder that numerous chapters, reviews, and books have been devoted to the development, standardization, and usage of predictive tests for mutagenicity/carcinogenicity. International guidelines indicate that a standard battery of genotoxicity tests, including the bacterial mutation assay, is normally required for new chemicals to assess their ability to cause genetic damage. During the past thirty years, bacterial systems have been extensively employed and modified for their ability to detect genotoxic potential of chemicals and drugs. The bacterial mutation assay is a reliable and widely used short-term assay for initial screening of chemicals for their potential mutagenic/carcinogenic activity. The assay has been recommended and accepted by various regulatory agencies for registration and acceptance of many chemicals. Although short-term tests are useful, they have their own advantages and limitations. This chapter provides an overall outline on the utilization of bacterial systems for rapidly screening/detecting mutagenic/carcinogenic chemicals, by their ability to induce single gene mutations. In addition, it provides procedures and recommendations for conducting the tests.

4.2   HISTORICAL PERSPECTIVE

Chemical mutagenesis and carcinogenesis have been known for many years and are well documented. Previously, potential carcinogenic/mutagenic chemicals have been identified based on their known association with human cancers and hereditary disorders and also by their ability to produce tumors in laboratory animals. Due to the lengthy, complex, and expensive nature of these studies and limited resources, attention has been focused on the development of "short-term tests" for detecting chemical carcinogens, using biological systems rather than whole mammals. Numerous short-term tests have been developed and are being used; such assays need less time than classical long-term studies.

The bacterial mutation assay is a widely used short-term test based on the principle of detecting chemicals that induce reverse mutations and restore the functional competence of a bacterial strain that is defective in synthesizing a vital amino acid. Chemical mutagens and/or carcinogens act directly on DNA, inducing irreversible genetic damage and cancers. However, the majority of chemicals are not biologically active until they are metabolized or enzymatically converted into reactive molecules, generally in the liver. Since bacteria are unable to metabolize chemicals as in mammals and other vertebrates, early attempts to demonstrate the potential mutagenicity/carcinogenicity of chemicals using bacterial assays failed to show responsiveness to various chemical mutagens.

In the 1950s, chemicals were tested for mutagenicity in *Escherichia coli* using suspension and plate (spot) tests or its variation. Due to the relative insensitivity of *E. coli* mutation in reverting from streptomycin dependence to streptomycin independence and lack of knowledge of metabolic activation of mutagens, this test was not well recognized. In suspension assay, cells are treated in suspension. In the spot test, a small amount of the test chemical is applied directly to the center of a selective agar medium plate seeded with the test organism. As the chemical diffuses into the agar, a concentration gradient is formed and will give rise to a ring of revertant colonies surrounding the area where the chemical is applied [1].

In 1971, Ames [2] initially used the same spot test method for screening mutagens using a large collection of *Salmonella typhimurium* histidine mutant strains. At the same time, Yanofsky [3] presented a number of *E. coli* tryptophan mutants that could also be used for detection of mutagens. The concept of metabolic activation of chemicals by mammalian liver was introduced by Miller and co-workers [4–6]. This was supported by Heinrich Malling's [7] report on the *in vitro* activation of dimethylnitrosamine to a mutagen for *Salmonella*, by incorporating a mouse liver homogenate with the cells in a suspension assay. This was further supported by a publication by Garner et al. [8] showing that liver microsomes could activate afla-toxin B1 to a product that was toxic to the *Salmonella* tester strains. Following the concepts of liver homogenate, Ames et al. [9] prepared a supernatant of liver homogenate by centrifugation at 9000*g*, called it S9, and incorporated it into a top agar containing a tester bacterial strain and a test chemical, thereby producing the plate test, which is more sensitive and quantitative than the spot test. The first com-prehensive validation of bacterial tests for detecting carcinogens was conducted by Ames and colleagues [10], using a combination of bacteria (*Salmonella*) and mam-malian microsomal enzymes. A series of studies from Ames's laboratory and other laboratories have demonstrated that *Salmonella* mutagens were rodent carcinogens, and almost all carcinogens were mutagens [11, 12]. Green and Muriel [13] first reported the *trp*+ (tryptophan) reversion assay using *E. coli* WP2 strain for routine screening of chemicals. It detects *trp*− to *trp*+ reversion at a site blocking a step in the biosynthesis of tryptophan prior to the formation of anthranilic acid. This assay is used by some laboratories in combination with the *Salmonella* assay to screen chemicals for mutagenic activity. Over the years, modifications to the standard plate incorporation assay have been developed by different researchers and additional mutations were engineered into the strains of *Salmonella* and *E. coli* that enhanced the sensitivity of the test and allowed testing of a wider range of chemicals. It is noteworthy that multiple tester strains are necessarily used in the bacterial mutation assay because of the differences in their sensitivity.

4.3   PRINCIPLES AND STRATEGIES OF THE ASSAY

The bacterial mutagenicity assay is a widely used short-term genetic toxicology assay designed to screen a wide range of chemical substances and drugs for their mutagenic or carcinogenic potential [10, 14]. It is also known as the bacterial reverse mutation test. In principle, the test employs several amino-acid-requiring strains of *Salmonella typhimurium/Escherichia coli (E. coli)*, carrying a different mutation in various genes involved in the histidine/tryptophan biosynthetic pathway [13, 15]. Hence, they are dependent on amino acid supplementation in culture medium in order to grow. Chemicals that induce mutations revert those mutations already present in the bacteria (back mutation) and restore the functional capacity of the bacteria to synthesize a particular amino acid, which is detected by the bacteria's ability to grow and form colonies in the absence of that amino acid. The number of spontaneously induced revertant colonies per plate is relatively constant. However, when a mutagen is added to the plate, the number of revertant colonies per plate is increased, usually in a dose-related manner. Figure 4.1 shows control and mutagen-treated bacterial plates.

Bacterial test systems fall into three main classes: namely, those that detect backward mutations, those that detect forward mutations, and those that rely on a DNA repair deficiency. However, the most widely exploited method is the induction of backward or reverse mutations in *Salmonella typhimurium* and less frequently in *Escherichia coli*. The objective of this assay is to evaluate the mutagenic potential of test chemicals by studying their effect on one or more histidine (auxotrophic) requiring strains of *Salmonella typhimurium* in the absence and in the presence of a liver metabolizing system. When the cultures are exposed to a mutagen, some of the bacteria undergo genetic changes due to chemical interactions, resulting in reversion of the bacteria to a non-histidine-requiring state. The reverted bacteria will then grow in the absence of exogenous histidine, thus providing an indication of the potential of the chemical to cause mutation.

Bacteria are single-celled organisms. They divide rapidly and are relatively easy to grow in large numbers in a few hours. However, mutations occur naturally at a

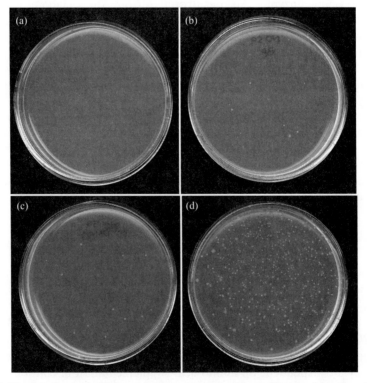

FIGURE 4.1   (a) Control, (b) benzopyrene treated without S9 mix, (c) solvent (DMSO) control with S9 mix, and (d) benzopyrene treated with S9 mix.

specific locus in less than one in a million bacteria at each cell division. As the biochemistry and genetics of bacteria are well established, it has been possible to develop special strains that are sensitive to a wide range of mutagens. Since different strains are mutated by different classes of compounds, multiple tester strains are necessarily used. Different amino acid requiring bacterial strains could also be used; however, the basis of the test is very similar, except that the bacteria have a requirement for a different amino acid.

To increase the test's sensitivity, bacterial strains have been modified genetically and made more susceptible to mutagens by changing the structure of their cell walls, so that they become more permeable to large fat-soluble molecules. Another genetic manipulation introduces plasmids (small DNA molecules) that carry genes that interfere with DNA repair, making the host bacteria even more susceptible to the mutagenic effects of chemicals. The possibility of a chemical mutagen hitting the mutational site of the tester strain in order to reverse mutate is increasingly achieved by using several strains of the same species of bacterium, each carrying a different preexisting mutation (targets) in the same amino acid gene. For example, there are several strains of *S. typhimurium*, each carrying different mutations in the histidine gene but commonly sharing other traits, like DNA-repair defects and cell-wall defects that improve the strain's sensitivity.

As mentioned previously, unlike mammalian cells, bacteria lack the ability to metabolize chemicals; hence, the test requires use of an exogenous source of metabolic activation [16]. The enzymes are therefore added in the form of a liver extract prepared from laboratory animals, usually rats. The rats are given chemicals ("inducers") that increase the amount of metabolic-activation enzymes in the liver. Subsequently, the liver homogenate is subjected to centrifugation at a speed of $9000g$ so as to collect the supernatant containing the metabolic enzymes and this is called S9 (short for "$9000g$ supernatant"). The most widely used inducer is Aroclor 1254, a mixture of polychlorinated biphenyls. Phenobarbital plus 5,6-benzoflavone is also used for induction.

In the bacterial mutation assay, the amino acid deficient bacteria, his^- bacteria, are mixed with S9 and several doses of the test chemical with very limited supply of histidine and are allowed to divide. A chemical that induces mutation either by itself or by its metabolites (by the action of S9) is detected by its ability to transform bacteria into those that can grow into a colony even when the supply of histidine has been used up. These transformed bacteria/revertants restore the ability to synthesize histidine from inorganic nitrogen and can grow without supplementation of histidine. Results are expressed as the number of revertant colonies per plate (Fig. 4.2).

4.4 SIGNIFICANCE AND LIMITATIONS OF THE ASSAY

The bacterial mutation assay is a rapid, reliable, and economical method for screening many types of substances for their potential genotoxic activity. It is widely used as an early screening tool, due to its procedural simplicity, and has demonstrated a positive correlation between bacterial mutagenicity and carcinogenicity in mammals. Many chemicals that are positive in this test are genotoxic in other tests as well. Bacterial tests have the advantage of testing millions of cells with a relatively short

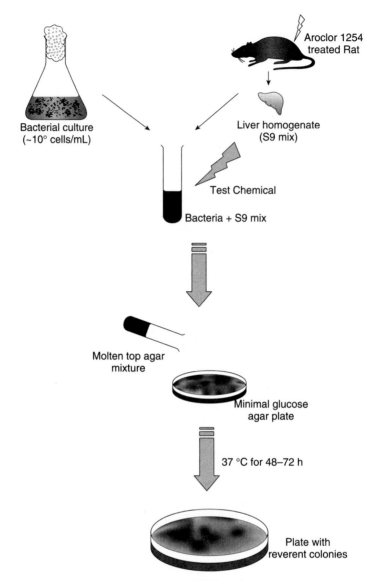

FIGURE 4.2   Diagrammatic procedural outline: bacterial mutation assay.

generation time. The rapidly dividing nature of a bacterial system and the rare occurrence of natural mutations at a specific locus makes it suitable for mutagenicity testing. Unlike higher organisms, in which the DNA is organized into complex chromosomal structures, bacteria contain a single circular molecule of DNA that is readily accessible to chemicals that can penetrate the cell wall. The biochemical and genetic nature of the bacteria is well recognized and has led to the possibility of developing special strains of bacteria that are sensitive to a wide range of mutagens. Each strain is specific and provides information on the types of mutations induced by genotoxic agents. Bacterial mutation assays are used in a large number of laboratories throughout the world. A database of the results for a wide variety of chemical structures is available for bacterial reverse mutation tests. The results obtained may be combined and correlated with the results of other tests (e.g., *in vitro* mammalian cell assays and *in vitro* cytogenetic assays) to evaluate the possible mutagenic risk of a test chemical. Thus, bacterial mutation assays give the best overall performance, producing reliable results in a large number of laboratories, and are confirmed as the first choice as an initial screening test. Furthermore, bacterial tests have been validated in far greater detail than any other tests currently used in genetic toxicology.

Although bacterial mutation tests have lots of advantages, they also have some limitations. Bacteria, being prokaryotic cells, differ from mammalian cells in factors such as uptake, metabolism, chromosome structure, and DNA-repair processes. Only gene mutations can be detected using a bacterial system. Bacteria do not or insufficiently possess enzyme systems responsible for metabolic processes. Hence, the test requires the use of an exogenous source of metabolic activation (S9), which does not represent the complicated enzyme network in mammalian tissue. The information obtained through the test, on the mutagenic and carcinogenic potency of a substance in mammals, is not always promising. The test may not provide sufficient information on the genotoxicity potential of compounds that are excessively toxic to bacteria, such as antibiotics, and compounds that are known to interfere with the mammalian cell replication system (e.g., topoisomerase inhibitors, nucleoside analogues, or inhibitors of DNA metabolism). The test also cannot detect chemical carcinogens that act by nongenotoxic (without causing DNA damage) mechanisms (e.g., asbestos, nickel, arsenic, and hormone-like chemicals such as diethylstilbestrol). Despite these limitations, bacterial mutation tests have been found to be extremely valuable as the first in a series of tests for screening chemicals for potential mutagenic and carcinogenic activity.

4.5   ASSAY PROCEDURES AND EXPERIMENTAL DESIGN

4.5.1   Procedural Outline

The bacterial mutation assay is used to assess the chemical's ability to induce point mutations in the bacteria, which are deficient in synthesizing an amino acid (due to the mutation present in the amino acid synthesizing gene), thus reverting the mutation and restoring the capacity to synthesize the amino acid and to grow without amino acid supplementation. In general, bacterial cultures are exposed to the test substance in the presence and absence of an exogenous metabolic activation system and are plated onto minimal agar medium. After 2–3 days of incubation, revertant colonies are counted and compared with that of the negative or solvent control plates. Statistical analysis of the counts are carried out, and the results for mutagenicity are assessed. This is one of several genotoxicity assays required for product safety testing.

Numerous procedures have been described for performing a bacterial mutation assay. The two basic and commonly used methods are the plate incorporation method and the preincubation method. The plate incorporation method is the most commonly used method; however, the preincubation method is recommended for some chemical classes such as azo dyes, aliphatic *N*-nitroso compounds, and alkaloids [17]. Other procedures include the fluctuation method and the suspension method. In the plate incorporation method, bacterial cultures are exposed to the test chemical in either the presence or absence of a metabolic activation system, combined with molten overlay agar, and plated immediately onto minimal agar medium [18–20]. In the case of the preincubation method, the treatment mixture is preincubated at 37 °C for 20–60 minutes and mixed with the overlay agar before plating onto minimal agar medium [19]. Minimal agar medium contains salts and a carbon source that is sufficient to support growth. The top agar/overlay agar contains a trace amount of amino acid that is sufficient to promote the limited growth of the nonrevertant bacteria. This is important for several reasons, which are discussed in later sections. Establishment of consistent methods for every phase of the experiment is a prerequisite [21]; hence, the parameters and the procedural details that influence the specificity and fidelity of the assay are discussed next.

4.5.2 Bacteria

Healthy growing bacterial cultures with high titer of viable bacteria should be used for the experiments. Viable cell numbers could be determined by a plating experiment. Bacterial cultures should be grown up to the late exponential or early stationary phase of growth (approximately 10^9 cells/mL). It is noteworthy that cultures in late stationary phase should not be used. For overnight cultures, excessive aeration and shaking exceeding 120 rpm should be avoided [30]. The culture temperature should be maintained at 37 °C. Although all *Salmonella* strains are histidine dependent, various strains of bacteria are available that differ in their sensitivity to various classes of mutagens. Some chemicals are strain specific, whereas others may be detected in several strains. The five recommended combination and commonly used strains of *S. typhimurium* are TA100, TA1535, TA102, TA98, and TA1537 or TA97. These strains, except TA102, have GC base pairs at the primary reversion site and detect a majority of mutagens [17] but not certain oxidizing mutagens, crosslinking agents, and hydrazines. Such substances may be detected by DNA repair-proficient strains of *E. coli* (e.g., *E. coli* WP2 or *E. coli* WP2 (pKM101)). *Escherichia coli* WP2 or *S. typhimurium* TA102 have an AT base pair at the primary reversion site [12]. Thus, on the basis of the chemical class or structure, alternative strain(s) should be considered.

Furthermore, additional mutations/genetic alterations have been introduced to increase the sensitivity of the tester strains to chemical mutagens: for example, *uvrA* gene mutation in *E. coli* and *uvrB-bio* gene mutation in *S. typhimurium*, which eliminate the accurate excision repair mechanism, thereby allowing more DNA lesions to be repaired by the error-prone DNA-repair mechanism. Furthermore, the deletion through the biotin gene makes the bacteria biotin dependent. *rfa* mutations lead to a defective lipopolysaccharide (LPS) layer that coats the bacterial surface, making the bacteria more permeable to bulky chemicals [16]. Introduction of plasmid pKM101 in strains enhances chemical and UV-induced mutagenesis via an increase in the error-prone recombinational DNA-repair pathway [22]. The plasmid confers ampicillin resistance, which is a convenient marker to detect the presence of the plasmid. Introduction of multicopy plasmid pAQ1 with a *hisG428* mutation amplifies the number of target sites.

In order to maintain experimental quality and reliability, bacterial strains should regularly be checked for their characteristic genetic traits, including amino acid requirement, background mutation, induced mutation with reference mutagens, presence of plasmids where appropriate, and presence of cell-wall and DNA-repair mutations. Furthermore, it is also necessary that the strains should yield spontaneous revertant colony counts within the frequency ranges expected from the laboratory's historical control data and preferably within the range reported in the literature. Stock cultures should be stored at a temperature below −70 °C. Overnight cultures for routine assays should be prepared by inoculation from stock cultures— never from a previously used overnight culture. The overnight culture should contain at least 10^9 viable bacteria/mL and should be freshly prepared for each experiment.

4.5.3   Storage and Reisolation

Frozen stocks of strains are stored at −80 °C. They are prepared from fresh overnight cultures to which 10% (v/v) DMSO or glycerol is added as a cryoprotective agent. Usually fresh oxoid nutrient broth culture is grown to a density of $1–2 \times 10^9$ bacteria/mL. For each 1 mL of culture, 0.09 mL of high purity grade DMSO is added. For preparing multiple frozen tubes, combine the culture and DMSO in a sterile tube, flask, or bottle, mix gently until the DMSO is dissolved, and distribute the culture aseptically into sterile 1.2 mL cryotubes that have been labeled appropriately. All the tubes are placed in a bed of crushed dry ice until the cultures are frozen solid and subsequently transferred to −80 °C freezer/liquid nitrogen.

Tester strains are reisolated from the frozen stock by streaking the bacteria on minimal glucose agar plates enriched with histidine and biotin. Dip a sterile wooden stick into a stock culture (or scrape the bacteria from the surface of the frozen culture) and make a single streak across the surface onto the agar plate. Cross streak the culture using sterile platinum wire. Incubate the plate for 48 h at 37 °C; pick a well isolated colony for overnight growth in oxoid nutrient broth. It should be noted that frequent thawing and refreezing of tester strains may result in reduced viability.

4.5.4   Medium

An appropriate minimal agar medium containing Vogel–Bonner minimal medium E, 0.5–2% glucose [23], and 1.5% agar (w/v) is generally used and is referred to as glucose minimal agar medium. Minimal agar plates contains 25 mL of solidified medium and are stored in sealed plastic bags at 4 °C either in a refrigerator or cold room, to avoid dehydration. Overlay agar or top agar containing 0.6% agar and 0.6% NaCl with a trace amount of amino acid such as histidine or biotin at a concentration of 0.05 mM (for *S. typhimurium*) or tryptophan (for *E. coli*), which is sufficient to promote a few cell divisions, should be used. The *uvrB* deletion extends through the biotin gene—hence the need for biotin in those strains possessing the *uvrB* mutation. These essential components can be added to minimal glucose agar before the test plates are poured or they can be applied to the surface of minimal glucose agar plates and incorporated into the plates using a glass spreader.

4.5.5   Metabolic Activation and Preparation of S9 Mix

Unlike mammalian cells, bacteria lack the ability to metabolize chemicals. To compensate for this, bacteria should be exposed to the test substance in both the presence and absence of an appropriate exogenous metabolic activation system. The most commonly used system is a cofactor-supplemented postmitochondrial fraction (S9) prepared from the livers of rodents (usually rats) treated with enzyme-inducing agents such as Aroclor 1254 (500 mg/kg body weight). Other inducers are phenobarbital and β-naphthoflavone [14, 24]. The animals should be free of disease and infection, kept at a reasonable temperature, and should not be stressed by careless handling. Dosing with inducing agents should be consistent from one batch of animals to the next. Animals should be killed humanely and the livers removed and chilled as soon as possible. A 9000*g* supernatant (S9) is prepared from pooled, homogenized livers of the treated animals. S9 should be stored at or below −70 °C in aliquots in order to avoid contamination. In order to maintain the activity of the S9 fraction, it should always be kept on ice during the experiment or kept frozen when not in use.

There are two widely accepted methods of using S9 mix. (1) S9 mix is mixed with the top agar, bacteria, and test substance, and the whole mixture is immediately poured onto the surface of the bottom agar. (2) In the preincubation method, the test substance, bacteria, and S9 mix are mixed and incubated for 30 min; top agar is then added, and the mixture is poured onto the bottom agar. The postmitochondrial supernatant fraction is usually used at concentrations in the range of 10–30% v/v in the S9 mix. The choice and concentration of a metabolic activation system may depend on the class of chemical being tested. In some cases, it may be appropriate to utilize more than one concentration of postmitochondrial fraction. Nevertheless, for optimal mutagenesis with a particular compound, the amount of S9 per plate is critical. Too much as well as too little S9 can drastically lower the sensitivity. Each new batch of S9 prepared should be routinely checked with known mutagenic compounds such as benzo[*a*]pyrene and aflatoxin B1. The optimum S9 level for a given compound should therefore be checked. The amount of S9 per plate is best expressed as milligram liver protein per plate calculated from the protein concentration of the S9.

Rodent liver homogenate should be supplemented with NADP and cofactor for NADPH-supported oxidation and with FMN for reductive metabolism of chemicals [23]. A reductive metabolic activation system may be more appropriate for azo dyes and diazo compounds. In addition, glucose-6-phosphate (for providing energy) and phosphate buffer (to maintain pH), including magnesium and potassium salts, are added. Liver S9 should be prepared using aseptic techniques so that subsequent filter sterilization could be avoided. Filtration of the S9 or S9 mix may lead to loss of enzyme activity. Each batch of S9, whether produced by the testing laboratory or obtained commercially, should be tested for sterility and discarded if contaminated.

To prepare S9 mix, rats weighing 200 g are exposed to a single intraperitoneal (IP) injection of Aroclor 1254 at a concentration of 500 mg/kg body weight. Aroclor is diluted in corn oil to a concentration of 200 mg/mL and is administered to each rat for 5 days before being sacrificed. Rats are provided with unlimited drinking water and chow until 12 h before killing. After the treatment period, rats are killed and the livers must be removed aseptically using sterile surgical tools. All the steps of the procedure are carried out at 0–4 °C using cold sterile solutions and glassware. The freshly excised livers are washed several times in fresh chilled 0.15 M KCl solution to ensure sterile preparation and to remove hemoglobin. Washed livers are placed in preweighed beakers containing approximately 3 mL of chilled 0.15 M KCl/g of wet liver and are minced with sterile scissors and homogenized using a homogenizer. The liver homogenate is centrifuged for 10 min at 9000g and the supernatant is decanted and assayed. Sterility of the preparation is determined by plating 0.1 mL on minimal agar containing histidine and biotin. Generally, the protein concentration of S9 is ~40 mg/mL. S9 mix consists of 1 mL of S9 fraction, 1 mL NADP (40 mM), 1 mL of glucose-6-phosphate (40 mM), 1 mL of $MgSO_4$ (70 mM), 5 mL of 0.1 M phosphate buffer (pH 7.4), and 1 mL water. This mixture is filtered through a millipore filter (0.45 µm) kept at 0 °C. Next, 2.5 mL of S9 mix is added to 10 mL of diluted bacterial cultures. Different sources of S9 and conditions of incubation can lead to qualitative and quantitative differences. To avoid frequent freezing and thawing cycles and contamination, it is advisable to aliquot into 1–2 mL and store at −80 °C.

4.5.6 Controls

Each experiment or assay should include a negative control (solvent control) in order to check the background mutation and positive controls (reference/known mutagen control). Possibly, the chemicals selected as positive controls should be structurally related to the compound under test. Concentrations that demonstrate the effective performance of each assay should be selected. Concurrent strain-specific positive and negative (solvent or vehicle) controls, both with and without metabolic activation, should be included in each assay. Some of the examples of strain-specific positive controls are: for strains TA1535 and TA100, sodium azide; for strain TA98, 2-nitrofluorene (without activation) and 2-anthramine (with activation); for TA1537, 9-aminoacridine; and for TA98, benzopyrene (with activation). Negative controls, consisting of solvent or vehicle alone, should be included without test substance and otherwise treated in the same way as the treatment groups. In addition, untreated controls should also be used unless there is historical control data demonstrating that no deleterious or mutagenic effects are induced by the chosen solvent.

4.5.7 Test Material and Solvents

Solid test substances should be dissolved or suspended in appropriate solvents or vehicles and diluted prior to treatment of the bacteria. Liquid test substances may be added directly to the test systems and/or diluted prior to treatment. Fresh preparations should be employed unless stability data demonstrate the acceptability of storage; unused portions should be discarded. Sterile distilled water is the good choice of solvent. However, chemicals that do not dissolve in water should be dissolved in dimethyl sulfoxide (DMSO). It dissolves numerous different kinds of chemicals, is miscible with water, and, at the amount used in the test (0.1 mL or less), is not toxic to bacteria. In cases where it is unsuitable, other solvents may be used, such as acetone, ethyl alcohol, diethyl formamide, and methyl ethyl ketone. It is noteworthy that the solvent/vehicle should not be suspected of chemical reaction with the test substance and the concentration used should be compatible with the survival of the bacteria and the S9 activity [25].

All data available on the substance to be tested should be provided and recorded, including its lot or batch number, physical appearance, chemical structure, purity, solubility, reactivity in aqueous and nonaqueous solvents, temperature and pH stability, and sensitivity to light. A sample of each substance to be assayed for mutagenicity should be retained for reference purposes. The proposed uses of the test substance should be known, since antibiotics, surfactants, preservatives, and biocides pose special problems in bacterial mutation assays. Gaseous or volatile substances should be tested by appropriate methods, such as in sealed vessels or in glass desiccators [26, 27].

Among the criteria to be taken into consideration when determining the highest amount of test substance to be used are cytotoxicity and solubility in the final treatment mixture. Cytotoxicity may be detected by a reduction in the number of revertant colonies or by a clearing or attenuation of the background lawn. The cytotoxicity of a substance may be altered in the presence of metabolic activation systems. Insolubility should be assessed as precipitation in the final mixture under the actual test conditions. The recommended maximum test concentration for soluble noncytotoxic substances is 5 mg/plate or 5 μL/plate. For noncytotoxic substances that are not soluble at 5 mg/plate or 5 μL/plate, one or more concentrations tested should be insoluble in the final treatment mixture. Test substances that are cytotoxic below 5 mg/plate or 5 μL/plate should be tested up to a cytotoxic concentration. For volatile liquids, 0.5–5 mL should be used as the low and high dose, respectively. At least five to eight different analyzable concentrations of the test substance should be used with approximately half-log (i.e., $\sqrt{10}$) intervals between test points for an initial experiment. For most mutagens, there is a linear dose–response over a certain concentration range. The highest concentration of test substance is desired to show evidence of significant toxicity. If precipitate is present on any of the plates, it may interfere with automatic counting of the colonies. In such a situation, all plates in that series of doses and controls should be counted by hand.

4.6 EXPERIMENTAL PROCEDURE/DESIGN OF EXPERIMENTS

In the plate incorporation method, each bacterial strain is grown in nutrient broth, supplemented with antibiotics for 15–18 h, and contains about 1×10^9 bacteria/mL. One hundred microliters (0.1 mL) of bacterial culture is added to 2.0 mL of 45 °C molten top agar, containing histidine and trace amounts of biotin, 0.05–0.1 mL of the test compound (a range of doses) or solvent, and 0.5 mL of sodium phosphate buffer (1 M, pH 7.4) or S9 mix. S9 mix consists of S9 (usually between 4% and 30% by volume) [15, 25] to which has been added nicotinamide-adenine dinucleotide phosphate (NADP) and glucose-6-phosphate (which together provide energy for metabolism), phosphate buffer to maintain pH, and salts of magnesium and potassium. A set of tubes is also prepared without S9. This is to check whether the test chemical can cause mutation without the need for metabolic activation. Chemicals of this type are directly acting mutagens: certain directly acting mutagens can be made nonmutagenic by S9. The additions of bacteria, test chemical, and S9 mix are made in rapid succession, in order to avoid the potentially harmful effects of the rather high temperature (45 °C) necessary to keep the soft agar molten. As soon as possible after mixing, the molten top agar mixture is poured onto 25–30 mL of solid 1.5% minimal glucose agar plates. The plate is shaken to distribute the top agar in a thin, even layer over the bottom agar and is placed on a level surface. As the top agar cools and solidifies, the plates are inverted and incubated for 48–72 hours at 37 °C; revertant colonies are then counted either manually or by an automatic colony counter. During the first few hours of incubation, all the *his⁻* bacteria will grow, since there is a trace of histidine present. When all the histidine has been used up, the bulk of bacteria will stop dividing, and a thin, visible confluent lawn of bacteria will be formed in the soft agar. However, bacteria that have sustained DNA damage leading to a mutation with the effect of reverting *his⁻* gene to *his⁺* will continue to divide, since they can now synthesize their own histidine from the ammonium salts in the bottom agar. Several tubes are set aside to act as "controls," that is, tubes that will receive the solvent but not the test chemical and will therefore indicate the background (spontaneous) level of mutation. If the spontaneous revertant colonies are more than 200 colonies/plate or chemical discolors the agar or when precipitate is present on the plate, it is better to use hand counting rather than automatic counting. All chemicals should be tested twice with triplicate plates for all doses and solvent controls for an adequate estimate of variation. Test dose levels are selected based on the known literature of the chemical or a structurally related substance. Several doses ranging from submicrogram to milligram levels of the test chemical should be tested at intervals, together with positive and solvent controls. The experiment should be repeated until a consistent picture emerges.

For the preincubation method, the test substance/test solution (usually 0.05 or 0.1 mL) is preincubated in liquid environment with the tester strain (0.1 mL, containing approximately 10^9 viable cells) and sterile buffer (0.5 mL) or the metabolic activation system (0.5 mL) usually for 20 min or more at 30–37 °C prior to mixing with the overlay agar (2.0 mL) and pouring onto the surface of a minimal agar plate. Tubes are usually aerated during preincubation by using a shaker.

For testing gases, the tester strains are precultured with the nutrient broth. The reaction mixture, containing phosphate buffer, S9, cofactors, and the preculture strain, is poured into the agar plates and placed upside down, without their lids, in a plate holder. The plate holder is then placed in a 10 L tedlar bag/desiccator through an opening on one side of the bag made by scissors. The bag is then closed by folding the opening two or three times and sealing it with adhesive tape. Air in the bag is removed and then the gas is released at a fixed amount per plate. The bacterial plates in the bag are kept at 37 °C for a time period. After termination of the exposure, the test substance (gas) in the bag is removed. The tape is peeled off and the bag is left to stand for 30 min, then covered with a lid and incubated for 24 h. Next, the revertant colonies are counted [17]. The results are expressed as number of revertants per plate based on moles of gas used. Volatile materials can be tested at reduced temperatures or at raised pressure. Alternatively, if the chemicals are volatile, the plates are exposed to known concentrations (v/v) of the compound and are incubated in closed systems or glass desiccators. However, bactericidal substances may be studied using the liquid suspension assay method. A treat-and-wash bacterial mutation test is employed to evaluate the mutagenicity of soluble biological material, capable of releasing histidine and tryptophan. Histidine and tryptophan can cause overgrown background bacterial lawns. In such cases, the procedure is modified to include a longer preincubation step for 90 min followed by a washing step to remove the amino acids prior to plating so as to prevent overgrown lawns. After the 90 min of preincubation, 15 mL of wash solution of oxoid nutrient broth in phosphate buffered saline (1:7) is added. The washed bacterial pellet is collected by centrifugation at 2000g for 30 min. Supernatant is discarded and the bacterial pellet is resuspended in the residual supernatant (~0.7 mL of the supernatant) prior to plating [28].

It should be noted that all plates in a given assay should be incubated at 37 °C for 2 or 3 days before being scored for the number of revertant colonies per plate. It is important to ensure that volatile test compounds and gases are incubated in closed systems or glass desiccators. After the incubation period, it is essential to check the background lawn of both treated and control plates for toxic effects (thinning of the lawn) or excess growth, which may indicate the presence of amino acids in the test material. All plates within a given experiment should be incubated for the same time period. If a clear positive response is obtained in the first experiment, then a second or confirmatory experiment may not be required. If a negative response or ambiguous response occurs, it may be necessary to perform a second experiment or additional experiments. The result of a bacterial mutation assay, whether positive or negative, is expressed as mean revertants per plate and standard deviation. Statistics are used to support the interpretation of the data.

4.7   CRITICAL FACTORS IN THE PROCEDURE

The bacterial mutation test forms the basis of all screening programs. There are several conditions that must be met in order to ensure a satisfactory test. It is essential that a baseline protocol should be written before starting a screening program. Methods for the preparation and storage of S9 and bacterial strains and other procedures should be thoroughly checked by performing assays with reference mutagens and authenticated bacterial strains, under conditions prescribed by the chosen protocol. Bacterial strains should be checked regularly for their characteristic genetic traits, including amino acid requirement, background mutation, induced mutation with reference mutagens, presence of plasmids where appropriate, and presence of cell-wall and DNA-repair mutations [29, 30]. Advice should be sought from experienced investigators. The strains should also yield spontaneous revertant colony counts within the frequency ranges expected from the laboratory's historical control data and preferably within the range reported in the literature. Deviations from standard procedures need to be scientifically justified. The following technical details are not intended as a defined recommended protocol, but represent good current practice and good criteria for successful bacterial tests.

4.8   TROUBLESHOOTING

4.8.1   Background Lawn

A faint background lawn of bacteria indicates the presence of trace amounts of histidine in the agar, which allows all the bacteria to undergo several divisions, producing a faint background lawn of bacteria. Since dividing cells are more suitable for mutation during DNA replication, the background lawn serves as a good indicator. If the amount of histidine in the agar is increased, mutagenesis may be enhanced but will also cause a heavy growth of the background lawn, obscuring the revertants. Plate without background lawn, but with colonies, may not contain true revertants, as they arise due to the surviving bacteria that live on the histidine present in the agar and therefore should not be scored. If the background lawn is thin compared to the control, it indicates toxicity of the chemical to the bacteria. To check whether colonies are true revertants, they should be streaked out onto minimal plates containing biotin but no histidine. True revertants will be able to grow, whereas microcolonies arising due to toxicity will not.

4.8.2   Spontaneous Reversion

Spontaneous reversion (to histidine independence) can be measured and expressed as the number of spontaneous revertants per plate. The number of spontaneous revertants is dependent on two populations: (1) pre-existing mutants in the inoculum and (2) mutants arising following divisions on the plate. Each tester strain should revert spontaneously at a frequency that is characteristic of the strain. Also, each laboratory should establish its own historical range, as these ranges are likely to vary from laboratory to laboratory. Any deviation from historical range may be due to altered characteristics of the strain and should be tested. It should also be noted that the number of spontaneous revertants varies between experiments; therefore, it is recommended that at least three control plates be included for each strain in a mutagenicity assay.

Abnormal high spontaneous reversion may indicate contamination or the accumulation of back mutations by repeated subculturing. If this occurs, the strain should be recovered by reisolation from the frozen master copy. Spontaneous reversions are influenced by histidine concentration in agar and also by the mutagens in the environment of the bacteria, such as the reagents used to perform the assay—for example, ethylene oxide used to sterilize plastic ware. If a test substance is derived from biological material that causes an increase in mutant colonies in a bacterial mutagenicity test, it is possible that such an increase may be due to the presence of amino acids or peptides in the test substance, at levels that interfere with standard procedure. In such situations, testing of amino-acid-free extracts of the test substance, with appropriate controls, is necessary. Abnormal test results may also be due to changes in the strain's characteristics.

4.8.3   Criteria for Checking Strain Characteristics

His⁻ Character. The *his⁻* character of the tester strains should be confirmed by demonstrating the histidine requirement for growth on selective agar plates.

TrpE Marker. Trypton auxotrophy of *E. coli* strain should be confirmed by streaking a overnight culture across the surface of glucose minimal defined agar plates with and without excess tryptophan (10–20 µg/mL). After overnight incubation at 37 °C, no growth should be observed on the plate without tryptophan, while full growth should be observed on the plate supplemented with tryptophan.

uvr⁻. uvrA mutation in *E. coli* and *uvrB* mutation in *S. typhimurium* should be confirmed by demonstrating sensitivity to UV light. The *uvrB⁻* deletion extends through the biotin gene, hence the need for biotin in those strains possessing the *uvrB* mutation. A sample of the cultures is streaked across a biotin control plate and then a histidine–biotin plate. The plates are incubated overnight at 37 °C and examined for growth on the histidine–biotin plates. There should be no growth on the control plates.

rfa Character. The *rfa* mutation permits large molecules, such as crystal violet, to enter and kill the bacteria. The *rfa* character of the tester strains is confirmed by determining crystal violet sensitivity. Crystal violet, added to the center of a sterile paper disk, is pressed lightly against the seeded plates to embed. The plate is then inverted and incubated. A clear zone of inhibition appears around the disk, indicating the presence of the *rfa* mutation.

R factor. Ampicillin resistance is a convenient marker enabling testing for the presence of the plasmid. The ampicillin resistant R factor is somewhat unstable and can be lost from the bacteria and hence should be checked routinely. This could be done by cross-streaking the culture to be tested against an ampicillin solution coated nutrient agar plate and allowing it to grow by incubating for 12–24 hours at 37 °C. Strains that contain the R factor will grow.

4.9   INTERPRETATION OF DATA AND REPORTING

If the test chemical causes an increase in revertant colonies, by inducing mutations in the genome of either *Salmonella typhimurium* and/or *Escherichia coli*, it indicates that the results are positive or the chemical is mutagenic in the species tested. In contrast, no colonies or very few colonies indicates the results are negative or the chemical is non-mutagenic. If the test chemical under investigation is found to be positive, there is no need to verify by additional testing. However, if it shows marginal or weak positive response, it should be further verified by additional testing.

Most experiments will give clear positive or negative results. However, in a few cases it is difficult to judge the nature of the test chemical. Hence, in the case of ambiguous results, further testing is necessary using different experimental conditions, such as modifying the concentrations or method of treatment (plate incorporation or liquid preincubation) or by adjusting metabolic activation conditions (source and concentration of S9 in the mix). Nevertheless, if the results are ambiguous or questionable even after repeated testing with modified protocols, it is advisable to carry out additional testing protocols using different test systems. Furthermore, negative results could also be confirmed by repeated testing using modified protocols. A test substance for which the results do not meet the above criteria is considered non-mutagenic in this test.

In general, data should be presented as the number of revertant colonies per plate. Individual plate counts, the mean number of revertant colonies per plate, and the standard deviation (mean revertant colonies per plate ± the SD or SEM) should be presented for each dose of the test substance, with positive (known mutagen) and negative (untreated and/or solvent) controls. Appropriate statistical methods may be used as an aid in evaluating the test results. There are several criteria for determining a positive result, one of which is a statistically significant dose-related increase in the number of revertants.

Minimum fold increase is another method, expressed as a two- or threefold increase of revertants. However, this is insensitive for strains with relatively high reversion frequencies and is too sensitive for chemicals with low reversion frequencies [31]. Another criterion is based on the mutant frequency, which is expressed as the quotient of the number of revertant colonies over the number of colonies in the negative control. A mutagenic potential of a test item is assumed if the mutant frequency is 2.0 or higher. A possible mutagenic potential is assumed if the quotient ranges between 1.7 and 1.9. No mutagenic potential is assumed if all quotients range between 1.0 and 1.6.

4.10   DISCUSSION

Although the bacterial mutation assay is known for its simplicity, there are many critical factors that can influence the validity of the data, and close attention to every aspect of the experimental procedure is required. Establishment of consistent methods for every phase of the experiment is a prerequisite for obtaining reliable results and for running large numbers of tests in routine screening programs. A deficiency in just one area will jeopardize the whole enterprise. A bacterial mutagenicity assay simply determines whether the substance under investigation is or is not a bacterial mutagen in the presence and/or absence of an exogenous metabolizing system derived from a mammal (S9). Such a test cannot determine whether the test substance is mutagenic and/or carcinogenic in any other species. However, it may be concluded that a substance found to be mutagenic in properly conducted bacterial mutation assays should be regarded as potentially mutagenic or carcinogenic in mammals (including humans) until further evidence indicates otherwise.

4.11   SAFETY CONSIDERATIONS

As mentioned in earlier sections, the bacterial mutation assay is a simple and easy to perform assay. However, there are two important factors to be considered while performing such assays or in designing laboratories for bacterial assays: (1) prevention of contamination of cultures by other microorganisms and (2) protection of staff against exposure to hazardous test chemicals. Hence, experimental procedures should be conducted in appropriate biological safety cabinets in which a curtain of filter-sterilized air protects the worker from chemical exposure and the cultures from contamination.

Mutagen contamination should be avoided. Assays should be performed in a well-ventilated fume hood designated solely for this purpose. Air from the cabinets should be extracted outside the building through appropriate filters to prevent environmental contamination. Incubators should have precise temperature control, and those used for testing purposes should be in an area where the ventilation system removes any hazardous vapors from volatile test chemicals, when incubator doors are opened.

Culture media may be either purchased as ready-poured plates or prepared in the laboratory from basic ingredients. In the latter case, a clean working area must be available for pouring and drying plates. Using disposable test tubes, petri plates, and micropipetters with disposable tips and autoclaving of used materials before washing is highly recommended to avoid recirculation of contamination. During experimentation, the wearing of gowns, eye glasses, and gloves is advisable. Either manual or electronic devices are used for counting bacterial colonies.

Most importantly, a safe means of disposal of cultures should be provided; for example, they should be sealed in plastic or paper sacks in the laboratory and then incinerated. Furthermore, it is essential to devise operating procedures that minimize the hazards from storage, handling, weighing, pipetting, and disposing of mutagens/carcinogens and that deal with accidental contamination. Laboratories performing the test should follow the guidelines. Closed chambers or desiccators are recommended for testing highly volatile chemicals and gases [32].

4.12 CONCLUSION

Point mutations are the cause of many human genetic diseases and there is substantial evidence that point mutations in oncogenes and tumor suppressor genes of somatic cells are involved in tumor formation in humans and experimental animals. The bacterial mutation assay utilizes bacterial strains to detect point mutations. Therefore, chemicals that are mutagenic in bacteria are more likely to cause cancer than chemicals that are not mutagenic. Furthermore, the test has proved to be a valuable component for assessing mutagenic/carcinogenic potential.

ACKNOWLEDGMENT

Grateful thanks to Dr. Mayumi Ishizuka for generously providing the photographs.

REFERENCES

1. Iyer VN, Szybalski W. Two simple methods for the detection of chemical mutagens. *Appl Microbiol* 1958;6:23–29.
2. Ames BN. The detection of chemical mutagens with enteric bacteria. In *Chemical Mutagens: Principles and Methods for Their Detection*. New York: Plenum Press; 1971, Vol 1, pp 267–282.
3. Yanofsky C. Mutagenesis studies with *Escherichia coli* mutants with known amino acid (and base-pair) changes. In *Chemical Mutagens: Principles and Methods for Their Detection*. New York: Plenum Press; 1971, Vol 1, pp 283–287.
4. Gelboin HV, Miller JA, Miller EC. The *in vitro* formation of protein-bound derivatives of aminoazo dyes by rat liver preparations. *Cancer Res* 1959;19:975–985.
5. Miller EC, Miller JA. Mechanisms of chemical carcinogenesis: nature of proximate carcinogens and interactions with macromolecules. *Pharmacol Rev* 1966;18:805–838.

6. Miller EC, Miller JA. Studies on the mechanism of activation of aromatic amine and amide carcinogens to ultimate carcinogenic electrophilic reactants. *Ann NY Acad Sci* 1969;163:731–750.

7. Malling HV. Dimethylnitrosamine: formation of mutagenic compounds by interaction with mouse liver microsomes. *Mutat Res* 1971;13:425–429.

8. Garner RC, Miller EC, Miller JA, Garner JV, Hanson RS. Formation of a factor lethal for *S. typhimurium* TA1530 and TA1531 on incubation of aflatoxin B1 with rat liver microsomes. *Biochem Biophys Res Commun* 1971;45:774–780.

9. Ames BN, Durston WE, Yamasaki E, Lee FD. Carcinogens are mutagens: a simple test system combining liver homogenates for activation and bacteria for detection. *Proc Natl Acad Sci USA* 1973;70:2281–2285.

10. McCann J, Choi E, Yamasaki E, Ames BN. Detection of carcinogens in the *Salmonella*/ microsome test: assay of 300 chemicals. *Proc Natl Acad Sci USA* 1975;72:5135–5139.

11. Sugimura T, Sato S, Nagao M, Yahagi T, Matsushima T, Seino Y, Takeuchi M, Kawachi T. Overlapping of carcinogens and mutagens. In *Fundamentals of Cancer Prevention*. Baltimore: University Park Press; 1976, pp 191–215.

12. Purchase IF, Longstaff E, Ashby J, Styles JA, Anderson D, Lefevre PA, Westwood FR. An evaluation of 6 short-term tests for detecting organic chemical carcinogens. *Br J Cancer* 1978;37:873–903.

13. Green MH, Muriel WJ. Mutagen testing using TRP[+] reversion in *Escherichia coli*. *Mutat Res* 1976;38:3–32.

14. McCann J, Ames BN. Detection of carcinogens as mutagens in the *Salmonella*/microsome test: assay of 300 chemicals: discussion. *Proc Natl Acad Sci USA* 1976;73:950–954.

15. Ames BN, McCann J, Yamasaki E. Methods for detecting carcinogens and mutagens with the *Salmonella*/mammalian microsome mutagenicity test. *Mutat Res* 1975;31:347–364.

16. Ames BN, Lee FD, Durston WE. An improved bacterial test system for the detection and classification of mutagens and carcinogens. *Proc Natl Acad Sci USA* 1973;70:782–786.

17. Yahagi T, Degawa M, Seino Y, Matsushima T, Nagao M. Mutagenicity of carcinogenic azo dyes and their derivatives. *Cancer Lett* 1975;1:91–96.

18. Kier LD, Brusick DJ, Auletta AE, Von Halle ES, Brown MM, Simmon VF, et al. The *Salmonella typhimurium*/mammalian microsomal assay: a report of the U.S. Environmental Protection Agency Gene-Tox Program. *Mutat Res* 1986;168:69–240.

19. Gatehouse D, Haworth S, Cebula T, Gocke E, Kier L, Matsushima T, et al. Recommendations for the performance of bacterial mutation assays. *Mutat Res* 1994;312:217–233.

20. Aeschbacher HU, Wolleb U, Porchet LJ. Liquid preincubation mutagenicity test for foods. *Food Safety* 1987;8:167–177.

21. OECD. *Guidelines for Testing of Chemicals*. Paris: Organization for Economic Co-operation and Development; 1997, pp 1–11.

22. Shanabruch WG, Walker GC. Localization of the plasmid (pKM101) gene(s) involved in recA[+] lexA[+]—dependent mutagenesis. *Mol Gen Genet* 1980;179:289–297.

23. Vogel HJ, Bonner DM. Acetylornithinase of *E. coli*; partial purification and some properties. *J Biol Chem* 1956;218:97–106.

24. Elliott BM, Combes RD, Elcombe CR, Gatehouse DG, Gibson GG, Mackay JM, Wolf RC. Alternatives to Aroclor 1254-induced S9 in *in vitro* genotoxicity assays. *Mutagenesis* 1992;7:175–177.

25. Maron D, Katzenellenbogen J, Ames BN. Compatibility of organic solvents with the *Salmonella*/microsome test. *Mutat Res* 1981;88:343–350.

26. Prival MJ, Bell SJ, Mitchell VD, Peiperl MD, Vaughan VL. Mutagenicity of benzidine and benzidine-congener dyes and selected monoazo dyes in a modified *Salmonella* assay. *Mutat Res* 1984;136:33–47.

27. Araki A, Noguchi T, Kato F, Matsushima T. Improved method for mutagenicity testing of gaseous compounds by using a gas sampling bag. *Mutat Res* 1994;307:335–344.

28. Thompson C, Morley P, Kirkland D, Proudlock R. Modified bacterial mutation test procedures for evaluation of peptides and amino acid-containing material. *Mutagenesis* 2005;20:345–350.

29. Zeiger E, Pagano DA, Robertson IGC. A rapid and simple scheme for confirmation of *Salmonella* tester strain phenotype. *Environ Mutagen* 1981;3:205–209.

30. Maron DM, Ames BN. Revised methods for the *Salmonella* mutagenicity test. *Mutat Res* 1983;113:173–215.

31. Cariello NF, Piegorsch WW. The Ames test: the twofold rule revisited. *Mutat Res* 1996;369:23–31.

32. Hughes TJ, Simmons DM, Monteith LG, Claxton LD. Vaporization technique to measure mutagenic activity of volatile organic chemicals in the Ames/*Salmonella* assay. *Environ Mutagen* 1987;9:421–441.

5

IN VITRO MAMMALIAN CELL MUTATION ASSAYS*

C. Anita H. Bigger,[1] Martha M. Moore,[2] and
Robert H. Heflich[2]

[1]*U.S. Food and Drug Administration, Center for Drug Evaluation and Research, Silver Spring, Maryland*
[2]*U.S. Food and Drug Administration, National Center for Toxicological Research, Jefferson, Arkansas*

Contents

*The views expressed in this chapter do not necessarily reflect FDA policy.

Preclinical Development Handbook: Toxicology, edited by Shayne Cox Gad
Copyright © 2008 John Wiley & Sons, Inc.

5.1   INTRODUCTION

The *in vitro* mammalian cell mutation assays used for preclinical safety testing detect forward mutations at the following target genes: (1) the thymidine kinase gene (*Tk*), (2) the hypoxanthine–guanine phosphoribosyl transferase gene (*Hprt*), and (3) the *E. coli* xanthine–guanine phosphoribosyl transferase gene (*xprt* or *gpt*), integrated into mammalian cell DNA as a stable bacterial transgene [1]. All three target genes detect base substitutions, frameshifts, deletions, insertions, and rearrangements within the locus; however, assays employing the *Tk* gene and the *xprt* transgene offer the additional advantage of detecting mutations involving multi-locus deletion. The *Tk* gene also detects translocation, as well as mutations requiring two alleles, such as mitotic recombination, gene conversion, and chromosome non-disjunction [1–11].

Commonly used cell lines for *in vitro* mammalian cell mutation assays are L5178Y mouse lymphoma cells, Chinese hamster ovary (CHO), AS52, and V79 cell lines derived from Chinese hamsters, and TK6 human lymphoblastoid cells [1]. At this time, by far the most frequently used *in vitro* cell mutation assay in drug development is the Mouse Lymphoma Assay (MLA), utilizing L5178Y mouse lymphoma cells and the *Tk* target gene. This is primarily because the MLA, in addition to being capable of detecting the broadest spectrum of types of genetic damage of the *in vitro* genetic toxicology assays [1–11], is one of the assays in the standard battery of genotoxicity tests agreed upon by the International Conference on Harmonisation of Technical Requirements for Registration of Pharmaceuticals for Human Use (ICH) [12]. The ICH *Guidance for Industry S2B Genotoxicity: A Standard Battery for Genotoxicity Testing of Pharmaceuticals* (ICH S2B) [12] also describes conditions under which the *Hprt* or *xprt* target genes in any of the cell lines mentioned above might be appropriate for assessment of the genotoxic potential of pharmaceuticals.

This chapter provides the following: (1) discussion of regulatory guidance for the use of *in vitro* mammalian cell mutation assays, as well as the role of *in vitro* mammalian cell mutation assays in the evaluation of pharmaceuticals for genetic toxicity; (2) comments on the validated and internationally accepted protocol guidelines available for these assays; (3) discussion of the advantages and disadvantages of the assays for determining the nature of the genotoxicity elicited by pharmaceuticals; and (4) study designs for the MLA, CHO/*Hprt*, and AS52/*xprt* assays, including recent changes to the MLA protocol, test criteria, and evaluation of results.

5.2   REGULATORY GUIDANCES AND PROTOCOL GUIDELINES FOR *IN VITRO* MAMMALIAN CELL MUTATION ASSAYS

5.2.1   Regulatory Guidances

The two primary ICH guidances devoted to genetic toxicology testing of pharmaceuticals are *Guideline for Industry: Specific Aspects of Regulatory Genotoxicity Tests for Pharmaceuticals* (ICH S2A) [13] and *Guidance for Industry S2B Genotoxicity: A Standard Battery for Genotoxicity Testing of Pharmaceuticals* (ICH S2B) [12].

ICH S2A provides guidance and recommendations on conducting the tests and evaluating the test results. The S2A defines the top concentration, cytotoxicity levels, and a strategy for testing poorly soluble compounds with *in vitro* mammalian cell mutation assays. ICH S2A also provides general guidance for the evaluation of assay results.

ICH S2B defines the standard test battery for pharmaceuticals as: (1) a test for gene mutation in bacteria; (2) an *in vitro* test for the cytogenetic evaluation of chromosomal damage in mammalian cells or an *in vitro* MLA measuring *Tk* gene mutation; and (3) an *in vivo* test for chromosomal damage using rodent hematopoietic cells. Other regulatory agencies also recommend this battery of tests for screening chemicals [14]. During the early ICH discussions of the standard battery, some parties preferred a four-test battery that included both of the *in vitro* mammalian assays that are listed in the three-test battery as alternates. The ICH Expert Working Group (EWG), however, reviewed additional studies, some of which were specifically designed to address this issue. The EWG compared results in the two *in vitro* mammalian cell tests for compounds that were considered genotoxic but gave negative results in the bacterial test. These studies demonstrated a high level of congruence between the *in vitro* mammalian cell assays, leading the EWG to conclude that the MLA and the *in vitro* mammalian cell chromosomal damage test could be used interchangeably in the standard battery (see ICH S2B III(ii), Notes 3 and 4). Based on this evidence, the EWG compromised with a three-test battery in which either the *in vitro* mammalian cell cytogenetics assay or the *in vitro* MLA satisfied the second element of the battery.

The ICH S2B also allows modifications of the three-test battery (ICH S2B IV) to include *in vitro* mammalian cell mutation assays other than the MLA. For example, for compounds that are extremely toxic to bacteria or for compounds that interfere with the mammalian cell replication system, the guidance suggests employing two *in vitro* mammalian cell tests. The two tests should use different cell lines and different endpoints, that is, gene mutation and chromosomal damage (ICH S2B IV A). ICH S2B (Note 1) also lists the currently accepted target loci and cell lines for *in vitro* mammalian cell mutation assays: (1) for the *Tk* gene, mouse lymphoma L5178Y cells or human lymphoblastoid TK6 cells; (2) for the *Hprt* gene, CHO cells, V79 cells, or L5178Y cells; and (3) for the *xprt* gene, AS52 cells.

The ICH S2B defines standard procedures for *in vitro* mammalian cell mutation tests other than the MLA (ICH S2A V) and indicates that a range-finding test can substitute for a complete repeat of the assay, as long as certain criteria are met (ICH S2B Note 10). For the MLA, the guidance states that the protocol must include testing with and without exogenous metabolic activation, with appropriate controls, and with treatment for 3 or 4 hours. If the short treatment without metabolic activation is negative, then that arm of the test should be repeated with treatment for 24 hours. An acceptable MLA also includes positive controls that induce small colonies and colony sizing for both positive and negative controls and at least one positive test compound dose, if present.

Both ICH S2A and ICH S2B were finalized approximately a decade ago. At the present time, there is discussion of revising these two guidances through the ICH Maintenance Procedure. That process, however, is likely to require years of discussion to achieve an agreed upon, finalized guidance to replace S2A and S2B. In the interim, possible changes to the guidances are discussed at international genetic toxicology meetings and conclusions are disseminated through publications in the literature. For example, the ICH S2B states that the microwell (or microtiter) method for the MLA is preferred over the agar method for use in the standard battery (ICH S2B Note 4). After extensive discussion, an informal agreement was reached between all the parties to the ICH EWG for genetic toxicology that both versions of the assay are acceptable for regulatory purposes. This information was made public through several publications [15, 16].

Other ICH guidances that govern the regulatory use of *in vitro* mammalian cell mutation assays are: (1) *ICH M3 Guidance: Non-clinical Safety Studies for the Conduct of Human Clinical Trials for Pharmaceuticals* [17]; (2) *ICH S1B Guidance: Testing for Carcinogenicity of Pharmaceuticals* [18]; (3) *ICH Q3A Guidance: Impurities in New Drug Substances* [19]; and (4) *ICH Q3B Guidance: Impurities in New Drug Products* [20].

ICH M3 states that, prior to the first human exposure to a pharmaceutical, *in vitro* assays should be performed to evaluate the ability of the pharmaceutical to induce mutations and chromosomal damage. The MLA is one option for addressing this recommendation.

ICH S1B states that additional genetic toxicology testing may be warranted in cases where the compound was negative in the standard battery but was positive in a carcinogenicity test with no evidence of an epigenetic mechanism. Additional tests could include changing the metabolic activation system used in the *in vitro* assays.

The decision trees for ICH Q3A and Q3B include a minimum screen for the genotoxic potential of impurities. The minimum screen consists of two *in vitro* studies, one to detect point mutations and one to detect chromosomal aberrations.

In addition to ICH guidances, regulatory agencies also may provide guidance to industry. The U.S. Food and Drug Administration (FDA) recently issued *Guidance for Industry and Review Staff: Recommended Approaches to Integration of Genetic Toxicology Study Results* [21]. The purpose of this guidance is to inform industry how the FDA Center for Drug Evaluation and Research (CDER) views positive genetic toxicology findings. The guidance gives recommendations on how to proceed with clinical studies when the results of genetic toxicology assays indicate the pharmaceutical may be capable of inducing genetic damage and cancer. The guidance recommends a number of options when one or more of the three assays in the ICH standard battery of genetic toxicology tests are positive. With respect to *in vitro* mammalian cell mutation assays, if any one of the three assays in the standard battery is positive, the guidance recommends first performing the fourth test in the standard battery and then applying a weight of evidence evaluation of the data. For example, a positive finding in an *in vitro* chromosomal aberration assay should be corroborated by positive findings in the MLA using the same exposure regimen. If the results of the MLA assay are negative, then doubt is cast on the significance of the positive finding in the *in vitro* chromosomal aberration assay. The guidance also emphasizes the need to carefully control cytotoxicity levels in the *in vitro* assays in order to avoid a secondary genotoxic effect that is not directly related to treatment with the test compound.

5.2.2   Protocol Guidelines

The following protocol guidelines are available for *in vitro* mammalian cell mutation assays: (1) *OECD Guideline for the Testing of Chemicals: In Vitro Mammalian Cell Gene Mutation Test* [22]; (2) *EPA Health Effects Test Guidelines OPPTS 870.5300:*

In Vitro Mammalian Cell Gene Mutation Test [23]; (3) Reports from the MLA Workgroup of the International Workshop on Genotoxicity Testing (IWGT) from meetings in Washington, District of Columbia, in 1999 [16], New Orleans, Louisiana, in 2000 [24], Plymouth, England in 2002 [25], Aberdeen, Scotland in 2003 [26], and in San Francisco, California, in 2005 [27]; and (4) *FDA CFSAN Redbook 2000: IV.C.1.c. Mouse Lymphoma Thymidine Kinase Gene Mutation Assay* [28].

The Organization for Economic Cooperation and Development (OECD) and the U.S. Environmental Protection Agency (EPA) guidelines on the *in vitro* mammalian cell gene mutation test are similar and both give general recommendations covering all the target genes and cell lines used for *in vitro* mammalian cell gene mutation testing. However, there are significant differences between the MLA and the other *in vitro* mammalian cell mutation assays employing the *Hprt* and *xprt* genes, and these guidelines do not address those differences in adequate detail for practical use.

The IWGT convened the MLA Workgroup to address a number of issues concerning the MLA. Through a series of meetings beginning in 1999, the Workgroup reached consensus on five areas: (1) acceptable versions of the assay, the soft agar [29], and microwell versions [30, 31]; (2) a common cytotoxicity measure for both versions of the assay; (3) acceptability of a 24 hour treatment arm; (4) microwell sizing and colony counting; and (5) criteria for data acceptance and approaches for data evaluation. At the first meeting in Washington, DC, the Workgroup agreed that both versions of the assay are equally acceptable and formulated a strategy for reaching consensus on the other four issues. Since the Workgroup agreed that more data were necessary before decisions could be made, data were gathered in ten laboratories for analysis and discussion at the subsequent meetings. Since the first meeting, the MLA Workgroup has reached consensus for all areas of focus and has published its recommendations for conducting the assay in five publications [16, 24–27].

The FDA CFSAN Redbook 2000 published a chapter on the MLA in October 2001. This chapter presented a detailed protocol for the assay; however, because it was published before the IWGT MLA Workgroup had completed its work, the chapter did not contain all of the MLA Workgroup recommendations. A recent update of the Redbook 2000 (April 2006) includes the IWGT MLA Workgroup recommendations through reference to the MLA Workgroup publications.

5.3 ENDPOINTS AND UNIQUE CHARACTERISTICS OF *IN VITRO* MAMMALIAN CELL MUTATION ASSAYS

5.3.1 Differences in the Spectra of Genetic Events Detected by *In Vitro* Mammalian Cell Mutation Assays

As indicated previously, the *in vitro* mammalian cell assays employing the *Tk, Hprt*, and *xprt* genes all detect base pair substitutions, frameshifts, deletions, insertions, and rearrangements within the locus; however, the MLA offers the additional advantage of being able to detect mutations involving the loss of multiple genes and recombination between chromosome homologs. This is because the *Tk* gene in the MLA cell line (L5178Y *Tk*$^{+/-}$-3.7.2C) is on an autosome (mouse chromosome 11) and it is heterozygous; that is, one of its alleles is wild-type while the other is a nonfunctional mutant. The same is true of the *TK* gene in TK6 cells, although the *TK* gene lies on chromosome 17 in human cells, and the inactivating mutations in the negative alleles of L5178Y *Tk*$^{+/-}$ and TK6 cells are different. In contrast, the hemizygous (or functionally hemizygous) location of the *Hprt* gene on the X chromosome makes it unlikely that mutations involving multilocus deletion or recombination will be recovered in assays employing this target gene [4].

In order to facilitate the identification of mammalian cells that have undergone a mutation, gene targets have been chosen so that single mutations can confer a selectable phenotype to the cells. One way to do this is to choose a target gene that is located on the X chromosome. This was the strategy used for the development of the CHO/*Hprt* assay and other assays employing the *Hprt* gene. Another approach, and the one used for the development of the MLA, is to create a cell strain in which one of the alleles of an autosomal target gene is a nonfunctional mutant. This is the case for the L5178Y *Tk*$^{+/-}$-3.7.2C strain. A major (theoretical) difference between these two types of mutational targets relates to their ability to detect multilocus deletions. The function of genes vital to the survival of the cell that flank the *Tk* gene can be provided by their homologs on the *Tk*$^{-}$ chromosome; thus, mouse lymphoma cells will survive even if the *Tk*$^{+}$ allele and vital surrounding genes are deleted from the *Tk*$^{+}$ chromosome. In the case of the *Hprt* gene, large deletions may never be seen because there is no back-up in the cell to provide the function of vital genes eliminated along with the *Hprt* gene; there is only one functional copy of each gene on the X chromosome, even in female cells. The presence of two functional alleles allows the MLA to detect mitotic recombination/gene conversion and those chromosomal events that typically are detected by cytogenetics assay, such as large structural deletions, translocations, and aneuploidy. None of these are detected by the CHO/*Hprt* assay or other assays employing the *Hprt* gene [7–11]. These theoretical considerations form the mechanistic rationale for treating the MLA and *in vitro* chromosomal damage assays as equal alternatives in regulatory testing batteries.

An additional feature of the MLA is that the mutant colonies that are detected in the assay fall into two size categories: small colonies with a slow growth rate and large colonies with a wild-type growth rate. The molecular and cytogenetic nature of small and large colonies has been studied extensively over the years [7–9, 32, 33], but the reasons underlying these growth phenotypes still are incompletely understood. In general, small colony mutants are induced by chemicals that are regarded as clastogens; that is, they have the ability to break chromosomes [34]. In contrast, large colony mutants are more likely to be induced by chemicals that induce small genetic lesions, such as point mutations. Thus, the mutagenic mechanism of a test article can be inferred from the proportion of small and large colonies induced by that test article.

The AS52 cell assay uses a CHO cell line that has a nonrevertable *Hprt* deletion mutation, but that carries a single, expressed copy of the bacterial *xprt* (or *gpt*) gene on one of its autosomes [35, 36]. The *xprt* gene is the functional equivalent of the *Hprt* gene so that *xprt* mutants are selected by 6-thioguanine (TG) in the AS52 assay similarly to how *Hprt* mutants are selected in the CHO/*Hprt* assay (see below for a description of mutant selection). The AS52 assay has some of the theoretical advantages of the MLA for detecting mutations: because the *xprt* gene is on an autosome, multilocus deletions that include the *xprt* gene are not necessarily lethal. Comparative analyses of the *Hprt* and AS52 cell assays indicate that a higher percentage of mutations with deletions are detected by the AS52 cell assay and that AS52 cells are more sensitive to the mutagenicity of clastogenic agents [37–41]. Because AS52 cells contain only one copy of the *xprt* gene, however, the AS52 cell assay does not detect mutations requiring two alleles (e.g., mitotic recombination) as does the MLA.

5.3.2 Differences in the Spectra of Genetic Events Detected by the MLA, the *In Vitro* Chromosomal Aberrations Assays, and the Ames Test

The MLA detects mutations that do not compromise the viability of the cell; that is, the assay detects only heritable changes in DNA sequence. Besides relatively small changes within the *Tk* gene, these mutations include large alterations (e.g., translocations, deletions) that also can be detected cytogenetically. The *in vitro* chromosomal aberration assay detects only microscopically visible (i.e., relatively large) chromosome alterations, many of which are not heritable to daughter and granddaughter cells because they are lethal events. Like the MLA, the Ames test detects only heritable alterations in DNA. However, the Ames test employs a series of specifically designed mutant tester strains, and each tester strain detects a limited spectrum of either base pair substitution or frameshift mutations. Because sequence context can cause striking differences in mutagenic frequencies at a given site [42], the specificity of the mutational target and the use of a bacterial chromosome rather than eukaryotic chromosomes as the target for mutation severely restricts the spectrum of point mutations detected in the Ames test. Unlike the MLA, the Ames test is incapable of detecting mutations larger than frameshifts, including mutations requiring chromosome homologs and sequence alterations generally considered chromosome-type mutations. Finally, the mutations that are detected by both the MLA and the Ames test alter the phenotype of the test cell. For the MLA, only mutations that inactivate the Tk^+ allele will be identified, while only mutations that restore the wild-type function of the target sequence will be scored as mutants in the Ames test. The only limitation on scoring sequence changes in cytogenetic assays is that they be visible microscopically.

5.3.3 Correlation of *In Vitro* Mammalian Cell Mutation Assays with Rodent Bioassays

Early in the development of the field of genetic toxicology, the various assays were claimed to be short-term tests that could be used to identify carcinogens. Over the years, a number of studies have been conducted to assess the ability of the assays to predict whether a chemical is a carcinogen. A very influential study conducted by the National Toxicology Program (NTP) used data generated by contractors specifically for the analysis [43]. More recently, Kirkland et al. [44, 45] and Matthews et al. [46, 47] have used extensive genetic toxicology databases compiled from a variety of sources with the goal of obtaining a more current assessment. All of these studies report that *in vitro* mammalian mutation assays have relatively low predictive ability for rodent carcinogenicity.

Unfortunately, the assays, particularly the MLA and the *in vitro* aberration assays, have evolved over the years, not only with respect to their protocols, but also in the acceptance criteria and the evaluation of data. This has resulted in a large number of assays that do not meet the current guidelines being included in the databases used for these studies of assay predictive ability. With the exception of the EPA Gene-Tox Expert Committee reports conducted in the 1980s [48], there has been no expert panel review of the databases. It should be noted that the MLA Gene-Tox panel placed a large number of chemicals (particularly from the NTP studies) into a category of insufficient data to determine whether the response was positive or negative [48]. The major reasons for this situation were that the dose selection process used for the NTP studies often did not provide data in the critical portion of the dose–response curve and that the NTP used a unique set of criteria for their positive and negative calls.

Because there currently is no adequate database for the MLA and chromosome aberration assay, it is unclear as to how well these assays actually predict the carcinogenicity of chemicals. Furthermore, in interpreting the data from genotoxicity studies, including *in vitro* mammalian cell mutation assays, it is important to keep in mind that cancer is a multistep process, having multiple modes of action, and that mutation is only one of the possible key events involved in the etiology of tumors.

5.4   CRITICISMS OF *IN VITRO* MAMMALIAN CELL ASSAYS

5.4.1   False Positives, High Concentrations, and Cytotoxicity Criteria

There is currently a lively debate in the regulatory community concerning the issue of too many "false positives" in the *in vitro* mammalian assays, specifically the MLA and the chromosome aberration test. This statement often is made based on the fact that the Ames test and the *in vivo* micronucleus (MN) assays for a test agent are negative while the *in vitro* mammalian assays are positive. There are several factors that may contribute to the generation of these "false positives."

First, as already indicated, it is expected that there will be chemicals that are positive in the *in vitro* mammalian assays and negative in the Ames test. In particular, chemicals that exclusively cause chromosomal damage (clastogens) will only be detected in assays capable of detecting chromosomal alterations; they would be expected to be negative in the Ames test. Furthermore, the *in vivo* MN assay detects only those events that result in micronuclei, which are not representative of the full spectrum of genetic damage. In addition, the rodent hematopoietic system target in this assay may not be reflective of other tissues. Finally, adequate concentrations of the test agent may not reach the bone marrow target for MN formation.

Second, the term "false positive" is often applied when a chemical is positive in a genetic toxicology assay and negative in the cancer bioassay. This should not be an unanticipated finding; the induction of mutation is only one of the possible modes of action for tumor induction. It would be more appropriate to judge the *in vitro* mutation assays for their ability to predict the induction of *in vivo* mutation.

Third, *in vitro* assays are criticized for the use of test agent concentrations higher than those that can be achieved *in vivo*. It is important to understand that by design the *in vitro* assays have properties that are unique to the *in vitro* test conditions. These properties make it possible to use high concentrations of test article and very short treatment times compared to those used *in vivo* (e.g., cancer bioassays typically are conducted using 2-year exposures). High test article concentrations and short treatment times are consistent with the role of *in vitro* assays in risk assessment, which is hazard identification. The use of high doses for short durations is intended to reveal potential test-article-induced toxicities before the drug is administered *in vivo* for longer durations at lower doses. In addition, high concentrations may be necessary to ensure assay validity. During the development of the MLA, a panel of known carcinogens was tested to determine what concentrations would be necessary to achieve a positive result in this assay [49]. This study revealed that the lowest effective concentration ranged from less than 1 μg/mL to over 10 mg/mL. Recent studies [44, 45], using reevaluated MLA data, found a similar broad range (<1 to >10,000 μM) for producing a positive response in the MLA. Importantly, these studies reported that, if positive results were included only when obtained below 10 mM, currently the internationally agreed upon limit dose for MLA [13], 5 out of 29 rodent carcinogens would not be found positive in the MLA.

Fourth, the *in vitro* assays are criticized for using high cytotoxicity levels. It is important to note that the criteria for cytotoxicity levels in the *in vitro* mammalian cell assays were established in the same manner as those establishing the maximum high concentration: that is, tests of panels of known carcinogens established appropriate cytotoxicity levels [49]. The ICH S2A (II.A.2.b.iii) [13] recommendation that the highest concentration should produce at least 80% toxicity reflects the high levels of cytotoxicity necessary to detect some carcinogens in these assays.

However, high doses of the test materials can result in nonphysiological alterations of osmolality and pH, leading to false-positive responses [13, 29]. Secondary effects from too much cytotoxicity also can cause increases in mutant frequency or chromosome aberrations. This raises the issue of biologically irrelevant responses (false positives) that may be obtained *in vitro*. Such positive responses would be expected to be observed only at the "higher" cytotoxicity levels, levels that may not be reached *in vivo*. In order to reduce/minimize the number of these biologically irrelevant "positive" responses, the ICH S2A (II.A.2.b.iii) [13] recommends caution with positive results obtained at levels of survival lower than 10% and requires demonstrating that osmolality and pH are maintained at appropriate levels during testing. For this reason, the IWGT MLA Workgroup set the maximum cytotoxicity level for the MLA, based on relative total growth (RTG), at 10%. As explained in more detail later, RTG is calculated by multiplying the relative suspension growth by the relative plating efficiency at the time of cloning for mutant selection. It is important to note that this DOES NOT represent killing 90% of the cells. For example, if a treated culture grows 50% as well as the negative control over the 2 day suspension growth period and plates 30% as well as the negative control during mutant selection, the RTG will be 15% (50% × 30%).

Despite the rationale for high concentrations and cytotoxicity levels and criteria for assay validity that set limit levels for both concentration and cytotoxicity, there is a "gray" zone where the concentration and/or cytotoxicity are close to the limit levels and the positive response in the assay is very weak. The biological relevance of such results to hazard identification is questionable. It is this "gray" zone that is driving much of the current debate on whether or not concentrations and cytotoxicity levels in the *in vitro* assays should be lowered and, if so, by what criteria. Since Kirkland et al. [44, 45] have shown that the current high concentration of 10 mM will not detect some rodent carcinogens, there also is concern that altering the test criteria by further lowering the top concentration or reducing the cytotoxicity limit will compromise safety assessments of drugs in development.

5.4.2 Hazard Identification and Risk Assessment

For preclinical safety evaluation, the *in vitro* mammalian (and other) genotoxicity assays are used to identify compounds that pose a hazard to exposed humans, specifically a hazard to the genetic material. The assays also are used as a part of the weight of the evidence evaluation for whether a chemical is a carcinogen and to make other safety assessments as a part of the drug approval process. Currently, the *in vitro* mammalian cell mutation assays are not used for establishing a safe human dose because the *in vitro* conditions of these tests do not sufficiently mimic *in vivo* physiological conditions, such as endogenous metabolism and detoxification systems, and do not provide information on the targeting of specific tissues by a drug. Although the drug approval process generally does not include a quantitative risk assessment for compounds that are genotoxicants, it should be noted that genotoxicity assays play a key role in such evaluations in other regulatory contexts (e.g., the setting of allowable limits for drinking water, air, and food contaminants), where the public has little choice in exposure to hazardous substances [50].

5.5 PROTOCOLS FOR *IN VITRO* MAMMALIAN CELL MUTATION ASSAYS

5.5.1 Commonalities and Differences in Protocols for *In Vitro* Mammalian Cell Mutation Assays

All of the assays include (1) cell preparation; (2) a preliminary cytotoxicity test to determine initial doses for the definitive assays; (3) the use of an exogenous metabolic activation system in one arm of treatment; (4) an expression period that allows fixation of DNA damage generated by the test article and depletion of the wild-type enzyme produced by the target gene; (5) a selection period during which the cells are treated with an agent that is toxic to nonmutant cells; (6) collection of data on the number of mutant versus wild-type cells, the level of cytotoxicity, and the cloning efficiency; (7) data analyses to determine cytotoxicity, cloning efficiency, and mutant frequency; and (8) evaluation of the validity of the test and the response to the test article.

The assays differ procedurally in a number of ways: the methods used for culturing and cloning of cells, the length of the expression period, the agents used for selection of mutants, and the manner of data collection. For example, the CHO/*Hprt* assay uses attached monolayer cultures and single-cell cloning of attached cells, while the MLA uses cultures of unattached cells in suspension and cloning either by immobilization in agar or by plating at limiting-dilutions in 96-well microtiter plates. However, the major difference in the assays stems from the differences in the target genes for mutation detection, as exemplified by the two most commonly used mammalian cell mutation assays, the MLA and the CHO/*Hprt* assay.

The *Tk* target gene used for the MLA is located on mouse chromosome 11 and codes for thymidine kinase (Tk), an enzyme involved in thymidine triphosphate synthesis [49, 51]. Thymidine triphosphate can be generated through metabolism of deoxyuridine monophosphate by thymidylate synthetase (*de novo* pathway) or by phosphorylation of exogenous thymidine by Tk (pyrimidine salvage pathway). The pyrimidine analogue trifluorothymidine (TFT) is also a substrate for Tk. However, phosphorylation of TFT makes cells vulnerable to its cytotoxic and cytostatic effects. Thus, TFT can be used as a selective agent for mouse lymphoma cells that have been mutated (either spontaneously or by the the test article) from $Tk^{+/-}$ (Tk-proficient) to $Tk^{-/-}$ (Tk-deficient) [52]. Mutation of the Tk^+ allele to Tk^- renders the cell resistant to the toxic effects of TFT; the cells remain viable because DNA synthesis can still be carried out by the *de novo* synthetic pathway. When test-article-exposed cells subsequently are grown in medium containing TFT, only $Tk^{-/-}$ cells can grow and the mutant frequency can be determined from the number of clones appearing in TFT-containing medium. Because cells in culture do not clone with 100% efficiency, the mutant frequencies are calculated by adjusting the number of clones observed in the presence of TFT with the cloning efficiency of cells from the same culture in medium without TFT.

The X-chromosome-linked *Hprt* target gene used for the CHO/*Hprt* assay codes for an enzyme in another salvage pathway, one involved in purine nucleotide synthesis [53, 54]. The Hprt enzyme catalyzes the transfer of a phosphoribosyl moiety to guanine or hypoxanthine, thereby creating a purine mononucleotide. The purine analogue 6-thioguanine (TG) is also a substrate for Hprt, generating 6-thioguanine monophosphate (TGMP). TGMP inhibits purine nucleotide biosynthesis through a feedback mechanism and is, in addition, toxic to the cell through incorporation into DNA and RNA. Thus, as was the case with TFT and the MLA, TG can be used to select cells in which the enzyme coded by the *Hprt* target gene has been mutated and rendered inactive. Mutated cells remain viable in the presence of toxic concentrations of TG because purine nucleotides continue to be produced via an endogenous *de novo* pathway that does not involve Hprt.

As indicted earlier, the product of the *xprt* transgene of AS52 cells is the functional equivalent of Hprt, the only difference being that xprt will phosphorylate xanthine as well as guanine and hypoxanthine [35]. From a methodological standpoint, TG can be used to select xprt-deficient AS52 cell mutants using the same methods developed for selecting Hprt-deficient mutants in the CHO/*Hprt* assay [55].

5.5.2   Detailed Protocols

MLA

1. *Principle of the Assay.* The purpose of the MLA is to determine the ability of a test article to induce forward mutations in the L5178Y $Tk^{+/-}$ mouse lymphoma cell line. The mutations are detected by growth of colonies in the presence of TFT.

2. *Soft Agar Versus Microwell Versions of the MLA.* There are two equally acceptable methods for conducting the MLA: (1) the soft agar method [29] and the microwell (or microtiter) method [30, 31]. The principal difference between these two methods is the technique used for cloning. In the first method, single cells are immobilized in soft agar medium in petri dishes, allowed to grow into clones, and counted. In the microwell method, cells are cloned by limiting dilution in 96-well

microwell plates. Over the years, some additional differences between the two methods developed, mainly involving the calculation of mutant frequency and the determination of cytotoxicity. Since 1999, the IWGT MLA Workgroup has been bringing the two methods into alignment with the goal of developing an internationally harmonized guideline for the conduct and interpretation of the assay. The consensus agreements [16, 24–27] for protocol changes in the MLA are included below. Additional updated descriptions of the protocol can be found in the FDA CFSAN RedBook 2000 [28] and in Chen and Moore [56].

3. *Cells.* It is important that the $Tk^{+/-}$-3.7.2C subline of L5178Y mouse lymphoma cells, the subline used to develop and validate the assay, be used for the MLA. Cells should be checked periodically for mycoplasma contamination and karyotype stability. Both a banded and spectral karyotype for the cell line have been published [10,11,57]. Attention should be paid to population doubling time (between 8 and 10 hours) when developing master stocks. Cells should be maintained in log-phase culture for no longer than approximately 3 months; at which time, a new working stock culture should be initiated. Some laboratories prefer to use a freshly thawed vial of cells for each experiment. The cells are used for the assay after they have recovered from the thawing and are growing normally.

4. *Media and Culture Conditions.* Both Fischer's Medium for Leukemic Cells of Mice and RPMI 1640 medium are appropriate for the MLA assay but these two media are used somewhat differently, as detailed in Chen and Moore [56]. It is important that the culture conditions promote optimal growth during the expression period and maximize colony forming ability for both mutant and nonmutant cells. In addition, the culture conditions must ensure optimal growth of small colony *Tk* mutants. In particular, different lots of horse serum should be tested for their ability to support optimal growth in suspension culture, high plating efficiency, and high small colony mutant recovery.

Maintenance of pH and osmolality in the physiological range (pH 7.0 ± 0.4 and 300 ± 20 mOsm) is critical for avoiding false-positive results [29].

5. *Preparation of Cultures.* Cells from stock cultures are seeded into culture medium and incubated at $37\,^{\circ}$C. Before use in the assay, the cells are cleansed of preexisting mutants by growth in a medium containing methotrexate, thymidine, hypoxanthine, and guanine so that Tk-deficient cells are inhibited while Tk-competent cells grow optimally [29].

6. *Metabolic Activation.* Cells lose metabolic competence after a few passages as a cell line. Since many chemicals require metabolism to show genotoxic potential, test articles must be tested in the presence and absence of an exogenous metabolic activation system. The most commonly used metabolic activation system contains a postmitochondrial supernatant (S9) prepared from the livers of Aroclor-1254-induced male rats supplemented with a standard mixture of cofactors. The amount of S9 varies from 1% to 10% v/v in the final test medium. The standard S9 is available commercially or can be produced by published methods [29]. Alternative metabolic activation systems such as the use of S9 from another species or the use of hepatocytes [58, 59] should be justified scientifically.

7. *Solvent/Vehicle.* The solvent/vehicle is chosen principally on the basis of its ability to dissolve the test article. The solvent/vehicle also must not reduce cell survival or S9 activity or react with the test article. An aqueous solvent (water or culture

medium) is preferred, but organic solvents, such as dimethyl sulfoxide (DMSO), acetone, or ethyl alcohol, can be used in the MLA when necessary to achieve sufficient solubility of the test article.

8. *Dose Selection.* Dose selection is based on the cytotoxicity and solubility of the test article, and the criteria for determining the highest dose described in ICH S2A [13]. For *in vitro* mammalian cell mutation assays, ICH S2A (II.2) defines the top concentration for freely soluble, nontoxic compounds as 5 mg/mL or 10 mM, whichever is lower. ICH S2A recognizes that some genotoxic compounds are active in *in vitro* mammalian cell mutation assays only at cytotoxic doses and that excessive cytotoxicity can induce secondary genotoxic events unrelated to the drug being tested. Keeping these facts in mind, the ICH EWG agreed that *in vitro* mammalian cell mutation assays should produce at least 80% cytotoxicity (i.e., no more than 20% survival), but that positive results obtained at survival levels below 10% are suspect and generally do not serve as a basis for the evaluation of test results. The IWGT MLA Workgroup also agreed on circumstances under which a test article could be deemed nonmutagenic when there is no test culture with an RTG (a measure of cytotoxicity; see below for definition) between 10% and 20% [24]: (1) there is no evidence of mutagenicity in a series of data points falling between 20% and 100% RTG and there is one negative data point between 20% and 25% RTG; (2) there is no evidence of mutagenicity in data points falling between 25% and 100% RTG and there is a negative data point between 1% and 10% RTG.

The IWGT MLA Workgroup addressed the issue that the two versions of the assay (agar and microwell) had evolved to use different cytotoxicity measures [16, 24]. The cytotoxicity measure commonly used for the microwell method was the relative survival (RS), determined by cloning cells immediately after treatment. This measurement was not made in laboratories using the soft agar method. The cytotoxicity measure for the soft agar method was the relative total growth (RTG), which is a combination of cell loss after treatment, reduction in growth rate during the expression period, and reduction in the cloning efficiency determined when the cells are plated for mutant selection. Another cytotoxicity measure, relative suspension growth (RSG), also was widely used for the selection of doses for the full mutation assay. The situation was further confounded by the use of two slightly different protocols for the microwell method, which resulted in different calculations of the RS, RSG, and RTG, such that a comparison of results between the two methods was not reliable. After additional data analysis and discussion, the Workgroup reached a consensus that the RTG would be the cytotoxicity measure for both the soft agar and microwell methods and that an adjustment—that includes any cytotoxicity that occurs during the treatment phase of the assay—would be applied to one of the two microwell method protocols. This adjustment makes the RS, RSG, and RTG values from both microwell methods and the soft agar version comparable.

The ICH S2A [13] also addressed the problems associated with testing insoluble compounds with *in vitro* mammalian mutagenesis assays. While recognizing that there is evidence that insoluble compounds may induce dose-related genotoxic activity in the insoluble range, precipitates may interfere with the scoring of the endpoint, render dose exposure uncontrollable, and make the compound unavailable to the cells. In the case of the MLA, cells are grown in suspension and are normally pelleted by centrifugation at the end of the treatment period and resuspended in fresh medium to remove the test article. If the test article precipitates, it will be pelleted with the cells and taken up with them into fresh medium, thereby extending the treatment time and possibly interfering with scoring mutant colonies. The ICH S2A recommends the following approach for testing insoluble compounds. If evidence of cytotoxicity is missing, the lowest precipitating concentration in the final treatment medium should be designated the high concentration as long as it does not exceed the 5 mg/mL or 10 mM maximum for testing with mammalian cell lines.

A dose range-finding experiment may be used to determine appropriate doses to achieve optimum cytotoxicity levels in the definitive tests. For this preliminary assay, cells are treated in the presence and absence of exogenous metabolic activation for 3 or 4 hours. Sufficient doses (e.g., nine or more) are used to cover a wide dose range (e.g., 4-log dose range) up to the limit of solubility or to the limit dose (5 mg/mL or 10 mM). After suspension growth for 24 hours, cells from test-article-treated and solvent control cultures are counted and diluted. After another 24 hours of suspension growth, cells from all cultures are again counted. The cell counts are used to determine cytotoxicity based on total suspension growth over the 48 hours of culture as compared to the solvent control cultures. The results are used to select doses for the definitive assay.

9. *Controls.* Positive and negative controls should be included in each experiment. The negative control should be exposed to the solvent/vehicle in the same manner as cultures receiving the test article. Untreated controls also should be included if there are no data on the responses produced by the solvent/vehicle in the assay.

The positive control should demonstrate the induction of small colony mutants and one positive control should require metabolic activation to serve as a control for S9 activity. Cyclophosphamide, benzo[*a*]pyrene, and 3-methylcholanthrene are appropriate controls for the metabolic activation arm of the test. Methyl methanesulfonate is appropriate for the arm without metabolic activation.

10. *Treatment with Test Article.* For the definitive assay, single or duplicate cultures may be used, as long as a sufficient number of concentrations are used to ensure that the appropriate dosing range has been covered. Logarithmically growing cells in suspension are treated with the test article in the presence and absence of metabolic activation for 3 or 4 hours. If the test article is particularly insoluble, a longer time may be warranted. ICH S2B (V and Note 4) [12] recommends a 24 hour treatment in the absence of metabolic activation for all test articles testing negative with the 3 or 4 hour treatment. ICH S2B also states that the detection of aneugens is enhanced by the use of a 24 hour treatment using the microwell method. The IWGT MLA Workgroup considered the usefulness of this requirement and published a consensus report on its findings [27]. After analyzing 990 datasets, the group found that less than 2% of the chemicals were uniquely positive at 24 hours. They found that the 24 hour treatment was effective for insoluble chemicals that could not be tested at adequate levels of cytotoxicity. The group also found evidence that some (but not all) aneugens require the longer treatment time. Based on these data, the group agreed to continue supporting the ICH recommendation that a 24 hour treatment be used when short treatment results are negative or equivocal.

11. *Expression Time and Measurement of Mutant Frequency.* After treatment, the cells are pelleted by centrifugation and washed to remove the test article by suspension in fresh media and recentrifugation. Cultures are grown for 2 days to allow expression of the mutant phenotype [60]. Cells are then cloned in the presence and absence of TFT [52], using either the soft agar or microwell method [16], in order to determine the cloning efficiency of cells in the presence and absence of mutant selection. Plates with seeded cells are incubated for 11–14 days, followed by colony counting and sizing.

The two cloning efficiencies (with and without TFT) are used to calculate the mutant frequency for each treatment. Mutant frequencies are calculated differently when using the soft agar method and the microwell method. For the soft agar method, mutant frequency (MF) is calculated by dividing the number of TFT-resistant colonies by the number of cells plated for selection, corrected for the plating efficiency (PE) of the cells. PE is determined from the cloning efficiency of cells from the same culture grown in the absence of TFT. This calculation can be expressed as MF = (number of mutants/number of cells plated) × PE. For the microwell method, the Poisson distribution is used to calculate PEs for cells cloned without TFT and with TFT selection. From the zero term of the Poisson distribution, the probable number of clones/well (P) is equal to −ln(negative wells/total wells) and PE = P/(Number of cells plated per well). Mutant frequency is then calculated as MF = (PE(TFT selected)/PE(unselected)). Mutant frequency usually is expressed as TFT-resistant mutants per 10^6 clonable cells or per 10^6 survivors.

12. *Mutant Colony Sizing.* For the soft agar method, colonies are counted and sized using an automatic colony counter capable of evaluating the size of the colonies.

For the microwell method, colonies are identified by eye or low power microscope. Small colonies are less than one-quarter of the diameter of the well, while large colonies are more than one-quarter of the diameter of the well (standard 96-well flat-bottomed culture plate).

If the test article is positive, colony sizing should be performed on mutant colonies from at least one of the treated cultures, preferably from the highest acceptable concentration, and on mutant colonies from the negative and positive controls. If the test article is negative, colony sizing should be performed on mutant colonies from the negative and positive controls. The assay, and a negative evaluation, is not valid unless the positive control demonstrates the ability to induce small colony mutants. Colony sizing of the negative control will demonstrate that large colonies are able to grow appropriately.

13. *Assay Validity Criteria.* Data should include pH and osmolality determinations, information on test article solubility, test article concentrations in dosing solutions, PE and cell count determinations, colony counts and mutant frequencies for control and treated cultures, RS, RTG, and RSG determinations, and the results of colony sizing of mutant colonies from at least one concentration of the test article for a positive response and of mutant colonies from the negative and positive controls regardless of outcome. These data must demonstrate that appropriate physiological conditions were maintained during the test, that the test concentrations were appropriate in that either a positive mutant frequency response or an 80% reduction in RTG or a persistent precipitate was achieved, and that the assay was able to

recover small colony mutants. In addition, acceptance criteria (see below) for the negative/vehicle and positive controls must be met.

Criteria for Negative/Vehicle and Positive Controls   The IWGT MLA Workgroup [26] reached consensus on acceptance criteria for the soft agar and microwell method negative/vehicle control parameters using the 3 or 4 hour treatment, as shown in the following table.

Parameter	Soft Agar Method	Microwell Method
Mutant frequency	$35–140 \times 10^{-6}$	$50–170 \times 10^{-6}$
Cloning efficiency	65–120%	65–120%
Suspension growth	8–32-fold	8–32-fold

In establishing these criteria, the Workgroup decided to include a measure of how well the negative/vehicle control cells grow during the 2 day expression phase. Suspension growth reflects the number of times the cell number increases from the starting cell density. Cells in stock cultures generally should undergo a 5-fold increase in number every 24 hours. Thus, over a 2 day period, there would theoretically be a 25-fold increase. The group was particularly concerned about poorly growing cultures and therefore set a minimum of an 8-fold increase. The maximum of 32-fold provides for reasonable errors in cell dilution and for a slightly variable rate in cell number increases.

The IWGT MLA Workgroup [27] also reached consensus on acceptance criteria for the soft agar and microwell method negative/vehicle control parameters for the 24 hour treatment, as shown in the following table. Suspension growth values were changed for the longer treatment time because it involves 3 days of suspension growth, rather than the 2 days for the 3 or 4 hour treatment.

Parameter	Soft Agar Method	Microwell Method
Mutant frequency	$35–140 \times 10^{-6}$	$50–170 \times 10^{-6}$
Cloning efficiency	65–120%	65–120%
Suspension growth	32–180-fold	32–180-fold

The IWGT MLA Workgroup [27] reached consensus on two equally appropriate criteria for an acceptable positive control response for both the short and long treatment times. (1) The positive control produces an induced mutant frequency (total mutant frequency minus concurrent negative control mutant frequency) of at least 300×10^{-6} with at least 40% of the colonies being small colonies. (2) The positive control produces an induced small colony mutant frequency of at least 150×10^{-6}. For both approaches, the RTG must be greater than 10%. Some laboratories prefer to use more than one dose of their positive control. In particular, they prefer to use a dose that gives only small increases in mutant frequency. These laboratories can meet the positive control criteria by selecting at least two doses for the positive control (one of which meets the criteria).

Confirmatory tests   There is no requirement for verification of a clear positive response in the MLA. Experiments that do not provide enough information to determine whether the chemical is positive or negative should be clarified by further testing, preferably by modifying the test concentrations or metabolic activation conditions. Negative results achieved using the 3 or 4 hour treatment should be confirmed by repeat testing using 24 hour treatment in the absence of S9 activation (ICH S2B (V and Note 4)) [12]. However, performing only a 24 hour treatment (i.e., with no 3 or 4 hour treatment) in the absence of S9 activation is not acceptable unless the highest concentration is a precipitating concentration or the limit concentration. The reason for performing a 3 or 4 hour treatment is that higher concentrations can be used than are generally tolerated when cells are treated for 24 hours.

14. *Assay Evaluation Criteria.* There have been several different approaches to defining a positive result in the MLA. All involve a concentration-dependent or reproducible increase in mutant frequency, but the absolute increase in mutant frequency that differentiates a positive response from a negative response varies. In some laboratories, a twofold increase in mutant frequency over background is considered a positive response. In other laboratories, the approach developed by the U.S. EPA MLA Gene-Tox Workgroup [48] is used as guidance in interpreting data. Also, the United Kingdom Environmental Mutagen Society developed a statistical program for determining a positive or negative result in the microwell version of the assay [61].

Recently, the IWGT MLA Workgroup recommended the adoption of a global evaluation factor (GEF) and an appropriate statistical trend analysis to define positive and negative results in the MLA [24–27]. This approach also takes into account the recommendation in previous guidance documents [22, 28] that biological relevance should be a factor in data evaluation.

To arrive at a GEF, the Workgroup analyzed distributions of negative/vehicle mutant frequencies for the agar and microwell versions of the MLA that they gathered from ten laboratories. The Workgroup defined the GEF as the mean of the negative/vehicle mutant frequency distribution plus one standard deviation. Applying this definition to the data, the Workgroup arrived at a GEF of 90 for the agar method and of 126 for the microwell method. The GEF is applied in the following manner. If the mutant frequency of the negative control in a soft agar assay is 100×10^{-6}, then one treatment group must have a mutant frequency of at least 190×10^{-6} (100 plus GEF of 90) to be called positive. In addition to evaluating the data against the GEF, the Workgroup recommended that the data be evaluated for the presence of a positive trend.

Following these recommendations, a test article is positive in the MLA if both the induced mutant frequency meets or exceeds the GEF and a trend test using the data is positive. A test article is negative if the induced mutant frequency is below the GEF and the trend test is negative.

Situations where either the GEF test or the trend test is positive should be considered on a case-by-case basis. Additional testing may be helpful to better define the assay response, particularly if the RTG is in the 10–30% range. While additional testing, which includes refining the dose range selection, will generally provide data for a definitive call, there will be some situations where the response will either vary between well-designed experiments or fluctuate within an experiment. Fluctuation within an experiment can occur when closely spaced doses are used to provide extensive coverage of an important part of the dose response for a test article. Either of these outcomes can result in an "equivocal" (equal voice) determination for the MLA. In such a situation, the MLA results should be evaluated in the context of other information as a part of a weight of the evidence assessment of the potential hazard posed by the test chemical.

CHO*/Hprt *Assay   Compared with the extensive guidance available for conducting and interpreting the MLA, there is very little published material that specifically relates to the use of the CHO/*Hprt* assay (and the AS52 assay) for preclinical testing. This most likely is due to the secondary status accorded the CHO/*Hprt* assay in the ICH test battery and the subsequent lack of emphasis placed on the assay by the IWGT. The following protocols for the CHO/*Hprt* and AS52 assays were derived from original research reports using the assays, literature reviews of assay performance, including that of the EPA Gene-Tox Program for the CHO/*Hprt* assay, and the authors' experience with these assays in their own laboratories.

1. *Principle of the Assay.* The purpose of the CHO/*Hprt* assay is to determine the ability of a test article to induce forward mutations in the *Hprt* gene of CHO cells. The mutations are detected by growth of colonies in the presence of TG (or, in rare instances, 8-azaguanine (AG)).

2. *Cells.* CHO-K$_1$-BH$_4$ cells [62] are the standard cells used in this assay. This cell line is a proline auxotroph with a modal chromosome number of 20 and a population doubling time of 12–14 hours [53]; some CHO cell lines may have slightly longer doubling times. Cells should be checked periodically for mycoplasma contamination, genetic markers, and karyotypic stability.

3. *Media and Culture Conditions.* Ham's nutrient mixture F12 containing 5–10% heat-inactivated fetal bovine serum (FBS) is used for growing stock cultures. The medium is adjusted to pH 6.8–7.2 before the addition of cells. While most parts of the assay are performed with F12 plus FBS, hypoxanthine-free nutrient mixture F12 is used for selection of TG-resistant mutants. In addition, the medium used for selection is often prepared with dialyzed FBS. Osmolality should be maintained in the physiological range (300 ± 20 mOsm) when cells are treated with a test article.

Cells are typically plated at a concentration of 1×10^6/100-mm dish or 5×10^5/25-cm^2 T-flask and subcultured every 2–3 days to maintain exponential growth. Trypsin (0.05%) is generally used for cell detachment for subculturing.

4. *Preparation of Cultures.* Frozen cell stocks are prepared from exponentially growing cells that were cleansed of preexisting *Hprt* mutants in medium supplemented with hypoxanthine, aminopterin, and thymidine. Freshly thawed cells are plated in growth medium and incubated at 37°C for 16–24 hours to allow time for cell attachment and growth to approximately 1×10^6 cells/25-cm^2 surface area.

5. *Metabolic Activation.* The rationale for using exogenous metabolic activation in the assay is the same as for the MLA. Also like the MLA, the most commonly used metabolic activation system uses an S9 prepared from the livers of Aroclor-1254-induced male rats. The standard S9 is available commercially or can be produced by published methods [29]. The S9 is supplemented with a standard mixture of cofactors as described by Machanoff and co-workers [63] and used at a concentration of 1–10% v/v in the final test medium. The concentration of S9 is determined

by preliminary tests of the cytotoxicity of the S9 and its ability to activate known metabolism-dependent mutagens (see below for activation-dependent controls). Alternative metabolic activation systems such as the use of S9 from another species or the use of hepatocytes should be justified scientifically.

6. *Solvent/Vehicle.* The solvents appropriate for this test system include but are not limited to the following, in order of preference: FBS-free F12, distilled water, DMSO, ethanol, and acetone. Nonaqueous solvent concentrations should not be greater than 1% and should be identical in all test cultures. The choice of the solvent principally depends on its ability to dissolve the test article. However, the suitability of the proposed solvent also should be evaluated by determining the effect of the dissolved agent on the pH and osmolality of the treatment medium, as well as by determining if the solvent reacts with the test article, the culture vessel, or the cells.

7. *Dose Selection.* As described for the MLA, dose selection is based on the cytotoxicity and solubility of the test article, and the criteria for determining the highest test dose described in ICH S2A [13]. For *in vitro* mammalian cell mutation assays, ICH S2A (II.2) defines the top concentration for freely soluble, nontoxic compounds as 5 mg/mL or 10 mM, whichever is lower. Thus, a preliminary cytotoxicity test should include a range of doses with a high dose of 5 mg/mL or 10 mM, unless limited by pH, osmolality, or solubility. Cells are seeded and allowed to grow for 18–24 hours followed by treatment with the solvent or the test article in the presence and absence of exogenous metabolic activation for 5 hours. Depending on how the mutagenicity assay is conducted (see later discussion), either immediately after the treatment or on the next day, the cells are trypsinized and reseeded into new plates at cloning density (100–200 cells/25-cm^2 T-flask or 60-mm plate). After incubation for 7–10 days, the colonies are fixed with absolute methanol, stained with methylene blue, and counted. Cytotoxicity is expressed as the cloning efficiency of test-article-treated cells relative to the cloning efficiency of the solvent control. When possible, the high dose is chosen to give a cell survival of 10–20%.

8. *Controls.* Appropriate negative controls are culture medium for the untreated control and solvent/vehicle for the solvent control. Appropriate positive controls are ethyl methanesulfonate or *N*-methyl-*N'*-nitro-*N*-nitrosoguanidine for direct-acting mutagens and 7,12-dimethylbenz[*a*]anthracene, benzo[*a*]pyrene, dimethylnitrosamine, or 2-acetylaminofluorene for promutagens requiring metabolic activation.

9. *Treatment with Test Article.* Exponentially growing cells are seeded into plates at a density of approximately 1×10^6 cells/55 cm^2 and incubated for 18–24 hours to achieve an approximate doubling of cell number. Next, the plates are washed with FBS-free F12 or Hank's Balanced Salt Solution (HBSS) and exposed to the test article or controls for 5 hours, generally with and without S9 activation. Duplicate cultures and three to five concentrations of the test article typically are used. After the treatment, the media are aspirated and the cells are washed with HBSS.

10. *Expression Time and Measurement of Mutant Frequency.* After the treatment, most laboratories culture the cells in complete F12 medium for 16–24 hours (overnight) before subculturing. This allows the various steps of the assay to be completed easily within an 8 hour working day. Alternatively, the cells can be subcultured immediately after treatment, a procedure viewed as giving more "accurate"

cytotoxicity data [54]. The posttreatment subculture involves establishing two sets of cultures from each treatment: one (100–200 cells/60-mm dish in triplicate) is incubated 7–10 days and used to determine cytotoxicity, while the second (no more than 1×10^6 cells/100-mm dish) is cultured for the expression of mutants. During the 7–9 day expression period, the cells are subcultured at 2–3 day intervals. At the end of the expression period, the cells are again split into two subcultures. One subculture is designated for the selection of mutant cells: 2×10^5 cells are plated in each of five (or more) 100-mm dishes using hypoxanthine-free F12 medium containing 10 µM TG. The other subculture is used for the determination of cloning efficiency: 100–200 cells are plated in 100-mm dishes using medium free of TG. After incubating both sets of dishes 7–10 days, the colonies are fixed, stained, and counted.

Cytotoxicity is determined from the plates seeded at cloning density up to 1 day after the treatment and is expressed as the cloning efficiency of the treated cultures relative to the solvent control. Mutant frequency is calculated by dividing the total number of mutant colonies by the total number of cells seeded into selection plates, corrected by the cloning efficiency of the cells seeded at the time of selection into plates without TG. Mutant frequency usually is expressed as TG-resistant mutants per 10^6 clonable cells or per 10^6 survivors.

11. *Assay Validity Criteria.* The cloning efficiency of the untreated and solvent controls must be greater than 50%. Spontaneous mutant frequency in the solvent and untreated controls may vary in different laboratories but should fall within 0–20 mutants per 10^6 clonable cells [54, 64]. Assays with slightly higher spontaneous mutant frequencies may be acceptable, especially when the test agent produces a clear increase in mutant frequency; higher spontaneous mutant frequencies, however, may prevent the detection of weak mutagens. The positive control must induce a mutant frequency sufficiently greater than the mutant frequency of the solvent control—for example, three times that of the solvent control—and should exceed the minimum mutant frequency considered to be a positive result. The high dose for noncytotoxic, soluble test articles must be 5 mg/mL or 10 mM (whichever is lower). Alternatively, the high dose may be limited by either the test agent's solubility in the treatment medium or by a maximum cytotoxicity of approximately 10–20% relative cloning efficiency measured up to one day after exposure.

12. *Assay Evaluation Criteria.* Data should be reproducible for both positive and negative responses. However, an abbreviated preliminary or confirmatory assay coupled with a full (definitive) assay may be sufficient for demonstrating reproducibility [54]. ICH S2B V [12] states that a range-finding test may be a satisfactory substitute for a complete repeat of an *in vitro* mammalian cell mutation assay other than the MLA, if the range-finding test is performed with and without metabolic activation, with appropriate positive and negative controls, and with quantification of mutants. Positive compounds should exhibit a concentration-related increase over at least 2 or 3 concentrations. Because the spontaneous mutant frequency can vary from 0 to 20 mutants per 10^6 cells, evaluation of the response in terms of a fold-increase in mutant frequency relative to the background mutant frequency is not reliable. Some laboratories use a minimum mutant frequency for a response to be considered positive, for example, greater than 40 or 50 mutants per 10^6 clonable

cells [65]. A statistical method may also be employed, although no single method has been agreed upon [53].

AS52/xprt Assay The procedure for conducting the AS52/*xprt* assay is nearly identical to that described above for the CHO/*Hprt* assay. Both assays are based on the same parent cell line: AS52 cells are derived from CHO-K1-BH$_4$ cells [35], and hence CHO cells and AS52 cells have similar growth and cloning characteristics. In addition, the expression and selection of *xprt* mutant AS52 cells and *Hprt* mutant CHO cells can be conducted using the same protocol [55].

A major difference between the two assays is that AS52 cells should be grown in MPA medium (nutrient mixture F12 supplemented with 5% FBS, 250 μg/mL xanthine, 25 μg/mL adenine, 50 μM thymidine, 3 μM aminopterin, and 10 μM mycophenolic acid) right up to the time of treating cells in the assay. MPA medium not only cleanses the cultures of *xprt* mutants (minimizing the background mutant frequency), but also ensures that cells that have lost their transgene (and will be selected as mutants) are not included in the assay. Assays conducted with MPA cleansing have spontaneous mutant frequencies only somewhat higher than that seen in the CHO/*Hprt* assay [37, 41, 55, 66], but culturing cells in the absence of MPA cleansing can result in background mutant frequencies of several hundred per 10^6 cells [67].

REFERENCES

1. Moore MM, DeMarini DM, DeSerres FJ, Tindall KR, Eds. *Banbury Report 28: Mammalian Cell Mutagenesis*. Cold Spring Harbor, NY: Cold Spring Harbor Laboratory; 1987.
2. Chu EHY, Malling HV. Mammalian cell genetics. II. Chemical induction of specific locus mutations in Chinese hamster cells *in vitro*. *Proc Natl Acad Sci USA* 1968;61: 1306–1312.
3. Liber HL, Thilly WG. Mutation assay at the thymidine kinase locus in diploid human lymphoblasts. *Mutat Res* 1982;94:467–485.
4. Moore MM, Harrington-Brock K, Doerr CL, Dearfield KL. Differential mutant quantitation at the mouse lymphoma TK and CHO HGPRT loci. *Mutagenesis* 1989;4:394–403.
5. Aaron CS, Stankowski LF Jr. Comparison of the AS52/XPRT and the CHO/HPRT assays: evaluation of six drug candidates. *Mutat Res* 1989;223:121–128.
6. Aaron CS, Bolcsfoldi G, Glatt HR, Moore M, Nishi Y, Stankowski L, Theiss J, Thompson E. Mammalian cell gene mutation assays working group report. Report of the International Workshop on Standardisation of Genotoxicity Test Procedures. *Mutat Res* 1994;312:235–239.
7. Applegate ML, Moore MM, Broder CB, Burrell A, Juhn G, Kasweck KL, Lin P, Wadhams A, Hozier JC. Molecular dissection of mutations at the heterozygous thymidine kinase locus in mouse lymphoma cells. *Proc Natl Acad Sci USA* 1990;87:51–55.
8. Hozier J, Sawyer J, Moore M, Howard B, Clive D. Cytogenetic analysis of the L5178Y/ TK$^{+/-}$ → TK$^{-/-}$ mouse lymphoma mutagenesis assay system. *Mutat Res* 1981;84: 169–181.
9. Moore MM, Clive D, Hozier JC, Howard BE, Batson AG, Turner NT, Sawyer J. Analysis of trifluorothymidine-resistant (TFT^r) mutants of L5178Y/TK$^{+/-}$ mouse lymphoma cells. *Mutat Res* 1985;151:161–174.

10. Sawyer JR, Moore MM, Hozier JC. High-resolution cytogenetic characterization of the L5178Y TK$^{+/-}$ mouse lymphoma cell line. *Mutat Res* 1989;214:181–193.

11. Sawyer J, Moore MM, Clive D, Hozier J. Cytogenetic characterization of the L5178Y TK$^{+/-}$ 3.7.2C mouse lymphoma cell line. *Mutat Res* 1985;147:243–253.

12. ICH Guidance for Industry S2B: Genotoxicity: A standard battery for genotoxicity testing of pharmacuticals (July 1997). *Federal Register, 62 FR 62472* (http://www.fda.gov/cder/guidance/index.htm).

13. ICH Guideline for Industry S2A: Specific aspects of regulatory genotoxicity tests for pharmaceuticals (April 1996). *Federal Register, 61 FR 18199* (http://www.fda.gov/cder/guidance/index.htm).

14. Dearfield KL, Auletta AE, Cimino MC, Moore MM. Considerations in the U.S. Environmental Protection Agency's testing approach for mutagenicity. *Mutat Res* 1991;258:259–283.

15. Müller L, Kikuchi Y, Probst G, Schechtman L, Shimada H, Sofuni T, Tweats D. ICH-harmonised guidances on genotoxicity testing of pharmaceuticals: evolution, reasoning and impact. *Mutat Res* 1999;436:195–225.

16. Moore MM (Chair), Honma M (Co-Chair), Clements J (Rapporteur), Awogi T, Bolcsfoldi G, Cole J, Gollapudi B, Harrington-Brock K, Mitchell A, Muster W, Myhr B, O'Donovan M, Ouldelhkim M-C, San R, Shimada H, Stankowski LF Jr. The mouse lymphoma thymidine kinase locus (tk) gene mutation assay: International Workshop on Genotoxicity Test Procedures (IWGTP) Workgroup Report. *Environ Mol Mutagen* 2000;35:185–190.

17. ICH M3 Guidance for Industry: Nonclinical safety studies for the conduct of human clinical trials for pharmaceuticals (July 1997). *Federal Register, 62 FR 62922* (http://www.fda.gov/cder/guidance/index.htm).

18. ICH S1B Guidance for Industry: Testing for carcinogenicity of pharmaceuticals (July 1997). *Federal Register, 63 FR 8983* (http://www.fda.gov/cder/guidance/index.htm).

19. ICH Q3A Guidance for Industry: Impurities in new drug substances (February 2003). (http://www.fda.gov/cder/guidance/index.htm).

20. ICH Q3B (R2) Guidance for Industry: Impurities in new drug products (July 2006). (http://www.fda.gov/cder/guidance/index.htm).

21. FDA CDER Guidance for Industry and Review Staff: Recommended approaches to integration of genetic toxicology study results (January 2006). (http://www.fda.gov/cder/guidance/index.htm).

22. OECD Guideline for the testing of chemicals: *In vitro* mammalian cell gene mutation test. OECD Guideline 476, July 1997.

23. EPA Health effects test guidelines OPPTS 870.5300: *In vitro* mammalian cell gene mutation test. EPA Guideline 870.5300, August 1998.

24. Moore MM, Honma M, Clements J, Harrington-Brock K, Awogi T, Bolcsfoldi G, Cifone M, Collard D, Fellows M, Flanders K, Gollapudi B, Jenkinson P, Kirby P, Kirchner S, Kraycer J, McEnaney S, Muster W, Myhr B, O'Donovan M, Oliver J, Ouldelhkim M-C, Pant K, Preston R, Riach C, San R, Shimada H, Stankowski L Jr. Mouse lymphoma thymidine kinase gene mutation assay: follow-up International Workshop on genotoxicity test procedures, New Orleans, Louisiana, April 2000. *Environ Mol Mutagen* 2002; 40:292–299.

25. Moore MM, Honma M, Clements J, Bolcsfoldi G, Cifone M, Delongchamp R, Fellows M, Gollapudi B, Jenkinson P, Kirby P, Kirchner S, Muster W, Myhr B, O'Donovan M, Ouldelhkim M-C, Pant K, Preston R, Riach C, San R, Stankowski L Jr, Thakur A, Wakuri S, Yoshimura I. Mouse lymphoma thymidine kinase locus gene mutation assay: International Workshop (Plymouth, England) on genotoxicity test procedures workgroup report. *Mutat Res* 2003;540:127–140.

26. Moore MM, Honma M, Clements J, Bolcsfoldi G, Burlinson B, Cifone M, Clarke J, Delongchamp R, Durward R, Fellows M, Gollapudi B, Hou S, Jenkinson P, Lloyd M, Majeska B, Myhr B, Omori T, Riach C, San R, Stankowski L Jr, Thakur A, Van Goethem F, Wakuri S, Yoshimura I. Mouse lymphoma thymidine kinase gene mutation assay: follow-up meeting of the International Workshop on genotoxicity tests—Aberdeen, Scotland, 2003—Assay acceptance criteria, positive controls, and data evaluation. *Environ Mol Mutagen* 2006;47:1–5.

27. Moore MM, Honma M, Clements J, Bolcsfoldi G, Burlinson B, Cifone M, Clarke J, Clay P, Doppalapudi R, Fellows M, Gollapudi B, Hou S, Jenkinson P, Muster W, Pant K, Kidd D, Lorge E, Lloyd M, Myhr B, O'Donovan M, Riach C, Stankowski L Jr, Thakur A, Van Goethem F. Mouse lymphoma thymidine kinase gene mutation assay: meeting of the International Workshop on Genotoxicity Testing—San Francisco 2005—Recommendations for 24-h treatment. *Mutat Res*, 2007;627:36–40.

28. FDA CFSAN Redbook 2000: IV.C.1.c. Mouse lymphoma thymidine kinase gene mutation assay. http://www.cfsan.fda.gov/guidance.html.

29. Turner NT, Batson AG, Clive D. Procedures for the L5178Y/TK$^{+/-}$ to TK$^{-/-}$ mouse lymphoma assay. In Kilbey BJ, Legator M, Nichols W, Ramel C, Eds. *Handbook of Mutagenicity Test Procedures*, 2nd eds. Amsterdam: Elsevier; 1984, pp 239–268.

30. Cole J, Arlett CF, Green MHL, Lowe J, Muriel W. A comparison of the agar cloning and microtitration techniques for assaying cell survival and mutation frequency in L5178Y mouse lymphoma cells. *Mutat Res* 1983;111:371–386.

31. Cole J, Muriel WJ, Bridges BA. The mutagenicity of sodium fluoride to L5178Y (wild-type and TK$^{+/-}$ 3.7.2C) mouse lymphoma cells. *Mutagenesis* 1986;1:157–167.

32. Hozier J, Sawyer J, Clive D, Moore M. Cytogenetic distinction between the TK$^+$ and TK$^-$ chromosomes in the L5178Y TK$^{+/-}$ 3.7.2C mouse-lymphoma cell line. *Mutat Res* 1982;105:451–456.

33. Hozier J, Sawyer J, Clive D, Moore MM. Chromosome 11 aberrations in small colony L5178Y TK$^{-/-}$ mutants early in their clonal history. *Mutat Res* 1985;147:237–242.

34. Moore MM, Doerr CL. Comparison of chromosome aberration frequency and small-colony TK-deficient mutant frequency in L5178Y/TK$^{+/-}$-3.7.2C mouse lymphoma cells. *Mutagenesis* 1990;5:609–614.

35. Tindall KR, Stankowski LF Jr, Machanoff R, Hsie AW. Detection of deletion mutations in pSV2*gpt*-transformed cells. *Mol Cell Biol* 1984;4:1411–1415.

36. Michaelis KC, Helvering LM, Kindig DE, Garriott ML, Richardson KK. Localization of the xanthine guanine phosphoribosyl transferase gene (*gpt*) of *E. coli* in AS52 metaphase cells by fluorescence *in situ* hybridization. *Environ Mol Mutagen* 1994;24:176–180.

37. Stankowski LF Jr, Tindall KR. Characterization of the AS52 cell line for use in mammalian cell mutagenesis studies. In Moore MM, DeMarini DM, DeSerres FJ, Tindall KR, Eds. *Banbury Report 28*. Cold Spring Harbor, NY: Cold Spring Harbor Laboratory; 1987, pp 71–79.

38. Hsie AW, Xu ZD, Yu YJ, Sognier MA, Hrelia P. Molecular analysis of reactive oxygen-species-induced mammalian gene mutation. *Teratog Carcinog Mutagen* 1990;10:115–124.

39. Hsie AW, Xu Z, Yu Y, An J, Meltz ML, Schwartz JL, Hrelia P. Quantitative and molecular analyses of genetic risk: a study with ionizing radiation. *Environ Health Perspect* 1993;101(Suppl 3):213–218.

40. Li AP, Aaron CS, Auletta AE, Dearfield KL, Riddle JC, Slesinski RS, Stankowski LF Jr. An evaluation of the roles of mammalian cell mutation assays in the testing of chemical genotoxicity. *Regul Toxicol Pharmacol* 1991;14:24–40.

41. Oberly TJ, Huffman DM, Scheuring JC, Garriott ML. An evaluation of 6 chromosomal mutagens in the AS52/XPRT mutation assay utilizing suspension culture and soft agar cloning. *Mutat Res* 1993;319:179–187.

42. Bigger CAH, Ponten I, Page JE, Dipple A. Mutational spectra of polycyclic aromatic hydrocarbons. *Mutat Res* 2000;450:75–93.

43. Tennant RW, Margolin BH, Shelby MD, Zeiger E, Haseman JK, Spalding J, Caspary W, Resnick M, Stasiewicz S, Anderson B, Minor R. Prediction of chemical carcinogenicity in rodents from *in vitro* genetic toxicity assays. *Science* 1987;236:933–941.

44. Kirkland D, Aardema M, Henderson L, Müller L. Evaluation of the ability of a battery of three *in vitro* genotoxicity tests to discriminate rodent carcinogens and non-carcinogens I. Sensitivity, specificity and relative predictivity. *Mutat Res* 2005;584:1–256.

45. Kirkland D, Aardema M, Müller L, Hayashi M. Evaluation of the ability of a battery of three *in vitro* genotoxicity tests to discriminate rodent carcinogens and non-carcinogens II. Further analysis of mammalian cell results, relative predictivity and tumour profiles. *Mutat Res* 2006;608:29–42.

46. Matthews EJ, Kruhlak NL, Cimino MC, Benz RD, Contrera JF. An analysis of genetic toxicity, reproductive and developmental toxicity, and carcinogenicity data: I. Identification of carcinogens using surrogate endpoints. *Regul Toxicol Pharmacol* 2006;44:83–96.

47. Matthews EJ, Kruhlak NL, Cimino MC, Benz RD, Contrera JF. An analysis of genetic toxicity, reproductive and developmental toxicity, and carcinogenicity data: II. Identification of genotoxicants, reprotoxicants, and carcinogens using *in silico* methods. *Regul Toxicol Pharmacol* 2006;44:97–110.

48. Mitchell AD, Auletta AE, Clive D, Kirby PE, Moore MM, Myhr BC. The L5178Y/tk$^{+/-}$ mouse lymphoma specific gene and chromosomal mutation assay: a phase III report of the US Environmental Protection Agency Gene-Tox Program. *Mutat Res* 1997;394:177–303.

49. Clive D, Johnson KO, Spector JFS, Batson AG, Brown MMM. Validation and characterization of the L5178Y TK$^{+/-}$ mouse lymphoma mutagen assay system. *Mutat Res* 1979;59:61–108.

50. Dearfield KL, Moore MM. Use of genetic toxicology information for risk assessment. *Environ Mol Mutagen* 2005;46:236–245.

51. Clive D, Caspary W, Kirby PE, Krehl R, Moore M, Mayo J, Oberly TJ. Guide for performing the mouse lymphoma assay for mammalian cell mutagenicity. *Mutat Res* 1987;189:143–156.

52. Moore-Brown MM, Clive D, Howard BE, Batson AG, Johnson KO. The utilization of trifluorothymidine (TFT) to select for thymidine kinase-deficient (TK$^{-/-}$) mutants from L5178Y/TK$^{+/-}$ mouse lymphoma cells. *Mutat Res* 1981;85:363–378.

53. Hsie AW, Casciano DA, Couch DB, Krahn DF, O'Neill JP, Whitfield BL. The use of Chinese hamster ovary cells to quantify specific locus mutation and to determine mutagenicity of chemicals. A report of the Gene-Tox Program. *Mutat Res* 1981;86:193–214.

54. Li AP, Carver JH, Choy WN, Hsie AW, Gupta RS, Loveday KS, O'Neill JP, Riddle JC, Stankowski LF Jr, Yang LL. A guide for the performance of the Chinese hamster ovary cell/hypoxanthine-guanine phosphoribosyl transferase gene mutation assay. *Mutat Res* 1987;189:135–141.

55. Stankowski LF Jr, Tindall KR, Hsie AW. Quantitative and molecular analyses of ethyl methanesulfonate- and ICR 191-induced mutation in AS52 cells. *Mutat Res* 1986;160:133–147.

56. Chen T, Moore MM. Screening for chemical mutagens using the mouse lymphoma assay. In Yan Z, Caldwell GW, Eds. *Methods in Pharmacology and Toxicology Optimization in Drug Discovery: In Vitro Methods.* Totowa, NJ: Humana Press; 2004, pp 337–352.

57. Sawyer JR, Binz RL, Wang J, Moore MM. Multicolor spectral karyotyping of the L5178Y TK$^{+/-}$-3.7.2C mouse lymphoma cell line. *Environ Mol Mutagen* 2006;47:127–131.

58. Brock KH, Moore MM, Oglesby LA. Development of an intact hepatocyte activation system for routine use with the mouse lymphoma assay. *Environ Mutagen* 1987;9:331–341.

59. Oglesby LA, Harrington-Brock K, Moore MM. Induced hepatocytes as a metabolic activation system for the mouse-lymphoma assay. *Mutat Res* 1989;223:295–302.

60. Moore MM, Clive D. The quantitation of TK$^{-/-}$ and HGPRT-mutants of L5178Y/TK$^{+/-}$ mouse lymphoma cells at varying times post treatment. *Environ Mutagen* 1982;4:499–519.

61. Robison WD, Green MHL, Cole J, Healy MJR, Garner RC, Gatehouse D. Statistical evaluation of bacterial/mammalian fluctuation tests. In Kirkland DJ, Ed. *Statistical Evaluation of Mutagenicity Test Data*. Cambridge, UK: Cambridge University Press; 1989, pp 102–140.

62. Hsie AW, Brimer PA, Mitchell TJ, Gosslee DG. The dose–response relationship for ethyl methanesulfonate-induced mutations at the hypoxanthine–guanine phosphoribosyl transferase locus in Chinese hamster ovary cells. *Somatic Cell Genet* 1975;1:247–261.

63. Machanoff R, O'Neill JP, Hsie AW. Quantitative analysis of cytotoxicity and mutagenicity of benzo[*a*]pyrene in mammalian cells (CHO/HGPRT system). *Chem-Biol Interact* 1981;34:1–10.

64. Li AP, Gupta RS, Heflich RH, Wassom JS. A review and analysis of the Chinese hamster ovary/hypoxanthine guanine phosphoribosyl transferase assay to determine the mutagenicity of chemical agents; a report of Phase III of the U.S. Environmental Protection Agency Gene-Tox Program. *Mutat Res* 1988;196:17–36.

65. Putman DL, San RHC, Bigger CAH, Jacobson-Kram D. Genetic toxicology. In Derelanko MJ, Hollinger MA, Eds. *CRC Handbook of Toxicology*. New York: CRC Press; 1995, pp 337–355.

66. Tindall KR, Stankowski LF Jr, Machanoff R, Hsie AW. Analysis of mutation in PSV2*gpt*-transformed CHO cells. *Mutat Res* 1986;160:121–131.

67. Li AP. Spontaneous frequency of 6-thioguanine resistant mutants in CHO-AS52 cells after prolonged culturing in the absence of selective agents. *Environ Mol Mutagen* 1990;15:214–217.

6

IN VITRO MAMMALIAN CYTOGENETIC TESTS

R. JULIAN PRESTON

National Health and Environmental Effects Research Laboratory, U.S. Environmental Protection Agency, Research Triangle Park, North Carolina

Contents

Preclinical Development Handbook: Toxicology, edited by Shayne Cox Gad
Copyright © 2008 John Wiley & Sons, Inc.

6.1 PURPOSE OF CYTOGENETIC TESTS

The first step in any cancer risk assessment process for exposures to environmental chemicals is *hazard identification*. Thus, in order for new products to be registered for the first time or to be reregistered, an assessment of whether or not they present a potential hazard has to be conducted. This applies equally to products for agricultural, pharmaceutical, or consumer use. In the present context, a hazard is considered to be represented by genetic alterations assessed as gene mutations or chromosomal alterations. In particular, this chapter concentrates on the induction of chromosomal alterations, both numerical and structural ones.

6.2 HISTORY OF CYTOGENETIC TESTING PROTOCOLS

The analysis of chromosomal alterations in cells exposed to environmental agents, particularly ionizing radiation, has a long history, starting in a quantitative fashion with the pioneering work of Karl Sax [1] using pollen grains of *Tradescantia*. These studies provided information on the dose response for X-ray- and neutron-induced chromosome aberrations and the relative effectiveness of acute, chronic, and fractionated exposures. These types of studies were expanded over the next decade or so to include the assessment of the cytogenetic effects produced by chemicals. The types of assay available for cytogenetic analysis were greatly expanded by the ability to grow mammalian cells *in vitro*, either as primary cultures or as transformed cell lines. This capability was further enhanced to include the use of readily available human cells following development of the *in vitro* culture of human lymphocytes by Moorhead et al. [2]. This method relied on the use of phytohemagglutinin to stimulate peripheral lymphocytes to reenter the cell cycle, thereby allowing for metaphase cells to be obtained. At this time, it was necessary to obtain metaphase cells because all cytogenetic assays relied on microscopic evaluation of chromosomes at metaphase. The use of colcemid to inhibit cells at metaphase and of hypotonic solutions to swell the cells for easy analysis of chromosomal alterations also made cytogenetic tests much more reliable, repeatable, and technically straightforward [3].

The standardization of approaches for visualizing chromosomes for assessing structural and numerical alterations following exposure to radiation or chemicals led to the development of cytogenetic assays for testing chemicals for potential hazard to humans. A plethora of different test systems became available, and there was unique merit to many of these. With fairly extensive validation studies, the assays that were considered to be the most straightforward to conduct and provided the more reliable predictions of clastogenicity (chromosome breakage) for carcinogens and noncarcinogens were incorporated into testing guidelines. This history is concisely described in Chapter 1 of the *Evaluation of Short-Term Tests for Carcinogens: Report of the International Collaborative Program* [4]. These *in vitro* cytogenetic assays incorporate chromosome alterations, sister chromatid exchanges (SCEs), or micronuclei as endpoints, and permanent cell lines (especially Chinese hamster) as the test cells. Based on the selection of the highest performing assays as regards carcinogen/noncarcinogen predictions, a number of national and international organizations developed test batteries that could further enhance predictive value. Typically, these include a bacterial reverse mutation assay, an *in vitro* cytogenetic assay in mammalian cell cultures and/or an *in vitro* gene mutation assay in mammalian cell cultures, and an *in vivo* cytogenetic assay in rodent bone marrow cells.

This standard battery of genotoxicity tests can satisfy the requirements of various global regulatory bodies. For example, several national and international regulatory agencies have presented minimum data requirements for regulatory reviews of commercial chemicals, and these include the use of a standard battery of genotoxicity tests as described above [5]. Although there have been some modifications to these basic assays for improving overall sensitivity and predictivity, the basic principles underlying the assays remain the same, as discussed in Sections 6.5 and 6.6.

Recent advances in chromosomal imaging techniques, based on the development of sophisticated fluorescence *in situ* hybridization (FISH) methods, have significantly enhanced the understanding of the mechanisms of chromosome aberration induction and the ability to identify specific aberration types (e.g., reciprocal translocations). These techniques have generally remained in the purview of mechanistic studies and have not been incorporated into cytogenetic tests for assessing carcinogens.

6.3 DESCRIPTION OF ENDPOINTS

6.3.1 Chromosomal Structural Alterations

A broad range of structural alterations can be observed in metaphase cells using either conventional cytogenetic techniques or fluorescence *in situ* hybridization (FISH). The types of structural alterations produced by treatment with chemicals and radiation are the same as those observed in untreated cells. Thus, treatment with a clastogenic agent enhances the frequencies of chromosomal alterations but does not produce a different spectrum of types. A comprehensive description of the classes of structural chromosomal alterations can be found in Savage [6]. In general terms, structural alterations can be subdivided into *unstable* (generally nontransmissible) and *stable* (transmissible to daughter cells at division). Within these two broad categories, an important distinction is made between chromosomal alterations produced prior to DNA replication (G_1) and those produced during (S) or after (G_2) replication. The former are called *chromosome-type* aberrations because they involve both chromatids of a chromosome and the latter are called *chromatid-type* because they involve one of the two chromatids. An exception is the so-called isochromatid aberration that is produced in S or G_2 of the cell cycle but involves both chromatids. Within each of these two classes, chromosomal alterations can be described as *deletions* (loss of chromosomal material) and *exchanges* (between or within chromosomes). Deletions are generally unstable alterations and exchanges can be stable (reciprocal exchanges) or unstable (dicentrics). For the purposes of most mammalian cytogenetic tests that are used for hazard identification, this level of definition of the range of structural alterations is generally sufficient.

6.3.2 Chromosomal Numerical Alterations (Aneuploidy)

There are chemicals that can alter the normal process of cell division either resulting in chromosomes failing to separate at metaphase or preventing one or more chromosomes attaching to the mitotic spindle. The results are that daughter cells will have either additional chromosomes beyond the normal diploid number (hyperploidy) or fewer chromosomes than the diploid number (hypoploidy). Because of possible artifacts produced during the preparative stages of cells for cytogenetic analysis that can result in chromosome loss, the general approach for assessing aneuploidy is to place greater emphasis on hyperploidy.

6.3.3   Sister Chromatid Exchanges (SCEs)

During the course of DNA replication, errors can occur that lead to the reciprocal exchange between the two sister chromatids of a chromosome. The result is the so-called sister chromatid exchange. While such exchanges had been identified by genetic methods for decades and using radioisotopes in the 1950s, it was not until the 1970s that a simple cytogenetic method was developed for direct observation of SCE [7, 8]. This method relied in general terms on differential staining of the sister chromatids—one being lightly stained with Giemsa and the other darkly stained. Exchanges between the sister chromatids could readily be seen in metaphase cells as light–dark switches. The principle behind the method was the preferential elution of DNA from one chromatid based on incorporation of bromodeoxyuridine (BrdU), binding of a BrdU-sensitive fluorescence dye to asymmetrically BrdU-labeled chromatids, and the subsequent preferential breakage of the DNA containing the dye by fluorescent light and its elution by warm saline sodium citrate. The chromatid with more DNA stains dark with Giemsa and that with less DNA stains lighter [7]. More recently, fluorescent antibodies to BrdU have been used for sister chromatid differentiation [9].

It has been demonstrated that a wide range of chemicals can increase the frequency of SCEs in a broad range of cell types [10]. There is a background level of SCEs that varies with cell type and concentration of BrdU; these SCEs are a consequence of the BrdU incorporation into the DNA. The analysis of SCEs can be a useful component of hazard identification, although it needs to be noted that there is no adverse phenotypic outcome known to be associated with the induction of SCEs. There is, however, a high frequency of SCEs in cells from individuals with Bloom syndrome that is a reflection of error-prone DNA replication of the BrdU-containing template [11]. Thus, SCE increases probably reflect an enhancement of errors in DNA replication, induced, for example, by a clastogen that produces DNA adducts. An advantage of the SCE assay is its high level of sensitivity of detecting chromosomal effects that are produced by S-phase-dependent mechanisms.

6.3.4   Micronuclei

The analysis of structural chromosomal alterations by standard metaphase analysis requires a high level of expertise and is time consuming. For hazard identification purposes, the analysis of micronuclei can be equally informative. Micronuclei are membrane-bounded structures that form either from acentric pieces of DNA (deletions) or whole chromosomes that are not incorporated into daughter nuclei. It is possible to distinguish between acentric fragments and whole chromosomes using an antibody to the kinetochore component of the centromere; a positive stain represents a micronucleus containing a whole chromosome [12]. Thus, the micronucleus assay can be used for the assessment of structural and numerical chromosomal alterations. While the micronucleus assay does not provide the detail for all types of chromosomal alterations induced by a clastogen that would be obtained by metaphase analysis, it is a robust assay for the identification of a clastogen.

6.4 DESCRIPTION OF CELL TEST SYSTEMS

6.4.1 Established Cell Lines

It is possible to use any permanent cell line that is cycling for cytogenetic tests. However, it is considerably easier for analysis of the data to use cell lines that have a stable karyotype that is close to the diploid number for the particular species. Chinese hamster cell lines (CHO and V79) have frequently been used because of their low near-diploid number of chromosomes ($2n$ is normally 22). Primary human cell lines or virally transformed ones can be used, but they have a relatively low mitotic index that makes analysis more burdensome than with rapidly dividing cells. Thus, any cell line with a stable karyotype and a high mitotic index is most suitable for cytogenetic tests. Human lymphocytes can be virally transformed to produce lymphoblastoid cell lines that generally have a stable karyotype close to the diploid number, but have the advantage of a relatively high mitotic index.

6.4.2 Human Lymphocyte Cultures

Human peripheral blood lymphocytes are nondividing cells but can be stimulated to reenter the cell cycle by use of a mitogen such as phytohemagglutinin. The stimulated cells move somewhat synchronously through the first cell cycle, so that cells can be treated in G_1, S, and/or G_2 either by selection of the appropriate treatment time after stimulation or by selection of an appropriate time after treatment for cell sampling and fixation. Mitogen stimulated cells have a relatively high mitotic index, especially at the first metaphase, and being primary cultures they have a stable diploid karyotype when sampled from a normal individual. A concern with their routine use is that blood samples have to be obtained from suitable volunteers and this requires some form of informed consent. However, the process for meeting the consent requirement can quite readily be met.

6.5 REQUIREMENTS FOR CYTOGENETIC ASSAYS

While it is possible to use any cycling cell system for cytogenetic analysis, it is highly advantageous to use one that has a stable diploid or near-diploid karyotype. Again, as noted previously, a high mitotic index is also greatly advantageous, if nothing else because this reduces the time to search for analyzable metaphase cells. Primary human lymphocyte cultures are very suitable for meeting both of these needs.

The great majority of chemical clastogens produce structural aberrations by inducing errors of DNA replication (e.g., from an induced DNA adduct) and so treatment with a test chemical has to be for cells in the S phase or that pass through the S phase between treatment and analysis at metaphase [13]. For maximum sensitivity, treatment in S phase is required such that repair of induced DNA damage prior to replication is minimized. Also, for maximal sensitivity of the assay for structural changes, analysis should be conducted on cells at their first metaphase after treatment. As noted in Section 6.3, a number of structural alterations are not transmitted to daughter cells, and many are cell lethal events. Thus, analysis at the second or subsequent metaphase after treatment will be much less sensitive than at the first metaphase.

For SCE, aneuploidy, and micronucleus assays, analysis has to be at the second or subsequent metaphase after treatment (SCE and aneuploidy) or during the second cell cycle after treatment (micronucleus) because either cell division produces the event (aneuploidy and micronuclei) or the assay itself relies on two cell cycles for observation of the endpoint (SCE). The maximum frequency for induced micronuclei will be observed during the second cell cycle after the start of treatment, and so a method has been developed to ensure that this requirement will be met. Cytochalasin B inhibits the process of cytokinesis (cell division) and so at division the cell itself will not divide in the presence of cytochalasin B but its nucleus will, and so a binucleate cell will be produced. Thus, micronuclei can be exclusively analyzed in binucleate cells to maximize the sensitivity of the assay [14].

There are other features of assays that more generally fall under the category of personal laboratory preferences rather than requirements. These modifications can be found in individual research papers or study reports [15].

6.6   DESCRIPTION OF ASSAYS

There are, of course, a wide range of protocols available for the conduct of *in vitro* cytogenetic assays. Some of these provide a required format for regulatory purposes (e.g., U.S. Environmental Protection Agency (EPA), U.S. Food and Drug Administration (FDA), and the European Union (EU) regulatory requirements). Others follow best practices and serve as guidelines (e.g., Organization for Economic Cooperation and Development (OECD) and the International Conference on Harmonization of Technical Requirements for Registration of Pharmaceuticals for Human Use (ICH)). These all address the requirements described in Section 6.5 but do differ in some of the specific technical details of the tests. These specific details can be found in the individual publications and reports from these organizations. Pertinent information to be used as a starting point for testing guidelines can be found in the review by Muller et al. [16]. Many of the components of *in vitro* assays are the same for the different cytogenetic endpoints whereas some are endpoint specific. In this latter case, the requirements for each assay are presented separately in the following sections.

6.6.1   Cell Growth and Maintenance

Any mammalian cell type that can be grown in tissue culture medium *in vitro* is acceptable for cytogenetic testing. As noted previously, a stable diploid or near-diploid karyotype is advantageous, as is a high mitotic index. Stocks of cells should be stored in liquid nitrogen until needed for a test rather than maintained in culture all the time. At the time of use for a test, cells should be in logarithmic growth phase. Cells should be checked routinely for mycoplasma contamination and not used if contaminated. Appropriate culture medium recommended for the routine growth of specific cell lines should be used. Culture conditions should be standardized for CO_2 concentration, temperature, and humidity. Besides routinely checking the karyotype of the cells to be used, a routine check of cell-cycle time under the standard culture conditions should be made.

6.6.2   Metabolic Activation

A broad range of chemicals require some form of metabolic activation to convert the parent compound into its active metabolites. The majority of cultured cells do not have endogenous metabolic capability and so some form of exogenous metabolic activation needs to be incorporated into the assay. A test is typically conducted with and without metabolic activation to establish whether or not such activation is required for clastogenicity. The most frequently used metabolic activation system is a cofactor-supplemented postmitochondrial fraction (S9) prepared from the livers of rodents treated with metabolism enzyme-inducing agents such as Aroclor 1254 [17]. The choice of concentration of S9 can be dependent on the particular chemical class under test. There have been proposals to use an appropriate species for the formulation of the S9 dependent on the species of the test cells used. For routine testing this has not been a general recommendation. In addition, specific cell lines have been engineered to express specific metabolic activating enzymes, providing an endogenous metabolizing system [18]. This has some potential advantages but knowledge of the metabolism of the test chemical is required so that the appropriate transgenic cell line can be used in a test. There clearly is room for improving the process whereby metabolic activation is incorporated into an assay, but for the present the use of S9 is reasonable.

6.6.3   Control Groups

The inclusion of appropriate control groups is an essential component of any assay system. At a minimum, it is necessary to have a control sample that does not include the test chemical but does include the solvent or vehicle used for the test chemical. These vehicle controls should include samples with and without the metabolic activation system. In addition, a negative control should be included for every cell sampling time used in an assay.

A positive control must be used and should be a known clastogen at treatment concentration levels that are known to give a reproducible and detectable increase over the historic background level for the cytogenetic endpoint being assayed. In this way the positive control demonstrates the sensitivity of the test system at the particular time of the test. If metabolic activation is used, then the positive control should be a clastogen that requires metabolic activation for its effectiveness.

It has been quite common for positive controls to be used at high concentrations that give a very potent positive response. However, this usually means that the slide analyzer will immediately recognize the positive control samples and this can provide a potential bias to the analysis. Positive control concentrations should produce a clear positive effect but not an excessive amount of chromosomal damage.

Several positive controls are used quite frequently and include the following:

Metabolic Activation Condition	Chemical	CAS Number
Absence of exogenous metabolic activation	Methyl methanesulfonate	[66-27-3]
	Ethyl methanesulfonate	[62-50-0]
	Ethylnitrosourea	[759-73-9]
	Mitomycin C	[50-07-7]
	4-Nitroquinoline-*N*-oxide	[56-57-5]
Presence of exogenous metabolic activation	Benzo[*a*]pyrene	[50-32-8]
	Cyclophosphamide	[50-18-01]

6.6.4   Test Chemicals

Solid test substances need to be dissolved or suspended in appropriate solvents or vehicles. If feasible, they may be prepared in tissue culture medium (without serum). In general, it is recommended that such chemical preparation be performed shortly prior to use in a test. In specific instances where stability of the test chemical in its dissolved state has been established, longer term storage might be used. The treatment solution or suspension should be diluted to the desired concentrations for test use. The vehicle itself should be at an amount in the cell culture that does not affect cell viability or growth rate.

6.6.5   Exposure Concentrations

The chemical should be tested over a range of concentrations that will allow for the assessment of a concentration–response relationship. If feasible, the highest test substance concentration tested with and without metabolic activation should show evidence of cytotoxicity or reduced mitotic activity. In addition, the highest concentration selected should be consistent with solubility issues and should not result in significant changes in pH or osmolality. The concentration range selected is based on preliminary cytotoxicity data and should include concentrations that induce substantial cytotoxicity (about 60%), intermediate cytotoxicity, and low or no cytotoxicity. In those cases where cytotoxicity is not observed in preliminary studies, the highest concentration should be of the order of 0.01 M, 5 mg/mL, or 5 µL/mL. Gases or volatile liquids should be tested in sealed vessels.

6.6.6   Treatment with Test Substances

Duplicate cultures should be used for each dose level, harvest time, or other experimental subdivision. For cell lines and strains, cells in the exponential phase should be treated with the test substance, with and without an exogenous metabolizing system. Human lymphocytes that have been stimulated to reenter the cell cycle with a mitogen can be similarly treated.

For chromosome aberration studies, there are a number of different rationales covering the timing of the start of treatment and the duration of treatment [17]. Given the broad need for cells to be treated at some point of the total treatment in the S phase of the cell cycle, an acute treatment of about 3 h with sampling some 3–6 h afterwards for the great majority of cell lines and 6–12 h for stimulated human lymphocytes will meet this requirement. For lymphocytes, treatment should start about 36 h after mitogenic stimulation, or earlier if longer treatment times are desired. The only exception would be for high concentrations when extensive cell cycle delay is induced. In this case, a repeat experiment using longer times between the end of treatment and sampling might be necessary. Variations in treatment duration and sampling time are recommended for different protocols. Continuous treatment throughout one cell cycle can also be used, provided a balance is maintained between cytotoxicity and mitotic index to obtain a sufficient number of analyzable metaphase cells.

For SCE or micronucleus studies, longer treatment times are recommended based on the requirement for a cell division (micronuclei) or two DNA replications (SCE) between the start of treatment and observation. For cell lines, treatment can be continuous for about two cell cycles in duration, or it can be more acute (3h) with a sampling of about two cell cycles from the start of treatment. For the micronucleus assay, cytochalasin B should be added during the first cell cycle of treatment with cells being harvested before the second mitosis. For lymphocytes, treatment can start at about 24h after mitotic stimulation and last for about two cell cycles until harvesting. Alternatively, an acute treatment of about 12h can be used starting also at 24h after mitotic stimulation. For the micronucleus assay, cytochalasin B is typically added at about 44h after mitotic stimulation with cell harvesting at 72h after stimulation.

6.6.7 Culture Harvest Times

The harvest times for established cell lines and for human lymphocytes are basically covered in Section 6.6.6, because these times are related to the start and end of treatment. An additional major requirement is that the majority of cells to be analyzed at metaphase (chromosome aberrations and SCEs) or as binucleate cells (micronuclei) have spent a significant proportion of the total treatment time in the S phase of the cell cycle. To ensure that this occurs and also to ensure sufficient mitotic cells or binucleate cells for analysis, either multiple sampling times or a single harvest time with supporting data for its selection can be used.

A spindle inhibitor, such as colchicine or colcemid, is added to the culture 2–3h prior to harvest to facilitate accumulation of metaphase cells and to produce contracted metaphase chromosomes that are particularly suitable for analysis purposes.

6.6.8 Chromosome Preparations

There is a fairly wide selection of methods available for obtaining cells suitable for chromosome aberration, SCE, or micronucleus analysis. There are some essential components and some that are individual preferences. For chromosome aberration and SCE analysis, cells need to be swollen with a hypotonic solution and gently fixed (e.g., with glacial acetic acid and alcohol) to avoid cell rupture. Ideal preparations for analysis have well-spread metaphase chromosomes with no overlaps but with minimal probability of chromosome loss as a result of the chromosome spreading technique. For micronuclei, the cytoplasm should be maintained (a hypotonic solution is not generally used) for the most reliable identification of micronuclei and for identification of binucleate cells.

The slides can be stained by a variety of methods with the requirement that clear definition of centromeres and differential chromatid staining are obtained where appropriate. Giemsa staining is generally the standard for metaphase analysis for chromosome aberrations and SCE. More recently, chromosome-specific fluorescent probes have been used for the assessment of reciprocal translocations but this is not generally a part of a standard battery of tests for hazard identification. For micronucleus analysis, fluorescent DNA-specific dyes are preferred, because these are able to facilitate the detection of even very small micronuclei. Anti-kinetochore antibodies or FISH with pancentromeric DNA probes can be used to establish whether not micronuclei contain whole chromosomes or chromosomal acentric fragments [12].

6.6.9   Analysis of Cytogenetic Alterations

A very important component of analysis is that it be conducted without the microscopist having knowledge of the treatment status of the material being analyzed. This can be accomplished by coding all the slides prior to microscopic analysis.

The number of cells to be analyzed for the different cytogenetic endpoints varies somewhat among the different guidelines and protocols: the following is a general guidance. For chromosome aberrations, it is reasonable for subsequent statistical analysis to analyze 100 cells from each of two duplicate cultures for each treatment group. For SCE analysis, 25 cells per duplicate sample per treatment group is reasonable and for micronuclei, 1000 binucleate cells from each of the duplicate cultures for each treatment is appropriate. For all endpoints, an assessment of cytotoxicity using a cell proliferation index or mitotic index is appropriate.

As general guidance, for human lymphocytes, chromosome aberration and SCE analysis should be performed for cells that have a centromere number of 46. For cell lines, it is frequently recommended that cells with ±2 centromeres from the modal number can be analyzed. This perhaps indicates a less than stable karyotype and it might be more appropriate to use a cell line that has a tight modal number of centromeres so that ±1 from this mode would be the recommended range for analysis.

6.6.10   Statistical Analysis and Evaluation of Results

There are many different statistical approaches that have been applied to *in vitro* cytogenetic data and it is not possible to discuss these and their relative merits in this short chapter. The reader is directed to two comprehensive discussions of the issues to be addressed by statistical analysis of these types of data and approaches for the conduct of the appropriate analysis. The reviews are by Margolin et al. [19] and Kim et al. [20].

Similarly, there has been much guidance on the criteria for establishing a positive or a negative result for *in vitro* cytogenetic data. The following is taken from the ICH Guidance presented in Muller et al. [16] since this provides a very informative set of questions to be addressed for evaluating datasets. (Note: Reference to other parts of the manuscript have been deleted from this quote)

2.3.1. *Guidance on the evaluation of in vitro test results*

2.3.1.1. *In vitro positive results*
The scientific literature gives a number of conditions which may lead to a positive in vitro result of questionable relevance. Therefore, any in vitro positive test result should be evaluated for its biological relevance taking into account the following considerations (this list is not exhaustive, but is given as an aid to decision-making):
(i) Is the increase in response over the negative or solvent control background regarded as a meaningful genotoxic effect for the cells?
(ii) Is the response concentration-related?
(iii) For weak/equivocal responses, is the effect reproducible?
(iv) Is the positive result a consequence of an in vitro specific metabolic activation pathway/active metabolite?
(v) Can the effect be attributed to extreme culture conditions that do not occur in in vivo situations, e.g., extremes of pH; osmolality; heavy precipitates especially in cell suspensions?
(vi) For mammalian cells, is the effect only seen at extremely low survival levels?
(viii) Is the positive result attributable to a contaminant (this may be the case if the compound shows no structural alerts or is weakly mutagenic or mutagenic only at very high concentrations)?
(viii) Do the results obtained for a given genotoxic endpoint conform to that for other compounds of the same chemical class?

2.3.1.2. *In vitro negative results*
For in vitro negative results, special attention should be paid to the following considerations (the examples given are not exhaustive, but are given as an aid to decision-making): Does the structure or known metabolism of the compound indicate that standard techniques for in vitro metabolic activation (e.g., rodent liver S9) may be inadequate? Does the structure or known reactivity of the compound indicate that the use of other tests methods/systems may be appropriate?

Based on adherence to a standard protocol and the availability of experience with a particular assay, it would be expected that a test can be described as clearly positive or clearly negative. However, this is certainly not always the case: test results sometimes do not fit the predetermined criteria for a positive or negative decision and therefore have to be described as "equivocal." It is thus assumed that neither biological interpretation nor statistical methods can resolve this situation. In such cases, further testing is usually required to resolve equivocal results. Such tests might involve a different concentration range, treatment times, and/or harvest times depending on available data that might indicate the appropriate experimental design.

6.6.11 Test Conclusions

It is important that the conclusions from *in vitro* cytogenetic assays be stated within the specific confines of the particular assay. For example, *positive results in the in vitro cytogenetic assay indicate that under the test conditions the test substance induces chromosomal aberrations* (or *SCE* or *micronuclei*) *in cultured mammalian somatic cells* (or *human lymphocytes*). Similarly, *negative results indicate that under the test conditions the test substance does not induce chromosomal aberrations* (or *SCE or micronuclei*) *in cultured mammalian somatic cells* (or *human lymphocytes*).

6.6.12 Test Report

The OECD Guideline for the Testing of Chemicals Draft Proposal for a New Guideline 487: *In Vitro* Micronucleus Test (found at http://www.oecd.org/dataoecd/60/28/32106288.pdf) provides a comprehensive summary of the information that constitutes a complete report for an *in vitro* cytogenetic test. This guideline is for the micronucleus assay but generally applies to other *in vitro* cytogenetic tests. The information to be included is covered in Sections 6.6.1–6.6.11.

6.7 FUTURE DIRECTIONS

The field of cytogenetics has changed quite significantly over the past decade or so with the development of a range of FISH techniques [21]. These can be used to measure specific events such as reciprocal translocations and genomic alterations associated with tumors, as examples. While these can provide significant input for understanding the underlying mechanisms of disease formation, particularly for tumors, and for use in quantitative risk assessments, they have not significantly enhanced the process of hazard identification. Given the added cost of FISH methods, their use in standard *in vitro* cytogenetic tests for hazard identification remains fairly limited.

There is an increasing interest in the role of stem cells in the initiation of disease processes and at the same time an increased availability of long-term adult stem cell *in vitro* cultures [22]. It is generally desirable, where possible, to use the most relevant cell types for *in vitro* cytogenetic assays, and so it is anticipated that human adult stem cell cultures will be incorporated into protocols.

There might also be further development of automated analysis systems for chromosomal alterations, SCEs, and micronuclei. Certainly, flow cytometry has been employed for micronucleus analysis with some success and is gaining in popularity [23]. Automated chromosome analysis systems are less reliable and very much in the development phase. Their improvement to join the arsenal of automated analysis tools would be a significant step in regard to time and cost savings.

ACKNOWLEDGMENTS

I wish to thank Dr. Andrew Kligerman and Dr. James Allen for their valuable review of this chapter. This chapter has been reviewed by the U.S. Environmental Protection Agency and approved for publication but it does not necessarily reflect Agency policy.

REFERENCES

1. Sax K. Induction by X-rays of chromosome aberrations in *Tradescantia* microspores. *Genetics* 1938;23:494–516.

2. Moorehead PS, Nowell PC, Mellman WJ, Battips DM, Hungerford DA. Chromosome preparations of leukocytes cultured from human peripheral blood. *Exp Cell Res* 1996;20:613–616.

3. Hsu TC. *Human and Mammalian Cytogenetics: An Historical Perspective*. New York: Springer-Verlag; 1979.

4. deSerres FJ, Ashby, J Eds. *Evaluation of Short-Term Tests for Carcinogens: Report of the International Collaborative Program. Progress in Mutation Research*, Volume 1. New York: Elsevier/North Holland; 1981.

5. Gollapudi BB, Krishna, G. Practical aspects of mutagenicity testing strategy: an industrial perspective. *Mutat Res* 2000;455:21–28.

6. Savage JR. Classification and relationships of induced chromosomal structural changes. *J Med Genet* 1976;13:103–122.

7. Latt SA. Microfluorometric analysis of deoxyribonucleic acid replication kinetics and sister chromatid exchanges in human chromosomes. *J Histochem Cytochem* 1974;22: 478–491.

8. Perry P, Evans HJ. Cytological detection of mutagen–carcinogen exposure by sister chromatid exchange. *Nature* 1975;258:121–125.

9. Tucker JD, Christensen ML, Strout CL, Carrano AV. Determination of the baseline sister chromatid exchange frequency in human and mouse peripheral blood lymphocytes using monoclonal antibodies and very low doses of bromodeoxyuridine. *Cytogenet Cell Genet* 1986;43:38–42.

10. Tucker JD, Auletta A, Cimino MC, Dearfield KL, Jacobson-Kram D, Tice RR, Carrano AV. Sister-chromatid exchange: second report of the Gene-Tox program. *Mutat Res* 1993;297:101–180.

11. Shiraishi Y, Ohesuki Y. SCE levels in Bloom-syndrome cells at very low bromodeoxyuridine (BrdU) concentrations: monoclonal anti-BrdU antibody. *Mutat Res* 1987; 176:157–164.

12. Schriever-Schwemmer G, Adler ID. Differentiation of micronuclei in mouse bone marrow cells: a comparison between CREST staining and fluorescent *in situ* hybridization with centromeric and telomeric probes. *Mutagenesis* 1994;9:333–340.

13. Preston RJ. Mechanisms of induction of chromosomal alterations and sister chromatid exchanges: presentation of a generalized hypothesis. In Li AP, Heflich RH, Eds. *Genetic Toxicology: A Treatise*. Telford Press: Caldwell, NJ 1991; Chap 3, pp 41–66.

14. Fenech M. The *in vitro* micronucleus techniques. *Mutat Res* 2000;455:81–95.

15. Bonassi S, Fenech M, Lando C, Lin YP, Ceppi M, Chang WP, Holland N, Kirsch-Volders M, Zeiger E, Ban S, Barale R, Bigatti MP, Bolognesi C, Jia C, DiGiorgio M, Ferguson LR, Fucic A, Lima OG, Hrelia P, Krishnaja AP, Lee TK, Migliore L, Mikhalevich L, Mirkova E, Mosesso P, Muller WU, Odagiri Y, Scarffi MR, Szabova E, Vorbtsova I, Vral A, Zijno A. HUman MicroNucleus project: international database comparison for results with the cytokinesis-block micronucleus assay in human lymphocytes: I. Effect of laboratory protocol, scoring criteria, and host factors on the frequency of micronuclei. *Environ Mol Mutagen* 2001;37:31–45.

16. Muller L, Kikuchi Y, Probst G, Schechtman L, Shimada H, Sofuni T, Tweats, D. ICH-Harmonized guidances on genotoxicity testing of pharmaceuticals: evolution, reasoning and impact. *Mutat Res* 1999;436:195–225.

17. Galloway SM, Aardema MJ, Ishidate M Jr, Ivett JL, Kirkland DJ, Morita T, Mosesso P, Sofuni T. Report from working group on *in vitro* tests for chromosomal aberrations. *Mutat Res* 1994;312:241–261.

18. Doherty AT, Ellard S, Perry EM, Parry JM. An investigation into the activation and deactivation of chlorinated hydrocarbons to genotoxins in metabolically competent human cells. *Mutagenesis* 1996;11:247–274.

19. Margolin BH, Resnick MA, Rimpo JY, Archer P, Galloway SM, Bloom AD, Zeiger E. Statistical analyses for *in vitro* cytogenetic assays using Chinese hamster ovary cells. *Environ Mutagen* 1986;8:183–204.

20. Kim BS, Zhao B, Kim HJ, Cho M. The statistical analysis of the *in vitro* chromosome aberration assay using Chinese hamster ovary cells. *Mutat Res* 2000;469:243–252.

21. Speicher MR, Carter NP. The new cytogenetics: blurring the boundaries with molecular biology. *Nat Rev Genet* 2005;6:782–792.

22. Li L, Neaves WB. Normal stem cells and cancer stem cells: the niche matters. *Cancer Res* 2006;66:4553–4557.

23. Dertinger SD, Bishop ME, McNamee JP, Hayashi M, Zuzuki T, Asano N, Nakajima M, Moore M, Torous DK, Macgregor JT. Flow cytometric analysis of micronuclei in peripheral blood reticulocytes: I. Intra- and inter-laboratory comparison with microscopic scoring. *Toxicol Sci* 2006;94:83–91.

7

IN VIVO GENOTOXICITY ASSAYS

ANDREAS HARTMANN,[1] KRISTA L. DOBO,[2] AND HANS-JÖRG MARTUS[1]
[1]Novartis Pharma AG, Basel, Switzerland
[2]Pfizer Global R&D, Groton, Connecticut

Contents

7.1 INTRODUCTION

The preclinical safety assessment of drug candidates includes conduct of assays intended to identify genotoxic hazards. Experience with genetic toxicology testing over the past several decades has demonstrated that no single assay is capable of detecting all genotoxic effects. Therefore, the potential for a chemical to cause genotoxicity is typically determined through a battery of tests conducted *in vitro* and *in vivo*. Genotoxicity tests are typically conducted early in the development of

Preclinical Development Handbook: Toxicology, edited by Shayne Cox Gad
Copyright © 2008 John Wiley & Sons, Inc.

a drug candidate as they are relatively short in duration and inexpensive and provide an early means to identify potential genotoxic carcinogens, which otherwise would not be detected until the completion of 2 year cancer bioassays. Current internationally harmonized guidance [1] recommends the conduct of both *in vitro* and *in vivo* genotoxicity assays, which together detect the potential of a drug candidate to induce small genetic mutations and chromosomal scale damage.

Compared to *in vitro* testing, an *in vivo* test system provides a model that takes into account important factors such as absorption, distribution, metabolism, and excretion that may influence the genotoxic activity of a compound. In addition, an *in vivo* test may detect chemicals that only act *in vivo*, although experience has shown that such compounds are rare. A small number of genotoxic carcinogens, including procarbazine, hydroquinone, urethane, and benzene, are reliably detected using bone marrow tests for chromosomal damage, whereas *in vitro* tests yield negative, weak, or conflicting results [2]. Thus, data from one *in vivo* test is valuable in that it can provide additional reassurance that a drug candidate does not possess genotoxic potential, beyond initial conclusions derived from *in vitro* testing.

Internationally harmonized guidance, ICH M3 [3], outlines which nonclinical safety studies are required to support the various stages of clinical development. Since Phase I clinical trials are usually limited to a few volunteers for a short duration of treatment, it is considered acceptable to limit genotoxicity testing for Phase I studies to the generally more sensitive *in vitro* tests of the standard battery consisting of a bacterial mutagenicity test and a clastogenicity test in cultured mammalian cells. Expansion of clinical investigations into larger populations with longer treatment duration, that is, Phase II and III studies, requires an *in vivo* cytogenetic assessment prior to the initiation of such trials. This *in vivo* assay can either be an analysis of chromosomal aberrations in bone marrow cells or an analysis of micronuclei in bone marrow or peripheral blood erythrocytes. Only under specific circumstances, that is, for compounds that are not systemically absorbed and do not provide for adequate target tissue exposure, may an assessment be based on *in vitro* data alone [1].

It is important to note that there are specific circumstances under which the ICH S2B guidance [1] recommends both *in vivo* and *in vitro* genotoxicity testing be complete prior to initiating clinical trials, including the following: (1) prior to clinical testing in women of childbearing potential, pregnant women, or in children; and (2) for compounds bearing structural alerts for genotoxic activity. Structurally alerting compounds as defined in the literature [4] or with *in silico* systems may have to be further investigated using appropriate tests if the standard tests yield negative results. (3) In the case of positive or equivocal findings *in vitro, in vivo* genotoxicity testing is required prior to clinical Phase I studies for the purpose of risk assessment [5]. A negative result in a standard *in vivo* test for chromosomal damage in rodent hematopoietic cells will not provide sufficient data to conclude that the compound is inactive in somatic cells *in vivo*. Rather, the *in vivo* relevance of positive *in vitro* genotoxicity data needs to be assessed in at least one additional *in vivo* genotoxicity test utilizing a different tissue.

Finally, an alternative approach to assessing genotoxicity prior to the initiation of clinical investigations has been outlined recently in an FDA draft guidance on exploratory investigational new drug (exploratory IND) applications. In the case of clinical investigations in which volunteers will receive a low number of doses of an investigational drug at relatively low doses, with the intent of collecting limited but critical information to determine feasibility of drug development (e.g., pharmacokinetics), a more limited nonclinical safety assessment is considered acceptable. With regard to genetic toxicology testing, it is acceptable to conduct a standard bacterial mutation assay as well as a test for chromosomal aberrations either *in vitro* or *in vivo*. Furthermore, according to the draft guidance it is acceptable to perform the *in vivo* cytogenetic assessment in conjunction with the repeated dose toxicity study in the rodent [6].

This chapter provides an overview of the standard *in vivo* cytogenetic assays that are commonly used as part of the genotoxicity test battery intended for hazard identification. In addition, exploratory *in vivo* assays are discussed that are utilized to follow up on positive genotoxicity results obtained in the standard battery or to assess a contribution of genotoxicity to preneoplastic/neoplastic changes detected in long-term tests in rodents.

7.2   STANDARD *IN VIVO* TESTS FOR CHROMOSOMAL DAMAGE IN RODENT HEMATOPOIETIC CELLS

The most commonly applied *in vivo* cytogenetic test is the evaluation of micronucleus formation in bone marrow or peripheral blood erythrocytes. Micronuclei are small, round remnants of nuclear chromatin that result from the induction of chromosome breakage or aberrant mitotic division. With the expulsion of the main nucleus during erythrocyte maturation, micronuclei are easily detected in the otherwise anucleate erythrocytic cells (Fig. 7.1). A less commonly applied, but equally acceptable approach for *in vivo* cytogenetic assessment is metaphase chromosome

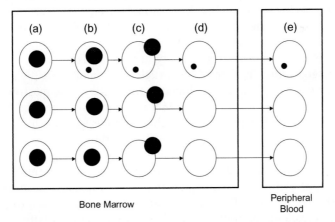

Bone Marrow   Peripheral Blood

FIGURE 7.1   Micronucleated erythrocyte formation. (**a**) Rapidly dividing erythroblast precursor cells in the bone marrow are exposed to test article capable of causing chromosome breakage or abnormal chromosomal segregation. (**b**) In the subsequent interphase erythroblast cells that were subject to chromosome breakage or loss contain micronuclei in addition to the main nucleus. (**c**) Expulsion of the main nucleus during erythrocyte maturation. (**d**) Micronuclei formed in susceptible erythroblast precursor cells remain in otherwise anucleate erythrocytes. (**e**) Migration of normal and micronucleated erythrocytes from the bone marrow to the peripheral blood.

aberration analysis in rodent bone marrow. Using this assay, the frequency and types of structural chromosomal damage observed in bone marrow cells are assessed. In general, metaphase analysis is much more tedious and time consuming and requires a highly skilled cytogenetic experimenter to complete. Furthermore, unlike the *in vivo* micronucleus assay that can detect clastogenicity and aneugenicity, metaphase analysis is limited to assessment of chromosome breakage.

ICH guidelines for genotoxicity testing [1, 6] provide general recommendations regarding the use of *in vivo* cytogenetic assays for the purposes of detecting genotoxic hazards. In addition, OECD guidelines 474 [7] and 475 [8] provide an overview of major methodological considerations for the design, conduct, analysis, and reporting of *in vivo* cytogenetic tests. Subsequent sections of this chapter review key aspects of study design, conduct, interpretation, and reporting of standard *in vivo* cytogenetic assays in the context of use for hazard identification.

7.2.1   *In Vivo* Micronucleus Assessment in Rodent Hematopoietic Tissue

Developed as a rapid alternative to chromosome aberration assessment in rodent bone marrow [9], the rodent micronucleus (MN) assay in erythrocytes is currently the most widely utilized *in vivo* genotoxicity test for assessing induction of cytogenetic damage. The basis of the *in vivo* MN assay is that actively dividing cells exposed to a test article capable of causing chromosome breakage or loss will induce the formation of micronuclei, which are readily identified in progeny cells (i.e., cells in the subsequent division). Immature or newly formed erythrocytes provide an ideal cell population for MN assessment as the erythroblast precursor cells are rapidly dividing in the bone marrow, with the nucleus extruded from the cell a few hours after final mitosis. Providing that there is sufficient time between exposure to the test article and recovery of erythrocytes for analyses, micronuclei that result from induction of chromosomal breakage or malsegregation in erythroblast precursor cells can easily be detected in the newly formed anucleate erythrocyte population. Furthermore, assessment of MN induction in the immature erythrocyte population provides a high assay sensitivity, as these cells were susceptible to chromosome damage during the time of test article treatment.

The MN assay was originally developed in the mouse bone marrow [9] and later it was demonstrated that assessment of MN induction in peripheral blood of mice was equally sensitive [10]. However, given that the rat is typically utilized in preclinical toxicology assessments of acute and subchronic duration, it is more practical to use the rat for *in vivo* cytogenetic safety assessment. Consequently, more recently, greater effort has been applied to investigations and developments using the rat.

Characteristics of the drug candidate that are established in initial toxicology studies, which help facilitate the design of an acceptable *in vivo* micronucleus test, include drug formulation, route of administration, toxicokinetics, and toxicity. Careful consideration of all available data for the drug candidate at the time of protocol design will help maximize the value of the *in vivo* MN study. In the absence of data from prior studies, a dose-range finding study may be conducted to gain this experience.

There is a large body of scientific data contained in the public literature regarding the design and conduct of *in vivo* MN studies. Major methodological considerations of *in vivo* MN study design have been the topic of numerous meetings of the International Workshop on Genotoxicity Test Procedures (IWGTP) [11, 12]. In addition, the Collaborative Study Group for the Micronucleus Test (CSGMT) has coordinated investigations directed at understanding the importance of specific elements of study design and methodology [13–19]. These efforts, in addition to contributions from a large number of investigators, have established current practices considered acceptable for the design and conduct of *in vivo* MN assays. Some specific aspects studied in detail include rodent species [18], sex [13, 20], strain [14, 21], treatment route [22], treatment regimen [15, 19, 23, 24], sampling times, sensitivity of blood versus bone marrow [18, 19, 25–27], and development and validation of automated analysis [28–35]. Important methodological aspects of the *in vivo* MN study are reviewed in the following sections. However, more detailed information may be found in the relevant cited references.

Species, Strain, Sex, and Number of Animals   In preclinical drug development the most commonly applied species of animals for the conduct of *in vivo* cytogenetic assessment are rat and mouse. In selecting a species and strain of test animal, several considerations should be made. First, the availability of historical control data for the strain and species intended for use is important for the selection of statistical methods and the interpretation of data. Another factor to consider is the availability of drug candidate toxicity data in a rodent species and strain that can be employed for the MN assay, as this can greatly facilitate the design of the study. Furthermore, if the same strain of animal is used for the conduct of long-term toxicology studies or carcinogenicity studies, the MN data may be valuable in assessing the relevance of other findings later in the development of the drug candidate. Given that the rat is the primary rodent species utilized in preclinical toxicology studies, the rat is often the species of choice for the conduct of *in vivo* MN assessment. In the absence of any special requirements for a particular age, young adult animals should be used.

The use of one sex is generally accepted based on studies that have demonstrated that sensitivity to MN induction is similar between male and female rodents [13, 20]. However, if there are data that suggest significant differences in toxicity, toxicokinetics, or metabolism between male and female animals, then both sexes should be utilized. In the case of MN studies that are integrated with toxicology studies, both male and female rodents will be on test by default. In such cases, it is recommended that samples from both sexes be prepared for analysis. However, it is considered acceptable to limit the conduct of MN analyses to a single gender [12]. Each treatment and control group should include at least five analyzable animals. Therefore, if mortality is expected at the high dose, additional animals should be included. Additional animals may also be included for the negative and test treatment groups for plasma drug concentration determination.

Treatment Regimen and Route of Administration   The route and schedule of administration of test articles should be determined based on consideration of the bioavailability and pharmacokinetics of the drug candidate being evaluated. It is imperative that the study be designed such that the hematopoietic tissue is exposed to significant concentrations of the drug candidate, otherwise the conduct of the study will add little value to the nonclinical safety assessment. In general, test substance should be administered at least once each day unless the half-life justifies otherwise. Therefore, in the case of drug candidates with short half-lives, multiple daily treatments may be necessary to maintain sufficiently high blood levels. Doses or formulations that require large volume administration to deliver the test article may also justify the need for multiple daily treatments. Challenges associated with drug candidates having short half-lives or limited oral bioavailability may be overcome by considering administration by continuous infusion or the parenteral route, respectively. Ultimately, the route and schedule of administration should be designed keeping in mind that the hematopoietic tissue is the target of exposure and subsequent evaluation.

Acute Treatment Protocols and Tissue Sampling   Studies of acute duration (i.e., 1 or 2 days) are typically designed as independent protocols. The application of acute treatment protocols in the mouse with assessment of MN induction in bone marrow or peripheral blood has been widely utilized, as well as in the rat with MN induction being evaluated in bone marrow. Due to early investigations in the rat demonstrating the ability of the spleen to capture and destroy micronucleated erythrocytes from the peripheral blood [36], assay sensitivity in this tissue has been a concern. Although the efforts of numerous investigators have resulted in the compilation of a significant body of data demonstrating that rat peripheral blood is also sensitive to the detection of aneugens and clastogens [18, 19, 25–27, 37] its use is not widely accepted.

For 1 day treatment protocols, tissue samples (i.e., bone marrow and/or blood) are typically collected and evaluated at two time points. For bone marrow, samples should be collected at ~24 and 48 hours post-treatment, whereas blood samples should be collected at ~48 and 72 hours post-treatment. In the case of 2 day treatment, tissues are typically sampled at a single time point, with bone marrow and/or blood collected at ~24 hours following the final administration.

Subchronic Treatment Protocol and Tissue Sampling   The incorporation of MN assessment into subchronic general toxicity studies is an attractive alternative to the acute protocol, as it can reduce animal usage with genotoxicity data generated in parallel with general toxicity and pharmacokinetic data. Treatment protocols that specify up to 4 weeks of treatment are considered acceptable study designs for both mouse and rat [12]. This is based on the outcome of studies in which repeated daily treatments with subchronic duration of exposures were shown to produce similar results (magnitude of response) in comparison to acute treatment in the majority of cases [19, 23, 38–41]. The use of a subchronic versus acute treatment protocol should be given special consideration for drug candidates that induce a positive response in vitro. In such cases an acute protocol should be used if higher systemic exposures can be achieved. As is the case for short duration studies, both bone marrow and blood are acceptable tissues for MN assessment in mouse and bone marrow for MN assessment in rat. For subchronic studies, tissue sampling (bone marrow and/or blood) should take place at one time point, approximately 24 hours following the last treatment.

Negative Controls   A concurrent negative control group should be included for each gender and for every sampling time. Negative control animals should be treated with the solvent or vehicle formulation, delivered via the same route of administration as test article, with animals receiving a volume equivalent to the test-article-treated animals. This control is used to help discriminate test-substance effects from effects of the solvent or vehicle alone (the vehicle should not produce toxicity at the doses used to administer drug). In addition, inclusion of a concurrent untreated control group should also be considered. In the absence of historical or published data demonstrating lack of confounding or mutagenic effects of the solvent or vehicle being used to deliver the test article, untreated control animals should be included in the study. If MN induction is being assessed in peripheral blood, untreated control data can be generated by collecting blood samples immediately prior to the initiation of the study (i.e., prior to the first dose of test article).

Positive Controls   The requirement for including a concurrent positive control group is dependent on a number of other aspects of the study design. However, at a minimum, positive control samples must be included as part of microscopic analysis to control for staining and scoring procedures. Omission of a concurrent positive control group may be considered acceptable if (1) verification of test article concentration and stability is conducted according to Good Laboratory Practice (GLP) guidance, and (2) systemic exposure is demonstrated under the experimental conditions used for the study, especially in the case of test articles that are expected to be relatively nontoxic *in vivo* or have demonstrated clastogenicity *in vitro*. If these conditions are not met, a concurrent positive control group should be included. Several examples of positive control substances include cyclophosphamide, mitomycin C, ethyl methanesulfonate, ethyl nitrosourea, and triethylenemelamine. The dose of positive control administered should create an increase in micronucleated cells that is clearly elevated, but not immediately evident to a technician conducting microscopic analysis. The route of administration of the positive control article may differ from that of the test article and a single treatment is acceptable with cells harvested at the appropriate time post-treatment. For example, in a bone marrow MN study conducted with test article treatment for 14 days, positive control animals may receive a single administration of cyclophosphamide on day 14, with cell harvest conducted approximately 24 hours post-treatment, concurrently with the harvest of samples from negative control and test-article-treated groups.

Dose Selection   For drug candidates that induce toxicity, the highest dose selected should be the maximum tolerated dose (MTD), that is, the dose that produces signs of toxicity, such that higher doses would result in lethality. Bone marrow toxicity, as evidenced by a reduction in the ratio of polychromatic erythrocytes (PCEs) to normochromatic erythrocytes (NCEs), can also be used to define the upper dose limit and provides an excellent confirmation that the target cells were exposed to the test article. In the absence of test compound toxicity, the highest dose may be limited to the maximum practical dose (MPD), which is defined as 2000 mg/kg/day for studies of acute duration (14 days or less) and 1000 mg/kg/day for studies greater than 14 days duration [11]. Three dose levels should be used and ideally cover a range from clear toxicity to little or no toxicity. Twofold dose spacing [11, 42] and log-type dose spacing [43] have been recommended. However, consideration should be given to all available toxicity data in selection of doses.

Sample Preparation and Analysis   Methodology for the preparation of hematopoietic tissue for microscopic analyses is detailed in the scientific literature [44, 45]. In brief, if MN assessment is to be conducted in bone marrow cells, the samples should be collected from the femurs and/or tibia of rodents immediately following sacrifice. Cells from bone marrow are flushed out using fetal serum. Subsequently, bone marrow samples are concentrated by centrifugation and then spread onto standard microscope slides. A column filtration method may be used to concentrate anucleated cells [46]. Once dry, the slides are fixed for several minutes in absolute methanol. Peripheral blood samples can be obtained from the tail vein or any other blood vessel.

Samples are then stained such that immature or polychromatic erythrocytes (PCEs), which contain RNA, can be differentiated from mature or normochromatic erythrocytes (NCEs), which are devoid of RNA. There are a number of staining methods that differentiate these cell populations while also facilitating the visualization of micronuclei. Blood samples may be stained supravitally by placing a small sample of blood onto a slide that has been previously coated with acridine orange [47]. Alternatively, blood smears may be prepared, air-dried, and fixed in absolute methanol. Fixed samples of bone marrow and blood can be stained using DNA-specific stains including acridine orange (Fig. 7.2) [48] or Hoechst 33258 and pyronin Y [49]. The non-DNA-specific stain Giemsa may also be utilized; however, it is not recommended for the preparation of bone marrow samples obtained from rat, due to the presence of mast cell granules, which can be mistaken for micronuclei.

All slides including positive and negative controls are coded prior to microscopic analysis. As a measure of toxicity to the hematopoietic tissue, the proportion of immature or polychromatic erythrocytes (PCEs) among total erythrocytes is determined for each animal by scoring 200 erythrocytes in the bone marrow or 1000

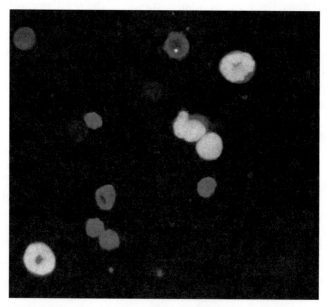

FIGURE 7.2   Rat bone marrow smear stained with acridine orange. Immature erythrocytes (PCEs) are anucleate, contain residual RNA, and appear bright red using fluorescent microscopy. Mature erythrocytes (NCEs) contain no RNA and do not stain with acridine orange, yet are readily visible. A micronucleated PCE appears as an anucleate red cell, containing a small, round, yellow nuclear fragment (top center). Nucleated cells with large yellow nuclei are also present in the bone marrow smear.

erythrocytes in peripheral blood. Two thousand PCEs per animal are scored for the frequency of micronucleated cells. In the mouse, supplementary information may also be obtained by scoring micronuclei in the mature erythrocyte population, as these cells have a relatively long lifetime and are not removed by the spleen.

Due to the tedious and time-consuming nature of microscopic analysis, a number of automated methods for MN quantification have been developed, including automated microscope slide reading [28] or flow cytometry based approaches [29–34]. This is a significant advancement, as the high analysis rates of flow cytometry allow tens of thousands of erythrocytes to be analyzed in several minutes. Both OECD and ICH guidances indicate that automated methods of MN assessment are acceptable as long as there is sufficient validation [1, 7]. The most widely investigated and validated flow cytometric method available to date is that developed by Dertinger et al. [31, 32]. This method uses anti-CD71-FITC labeling to differentiate immature (CD71+) from mature (CD71−) erythrocytes. In addition, RNA degradation and propidium iodide staining of DNA allows discrimination of erythrocytes with and without micronuclei. By using a single laser to excite both fluorochromes, the immature and mature erythrocytes with and without micronuclei are then readily differentiated into four discrete populations (Fig. 7.3). Typically, when flow cytometry is used to quantify MN frequencies, 20,000 immature erythrocytes are evaluated for the frequency of micronucleated cells. Similar to microscopic analysis, the proportion of immature erythrocytes among total erythrocytes is also determined and utilized as a measure of toxicity to the hematopoietic tissue.

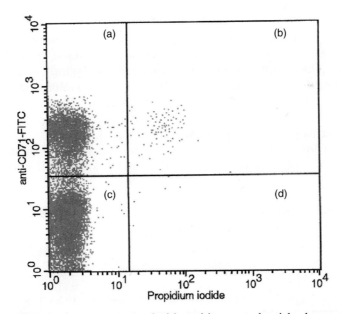

FIGURE 7.3 Dot plot from a rat treated with positive control article, demonstrating application of MicroFlow® flow cytometric method for enumeration of micronucleated erthyrocytes. (a) Immature erythrocytes, without micronuclei (CD71+, no PI stain). (b) Immature erythrocytes, with micronuclei (CD71+, containing PI stain). (c) Mature erythrocytes, without micronuclei (CD71−, no PI stain). (d) Mature erythrocytes, with micronuclei (CD71−, containing PI stain).

Reporting of Data Details of study design, study conduct, tissue preparation, sample analysis, and results should be reported in accordance with expectations outlined in OECD guidance 474 [7]. Data obtained from microscopic or cytometric analysis should be presented in tabular form and listed separately for each animal. Data points should include the numbers of immature erythrocytes scored, the numbers of micronucleated immature erythrocytes observed, and the numbers of immature erythrocytes among total erythrocytes. If micronuclei are scored in the mature erythrocyte population, then this data should be presented as well. Calculated values should also be presented, including the proportion of immature erythrocytes among total erythrocytes, the percentage of micronucleated immature erythrocytes, group mean values, and standard errors.

Data Analysis and Interpretation of Results Data should be analyzed using statistical methods [11, 50–53]; however, the biological relevance of statistically significant results should be taken under consideration when interpreting data and making a conclusion. Both trend tests and pairwise comparison tests are appropriate for the statistical analysis of results obtained from *in vivo* MN assessment, with numerous methods considered equally acceptable [50].

The use of negative historical control data in the evaluation and interpretation of study results is also valuable. For example, concurrent negative control data can be compared to the historical negative control data to confirm the acceptability of the study. The historical data can also be used to understand the biological relevance of statistically significant increases in micronuclei. For example, consider study results in which all concurrent negative control and test-article-treated animals generate MN frequencies within the historical control range, yet the trend test indicates statistical significance (Tables 7.1 and 7.2). In this case, comparison of the study data to the negative historical control data indicates that the statistically significant result produced by the trend test is not indicative of a biologically relevant response to drug treatment. With regard to biological relevance and interpretation of results, it is also worth noting that a number of confounding factors have been demonstrated to induce increases in micronucleated erythrocytes including hypothermia [54, 55], induction of hematopoiesis [56], and malnutrition [57].

The criteria for a positive, negative, and equivocal response should be clearly defined prior to initiation of the study (i.e., in the study protocol). A positive

TABLE 7.1 Representative Historical Control Data Compiled from Bone Marrow Micronucleus Studies Conducted in Male Rats

Control Type	Number[a]	% PCE Mean ± SD[b]	Range (%)[c]	% MN-PCE Mean ± SD[d]	Range (%)[e]
Negative	412	64.8 ± 13.2	34.0–94.7	0.11 ± 0.09	0.00–0.60
Positive	115	54.4 ± 15.6	16.4–89.0	4.18 ± 2.28	0.50–9.30

[a]The total number of animals evaluated.
[b]The mean percentage of PCEs among total erythrocytes observed in control animals ± the standard deviation.
[c]The range of percent PCE frequencies observed among control animals.
[d]The mean percentage of micronucleated PCEs observed in control animals ± the standard deviation.
[e]The range of percent micronucleated-PCE frequencies observed among control animals.

TABLE 7.2   Representative Example of Summary Study Data from Rat Micronucleus Assay (Male Rat)

Compound	Animal Number	% PCE[a]	% MN PCE[b]
Vehicle control	1	65.8	0.00
	2	60.5	0.05
	3	67.9	0.05
	4	60.0	0.10
	5	62.6	0.10
	Mean	*63.4*	*0.06*
	SD ±	*3.4*	*0.04*
Positive control	7	39.3	3.95
	8	51.4	3.45
	9	46.9	3.15
	10	42.0	3.90
	11	58.6	4.40
	Mean	*47.6*	*3.77*
	SD ±	*7.7*	*0.48*
Test article, 500 mg/kg	19	66.0	0.00
	20	54.6	0.00
	21	51.8	0.05
	22	61.4	0.15
	23	42.2	0.00
	Mean	*55.2*	*0.04*
	SD ±	*9.2*	*0.07*
Test article, 1000 mg/kg	25	56.2	0.10
	26	59.8	0.05
	27	58.6	0.10
	28	61.1	0.05
	29	52.3	0.15
	Mean	*57.6*	*0.09*
	SD ±	*3.5*	*0.04*
Test article, 2000 mg/kg	31	40.5	0.25
	32	36.0	0.05
	33	60.8	0.20
	34	54.9	0.05
	35	42.9	0.15
	Mean	*47.0*	*0.14*
	SD ±	*10.4*	*0.09*

[a]Percentage of PCEs among total erythrocytes.
[b]Percentage of micronucleated PCEs.

response may be defined by a number of criteria. For example, test results may be considered positive when statistical significance is observed from trend test analysis, with concurrent observation of MN frequencies outside the historical control range for at least one treatment group. Alternatively, a clear increase in micronucleated cells in a single treatment group at a single sampling time may also define a positive response. The observation of a positive response in the *in vivo* MN assay indicates that the drug candidate has the potential to induce clastogenic or aneugenic effects in the hematopoietic tissue. Negative results indicate that the drug candidate does not induce such effects under the test conditions utilized. When the results of an *in vivo* MN assay are equivocal, conduct of a subsequent study to clarify the finding should be considered, preferably using a modification to the original experimental design (e.g., refined dose selection or treatment regimen).

7.2.2 *In Vivo* Rodent Bone Marrow Chromosomal Aberration Assay

An equally accepted [1, 5] but much less utilized method for identifying the potential of a drug candidate to induce clastogenicity *in vivo* is the evaluation of chromosomal aberrations in rodent bone marrow metaphase cells. Bone marrow is the target tissue for this assay as the cells are rapidly dividing, thereby making the tissue susceptible to the genotoxic effects of chemical treatment. In contrast to the quantification of micronuclei in erythrocytes, the assessment of chromosomal damage via aberration analysis in metaphase cells is tedious and requires a highly skilled experimenter to complete. In addition, chromosome analysis does not provide ready analysis of aneugenic mechanisms, as in the case of the MNT recommendations regarding major methodological aspects of study design, conduct, analysis, and reporting published in OECD guidance 475 [8]. Additional detail regarding minimal requirements for the design and conduct of scientifically valid and practical studies has also been published [58]. The previous discussions regarding optimal study design for *in vivo* MN assays are largely applicable to the design of bone marrow aberration assays. Therefore, the following overview focuses on those aspects of the aberration assay study design, conduct, analysis, and reporting that differ from the MN assay or are unique to the chromosomal aberration assay.

Overview of the Study Design of the **In Vivo** ***Chromosome Aberration Assay***   Mouse and rat are the most commonly utilized rodent species for the conduct of the bone marrow chromosome aberration assay, based on their widespread use in general toxicity studies. Similar to the micronucleus (MN) assay, young adult animals should be utilized with a minimum of 5 analyzable animals per treatment group. A single sex may be tested unless data demonstrate differences in toxicity or pharmacokinetics between male and female animals. Concurrent negative vehicle control groups should be included for each sex and sampling time. A concurrent positive control group should be included for each sex as well, but a single sampling time is acceptable. The positive control substances suggested for use in the *in vivo* MN assay are also applicable for the aberration assay.

Acute and Subchronic Treatment Protocols and Sampling Times   Important considerations for selecting route of administration and treatment regimen, such that exposure to the hematopoietic tissue is optimized, were previously discussed for *in vivo* MN study design and are applicable to the design of a bone marrow chromosome aberration assay. Both acute and subchronic treatment protocols can be utilized. Acute treatment protocols of 1 day should be followed by two sample collections. Sample collection is scheduled such that cells are in the first metaphase after exposure to drug. Therefore, the first sample collection should occur between 12 and 18 hours following treatment, which corresponds to approximately 1.5 cell cycles. The second collection should occur 24 hours following the first. The second sampling collection is intended to account for treatment-related cell cycle delay or slow rates of drug uptake and metabolism. In order to enrich the population of metaphase cells in the bone marrow prior to harvest, animals are administered a metaphase arresting compound (e.g., colchicine) intraperitoneally about 3–5 hours prior to sacrifice. For studies in which drug is administered for multiple days, only one sample collection is necessary and should occur at 12–18 hours following the final treatment.

Dose Selection   The recommendations for dose selection are similar to those of the *in vivo* MN assay. The highest dose tested should be the maximum tolerated dose (MTD), or one that induces bone marrow toxicity, such that there is a significant reduction of the mitotic index in test-article-treated animals in comparison to the concurrent negative controls. Alternatively, for nontoxic drug candidates, the maximum practical dose (MPD) can be used to define the upper dose limit (2000 mg/kg/day for 1–14 days; 1000 mg/kg/day for greater than 14 days). Three test-article-treated groups should be included with twofold or log-type dose spacing.

Sample Preparation and Analysis   Bone marrow is collected from the femur and/or tibia immediately following sacrifice. Samples are prepared by exposure to a hypotonic solution and then fixative. Fixed samples are dropped onto slides and stained. Slides from all treatment groups are blind coded prior to microscopic evaluation. Sample analysis includes determination of the mitotic index by scoring 1000 cells/animal for the frequency of metaphase cells, and quantification of chromosome aberrations by scoring a minimum of 100 metaphase cells/animal. In selecting cells for chromosome aberration analysis, it is considered acceptable to score metaphase cells with a total centromer count of $2n \pm 2$, where n is equal to the haploid number of chromosomes for the species being tested. During analysis, the number and types of aberrations observed in each cell should be recorded. The minimal classes of aberrations that should be differentiated when collecting data include chromatid-type and chromosome-type gaps, breaks, and rearrangements. It is also recommended that a polyploidy index be determined for all bone marrow samples by assessing 200 metaphase cells for the frequency of polyploidy and endoreduplicated cells [58]. Increases in polyploid or endoreduplicated cells in treated animals may be indicative of aneugenic potential.

Reporting of Data   Details of study design, study conduct, tissue preparation, sample analysis, and results should be reported in accordance with expectations outlined in OECD guidance 475 [8]. Data should be reported in tabular form for each animal including the number of cells scored, the number of aberrations per cell, and the percentage of cells with structural aberrations. Structural chromosome aberrations should be listed according to their classification with the number and frequency for treated and control groups. Gaps should also be reported in tabular form but not included in the tally of aberrant cells.

Data Analysis and Interpretation of Results   The use of statistical analysis in the evaluation and interpretation of chromosome aberration assay data is recommended, along with consideration of historical control data and biological relevance [58]. As with the *in vivo* MN assay, commonly utilized and acceptable methods of statistical analysis include the application of trend and/or pairwise comparison tests. For example, data can be analyzed to assess the occurrence of a statistically significant dose–response relationship by conducting a trend test such as the Cochran–Armitage trend test. Alternatively, or in addition, pairwise comparisons may also be conducted (e.g., Fisher's exact test) to assess significant increases at each individual dose group. Historical control data is also valuable for evaluation and interpretation of data in that it can be used to assess the acceptability of the response observed in the concurrent control, and also for considering the biological relevance of responses that are flagged as statistically significant.

Several criteria can be used for concluding a result is positive; a reasonable example is observation of a dose-related increase in aberrant cells with a concurrent statistically significant increase in at least one dose group. The observation of equivocal results should be clarified by conducting further testing, preferably using a modification of the experimental conditions used in the first study. Positive results in the chromosomal aberration assay indicate that the drug candidate induces clastogenic effects under the test conditions, whereas negative results indicate that the drug candidate is not clastogenic. Finally, increases in polyploidy may be indicative of aneugenic potential; however, polyploidy can also be the result of cytotoxicity.

7.3   SUPPLEMENTAL *IN VIVO* GENOTOXICITY ASSAYS

Supplemental *in vivo* genotoxicity studies are used (1) to follow up on positive findings in one or more tests of the standard genotoxicity battery; (2) to elucidate a potential contribution of genotoxicity to the induction of preneoplastic and/or neoplastic changes detected in long-term tests in rodents; and (3) to elucidate mechanisms of micronucleus formation to differentiate clastogenic from aneugenic effects. Since aneugenicity is well accepted to result from mechanisms of action for which thresholds exist, demonstration that micronucleus formation is a result of chromosome loss should allow an acceptable level of human exposure to be defined [59]. No matter the trigger for conducting supplemental *in vivo* genotoxicity testing, it is critical that the approach utilized—for example, the endpoint and target tissue assessed—is scientifically valuable, such that the results will aid in interpreting the relevance of the initial finding of concern. Ultimately, the goal of supplemental genotoxicity testing is to determine if a genotoxic risk is posed to patients under intended conditions of treatment.

Follow-up Testing of Drug Candidates Positive in the Standard Genotoxicity Test Battery   It has been reported that approximately 30% of pharmaceuticals produce positive genotoxicity results *in vitro* [60]. In contrast, results from bone marrow cytogenetic assays are frequently negative, even for those compounds that produce positive results *in vitro*. This discrepancy may result from a number of major differences that exist when testing in cultured cells versus intact animals. For example, differing metabolic pathways can exist *in vitro* and *in vivo*, metabolic inactivation can occur in the intact animal, parent compound or active metabolite may not reach the target cell *in vivo*, rapid detoxification and elimination may occur, or plasma levels *in vivo* may not be comparable to concentrations that generate positive responses in the *in vitro* assay, which is often accompanied by high levels of cytotoxicity. It is also worth noting that positive results generated *in vitro* may be secondary to effects, such as cytotoxicity, which may never be achieved under *in vivo* exposure conditions. Data from *in vivo* experiments are therefore essential before definitive conclusions are drawn regarding the potential mutagenic hazard to humans from chemicals that produce positive results in one or more *in vitro* tests.

Follow-up Testing of Tumorigenic Drug Candidates Negative in the Standard Genotoxicity Test Battery   Carcinogenicity testing of pharmaceutical drug candidates negative in the standard *in vitro* and *in vivo* genotoxicity assays may yield evidence of a tumorigenic response in rodents. The ICH guidance S2B [1] stipulates that such compounds shall be investigated further in supplemental genotoxicity tests, if rodent tumorigenicity is not clearly based on a nongenotoxic mechanism. Typically, supplemental *in vivo* genotoxicity tests should be performed with cells of the respective tumor target organ to distinguish between genotoxic and nongenotoxic mechanisms of tumor induction.

Endpoints Assessed in Supplemental Assays   In section 7.3.1, commonly applied test systems are described that are used as supplemental genotoxicity assays. These assays differ with respect to the endpoints assessed:

1. Induction of primary DNA lesions, that is, measurement of exposure, uptake, and reactivity to DNA via the comet assay or ^{32}P-postlabeling assay.
2. Measurement of the repair of DNA lesions using the unscheduled DNA synthesis (UDS) test.
3. Measurement of induction of genetic changes using transgenic animal assays for point mutations or the mouse spot test.

7.3.1   *In Vivo* Genotoxicity Tests for the Assessment of Primary DNA Lesions

Primary DNA lesions are detected with so-called indicator tests. These tests do not directly measure consequences of DNA interaction (i.e., mutation) but do detect effects related to the process of mutagenesis, such as DNA damage, recombination, and repair. Results from indicator tests can provide additional useful information in the context of extended genotoxicity testing. However, primary DNA lesions may be repaired error-free and do not necessarily result in formation of mutations. The most commonly utilized assays in pharmaceutical development are the ^{32}P-postlabeling assay and the comet assay. Further methods such as the alkaline elution or unwinding assays will not be described here. However, comprehensive data for these tests and descriptions of the assays have been published [61, 62]. A comparison of different aspects of the methods described in the text is depicted in Table 7.3. Basic aspects regarding optimal study design for *in vivo* micronucleus assays are largely applicable to the design of supplemental *in vivo* assays. Specific or unique aspects on study protocols are described more extensively where appropriate.

Comet Assay for the Detection of DNA Damage   The *in vivo* comet assay (single-cell gel electrophoresis) is increasingly being used as a supplemental genotoxicity test for drug candidates [63, 64]. There are general review articles on the comet assay [65, 66] and a general guideline for test conductance has been published as a result of the International Workshop on Genotoxicity Test Procedures (IWGTP) [67].

TABLE 7.3   Overview on Key Aspects of Exploratory In Vivo Genotoxicity Assays

Aspect	Comet Assay	DNA Adducts	UDS Test (Liver)	Transgenic Gene Mutation
Test definition (accepted protocol)	Yes	No	Yes	Yes
Regulatory acceptance/use	Yes	Yes	Yes	Yes
Relevance of endpoint	Moderate	Moderate	Moderate	High
Technical demands	Low–moderate	Moderate–high	Moderate	High
Widespread use	Yes	No	Yes	No
Applicable to most tissues?	Yes	Yes	No	Yes
Dependence of cell turnover	No	No	No	Yes
Cost	Low–moderate	Moderate–high	Low	High

More specific recommendations with the goal of gaining more formal regulatory acceptance of the comet assay were published following the 4th International Comet Assay Workshop [68]. An updated position paper on specific aspects of test conditions and data interpretation was prepared following the IWGT in 2005 [69].

Principle of the Method   The basic principle of the comet assay is the migration of DNA in an agarose matrix under electrophoretic conditions (Fig. 7.4). When viewed through the microscope, a cell has the appearance of a comet, with a head (the nuclear region) and a tail containing DNA fragments or strands migrating in the direction of the anode (Fig. 7.5). Among the various versions of the comet assay, the alkaline (pH of the unwinding and electrophoresis buffer ≥13) method enables detection of the broadest spectrum of DNA damage and is therefore recommended (in the first instance) for regulatory purposes [67, 68]. The alkaline version detects DNA damage such as strand breaks, alkali-labile sites (ALS), and single strand breaks associated with incomplete excision repair. Under certain conditions, the assay can also detect DNA–DNA and DNA–protein crosslinking, which (in the absence of other kinds of DNA lesions) appears as a relative decrease in DNA migration compared to concurrent controls. In contrast to other DNA alterations, crosslinks may stabilize chromosomal DNA and inhibit DNA migration [70, 71]. Thus, reduced DNA migration in comparison to the negative control (which should show some degree of DNA migration) may indicate the induction of crosslinks, which are relevant lesions with regard to mutagenesis and should be further investigated. Increased DNA migration indicates the induction of DNA strand breaks and/or ALS. Furthermore, enhanced activity of excision repair may result in increased DNA migration. DNA excision repair can influence comet assay effects in a complex way [72, 73]. While DNA repair generally reduces DNA migration by eliminating DNA lesions, ongoing excision repair may increase DNA migration due to incision-related DNA strand breaks. Thus, the contribution of excision repair to the DNA

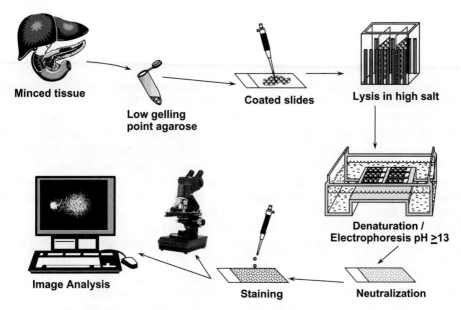

FIGURE 7.4   Flow diagram for performing a comet assay.

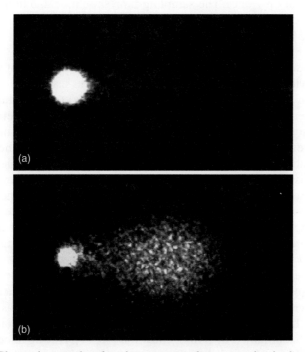

FIGURE 7.5   Photomicrographs of rat hepatocytes after processing in the comet assay: (a) hepatocyte of vehicle control animal and (b) hepatocyte of rat dosed once orally with 40 mg/kg methyl methanesulfonate, exhibiting increased DNA migration.

effects seen in the comet assay depends on the types of induced primary DNA damage and the time point of analysis [73].

Test Procedure   Aspects regarding test animals, test substance, use of concurrent negative and positive control animals, as well as dose selection for the design of a cytogenetic assay, as described in detail previously, are largely applicable to the design of an *in vivo* comet assay. In addition, more specific details can be found in an earlier publication [68]. A single treatment or repeated treatments (generally at 24 hour intervals) are equally acceptable. In both experimental designs, the study is acceptable as long as a positive effect has been demonstrated or, for a negative result, as long as an appropriate level of animal or tissue toxicity has been demonstrated or the limit dose with appropriate tissue exposure has been used. For repeated treatment schedules, dosing must be continued until the day of sampling. On a daily basis, test substances may be administered as a split dose (i.e., two treatments separated by no more than a few hours), to facilitate administering a large volume of material. The test may be performed in two ways. If animals are treated with the test substance once, then tissue/organ samples are obtained at 2–6 hours and 16–26 hours after dosing. The shorter sampling time is considered sufficient to detect rapidly absorbed as well as unstable or direct acting compounds. In contrast, the late sampling time is intended to detect compounds that are more slowly absorbed, distributed, and metabolized. When a positive response is identified at one sampling time, data from the other sample time need not be collected. Alternatively, if multiple treatments at 24 hour intervals are used, tissue/organ samples need be collected only once. The sampling time should be 2–6 hours after the last administration of the test substance. Alternative sampling times may be used when justified on the basis of toxicokinetic data.

Selection of Tissues and Cell Preparation   In principle, any tissue of the experimental animal, provided that a high quality single cell/nucleus suspension can be obtained, can be used for a comet assay. Selection of the tissue(s) to be evaluated should be based, wherever possible, on data from absorption, distribution, metabolism, excretion studies, and/or other toxicological information. A tissue should not be evaluated unless there is evidence of, or support for, exposure of the tissue to the test substance and/or its metabolite(s). In the absence of such information and unless scientifically justified, two tissues should be examined. Recommended tissues are liver, which is the major organ for the metabolism of absorbed compounds, and a site of first contact tissue—for example, gastrointestinal for orally administered substances, respiratory tract for substances administered via inhalation, or skin for dermally applied substances. Which tissue is evaluated first is at the discretion of the investigator and both tissues need not be evaluated if a positive response is obtained in the first tissue evaluated.

   Single-cell suspensions can be obtained from solid tissue by mincing briefly with a pair of fine scissors [74], incubation with digestive enzymes such as collagenase or trypsin [75], or by pushing the tissue sample through a mesh membrane. In addition, cell nuclei can be obtained by homogenization [76, 77]. During mincing or homogenization, EDTA can be added to the processing solution to chelate calcium/magnesium and prevent endonuclease activation. In addition, radical scavengers (e.g., DMSO) can be added to prevent oxidant-induced DNA damage. Any cell dissociation method is acceptable as long as it can be demonstrated that the process is not associated with inappropriate background levels of DNA damage.

Cytotoxicity—A Potential Confounding Factor   A general issue with DNA strand break assays such as the comet assay is that indirect mechanisms related to cytotoxicity may lead to enhanced strand break formation. However, since DNA damage in the comet assay is assessed on the level of individual cells, dead or dying cells may be identified on microscopic slides by their specific image. Necrotic or apoptotic cells can result in comets with small or nonexistent head and large, diffuse tails [78] as observed *in vitro* upon treatment with cytotoxic, nongenotoxic articles [79–81]. However, such microscopic images are not uniquely diagnostic for apoptosis or necrosis since they may also be detected after treatment with high doses of radiation or high concentrations of strong mutagens [82]. For the *in vivo* comet assay, only limited data are available to establish whether cytotoxicity results in increased DNA migration in tissues of experimental animals. Despite necrosis or apoptosis in target organs of rodents such as kidneys [83], testes [84], liver, or duodenum [63], no elevated DNA migration was observed. However, enhanced DNA migration was seen in homogenized liver tissue of mice dosed with carbon tetrachloride [85] when histopathological examination showed evidence of necrosis in the liver. Therefore, to avoid potential false-positive effects resulting from cytotoxicity, recommendations regarding a concurrent assessment of target organ toxicity have been made, including dye viability assays, histopathology, and a neutral diffusion assay [67, 68].

Biological Significance of Lesions Detected   DNA lesions leading to effects in the comet assay can be strand breaks which may be relevant to the formation of chromosome aberrations or DNA modifications such as abasic sites (AP sites) with relevance to the induction of gene mutations. However, primary lesions detected by the comet assay may also be correctly repaired without resulting in permanent genetic alterations. Neither the magnitude of DNA migration in the comet assay nor the shape of the comet can reveal the types of DNA damage causing the effect or their biological significance, that is, their mutagenic potential. Therefore, conclusions regarding the mutagenicity of a test compound cannot be made solely on the basis of comet assay effects. There are a few limitations of the comet assay with regard to its application and interpretation of test results. For example, short-lived primary DNA lesions such as single strand breaks, which may undergo rapid DNA repair, could be missed when using inadequate sampling times. However, an appropriate study design including one early preparation time point (i.e., at 3–6h) is considered sufficient to ensure that these lesions are captured—in particular at higher dose levels, where DNA repair may be significantly delayed or even overwhelmed. In any case, it should be kept in mind that a negative comet result can be considered as a strong indicator for the absence of a mutagenic potential.

Advantages   The advantages of this assay for use in genotoxicity testing of drug candidates include its applicability to various tissues and/or special cell types, its sensitivity for detecting low levels of DNA damage, its requirement for small numbers of cells per sample, the general ease of test performance, the short time needed to complete a study, and its relatively low cost. The comet assay can be applied to any tissue in the given *in vivo* model, provided that a single cell/nuclei suspension can be obtained. Therefore, the comet assay has potential advantages over other *in vivo* genotoxicity test methods, which are reliably applicable to rapidly proliferating cells only or have been validated preferentially in a single tissue only. The comet assay may detect a broader spectrum of primary DNA lesions, including single strand breaks and oxidative base damage, which may not be detected in the UDS test because they are not repaired by nucleotide excision repair [86]. The advantages of the comet assay over the alkaline elution test include the detection of DNA damage on a single-cell level and the requirement for only small numbers of cells per sample. In contrast, when using the alkaline elution assay, large quantities of cells are necessary for the determination of genotoxic effects, and, therefore, only a limited number of organs/tissues can be evaluated using this technique. In particular, this seems important for investigation of suspected tissue-specific genotoxic activity, which includes "site-of-contact" genotoxicity (cases of high local versus low systemic exposure).

Limitations   Experimental variability is an important issue and should be kept to a minimum to ensure reliable interpretation and comparability of the data obtained with other *in vivo* comet experiments. Experimental variability may result from shortcomings with regard to number of doses tested, number of animals per dose, number of slides per animal, number of cells analyzed, lack of sufficient DNA migration in cells of concurrent controls, and deviation from minimum time for treatment of slides with alkaline buffer. Shortcomings regarding technical details apply, for example, to the most comprehensive overview on *in vivo* comet assay test results published so far [87]. This paper provides data on more than 200 compounds tested in rodents, all of which was produced before specific recommendations on assay conduct [67] were available. Therefore, although a valuable resource with very relevant data, the paper by Sasaki et al. [87] has areas where technical aspects of the assay differ from the current minimal requirements recommended [67, 68]. Considering these discrepancies, the data of the comprehensive study [87], as well as other study reports not in agreement with the current recommendations, should be interpreted with caution. This point was highlighted recently in a position paper on the use and status of the *in vivo* comet assay in genotoxicity testing [64], which critically assessed published data produced under test conditions not fully in agreement with the minimal requirements for an acceptable test [67, 68]. For example, it was noted that positive comet assay data were published for compounds that have been assessed before to be neither genotoxic nor carcinogenic, such as food additives [88]. Such isolated positive comet assay results should be critically evaluated in the light of current recommendations [67, 68] to exclude methodological shortcomings and potential artifacts. In cases where negative carcinogenicity data are already available and the *in vivo* comet assay result represents an isolated positive finding in the context of existing genotoxicity data, the biological significance of the effect seen in the comet assay should be assessed with caution.

Determination of DNA Adduct Formation   The assessment of DNA adducts in target organs of toxicity is an effective molecular dosimeter of genotoxic exposure and may facilitate differentiation of genotoxic and nongenotoxic agents [89]. The role of DNA adducts in mutagenesis is well documented [90]. However, the relationship between DNA adduct formation, mutagenesis, and subsequent carcinogenesis is complex. For example, comparative investigations have shown that there is not always a clear relationship between DNA adduct levels as an early event and the induction of mutations in marker genes [91, 92]. Thus, some DNA adducts are of greater significance with respect to mutagenesis or carcinogenesis with some adducts being efficiently removed, while other types, or the same adducts at different DNA locations, remain unrepaired. In some cases, the presence of unrepaired adducts may lead to mutations via mispairing during replication. Alternatively, the removal of adducts, particularly if DNA resynthesis is involved, may not be error-free and may lead to mutations. Attempts to elucidate the relationship between specific primary DNA alterations and mutations are limited and influenced by confounding factors [93, 94].

The ^{32}P-Postlabeling Assay   The ^{32}P-postlabeling assay has widely been used to measure covalent DNA–xenobiotic adducts [95–97]. In the ^{32}P-postlabeling assay, DNA is hydrolyzed enzymatically to 3′-monophosphates and DNA adducts are enriched by the selective removal of normal nucleotides [98]. The DNA adducts are then labeled with [^{32}P]phosphate and the resulting ^{32}P-labeled DNA adducts are usually separated by thin-layer chromatography or high performance liquid chromatography (HPLC). Radioactivity of DNA adducts is detected by autoradiography and liquid scintillation counting, imaging analysis, or a liquid scintillation analyzer.

Advantages and Limitation   The 32P-postlabeling technique is the most sensitive method for the detection of a wide range of large hydrophobic compounds bound to DNA and can potentially detect one DNA adduct, such as those derived from polycyclic aromatic compounds in 10^9–10^{10} bases. As a result of an IWGTP conference in 1999, recommendations on the use of the postlabeling assay have been issued [96]. The assay allows the detection of adducts from different chemicals with diverse chemical structures, such as polycyclic aromatic hydrocarbons, aromatic amines, heterocyclic amines, alkenylbenzene derivatives, benzene and its metabolites, styrene, mycotoxins, simple alkylating agents, unsaturated aldehydes from lipid peroxidation, pharmaceuticals, reactive oxygen species, and UV radiation. One unique strength of the assay is that it has been useful for the detection of adducts from complex mixtures [99, 100]. The assay can be applied to measure adducts after multiple dosing in any tissue or to examine the removal of adducts after cessation of exposure. However, one of the major challenges or limitations of using the postlabeling assay for investigating new drug candidates is selection of appropriate methods in the absence of knowing what adducts are or are not formed. The chances of adduct detection may be severely limited as applied methods of chromatography may not be appropriate for the adduct being formed [96]. The assay could give false-negative results due to loss of adducts. In addition, false-negative results are more likely to occur with nonaromatic versus aromatic adducts due to the lower sensitivity of the assay for nonaromatic adducts. Furthermore, polynucleotide kinase can label non-nucleic-acid components, such as some hydroxylated metabolites, leading to false-positive results [101]. Finally, endogenous DNA adducts called I-compounds [102] can interfere with the detection of adducts formed from a test compound exposure. Some I-compounds are present at levels of 1 adduct in 10^7 or more DNA nucleotides and migrate on chromatography plates similar to adducts derived from aromatic carcinogens [102].

Mass Spectrometry Mass spectrometry methods for measuring DNA adducts have been introduced more recently. Of the physicochemical methods used to detect DNA binding, mass spectrometry has the greatest potential because of its high chemical specificity that allows for unequivocal characterization of the DNA binding products [103]. Thus, genuine DNA adducts derived from the chemical being tested may be distinguished from unrelated adducts and from products of endogenous DNA damage, which is not possible with the postlabeling assay. Detailed structural information on DNA adducts may also be obtained. Accelerator mass spectrometry (AMS) has been used to measure radiocarbon isotope with attomole (10^{-18} mol) sensitivity [104]. Because of the extraordinary sensitivity of AMS, only trace levels of radioactivity are required. However, this technique requires that the isolated DNA be devoid of noncovalently bound radioactivity to assure accurate estimates of DNA adduct levels. Although structural information is not provided by this technique, the use of HPLC in combination with AMS provides a greater degree of confidence in analyte identity. Soft ionization techniques such as matrix-assisted laser desorption ionization (MALDI) and electrospray ionization (ESI) have emerged as techniques to detect nonvolatile and thermally labile compounds [105]. The online coupling of HPLC with tandem mass spectrometry provides structural information of the adducts, and the incorporation of stable, isotopically labeled internal standards into the assay assures precision and accurate quantification of the DNA adducts [106]. Although tandem mass spectrometry is not as sensitive as those of ^{32}P-postlabeling or AMS, DNA adduct detection limits have been reported to range from 1 adduct per 10^7 to 10^9 bases using 100–500 µg of DNA [107].

7.3.2 Unscheduled DNA Synthsis (UDS) Assay for the Detection of DNA Repair

The unscheduled DNA synthesis assay is a widely used method to investigate chemically induced DNA excision repair. The induction of repair mechanisms is presumed to have been preceded by DNA damage. Measuring the extent to which DNA synthesis occurs offers indirect evidence of the DNA damaging ability of a test chemical. The recommended methodology is described in OECD test guideline 486 [108].

Principle of the Method The UDS assay measures DNA synthesis induced for the purposes of repairing an excised segment of DNA containing a region damaged by a test chemical. DNA synthesis is measured by detecting tritium-labeled thymidine (^{3}H-TdR) incorporation into DNA, preferably using autoradiography. The liver is generally used for analysis because, under normal circumstances, there is a low proportion of primary hepatocytes in the S phase of the cell cycle. Therefore, an increase in DNA synthesis can readily be attributed to repair of induced DNA damage, rather than DNA synthesis supporting normal cell division. The liver is also the site of first-pass metabolism for chemicals administered orally or by intraperitoneal injection. The larger the number of nucleotides excised and repaired, the greater is the amount of detectible ^{3}H-TdR incorporated into DNA. For this reason, the UDS assay is more sensitive in detecting DNA damage that is repaired through nucleotide excision repair (removal of up to 100 nucleotides) as compared to base excision repair (removal of 1–3 nucleotides) [108]. Test chemicals more prone to inducing nucleotide excision repair, such as those that form bulky DNA adducts, have a greater potential to cause detectible UDS. However, the UDS assay does not, in itself, indicate if a test chemical is mutagenic because it provides no information regarding the fidelity of DNA repair, and it does not identify DNA lesions repaired by mechanisms other than excision repair. The UDS assay is usually conducted using rats, although other species may be used if justified. Two dose levels are selected on the basis of preliminary toxicity testing, with the highest dose defined as that causing toxicity such that higher levels would be expected to produce lethality. At least three animals per group (typically males only) are administered the test chemical once by gavage. Intraperitoneal injection is not recommended because it could potentially expose the liver directly to the chemical. A group of animals is sacrificed at 2–4 h and another at 12–16 h after treatment. Cultures of hepatocytes are prepared and incubated for 3–8 h in ^{3}H-TdR. Slides are prepared and processed for autoradiography using standard techniques. At least 100 cells per animal are examined and both nuclear and cytoplasmic grains should be counted to determine the net nuclear grain count (cytoplasmic grains subtracted from nuclear grains). Chemicals inducing a significant increase in net nuclear grain count for at least one treatment group are considered to have induced UDS [109].

Advantages and Limitations   Basically, any tissue with a low proportion of cells in the S phase can be used for analysis. However, the *in vivo* UDS test has been validated only in the liver, whereas alternative tissues have been investigated to a limited extent [110]. Because UDS is measured in the whole genome, it is potentially much more sensitive than assays examining only specific loci. However, the extent of UDS gives no indication of the fidelity of the repair process. For that reason, UDS does not provide specific information on the mutagenic potential of a test chemical, but only information suggesting it does or does not induce excision repair. Despite this limitation, a positive response in the *in vivo* liver UDS assay has very high correlation with rodent hepatocarcinogenicity. However, an important limitation of the UDS test is the comparatively low sensitivity for DNA lesions being repaired by base excision repair [108].

7.3.3 *In Vivo* Gene Mutation Assays

Transgenic Rodents for the Analysis of Somatic Mutations   Few endogenous genes lend themselves to the analysis of gene mutations *in vivo*. Due to the fact that vertebrates are diploid organisms, only hemizygous genes are amenable to the detection of mutations occurring in one chromosome, which normally is only the case with genes residing on sex chromosomes. Furthermore, to detect mutations, which are rare events, the necessity exists to propagate cells in order to select phenotypically for mutants among a vast excess of unmutated cells. This limits the use of endogenous genes to only a few cell types or developmental stages, such as color coat genes in the case of the mouse spot test, or the *hprt* gene of lymphoid cells.

Finally, endogenous genes generally serve a biological purpose, so that in many cases the mutation of such a gene may result in a selective disadvantage for the affected cells, leading to the risk of elimination of mutations with an obvious probability to underestimation of true mutation frequencies.

The use of shuttle vectors as mammalian mutagenesis test systems was first proposed *in vitro* by Glazer et al. [111], and later by Malling and Burkhart [112], *in vivo*, where they described the use of λsufF and ΦX174 or shuttle vectors, respectively, as mammalian mutation systems. The first assay that came into wider use was that of Gossen et al. [113], who placed the bacterial *lacZ* gene, encoding for β-galactosidase, in a λgt10 vector. This model is now commercially available as Muta™-Mouse (Covance, www.covance.com). Shortly thereafter, similar transgenic mice were introduced by Kohler et al. [114, 115], utilizing the bacterial *lacI* gene embedded in a λLIZ vector, which codes for the repressor of the *lacZ* gene, as the mutational target *in vivo*. This model, which is now commercially available as BigBlue®, can also be obtained on a rat background (Stratagene www.stratagene.com). Those novel lambda vectors share the advantages of being forward mutation systems with hundreds of inactivating target sequences, which, in contrast to the reverse mutation ΦX174 type, allows the detection of many kinds of different mutagenic events.

All these models utilize the so-called shuttle vector principle for mutation analysis, which describes a method in which the transgenes are mutated in the animal body, whereas mutation analysis occurs after specific retrieval of the transgene and subsequent transfer of the mutational target gene into suitable bacterial hosts. Mutation analysis is carried out by extracting high molecular weight genomic DNA from the tissue of interest, packaging the lambda shuttle vector *in vitro* into lambda phage heads, and testing for mutations that arise in the transgene sequences following infection of an appropriate bacterial strain. Packaging extract, which contains the catalytic and structural proteins needed for excising single transgene copies from the genomic DNA and packaging them individually into phage heads, can either be obtained commercially or prepared with standard laboratory methods. A key prerequisite of those systems has been the use of methylation-restriction-deficient host strains such as *E. coli* C, which allow the rescue of the nontranscribed and therefore highly methylated transgenic DNA without any host defense [116].

Later, accumulating evidence indicated that those lacZ or lacI bacteriophage lambda models are insufficiently sensitive for events that involve large genomic rearrangements such as deletions, insertions, or recombinations [117, 118]. Therefore, models were developed to overcome these limitations, such as the pUR288 or the gpt-delta mouse. Those models are described later in more detail.

One key assumption in this approach is that the bacterial target gene behaves similar with respect to mutation induction to endogenous genes, which are causally related to tumor initiation. Several differences between transgenes and native genes can be assumed or have been experimentally demonstrated, which have the potential to affect the relative magnitude of the mutagenic response observed. Thus, prokaryotic transgenes possess attributes that differ from most mammalian genes, which include higher GC content, higher density of the dinucleotide "CpG" and associated 5-methylcytosine, which is a mutation hotspot after spontaneous desamination [119], and existence of the transgenic cluster as a nontranscribed multicopy, head-to-tail concatemer, which is hypermethylated and lacks transcription-coupled repair. While these differences do not preclude the utility of transgenic assays as general mutation analysis tools, they should be taken into consideration when interpreting assay results. On the other hand, it should be kept in mind that every mutation assay, whether transgenic or not, has its own spectrum of detectable mutations, and, accordingly, some differences are to be expected between any two assays compared. For the transgenic systems, a large body of evidence has been accumulated, which demonstrates that mutation induction in those transgenes strongly resembles the one in endogenous genes [120] and that those models therefore will deliver relevant and valid results.

A number of transgenic systems have been generated and used for mutation experiments *in vivo*, which are described in detail later. Generally, these systems offer the opportunity to study gene mutations, which is considered to be a relevant toxicological endpoint indicative of a tumorigenic potential, in all organs or tissues of mice and rats from which high molecular weight genomic DNA can be obtained. A huge body of experimental data exists that demonstrates the suitability of these systems to study mutation induction *in vivo*, and that shows the relevance of the results obtained (for a detailed review see Ref. 121). However, of the models available, mostly the two commercially available bacteriophage lambda models Muta™Mouse and Big Blue®, and with restrictions the pUR288 and the gpt-delta mouse, can be considered sufficiently validated to be recommended for regulatory purposes. Commercial models have the advantage that there is professional support in the case of experimental problems, and that there is a high quality supply of all necessary material, which may be a problem for the less frequently used systems. Standards for the conductance of transgenic assays for regulatory purposes have been defined in international workshops [122, 123]. Generally, repeated dosing of at least 28 days is advised in order to allow for the detection of weak effects. Different tissues should be analyzed, guided by information such as metabolism or distribution of the test compound and also known biological mechanisms or toxicity target organs. Generally, it can be concluded that at present those systems represent the most reliable method of analyzing *in vivo* gene mutations and therefore can be considered to be the systems of choice for the *in vivo* clarification of gene mutagenic effects observed in other (*in vitro*) systems.

Bacteriophage Lambda-Based Models (lacZ or lacI)   The two most popular and widely used transgenic models are Muta™Mouse and Big Blue®, employing the bacterial *lacZ* and *lacI* genes, respectively, as mutational targets [131, 114, 122, 123]. In those animals a recombinant bacteriophage lambda is used as the transgenic shuttle vector. Genomic DNA is extracted from any organ or tissue of interest by proteinase K digestion, followed by phenol/chloroform extraction, ethanol precipitation of the total genomic DNA, and subsequent resuspension in the appropriate buffer. For all bacteriophage lambda models, highly intact unfragmented genomic DNA is an essential element for a sufficiently high rescue efficiency, so that alternative DNA extraction methods such as columns have not been shown to be feasible so far. However, dialysis procedures have been described to yield good quality genomic DNA [124]. Subsequently, bacteriophage particles containing single copies of the recombinant phages are produced by *in vitro* lambda packaging using a commercial or self-made packaging extract. Phage DNA is brought into suitable host bacteria by infection with the reconstituted lambda particles, after which the cells are plated either on plates containing a chromogenic substrate (lacI or the earlier lacZ method) or using a P-Gal selection system (lacZ). Advantages of both methods are the robustness of the experimental procedure, the vendor support that is provided as for other commercially available systems, which can be very helpful in the case of experimental problems, and the extensive body of experimental data and experience in the literature and the scientific community. Disadvantages of the models are that experiments are relatively expensive and laborious to perform, which is, however, the case for all gene mutation assays *in vivo*. Furthermore, in all lambda models a relatively high quality high molecular genomic DNA is essential for an efficient rescue of the transgenic phage, and both have shown to be not very sensitive for mutations involving large DNA rearrangements, such as deletions.

Muta™*Mouse*   Transgenic lacZ mice were produced by microinjection of ~150 copies of the monomeric λgt10lacZ vector into the male pronucleus of fertilized eggs of (BALB/c × DBA/2) CD2F1 mice [113]. From the offspring, strain 40.6 was used to generate the commercially available Muta™Mouse model. In this strain, ~40 copies of the transgene per haploid genome are integrated at a single site on chromosome 3 [125]. As basically always, the transgene is integrated as a concatemeric cluster, in a head-to-tail fashion. The *lacZ* gene, which serves as the mutational target, has a size of ~3100 base pairs, whereas the lambda vector is about 47 kb large. To assess mutation, the λgt10lacZ shuttle vectors are excised from genomic DNA and packaged into phage heads by using an *in vitro* packaging extract, as described earlier. The resultant reconstituted phage particles are used to infect *E. coli* C (lacZ⁻) cells. Originally, bacteria were plated onto agar plates containing the chromogenic X-Gal (a substrate for β-galactosidase that yields an insoluble blue reaction product). Blue plaques containing wild-type *lacZ* genes were distinguished visually from white plaques containing mutant *lacZ* genes. Subsequently, a simpler and faster selective system was developed in which an *E. coli* C (galE⁻lacZ⁻) host is used for phage infection [126]. In this system, a small proportion of the bacterial suspension is on nonselective titer plates, whereas the majority is seeded on selection plates containing P-Gal medium. Phospho-P-Gal accumulates to toxic concentrations in galE⁻ cells that express a functional *lacZ* gene; thus, only phage that harbors a mutated *lacZ* will be able to form plaques on P-Gal medium. The *lacZ* mutant frequency is determined by calculating the proportion of plaques on both plate types [127]. As usual, genomic DNA is isolated from the tissue of interest by phenol/chloroform extraction of proteinase K-digested tissue followed by ethanol precipitation, and as for all bacteriophage lambda models, it is critical to obtain high molecular DNA, which has not been overly sheared during preparation. One major advantage of the lacZ model over the lacI model lies in the availability of a functional selection system, which allows the analysis of a high number of rescued copies with relative ease, whereas the lacI system needs a visual identification of colored plaques among the excess of colorless plaques (see later discussion). On the other hand, if sequencing of mutants is a goal, the ~3 kb *lacZ* gene is more laborious to sequence than the *lacI* gene, which is roughly one-third in size.

Big Blue®   The Big Blue mouse and rat transgenic systems are based on the bacterial *lacI* gene. The λLIZα shuttle vector, which carries the bacterial *lacI* gene (1080 bp) as a mutational target, together with the *lacO* operator sequences and *lacZ* gene, was injected into a fertilized oocyte of C57BL/6 mice. The transgenic

C57Bl/6 A1 line was also crossed with an animal of the C3H line to produce a transgenic B6C3F1 mouse with the same genetic background as the National Toxicology Program bioassay test strain. The 45.6 kb λlacI construct is integrated as approximately 40 copies per genome, with integration occurring at a single locus on chromosome 4, in a head-to-tail arrangement. In the meantime, a lacI transgenic rat was produced in a Fisher 344 background [128]. Mutations arising in the rodent genome *in vivo* are scored in *E. coli* SCS-8 cells (lacZΔM15) following *in vitro* packaging of the λLIZα phage. As the BigBlue vector utilizes the lac repressor (*lacI*) gene as the mutational target, white (colorless) plaques will arise from phage bearing wild-type lacI when the SCS-8 host is plated on X-Gal medium. Mutations inactivating lacI will produce a lac repressor that is unable to bind to the lac operator so that *lacZ* transcription is derepressed and β-galactosidase will cleave X-Gal, producing a blue plaque. The proportion of blue plaques among the total number of plaques is a measure of mutant frequency. To date, there has not been an effective positive selection method for *lacI⁻* mutants developed for the Big Blue mouse or rat systems. Due to its smaller size, the *lacI* gene is easier to sequence than the three times bigger *lacZ* gene.

cII System   For all bacteriophage lambda models, an assay has been developed that utilizes the *cII* gene within the lambda molecule. As discussed, both the *lacI* and *lacZ* genes are of considerable size (~1 and 3 kb, respectively), which makes sequencing in order to obtain molecular information on mutagenic events relatively laborious. The *cII* gene is a component of the lysogenic life cycle of bacteriophage lambda, and phages containing an inactivating forward mutation in this gene are selected for in *hfl⁻* bacterial host strains [129, 130], which are commercially available. This gene, with a size of 294 base pairs, is substantially easier to sequence than *lacI* or *lacZ*, so that this model shows advantage over the traditional MutaMouse or Big Blue when sequencing is an experimental goal. However, this target gene has not been as extensively validated as *lacI* or *lacZ*.

Conductance of a Transgenic Study   Of the previously described models, MutaMouse, Big Blue mouse and rat, and, with some restrictions, the lacZ plasmid mouse and the gpt-delta mouse have a sufficient quantity of experimental data associated with them to refer to them as sufficiently validated for drug safety objectives. Comprehensive recommendations for transgenic studies for regulatory purposes were formulated during the IWGT (International Workshops on Genotoxicity Tests) held 1999 in Washington, DC, and 2001 in Plymouth, UK. In these workshops, advice was given on how a transgenic mutation study should be designed in order to provide the maximum confidence in a negative result, that is, exclusion of a mutagenic potential under the chosen experimental conditions [122, 123]. By their nature, transgenic mutation assays are comparably insensitive to biological artifacts, which may mimic a mutagenic response, as happens for other endpoints, due to the fact that the endpoint assessed, the gene mutation, is the result of specific sequential events that are not mimicked by cytotoxic effects, as occurs with other endpoints. A number of experimental artifacts may exist, such as the carryover of DNA adducts into bacteria with subsequent *ex vivo* mutagenesis in bacteria. However, the large body of evidence indicates that the mutations measured in these systems arise predominantly in the rodent tissues [122]. Also, one of the main confounders to contribute to the apparent mutant frequency is the spontaneous desamination of methylated cytosine, which occurs preferentially at GpC sites within the gene. Therefore, the spontaneous mutant frequency is relatively high, which means that it is basically difficult to detect weak increases. However, gene mutations, particularly those in selectively neutral transgenes, accumulate linearly in most tissues unless cells are eliminated by cell turnover, which should occur at the same rate for mutated and unmutated cells. Therefore, a repeated (daily) dosing is recommended for most situations, and cessation of treatment should be at or shortly before tissue sampling (see later discussion).

A number of influence factors should be considered when designing a transgenic study. Some of those, such as species (if available), route of administration, or gender, follow the same lines of argumentation as would be used for other *in vivo* assays. Thus, species- or gender-specific metabolism or other PK parameters may guide the choice of species or gender, where it has to be kept in mind that, apart from Big Blue or gpt-delta rats, the mouse will be the species of choice in all cases. Information from other toxicity studies can be used for decision making, and as a general rule the use of one gender is considered sufficient if no toxicity or pharmacokinetic differences are observed between males and females. Thus, unless scientific evidence commands otherwise, the following features should characterize a transgenic rodent study used for regulatory purposes [122, 123]: 5 animals per gender (if a gender difference in factors such as metabolism or toxicity is known or suspected), or 7 animals of one gender, normally males, are used. Scenarios such as a gender-specific therapeutic use of a test substance may guide the choice of gender. Generally, the animals are treated daily for 28 consecutive days and tissues are sampled 3 days after the final treatment. Also, slightly differing recommendations have been formulated [131], and one may deviate from this scheme in cases where the human treatment schedule is strongly different. However, there is consensus that, unless there is a strong mutagenic effect to be expected, a repeated daily dosing for 4 weeks is sufficient to detect most mutagens. Obviously, this recommendation could be modified by reducing or increasing the number of treatments or the length of the treatment period, when scientifically justified. Normally, at least one rapidly proliferating and one slowly proliferating tissue should be sampled. Scientific arguments such as metabolism, accumulation or disposition, or site-of-contact considerations should guide the choice of tissue to be analyzed. For statistical reasons, 124,000–300,000 plaques or colonies should be analyzed per tissue sample, and three doses are used, whereas not all doses need to be analyzed, should the top dose yield a negative result. At sampling, tissues should be flash frozen, after which they can be stored at −80 °C for prolonged times. Likewise, isolated genomic DNA can be stored at 4 °C, although not as long as deep frozen tissues. Although sequencing data are not normally required, they might provide useful additional information in specific circumstances. However, they are mainly used to identify and correct for clonal expansion (i.e., an artificially elevated mutant frequency), and in some cases to determine a mechanism associated with a positive response, although owing to the significant variation in background mutant spectra the power of this tool may be limited. A schematic overview of a transgenic study is given in Fig. 7.6.

Advantages and Limitations   Thus, in summary, the advantages of transgenic mutation assays lie in the analysis of gene mutations, an endpoint that can be considered

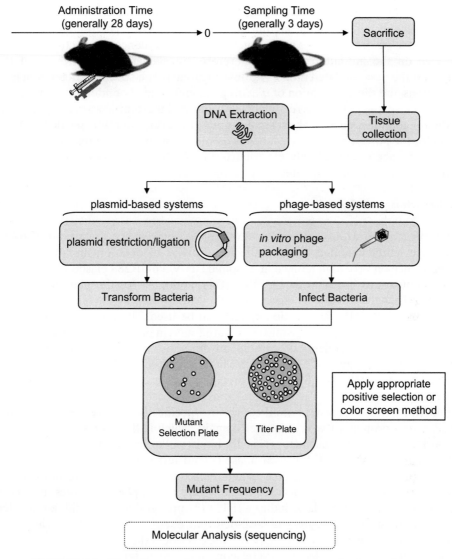

FIGURE 7.6   Flow diagram for performing a transgenic animal experiment.

as very relevant for tumor induction, in basically any tissue of interest in mice and some rat models. Obviously, the analysis is limited to those strains where specific models have been generated. The fixed gene mutations are definitive endpoints that accumulate in most organs so that an increased sensitivity can be achieved by repeated dosing. Thus, when using the recommended 4 week treatment schedule, it can be expected that even weak mutagens are detected reliably [121–123]. Also, gene mutation induction in those models is not subject to artifactual conditions such as cellular toxicity, so that a positive result can be regarded as a very relevant indicator of an *in vivo* mutagenicity. These assays permit the screening of a large number of copies of a locus and provide statistically reliable results on the frequency of mutations in an animal or tissue. Furthermore, the mutants can be sequenced so that the molecular nature of the mutation can be analyzed. The transgenic loci are expected to be genetically neutral, which avoids the influence of selective pressures *in vivo* on the mutant frequency. Therefore, transgenic models provide at this moment the best validated models for investigating tissue-specific induction of gene mutations and the clarification of *in vitro* gene mutagenicity findings. The disadvantage of these assays lies in a relatively laborious and therefore expensive procedure with a recommended 4 week treatment time. However, the effort needed, particularly for the postmortem phase, depends on the know-how of the respective laboratory, and, once used routinely, experience shows that the assays can be conducted with relative ease and high efficiency.

Other Transgenic Models

pUR288 Plasmid Mouse   In order to overcome some of the limitations of bacteriophage lambda models, such as the insensitivity to deletion mutations or the dependence on very high molecular genomic DNA, a pUR288 plasmid-based transgenic mouse was introduced [132, 133]. This model carries the plasmid pUR288, which utilizes the same lacZ sequence as the MutaMouse as the mutational target, and therefore the P-Gal selection system can be used. The mice were made on a C57Bl/6J background, and plasmid copies are found in line 60, the line that has been used for most experiments, integrated on chromosomes 3 and 4 [134]. Plasmid rescue from total genomic DNA, which can be prepared by classical phenol/chloroform extraction followed by ethanol precipitation, or alternatively by using commercially available DNA isolation columns, is done by digesting the DNA with HindIII. From this digest, plasmid copies are specifically retrieved by using a lacI/lacZ fusion protein, of which the lacI domain, which is the repressor for the *lacZ* gene located on the plasmid, specifically binds to the operator sequence of lacZ. Rescue is done with anti-β-galactosidase-coated ferromagnetic beads, which bind the lacZ domain of the fusion protein and thus couple it to the surface of the beads. After removing the excess of unbound genomic DNA, plasmid copies are eluted from the beads with the lacZ inducer IPTG (isopropyl thiogalactoside), relegated, and electroporated into galE and lacZ-deficient *E. coli* C host bacteria. Then 0.1% of the transformants are plated on titer plates to assess the overall rescue efficiency, whereas 99.9% are seeded on P-Gal containing selection plates on which only mutants can grow. Mutant frequency is determined by the colony ratio on both plates times the dilution factor. Experiments using this model have shown that indeed it is able to detect mutations induced by typical clastogens such as X-ray [132] or age-dependent mutation accumulation, and that even large mutations ranging into the mouse genome are recovered, owing to the existence of HindIII sites in the mouse genomic DNA [134]. Other data show that part of the spontaneous mutation spectrum is generated by a residual star activity of HindIII, but generally it is assumed that this effect does not contribute significantly to the overall mutant frequency [135].

gpt-Delta Mouse and Rat   Another transgenic system, which was constructed to overcome the relative insensitivity of bacteriophage lambda models of the *lacI* and *lacZ* type for clastogenic events, is the *gpt*-delta mouse [136]. This model carries the bacteriophage lambda EG10 as the transgene. Similar to lambda systems, the phage is rescued from total genomic DNA by an *in vitro* packaging method. The novel feature of this system is the use of two distinct selection methods, namely, 6-thioguanine for the selection of point mutations and Spi⁻ selection for larger rearrangements such as deletions. The 6-thioguanine selection used the *gpt* gene of *E. coli* as the selection marker, which is known to be sensitive for point mutations and, due to its relatively small size of 456 base pairs, is also convenient to sequence. The second selection principle uses a system that relies on the loss of two distinct genes, *red* and *gam*, to allow for a positive selection by plaque formation on P2 lysogens of *E. coli*. Spi⁻ selection utilizes the restricted growth of wild-type lambda phage in P2 lysogens [137, 138]. Only mutant lambda phages that are deficient in the functions of both the *gam* and *redBA* genes can grow well in P2 lysogens and display the Spi⁻ phenotype. Simultaneous inactivation of both the *gam* and *redBA* genes, the prerequisite for plaque formation, happens generally only in the case of large deletions. Experiments with this model indeed have shown that typical point mutagens (e.g., ethylnitrosourea) or clastogens (e.g., gamma irradiation, mitomycin C) induce the expected effects [139]. In between, this model is also available on a rat background [140]. Obviously, this system is somewhat more laborious than a system that uses only one selective principle. However, without sequencing, the two parallel selection methods reveal some fundamental information about possible mutagenic mechanisms.

ΦX174 Mouse   The ΦX174 am3 model was presented by Burkhardt et al. [141]. The bacteriophage ΦX174, which is about 5 kb in size, is chromosomally integrated at about 50 copies per haploid genome of inbred C57Bl/6 mice. Phage recovery from the mouse genome is done from proteinase K digested, phenol/choloroform extracted, and ethanol precipitated total genomic DNA by a PstI and Sau3A restriction digest, followed by filtration on Sephacryl® S-1000 gel filtration columns to remove genomic DNA and RNA. The DNA is ligated and electroporated into competent cells, where mutant frequency determination is done by a single burst method using *E. coli* CQ2 (sup⁺) cells to determine the titer of totally recovered phage copies, whereas mutations at the A:T target site at the nonsense mutation in the am3 stop codon are selected for in *E. coli* C (sup⁻) cells. In this system, reversion of the am3 target codon can occur via two transversions and one transition, which means that only certain types of mutations can be detected. On the other hand, the specificity of this site prevents a major type of mutation, which, in the bacteriophage lambda systems, stems from spontaneous desamination of 5-methylcytosin at GpC sites, which in those models contributes significantly to the background mutation load.

A few other transgenic systems have been described. One of the earlier models introduced was a supF gene-based bacteriophage lambda mouse, which, after *in vitro* lambda packaging from mouse genomic DNA and infection of suitable host bacteria, mutations in the supF gene are selected for by growth on lacI(amber) *E. coli* in the presence of X-Gal [111]. Another model used the plasmid pML4 as the shuttle vector, present at relatively high copy numbers (several hundred per genome, depending on the mouse line [142]). After restriction digest and direct ligation of genomic DNA, followed by electroporation of kanamycin-resistant and streptomycin-sensitive *E. coli* host cells, mutations in the *rspL* gene are detected by plating on kanamycin- and streptomycin-containing plates. Also, an *in situ* model was presented that held the promise of mutation detection *in situ*, which would allow an analysis at the single-cell level [143]. However, those systems have so far not advanced to a state where more than one or a few laboratories have used them, so that the basis for experimental data is insufficient to draw conclusions on their performance.

Mouse Spot Test   The mouse spot test is an *in vivo* assay capable of detecting genetic effects of several kinds, including intragenic mutations, minute deficiencies, deletions (through breakage or nondisjunction) of various amounts of chromosomal material, and somatic crossing-over [144, 145]. The assay involves treatment of mouse embryos, which are heterozygous for different recessive coat color genes and are treated *in utero* at gestation day 9–11 with the test substance. The exposed embryo at gestation day 10 contains about 150–200 melanoblasts and each melano-blast has 4 coat color genes that are studied [145, 146]. The *in utero* exposure may result in an alteration or loss of a specific wild-type allele in a pigment precursor cell, resulting in a color spot in the coat of the adult animal. The frequency of spots is compared with the frequency in negative controls [145, 146]. In the mouse spot test there are four possible mechanisms by which the recessive coat color alleles can be expressed: gene mutation in the wild-type allele, deficiency (large or small) of a chromosomal segment involving the wild-type allele, nondisjunctional (or other) loss of the chromosome carrying the wild-type allele, and somatic recombina-tion (using a marker gene that then becomes homozygous after recombination). Mutagenic but also clastogenic effects are detected by this test system [147, 148].

The mouse spot test is not a very frequently employed genotoxicity assay for the detection of somatic mutations; however, an OECD guideline exists [149]. The test was suggested as a complementary *in vivo* test to the bacterial mutagenicity assay for detection of mutagenic substances and as a confirmatory test for the identifica-tion of carcinogens [145]. However, the infrequent use of the spot test may partly be due to considerations of cost effectiveness and the number of animals needed for testing and also for toxicological considerations. The usefulness of the mouse spot test in toxicology is limited by restrictions in toxicokinetics, sensitivity, target cell/organ, and molecular genetics. The test may be used to further investigate spe-cific issues such as compounds demonstrating effects in the *in vitro* bacterial muta-tion assay but not in clastogenicity tests *in vitro* and *in vivo*. One such example is the antiviral pryrimidine nucleoside analogue 5-(2-chloroethyl)-2′-deoxyuridine [150]. However, for the detection of gene but not chromosome mutations *in vivo*, the mouse spot test should likely be replaced by the transgenic mouse assays, which were shown to be of comparable sensitivity [151].

Other Assays for Somatic Cell Gene Mutations   Various other assays exist that investigate endogenous genes. These tests are rarely used for testing purposes because they are cumbersome and generally not suitable for routine use. Some promising mutation tests using endogenous genes have been developed. These endogenous gene mutation assays include RetinoBlast, Hprt, Aprt, Tk$^{+/-}$, and Dlb-1. A comprehensive review outlining the current status of these test has recently been published [121].

7.4 *IN VIVO* GENOTOXICITY TESTS FOR INVESTIGATING GERMLINE CELLS

Thus far, all established germ cell mutagens have been shown also to produce positive results in bone marrow assays. There is no current evidence for germ-cell-specific mutagens [152]; however, the reverse is not true. Not all somatic cell mutagens can be demonstrated to be germ cell mutagens, which indicates mechanisms exist that protect germ cells against genotoxic exposure of induction of DNA damage. However, for most compounds identified as *in vivo* somatic cell mutagens, no specific genotoxicity testing in germ cells will be needed since these compounds will be assumed to be both potential genotoxic carcinogens and potential germ cell mutagens, unless the exposure of germ cells can be reliably excluded, which will be difficult in most cases. Data on the mutagenic effects in germ cell DNA are needed before any definite conclusions can be drawn relating to the mutagenic hazard of a chemical specifically to germ cells. There may be justified cases in which germ cell studies will be undertaken for the specific purpose of demonstrating whether an identified *in vivo* somatic cell mutagen is a germ cell mutagen as well. However, none of these assays provide conclusive information as to whether the effects seen are heritable in future generations. The methods available for such risk assessments, such as the mouse heritable translocation test and the mouse specific locus test, involve the investigation of effects in subsequent generations bred from treated animals. In view of the very large number of animals used, these are not practical options and should only be considered in exceptional circumstances.

In principle, the methods described earlier in this chapter may be applied to investigate genotoxic effects in germ line cells. The transgenic animal systems may be used to investigate effects in germ cells [153], micronucleus induction may be detected in spermatocytes using appropriate staining methods, and induction of DNA lesions in germ cell DNA may be obtained from UDS [154–156], comet [157, 158], or postlabeling assays [159].

Specific germline cell tests are not very frequently applied; however, they are listed in ICH guidelines. A brief summary on the specific areas of use, advantages, and disadvantages of these test systems are provided. In general, the available methods involve measuring effects in the gonads of male rodents. Methods for investigating clastogenicity in mammalian spermatogonial cells are well established. There is an internationally recognized guideline (OECD No. 483) for this approach [160].

The dominant lethal assay may also be used to investigate clastogenicity or aneugenicity in germ cells [161]. There is an internationally recognized guideline, OECD No. 478, for this assay [162]. For this method, the endpoint is the production of embryo-lethal genetic changes measured as death of the conceptus as a blastoma or soon afterwards. Dominant lethal mutations are believed to be primarily due to structural or numerical chromosome aberrations. There are essentially two different dosing regimes that may be used in this assay. In one case, this involves repeated dosing of the males for a period covering spermatogenesis followed by mating with untreated females and examining the latter for dominant lethals after an appropriate period of gestation. In the other regime, single dosing is followed by sequential mating of females. The latter provides information on the various stages of the germ cell cycle that may be affected but uses very many more animals and the need for this additional information is rarely justified.

7.5 CONCLUSION

The assessment of a genotoxic potential of a drug candidate is typically determined through a battery of tests conducted *in vitro* and *in vivo*. Genotoxicity tests provide a means to identify potential genotoxic carcinogens relatively early in the development of a drug candidate. According to current internationally accepted guidance, the most appropriate initial *in vivo* test will be a bone marrow micronucleus assay unless the initial considerations indicate otherwise. Techniques for the assessment of whole chromosomes are appropriate if there is evidence of aneugenicity. If a genotoxic hazard is observed in any *in vitro* tests, further investigations are conducted to assess whether genotoxic activity observed *in vitro* can be expressed in somatic cells *in vivo*. For this purpose, supplemental tests utilizing other tissue(s) are conducted. The type of study needs to be considered on a case-by-case basis, taking into account the available information on the compound including the results from earlier tests. Studies that may be appropriate include, but are not limited to, the liver UDS assay, comet assay, ^{32}P-postlabeling assay, or assays using transgenic animals. Specific germline genotoxicity assays usually are not required since it can be assumed that drug candidates demonstrating *in vivo* genotoxicity will be both potential genotoxic carcinogens and germ cell mutagens. However, in some cases, germ cell studies may be undertaken to demonstrate that a somatic cell mutagen is not a germ cell mutagen, unless there is convincing evidence that the chemical does not dispose into the germ cell compartment. In such a case, most of the above listed supplemental assays can be applied to germline cells. However, it is important to note that none of these assays provide conclusive information as to whether genotoxic effects will be seen in future generations. Assays that facilitate such risk estimates include the heritable translocation test and the mouse specific locus test. However, these assays are not practical in view of the very large number of animals needed. Ultimately, the choice and design of *in vivo* genotoxicity assays needs to be scientifically justified and conducted in a way that adds value to the nonclinical safety assessment either in terms of initial genotoxic hazard identification or with regard to understanding the risk and relevance of positive results obtained from *in vitro* genotoxicity tests or rodent cancer bioassays.

REFERENCES

1. ICH S2B. *A Standard Battery for Genotoxicity Testing of Pharmaceuticals*. 1997. http://www.ich.org/.
2. Müller L, Blakey D, Dearfield KL, Galloway S, Guzzie P, Hayashi M, Kasper P, Kirkland D, MacGregor JT, Parry JM, Schechtman L, Smith A, Tanaka N, Tweats D, Yamasaki H. Strategy for genotoxicity testing and stratification of genotoxicity test results—report on initial activities of the IWGT Expert Group. *Mutat Res* 2003;540:177–181.
3. ICH M3(M). *Maintenance of the ICH Guideline on Non-clinical Safety Studies for the Conduct of Human Clinical Trials for Pharmaceuticals*. 2000. http://www.ich.org/.
4. Ashby J, Tennant RW. Definitive relationships among chemical structure, carcinogenicity and mutagenicity for 301 chemicals tested by the U.S. NTP. *Mutat Res* 1991; 257:229–308.
5. ICH S2A. *Specific Aspects of Regulatory Genotoxicity Tests*. 1995. http://www.ich.org/.

6. Food and Drug Administration. *Guidance for Industry, Investigators, and Reviewers. Exploratory IND Studies.* Draft Guidance. 2005.

7. OECD Guideline 474. *Guideline for the Testing of Chemicals. Mammalian Erythrocyte Micronucleus Test.* OECD; 1997.

8. OECD Guideline 475. *Guideline for the Testing of Chemicals. Mammalian Bone Marrow Chromosome Aberration Test.* OECD; 1997.

9. Heddle J. A rapid *in vivo* test for chromosome damage. *Mutat Res* 1973;18:187–190.

10. MacGregor JT, Wehr CM, Gould DH. Clastogen-induced micronuclei in peripheral blood erythrocytes: the basis of an improved micronucleus test. *Environ Mutagen* 1980;2:509–514.

11. Hayashi M, Tice RR, MacGregor JT, Anderson D, Blakey DH, Kirsch-Volders M, Oleson FB Jr, Pacchierotti F, Romagna F, Shimada H, Sutou S, Vannier B. *In vivo* rodent erythrocyte micronucleus assay. *Mutat Res* 1994;312:293–404.

12. Hayashi M, MacGregor JT, Gatehouse DG, Adler I-D, Blakey DH, Dertinger SD, Krishna G, Morita T, Russo A, Sutou S. *In vivo* rodent erythrocyte micronucleus assay. II. Some aspects of protocol design including repeated treatments, integration with toxicity testing, and automated scoring. *Environ Mol Mutagen* 2000;35:234–252.

13. CSGMT. Sex differences in the micronucleus test. *Mutat Res* 1986;172:151–163.

14. CSGMT. Strain differences in the micronucleus test. *Mutat Res* 1988;204:307–316.

15. CSGMT. Single versus multiple dosing in the micronucleus test: the summary of the fourth collaborative study by CSGMT/JEMS-MMS. *Mutat Res* 1990;234:205–222.

16. CSGMT. Micronucleus test with mouse peripheral blood erythrocytes by acridine orange supravital staining: the summary report of the 5th collaborative study by CSGMT/ JEMS-MMS. *Mutat Res* 1992;278:83–98.

17. CSGMT. Protocol recommended by the CSGMT/JEMS-MMS for the short-term mouse peripheral blood micronucleus test. *Mutagenesis* 1995;10:153–159.

18. Wakata A, Miyamae Y, Sato S, Suzuki T, Morita T, Asano N, Awogi T, Kondo K, Hayashi M. Evaluation of the rat micronucleus test with bone marrow and peripheral blood: summary of the 9th collaborative study by CSGMT/JEMS-MMS. *Environ Mol Mutagen* 1998;13:347–356.

19. Hamada S, Sutou S, Morita T, Wakata A, Asanami S, Hosoya S, et al. Evaluation of the rodent micronucleus assay by a 28-day treatment protocol: summary of the 13th collaborative study by the Collaborative Study Group for the Micronucleus Test (CSGMT)/ Environmental Mutagen Society of Japan (JEMS)–Mammalian Mutagenicity Study Group (MMS). *Environ Mol Mutagen* 2001;37:93–110.

20. Hamada S, Nakajima K, Namiki C, Serikawa T, Hayashi M. Sex differences in the chemical induction of micronuclei in the rat. *Environ Mutagen Res* 2003;25:33–37.

21. Hamada S, Yamasaki K-I, Nakanishi S, Omori T, Serikawa T, Hayashi M. Evaluation of the general suitability of the rat for the micronucleus assay: the effect of cyclophosphamide in 14 strains. *Mutat Res* 2001;495:127–134.

22. Hayashi M, Sutou S, Shimada H, Sato S, Sasaki Y-F, Wakata A. Difference between intraperitoneal and oral gavage application in the micronucleus test, the 3rd collaborative study by CSGMT/JEMS-MMS. *Mutat Res* 1989;23:329–344.

23. MacGregor JT, Wehr CM, Henika PR, Shelby MD. The *in vivo* erythrocyte micronucleus test: measurement at steady state increases assay efficiency and permits integration with toxicity studies. *Fundam Appl Toxicol* 1990;14:513–522.

24. Garriott ML, Brunny JD, Kindig DEF, Parton JW, Schwier LS. The *in vivo* rat micronucleus test: integration with a 14-day study. *Mutat Res* 1995;342:71–76.

25. Asanami S, Shimono K, Sawamoto O, Kurisu K, Uejima M. The suitability of rat peripheral blood in subchronic studies for the micronucleus assay. *Mutat Res* 1995;347:73–78.

26. Holder HE, Majeska JB, Studwell D. A direct comparison of mouse and rat bone marrow and blood as target tissues in the micronucleus assay. *Mutat Res* 1997; 391:87–89.

27. Torous DK, Hall NE, Murante FG, Gleason SE, Tometski CR, Dertinger SD. Comparative scoring of micronucleated reticulocytes in rat peripheral blood by flow cytometry and microscopy. *Toxicol Sci* 2003;74:309–314.

28. Frieauff W, Romagna F. Technical aspects of automatic micronucleus analysis in rodent bone marrow assays. *Cell Biol Toxicol* 1994;10:283–289.

29. Grawé J, Zetterbert G, Amneus H. Flow-cytometric enumeration of micronucleated polychromatic erythrocytes in mouse peripheral blood. *Cytometry* 1992;13:750–758.

30. Tometsko AM, Torous DK, Dertinger SD. Analysis of micronucleated cells by flow cytometry. 3. Advanced technology for detecting clastogenic activity. *Mutat Res* 1993;292:145–153.

31. Dertinger SD, Torous DK, Tometsko KR. Simple and reliable enumeration of micronucleated reticulocytes with a single-laser flow cytometer. *Mutat Res* 1996;371:283–292.

32. Dertinger SD, Torous DK, Tometsko KR. Flow cytometric analysis of micronucleated reticulocytes in mouse bone marrow. *Mutat Res* 1997;390:257–262.

33. Criswell K, Krishna G, Zielinski D, Urda G, Theiss J, Juneau P, Bleavins M. Use of acridine orange in flow cytometric assessment of micronuclei induction. *Mutat Res* 1998;414:63–75.

34. Torous DK, Hall NE, Dertinger SD, Diehl MS, Illi-Love AH, Cederbrant K, et al. Flow cytometric enumeration of micronucleated reticulocytes: high transferability among 14 laboratories. *Environ Mol Mutagen* 2001;38:59–68.

35. Torous DK, Hall NE, Illi-Love AH, Diehl MS, Cederbrant K, Sandelin K, et al. Interlaboratory validation of a CD71-based flow cytometric method (MicroFlow®) for scoring of micronucleated reticulocytes in mouse peripheral blood. *Environ Mol Mutagen* 2005;45:44–55.

36. Schlegel R, MacGregor JT. The persistence of micronucleated erythrocytes in the peripheral circulation of normal and splenectomized Fischer 344 rats: implications for cytogenetic screening. *Mutat Res* 1984;127:169–174.

37. Torous D, Dertinger S, Hall N, Tometsko C. Enumeration of micronucleated reticulocytes in rat peripheral blood: a flow cytometric study. *Mutat Res* 2000;465:91–99.

38. Schlegel R, MacGregor JT. A rapid screen for cumulative chromosomal damage in mice. Accumulation of circulating micronucleated erythrocytes. *Mutat Res* 1982;113:481–487.

39. Schlegel R, MacGregor JT. The persistence of micronuclei in peripheral blood erythrocytes: detection of chromic chromosome breakage in mice. *Mutat Res* 1983;104: 367–369.

40. Choy WN, MacGregor JT, Shelby MD, Maronpot RR. Induction of micronuclei by benzene in B6C3F1 mice: retrospective analysis of peripheral blood smears from the NTP carcinogenesis bioassay. *Mutat Res* 1985;143:55–59.

41. Krishna G, Urda G, Theiss J. Principles and practices of integrating genotoxicity evaluation into routine toxicology studies: a pharmaceutical industry perspective. *Environ Mol Mutagen* 1998;32:115–120.

42. MacGregor JT, Heddle JA, Hite M, Margolin BH, Ramel C, Salamone MF, Tice RR, Wild D. Guidelines for the conduct of micronucleus assays in mammalian bone marrow erythrocytes. *Mutat Res* 1987;189:103–112.

43. Mackay JM, Elliott BM. Dose-ranging and dose-settings for *in vivo* genetic toxicology studies. *Mutat Res* 1992;271:97–99.

44. Schmid W. The micronucleus test for cytogenetic analysis. In Hollaender A, Ed. *Chemical Mutagens*, Vol 4. New York: Plenum Press; 1976, pp 31–53.

45. Salamone MF, Heddle JA. The bone marrow micronucleus assay: rationale for a revised protocol. In Serres FJ, Ed. *Chemical Mutagens*, Vol 8. New York: Plenum Press; 1983, pp 111–149.

46. Romagna F. Improved method of preparing bone marrow micronucleus slides: fractionation of a pure PE and NE population from rodent bone marrow. *Mutat Res* 1988;206:307–309.

47. Hayashi M, Morita T, Kodama Y, Sofuni T, Ishidate M Jr. The micronucleus assay with mouse peripheral blood reticulocytes using acridine orange-coated slides. *Mutat Res* 1990;245:245–249.

48. Hayashi M, Sofuni T, Ishidate M. An application of acridine orange fluorescent staining to the micronucleus test. *Mutat Res* 1983;120:241–247.

49. MacGregor JT, Wehr CM, Langlois RG. A simple fluorescent staining procedure for micronuclei and RNA in erythrocytes using Hoechst 33258 and pyronin Y. *Mutat Res* 1983;120:269–275.

50. Kirkland DJ. Statistical evaluation of mutagenicity test data: recommendations of the UKEMS. *Environ Health Persp Suppl* 1994;102:43–47.

51. Yoshimura I, Sofuni T, Ishidate M Jr, Hayashi M. A procedure for data analysis of the rodent micronucleus test involving a historical control. *Environ Mol Mutagen* 1989;13:347–356.

52. Lovell DP. Anderson D, Albanese R, Amphlett GE, Clare G, Ferguson R, Richold M, Papworth DG, Savage JRK. Statistical analysis of *in vivo* cytogenetic assays. In Kirkland DJ, Ed. *Statistical Evaluation of Mutagenicity Test Data. UKEMS Sub-Committee on Guidelines for Mutagenicity Testing, Report, Part III*. New York: Cambridge University Press; 1989, pp 184–232.

53. Adler I-D, Bootman J, Favor J, Hook G, Schriever-Schwemmer G, Welzl G, Whorton E, Yoshimura I, Hayashi M. Recommendations for statistical designs of *in vivo* mutagenicity tests with regard to subsequent statistical analysis. *Mutat Res* 1998;417:19–30.

54. Asanami S, Shimono K. Hypothermia induces micronuclei in mouse bone marrow cells. *Mutat Res* 1997;393:91–98.

55. Asanami S, Shimono K. Effects of chemically- and environmentally-induced hypothermia on micronucleus induction in rats. *Mutat Res* 2000;471:81–86.

56. Hamada S, Nakajima K, Serikawa T, Hayashi M. The effect of aging on the results of the rat micronucleus assay. *Mutagenesis* 2003;18:273–275.

57. Ortiz R, Medina H, Rodriguez L, Gonzalez-Marquez H, Cortés E. Spontaneous and mitomycin C-induced micronuclei in peripheral blood reticulocytes from severely malnourished rats. *Environ Mol Mutagen* 2004;43:179–185.

58. Tice RR, Shelby MD. International Workshop on Standardisation of Genotoxicity Test Procedures. Report of *in vivo* subgroup. *Mutat Res* 1994;312:287–292.

59. Bentley KS, Kirkland D, Murphy M, Marshall R. Evaluation of thresholds for benomyl- and carbendazim-induced aneuploidy in cultured human lymphocytes using fluorescence *in situ* hybridization. *Mutat Res* 2000;464:41–51.

60. Kirkland DJ, Müller L. Interpretation of the biological relevance of genotoxicity test results: the importance of thresholds. *Mutat Res* 2000;464:137–147.

61. Ahnstrom G. Techniques to measure DNA single-strand breaks in cells: a review. *Int J Radiat Biol* 1988;54:695–707.

62. Elia MC, Storer RD, McKelvey TW, Kraynak AR, Barnum JE, Harmon LS, DeLuca JG, Nichols WW. Rapid DNA degradation in primary rat hepatocytes treated with diverse cytotoxic chemicals: analysis by pulsed field gel electrophoresis and implications for alkaline elution assays. *Environ Mol Mutagen* 1994;24:181–191.

63. Hartmann A, Schumacher M, Plappert-Helbig U, Lowe P, Suter W, Mueller L. Use of the alkaline *in vivo* comet assay for mechanistic genotoxicity investigations. *Mutagenesis* 2004;19:51–59.

64. Brendler-Schwaab S, Hartmann A, Pfuhler S, Speit G. The *in vivo* comet assay: use and status in genotoxicity testing. *Mutagenesis* 2005;20:245–254.

65. Tice RR. The single cell gel/comet assay: a microgel electrophoretic technique for the detection of DNA damage and repair in individual cells. In Phillips DH, Venitt S, Eds. *Environmental Mutagenesis*. Oxford, UK: Bios Scientific Publishers; 1995, pp 315–339.

66. Speit G, Hartmann A. The comet assay (single-cell gel test)—a sensitive genotoxicity test for the detection of DNA damage and repair. In Henderson DS, Ed. *Methods in Molecular Biology Volume 113: DNA Repair Protocols: Eucaryotic Systems*, 2nd ed. Totowa, NJ: Humana Press; 2005, pp 275–286.

67. Tice RR, Agurell E, Anderson D, Burlinson B, Hartmann A, Kobayashi H, Miyamae Y, Rojas E, Ryu J-C, Sasaki YF. The single cell gel/comet assay: guidelines for *in vitro* and *in vivo* genetic toxicology testing. *Environ Mol Mutagen* 2000;35:206–221.

68. Hartmann A, Agurell E, Beevers C, Brendler-Schwaab S, Burlinson B, Clay P, Collins AR, Smith A, Speit G, Thybaud V, Tice RR. Recommendations for conducting the *in vivo* alkaline comet assay. *Mutagenesis* 2003;18:45–51.

69. Burlinson B, Tice RR, Speit G, Agurell E, Brendler-Schwaab SY, Collins AR, Escobar P, Honma M, Kumaravel TS, Nakajma M, Sasaki YF, Thybaud V, Uno Y, Vasquez M, Hartmann A. In Vivo Comet Assay Workgroup, part of the Fourth International Workgroup on Genotoxicity Testing. *Mutat Res* 2007;627:31–35.

70. Pfuhler S, Wolf HU. Detection of DNA-crosslinking agents with the alkaline comet assay. *Environ Mol Mutagen* 1996;27:196–201.

71. Merk O, Speit G. Detection of crosslinks with the comet assay in relationship to genotoxicity and cytotoxicity. *Environ Mol Mutagen* 1999;33:167–172.

72. Speit G, Hartmann A. The contribution of excision repair to the DNA-effects seen in the alkaline single cell gel test (comet assay). *Mutagenesis* 1995;10:555–559.

73. Collins AR, Duthie SJ, Dobson VL. Direct enzymic detection of endogenous oxidative base damage in human lymphocyte DNA. *Carcinogenesis* 1993;14:1733–1735.

74. Tice RR, Andrews PW, Hirai O, Singh NP. The single cell gel (SCG) assay: an electrophoretic technique for the detection of DNA damage in individual cells. In Witmer CR, Snyder RR, Jollow DJ, Kalf GF, Kocsis JJ, Sipes IG, Eds. *Biological Reactive Intermediates IV, Molecular and Cellular Effects and Their Impact on Human Health*. New York: Plenum Press; 1991, pp 157–164.

75. Brendler-Schwaab SY, Schmezer P, Liegibel U, Weber S, Michalek K, Tompa A, Pool-Zobel BL. Cells of different tissues for *in vitro* and *in vivo* studies in toxicology: compilation of isolation methods. *Toxicol in Vitro* 1994;8:1285–1302.

76. Miyamae Y, Yamamoto M, Sasaki YF, Kobayashi H, Igarashi Soga M, Shimol K, Hayashi M. Evaluation of a tissue homogenization technique that isolates nuclei for the *in vivo* single cell gel electrophoresis (comet) assay: a collaborative study by five laboratories. *Mutat Res* 1998;418:131–140.

77. Sasaki YF, Tsuda S, Izumiyama F, Nishidate E. Detection of chemically induced DNA lesions in multiple mouse organs (liver, lung, spleen, kidney, and bone marrow) using the alkaline single cell gel electrophoresis (comet) assay. *Mutat Res* 1997;388:33–44.

78. Olive PL, Frazer G, Banath JP. Radiation-induced apoptosis measured in TK6 human B lymphoblast cells using the comet assay. *Radiat Res* 1993;136:130–136.

79. Henderson L, Wolfreys A, Fedyk J, Bourner C, Windebank S. The ability of the comet assay to discriminate between genotoxins and cytotoxins. *Mutagenesis* 1998;13:89–94.

80. Hartmann A, Kiskinis E, Fjaellman A, Suter W. Influence of cytotoxicity and compound precipitation on test results in the alkaline comet assay. *Mutat Res* 2001;497:199–212.

81. Kiffe M, Christen P, Arni P. Characterization of cytotoxic and genotoxic effects of different compounds in CHO K5 cells with the comet assay (single-cell gel electrophoresis assay). *Mutat Res* 2003;537:151–168.

82. Rundell MS, Wagner ED, Plewa MJ. The comet assay: genotoxic damage or nuclear fragmentation? *Environ Mol Mutagen* 2003;42:61–67.

83. Mensing T, Welge P, Voss B, Fels LM, Fricke HH, Bruning T, Wilhelm M. Renal toxicity after chronic inhalation exposure of rats to trichloroethylene. *Toxicol Lett* 2002;128:243–247.

84. Scassellati-Sforzolini G, Pasquini R, Moretti M, Villarini M, Fatigoni C, Dolara P, Monarca S, Caderni G, Kuchenmeister F, Schmezer P, Pool-Zobel BL. *In vivo* studies on genotoxicity of pure and commercial linuron. *Mutat Res* 1997;390:207–221.

85. Sasaki YF, Saga A, Akasaka M, Ishibashi S, Yoshida K, Su YQ, Matsusaka N, Tsuda S. Detection of *in vivo* genotoxicity of haloalkanes and haloalkenes carcinogenic to rodents by the alkaline single cell gel electrophoresis (comet) assay in multiple mouse organs. *Mutat Res* 1998;419:13–20.

86. Purschke M, Jacobi H, Witte I. Differences in genotoxicity of H_2O_2 and tetrachlorohydroquinone in human fibroblasts. *Mutat Res* 2002;513:159–167.

87. Sasaki YF, Sekihashi K, Izumiyama F, Nishidate E, Saga A, Ishida K, Tsuda S. The comet assay with multiple mouse organs: comparison of comet assay results and carcinogenicity with 208 chemicals selected from the IARC monographs and U.S. NTP Carcinogenicity Database. *Crit Rev Toxicol* 2000;30:629–799.

88. Sasaki YF, Kawaguchi S, Kamaya A, Ohshita M, Kabasawa K, Iwama K, Taniguchi K, Tsuda S. The comet assay with 8 mouse organs: results with 39 currently used food additives. *Mutat Res* 2002;519:103–119.

89. Phillips DH. Use of ^{32}P-postlabelling to distinguish between genotoxic and nongenotoxic carcinogens. In Vainio HJ, Magee PN, McGregor DB, McMichael JA, Eds. *Mechanisms of Carcinogenesis in Risk Identification*. Lyon, France: IARC Scientific Publications No. 116; 1992, pp 211–224.

90. Beland FA, Poirier MC. DNA adducts and their consequences. In Tardiff RG, Lohmann PHM, Wogan GN, Eds. *Methods to Assess DNA Damage and Repair: Interspecies Comparisons*. Chichester, UK: John Wiley & Sons; 1994, pp 29–55.

91. Vodicka P, Bastlova T, Vodickova L, Peterkova K, Lambert B, Hemminki K. Biomarkers of styrene exposure in lamination workers: levels of *O*6-guanine DNA adducts, DNA strand breaks and mutant frequencies in the hypoxanthine guanine phosphoribosyltransferase gene in T-lymphocytes. *Carcinogenesis* 1995;16:1473–1482.

92. Bastlova T, Vodicka P, Peterkova K, Hemminki K, Lambert B. Styrene oxide-induced HPRT mutations, DNA adducts and DNA strand breaks in cultured human lymphocytes. *Carcinogenesis* 1995;16:2357–2362.

93. Weinstein IB. The origins of human cancer: molecular mechanisms of carcinogenesis and their implications for cancer prevention and treatment. *Cancer Res* 1988;48:4135–4143.

94. Perera FP, Whyatt RM. Biomarkers and molecular epidemiology in mutation and cancer research. *Mutat Res* 1994;313:117–129.

95. Beach AC, Gupta RC. Human biomonitoring and the ^{32}P postlabeling assay. *Carcinogenesis* 1992;13:1053–1074.

96. Phillips DH, Farmer PB, Beland FA, Nath RG, Poirier MC, Reddy MV, Turteltaub KW. Methods of DNA adduct determination and their application to testing compounds for genotoxicity. *Environ Mol Mutagen* 2000;35:222–233.

97. Randerath K, Reddy MV, Gupta RC. ^{32}P-labeling test for DNA damage. *Proc Natl Acad Sci USA* 1981;78:6126–6129.

98. Reddy MV, Randerath K. Nuclease P1-mediated enhancement of sensitivity of ^{32}P-postlabelling test for structurally diverse DNA adducts. *Carcinogenesis* 1986;7:1543–1551.

99. Randerath K, Randerath E. ^{32}P-postlabelling methods for DNA adduct detection: overview and critical evaluation. *Drug Metab Rev* 1994;26:67– 85.

100. Phillips DH. Detection of DNA modifications by the ^{32}P-postlabelling assay. *Mutat Res* 1997;378:1–12.

101. Masento MS, Hewer A, Grover PL, Phillips DH. Enzyme-mediated phosphorylation of polycyclic hydrocarbon metabolites: detection of non-adduct compounds in the ^{32}P-postlabelling assay. *Carcinogenesis* 1989;10:1557–1559.

102. Randerath K, Li D, Moorthy B, Randerath E. I-compounds: endogenous DNA markers of nutritional status, ageing, tumour promotion and carcinogenesis. In Phillips DH, Castegnaro M, Bartsch H, Eds. *Postlabelling Methods for Detection of DNA Damage.* Lyon, France: IARC; 1993, pp 157–165.

103. Sweetman GMA, Shuker DEG, Glover RP, Farmer PB. Mass spectrometry in carcinogenesis research. *Adv Mass Spectrom* 1998;14:343–376.

104. Turteltaub KW, Dingley KH. Application of accelerated mass spectrometry (AMS) in DNA adduct quantification and identification. *Toxicol Lett* 1998;102–103:435–439.

105. Turesky RJ, Vouros P. Formation and analysis of heterocyclic aromatic amine–DNA adducts *in vitro* and in vivo. *J Chromatogr B* 2004;802:155–166.

106. Andrews CL, Vouros P, Harsch A. Analysis of DNA adducts using high-performance separation techniques coupled to electrospray ionization mass spectrometry. *J Chromatogr A* 1999;856:515–526.

107. Paehler A, Richoz J, Soglia J, Vouros P, Turesky RJ. Analysis and quantification of DNA adducts of 2-amino-3,8-dimethylimidazo[4,5-*f*]quinoxaline in liver of rats by liquid chromatography/electrospray tandem mass spectrometry. *Chem Res Toxicol* 2002; 15:551–561.

108. *OECD Guideline 486. Guidelines for Testing of Chemicals: Unscheduled DNA Synthesis (UDS) Test with Mammalian Liver Cells in Vitro.* OECD; 1997.

109. Madle S, Dean SW, Andrae U, Brambilla G, Burlinson B, Doolittle DJ, Furihata C, Hertner T, McQueen CA, Mori H. Recommendations for the performance of UDS tests *in vitro* and *in vivo. Mutat Res* 1994;312:263–285.

110. Burlinson B, Morriss S, Gatehouse DG, Tweats DJ, Jackson MR. Uptake of tritiated thymidine by cells of the rat gastric mucosa after exposure to loxtidine or omeprazole. *Mutagenesis* 1991;6:11–18.

111. Glazer PM, Sarker SN, Summer WC. Detection and anaylsis of UV-induced mutations in mammalian cell DNA using a λ phage shuttle vector. *Proc Natl Acad Sci USA* 1986;83:1041–1044.

112. Malling HV, Burkhart JG. Use of ΦX17 as a shuttle vector for the study of *in vivo* mammalian mutagenesis. *Mutat Res* 1989;212:11–21.

113. Gossen JA, de Leeuw WJF, Tan CHT, Lohman PHM, Berends F, Knook DL, Zwarthoff EC, Vijg J. Efficient rescue of integrated shuttle vectors from transgenic mice: a model for studying mutations *in vivo. Proc Natl Acad Sci USA* 1989;86:7981–7985.

114. Kohler SW, Provost GS, Kretz PL, Dycaico MJ, Sorge JL, Short JM. Develepoment of a short-term, *in vivo* mutagenesis assay: the effects of methylation on the recovery of a lambda phage shuttle vector from transgenic mice. *Nucl Acids Res* 1990;18:3007–3013.

115. Kohler SW, Provost GS, Kretz PL, Fieck A, Sorge JA, Short JM. The use of transgenic mice for short-term, *in vivo* mutagenicity testing. *Genet Anal Tech Appl* 1990; 7:212–218.

116. Gossen JA, Vijg J. *Escherichia coli* C: a convenient host strain for rescue of highly methylated DNA. *Nucl Acids Res* 1988;16:9343.

117. Suzuki T, Hayashi M, Sofuni T, Myhr BC. The concomitant detection of gene mutations and micronucleus induction by mitomycin C *in vivo* using lacZ transgenic mice. *Mutat Res* 1993;285:219–224.

118. Tao KS, Urlando C, Heddle JA. Comparison of somatic mutation in a transgenic versus host locus. *Proc Natl Acad Sci USA* 1993;90:10681–10685.

119. Duncan BK, Miller JH. Mutagenic deamination of cytosine residues in DNA. *Nature* 1980;287:560–561.

120. Casentino L, Heddle JA. Differential mutation of transgenic and endogenous loci *in vivo*. *Mutat Res* 2000;454:1–10.

121. Lambert IB, Singer T, Boucher S, Douglas GR. Detailed review of transgenic rodent gene mutation assays. *Mutat Res Rev* 2005;290:1–280.

122. Heddle JA, Dean J, Nohmi T, Boerrigter M, Casciano D, Douglas GR, Glickman BW, Gorelick NJ, Mirsalis JC, Martus HJ, Skopek TR, Thybaud VR, Tindall KR, Yajima N. *In vivo* transgenic mutation assays. *Environ Mol Mutagen* 2000;35:253–259.

123. Thybaud VS, Dean S, Nohmi T, deBoer J, Douglas GR, Glickman BW, Gorelick NJ, Heddle JA, Heflich RH, Lambert I, Martus HJ, Mirsalis JC, Suzuki T, Yajima N. *In vivo* transgenic mutation assays. *Mutat Res* 2003;540:141–151.

124. Winegar RA, Carr G, Mirsalis JC. Analysis of the mutagenic potential of ENU and MMS in germ cells of male C57BL/6 lacI transgenic mice. *Mutat Res* 1997;388:175–178.

125. Swiger RR, Myhr B, Tucker JD. The LacZ transgene in MutaMouse maps to chromosome 3. *Mutat Res* 1994;325(4):145–148.

126. Gossen JA, Molijn AC, Douglas GR, Vijg J. Application of galactose-sensitive *E. coli* strains as selective hosts for lacZ- plasmids. *Nucl Acids Res* 1992;20:32–54.

127. Vijg J, Douglas GR. Bacteriophage lambda and plasmid lacZ transgenic mice for studying mutations *in vivo*. In Pfeifer GP, Ed. *Technologies for Detection of DNA Damage and Mutations*. New York: Plenum Press; 1996, pp 391–410.

128. Dycaico MJ, Provost GS, Kretz PL, Ransom SL, Moores JC, Short JM. The use of shuttle vectors for mutation analysis in transgenic mice and rats. *Mutat Res* 1994;307:271–281.

129. Jakubczak JL, Merlino G, French JE, Muller WJ, Paul B, Adhya S, Garges S. Analysis of genetic instability during mammary tumor progression using a novel selection-based assay for *in vivo* mutations in a bacteriophage lambda transgene target. *Proc Natl Acad Sci USA* 1996;93:9073–9078.

130. Swiger RR. Quantifying *in vivo* somatic mutation using transgenic mouse model systems. In Keohavong P, Grant SG, Eds. *Methods in Molecular Biology, Volume 291, Molecular Toxicology Protocols*. Totowa NJ: Humana Press; 2005, pp 145–153.

131. Heddle JA, Martus HJ, Douglas GR. Treatment and sampling protocols for transgenic mutation assays. *Environ Mol Mutagen* 2003;41:1–6.

132. Gossen JA, Martus HJ, Wei JY, Vijg J. Spontaneous and X-ray-induced deletion mutations in a LacZ plasmid-based transgenic mouse model. *Mutat Res* 1995;331:89–97.

133. Boerrigter METI, Dolle MET, Martus HJ, Gossen JA, Vijg J. Plasmid-based transgenic mouse model for studying *in vivo* mutations. *Nature* 1995;377:657–659.

134. Dolle MET, Giese H, Hopkins CL, Martus H-J, Hausdorff JM, Vijg J. Rapid accumulation of genome rearrangements in liver but not in brain of old mice. *Nat Genet* 1997;17:431–434.

135. Dolle ME, Snyder WK, van Orsouw NJ, Vijg J. Background mutations and polymorphisms in LacZ-plasmid transgenic mice. *Environ Mol Mutagen* 1999;34:112–120.

136. Nohmi T, Katoh M, Suzuki H, Matsui M, Yamada M, Watanabe M, Suzuki M, Horiya N, Ueda O, Shibuya T, Ikeda H, Sofuni T. A new transgenic mouse mutagenesis test system using spi- and 6-thioguanine selections. *Environ Mol Mutagen* 1996;28:465–470.

137. Ikeda H, Shimizu H, Ukita T, Kumagai M. A novel assay for illegitimate recombination in *Escherichia coli*: stimulation of lambda biotransducing phage formation by ultraviolet light and its independence from RecA function. *Adv Biophys* 1995;31:197–208.

138. Shimizu H, Yamaguchi H, Ikeda H. Molecular analysis of lambda biotransducing phage produced by oxolinic acid-induced illegitimate recombination *in vivo*. *Genetics* 1995;140:889–896.

139. Nohmi T, Masumura K. Molecular nature of intra-chromosomal deletions and base substitutions induced by environmental mutagens. *Environ Mol Mutagen* 2005; 45:150–161.

140. Hayashi H, Kondo H, Masumura K, Shindo Y, Nohmi T. Novel transgenic rat for *in vivo* genotoxicity assays using 6-thioguanine and spi-selection. *Environ Mol Mutagen* 2003;41:253–259.

141. Burkhart JG, Winn RN, VanBeneden R, Malling HV. The ΦX174 bacteriophage shuttle vector for the study of mutagenesis. *Environ Mol Mutagen* 1992;19(Suppl 20):8.

142. Gondo Y, Shioyama Y, Nakao K, Katsuki M. A novel positive detection system of *in vivo* mutation in rpsL (strA) transgenic mice. *Mutat Res* 1996;360:1–14.

143. Deprimo SE, Stambrook PJ, Stringer JR. Human placental alkaline phosphatase as a histochemical marker of gene expression in transgenic mice. *Transgen Res* 1996; 5:459–466.

144. Fahrig R. A mammalian spot test: induction of genetic alterations in pigment cells of mouse embryos with X-rays and chemical mutagens. *Mol Gen Genet* 1975; 138:309–314.

145. Styles JA, Penman MG. The mouse spot test. Evaluation of its performance in identifying chemical mutagens and carcinogens. *Mutat Res* 1985;154:183–204.

146. Fahrig R. The mammalian spot test (Fellfleckentest) with mice. *Arch Toxicol* 1977;38:87–98.

147. Russell LB. Validation of the *in vivo* somatic mutation method in the mouse as a pre-screen for germinal point mutations. *Arch Toxicol* 1977;38:75–85.

148. Russell LB, Selby PB, von Halle E, Sheridan W, Valcovic L. Use of the mouse spot test in chemical mutagenesis: interpretation of past data and recommendations for future work. *Mutat Res* 1981;86:355–379.

149. *OECD Guideline 484. Guideline for the Testing of Chemicals. Genetic Toxicology: Mouse Spot Test.* OECD; 1986.

150. Suter W, Plappert-Helbig U, Glowienke S, Poetter-Locher F, Staedtler F, Racine R, Martus HJ. Induction of gene mutations by 5-(2-chloroethyl)-2′-deoxyuridine (CEDU), an antiviral pyrimidine nucleoside analogue. *Mutat Res* 2004;568:195–209.

151. Wahnschaffe U, Bitsch A, Kielhorn J, Mangelsdorf I. Mutagenicity testing with transgenic mice. Part II: Comparison with the mouse spot test. *J Carcinogen* 2005;4:4.

152. Shelby MD. Selecting chemicals and assays for assessing mammalian germ cell mutagenicity. *Mutat Res* 1996;352:159–169.

153. Douglas GR, Jiao J, Gingerich JD, Gossen JA, Soper LM. Temporal and molecular characteristics of mutations induced by ethylnitrosourea in germ cells isolated from seminiferous tubules and in spermatozoa of lacZ transgenic mice. *Proc Natl Acad Sci USA* 1995;92:7485–7489.

154. Sega GA. Unscheduled DNA synthesis in the germ cells of male mice exposed *in vivo* to the chemical mutagen ethyl methanesulfonate. *Proc Natl Acad Sci USA* 1974;71:4955–4959.

155. Sega GA. Unscheduled DNA synthesis (DNA repair) in the germ cells of male mice—its role in the study of mammalian mutagenesis. *Genetics* 1979;92:49–58.

156. Working PK, Butterworth BE. An assay to detect chemically induced DNA repair in rat spermatocytes. *Environ Mutagen* 1984;6:273–286.

157. Anderson D, Dobrzynka MM, Jackson LI, Yu TW, Brinkworth MH. Somatic and germ cell effects in rats and mice after treatment with 1,3-butadiene and its metabolites, 1,2-epoxybutene and 1,2,3,4-diepoxybutane. *Mutat Res* 1997;391:233–242.

158. Dobrzynska MM. The effects in mice of combined treatments to X-rays and antineoplastic drugs in the comet assay. *Toxicology* 2005;207:331–338.

159. Anderson D, Bishop JB, Garner RC, Ostrosky-Wegman P, Selby PB. Cyclophosphamide: review of its mutagenicity for an assessment of potential germ cell risks. *Mutat Res* 1995;330:115–181.

160. *OECD Guideline 483. Mammalian Spermatogonial Chromosome Aberration Test.* OECD; 1997.

161. Holmstrom LM, Palmer AK, Favor J. The rodent dominant lethal assay. In *Supplementary Mutagenicity Tests. UKEMS Report.* Cambridge, UK: Cambridge University Press; 1993, pp 129–156.

162. *OECD Guideline 478. Guideline for the Testing of chemicals. Genetic Toxicology: Rodent Dominant Lethal Test.* OECD; 1984.

8

REPEAT DOSE TOXICITY STUDIES

SHAYNE COX GAD

Gad Consulting Services, Cary, North Carolina

Contents

8.1 INTRODUCTION

In the broadest sense, subchronic and chronic studies for pharmaceutical products can incorporate any of the routes used to administer a therapeutic agent, use any of a number of animal models, and conform to a broad range of experimental designs. They can be two weeks long (what used to be called "subacute" studies because they were conducted at dose levels below those employed for single dose or acute studies) or last up to a year. Another name for these studies is repeat dose studies [1, 2]—that is, those studies whereby animals have a therapeutic agent

Preclinical Development Handbook: Toxicology, edited by Shayne Cox Gad
Copyright © 2008 John Wiley & Sons, Inc.

administered to them on a regular and repeated basis by one or more routes over a period of one year or less. There is great flexibility and variability in the design of such studies.

The first thing to note about repeat dose studies and their design are the priniciples of dose response—a governing general principle of toxicology:

The Three Dimensions of Dose Response

As dose increases:

- Incidence of responders in an exposed population increases.
- Severity of response in affected individuals increases.
- Time to occurrence of response or of progressive stage of response decreases.
- An implication is that as duration of dosing increases, NOEL/NOAEL decreases.

This chapter seeks to provide a firm grasp of the objectives for repeat dose studies, the regulatory requirements governing them, the key factors in their design and conduct, and the interpretation of their results.

8.2 OBJECTIVES

As with any scientific study or experiment (but especially for those in safety assessment), the essential first step is to define and understand the reason(s) for the conduct of the study—that is, its objectives. There are three major (scientific) reasons for conducting repeat dose toxicity studies, but the basic characteristic and objective of all but a few repeat studies needs to be understood. The repeat dose study is (as are most other studies in whole animal toxicology) a broad screen. It is not focused on a specific endpoint; rather, it is a broad exploration of the cumulative biological effects of the administered agent over a range of doses: so broad an exploration, in fact, that it can be called a "shotgun" study.

The objectives of the typical repeat dose study fall into three categories. The first is to broadly define the toxicity (and, if one is wise, the pharmacology and hyperpharmacology) of repeated doses of a potential therapeutic agent in an animal model [3, 4, 5]. This definition is both qualitative (what are the target organs and the nature of the effects seen) and quantitative (at what dose levels, or, more importantly, at what plasma and tissue levels, are effects definitely seen and not seen). It seeks to characterize the cumulative toxicity of the drug under study. Such cumulative toxicity is rarely predicted by single dose toxicity.

The second objective (and the one that in the pharmaceutical industry usually compels both timing and compromising of design and execution) is to provide support for the initiation of and/or continued conduct of clinical trials in humans [6, 7]. As such, repeat dose studies should provide not only adequate clearance (therapeutic margin) of initial dose levels and duration of dosing, but also guidance for any special measures to be made or precautions to be taken in initial clinical trials. Setting inappropriate dose levels (either too low or too high) may lead to the failure of a study. A successful study must both define a safe or "clean" dose level

TABLE 8.1   Duration of Treatment Supported by Preclinical Studies

Animal Study Length	Generally Allowed Human Dosing
2 weeks	Up to 3 doses (but could be as much as 12 consecutive doses)
1 month	Up to 30 days (though usually 28)
3 months	3 months
6 months (rodent); 9–12 months (dog)(U.S.)/6 months (EEC and Japan)	Unlimited

(one that is as high as possible, to allow as much flexibility as possible in the conduct of clinical studies) and demonstrate and/or characterize signs of toxicity at some higher dose. The duration of dosing issue is driven by a compromise between meeting established regulatory guidelines (as set out in Table 8.1) and the economic pressure to initiate clinical trials as soon as possible.

The third objective is one of looking forward to later studies. The repeat dose study must provide sufficient information to allow a prudent setting of doses for later, longer studies (including, ultimately, carcinogenicity studies). At the same time, the repeat dose study must also provide guidance for the other (than dose) design features of longer-term studies (such as what parameters to measure and when to measure them, how many animals to use, and how long to conduct the study).

These objectives are addressed by the usual repeat dose study. Some repeat dose studies, however, are unusual in being conceived, designed, and executed to address specific questions raised (or left unanswered) by previous preclinical or early clinical studies. Such a special purpose is addressed separately. Common study durations are 2, 4, and 13 weeks (all species), 26 weeks (rodent chronic toxicity), 39 or 52 weeks (nonrodent chronic toxicity), and 2 years (rodent carcinogenicity).

Chronic studies (those that last six or nine months or a year) may also be conducted for the above purposes but are primarily done to fulfill registration requirements for drugs that are intended for continuous long-term (lifetime) use or frequent intermittent use.

8.3   REGULATORY CONSIDERATIONS

Much of what is done (and how it is done) in repeat dose studies is a response to a number of regulations. Three of these have very broad impact. These are the Good Laboratory Practices requirements, Animal Welfare Act requirements, and regulatory requirements that actually govern study design.

8.3.1   Good Laboratory Practices (GLPs)

Since 1978, the design and conduct of preclinical safety assessment studies for pharmaceuticals in the United States (and, indeed, internationally) have been governed and significantly influenced by GLPs. Strictly speaking, these regulations cover qualifications of staff and facilities, training, record-keeping, documentation, and actions required to ensure compliance with and the effectiveness of these steps. Although the initial regulations were from the U.S. FDA [8], they have always extended to cover studies performed overseas [9]. Most other countries have adopted similar regulations. A discussion of these regulations is beyond the scope of the current chapter, but several aspects are central to this effort. Each technique or methodology to be employed in a study (such as animal identification, weighing and examination, blood collection, and data recording) must be adequately described in a standard operating procedure (SOP) before the study begins. Those who are to perform such procedures must be trained in them beforehand. The actual design of the study, including start date and how it is to be ended and analyzed, plus the principal scientists involved (particularly the study director), must be specified in a protocol that is signed before the study commences. Any changes to these features must be documented in amendments once the study has begun. It is a good idea that the pathologist who is to later perform or oversee histopathology be designated before the start of the study, and that the design be a team effort involving the best efforts of the toxicologist, pathologist, and (usually for subchronic studies) the drug metabolism scientist [10].

8.3.2   Animal Welfare Act

Gone are the days when the pharmaceutical scientist could conduct whatever procedures or studies that were desired using experimental animals. The Animal Welfare Act [11] (and its analogues in other countries) rightfully requires careful consideration of animal usage to ensure that research and testing uses as few animals as possible in as humane a manner as possible. As a start, all protocols must be reviewed by an Institutional Animal Care and Use Committee. Such review takes time but should not serve to hinder good science. When designing a study or developing a new procedure or technique, the following points should be kept in mind:

1. Will the number of animals used be sufficient to provide the required data yet not constitute excessive use? (It ultimately does not reduce animal use to utilize too few animals to begin with and then have to repeat the study.)
2. Are the procedures employed the least invasive and traumatic available? This practice is not only required by regulations but is also sound scientific practice, since any induced stress will produce a range of responses in test animals that can mask or confound the chemically induced effects.

8.3.3   Regulatory Requirements for Study Design

The first consideration in the construction of a study is a clear statement of its objectives, which are almost always headed by meeting regulatory requirements to support drug development and registration. Accordingly, the relevant regulatory requirements must be analyzed, which is complicated by the fact that new drugs are no longer developed for registration and sale in a single-market country. The expense is too great, and the potential for broad international sales too appealing. While each major country has its own requirements as to study designs and studies required (with most of the smaller countries adhering to the regulations of one of the major players), harmonization has done much to smooth these differences [12]. Meeting these regulatory requirements is particularly challenging for several reasons. First, the only official delineation of general requirements in the Untied States is dated

[13], and recently special cases have arisen (anti-HIV agents, biotechnologically derived agents, therapeutic agents for neonates and the very elderly, etc.) that try the utility of these requirements. These needs have led to a stream of points-to-consider, which seek to update requirements. Second, the term "guidelines" means different things in different countries (in the United States it means "requirements," and in Japan, "suggestions").

Agents intended to treat or arrest the progress of rapidly spreading life-threatening diseases (such as AIDS) are subject to less stringent safety assessment requirements prior to initial clinical evaluations than are other drugs. However, even though approval (if clinical efficacy is established) for marketing can be granted with preclinical testing still under way, all applicable safety assessments (as with any other class of drugs) must still be completed [14].

Drugs intended for use in either the elderly or the very young have special additional requirements for safety evaluation, in recognition of the special characteristics and potential sensitivities of these populations. For the elderly, these requirements call for special consideration of renal and hepatic effects [15]. Likewise, drugs intended for the young require special studies to be performed in neonates and juvenile animals (usually of 2–4 weeks' duration in rats).

In the last five to six years, a number of potentially important drugs have been produced by recombinant DNA technology. These biomacromolecules, which are primarily endogenously occurring proteins, present a variety of special considerations and concerns, including the following:

- Because they are endogenously occurring molecules, assessing their pharmacokinetics and metabolism presents special problems.
- One must determine if the externally commercially produced molecule is biologically equivalent to the naturally occurring one.
- Since they are proteins, there is the question of whether they are immunogenic or provoke neutralizing antibodies that will limit their usefulness.
- Because they are available only in very small quantities, the use of traditional protocols (such as those that use ever-increasing doses until an adverse effect is achieved) is impractical.
- Agents with such specific activity in humans may not be appropriately evaluated in rodents or other model species.

Each of these points must be addressed in any safety testing plan [16]. The requirements set out in this chapter are designed to do this (for repeat dose testing).

8.4   STUDY DESIGN AND CONDUCT

8.4.1   Animals

In all but a few rare cases, for pharmaceutical safety assessment, separate studies in at least two species are required. Regulations require that both species be mammalian, and one of these must be a nonrodent; practice and economics dictate that the other species will be a rodent. With extremely rare exception, the rodent species employed is the rat (although the mouse also sees significant use). There is considerably more variability in the nonrodent species, with a range of factors determining whether the dog (most common choice), a primate species (typically the rhesus or cynomolgus, although some others are used in particular cases), the pig (particularly in Europe), or some other animal (e.g., the ferret) is selected. The factors that should and do govern species selection are presented in detail in Gad and Chengelis [17]. The use of multiple species is a regulatory requirement arising from experience and the belief (going back to 1944 at least) that it will provide a better chance of detecting the full range of biological responses (adverse and otherwise) to the new molecular entity being evaluated. This belief has come under fire in recent years [18], but is unlikely to be changed soon. Along the same lines, unless an agent is to be used by only one sex or the other of humans, equal numbers of both sexes of an animal species are utilized in the studies, with the sexes being treated as unrelated for purposes of statistical analysis. Also except in rare cases, the animals used are young, healthy adults in the logarithmic phase of their growth curve. (The FDA specifies that rodents be less than 6 weeks of age at the initiation of dosing.)

Numbers of animals to be used in each dose group of a study are presented in Table 8.2. Although the usual practice is to use three different dose groups and at least one equal-sized control group, this number is not fixed and should be viewed as a minimum (see Section 8.4.6). Use of more groups allows for a reduction in the risk of not clearly defining effects and establishing the highest possible safe dose at a modest increase in cost. There must be as many control animals as are in the largest-size test group to optimize statistical power.

Animals are assigned to groups (test and control) by one or another form of statistical randomization. Prior to assignment, animals are evaluated for some period of time after being received in-house (usually at least 1 week for rodents and 2 weeks for nonrodents) to ensure that they are healthy and have no discernible abnormalities. The randomization is never pure; it is always "blocked" in some form or another (by initial body weight, at least) so that each group is not (statistically) significantly different from the others in terms of the "blocked" parameters.

Proper facilities and care for test animals are not only a matter of regulatory compliance (and a legal requirement), but also essential for a scientifically sound and valid study.

Husbandry requires clean cages of sufficient size and continuous availability of clean water and food (unless the protocol requires some restriction on their availability). Environmental conditions (temperature, humidity, and light–dark cycle) must be kept within specified limits. All of these must, in turn, be detailed in the

TABLE 8.2   Numbers of Animals for Chronic and Subchronic Study per Test Group

Study Length	Rats per Sex	Dogs per Sex	Primates per Sex
2–4 weeks	5–10	3–4	3
3 months[a]	20	6	5
6/9/12 months	30	8	5
Carcinogenicity (24 months)	50	10	10

[a]Starting with 1 month studies, one should consider adding animals (particularly to the high dose and control groups) to allow evaluation of reversal (or progression) of effects. The FDA is becoming more invested in this approach—to evaluate both recovery from effects and possible progression after dosing.

protocols of studies. The limits for these conditions are set forth in relevant NIH and USDA publications.

8.4.2   Routes and Setting Doses

Route (how an agent is administered to a test animal) and dose (how much of and how frequently an agent is administered) are inseparable in pharmaceutical safety assessment studies and really cannot be defined independently. The selection of both begins with an understanding of the intended use of the drug in humans. The ideal case is to have the test material administered by the same route, at the same frequency (once a day, three times a day, etc.), and for the same intervals (continuously, if the drug is an intravenously infused agent, for example) as the drug's eventual use in people. Practical considerations such as the limitations of animal models (i.e., there are some things you can't get a rat to do), limitations on technical support,[1] and the like, and regulatory requirements (discussed below as part of dose setting) frequently act or interact to preclude this straightforward approach.

Almost 30 routes exist for administration of drugs to patients, but only a handful of these are commonly used in preclinical safety studies [19]. The most common deviation from what is to be done in clinical trials is the use of parenteral (injected) routes such as IV (intravenous) and SC (subcutaneous) deliveries. Such injections are loosely characterized as bolus (all at once or over a very short period, such as 5 minutes) and infusion (over a protracted period of hours, days, or even months). The term *continuous infusion* implies a steady rate over a protracted period, requiring some form of setup such as an implanted venous catheter or infusion port.

It is rare that the raw drug itself is suitable (in terms of stability, local tissue tolerance, and optimum systemic absorption and distribution) for direct use as a dosage form. Either it must be taken into a solution or suspension in a suitable carrier, or a more complex formulation (a prototype of the commercial form) must be developed. Gad and Chengelis [20] should be consulted for a more complete discussion of dose formulation for animals or humans. One formulation or more must be developed (preferably the same one for both animals and humans) based on the specific requirements of preclinical dosage formulation. For many therapeutic agents, limitations on volumes that can be administered and concentrations of active ingredient that can be achieved impact heavily on dose setting.

Setting of doses for longer-term toxicity studies is one of the most difficult tasks in study design. The doses administered must include one that is devoid of any adverse effect (preferably of *any* effect) and yet still high enough to "clear" the projected clinical dose by the traditional or regulatory safety factors. Such safety or uncertainty factors are currently predictions on the FDA HED guidance [21]. At the same time, if feasible, at least one of the doses should characterize the toxicity profile associated with the agent (for some biotechnologically derived agents, particularly those derived from endogenous human molecules, it may only be possible to demonstrate biological effects in appropriate disease models, and impossible to

---

[1] Many antiviral agents, particularly some anti-HIV agents, have rather short plasma half-lives, which requires frequent oral administration of the agent. Thirteen week studies have been conducted with tid (3x/day) dosing of rats and monkeys, requiring around-the-clock shift work for technical staff of the laboratory.

demonstrate toxicity). Because of limitations on availability of protodrugs, it is generally undesirable to go too high to achieve this second (toxicity) objective.

Traditionally, studies include three or more dose groups to fulfill these two objectives. Based on earlier results (generally single dose or two week studies), doses are selected. It is, by the way, generally an excellent idea to observe the "decade rule" in extrapolation of results from shorter to longer studies; that is, do not try to project doses for more than an order-of-magnitude-longer study (thus the traditional progression from single dose to 14 day to 90 day studies). Also, one should not allow the traditional use of three dose groups plus a control to limit designs. If there is a great deal of uncertainty, it is much cheaper in every way to use four or five dose groups in a single study than to have to repeat the entire study. Finally, remember that different doses may be appropriate for the different sexes.

It should also be kept in mind that formulating materials may have effects of their own, and a "vehicle" control group may be required in addition to a negative control group.

8.4.3 Parameters to Measure

As stated earlier, repeat dose studies are "shotgun" in nature; that is, they are designed to look at a very broad range of endpoints with the intention of screening as broadly as possible for indications of toxicity. Meaningful findings are rarely limited to a single endpoint—rather, what typically emerges is a pattern of findings. This broad search for components of toxicity profile is not just a response to regulatory guidelines intended to identify potentially unsafe drugs. An understanding of all the indicators of biological effect can also frequently help one to understand the relevance of findings, to establish some as unrepresentative of a risk to humans, and even to identify new therapeutic uses of an agent.

Parameters of interest in the repeat dose study can be considered as sets of measures, each with its own history, rationale, and requirements. It is critical to remember, however, that the strength of the study design as a scientific evaluation lies in the relationships and patterns of effects that are seen in looking at each of these measures (or groups) not as independent findings but rather as integrated profiles of biological effects.

Body Weight Body weight (and the associated calculated parameter of body weight gain) is a nonspecific, broad screen for adverse systemic toxicity. Animals are initially assigned to groups based on a randomization scheme that includes each group varying insignificantly from one another in terms of body weight. Weights are measured prior to the initial dose, then typically 1, 3, 5, 7, 11, and 14 days thereafter. The frequency of measurement of weights goes down as the study proceeds; after 2 weeks, weighing is typically weekly through 6 weeks, then every other week through 3 months, and monthly thereafter. Because the animals used in these studies are young adults in the early log phase of their growth, decreases in the rate of gain relative to control animals is a very sensitive (albeit nonspecific) indicator of systemic toxicity [22].

Food Consumption Food consumption is typically measured with one or two uses in mind. First, it may be explanatory in the interpretation of reductions (either absolute or relative) in body weight. In cases where administration of the test compound is via diet, it is essential to be able to adjust dietary content so as to accurately maintain dose levels. Additionally, the actual parameter itself is a broad and nonspecific indicator of systemic toxicity. Food consumption is usually measured over a period of several days, first weekly and then on a once-a-month basis. Water consumption, which is also sometimes measured, is similar in interpretation and use [23, 24].

Clinical Signs   Clinical signs are generally vastly underrated in value, probably because insufficient attention is paid to care in their collection. Two separate levels of data collection are actually involved here. The first is the morbidity and mortality observation, which is made twice a day. This generally consists of a simple cage-side visual assessment of each animal to determine if it is still alive, and, if so, whether it appears in good (or at least stable) health. Historically, this regulatory required observation was intended to ensure that tissues from intoxicated animals were not lost for meaningful histopathologic evaluation due to autolysis [25].

The second level of clinical observation is the detailed hands-on examination analogous to the human physical examination. It is usually performed against a checklist (e.g., see Ref. 20) and evaluation is of the incidence of observations of a particular type in a group of treated animals compared to controls. Observations range from being indicative of nonspecific systemic toxicity to fairly specific indicators of target organ toxicity. These more detailed observations are typically taken after the first week of a study and on a monthly basis thereafter.

Ophthalmologic examinations are typically made immediately prior to initiation of a study (and thus serve to screen out animals with preexisting conditions) and toward the end of a study.

Particularly when the agent under investigation either targets or acts via a mechanism likely to have a primary effect on a certain organ for which functional measures are available, an extra set of measurements of functional performance should be considered. The organs or organ systems that are usually of particular concern are the kidneys, liver, and cardiovascular, nervous, and immune systems. Special measures (such as creatinine clearance as a measure of renal function) are combined with other data already collected (organ weights, histopathology, clinical pathology, etc.) to provide a focused "special" investigation or evaluation of adverse effects on the target organ system of concern. In larger animals (dogs and primates) some of these measures (such as ECGs) are made as a matter of course in all studies.

Clinical Pathology   Clinical pathology covers a number of biochemical and morphological evaluations based on invasive and noninvasive sampling of fluids from animals that are made periodically during the course of a subchronic study. These evaluations are sometimes labeled as clinical (as opposed to anatomical) pathology determinations. Table 8.3 presents a summary of the parameters measured under the headings of clinical chemistry, hematology, and urinalysis, using samples of blood and urine collected at predetermined intervals during the study. Conventionally, these intervals are typically at three points evenly spaced over the course of the study, with the first being 1 month after study initiation and the last being immediately prior to termination of the test animals. For a 3 month study, this means that

TABLE 8.3   Clinical Pathology Measures

Clinical Chemistry	Hematology	Urinalysis
Albumin	Erythrocyte count (RBC)	Chloride
Alkaline phosphatase (ALP)	Hemoglobin (HGB)	Bilirubin
Blood urea nitrogen (BUN)	Hematocrit (HCT)	Glucose
Calcium	Mean corpuscular hemoglobin (MCH)	Occult blood
Chloride	Mean corpuscular volume (MCV)	pH
Creatine	Platelet count	Phosphorus
Creatine phosphokinase (CPK)	Prothrombin time	Potassium
Direct bilirubin	Reticulocyte count	Protein
γ-Glutamyltransferase (GGT)	White cell count (WBC)	Sodium
Globulin	White cell differential count	Specific gravity
Glucose		Volume
Lactic dehydrogenase (LDH)		
Phosphorus		
Potassium		
Serum glutamic-oxaloacetic trans-aminase (SGOT)		
Serum glutamic-pyruvic transaminase (SGPT)		
Sodium		
Total bilirubin		
Total cholesterol		
Total protein		
Triglycerides		

samples of blood and urine would be collected at 1, 2, and 3 months after study initiation (i.e., after the first day of dosing of the animals). There are some implications of these sampling plans that should be considered when the data are being interpreted. Many of the clinical chemistry (and some of the hematologic) markers are really the result of organ system damage that may be transient in nature (see Table 8.4 for a summary of interpretations of clinical chemistry findings and Table 8.5 for a similar summary for hematologic findings). The samples on which analysis is performed are from fixed points in time, which may miss transient changes (typically increases) in some enzyme levels.

Pharmacokinetics and Metabolism   Pharmaceutical subchronic toxicity studies are always accompanied by a parallel determination of the pharmacokinetics of the material of interest administered by the same route as that used in the safety study. This parallel determination consists of measuring plasma levels of the administered agent and its major metabolites either in animals that are part of the main study or in a separate set of animals (in parallel with the main study) that are dosed and evaluated to determine just these endpoints. The purpose of these determinations is both to allow a better interpretation of the findings of the study and to encourage the most accurate possible extrapolation to humans. The first data of interest are the absorption, distribution, and elimination of the test material, but a number of other types of information can also be collected [26, 27, 28]. For nonparenteral

TABLE 8.4 Association of Changes in Biochemical Parameters with Actions at Particular Target Organs

| Parameter | Organ System | | | | | | | | Notes |
	Blood	Heart	Lung	Kidney	Liver	Bone	Intestine	Pancreas	
Albumin				↓	↓				Produced by the liver. Very significant reductions indicate extensive liver damage.
ALP (alkaline phosphatase)					↑	↑	↑		Elevations usually associated with cholestasis. Bone alkaline phosphatase tends to be higher in young animals.
Bilirubin (total)	↑				↑				Usually elevated due to cholestasis either due to obstruction or hepatopathy.
BUN (blood urea nitrogen)				↑	↓				Estimates blood-filtering capacity of the kidneys. Doesn't become significantly elevated until kidney function is reduced 60–75%.
Calcium				↑					Can be life threatening and result in acute death.
Cholinesterase				↑	↓				Found in plasma, brain, and RBCs.
CPK (creatine phosphokinase)		↑							Most often elevated due to skeletal muscle damage but can also be produced by cardiac muscle damage. Can be more sensitive than histopathology.
Creatine				↑					Also estimates blood-filtering capacity of kidney as BUN does. More specific than BUN.

223

TABLE 8.4 *Continued*

Parameter	Organ System								Notes
	Blood	Heart	Lung	Kidney	Liver	Bone	Intestine	Pancreas	
Glucose								↑	Alterations other than those associated with stress are uncommon and reflect an effect on the pancreatic islets or anorexia.
GGT (γ-glutamyltransferase)					↑				Elevated in cholestasis. This is microsomal enzyme and levels often increase in response to microsomal enzyme induction.
HBDH (hydroxybutyric dehydrogenase)		↑			↑				Most prominent in cardiac muscle tissue.
LDH (lactic dehydrogenase)		↑	↑	↑	↑				Increase usually due to skeletal muscle, cardiac muscle, and liver damage. Not very specific unless isozymes are evaluated.
Protein (total)				↑	↑				Absolute alterations are usually associated with decreased production (liver) or increased loss (kidney).
SGOT (serum glutamic-oxaloacetic trans-aminase); also called AST (aspartate aminotransferase)		↑		↑	↑			↑	Present in skeletal muscle and heart and most commonly associated with damage to these.
SGPT (serum glutamic-pyruvic transaminase); also called ALT (alanine aminotransferase)					↑				Evaluations usually associated with hepatic damage or disease.
SDH (sorbitol dehydrogenase)					↑ or ↓				Liver enzyme that can be quite sensitive but is fairly unstable. Samples should be processed as soon as possible.

TABLE 8.5   Some Probable Conditions Affecting Hematological Changes

Parameter	Elevation	Depression

Red blood cells	1. Vascular shock
	2. Excessive diuresis
	3. Chronic hypoxia
	4. Hyperadrenocorticism
		1. Anemias
		  (a) Blood loss
		  (b) Hemolysis
		  (c) Low RBC production

Hematocrit	1. Increased RBCs
	2. Stress
	3. Shock
	  (a) Trauma
	  (b) Surgery
	4. Polycythemia
		1. Anemias
		2. Pregnancy
		3. Excessive hydration

Hemoglobin	1. Polycythemia (increase in production of RBCs)	1. Anemias 2. Lead poisoning
Mean cell volume	1. Amemias 2. Vitamin B_{12} deficiency	1. Iron deficiency
Mean corpuscular hemoglobin	1. Reticulocytosis	1. Iron deficiency
White blood cells	1. Bacterial infections 2. Bone marrow stimulation	1. Bone marrow depression 2. Cancer chemotherapy 3. Chemical intoxication 4. Splenic disorders
Platelets		1. Bone marrow depression 2. Immune disorder
Neutrophilis	1. Acute bacterial infections 2. Tissue necrosis 3. Strenuous exercise 4. Convulsions 5. Tachycardia 6. Acute hemorrhage	1. Viral infections
Lymphocytes	1. Leukemia 2. Malnutrition 3. Viral infections	
Monocytes	1. Protozoal infections	
Eosinophils	1. Allergy 2. Irradiation 3. Pernicious anemia 4. Parasitism	
Basophils	1. Lead poisoning	

routes it is essential to demonstrate that systemic absorption and distribution of the test material did occur; otherwise, it is open to question whether the potential safety of the agent in humans has been adequately addressed (not to mention the implication for potential human therapeutic efficacy).

Both clinical chemistry, pathology, and pharmacokinetics have in common the requirement to collect blood. There are species-specific limitations on how this may be done and how much can be collected without compromising the test animals. These are summarized in Tables 8.6 and 8.7.

TABLE 8.6   Blood Sample Requirements

Species	Body Weight (kg)	Blood Volume (mL)	Sample / Time Point (mL)
Mouse	0.03	2	0.075
Rat	0.3	20	1
Dog	12	1000	50
Cynomolgus monkey	3	200	10
Rabbit	3	200	10

TABLE 8.7   Blood Sampling Techniques

Species	Techniques
Mouse	Orbital sinus, cardiac puncture
Rat	Sublingual, orbital sinus, jugular vein, cardiac puncture, tail vein
Dog	Jugular vein, cephalic vein
Cynomolgus monkey	Femoral vein/artery, cephalic vein
Rabbit	Jugular vein, marginal ear vein, cardiac puncture

8.4.4   Other In-Life Endpoints for Evaluation

Ophthalmology   Ophthalmological examination of all animals in study (particularly nonrodents) should be performed both before study initiation and at the completion of the period for which the drug is administered. This should be performed by an experienced veterinary ophthalmologist.

Cardiovascular Function   Particularly in light of recent concerns with drug-induced arrhythmias, careful consideration must be given to incorporating adequate evaluation of drug-induced alterations on cardiovascular function. This is usually achieved by measuring blood pressure, heart rate, and an EKG prestudy and periodically during the course of the study (usually at least one intermediate period and at the end of the study) in the nonrodent species being employed.

Neurotoxicology   Table 8.8 presents the FDA's current draft criteria [3, 4] for endpoints to be incorporated in studies as a screen for neurotoxicity. In practice, a functional observation battery is employed at several endpoints (usually 1 and 3 months into the study) to fill these requirements.

Immunotoxicology   In response to concerns about potential effects of drugs on the immune system, the FDA [4] has proposed that a basic set of criteria (Table 8.9) be evaluated and considered in standard subchronic and chronic studies. It should be noted that most of these endpoints are already collected in traditional subchronic designs.

Pharmacokinetics   All subchronic and chronic toxicity studies now incoprorate (either in the study itself or in a parallel study) evaluation of the basic pharmacokinetics of a compound [29].

TABLE 8.8   FDA Draft Criteria for a Neurotoxicity Screen as a Component of Short-Term and Subchronic Studies

- Histopathological examination of tissues representative of the nervous system, including the brain, spinal cord, and peripheral nervous system.
- Quantitative observations and manipulative test to detect neurological, behavioral, and physiological dysfuntions. These may include:
  General appearance
  Body posture
  Incidence and severity of seizure
  Incidence and severity of tremor, paralysis, and other dysfunction
  Level of motor activity and arousal
  Level of reactivity to stimuli
  Motor coordination
  Strength
  Gait
  Sensorimotor response to primary sensory stimuli
  Excessive lacrimation or salivation
  Piloerection
  Diarrhea
  Ptosis
  Other signs of neurotoxicity deemed appropriate

TABLE 8.9 FDA Draft Recommendations for Type I Immunotoxicity Test that Can Be Included in Repeat Dose Toxicity Studies

Hematology
- White blood cell counts
- Differential white blood cell counts
- Lymphocytosis
- Lymphopenia
- Eosinophilia

Histopathology
- Lymphoid tissues
- Spleen
  Lymph nodes
  Thymus
  Peyer's patches in gut
  Bone marrow
- Cytology (if needed)[a]
  Prevalence of activated macrophages
  Tissue prevalence and location of lymphocytes
  Evidence of B-cell germinal centers
  Evidence of T-cell germinal centers
- Necrotic or proliferative changes in lymphoid tissues

Clinical chemistry
- Total serum production
- Albumin
- Albumin-to-globulin ratio
- Serum transaminases

[a]More comprehensive cytological evaluation of the tissues would not be done unless there is evidence of potential immunotoxicity from the preceding evaluations.

8.4.5   Histopathology

Histopathology is generally considered the single most significant portion of data to come out of a repeat dose toxicity study. It actually consists of three related sets of data (gross pathology observations, organ weights, and microscopic pathology) that are collected during the termination of the study animals. At the end of the study, a number of tissues are collected during termination of all surviving animals (test and control). Organ weight and terminal body weights are recorded at study termination, so that absolute and relative (to body weight) values can be statistically evaluated.

These tissues, along with the organs for which weights are determined, are listed in Table 8.10. All tissues collected are typically processed for microscopic observation, but only those from the high dose and control groups are necessarily evaluated microscopically. If a target organ is discovered in the high dose group, then successively lower dose groups are examined until a "clean" (devoid of effect) level is discovered [30].

In theory, all microscopic evaluations should be performed blind (without the pathologist knowing from which dose group a particular animal came), but this is difficult to do in practice and such an approach frequently degrades the quality of the evaluation. Like all the other portions of data in the study, proper evaluation benefits from having access to all data that addresses the relevance, severity, timing, and potential mechanisms of a specific toxicity. Blind examination is best applied in peer review or consultations on specific findings.

In addition to the "standard" set of tissues specified in Table 8.10, observations during the course of the study or in other previous studies may dictate that additional tissues be collected or special examinations (e.g., special stains, polarized light or electron microscopy, immunocytochemistry, or quantitative morphometry) be

TABLE 8.10   Tissues for Histopathology

Adrenals[a]	Mainstream bronchi
Body and cervix	Major salivary glands
Brain, all three levels[a]	Mesenteric lymph nodes
Cervical lymph nodes	Ovaries and tubes
Cervical spinal cord	Pancreas
Duodenum	Pituitary
Esophagogastric junction	Prostate
Esophagus	Skeletal muscle from proximal hind limb
Eyes with optic nerves	Spleen[a]
Femur with marrow	Sternebrae with marrow
Heart	Stomach
Ileum	Testes with epididymides[a]
Kidneys[a]	Thymus and mediastinal contents[a]
Large bowel	Thyroid with parathyroid[a]
Larynx with thyroid and parathyroid	Trachea
Liver[a]	Urinary bladder
Lungs[a]	Uterus including horns

[a]Organs to be weighed.

undertaken to evaluate the relevance of, or to understand the mechanisms underlying, certain observations.

Histopathology testing is a terminal procedure, and, therefore, sampling of any single animal is a one-time event (except in the case of a tissue collected by biopsy). Because it is a regulatory requirement that the tissues from a basic number of animals be examined at the stated end of the study, an assessment of effects at any other time course (most commonly, to investigate recovery from an effect found at study termination) requires that satellite groups of animals be incorporated into the study at start-up. Such animals are randomly assigned at the beginning of the study, and otherwise treated exactly the same as the equivalent treatment (or control) animals.

8.4.6 Study Designs

The traditional design for a repeat dose toxicity study is very straightforward. The appropriate number of animals of each sex are assigned to each of the designated dose and control groups. Unfortunately, this basic design is taken by many to be dogma, even when it does not suit the purposes of the investigator. There are many possible variations to study design, but four basic factors should be considered: controls, the use of interval and satellite groups, balanced and unbalanced designs, and staggered starts.

Classically, a single control group of the same size as each of the dose groups is incorporated into each study. Some studies incorporate two control groups (each the same size as the experimental groups) to guard against having a statistically significant effect due to one control group being abnormal for one or more parameters (a much more likely event when laboratory animals were less genetically homogeneous than they are now). The belief is that a "significant" finding that differs from one (but not both) of the concurrent control groups, and does not differ from historical control data, can be considered as not biologically significant. This is, however, an indefensible approach. Historical controls have value, but it is the concurrent control group(s) in a study that is of concern.

Interval or satellite groups have been discussed at two earlier points in this chapter. They allow measurement of termination parameters at intervals other than at termination of the study. They are also useful when the manipulation involved in making a measurement (such as the collection of an extensive blood sample), while not terminal, may compromise (relative to other animals) the subject animals. Another common use of such groups is to evaluate recovery from some observed effect at study termination.

Usually, each of the groups in a study is the same size, with each of the sexes being equally represented. The result is called a balanced design, with statistical power for detection of effects optimized for each of the treatment groups. If one knows little about the dose–toxicity profile, this is an entirely sound and rational approach. However, there are situations when one may wish to utilize an unbalanced design—that is, to have one or more dose groups larger than the others. This is usually the case when either greater sensitivity is desired (typically in a low dose group), or an unusual degree of attrition of test animals is expected (usually due to mortality in a high dose group), or as a guard against a single animal's idiopathic response being sufficient to cause "statistical significance."

As it is normal practice to have a balanced design, it is also traditional to initiate treatment of all animals at the same time. This may lead to problems at study termination, however. It is a very uncommon toxicology laboratory that can "bring a study down" on a single day. In fact, there are no labs that can collect blood and perform necropsies in a single day on even the 48–80 dogs involved in a study, much less the 160–400+ rats in the rodent version. Starting all animals in a study on the same day presents a number of less than desirable options. The first is to terminate as many animals as can be done each day, continuing to dose (and therefore further affect) the remaining test animals. Assuming that the animals are being terminated in a random, balanced manner, this means that the last animals terminated will have received from 3 to 10 additional days of treatment. At the least, this is likely to cause some variance inflation (and therefore both decrease the power of the study design and possibly confound interpretation). If the difference in the length of treatment of test animals is greater than 3% of the intended length of the study, one should consider alternative designs.

An alternative approach to study design that addresses this problem employs one of several forms of staggered starts. In these, distinct groups of animals have their dosing initiated at different times. The most meaningful form recognizes that the two sexes are in effect separate studies anyway (they are never compared statistically, with the treatment groups being compared only against the same-sex control group). Thus, if the termination procedure for one sex takes 3–5 days, then one sex should be initiated on dosing one week and the other on the following week. This maximizes the benefits of common logistical support (such as dose formulation) and reduces the impact of differential length of dosing on study outcome.

Another variation recognizes that any repeat dose study using both males and females is really two studies. The different sexes are considered separately and, except for ending up in a single report, are treated as separate studies. Accordingly, each sex can be started on a different day without increasing variability.

A further variation on this is to stagger the start-up either of different dose groups, or of the satellite and main study portions of dose groups. The former is to be avoided (it will completely confound study outcome), while the latter makes sense in some cases (pharmacokinetics and special measures) but not others (recovery and interval sacrifice).

8.5   STUDY INTERPRETATION AND REPORTING

For a successful repeat dose study, the bottom line is the clear demonstration of a no-effect level, characterization of a toxicity profile (providing guidance for any clinical studies), enough information on pharmacokinetics and metabolism to scale dosages to human applications, and at least a basic understanding of the mechanisms involved in any identified pathogenesis. The report that is produced as a result of the study should clearly communicate these points—along with the study design and experimental procedures, summarized data, and their statistical analysis—and it should be GLP compliant, suitable for FDA submission format.

Interpretation of the results of a study should be truly scientific and integrative. It is elementary to have the report state only each statistically and biologically significant finding in an orderly manner. The meaning and significance of each in relation to other findings, as well as the relevance to potential human effects, must be evaluated and addressed.

The author of the report should ensure that it is accurate and complete, but also that it clearly tells a story and concludes with the relevant (to clinical development) findings.

REFERENCES

1. Ballantyne B. Repeated exposure toxicity. In Ballantyne B, Marrs T, Syversen T, Eds. *General and Applied Toxicology*. London: MacMillan; 2000, pp 55–66.

2. Wilson NH, Hardisty JF, Hayes JR. Short-term, subchronic and chronic toxicity studies. In Hayes AW, Ed. *Principles and Methods of Toxicicology*, 4th ed. Philadelphia: Taylor & Francis; 2001, pp 917–958.

3. FDA. *Toxicological Principles for the Safety Assessment of Direct Food Additives and Color Additives Used in Food*, Redbook II, p 86. Washington, DC: Center for Food Safety and Applied Nutrition, FDA; 1993.

4. FDA. *Toxicological Principles for the Safety of Food Ingredients*, Redbook 2000. Washington, DC: Center for Food Safety and Applied Nutrition, FDA; 2000.

5. OECD. *Guidance Notes for Analysis and Evaluation of Chronic Toxicity and Carcinogenicity Studies* 1998.

6. O'Grady J, Linet OI. *Early Phase Drug Evaluation In Man*. Boca Raton, FL: CRC Press; 1990.

7. Smith CG. *The Process of New Drug discovery and Development*. Boca Raton, FL: CRC Press; 1992.

8. Food and Drug Administration (FDA). Good Laboratory Practices for Nonclinical Laboratory Studies. *CFR* 21 Part 58, March 1983.

9. Food and Drug Administration (FDA). Good Laboratory Practices. *CFR* 21 Part 58, April 1988.

10. OECD. *Principles of Good Laboratory Practice* 1997.

11. Animal and Plant Health Inspection Service (APHIS). United States Department of Agriculture (31 August 1989). *Fed Reg* 1989;54(168):36112–36163.

12. Alder S, Zbinden G. *National and International Drug Safety Guidelines*. Zollikon, Switzerland: M.T.C. Verlag; 1988.

13. Food and Drug Administration (FDA). *FDA Introduction to Total Drug Quality*. Washington, DC: US Government Printing Office; 1971.

14. Food and Drug Administration (FDA). Investigational new drug, antibiotic, and biological drug product regulations, procedures for drugs intended to treat life-threatening and severely debilitating illness. *Fed Reg* 1988;53(204):41516–41524.

15. Center for Drug Evaluation and Research (CDER). *Guideline for the Study of Drugs Likely to Be Used in the Elderly*. FDA; November 1989.

16. Weissinger J. Nonclinical pharmacologic and toxicologic considerations for evaluating biologic products. *Regul Toxicol Pharmacol* 1989;10:255–263.

17. Gad SC, Chengelis CP. *Animal Models in Toxicology*. New York: Marcel Dekker; 1992.

18. Zbinden G. The concept of multispecies testing in industrial toxicology. *Regul Toxicol Pharmacol* 1993;17:84–94.

19. Gad SC. Routes in safety assessment studies. *J Am Coll Toxicol* 1994;13:1–17.

20. Gad SC, Chengelis CP. *Acute Toxicology*, 2nd ed. San Diego, CA: Academic Press; 1999.

21. CBER. *Estimating the Safe Starting Dose in Clinical Trials for Therpeutics in Adult Healthy Volunteers*. 2005. http://www.fda.gov/cber/gdlns/dose.htm.

22. Allaben WT, Hart RW. Nutrition and toxicity modulation: the impact of animal body weight on study outcome. *Int J Toxicol* 1998;17(Suppl 2):1–3.

23. CPMS/SWP/2877/00 *Note for Guidance on Carcinogenic Potential*.

24. Ellaben WT, Hart RW. Nutrition and toxicity modulation: the impact of animal body weight on study outcome. *Int J Toxicol* 1998;17(Suppl 2):1–3.

25. Arnold DL, Grice HC, Krawksi DR. *Handbook of In Vivo Toxicity Testing*. San Diego, CA: Academic Press; 1990.

26. Yacobi A, Skelly JP, Batra VK. *Toxicokinetics and New Drug Development*. New York: Pergamon Press; 1989.

27. Tse FLS, Jaffe JM. *Preclinical Drug Disposition*. New York: Marcel Dekker; 1991.

28. EMEA. *Guideline on the Evaluation of Control, Samples for Toxicokinetics Parameters in Toxicology Studies: Checking for Contamination with the Test Substance*. 2004.

29. CPMP/ICH/384/95; ICH S3A. *Toxicokinetics: A Guidance Assessing Systematic Exposure in Toxicology Studies*.

30. Haschek WM, Rousseaup CG. *Handbook of Toxicology Pathology*. San Diego, CA: Academic Press; 1991.

9

IRRITATION AND LOCAL TISSUE TOLERANCE STUDIES IN PHARMACETICAL SAFETY ASSESSMENT

Shayne Cox Gad

Gad Consulting Services, Cary, North Carolina

Contents

Preclinical Development Handbook: Toxicology, edited by Shayne Cox Gad
Copyright © 2008 John Wiley & Sons, Inc.

9.1 INTRODUCTION

Both irritation and local tolerance studies assess the short-term hazard of pharmaceutical agents in the immediate region of their application or installation. In particular, these studies are generally performed to assess the potential for topically or parenterally administered drugs to cause damage at its site of application or administration. The point of administration is where tissues in patients or test animals' bodies experience the highest concentration exposure and therefore are subject to the greatest physiochemical, chemical, and pharmacologic challenge [1, 2].

Topical local tolerance effects are generally limited to irritation but may also include hematocompatability and pyrogenicity. Alhough this usually means dermal irritation, it can also be intracutaneous, mucosal, penile, perivascular, venous, vaginal, muscle, bladder, rectal, nasal, or ocular, depending on the route of drug administration (Table 9.1). All but ocular irritation use some version of a common subjective rating scale (see Table 9.2) to evaluate responses—the outcome of all of these tests, which primarily evaluate the response of the first region of tissue (which is exposed to the highest concentration) to an administered drug substance. In general, any factor that enhances absorption through this tissue is likely to decrease tissue tolerance.

TABLE 9.1   Irritation Tests—Types

Intracutaneous	Venous
Dermal	Penile
Ocular	Rectal
Mucosal	Bladder
Vaginal	Perivascular
Muscle (injection site)	Nasal

TABLE 9.2   Evaluation of Local Tissue Reactions in Tissue Irritation Studies

Skin Reaction	Value
Erythema and eschar formation	
No erythema	0
Very slight erythema (barely perceptible)	1
Well-defined erythema	2
Moderate to severe erythema	3
Severe erythema (beet redness) to slight eschar formation (injuries in depth)	4
Necrosis (death of tissue)	+N
Eschar (sloughing or scab formation)	+E
Edema formation	
No edema	0
Very slight edema (barely perceptible)	1
Slight edema (edges of area welldefined by definite raising)	2
Moderate edema (raised approximately 1 mm)	3
Severe edema (raised more than 1 mm and extending beyond the area of exposure)	4
Total possible score for primary irritation	8

For the skin, this scale is used in the primary dermal irritation test, which is performed for those agents that are to be administered to patients by application to the skin. As with all local tolerance tests, it is essential that the material be evaluated in "condition of use"—that is, in the final formulated form, applied to test animals in the same manner that the agent is to be used clinically.

9.2 PRIMARY DERMAL IRRITATION TEST

A. Rabbit Screening Procedure

1. A group of at least 8–12 New Zealand white rabbits are screened for the study.
2. All rabbits selected for the study must be in good health; any rabbit exhibiting sniffles, hair loss, loose stools, or apparent weight loss is rejected and replaced.
3. One day (at least 18 h) prior to application of the test substance, each rabbit is prepared by clipping the hair from the back and sides using a small animal clipper. A size No. 10 blade is used to remove long hair and then a size No. 40 blade is used to remove the remaining hair.
4. Six animals with skin sites that are free from hyperemia or abrasion (due to shaving) are selected. Skin sites that are in the telogen phase (resting stage of hair growth) are used; those skin sites that are in the anagen phase (stage of active growth, indicated by the presence of a thick undercoat of hair) are not used.

B. Study Procedure

1. As many as four areas of skin, two on each side of the rabbit's back, can be utilized for sites for administration.
2. Separate animals are not required for an untreated control group. Each animal serves as its own control.
3. Besides the test substance, a positive control substance (a known skin irritant—1% sodium lauryl sulfate in distilled water) and a negative control (untreated patch) are applied to the skin. When a vehicle is used for diluting, suspending, or moistening the test substance, a vehicle control patch is required—especially if the vehicle is known to cause any toxic dermal reactions or if there is insufficient information about the dermal effects of the vehicle.
4. The intact (free of abrasion) sites of administration are assigned a code number. Up to four sites can be used, as follows: (#1) test substance, (#2) negative control, (#3) positive control, and (#4) vehicle control (if required).
5. Application sites should be rotated from one animal to the next to ensure that the test substance and controls are applied to each position at least once.
6. Each test or control substance is held in place with a 1 in. × 1 in. 12-ply surgical gauze patch. The gauze patch is applied to the appropriate skin

site and secured with 1 in. wide strips of surgical tape at the four edges, leaving the center of the gauze patch nonoccluded.

7. If the test substance is a solid or a semisolid, a 0.5 g portion is weighed and placed on the gauze patch. The test substance patch is placed on the appropriate skin site and secured. The patch is subsequently moistened with 0.5 mL of physiological saline.

8. When the test substance is in flake, granule, powder, or other particulate form, the weight of the test substance that has a volume of 0.5 mL (after compacting as much as possible without crushing or altering the individual particles, such as by tapping the measuring container) is used whenever this volume is less than 0.5 g. When applying powders, granules, and the like, the gauze patch designated for the test sample is secured to the appropriate skin site with one of the four strips of the tape at the most ventral position of the animal. With one hand, the appropriate amount of sample measuring 0.5 mL is carefully poured from a glycine weighing paper onto the gauze patch that is held in a horizontal (level) position with the other hand. The patch containing the test sample is then carefully placed into position onto the skin and the remaining three edges are secured with tape. The patch is subsequently moistened with 0.5 mL of physiological saline.

9. If the test substance is a liquid, a patch is applied and secured to the appropriate skin site. A 1 mL tuberculin syringe is used to measure and apply 0.5 mL of test substance to the patch.

10. The negative control site is covered with an untreated 12-ply surgical gauze patch (1 in. × 1 in.).

11. The positive control substance and vehicle control substance are applied to a gauze patch in the same manner as a liquid test substance.

12. The entire trunk of the animal is covered with an impervious material (such as Saran Wrap) for a 24 h period of exposure. The Saran wrap is secured by wrapping several long strips of athletic adhesive tape around the trunk of the animal. The impervious material aids in maintaining the position of the patches and retards evaporation of volatile test substances.

13. An Elizabethan collar is fitted and fastened around the neck of each test animal. The collar remains in place for the 24 h exposure period. The collars are utilized to prevent removal of wrappings and patches by the animals, while allowing the animals food and water *ad libitum*.

14. The wrapping is removed at the end of the 24 h exposure period. The test substance skin site is wiped to remove any test substance still remaining. When colored test substances (such as dyes) are used, it may be necessary to wash the test substance from the test site with an appropriate solvent or vehicle (one that is suitable for the substance being tested). This is done to facilitate accurate evaluation for skin irritation.

15. Immediately after removal of the patches, each 1 in. × 1 in. test or control site is outlined with indelible marker by dotting each of the four corners. This procedure delineates the site for identification.

C. Observations

1. Observations are made of the test and control skin sites 1 h after removal of the patches (25 h postinitiation of application). Erythema and edema are evaluated and scored on the basis of designated values presented earlier in Table 9.2.
2. Observations are again performed 48 and 72 h after application and scores are recorded.
3. If necrosis is present or the dermal reaction is unusual, the reaction should be described. Severe erythema should receive the maximum score (4), and +N should be used to designate the presence of necrosis and +E the presence of eschar.
4. When a test substance produces dermal irritation that persists 72 h postapplication, daily observations of test and control sites are continued on all animals until all irritation caused by the test substance resolves or until day 14 postapplication.

D. Evaluation of Results

1. A *Subtotal Irritation Value* for erythema or eschar formation is determined for each rabbit by adding the values observed at 25, 48, and 72 h postapplication.
2. A *Subtotal Irritation Value* for edema formation is determined for each rabbit by adding the values observed at 25, 48, and 72 h postapplication.
3. A *Total Irritation Value* is calculated for each rabbit by adding the subtotal irritation value for erythema or eschar formation to the subtotal irritation value for edema formation.
4. The *Primary Dermal Irritation Index* is calculated for the test substance or control substance by dividing the sum of the Total Irritation Scores by the number of observations (3 days × 6 animals = 18 observations).
5. The categories of the Primary Dermal Irritation Index (PDII) are as follows (this categorization of dermal irritation is a modification of the original classification described by Draize et al. [3]):

PDII = 0.0	Nonirritant
> 0.0–0.5	Negligible irritant
> 0.5–2.0	Mild irritant
> 2.0–5.0	Moderate irritant
> 5.0–8.0	Severe irritant

Other abnormalities, such as atonia or desquamation, should be noted and recorded.

9.3   OTHER NONPARENTERAL ROUTE IRRITATION TESTS

The design of vaginal, rectal, and nasal irritation studies is less formalized, but follows the same basic pattern as the primary dermal irritation test. The rabbit is the preferred species for vaginal and rectal irritation studies, but the monkey and dog have also been used for these [4]. Both the rabbit and rat have commonly seen use for nasal irritation evaluations. Defined quantities (typically 1.0 mL) of test solutions or suspensions are instilled into the orifice in question. For the vagina or rectum, inert bungs are usually installed immediately thereafter to continue exposure for a defined period of time (usually the same period of hours as future human exposure). The orifice is then flushed clean, and 24 h after exposure it is examined and evaluated (graded) for irritation using the scale in Table 9.2.

9.4   FACTORS AFFECTING IRRITATION RESPONSES AND TEST OUTCOME

The results of local tissue irritation tests are subject to considerable variability due to relatively small differences in test design or technique. Weil and Scala [5] arranged and reported on the best known of several intralaboratory studies to clearly establish this fact. Although the methods presented earlier have proved to give reproducible results in the hands of the same technicians over a period of years [6] and contain some internal controls (the positive and vehicle controls in the PDI) against large variabilities in results or the occurrence of either false positives or negatives, it is still essential to be aware of those factors that may systematically alter test results. These factors are summarized next.

   A. In general, any factor that increases absorption through the stratum corneum, mucous membrane, or other outer barrier layers will also increase the severity of an intrinsic response. Unless this factor mirrors potential exposure conditions, it may, in turn, adversely affect the relevance of test results.

   B. The physical nature of solids must be carefully considered both before testing and in interpreting results. Shape (sharp edges), size (small particles may abrade the skin due to being rubbed back and forth under the occlusive wrap), and rigidity (stiff fibers or very hard particles will be physically irritating) of solids may all enhance an irritation response.

   C. Solids frequently give different results when they are tested dry than if wetted for the test. As a general rule, solids are more irritating if moistened (going back to Item A, wetting is a factor that tends to enhance absorption). Care should also be taken as to moistening agent—some (few) batches of U.S. Pharmacopeia physiological saline (used to simulate sweat) have proved to be mildly irritating to the skin and mucous membrane on their own. Liquids other than water or saline should not be used.

   D. If the treated region on potential human patients will be a compromised skin surface barrier (e.g., if it is cut or burned) some test animals should likewise have their application sites compromised. This procedure is based on the assumption that abraded skin is uniformly more sensitive to irritation. Experiments, however, have shown that this is not necessarily true; some materials produce more irritation on abraded skin, while others produce less [6, 7].

   E. The degree of occlusion (in fact, the tightness of the wrap over the test site) also alters percutaneous absorption and therefore irritation. One important quality control issue in the laboratory is achieving a reproducible degree of occlusion in dermal wrappings.

F. Both the age of the test animal and the application site (saddle of the back vs. flank) can markedly alter test outcome. Both of these factors are also operative in humans, of course [8], but in dermal irritation tests, the objective is to remove all such sources of variability. In general, as an animal ages, sensitivity to irritation decreases. For the dermal test, the skin middle of the back (other than directly over the spine) tends to be thicker (and therefore less sensitive to irritations) than that on the flanks.

G. The sex of the test animals can also alter study results, because both regional skin thickness and surface blood flow vary between males and females.

H. Finally, the single most important (yet also most frequently overlooked) factor that influences the results and outcome of these (and in fact most) acute studies is the training of the staff. In determining how test materials are prepared and applied and in how results are "read" against a subjective scale, both accuracy and precision are extremely dependent on the technicians involved. To achieve the desired results, initial training must be careful and all-inclusive. As important, some form of regular refresher training must be exercised—particularly in the area of scoring results. Use of a set of color photographic standards as a training and reference tool is strongly recommended; such standards should clearly demonstrate each of the grades in the Draize dermal scale.

I. It should be recognized that the dermal irritancy test is designed with a bias to preclude false negatives and therefore tends to exaggerate results in relation to what would happen in humans. Findings of negligible irritancy (or even in the very low mild irritant range) should therefore be of no concern unless the product under test is to have large-scale and prolonged dermal contact.

9.5   PROBLEMS IN TESTING (AND THEIR RESOLUTIONS)

Some materials, by either their physicochemical or toxicological natures, generate difficulties in the performance and evaluation of dermal irritation tests. The most commonly encountered of these problems are presented next.

A. *Compound Volatility.* One is sometimes required or requested to evaluate the potential irritancy of a liquid that has a boiling point between room temperature and the body temperature of the test animal. As a result, the liquid portion of the material will evaporate off before the end of the testing period. There is no real way around the problem; one can only make clear in the report on the test that the traditional test requirements were not met, although an evaluation of potential irritant hazard was probably achieved (for the liquid phase would also have evaporated from a human that it was spilled on).

B. *Pigmented Material.* Some materials are strongly colored or discolor the skin at the application site. This makes the traditional scoring process difficult or impossible. One can try to remove the pigmentation with a solvent; if successful, the erythema can then be evaluated. If use of a solvent fails or is unacceptable, one can (wearing thin latex gloves) feel the skin to determine if there is warmth, swelling, and/or rigidity—all secondary indicators of the irritation response.

C. *Systemic Toxicity.* On rare occasions, the dermal irritation study is begun only to have the animals die very rapidly after test material is applied.

9.6 OCULAR IRRITATION TESTING

Ocular irritation is significantly different from the other local tissue irritation tests on a number of grounds. For the pharmaceutical industry, eye irritation testing is performed when the material is intended to be put into the eye as a means or route of application for ocular therapy. There are a number of special tests applicable to pharmaceuticals or medical devices that are beyond the scope of this volume, since they are not intended to assess potential acute effects or irritation. In general, however, it is desired that an eye irritation test that is utilized by this group be both sensitive and accurate in predicting the potential to cause irritation in humans. Failing to identify human ocular irritants (lack of sensitivity) is to be avoided, but of equal concern is the occurrence of false positives.

The primary eye irritation test was originally intended to predict the potential for a single splash of chemical into the eye of a human being to cause reversible and/or permanent damage. Since the introduction of the original Draize test 50 years ago [3], ocular irritation testing in rabbits has both developed and diverged. Indeed, clearly there is no longer a single test design that is used and different objectives are pursued by different groups using the same test. This lack of standardization has been recognized for some time and attempts have been made to address standardization of at least the methodological aspects of the test, if not the design aspects.

One widely used study design, which begins with a screening procedure as an attempt to avoid testing severe irritants or corrosives in animals, goes as follows:

A. Test Article Screening Procedure

1. Each test substance will be screened in order to eliminate potentially corrosive or severely irritating materials from being studied for eye irritation in the rabbit.
2. If possible, the pH of the test substance will be measured.
3. A primary dermal irritation test will be performed prior to the study.
4. The test substance will not be studied for eye irritation if it is a strong acid (pH of 2.0 or less) or strong alkali (pH of 11.0 or greater), and/or if the test substance is a severe dermal irritant (with a PDII of 5–8) or causes corrosion of the skin.
5. If it is predicted that the test substance does not have the potential to be severely irritating or corrosive to the eye, continue to Section B, Rabbit Screening Procedure.

B. Rabbit Screening Procedure

1. A group of at least 12 New Zealand white rabbits of either sex are screened for the study. The animals are removed from their cages and placed in rabbit restraints. Care should be taken to prevent mechanical damage to the eye during this procedure.
2. All rabbits selected for the study must be in good health; any rabbit exhibiting sniffles, hair loss, loose stools, or apparent weight loss is rejected and replaced.

3. One hour prior to installation of the test substance, both eyes of each rabbit are examined for signs of irritation and corneal defects with a hand-held slit lamp. All eyes are stained with 2.0% sodium fluorescein and examined to confirm the absence of corneal lesions. *Fluorescein Staining:* Cup the lower lid of the eye to be tested and instill one drop of a 2% (in water) sodium fluorescein solution onto the surface of the cornea. After 15 seconds, thoroughly rinse the eye with physiological saline. Examine the eye, employing a hand-held long-wave ultraviolet illuminator in a darkened room. Corneal lesions, if present, appear as bright yellowish-green fluorescent areas.

4. Only 9 of the 12 animals are selected for the study. The 9 rabbits must not show any signs of eye irritation and must show either a negative or minimum fluorescein reaction (due to normal epithelial desquamation).

C. Study Procedure

1. At least 1 h after fluorescein staining, the test substance is placed in one eye of each animal by gently pulling the lower lid away from the eyeball to form a cup (conjunctival cul-de-sac) into which the test material is dropped. The upper and lower lids are then gently held together for 1 second to prevent immediate loss of material.

2. The other eye remains untreated and serves as a control.

3. For testing liquids, 0.01 mL of the test substance is used.

4. For solids or pastes, 100 mg of the test substance is used.

5. When the test substance is in flake, granular, powder, or other particulate form, the amount that has a volume of 0.01 mL (after gently compacting the particles by tapping the measuring container in a way that will not alter their individual form) is used whenever this volume weighs less than 10 mg.

6. For aerosol products, the eye should be held open and the substance administered in a single, 1 second burst at a distance of about 4 inches directly in front of the eye. The velocity of the ejected material should not traumatize the eye. The dose should be approximated by weighing the aerosol can before and after each treatment. For other liquids propelled under pressure, such as substances delivered by pump sprays, an aliquot of 0.01 mL should be collected and instilled in the eye as for liquids.

7. The treated eyes of six of the rabbits are not washed following the instillation of the test substance.

8. The treated eyes of the remaining three rabbits are irrigated for 1 minute with room temperature tap water, starting 20 seconds after instillation.

9. To prevent self-inflicted trauma by the animals immediately after installation of the test substance, the animals are not immediately returned to their cages. After the test and control eyes are examined and graded at 1 h post-exposure, the animals are returned carefully to their respective cages.

D. Observations

1. The eyes are observed for any immediate signs of discomfort after instilling the test substance. Blepharospasm and/or excessive tearing are indicative of

TABLE 9.3   Scale of Weighted Scores for Grading the Severity of Ocular Lesions[a]

Reaction Criteria	Score
I. Cornea	
A. Opacity degree of density (area that is most dense is taken for reading)	
1. Scattered or diffuse area, details of iris clearly visible	1
2. Easily discernible translucent area, details of iris slightly obscured	2
3. Opalescent areas, no details of iris visible, size of pupil barely discernible	3
B. Area of cornea involved	
1. One-quarter (or less) but not zero	1
2. Greater than one-quarter, less than one-half	2
3. Greater than one-half, less than whole area	3
4. Greater than three-quarters up to whole area	4

Scoring equals $A \times B \times 5$; total maximum = 80[b]

II. Iris	
A. Values	
1. Folds above normal, congestion, swelling, circumcorneal ingestion (any one or all of these or combination of any thereof), iris still reacting to light (sluggish reaction is possible)	1
2. No reaction to light, hemorrhage, gross destruction (any one or all of these)	2

Scoring equals $A \times B$ (where B is the area of the iris involved, graded as "under cornea"); total maximum = 10

III. Conjunctivae	
A. Redness (refers to palpebral conjunctivae only)	
1. Vessels definitely injected above normal	1
2. More diffuse, deeper crimson red, individual vessels not easily discernible	2
3. Diffuse beefy red	3
B. Chemosis	
1. Any swelling above normal (includes nictitating membrane)	1
2. Obvious swelling with partial eversion of the lids	2
3. Swelling with lids about half closed	3
4. Swelling with lids about half closed to completely closed	4
C. Discharge	
1. Any amount different from normal (does not include small amount observed in inner canthus of normal animals)	1
2. Discharge with moistening of the lids and hair just adjacent to the lids	2
3. Discharge with moistening of the lids and considerable area around the eye	3

Scoring $(A + B + C) \times 2$; total maximum = 20

[a]The maximum total score is the sum of all scores obtained for the cornea, iris, and conjunctivae. [b]All A $\times$ B = Σ (1–3) $\times$ Σ (1–4) for six animals.

irritating sensations caused by the test substance, and their duration should be noted. Blepharospasm does not necessarily indicate that the eye will show signs of ocular irritation.

2. Grading and scoring or ocular irritation are performed in accordance with Table 9.3. The eyes are examined and grades of ocular reactions are recorded.

3. If signs or irritation persist at day 7, readings are continued on days 10 and 14 after exposure or until all signs of reversible toxicity are resolved.

4. In addition to the required observation of the cornea, iris, and conjunctiva, serious effects (such as pannus, rupture of the globe, or blistering of the conjunctivae) indicative of a corrosive action are reported.

5. Whether or not toxic effects are reversible depends on the nature, extent, and intensity of damage. Most lesions, if reversible, will heal or clear within 21 days. Therefore, if ocular irritation is present at the 14 day reading, a 21 day reading is required to determine whether the ocular damage is reversible or nonreversible.

9.7 VAGINAL IRRITATION

Few if any products are administered via the vagina that are intended for systemic absorption. Thus, this route has not been as widely studied and characterized as others. On the other hand, large numbers of different products (douches, spermicides, antiyeast agents, etc.) have been developed that require introduction into the vagina in order to assert their localized effects. Increased research into different birth control and antiviral prophylaxis will result in more vaginal products in the future. All these must be assessed for vaginal irritation potential, and this serves as an example of the other tissue tolerance issues.

Considerable research [4, 9] has indicated that the rabbit is the best species for assessing vaginal irritation. There are those investigators, however, who consider the rabbit too sensitive and recommend the use of ovariectomized rats. Ovariectomy results in a uniformly thin, uncornified epithelium, which is more responsive to localized effects. This model is used when the results from a study with rabbits are questionable [9]. The routine progression of studies consists of first doing an acute primary vaginal irritation study, then a 10 day repeated dose study in rats. These protocols are summarized next. Longer-term vaginal studies have been conducted in order to assess systemic toxicity of the active agents, when administered by these routes (while the intended effects may be local, one cannot assume that there will be no systemic exposure).

9.7.1 Acute Primary Vaginal Irritation Study in the Female Rabbit

1. *Overview of Study Design.* One group of six adult rabbits receive a single vaginal exposure and are observed for 3 days with periodic examination (1, 24, 48, and 72 hours postdosing) of the genitalia. Animals are then euthanized and the vagina is examined macroscopically.

2. *Administration.*

   (a) Route: The material is generally introduced directly into the vagina using a lubricated 18 French rubber catheter attached to a syringe for quantification and delivery of the test material. Gentle placement of the catheter is important because one needs to ensure complete delivery of the dose without mechanical trauma. For rabbits, the depth of insertion is about 7.5 cm, and the catheter should be marked to about that depth. After delivery is completed, the tube is slowly withdrawn. No attempt is made to close or seal the vaginal orifice. Alternative methods may be used to administer more viscous materials. The most common is to backload a lubricated 1 mL tuberculin syringe, then warm the material to close to body temperature. The syringe is then inserted into the vagina and the dose administered by depressing the syringe plunger.

(b) Dosage: The test material should be one (concentration, vehicle, etc.) that is intended for human application.

(c) Frequency: Once.

(d) Duration: 1 day.

(e) Volume: 1 mL per rabbit.

3. *Test System.*

(a) Species, age, and weight range: Sexually mature New Zealand white rabbits are generally used, weighing between 2 and 5 kg. The weight is not as important as the fact that the animals need to be sexually mature.

(b) Selection: Animals should be multiparous and nonpregnant. Animals should be healthy and free of external genital lesions.

(c) Randomization: Because there is only one group of animals, randomization is not a critical issue.

4. *In-Life Observations.*

(a) Daily observations: At least once daily for clinical signs.

(b) Detailed physical examination: Once during the week prior to dosing.

(c) Body weight: Day of dosing.

(d) Vaginal irritation: Scored at 1, 24, 48, and 72 hours postdosing. Scoring criteria are shown in Table 9.4.

5. *Postmortem Procedures.* Rabbits are euthanized by lethal dose of a barbiturate soon after the last vaginal irritation scores are collected. The vagina is opened by longitudinal section and examined for evidence of mucosal damage such as erosion and localized hemorrhage. No other tissues are examined. No tissues are collected. After the macroscopic description of the vagina is recorded, the animal is discarded.

9.7.2 Repeated Dose Vaginal Irritation Study in the Female Rabbit

1. *Overview of Study Design.* Four groups of five adult rabbits each receive a single vaginal exposure daily for 10 days. The genitalia are examined daily. Animals are then euthanized and the vagina is examined macroscopically and microscopically.

2. *Administration.*

(a) Route: The test materials are introduced directly into the vagina using a lubricated 18 French rubber catheter, using the techniques described previously for acute studies.

(b) Dosage: The test material should be one (concentration, vehicle, etc.) that is intended for human application. There will also be a sham-negative control (catheter in place but nothing administered), a vehicle control, and a positive control (generally 2% nonoxynol-9).

(c) Frequency: Once daily.

TABLE 9.4   Scoring Criteria for Vaginal Irritation

Value	Irritation
	Erythema
0	No erythema
1	Very slight erythema (barely perceptible)
2	Slight erythema (pale red in color)
3	Moderate to severe erythema (definite red in color)
4	Severe erythema (beet or crimson red)
	Edema
0	No edema
1	Very slight edema (barely perceptible)
2	Slight edema (edges of area well defined by definite raising)
3	Moderate edema (raised approximately 1 mm)
4	Severe edema (raised more than 1 mm and extending beyond area of exposure)
	Discharge
0	No discharge
1	Very slight discharge
2	Slight discharge
3	Moderate discharge
4	Severe discharge (moistening of considerable area around vagina)

    (d) Duration: 10 days.

    (e) Volume: 1 mL per rabbit for each material.

3. *Test System.*

    (a) Species, age and weight range: Sexually mature New Zealand white rabbits are generally used, weighing between 2 and 5 kg. The weight is not as important as the fact that the animals need to be sexually mature.

    (b) Selection: Animals should be nulliparous and nonpregnant. Animals should be healthy and free of external genital lesions.

    (c) Randomization: At least 24 animals should be on pretest. Randomization to treatment groups is best done using a computerized blocking by body weight method or a random number generation method.

4. *In-Life Observations.*

    (a) Daily observations: At least once daily for clinical signs.

    (b) Detailed physical examination: Once during the week prior to dosing and immediately prior to necropsy.

    (c) Body weight: First, fifth, and last day of dosing.

    (d) Vaginal irritation: Scored once daily. Scoring criteria are shown in Table 9.4.

5. *Postmortem Procedures.* Rabbits are euthanized by lethal dose of a barbiturate soon after the last vaginal irritation scores are collected. The vagina is isolated using standard prosection techniques and then opened by longitudinal section and examined for evidence of mucosal damage such as erosion and

TABLE 9.5   Microscopic Scoring Procedure for Vaginal Sections

Section	Value
Epithelium	
Intact—normal	0
Cell degeneration or flattening of the epithelium	1
Metaplasia	2
Focal erosion	3
Erosion or ulceration, generalized	4
Leukocytes	
Minimal—<25 per high power field	1
Mild—25–50 per high power field	2
Moderate—50–100 per high power field	3
Marked—>100 per high power field	4
Injection	
Absent	0
Minimal	1
Mild	2
Moderate	3
Marked with disruption of vessels	4
Edema	
Absent	0
Minimal	1
Mild	2
Moderate	3
Marked	4

Source: From Ref. 2.

localized hemorrhage. No other tissues are examined. The vagina and cervix are collected and fixed in 10% neutral buffered formalin. Standard hematoxylin/eosin stained, paraffin-embedded histologic glass slides are prepared by routing methods. Three levels of the vagina (low, middle, and upper) are examined and graded using the scoring system shown in Table 9.5. Each level is scored separately and an average is calculated. Irritation is rated as follows:

Score	Rating
0	Nonirritating
1–4	Minimal irritation
5–8	Mild irritation
9–11	Moderate irritation
12–16	Marked irritation

The score for each rabbit is then averaged and acceptability ratings are given as follows:

Average Score	Acceptability Ratings
0–8	Acceptable
9–10	Marginal
11 or greater	Unacceptable

9.7.3   Repeated Dose Vaginal Irritation Study in the Ovariectomized Rat

This study is very similar in design to that described previously for rabbits, with the following (sometimes obvious) exceptions. Mature ovariectomized female rats can be obtained from a commercial breeder. A 15% surplus should be obtained. Ten animals per group should be used (40 total for the study). The vaginal catheter is placed to a depth of approximately 2.5 cm and the treatment volume should be 0.2 mL.

9.8   PARENTERAL IRRITATION/TOLERANCE

There are a number of special concerns about the safety of materials that are routinely injected (parenterally administered) into the body [10]. By definition, these concerns are all associated with materials that are the products of the pharmaceutical and (in some minor cases) medical device industries. Such parenteral routes include three major ones—IV (intravenous), IM (intramuscular), and SC (subcutaneous)—and a number of minor routes (such as intraarterial) that are not considered here.

These unusual concerns include irritation (vascular, muscular, or subcutaneous), pyrogenicity, blood compatibility, and sterility [11]. The background of each of these along with the underlying mechanisms and factors that influence the level of occurrence of such an effect are briefly discussed next.

Irritation   Tissue irritation upon injection, and the accompanying damage and pain, is a concern that must be addressed for the final formulation, which is to be either tested in humans or marketed, rather than for the active ingredient. This is because most irritation factors are either due to or influenced by aspects of formulation design (see Refs. 10 and 12 for more information on parenteral preparations). These factors are not independent of the route (IV, IM, or SC) that will be used and, in fact (as discussed later), are part of the basis for selecting between the various routes.

The lack of irritation and tissue damage at the injection site is sometimes called *tolerance*. Some of the factors that affect tolerance are not fully under the control of an investigation and are also unrelated to the material being injected. These include body movement, temperature, and animal age. Factors that can be controlled, but that are not inherent to the active ingredient, include solubility, tonicity, and pH. Finally, the active ingredient and vehicle can have inherent irritative effects and factors such as solubility (in the physiological milieu into which they are being injected), concentration, volume molecular size, and particle size must be considered. Gray [13] and Ballard [14] discuss these factors and the morphological consequences that may occur if they are not addressed.

Pyrogenicity   Pyrogenicity is the induction of a febrile (fever) response induced by the parenteral (usually IV or IM) administration of exogenous material. Pyrogenicity is usually associated with microbiological contamination of a final formulation, but it is now of increasing concern because of the growing interest in biosynthetically produced materials. Generally, ensuring sterility of product and process will guard against pyrogenicity for traditional pharmaceuticals. For biologically produced products, the FDA has promulgated the general guideline that no more than 5.0 units of endotoxin may be present per milligram of drug substance [38].

Blood Compatibility   It is important that cellular components of the blood are not disrupted and that serum- or plasma-based responses are not triggered by parenteral administration. Therefore, two mechanisms must be assessed regarding the blood compatibility of component materials. These include the material's effect on cellular components that cause membrane destruction and hemolysis and the activation of the clotting mechanism resulting in thromboembolism.

Many of the nonactive, ingredient-related physicochemical factors that influence irritation (e.g., tonicity, pH, and particle size) also act to determine blood compatibility. But the chemical features of a drug entity itself—its molecular size and reactivity—can also be of primary importance.

Sterility   Sterility is largely a concern to be answered in the process of preparing a final clinical formulation, and it is not addressed in detail in this chapter. However, it should be clear that it is essential that no viable microorganisms are present in any material to be parenterally administered (except for vaccines).

9.8.1   Parenteral Routes

There are at least 13 different routes by which to inject material into the body, including the following: (1) intravenous, (2) subcutaneous, (3) intramuscular, (4) intraarterial, (5) intradermal, (6) intralesional, (7) epidural, (8) intrathecal, (9) intracisternal, (10) intracardiac, (11) intraventricular, (12) intraocular, and (13) intraperitoneal.

Only the first three are discussed in any detail here. Most of these routes of administration place a drug directly or indirectly into systemic circulation. There are a number of these routes, however, by which the drug exerts a local effect; in which case, most of the drug does not enter systemic circulation (e.g., intrathecal, intraventricular, intraocular, intracisternal). Certain routes of administration may exert both local and systemic effects, depending on the characteristics of the drug and excipients (e.g., subcutaneous) [15].

The choice of a particular parenteral route will depend on the required time of onset of action, the required site of action, and the characteristics of the fluid to be injected, among other factors.

9.8.2   Bolus Versus Infusion

Technically, for all the parenteral routes (but in practice only for the IV route), there are two options for injecting a material into the body. The bolus and infusion methods are differentiated on the single basis of rate of injection, but they actually differ on a wide range of characteristics.

The most commonly exercised option is the bolus, or "push," injection, in which the injection device (syringe or catheter) is appropriately entered into the vein and a defined volume of material is introduced through the device. The device is then removed. In this operation, it is relatively easy to restrain an experimental animal and the stress on the animal is limited. Although the person doing the injection must be skilled, it takes only a short amount of time to become so. And the one variable to be controlled in determining dosage is the total volume of material injected (assuming dosing solutions have been properly prepared).

There are limitations and disadvantages to the bolus approach, however. Only a limited volume may be injected, which may prohibit the use of bolus when volumes to be introduced are high (e.g., due to low active compound solubility or a host of other reasons). Only two devices (syringe and catheter) are available for use in the bolus approach. If a multiple-day course of treatment is desired (say, every day for 15 days), separate injections must be made at discreet entry sites.

The infusion approach involves establishing a fixed entry point into the vein, then slowly passing the desired test material through that point over a period of time (30 minutes is about minimum, while continuous around-the-clock treatment is at least therapeutically possible). There are a number of devices available for establishing their entry point; catheter, vascular port [16], or osmotic pump [17]. Each of these must, in turn, be coupled with a device to deliver the dosing solution at a desired rate. The osmotic pump, which is implanted, is also its own delivery device. Other options are gravity driven "drips," hand–held syringes (not practical or accurate over any substantial period of time), or syringe pumps. Very large volumes can be introduced by fusion over a protracted period of time, and only a single site need be fitted with an entry device.

However, infusion also has its limitations. Skilled labor is required, and the setup must be monitored over the entire period of infusion. Larger animals must be restrained, while there are special devices that make this requirement unnecessary for smaller animals. Restraint and protracted manipulation are very stressful on animals. Over a period of time, one must regularly demonstrate patency of a device—that is, entry into the vascular system continues to exist. Finally, one is faced with having to control two variables in controlling the dose—total volume and rate.

When are the two approaches (bolus and infusion) interchangeable? And why select one over the other? The selection of infusion is usually limited to two reasons: (1) when a larger volume must be introduced than is practical in a bolus injection or (2) tolerance is insufficient if the dose is given all at once (i.e., an infusion will "clear" a higher daily dose than will a bolus injection). For safety studies, when a bolus can be used to clear a human infusion, dosing is a matter of judgment. If the planned clinical infusion will take less than a half hour, practicality dictates that the animal studies be accomplished by bolus. In other situations, pharmacokinetics (in particular, the half-life of the drug entity) should be considered in making the decision.

9.8.3   Test Systems for Parenteral Irritation

There are no regulatory guidelines or suggested test methods for evaluating agents for muscular or vascular irritation. Since such guidelines are lacking, but the evaluation is necessary, those responsible for these evaluations have tried to develop and employ the most scientifically valid procedures.

Hagan [18] first suggested a method for assessing IM irritation. His approach, however, did not include a grading system for evaluation of the irritation, and the method used the sacrospinalis muscles, which are somewhat difficult to dissect or repeatedly inject.

Shintani et al. [19] developed and proposed the methodology that currently seems to be more utilized. It uses the lateral vastus muscle and includes a methodology for evaluation, scoring, and grading of irritation. Additionally, Shintani and co-workers investigated the effects of several factors such as pH of the solution, drug concentration, volume of injection, the effect of repeated injections, and the time to maximum tissue response.

9.8.4 Acute Intramuscular Irritation in the Male Rabbit [20]

1. *Overview of Study Design.* Each rabbit is injected as follows:

Site	Treatment
(musculus vastus lateralis)	(1.0 mL/site)
Left	(Test article)
Right	(Vehicle)

Day 1: Injection of all treatment groups—9 rabbits.
Day 2: Sacrifice and evaluation: 24 h posttreatment group—3 rabbits.
Day 3: Sacrifice and evaluation: 48 h posttreatment group—3 rabbits.
Day 4: Sacrifice and evaluation: 72 h posttreatment group—3 rabbits.

2. *Administration.*
   (a) Route: The test article is injected into the musculus vastus lateralis of each rabbit.
   (b) Dose: The dose selected is chosen to evaluate the severity of irritation and represents a concentration that might be used clinically. This volume has been widely used in irritation testing.
   (c) Frequency: Once only.
   (d) Duration: 1 day
   (e) Volume: 1.0 mL per site.

3. *Test System.*
   (a) Species, age, and weight range: Male New Zealand white rabbits weighing 2–5 kg are used. The New Zealand white rabbit has been widely used in muscle irritation research for many years and is a reasonable sized, even-tempered animal that is well adapted to the laboratory environment.
   (b) Selection: Animals to be used in the study are selected on the basis of acceptable findings from physical examinations and body weights.
   (c) Randomization: Animals are ranked by body weight and assigned a number between one and three. The order of number assigned (e.g., 1-3-2)

TABLE 9.6   Scoring of Muscle Injection Site Irritation

Reaction Criteria	Score
No discernible gross reaction	0
Slight hyperemia	1
Moderate hyperemia and discoloration	2
Distinct discoloration in comparison with the color of the surrounding area	3
Brown degeneration with small necrosis	4
Widespread necrosis with an appearance of "cooked meat" and occasionally an abscess involving the major portions of the muscle	5

is chosen from a table of random numbers. Animals assigned number 1 are in the 24 h posttreatment group; those assigned number 2 are in the 48 h posttreatment group; and those assigned number 3 are in the 72 h posttreatment group.

4. *In-Life Observations.*
   (a) Daily observations: Once daily following dosing.
   (b) Physical examinations: Once within the 2 weeks before the first dosing day.
   (c) Body weight: Should be determined once before the start of the study.
   (d) Additional examinations may be done by the study director to elucidate any observed clinical signs.

5. *Postmortem Procedures.* Irritation is evaluated as follows. Three rabbits are sacrificed by a lethal dose of barbiturate at approximately 24, 48, or 72 h after dosing. The left and right lateral vastus muscles of each rabbit are excised. The lesions resulting from injection are scored for muscle irritation on a numerical scale of 0–5 as described in Table 9.6 [19]. The average score for the nine rabbits is calculated, and a category of irritancy assigned based on the following table:

Average Score	Grade
0.0–0.4	None
0.5–1.4	Slight
1.5–2.4	Mild
2.5–3.4	Moderate
3.5–4.4	Marked
4.5 or greater	Severe

9.8.5   Acute Intravenous Irritation in the Male Rabbit

The design here is similar to the intramuscular assay, except that injections are made into the veins in specific muscle masses.

1. *Overview of Study Design.* Rabbits are injected as follows:

Group	Number of Animals	Treatment Site	Evaluation
1	2	Musculus vastus lateralis (left) and cervicodorsal subcutis (left)	24 h
		Musculus vastus lateralis (right) and cervicodorsal subcutis (right)	24 h
2	2	Musculus vastus lateralis (left) and cervicodorsal subcutis (left)	72 h
		Musculus vastus lateralis (right) and cervicodorsal subcutis (right)	72 h
3	2	Auricular vein (left)	24 and 72 h evaluations
		Auricular vein (right)	

Day 1: Injection of all groups (6 rabbits).

Day 2: Evaluation of Group 3 (2 rabbits). Sacrifice and evaluation of Group 1 (2 rabbits).

Day 4: Evaluation of Group 3 (2 rabbits). Sacrifice and evaluation of Group 2 (2 rabbits).

2. *Administration.*

   (a) Intramuscular: Musculus vastus lateralis.

   (b) Subcutaneous: Cervicodorsal subcutis.

   (c) Intravenous: Auricular vein.

   (d) Dose: The doses and concentration selected are chosen to evaluate the severity of irritation. The dose volumes have been widely used in irritation testing.

   (e) Frequency: Once only.

   (f) Duration: 1 day.

   (g) Volume: Musculus vastus lateralis and cervicodorsal subcutis: 1.0 mL per site; auricular vein: 0.5 mL per site.

3. *Test System.*

   (a) Species, age, and weight range: Male New Zealand white rabbits, weighing 2–5 kg, are used.

   (b) Selection: Animals to be used in the study are selected on the basis of acceptable findings from physical examinations.

   (c) Randomization: Animals are ranked by body weight and assigned a number between 1 and 3. The order of numbers assigned (e.g., 1-3-2) is chosen from a table of random numbers. Animals assigned number 1 are in Group 1; those assigned number 2 are in Group 2; and those assigned number 3 are in Group 3.

TABLE 9.7   Muscle Irritation Scoring

Reaction Criteria	Score
No discernible gross reaction	0
Slight hyperemia and discoloration	1
Moderate hyperemia and discoloration	2
Distinct discoloration in comparison with the color of the surrounding area	3
Small areas of necrosis	4
Widespread necrosis, possibly involving the underlying muscle	5

4. *In-Life Observations.*
    (a) Daily observations: Once daily following dosing.
    (b) Physical examinations: Once within the 2 weeks before the first dosing day.
    (c) Body weight: Determined once before the start of the study.
    (d) Additional examinations may be done by the study director to elucidate any observed clinical signs.

5. *Postmortem Procedures.*
    (a) Intramuscular irritation is evaluated as follows. Rabbits are sacrificed by lethal dose of barbiturate approximately 24 and 72 h after dosing. The left and right lateral vastus muscles of each rabbit are excised. The reaction resulting from injection is scored for muscle irritation using the scale shown in Table 9.6.
    (b) Subcutaneous irritation is evaluated as follows. Rabbits are scarified by a lethal dose of barbiturate approximately 24 and 72 h after dosing. The subcutaneous injection sites are exposed by dissection, and the reaction is scored for irritation on a scale of 0–5 as in Table 9.7 [19].

Average Score per Site	Irritancy Grade
0.0–0.4	None
0.5–1.4	Slight
1.5–2.4	Mild
2.5–3.4	Moderate
3.5–4.4	Marked
4.5 or greater	Severe

    (c) Intravenous irritation is evaluated as follows. Rabbits are sacrificed by a lethal dose of barbiturate following the 72 h irritation evaluation. The injection site and surrounding tissue are grossly evaluated at approximately 24 and 72 h after dosing on a scale of 0–3 as in Table 9.8.

Average Score per Site	Irritancy Grade
0.0 to 0.4	None
0.5 to 1.4	Slight
1.5 to 2.4	Moderate
2.5 or greater	Severe

    (d) Additional examinations may be done by the study director to elucidate the nature of any observed tissue change.

TABLE 9.8 Venous Irritation Scoring

Reaction Criteria	Score
No discernible gross reaction	0
Slight erythema at injection site	1
Moderate erythema and swelling with some discoloration of the vein and surrounding tissue	2
Severe discoloration and swelling of the vein and surrounding tissue with partial or total occlusion of the vein	3

9.8.6 Alternatives

Intramuscular (IM) and intravenous (IV) injection of parenteral formulations of pharmaceuticals can produce a range of discomfort including pain, irritation, and/or damage to muscular or vascular tissue. These are normally evaluated for prospective formulations before use in humans by histopathologic evaluation of damage in intact animal models, usually the rabbit. Attempts have been made to make this *in vivo* methodology both more objective and quantitative based on measuring the creatine phosphokinase released in the tissue surrounding the injection site [21]. Currently, a protocol utilizing a cultured skeletal muscle cell line (L6) from the rat as a model has been evaluated in an interlaboratory validation program among 11 pharmaceutical laboratories. This methodology [22] measures creatine kinase levels in media after exposure of the cells to the formulation of interest and predicts *in vivo* IM damage based on this endpoint. It is reported to give excellent rank-correlated results across a range of antibiotics [23]. The current multilaboratory evaluation covers a broader structural range of compounds and has shown a good quantitative correlation with *in vivo* results for antibiotics and a fair correlation for a broader range of parenteral drug products. Likewise, Kato et al. [24] have proposed a model that uses cultured primary skeletal muscle fibers from the rat. Damage is evaluated by the release of creatine phosphokinase. An evaluation using six parenterally administered antibiotics (ranking their EC_{50} values) showed good relative correlation with *in vivo* results.

Another proposed *in vitro* assay for muscle irritancy for injectable formulations is the red blood cell hemolysis assay [25]. Water-soluble formulations in a 1:2 ratio with freshly collected human blood are gently mixed for 5 min. The percentage of red blood cell survival is then determined by measuring differential absorbance at 540 nm; this value is then compared to values for known irritants and nonirritants. Against a very small group of compounds (four), this assay reportedly accurately predicts muscle irritation.

9.9 PHOTOTOXICITY

The potential for sunlight (or selected other light frequencies) to transform a drug or product is both a useful tool for activating some drugs and a cause of significant adverse effects for others (such as the quinolone antibiotics [26, 27]).

9.9.1 Theory and Mechanisms

The portion of the solar spectrum containing the biologically most active region is from 290 to 700 mm.

The ultraviolet (UV) part of the spectrum includes wavelengths from 200 to 400 nm. Portions of the UV spectrum have distinctive features from both the physical and biological points of view. The accepted designations for the biologically important parts of the UV spectrum are UVA, 400–315 nm; UVB, 315–280 nm; and UVC, 280–220 nm. Wavelengths less than 290 nm (UVC) do not occur at the earth's surface because they are absorbed, predominantly by ozone in the stratosphere. The most thoroughly studied photobiological reactions that occur in skin are induced by UVB. The quinolones, for example, absorb light strongly in the 300–400 nm wavelength range. Although UVB wavelengths represent only approximately 1.5% of the solar energy received at the earth's surface, they elicit most of the known chemical phototoxic and photoallergic reactions. The visible portions of the spectrum, representing about 50% of the sun's energy received at sea level, includes wavelengths from 400 to 700 nm. Visible light is necessary for such biological events as photosynthesis, the regulation circadian cycles, vision, and pigment darkening. Furthermore, visible light in conjunction with certain chromophores (e.g., dyes, drugs, and endogenous compounds that absorb light and therefore "give" color) and molecular oxygen induces photodynamic effects.

Understanding the toxic effects of light impinging on the skin requires knowledge of both the nature of sunlight and the skin's optical properties. Skin may be viewed as an optically heterogeneous medium, composed of three layers that have distinct refractive indices, chromophore distributions, and light-scattering properties. Light entering the outermost layer, the stratum corneum, is in part reflected—4–7% for wavelengths between 250 and 300 nm [28]—due to the difference in refractive index between air and the stratum corneum. Absorption by urocanic acid (a deamination product of histidine), melanin, and proteins containing the aromatic amino acids tryptophan and tyrosine in the stratum corneum produces further attenuation of light, particularly at shorter UV wavelengths. Approximately 40% of UVB is transmitted through the stratum corneum to the viable epidermis. The light entering the epidermis is attenuated by scattering and, predominantly, absorption. Epidermal chromophores consist of proteins, urocanic acid, nucleic acids, and melanin. Passage through the epidermis results in appreciable attenuation of UVA and UVB radiation. The transmission properties of the dermis are largely due to scattering, with significant absorption of visible light by melanin, β-carotene, and the blood-borne pigments bilirubin, hemoglobin, and oxyhemoglobin. Light traversing these layers of the skin is extensively attenuated, most drastically for wavelengths less than 400 nm. Longer wavelengths are more penetrating. It has been noted that there is an "optical window"—that is, greater transmission—for light at wavelengths of 600–1300 nm, which may have important biological consequences.

Normal variations in the skin's optical properties frequently occur. The degree of pigmentation may produce variations in the attenuation of light, particularly between 300 and 400 nm, by as much as 1.5 times more in blacks than in Caucasians [29]. Alterations in the amount or distribution of other natural chromophores account for further variations in skin optical properties. Urocanic acid, deposited on the skin's surface during perspiration [28], and UV-absorbing lipids, excreted in sebum, may significantly reduce UV transmission through the skin. Epidermal thickness, which varies over regions of the body and increases after exposure to UVB radiation, may significantly modify UV transmission.

Certain disease states also produce alterations in the skin's optical properties. Alterations of the skin's surface, such as by psoriatic plaques, decrease transmitted light. The effect may be lessened by application of oils whose refractive index is similar to that of skin [28]. Disorders such as hyperbilirubinemia, porphyrias, and blue skin nevi result in increased absorption of visible light due to accumulation or altered distribution of endogenous chromophoric compounds.

The penetration of light into and through dermal tissues has important consequences. This penetration is demonstrated in Fig. 9.1. Skin, as the primary organ responsible for thermal regulation, is overperfused relative to its metabolic requirements [28].

It is estimated that the average cutaneous blood flow is 20–30 times that necessary to support the skin's metabolic needs. The papillary boundaries between epidermis and dermis allow capillary vessels to lie close to the skin's surface, permitting the blood and important components of the immune system to be exposed to light. The equivalent of the entire blood volume of an adult may pass through the skin, and potentially be irradiated, in 20 min. This corresponds to the time required to receive 1 or 2 MEDs (the MED is defined as the minimal dose of UV irradiation that produces definite, but minimally perceptible, redness 24 h after exposure). The accessibility of incident radiation to blood has been exploited in such regimens as phototherapy of hyperbilirubinemia in neonates, where light is used as a therapeutic agent. However, in general, there is a potential for light-induced toxicity due to irradiation of blood-borne drugs and metabolites.

9.9.2   Factors Influencing Phototoxicity/Photosensitization

There are a number of factors that can influence an agent acting either as a phototoxin or a photoallergen.

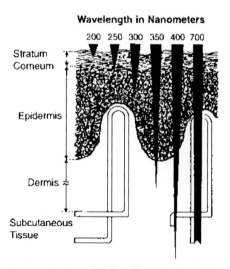

FIGURE 9.1   Schematic penetration of light of varying wavelengths into the skin.

1. The quantity and location of photoactive material present in or on the skin.
2. The capacity of the photoactive material to penetrate into normal skin by percutaneous absorption as well as into skin altered by trauma, such as maceration, irritation, and sunburn.
3. The pH, enzyme presence, and solubility conditions at the site of exposure.
4. The quantity of activating radiation to which the skin is exposed.
5. The capacity of the spectral range to activate the materials on or within the skin.
6. The ambient temperature and humidity.
7. The thickness of the horny layer.
8. The degree of melanin pigmentation of the skin.
9. The inherent "photoactivity" of the chemical. Does it weakly or strongly absorb light?

Basically, any material that has both the potential to absorb ultraviolet light (in the UVA or UVB regions) and the possibility of dermal exposure or distribution into the dermal region should be subject to some degree of suspicion as to potential phototoxicity. As shown in Table 9.9, a large number of agents have been identified as phototoxic or photoallergenic agents. Of these, tetrachlorosalicylanilide (TCSA) is the most commonly used as a positive control in animal studies.

9.9.3 Predictive Tests for Phototoxicity

Before we start on our description of the different methods, we first cover some basics on light dosimetry. The intensity of the irradiation used in phototoxicity testing is determined with a light meter, which provides output as watts per meter^2. The shelves on which the animals rest during the exposure periods are normally adjustable in order to control the dose of light to the exposure area. The irradiation from fluorescent lights will vary somewhat from day to day, depending on temperature, variations in line current, and so on. The dose the animals receive is generally represented as joules/centimeter^2. A joule is equal to 1 watt/second. Therefore, the dose of light is dependent on the time of exposure. For example, in their review, Lambert et al. [27] discuss dosages of light of 9 or $10 J/cm^2$ in the UVA spectral region. If the irradiation from the light is found to be $20 W/m^2$ at the exposure site, then the time of exposure required to obtain the target dose of light (in joules) is calculated as

$$\text{Time of exposure} = \frac{W \cdot s}{J} \frac{9 J}{cm^2} \frac{m^2}{20 W} \frac{10^4 cm^2}{m^2} \frac{min}{60 s} = 75 \, min$$

If, with the same set of lights, 2 weeks later the irradiation is determined to be $19 W/m^2$, then the exposure period would have to be 79 min.

There are three recommended protocols for assessing topical phototoxicity potential—rabbit, guinea pig, and mouse. Only the rabbit and guineapig are described.

TABLE 9.9   Known Phototoxic Agents

In Humans		In Animals	
Compounds	Route	Compound	Route
Aminobenzoic acid derivatives	Topical	Acradine	Topical
		Amiodarone	Oral
Amyldimethylamino benzoate, mixed *ortho* and *para* isomers	Topical	Anthracine	Topical
		Bergapten (5-methoxypsolaren)	Topical
Anthracene acridine	Topical	Bithionol	Topical
Bergapten (5-methoxypsoralen)	Topical	Chlorodiazepoxide	Intraperitoneal
Cadmium sulfide	Tattoo	Chlorprothiazide	Intraperitoneal
Chlorothiazides	Oral	Chlorpromazine	Topical
Coal tar (multicomponent)	Topical	Demeclocycline	Intraperitoneal
Dacarbazine	Infusion	Griseofulvin	Intraperitoneal
Disperse blue 35 (anthaquinone-based dye)	Topical	Kynuremic acid	Oral
Nalidixic acid	Oral	Nalidixic acid	Oral
Padimate A or Escolol 506 (amyl-*p*-dimethylamino benzoate)	Topical	Prochlorperazine	Intraperitoneal
		Quinokine methanol	Intraperitoneal
		Quinolone (antibacterial)	Oral
Psoralens	Oral, topical	Tetracyclines	Intraperitoneal, topical
Quinolone (antibacterial)	Oral	Xanthotoxin (8-methoxypsoralen)	Oral, intraperitoneal, intramuscular
Tetracyclines	Oral		
Xanthotoxin (8-methoxypsoralen)	Topical, oral		

Rabbit   The traditional methodology for a predictive test for phototoxicity has been an intact rabbit test [30]. This test is conducted as follows (and illustrated diagrammatically in Fig. 9.2):

A. Animals and Animal Husbandry

1. Strain/species: Female New Zealand white rabbits.
2. Number: 6 rabbits per test; 2 rabbits for positive control.
3. Age: Young adult.
4. Acclimation period: At least 7 days prior to study.
5. Food and water: Commercial laboratory feed and water are freely available.

B. Test Article

1. A dose of 0.5 mL of liquid or 500 mg of a solid or semisolid is applied to each test site.

Species: New Zealand white Rabbits
Test Group: 6 Rabbits
Positive Control: 2 Rabbits

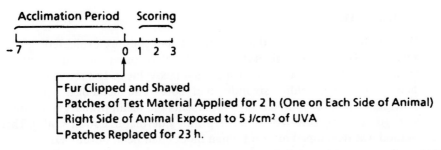

FIGURE 9.2 Line chart for the design and conduct of phototoxicity assay using rabbits.

2. Liquid substances are used undiluted.
3. For solids, the test article is moistened with water (500 mg test article/0.5 mL water or another suitable vehicle) to ensure good contact with the skin.
4. The positive control material is a lotion containing 1% 8-methoxypsoralen.

C. Experimental Procedures

1. Animals are weighed on the first day of dosing.
2. On the day prior to dosing, the fur of the test animals is clipped from the dorsal area of the trunk using a small animal clipper, then shaved clean with a finer bladed clipper.
3. On the day of dosing, the animals are placed in restraints.
4. One pair of patches (approximately 2.5 cm × 2.5 cm) per test article is applied to the skin of the back, with one patch on each side of the backbone.
5. A maximum of two pairs of patches may be applied to each animal and the patches must be at least 2 in. apart.
6. The patches are held in contact with the skin by means of an occlusive dressing for the 2 h exposure period.
7. After the 2 h exposure period, the occlusive dressing and the patches on the right side of the animal are removed (aluminum foil).
8. The left side of the animal is covered with opaque material.
9. The animal is then exposed to approximately 5 J/cm² of UVA (320–400 nm) light.
10. After exposure to the UVA light, the patches on the right side of the animal, as well as the occlusive dressing, are replaced.
11. The dressing is again removed approximately 23 h after the initial application of the test article. Residual test article is carefully removed, where applicable, using water (or another suitable vehicle).

12. Animals are examined for signs of erythema and edema and the responses are scored at 24, 48, and 72 h after the initial test article application according to the Draize reaction grading system previously presented in this volume.

13. Any unusual observation and mortality are recorded.

D. Analysis of Data

The data from the irradiated and nonirradiated sites are evaluated separately. The scores from erythema and eschar formation and edema at 24, 48, and 72 h are added for each animal (six values). The six values are then divided by 3, yielding six individual scores. The mean of the six individual animal irritation scores represents the mean primary irritation score (maximum score = 8, as in the primary dermal irritation study). This method was developed after a human model had been developed.

Guinea Pig Recently, a standardized protocol for using the guinea pig for phototoxicity testing has been proposed [31], which has been the subject of an international validation exercise. This is detailed in Fig. 9.3.

A. Animals and Animal Husbandry

1. Strain/species: Male Hartley guinea pigs.
2. Number: At least 10 (two groups). Irradiation control: 4 animals; test material treated: 6 animals.

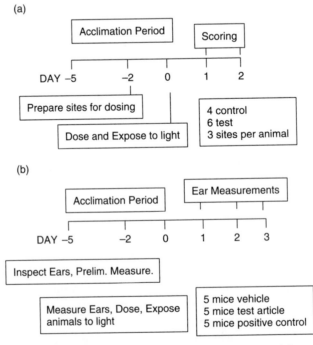

FIGURE 9.3 (a) Guinea pig and (b) mouse for phototoxicity testing.

3. Age: Young adult, 300–500 g.

4. Acclimation period: At least 5 days.

5. Feed/water: *Ad libitum.*

B. Test Material

1. Vehicle: Test assumes that material will be in solution. Use the most volatile, nonirritating organic solvent possible, for example, ethanol, acetone, dimethylacetamide, or some combination.

2. Treatment: There can be up to four sites per animal, each measuring 1.5 cm × 1.5 cm (2.25 cm^2). In general, one side should be for a vehicle control, and another for a positive control (8-methoxypsoralen (8-MOP), 0.005% in ethanol).

3. Dosage: A dose of 0.025–0.050 mL is applied using a micropipette to each site.

C. Experimental Procedure

1. Animals are weighed on the first day of dosing.

2. Preparation: Approximately 48 h prior to treatment, remove the hair from a 6 cm × 8 cm area on the back with a fine clipper. On the day of dosing, animals are dosed as described previously. Tests are situated as to prevent mixing of test solutions after application. No patches or wraps are used.

3. Immediately after the dose application, the animals are placed in a restraint while keeping the test sites uncovered. Prior to irradiation the heads are covered to prevent ocular damage from the light exposure.

4. Thirty minutes after dosing, animals are exposed to a nonerythmogenic dose of light in the UVA band (should have peak intensity between 335 and 365 nm). The dose of light should be 9 or 10 J/cm^2 for UVA and 0.1–0.3 J/cm^2 for UVB.

5. Immediately after light exposure, the animals are wiped clean if necessary and returned to their home cages.

6. Animals are inspected and scored at 24 and 48 h postexposure according to the following:

0	No reaction
1	Slight erythema
2	Moderate erythema
3	Severe erythema, with or without edema

The reader should note that this scoring scheme is the same one used for dermal sensitization scoring, whereas the scoring method for the rabbit model discussed previously is that used for dermal irritation studies.

7. Any unusual clinical signs noted during exposure should be documented. The following descriptive parameters can be calculated from the data.

$$\text{Phototoxic Irritation Index (PTII)} = \frac{(\text{Number of positive sites} \times 100)}{(\text{Number of exposure sites})}$$

$$\text{Phototoxicity Severity Index (PSI)} = \frac{\text{(Total of scores)}}{\text{(Total of observations)}}$$

Lovell and Sanders [32] had previously proposed a similar model of assessing topical phototoxicity potential in the guinea pig. Their model differed from the one proposed by Nilson et al. [31] with regard to the following:

Only one test site per animal was used.

Test sites were smaller (about $1.6\,cm^2$).

Amounts applied were less (about $10\,\mu L$).

Light intensity was set at $15\,J/cm^2$.

Their paper made no reference to the use of a restrainer.

Assessments were conducted at 4, 24, 48, and 72 h.

The scoring system was as follows:

0   Normal
2   Faint/trace erythema
4   Slight erythema
6   Definite erythema
8   Well-developed erythema

(Intermediate scores were indicated by odd numbers.)

They recommended the use of acidine (weak phototoxin) or anthracene (strong phototoxin) for positive controls.

9.9.4 Pyrogenicity

The United States Pharmacopeia describes a pyrogen test using rabbits as a model. This test, which is the standard for limiting risks of a febrile reaction to an acceptable level, involves measuring the rise in body temperature in a group of three rabbits for 3 h after injection of 10 mL of test solution.

Apparatus and Diluents   Render the syringes, needles, and glassware free of pyrogens by heating at 250 °F for not less than 30 min or by any other suitable method. Treat all diluents and solutions for washing and rinsing of devices or parenteral injection assemblies in a manner that will ensure that they are sterile and pyrogen-free. Periodically perform control pyrogen tests on representative portions of the diluents and solutions that are used for washing or rinsing of the apparatus.

Temperature Recording   Use an accurate temperature-sensing device, such as a clinical thermometer or thermistor or similar probe, that has been calibrated to ensure an accuracy of ± 0.1 °C and has been tested to determine that a maximum reading is reached in less than 5 min. Insert the temperature-sensing probe into the rectum of the test rabbit to a depth of not less than 7.5 cm and, after a period of time not less than that previously determined as sufficient, record the rabbit's temperature.

Test Animals   Use healthy, mature rabbits. House the rabbits individually in an area of uniform temperature (between 20 and 23 °C) free from disturbances likely to excite them. The temperature should vary no more than ±3 °C from the selected temperature. Before using a rabbit for the first time in a pyrogen test, condition it for not more than 7 days before use by a sham test that includes all of the steps as directed under Procedure, except injection. Do not use a rabbit for pyrogen testing more frequently than once every 48 h, nor prior to 2 weeks following a maximum rise in its temperature of 0.6 °C or more while being subjected to the pyrogen test, or following its having been given a test specimen that was determined to be pyrogenic.

Procedure   Perform the test in a separate area designated solely for pyrogen testing and under environmental conditions similar to those under which the animals are housed. Withhold all food from the test rabbits during the period of the test. Access to water is allowed at all times but may be restricted during the test. If probes measuring rectal temperature remain inserted throughout the testing period, restrain the rabbits with loose-fitting Elizabethan collars that allow the rabbits to assume a natural resting posture. Not more than 30 min prior to the injection of the test dose, determine the "control temperature" of each rabbit; this is the base for the determination of any temperature increase resulting from the injection of a test solution. In any one group of test rabbits, use only those rabbits whose control temperatures do not vary by more than 1 °C from each other, and do not use any rabbit having a temperature exceeding 39.8 °C.

Unless otherwise specified in the individual protocol, inject 10 mL of the test solution per kilogram of body weight into an ear vein of each of three rabbits, completing each injection within 10 min after the start of administration. The test solution is either the product, constituted if necessary as directed in the labeling, or the material under test. For pyrogen testing of devices or injection assemblies, use washings or rinsings of the surfaces that come in contact with the parenterally administered material or with the injection site or internal tissues of the patient. Ensure that all test solutions are protected from contamination. Perform the injection after warming the test solution to a temperature of 37 ± 2 °C. Record the temperature at 1, 2, and 3 h subsequent to the injection.

Test Interpretation and Continuation   Consider any temperature decreases as zero rise. If no rabbit shows an individual rise in temperature of 0.6 °C or more above its respective control temperature, and if the sum of the three individual maximum temperature rises does not exceed 1.4 °C, the product meets the requirements for the absence of pyrogens. If any rabbit shows an individual temperature rise of 0.6 °C or more, or if the sum of the three individual maximum temperature rises exceeds 1.4 °C, continue the test using five other rabbits. If not more than three of the eight rabbits show individual rises in temperature of 0.6 °C or more, and if the sum of the eight individual maximum temperature rises does not exceed 3.7 °C, the material under examination meets the requirements for the absence of pyrogens.

In Vitro *Pyrogenicity*   *In vitro* pyrogenicity testing (or bacterial endotoxin testing) is one of the great success stories for *in vitro* testing. Some fifteen years ago, the limulus amebocyte lysate (LAL) test was developed, validated, and accepted as an *in vitro* alternative [33, 34] to the rabbit test. An *in vitro* test for estimating the concentration of bacterial endotoxins that may be present in or on a sample of the article(s) to which the test is applied uses LAL that has been obtained from aqueous extracts of the circulating amebocytes of the horseshoe crab, *Limulus polyphemus*, and that has been prepared and characterized for use as an LAL reagent for gel-clot formation. The test's limitation is that it detects only the pyrogens of gram-negative bacteria. This is generally not significant, since most environmental contaminants that gain entrance to sterile products are gram-negative [35].

Where the test is conducted as a limit test, the specimen is determined to be positive or negative to the test judged against the endotoxin concentration specified in the individual monograph. Where the test is conducted as an assay of the concentration of endotoxin, with calculation of confidence limits of the result obtained, the specimen is judged to comply with the requirements if the result does not exceed (1) the concentration limit specified in the individual monograph and (2) the specified confidence limits for the assay. In either case the determination of the reaction endpoint is made with parallel dilutions of redefined endotoxin units.

Since LAL reagents have also been formulated to be used for turbidimetric (including kinetic) assays or colorimetric readings, such tests may be used if shown to comply with the requirements for alternative methods. These tests require the establishment of a standard regression curve and the endotoxin content of the test material is determined by interpolation from the curve. The procedure includes incubation for a preselected time of reacting endotoxin and control solutions with LAL reagent and reading the spectrophotometric light absorbance at suitable wavelengths. In the case of the turbidimetric procedure, the reading is made immediately at the end of the incubation period. In the kinetic assays, the absorbance is measured throughout the reaction period and rate values are determined from those readings. In the colorimetric procedure, the reaction is arrested at the end of the preselected time by the addition of an appropriate amount of acetic acid solution prior to the readings. A possible advantage in the mathematical treatment of results, if the test is otherwise validated and the assay suitably designed, could be the confidence interval and limits of potency from the internal evidence of each assay itself.

9.9.5 Blood Compatibility

The standard test (and its major modifications) currently used for this purpose is technically an *in vitro* one, but it requires a sample of fresh blood from a dog or other large donor animal. The test was originally developed by the National Cancer Institute for use in evaluating cancer chemotherapeutic agents [36] and is rather crude, though definitive.

The variation described here is one commonly utilized. It uses human blood from volunteers, eliminating the need to keep a donor colony of dogs. The test procedure is described next.

1. *Test System.* Human blood. Collect 30 mL heparinized blood for whole blood and plasma (three tubes) and 30 mL clotted blood for serum (two tubes) from each of six donors.

2. *Precipitation Potential.*
   (a) For each donor, set up and label eight tubes 1 through 8.
   (b) Add 1 mL serum to tubes 1 through 4.
   (c) Add 1 mL plasma to tubes 5 through 8.
   (d) Add 1 mL formulation to tubes 1 through 5.
   (e) Add 1 mL vehicle to tubes 2 and 6.
   (f) Add 1 mL physiological saline to tubes 3 and 7 (negative control).
   (g) Add 1 mL 2% nitric acid to tubes 4 and 8 (positive control).
   (h) Observe tubes 1 through 8 for qualitative reactions (e.g., precipitation or clotting) before and after mixing.
   (i) If a reaction is observed in the formulation tubes (tubes 1 and/or 5), dilute the formulation in an equal amount of physiological saline ($\frac{1}{2}$ dilution) and test 1 mL of the dilution with an equal amount of plasma and/or serum. If a reaction still occurs, make serial dilutions of the formulation in saline ($\frac{1}{4}$, $\frac{1}{8}$, etc.).
   (j) If a reaction occurs in the vehicle tubes (tubes 2 and/or 6), repeat in a manner similar to that in Step (i).

3. *Hemolytic Potential.*
   (a) For each donor, set up and label eight tubes 1 through 8.
   (b) Add 1 mL whole blood to each tube.
   (c) Add 1 mL formulation to tube 1.
   (d) Add 1 mL vehicle to tube 2.
   (e) Add 1 mL of 1/2 dilution of formulation in saline to tube 3.
   (f) Add 1 mL of 1/2 dilution of vehicle in saline to tube 4.
   (g) Add 1 mL of 1/4 dilution of formulation in saline to tube 6.
   (h) Add 1 mL of 1/4 dilution of vehicle in saline to tube 6.
   (i) Add 1 mL of physiological saline to tube 7 (negative control).
   (j) Add 1 mL of distilled water to tube 8 (positive control).
   (k) Mix by gently inverting each tube three times.
   (l) Incubate tubes for 45 min at 37 °C.
   (m) Centrifuge 5 min at 1000 g.
   (n) Separate the supernate from the sediment.
   (o) Determine hemoglobin concentrations to the nearest 0.1 g/dL on the supernate (plasma).
   (p) If hemoglobin concentrations of the above dilutions are 0.2 g/dL (or more) greater than the saline control, repeat the procedure, adding 1 mL of further serial dilutions ($\frac{1}{8}$, $\frac{1}{16}$, etc.) of formulation or vehicle to 1 mL of blood until the hemoglobin level is within 0.2 g/dL of the saline control.

There are two proposed, true *in vitro* alternatives to this procedure [37, 38], but neither has been widely evaluated or accepted.

REFERENCES

1. Gad SC, Chengelis CP. *Acute Toxicity: Principles and Methods*, 2nd ed. San Diego: CA: Academic Press; 1998.

2. Gad SC. Irritation and local tissue tolerance in pharmaceutical safety assessment. In *Drug Safety Evaluation*. Hoboken NJ: John Wiley & Sons; 2002, pp 367–403.

3. Draize JH, Woodard G, Calvery HO. Method for the study of irritation and toxicity of substances applied topically to the skin and mucous membranes. *J Reprod Fertil* 1944;20:85–93.

4. Eckstein P, Jackson M, Millman N, Sobero A. Comparison of vaginal tolerance test of spermical preparations in rabbits and monkeys. *J Reprod Fertil* 1969;20:85–93.

5. Weil CS, Scala RA. Study of intra- and interlaboratory variability in the results of rabbit eye and skin irritation tests. *Toxicol Appl Pharmacol* 1971;19:276–360.

6. Gad SC, Walsh RD, Dunn BJ. Correlation of ocular and dermal irritancy of industrial chemicals. *Ocular Dermal Toxicol* 1986;5(3):195–213.

7. Guillot JP, Gonnet JF, Clement C, Caillard L, Trahaut R. Evaluation of the cutaneous-irritation potential of 56 compounds. *Fundam Chem Toxicol* 1982;201:563–572.

8. Mathias CGT. Clinical and experimental aspects of cutaneous irritation. In Margulli FM, Maiback HT, Eds. *Dermatotoxicology*. New York: Hemisphere Publishing; 1983, pp 167–183.

9. Auletta C. Vaginal and rectal administration. *J Am Coll Toxicol* 1994;13:48–63.

10. Jochims K, et al. Local tolerance testing of parenteral drugs: how to put into practice. *Regul Toxicol Pharmacol* 2003;38:166–182.

11. Avis KE. Parenteral preparations. In Gennaro AR, Ed. *Remington's Pharmaceutical Sciences*. Easton, PA: Mack Publishing Company; 1985, pp 1518–1541.

12. Bacterial endotoxins test. *United States Pharmacopeia*. Rockville, MD: USP Convention; 1995, pp 1696–1697.

13. Gray JE. Pathological evaluation of injection injury. In Robinson J, Ed. *Sustained and Controlled Release Drug Delivery Systems*. New York: Marcel Dekker; 1978, pp 351–405.

14. Ballard BE. Biopharmaceutical considerations in subcutaneous and intramuscular drug administration. *J Pharm Sci* 1968;57:357–378.

15. Intracutaneous test. *United States Pharmacopoeia*. Rockville, MD: USP Convention; 1995, pp 1201–1202.

16. Garramone JP. *Vascular Access Port Model SLA. Users Manual*. Skokie, IL: Norfolk Medical Products; 1986.

17. Theeuwes F, Yum SI. Principles of the design and operation of generic osmotic pumps for the delivery of semisolid or liquid drug formulations. *Ann Biomed Eng* 1976;4:343–353.

18. Hagan EC. *Appraisal of the Safety of Chemicals in Foods, Drugs and Cosmetics*. Austin, TX: Association of Food and Drug Officials of the United States; 1959, p 19.

19. Shintani S, Yamazaki M, Nakamura M, Nakayama I. A new method to determine the irritation of drugs after intramuscular injection in rabbits. *Toxicol Appl Pharmacol* 1967;11:293–301.

20. Intramuscular irritation test. *United States Pharmacopeia*. Rockville, MD: USP Convention; 1985, pp 1180–1183.

21. Sidell FR, Calver DL, Kaminskis A. Serum creatine phosphokinase activity after intramuscular injection. *JAMA* 1974;228:1884–1887.

22. Young MF, Tobretta LD, Sophia JV. Correlative *in vitro* and *in vivo* study of skeletal muscle irritancy. *Toxicologist* 1986;6(1):1225.

23. Williams PD, Masters BG, Evans LD, Laska DA, Hattendorf GH. An *in vitro* model for assessing muscle irritation due to parenteral antibiotics. *Fundam Appl Toxicol* 1987;9:10–17.

24. Kato I, Harihara A, Mizushima Y. An *in vitro* method for assessing muscle irritation of antibiotics using rat primary cultured skeletal muscle fibers. *Toxicol Appl Pharmacol* 1992;117:194–199.

25. Brown S, Templeton D, Prater DA, Potter CC. Use of an *in vitro* hemolysis test to predict tissue irritancy in an intramuscular formation. *J Parenter Sci Technol* 1989;43:117–120.

26. Horio T, Kohachi K, Ogawa A, Inoue T, Ishirara M. Evaluation of photosensitizing ability of quinolones in guinea pigs. *Drugs* 1995;49(Suppl 2):283–285.

27. Lambert L, Warmer W, Kornhauser A. Animal models for phototoxicity tesing. *Toxicol Methods* 1996;2:99–114.

28. Anderson RR, Parrish JA. The optics of skin. *J Invest Dermatol* 1981;77:13–19.

29. Pathak MA. Photobiology of melanogenesis: biophysical aspects. In Montagna W, Uh F, Eds. *Advances in Biology of Skin, Volume 8, The Pigmentary System*. New York: Pergamon; 1967, pp 400–419.

30. Marzulli FM, Maibach HK. Perfume phototoxicity. *J Soc Cosmet Chem* 1970;21:685–715.

31. Nilsson R, Maurer T, Redmond N. A standard protocol for phototoxicity testing: results from an interlaboratory study. *Contact Dermatitis* 1993;28:285–290.

32. Lovell WW, Sanders DJ. Phototoxicity testing in guinea pigs. *Food Chem Toxicol.* 1992;30:155–160.

33. Cooper JF. Principles and applications of the limulus test for pyrogen in parenteral drugs. *Bull Parenter Drug Assoc* 1975;3:122–130.

34. Wearly M, Baker B. Utilization of the limulus amebocyte lysage test for pyrogen testing of large-volume parenterals, administration sets and medical devices. *Bull Parenter Drug Assoc* 1977;31:127–133.

35. Develeeshouwer MJ, Cornil MF, Dony J. Studies on the sensitivity and specificity of the limulus amebocyte lysate test and rabbit pyrogen assays. *Appl Environ Microbiol* 1985;50:1509–1511.

36. Prieur DJ, Young DM, Davis RD, Cooney DA, Homan ER, Dixon RL, Guarino AM. Procedures for preclinical toxicologic evaluation of cancer chemotherapeutic agents: protocols of the laboratory of toxicology. *Cancer Chemother Rep* 1973;4(Part 3):1–30.

37. Mason RG, Shermer RW, Zucker WH, Elston RC, Blackwelder WC. An *in vitro* test system for estimation of blood compatibility of biomaterials. *J Biomed Mater Res* 1974;8:341–356.

38. Kambic HE, Kiraly RJ, Yukihiko N. A simple *in vitro* screening test for blood compatibility of materials. *J Biomed Mater Res Sympos* 1976;7:561–570.

10

SAFETY ASSESSMENT STUDIES: IMMUNOTOXICITY

JACQUES DESCOTES

Poison Center and Claude Bernard University, Lyon, France

Contents

Preclinical Development Handbook: Toxicology, edited by Shayne Cox Gad
Copyright © 2008 John Wiley & Sons, Inc.

10.1   INTRODUCTION

Over the last three decades, immunotoxicology slowly grew into a significant component of the preclinical safety evaluation of xenobiotics. In the mid-1960s, infections and neoplasia were identified as complications of potent immunosuppressive drugs shortly after their introduction for clinical use in transplant patients [1, 2]. These clinical findings served as an impetus to conduct experimental studies that almost exclusively focused on immunosuppression. Most early studies, however, lacked sufficient awareness that conditions of exposure or adequately selected doses are absolutely essential to generate relevant results for extrapolation from animal to human. Even though immunotoxicology was seemingly for the very first time the sole theme of a workshop held in 1974 [3], the birth of this new discipline was heralded in 1979 [4]. The shift from immunology to toxicology led to the introduction of toxicological concepts in immunotoxicity evaluation as summarized in a special issue of the journal *Drug and Chemical Toxicology* [5]. A major advance was the concept of tiered protocols, which consisted of a screening phase (tier I) including a matrix of *in vitro* and *in vivo* assays to be selected initially, and then a mechanism phase (tier II) based on a list of additional assays to be conducted depending on the results of the first tier [6]. This rationalized approach culminated in the conduct of interlaboratory validation studies of which the most significant were the B6C3F$_1$ mouse immunotoxicology study under the auspices of the U.S. National Toxicology Program (NTP) [7], the Fisher 344 cyclosporine validation study [8], the modified 28-day rat study [9], and the ICICIS rat validation study [10].

After many years almost entirely devoted to immunosuppression—often misleadingly used as a synonym for immunotoxicity even today—the scope of immunotoxicology expanded to include autoimmunity, then allergy, and finally immunostimulation. The importance of autoimmunity was first highlighted by the withdrawal from the market of the β-blocking drug practolol, which was the cause of the so-called oculomucocutaneous syndrome [11]. Thereafter, two major epidemics, the Spanish toxic oil syndrome, which affected more than 20,000 persons in 1981–1982 and killed over 300 [12], and the eosinophilia-myalgia syndrome (EMS) in users of preparations containing L-tryptophan [13], showed that chemically induced autoimmunity can be a significant health issue. Despite the routine use of guinea pig models to assess contact sensitization—a prototypic immunoallergic reaction [14]—there was an implicit but unfounded consensus that allergic reactions cannot be predicted in animal studies. However, when drug allergies turned out to be a major cause of concern, efforts began to be paid to designing predictive models for use during drug development [15]. Last but not least, the introduction of the therapeutic cytokines demonstrated that enhancement of immune responses, that is, (unspecific) immunostimulation, is a relevant aspect of immunotoxicology [16].

Immunotoxic effects have often been subdivided into two broad categories, namely, immunosuppression and immunostimulation, the latter encompassing allergy and autoimmunity. As suggested long ago [17], categorization into immuno-suppression, immunostimulation, hypersensitivity, and autoimmunity should be preferred as it more closely reflects the distinction between clinically significant immunotoxic effects that involve different effector mechanisms and require differ-ent animal models and assays for identification during nonclinical immunotoxicity evaluation.

10.2 THE IMMUNE SYSTEM: AN OVERVIEW

The immune system is a complex network of cells and molecules that ensures the detection of self from nonself in order to defend the integrity of the body [18]. To achieve this goal, a wide variety of mechanisms, either nonspecific (innate or natural immunity) or specific (adaptive or acquired immunity), come into play. Coordinated immune responses require interactions between specialized immunocompetent cells and biologically active molecules [19]. Immunocompetence is under the control of many mechanisms with redundant effects or conflicting outcome. Redundancy is an essential feature, which contributes to the functional reserve capacity of the immune system. Thus, it may prove difficult to anticipate the consequences of isolated mor-phological changes or functional alterations induced by medicinal products because of compensatory mechanisms. Last but not least, immune responses can be detri-mental in certain circumstances, such as responses against self constituents of the host that result in autoimmune diseases, or reactivity against "innocent" foreign antigens (e.g., penicillin), leading to life-threatening systemic allergies.

10.2.1 Lymphoid Organs

Immunocompetent cells are found in the blood and almost all organs or tissues of the body, but they concentrate into specific anatomical structures, the lymphoid organs, which include central and peripheral lymphoid organs [20].

Central Lymphoid Organs   Central (or primary) lymphoid organs, where the pro-duction and/or maturation of lymphocytes take place, are lymphoepithelial struc-tures that develop early during organogenesis and independently of antigenic stimulations.

Bone Marrow   The bone marrow is the main hematopoietic organ in mammals and the equivalent of the bursa of Fabricius in birds. All blood cell types at various stages of maturation (except mature T lymphocytes) and their progenitors can be found in the medullary cavity of bones. A common multipotent progenitor cell gives rise to lymphoid and myeloid progenitor cells that follow differentiation pathways to produce a variety of blood cell types. Soluble factors released by the stroma or accessory cells, including interleukin-3 (IL-3), the macrophage-colony stimulating factor (M-CSF), granulocyte-macrophage-colony stimulating factor (GM-CSF), and granulocyte-colony stimulating factor (G-CSF), exert critical influences on these complex processes. B lymphocytes, which derive from lymphoid progenitor cells, mature in the bone marrow.

Thymus   The thymus is the main central lymphoid organ because T lymphocytes mature within the thymus. T lymphocytes at different stages of development can be identified from the expression of surface molecules (markers) denoted CD for cluster of differentiation. Triple negative bone marrow-derived thymocytes express none of the CD3, CD4, and CD8 major T lymphocyte markers. One subsequent step is the DP (double positive) thymocytes in the thymic cortex, which express both CD4 and CD8. Then, DP thymocytes migrate to the medulla to become single-positive T lymphocytes, either CD4$^+$CD8$^-$ or CD4$^-$CD8$^+$. They mature further and leave the thymus to populate organs and lymphoid tissues. T lymphocyte maturation is regulated by the epithelial microenvironment and thymic hormones. In the cortex, more than 95% of immature DP thymocytes are eliminated by apoptosis. Only those immature thymic T cells expressing receptors (TCRs) that recognize major histo-compatibility complex (MHC) class I or class II molecules and associated self-peptides with moderate affinity escape from apoptosis and continue to differentiate (positive selection).

Peripheral Lymphoid Organs   Antigens and immunocompetent cells come into contact in the peripheral (or secondary) lymphoid organs, which fully develop only after repeated antigenic stimulations. The lymphoid follicles are small clusters of B lymphocytes, either primary follicles prior to antigenic stimulation, or secondary follicles containing a germinative center where precursors of plasma cells, memory B lymphocytes, CD4$^+$ T lymphocytes, and macrophages can be seen.

Spleen   The spleen is a filter in the circulation and the site of immune responses against blood-borne antigens (e.g., opsonized microbes). The red pulp is the most prominent compartment containing macrophages, lymphocytes, and plasma cells. About 25% of all lymphocytes are located in the white pulp of the spleen, which consists of periarteriolar lymphoid sheaths with many T lymphocytes and adjacent follicles containing B lymphocytes. The white pulp plays a major role in immune responses against blood-borne antigens.

Lymph Nodes   The lymph nodes are grouped at sites connecting blood and lymph vessels to ensure direct contact between antigens and immunocompetent cells. They are comprised of cortical, paracortical, and medullary areas. Antigens are processed by macrophages in the medulla. In the paracortex, free or processed antigens are presented to T lymphocytes. The cortical area is the site where B lymphocytes encounter antigens.

MALT   The mucosa-associated lymphoid tissue (MALT) is located underneath the epithelium of the gut (gut-associated lymphoid tissue or GALT), the bronchopulmonary tract (bronchi-associated lymphoid tissue or BALT), and the upper airways (nasal-associated lymphoid tissue or NALT). GALT includes the Peyer's patches in the duodenum and jejunum, and the appendix of the large intestine. In addition to IgA-producing plasma cells and intraepithelial T lymphocytes, MALT contains the M cells, a particular type of epithelial cells that take up inhaled or ingested antigens by pinocytosis. Because of its role in mucosal immunity, MALT is considered to be a first line of the host's defense.

10.2.2 Immunocompetent Cells

All immune cells originate in the bone marrow from multipotent stem cells that mature along different pathways. The lymphoid cell lineage gives rise to lymphocytes, and the myeloid cell lineage to neutrophils, basophils and eosinophils, monocytes and macrophages, dendritic cells, and mast cells (Fig. 10.1).

Lymphocytes   Lymphocytes [21] constitute 10% of blood cells in pigs, 20–40% in humans and dogs, 40–65% in monkeys, 50–70% in mice, and >80% in rats. There are marked interindividual variations depending on the age, sex, and strain of the animals. As lymphocytes display no cytological or ultrastructural characteristics, surface markers are used to distinguish between lymphocyte populations. Lymphocytes include T and B lymphocytes and natural killer (NK) cells.

T Lymphocytes   Approximately 55–70% of circulating lymphocytes are T lymphocytes in humans and most mammals. They express the T-cell receptor (TCR), and CD2 and CD3 surface markers. T lymphocytes are subdivided into $CD4^+$ and $CD8^+$ T lymphocytes. $CD4^+$ (helper) T lymphocytes make up two-thirds of T lymphocytes in humans, rats, and dogs, but only one-half in monkeys. All $CD4^+$ T lymphocytes release IL-3, GM-CSF, and the tumor-necrosis factor-α (TNF-α). Depending on the profile of cytokines they secrete in certain circumstances, $CD4^+$ T lymphocytes are further divided into T_H1 and T_H2 lymphocytes, which primarily release IL-2 and interferon-γ (INF-γ), or IL-4, IL-5, and IL-10, respectively. The dichotomy between T_H1 and T_H2 lymphocytes is not a preexisting characteristic. Resting T_H0 lymphocytes are thought to be polarized to mount a T_H1 or a T_H2 response by ill-understood mechanisms. $CD4^+$ T lymphocytes control immune responses. $CD8^+$ (cytotoxic/effector) T lymphocytes recognize antigens presented by antigen-presenting cells (APCs) in association with MHC class I molecules. Activated $CD8^+$ T lymphocytes lyse target cells. Similar patterns of cytokine secretion have been shown so that $CD8^+$ T lymphocytes can also be subdivided into T_C1 and T_C2 lymphocytes.

B Lymphocytes   Approximately 10–20% of peripheral blood lymphocytes are B lymphocytes in all mammals. They develop in the fetal liver, then in the bone marrow. They are identified by the surface immunoglobulins IgM, IgD, IgG, IgA, or IgE, and various surface cell markers including CD19, CD22, CD23, and CD37. Following antigen encounter, B lymphocytes proliferate and this results in the formation of germinal centers in the spleen and lymph nodes. As a general rule, B lymphocytes cannot be activated by the antigen alone. A second accessory signal is normally required for B lymphocytes to be activated (thymus-dependent antigens).

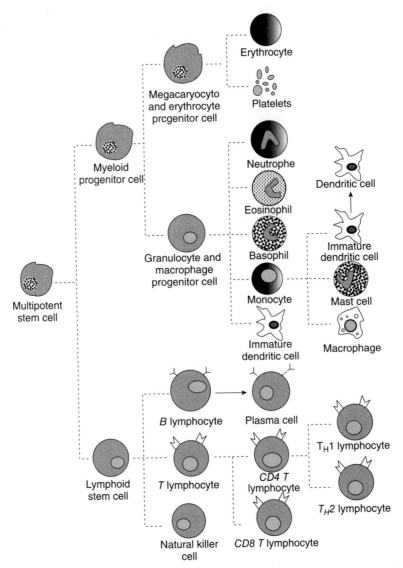

FIGURE 10.1 Cells of the immune system and differentiation pathways. All cells of the immune system derive from a common multipotent bone marrow progenitor. Differentiation pathways lead to the myeloid and lymphoid lineages, and then well-characterized cells.

At their final stage of maturation, B lymphocytes form antibody-secreting plasma cells.

Memory Lymphocytes Lymphocytes have been estimated to produce 10^{15} different antibodies and TCRs. Antigen-binding specificities correspond to the antigenic repertoire whose diversity is achieved by extensive gene rearrangements. Normally, only a few thousand lymphocytes are specific for a given antigen. Memory T and B lymphocytes can persist in the body in a resting state for many years to ensure a more vigorous and effective immune response upon reexposure to a previously encountered antigen.

NK Cells   Natural killer (NK) cells are large granular lymphocytes that account for 15% of all leukocytes in humans, but only 5% in rats [22]. They are $CD3^-CD56^+CD16^+$ cells. However, murine NK cells do not express CD56, and CD56 is not a suitable marker in monkeys. Most NK cells are non T cells, but a subset of T lymphocytes—the NKT cells—express characteristic markers of NK cells along with a TCR. The role of NK cells is primarily to kill virus-infected or tumor cells without prior sensitization through the release of stored cytoplasmic cytotoxic mediators (e.g., perforin and granzymes). Activation of NK cell cytotoxicity is the result of a balance between killer-activating and killer-inhibiting receptors that recognize HLA molecules. Normal nucleated cells express MHC class I molecules on their surface, but virus-infected cells and tumor cells lose this ability. As the inhibitory signals are lacking, NK cells can kill the abnormal target cells and contribute to the host's defense against viral infections and cancers.

Phagocytes   Phagocytosis is the process by which cells can ingest and eradicate microbial pathogens and foreign particles whose size exceeds 1 μm. The most effective phagocytozing cells are neutrophils and monocytes/ macrophages.

Neutrophils   Neutrophils constitute one-half of circulating white blood cells in most species and over 95% of PMNLs, but only 5–35% of rat leukocytes are neutrophils. Neutrophils contain two types of cytoplasmic granules: the primary (azurophil) granules that contain lytic enzymes (lysozyme, myeloperoxidase-derived substances, and cationic proteins), and the secondary (specific) granules that contain enzymes, such as lactoferrin and collagenases. Their half-life is 4–8 hours and because of this rapid turnover, they are particularly susceptible to toxic or immune-mediated insults. The primary function of neutrophils is phagocytosis so that patients with an innate or acquired decrease in neutrophil number or function can develop severe infections [23].

Monocytes/Macrophages   Monocytes constitute 5% of circulating leukocytes. Their life span in the circulation is between 8 and 70 hours; then, they migrate to tissues where they differentiate into macrophages. The vast majority of macrophages are found in tissues. In humans and pigs, but not in rodents and dogs, there are intravascular macrophages fixed to the capillary bed of the lungs and their *in situ* activation can result in lung injury. There is a wide morphological and functional polymorphism of macrophages depending on their location [24]. Monocytes and macrophages are phagocytozing cells, but they also play the role of APCs. Activated monocytes and macrophages release cytokines (IL-1, IL-6, TNF-α), and this can result in target-organ toxicity (e.g., hepatotoxicity).

Other Immunocompetent Cells   A number of other cell types are involved in immune responses.

Dendritic Cells   Immature dendritic cells (DCs) are scattered throughout the body. Because of their low phagocytic capacity, they degrade antigens by endocytosis to small peptides subsequently presented to T lymphocytes. So-called danger signals can activate DCs via specific receptors to endogenous or exogenous substances. DCs then mature, attract and cluster with T lymphocytes to present antigenic peptides. Mature DCs play a major role in immune regulation [25]. They direct antigen-specific T lymphocytes either to die by apoptosis or to become anergic, memory or effector T lymphocytes. They also trigger T lymphocyte proliferation. When mature DCs release IL-12, they skew the immune response toward a T_H1 response. DCs also regulate antigen-specific $CD8^+$ T cell cytotoxicity and NK cell activity.

Polymorphonuclear Leukocytes (PMNLs)   In addition to neutrophils, PMNLs include eosinophils and basophils [26]. Eosinophils account for 1–3% of peripheral blood leukocytes in humans and most animal species. Their cytoplasm contains specific granules where cationic proteins are stored. IL-5 controls the production of eosinophils in the bone marrow, and overproduction of IL-5 results in hypereosino-philia. Their half-life in blood is 8–18 hours. They distribute to tissues, especially the lungs and gut. Activated eosinophils release proinflammatory mediators including cationic proteins, newly synthesized eicosanoids, and cytokines. The major basic protein (MBP) accounts for 50% of all stored cationic proteins and is directly toxic to epithelial cells in the lungs. CD69 is a marker of activated eosinophils. Hypereo-sinophilia is typically noted in allergic diseases, inflammatory disorders, and hel-minth infections. Less than 1% of circulating leukocytes are basophils. They are stained by basic dyes, such as toluidine blue. After maturation in the bone marrow under the influence of IL-3, basophils circulate in the blood with a life span of several days. They express the high affinity receptor for IgE (FcεRI). Activation of basophils is induced by cross-linking of two adjacent FcεRI following binding of specific divalent antigen. CD63 is a marker of basophil activation. Activated baso-phils release preformed mediators stored in cytoplasmic granules including hista-mine, MBP, and tryptase. They also release newly formed mediators, such as leukotriene LTC_4, IL-4, and IL-13.

Mast Cells   Mast cells are long-lived cells preferentially found near blood vessels and under epithelial, serous, and synovial membranes in the skin, the lungs, and the gut [26]. Like basophils, they are characterized by dense cytoplasmic granules stained by toluidine blue. Mast cells do not circulate in blood. They express a variety of surface receptors including FcεRI and the C3a and C5a receptors. The main pre-formed mediators stored in cytoplasmic granules are histamine, the neutral prote-ases tryptase, chymase, carboxypeptidase, and cathepsin D, and the proteoglycans heparin and chondroitin sulfate E. Newly synthesized mediators including the eico-sanoids prostaglandin D2 and leukotriene LTC4, and TNF-α are also released by activated mast cells. The mechanism of mast cell activation is similar to that of basophils.

10.2.3   Innate Immunity

Immune responses are divided into innate (nonspecific) and adaptive (specific) immunity. Innate immunity, the first line of defense of the body against invading pathogens, involves a number of components and mechanisms [27].

Components of Innate Immunity

Epithelial Barriers   The body is protected by epithelial barriers in the skin and the respiratory, gastrointestinal, and urogenital tracts. Epithelial defenses include mechanical mechanisms (flow of air or mucus to entrap invading bacteria), chemical mechanisms (secretion of enzymes, such as lysozyme, or antimicrobial peptides), and microbial mechanisms (gut flora). When an epithelial barrier is breached by an invading pathogen, other mechanisms are brought into play.

Soluble Factors   Antimicrobial peptides are small polypeptides divided into three main families: the defensins, histatins, and cathelicidins [28]. The isolated peptides are very heterogeneous in length, sequence, and structure, but most of them are small, cationic, and amphipathic. They exhibit broad-spectrum activity against bacteria, yeasts, fungi, and enveloped viruses.

Complement   The complement is a complex system of more than 30 proteins with marked interspecies differences [29]. Several proteins are normally present in the circulation and tissues as functionally inactive molecules. Complement activation functions as an enzymatic cascade: inactive proteins are cleaved and activated, and then cleave and activate downstream proteins. Three activation pathways have been identified: the classical, alternative, and lectin-mediated pathways. The complement system serves important functions, as shown by the development of various pathological conditions in patients with primary or secondary complements deficiencies. Whatever the activation pathway, complement convertases cleave component C3 to C3a and C3b, which can bind covalently to the surface of pathogens. C3b-bound (opsonized) pathogens are more easily taken up and destroyed by phagocytes that bind C3b via the surface receptor CR1 (CD35). The small fragments C3a, C4a, and C5a—the anaphylatoxins—are formed during complement activation and can release inflammatory mediators from mast cells and basophils, which results in pseudoallergic reactions. The binding of the classical or alternative C3 convertase to C3b leads to the sequential cleavage of C5, C6, C7, and C8, and the polymerization of C9 to form the membrane-attack complex, which induces the formation of transmembrane pores in pathogens. The membrane-attack complex is also involved in the immunoallergic destruction of blood cells. The removal of circulating immune complexes is enhanced by complement activation. When immune complexes are not removed, they enlarge and precipitate at the basement membrane of small blood vessels, especially in the kidney glomeruli, a common feature in patients with systemic lupus erythematosus due to frequently associated deficiencies in the early complement components.

Acute-Phase Proteins   Acute-phase proteins are molecules whose concentrations increase in response to inflammation [30]. In addition to several complement components, they include C-reactive protein, serum amyloid A, fibronectin, antiproteases (α1-protease inhibitor, α1-antichymotrypsin), and coagulation proteins (fibrinogen, plasminogen, urokinase). Following infection, trauma, or stress, increased plasma concentrations of acute-phase proteins are associated with fever, behavioral changes (anorexia, somnolence), stimulation of the adrenal cortex, and anemia. Clinically, the most widely used indicator of an acute-phase response is C-reactive protein plasma concentration. The protective role of acute-phase proteins is still hypothetical.

Chemokines   Chemokines are small cytokines that facilitate the migration (chemotaxis) of lymphocytes, monocytes, neutrophils, and eosinophils [31]. Over 50 different chemokines have been identified. Depending on their structure, they are classified into CC, CXC, C, and CX3C chemokines. Over 20 distinct receptors are known. Functionally, chemokines are either inducible chemokines that recruit leukocytes in response to stress, or constitutive chemokines involved in the trafficking of leukocytes and the architecture of secondary lymphoid organs. Chemokines play a major role in cell migration, stimulate leukocyte degranulation, and promote angiogenesis. Recent data suggest that chemotaxis is not their sole function. Indeed, chemokines have been shown to play a significant role in various pathological conditions including cardiovascular diseases, allergy, transplantation, neuroinflammation, and cancer.

Proinflammatory Cytokines   In addition to their role in adaptive immunity, cytokines defend the body against infectious invaders. IFN-α and IFN-β produced by virus-infected cells inhibit virus replication and enhance antiviral defenses and NK cell activity. Activated macrophages release IL-1, IL-6, and TNF-α with a resulting increase in the production of acute-phase proteins.

Mechanisms of Innate Immunity   Inflammation defends the host against aggressions produced by physical or chemical agents, microbial pathogens, and various immune reactions. It is primarily characterized by the migration (chemotaxis) of leukocytes and the extravasation of serum proteins from the circulation. Thus, leukocytes can play their phagocytic role at the site of inflammation. The most effective phagocytozing cells are neutrophils and monocytes/macrophages. Under the influence of chemokines, phagocytes migrate to their targets and adhere to their surface nonspecifically (via lectins) or following opsonization. Then, phagocytes engulf their prey within phagosomes, where they release catalytic enzymes and free radicals. Soluble mediators involved in inflammatory reactions include free radicals, such as oxygen and nitrogen reactive species that induce direct tissue and cell injury or promote chain reactions, such as lipid peroxidation, leading to further tissue damage. Membrane lipids are the source of potent mediators, such as the prostaglandins and leukotrienes. Tissue injury is associated with the release of proteases that cause further tissue damage. Activation of the complement cascade can contribute to the inflammatory reaction via the formation of the membrane-attack complex or release of anaphylatoxins. Other important soluble mediators include the kinins, proinflammatory cytokines, and acute-phase proteins.

Recent evidence suggests that innate immunity facilitates specific immune responses. When pathogens breach the epithelial barrier, receptors, especially the toll-like receptors (TLRs) [32], recognize molecular patterns characteristic of particular classes of microorganisms as they are not found on self tissues. TLRs are mainly expressed by macrophages, neutrophils, and epithelial or endothelial cells. Recognition of pathogen-associated molecular patterns results in the activation of signaling pathways that drive and control specific immune responses.

10.2.4 Specific Immunity

Specific (adaptive) immunity comprises immune responses that are antigen-specific in contrast to innate immunity. Specific immune responses are subdivided into humoral and cell-mediated responses, both requiring close cell–cell interactions.

Humoral Immunity   Humoral immunity is the production of antigen-specific antibodies following contact with an antigen. Antibodies are heterodimeric glycoproteins, the immunoglobulins (Ig). In humans and most mammals, five classes of Ig have been identified, namely, the IgG, IgM, IgA, IgE, and IgD. The IgG class is further divided into four subclasses, IgG_{1-4} in humans; IgG_1, IgG_{2a}, IgG_{2b}, and IgG_{2c} in rodents. An Ig consists of two heavy (H) and two light (L) chains linked by disulfide bridges, which define domains (V_H, V_L, C_{1L}, C_{1H}, C_{2H}, and C_{3H}) in the amino acid sequence of the variable (V) and constant (C) regions of the H and L chains. The antibody site is formed by the variable domains. Each Ig molecule can be divided into two Fab fragments, which bind the antibody, and one Fc fragment involved in complement activation, opsonization, and placental transfer.

Antibody production requires the activation of B lymphocytes expressing the antigen-specific membrane Ig. Activated B lymphocytes proliferate and are transformed into lymphoblasts that give rise to memory B lymphocytes and antibody-secreting plasma cells. Following a first encounter with the antigen (primary response), antibody production starts after a latency period of 3–4 days, depending on the route of antigen entry and the dose and nature of the antigen (Fig. 10.2). Antibody titers subsequently grow exponentially and then decrease totally or to a residual level. In primary responses, IgM are first detected, then IgG. After a second encounter with the antigen (secondary response), antibody production is much earlier and more marked. Antibodies are primarily IgG with markedly higher affinity for the antigen and sustained antibody response.

Cell-Mediated Immunity   The immune system is a complex network where T lymphocytes play a pivotal role. Intercellular communications include the processing then the presentation of the antigen to T lymphocytes under strict genetic

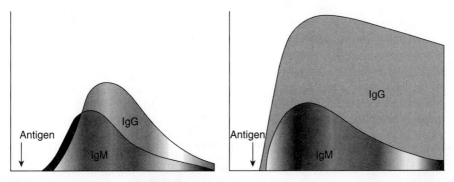

FIGURE 10.2   Primary and secondary antibody response. Primary antibody responses are characterized by a latency period of 3–4 days. Then IgM and IgG titers grow exponentially and decrease totally or to a residual level. In secondary responses, antibody (primarily IgG) production is much earlier and more marked.

control of MHC class I or II molecules. Activation of T lymphocytes is under the control of IL-2. For optimal activation, two signals are required: a TCR signal upon binding to the peptide–MHC on an antigen-presenting cell (APC), and an antigen-independent signal involving costimulatory molecules (Fig. 10.3). If both signals are provided, T lymphocytes can proliferate and secrete cytokines. In the absence of costimulatory signals, T lymphocytes become anergic or apoptotic. Surface immunoglobulins bound to B lymphocytes can recognize a wide range of antigens in their native form, but TCRs can only recognize antigens as peptides bound to MHC molecules at the surface of APCs. Thus, antigens must first be processed into small peptides to be recognized. When T lymphocytes encounter a peptide–MHC complex, the signal delivered through the TCR is insufficient to trigger activation. A second costimulatory signal is required via ligation of costimulatory molecules, for example, CD28-B7, CD40L-CD40, CD2-LFA-3 (CD48, CD58), and LFA-1-ICAM-1. The term immunological synapse is used to refer to these close interactions between APCs and T lymphocytes [33].

Cellular immune responses include delayed-type hypersensitivity (DTH) reactions, systemic responses to microbial pathogens, contact dermatitis, granulomatous reactions, allograft rejection, and graft-versus-host reactions. They are mediated by CD4$^+$ or CD8$^+$ T lymphocytes. CD4$^+$ T lymphocytes are mainly cytokine-secreting lymphocytes that trigger and control immune responses. A subset of CD4$^+$ T lymphocytes, the CD4$^+$CD25$^+$ (regulatory) T cells, control immune homeostasis [34]. CD8$^+$ T lymphocytes are primarily involved in T lymphocyte-mediated cytotoxicity to kill target cells. Cytokines, of which more than 150 have been identified to date, are polypeptides released by a variety of cells, which play a pivotal role in many responses including inflammation or specific immunity [35]. They include

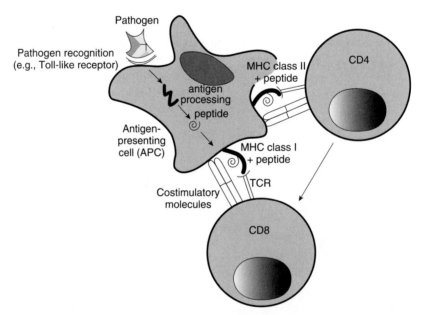

FIGURE 10.3 Schematic representation of interactions between an antigen-presenting cell and CD4$^+$ or CD8$^+$ T lymphocytes.

interleukins, chemokines, growth factors, and many other endogenous substances. A brief description of the main cytokines is given in Table 10.1. The cytokine network is extremely complex. One given cytokine often exerts effects on various target cell populations (pleiotropy) and several cytokines can exert similar effects on the same target cells (redundancy).

10.2.5   External Influences on the Immune System

External factors can interfere with immune responses. They include the central and autonomic nervous system, the neuroendocrine system, nutrition, and age. The role of external factors should not be overlooked when interpreting immune findings in

TABLE 10.1   Main Sources and Effects of Major Cytokines

Cytokine	Main Sources	Main Effects
IL-1α/β	Monocytes/macrophages, B cells, dendritic cells	Activation of T lymphocytes and APCs; induction of IL-2 production; synthesis of acute phase proteins
IL-2	T_H1 cells	Stimulation of T cells, B cells, and NK cells
IL-3	T_H cells, NK cells	Growth factor of bone marrow precursor cells; activation of mast cells
IL-4	T_H2 cells	Secretion of IgG_1 and IgE by B cells; inhibition of T_H1 cytokine production; proliferation of T cells
IL-5	T_H2 cells	Growth factor of eosinophils; proliferation and differentiation of B cells; synthesis of IgA
IL-6	B and T_H2 cells, fibroblasts, macrophages, endothelial cells	Differentiation of B cells into plasma cells; induction of acute-phase reaction
IL-7	Bone marrow and thymus stroma cells	Differentiation of stem cells, B and T cells, progenitor cells
IL-8	Macrophages, endothelial cells	Chemotactic factor of neutrophils
IL-10	T_H2 cells	Activation and proliferation of B cells, thymocytes, and mast cells; inhibition of IFN-γ production
IL-12	Macrophages, B cells	Stimulation of IFN-γ production; activation and differentiation of T_H1 cells; cytotoxicity
GM-CSF	T_H cells	Growth and differentiation of monocytes and dendritic cells
IFN-α	Leukocytes	Inhibition of viral replication; expression of MHC class I
IFN-γ	T_H1 and T_C cells, NK cells	Inhibition of viral replication; expression of MHC; proliferation of T_H2 cells
TGF-β	T cells, monocytes	Chemotaxis of monocytes/macrophages; IgA synthesis; activation of macrophages (IL-1 secretion)
TNF-α	Macrophages, NK cells	Cytokine expression; induction of tumor cell death

nonclinical studies. Immune responses can be altered by acute and chronic stress so that it can be difficult to differentiate immunosuppressive effects related to stress from a direct impact of the test article in animal studies. The thymus, spleen, lymph nodes, and MALT are innervated with neurotransmitter-containing fibers and many types of receptors have been demonstrated on immunocompetent cells including noradrenaline, adrenaline, dopamine, and serotonin receptors. There is a large body of evidence that cytokines exert effects on nonimmune tissues, such as the nervous and endocrine systems, and most hormones have immunomodulatory properties as well. Immune functions decline with age and aging-related changes contribute to more frequent diseases in elderly people. Both humoral and cellular immunity are affected, but cellular immunity is more markedly impaired due to physiologic thymic involution, which starts at puberty.

10.3 IMMUNOTOXIC EFFECTS

Even though this chapter is intended to review animal models and assays applicable to nonclinical immunotoxicity evaluation, a description of immunotoxic effects is helpful to select the most appropriate methods and interpret results adequately.

10.3.1 Clinical Consequences of Immunosuppression

Immunosuppression corresponds to decreased immune responsiveness. The difference between a total or partial inhibition of immune responsiveness—that is, immunosuppression and immunodepression, respectively—has never gained much attention despite obvious consequences in terms of risk assessment. Infections and virus-induced malignancies are the predominant clinical adverse effects associated with immunosuppression.

Infectious Complications   Immunocompromised human subjects typically present with more frequent, often more severe and relapsing, and sometimes atypical (opportunistic) infections. All pathogens including bacteria, viruses, fungi, and parasites can be involved. Even though all sites of the body can be affected, infections of the respiratory and gastrointestinal tracts, central nervous system, and skin are more frequent. Infectious complications have been described in patients treated with various immunosuppressive drug regimens, for instance, to prevent graft rejection [36], with corticosteroids to treat asthma, especially children [37], or with anti-TNF-α drugs used to treat rheumatoid arthritis and other autoimmune diseases [38]. Opportunistic infections, because they are caused by atypical pathogens and are located in uncommon sites, are generally easily attributed to marked immunosuppression. Clinically and microbiologically unremarkable infections may also develop in human subjects treated with less potent immunosuppressive (immunodepressive) drugs. Because these infections are unremarkable, only dedicated epidemiological studies can demonstrate an increased incidence in treated human subjects.

Virus-Associated Malignancies   Organ transplant patients are at a fourfold to 500-fold greater risk of developing malignancies, the most frequent being skin and lip cancers, lymphoproliferative disorders, and Kaposi's sarcomas [39]. The more profound is immunosuppression, the more frequent are malignancies. However, lymphoproliferative disorders have also been described in patients treated with low-dose methotrexate [40] or anti-TNF-α drugs [41], suggesting a mild-to-moderate level of immunosuppression may suffice. A latent viral infection due to a human herpesvirus or the Epstein–Barr virus has been suggested to be involved, which can explain the possible regression of lymphoproliferative disorders in those patients where discontinuation of the offending drug is acceptable.

10.3.2 Clinical Consequences of Immunostimulation

Adverse effects associated with the therapeutic use of recombinant cytokines are the best examples of the clinical consequences of immunostimulation [16]. In this context, immunostimulation refers not to an antigen-specific but to a "globally" stimulated immune response, so that the term unspecific immunostimulation (or immunoactivation) is sometimes used.

Flu-Like Reactions Mild-to-moderate fever (38–38.5 °C) with chills, arthralgias, and malaise can occur following initiation of treatment with immunostimulatory drugs or vaccination [42]. The reaction can, however, be much more severe with marked pyrexia (>40 °C), cardiovascular collapse or myocardial ischemia, obnubilation, and seizures. The suggested mechanism is the acute release of hypothalamic fever-promoting factors secondary to overproduction of IL-1 and TNF-α by activated monocytes/macrophages.

Autoimmune Diseases A variety of autoimmune diseases similar to spontaneous diseases are more frequent in patients treated with several recombinant cytokines, such as the interferons-α and rIL-2 [43]. The underlying mechanism is not elucidated in many instances. Preexisting pathological conditions, such as hepatitis C infection, may be a risk factor. Enhanced expression of major histocompatibility complex (MHC) class I and class II antigens and the immunomodulatory effects of cytokines are thought to play a critical, even though ill-understood role.

Hypersensitivity Reactions to Unrelated Allergens Treatments with immunostimulatory drugs can be associated with more frequent hypersensitivity reactions to unrelated allergens (e.g., asthma, rhinitis, or eczema). Interestingly, controlled clinical studies evidenced a greater risk of developing hypersensitivity reactions to radiocontrast media in rIL-2-treated cancer patients when compared to matched non-rIL-2-treated patients [44].

Inhibition of Drug-Metabolizing Enzymes A poorly recognized adverse effect of immunostimulatory drugs is their potential to inhibit drug-metabolizing enzymes [45]. Human studies showed a negative impact of the interferons-α, several viral vaccines, or BCG on drug-metabolizing enzymes at therapeutic doses, sometimes leading to clinically significant drug interactions. Loss of cytochromes P450 was shown to predominate at the level of gene expression.

10.3.3   Hypersensitivity Reactions

The term allergy is often used misleadingly, hence the preferred use of hypersensitivity. Hypersensitivity reactions are considered to be the most frequent immunotoxic effects of drugs in humans, even though their actual incidence is not known accurately [46]. A variety of mechanisms are suspected, but only few have been fully elucidated. This may explain current difficulties in the diagnosis of drug-induced immune-mediated hypersensitivity reactions [47]. After years of debate, it is widely accepted that hypersensitivity reactions are caused by either immune-mediated or nonimmune-mediated mechanisms [48].

Immune-Mediated Hypersensitivity Reactions   Immune-mediated hypersensitivity (immunoallergic) reactions result from an antigen-specific immune response against the parent drug molecule or its metabolites. Nearly every organ or tissue (e.g., the skin, blood cells, lungs, kidneys, and liver) can be affected [49]. The time course of the reaction can be acute or chronic. Specific IgE, IgG, IgM, or IgA antibodies as well as T lymphocytes can be involved. The Gell and Coombs classification into four pathogenic mechanisms (Types I–IV) is no longer recommended as only a limited number of drug-induced immune-mediated reactions are adequately covered by this classification [50].

Large foreign molecules, such as recombinant cytokines, therapeutic proteins, and monoclonal antibodies, can act as direct immunogens and trigger a specific immune response. In contrast, the majority of medicinal products are small-molecular-weight chemicals that can only induce sensitization by playing the role of haptens, which means they have to bind to carrier proteins to form immunogenic complexes. In most instances, they have minimal or no intrinsic chemical reactivity, and therefore highly reactive intermediate metabolites instead of the parent molecule are thought to be involved [51]. Recently, however, direct binding of several drugs or metabolites to T lymphocytes has been shown to occur, thus bypassing the haptenization step [52].

Nonimmune-Mediated Hypersensitivity Reactions   A prior sensitizing contact is an absolute prerequisite for any drug-induced immune-mediated hypersensitivity reaction to develop. Because patients with no history of prior contact can nevertheless develop clinically similar reactions, nonimmune-mediated (pseudoallergic) mechanisms have been hypothesized to be involved. Clinical similarities are linked to the involvement of the same mediators as in immune-mediated reactions, but their release is due to pharmacotoxicological instead of immunological mechanisms [53]. Direct (nonspecific) histamine release and complement activation are characterized by clinical features more or less reminiscent of an anaphylactic (IgE-mediated) reaction, but flush, redness of the skin, abdominal pain, cough, mild-to-moderate tachycardia, and blood pressure changes are often predominant. Two additional mechanisms are cyclo-oxygenase inhibition with the compensatory overproduction of leukotrienes, resulting in intolerance to aspirin and NSAIDs, and the accumulation of bradykinin normally cleaved into inactive fragments by the angiotensin-converting enzyme (ACE), leading to angioedema caused by ACE inhibitors and angiotensin II receptor antagonists.

10.3.4   Autoimmune Reactions

Autoimmune diseases are collectively frequent in the general population, but drug-induced autoimmune reactions seem to be rare [54]. Autoimmune diseases that develop more frequently in patients treated with certain immunoactivating drugs (see earlier discussion) must be clearly differentiated from drug-induced autoimmune reactions. In contrast to the first situation, where nearly every autoimmune disease can be observed, one given drug is usually associated with only one type of autoimmune reaction: for example, autoimmune hemolytic anemia and α-methyl dopa, or the lupus syndrome and hydralazine. In addition, the clinical and immunobiological features of systemic autoimmune reactions, such as the lupus syndrome, are dissimilar from those of the spontaneous disease, that is, systemic lupus erythematosus (SLE).

10.4   PRECLINICAL ASSESSMENT OF IMMUNOSUPPRESSION

Immunosuppression has been the main if not only focus of most immunotoxicologists for many years. Thus, quite a few animal models and assays have been designed, standardized, and validated so that unintended immunosuppressive drugs can reasonably be expected to be detectable provided adequate nonclinical studies are performed in due time.

10.4.1   Histology

Histological examination of the major lymphoid organs is routinely performed. Lymphoid organs are sites where immunocompetent cells, mainly lymphocytes and monocytes/macrophages, are found in an organized microenvironment. In fact, immunocompetent cells are disseminated in nearly every organ and tissue of the body. For practical purposes, histological examination is restricted to some key lymphoid organs and tissues.

Histological Technique   Typically, the lymphoid organs submitted to histological examination include the thymus, spleen, bone marrow, lymph nodes, and Peyer's patches [55]. Lymphoid organs must be carefully dissected and weighed unfixed. Although lymphoid organ weights have often been used as an index of immunotoxicity, there is considerable variation so that statistical significance between controls and treated animals is rarely attained. Decreases in the relative weight of the thymus often characterize a potential for immunosuppression, whereas the relevance of decreases in spleen weight is debatable. Changes in lymph node weight are rarely useful due to marked interindividual variability. The bone marrow collected from the sternum or the femur is processed to smears stained with conventional dyes. Cell suspensions can be prepared for cytological or flow cytometry analysis. GALT is obtained from rolled intestinal segments or "Swiss rolls" that are either fixed or frozen. BALT is best examined from lung sections. Sampling of blood and nonlymphoid organs including the skin, lungs, kidneys, and liver is also needed for comprehensive histological examination. Tissues and organs are fixed as quickly as possible after necropsy. Formalin fixation, paraffin embedding, and staining with hematoxylin and eosin are recommended to identify changes in the architecture of lymphoid tissues and the morphology of most immunocompetent cells. Electron microscopy requires special equipment and glutaraldehyde/paraformaldehyde fixatives. A description of best practice for routine pathology evaluation of the immune system was recently published by the Society of Toxicologic Pathology [56]. Interspecies variability must be taken into account when interpreting the results of histological examination [57].

Frank lesions, such as necrosis, fibrosis, and inflammation, are easily recognized, whereas changes in cell density, germinal center development, or prominence of high endothelial venules are often more subtle and require a skilled pathologist to differentiate abnormal findings from normal range. Structural changes are expected to be associated with modifications in the function of the affected organ, but it is as yet not established whether altered immune functions do correlate with structural changes. The term "enhanced pathology" was coined in the mid-1990s when standard histological examination of the lymphoid organs in rodents was first suspected to lack sufficient sensitivity. A number of new techniques have been introduced in toxicological pathology and are being considered for inclusion in nonclinical immunotoxicity evaluation. Immunohistochemistry detects proteins in tissue samples using specific polyclonal or monoclonal antibodies [58]. A secondary marker (e.g., a fluorochrome-conjugated antibody or streptavidin-biotin label) is used to visualize the binding of a primary antibody to specific epitopes. Nonfluorescent markers, such as immunoperoxidase and immunogold conjugates, are suitable for bright-field microscopy. A major limitation of immunohistochemistry is that it cannot be used for quantitative measurement, except cell proliferation. When antibodies are available commercially, a careful prevalidation is absolutely essential. When no antibodies are available, cross-reactivity across species is possible. In order to avoid diffusion in tissues, target molecules must be immobilized. Freezing following mild fixation (e.g., with acetone) is the preferred method as formalin-fixed, paraffin embedded tissue may not be appropriate due to antigen loss. Immunohistochemistry is used to detect changes in cell surface markers in response to inflammation or immunomodulation. Changes in the number or distribution of cell surface markers may be observed despite a lack of apparent changes in lymphoid tissue. However, the observed changes do not provide information on cellular function. Importantly, misinterpretation is possible due to the expression of the same cell surface marker by different subsets of immune cells. As standard histological examination can only provide a semiquantitative assessment of morphological changes, quantitative analysis may be necessary utilizing image analysis and stereological techniques that generate numerical values. *In situ* hybridization is based on the principle that labeled sequences of nucleic acids (probes) can specifically hybridize with cellular mRNA or DNA (gene) in tissues [59]. RNA probes offer the advantage of higher sensitivity, but they are labile and require technical skill. Labeling is achieved by radioisotopic methods using ^{35}S- and ^{33}P-labeled probes, or nonradioisotopic methods where probes are labeled with fluorochromes or the enzymes horseradish peroxidase and alkaline phosphatase. *In situ* hybridization is a valuable tool for the study of gene expression following drug administration, but its role in nonclinical immunotoxicity evaluation remains to be established.

Histology of the Bone Marrow   The bone marrow is distributed throughout the cavities of the skeleton. The hematopoietic tissue is progressively limited to the proximal epiphyses of long bones, central skeleton, and skull after birth. Fat constitutes 70–80% of the bone marrow in rodents and only 50% in larger animals. Hematopoiesis takes place in the convoluted extravascular spaces of sinuses lined by a single layer of endothelial cells interdigitating with other cell types including reticular and dendritic cells. Niches are formed in the extravascular spaces where hematopoietic and myelopoietic cells can be generated. Bone marrow evaluation from sections of the femur or sternum is based on the cytological examination of smears to measure cellularity of the erythroid, myeloid, lymphoid, and megakaryocytic lines, the maturation of cells, and the ratio of myeloid to nucleated erythroid cells [60]. In most species, the myeloid:erythroid ratio has a slight myeloid predominance. The interpretation of results requires a peripheral blood cell count. From the limited published database, histological examination of the bone marrow is more likely to serve as a tool to detect myelotoxic drugs, which should be subsequently considered for extensive immunotoxicological evaluation.

Histology of the Thymus The thymus is located in the anterosuperior mediastinum, except in the guinea pig, where it is located in the neck. It consists of two independent lobes attached by connective tissue. Each lobe is divided into lobules. Lobules are the basic thymic functional units enclosed by a fibrous capsule (Fig. 10.4). Three main areas can be identified: the subcapsular zone containing the earliest progenitor cells; the cortical area, which is packed with immature thymocytes undergoing selection; and the medulla, which is less densely populated by mature lymphocytes ready to leave. The thymus architecture is grossly similar across species

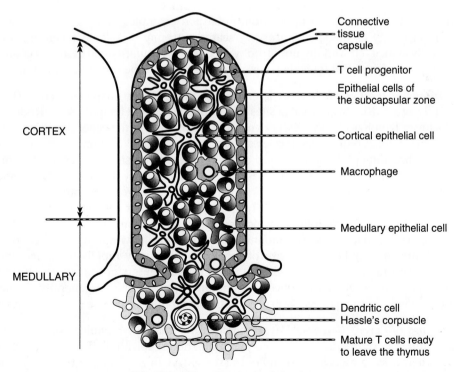

FIGURE 10.4 Histology of the thymus.

[57]. Blood vessels and closely related nerves enter the lobules at the corticomedullary junction and plunge into the cortex. The thymus develops early in fetal life and the peripheral immunologic repertoire is fully established at birth. The thymus size increases considerably after birth, peaks before puberty, and then involutes. Most of the parenchyma is progressively replaced by adipose tissue so that only sparse lymphoid islets are seen in aged animals. The reason for aging-associated thymus atrophy is not known. Involution of the thymus in response to stress can occur and is primarily due to an increased production of corticosteroid hormones. Acute involution is seen in the first few days after stress and regeneration starts very rapidly with proliferation of large thymocytes in the outer cortex. The size of the cortex gradually increases with a considerable reduction in size of the medulla. Transient hypertrophy can be seen. Systemic toxicity resulting in decreased food consumption, or stressful housing and handling of animals are possible causes of thymic involution. Most potent immunosuppressive drugs induce thymic atrophy in rodents.

Histology of the Spleen   The spleen is surrounded by a capsule of dense connective tissue that forms branched trabeculae extending into the parenchyma [61]. The red pulp is the most prominent compartment with large, irregular, thin-walled blood vessels—the splenic sinusoids—interposed between sheets of reticular connective tissue—the splenic cords of Billroth—containing many macrophages. In mice and to a lesser extent in rats, the red pulp is the site of extramedullary hematopoiesis. The white pulp consists of a central arteriole surrounded by periarteriolar lymphoid sheaths with many T cells—the thymo-dependent area—and adjacent follicles containing B cells. The marginal zone, easily identified in rats but absent in humans, is located at the border of the red and white pulps. Spleen weight is a relatively insensitive correlate of immunosuppression. Published examples of significant changes in the histology of the spleen are very scarce. Atrophy of splenic T cell areas is generally associated with thymus atrophy. Decreased cellularity and germinal center development in splenic follicular areas are considered to be sensitive parameters.

Histology of the Lymph Nodes   Lymph nodes have a bean-shaped structure (Fig. 10.5). They are usually grouped at sites connecting blood and lymph vessels. Rodents have fewer lymph nodes than larger animals or humans, but the general architecture is relatively consistent across species despite interindividual differences and pathogen-free breeding [57]. The structure of lymph nodes consists of the cortical, paracortical, and medullary areas. Antigens enter lymph nodes by the afferent lymphatic vessels, which end in the medulla. Free or processed antigens are presented to T lymphocytes in the paracortex and B lymphocytes encounter antigens in the cortical area containing primary follicles, which are aggregates of small resting B lymphocytes, and secondary follicles containing B lymphoblasts within germinal centers. Upon antigen stimulation, the size of lymph nodes is very rapidly increased and signs of hyperactivity with well-developed germinal centers appear. In the lymph nodes, histological changes induced by immunosuppressants are generally similar and concomitant to changes observed in other lymphoid organs (e.g., the thymus).

Histology of Peyer's Patches   Peyer's patches are areas of lymphoid tissue beneath the epithelium of the duodenum and jejunum. The organization of Peyer's patches and other mucosa-associated lymphoid tissue (MALT) is similar to that of lymph nodes [62]. A characteristic of MALT is that IgA is the predominant antibody pro-

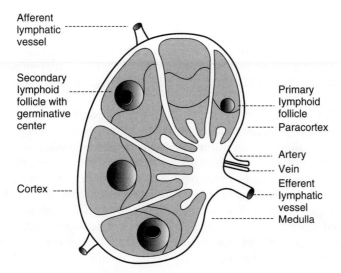

FIGURE 10.5   Histology of lymph nodes.

duced by mucosal B lymphocytes. Although histological examination of the Peyer's patches is often required, relevant endpoints need to be defined and very few examples of consistent histological changes induced by medicinal products have been reported.

10.4.2   Hematology and Immunology

Hematology endpoints are included in every toxicity study and some changes may be used as predictors of immunosuppression. Specific immunological endpoints can also be measured.

Hematology   Differential leukocyte counts enumerate neutrophils, lymphocytes, monocytes, eosinophils, and basophils in the peripheral blood. In general, statistically significant, dose-related changes of 10–20% from baseline values are considered relevant. Leukopenia, lymphopenia, neutropenia, and eosinophilia are suggestive of an immunosuppressive effect, but they may also be due to stress. Indeed, leukocytosis can be seen in excited or frightened animals. Neutrophilia is more frequent in dogs and lymphocytosis in rats. This should be carefully avoided by adequate handling of the animals. Neutrophilia can also reflect an inflammatory response to the technical procedure, such as catheter implantation or repeated injections. Neutropenia is generally a direct toxic effect of the test article. In contrast, lymphopenia, especially in rats where the number of lymphocytes is normally high, can suggest an immunosuppressive effect [63]. Hematopoietic cells from the bone marrow are exquisitely sensitive to cytotoxic effects. Bone marrow toxicity is primarily evidenced by colony-forming cell assays, but flow cytometry techniques are increasingly used [64]. A number of *in vitro* assays are available to investigate the effects of medicinal products on specific progenitor cell populations of rodents, dogs, and monkeys including CFU-E (erythroid), CFU-GM (granulocytic-macrophage), and CFU-MK (megakaryocytic) clonogenic assays.

Immunology

Serum Immunoglobulins   All classes of serum immunoglobulins can be assayed by ELISA in animals. In most instances, however, changes in serum immunoglobulins are not associated with consistent changes in other parameters.

Lymphocyte Subset Analysis   Flow cytometry is a powerful technique to analyze lymphocyte subsets [65]. Large populations of 10,000 or more single cells can be analyzed within a short period of time. Individual cells are passed in a fluid stream to be positioned through the path of a laser beam. The emitted light is gathered by detectors and then amplified by photomultiplier tubes. Information on cell size and density is obtained from the light scattered from each cell. Forward-angle light scatter is an approximate indicator of cell size used to distinguish viable from dead cells that exhibit lower forward-angle light scatter, whereas activated cells exhibit increased forward-angle light scatter. Side-angle light scatter correlates with granularity of the cell. Cell subsets can be recognized within complex cell populations using a combination of forward-angle and side-angle scatter. Fluorochromes (or fluorescent dyes), which interact with cells, enhance the power of flow cytometry. For instance, cells can be labeled with fluorochromes specific for surface markers (CDs). The resulting fluorescence is recorded cell by cell and quantified. The most recent cytometers can measure several fluorescence parameters simultaneously (multiparameter analysis). For lymphocyte subset analysis (immunophenotyping), lymphocytes are treated with a panel of monoclonal antibodies that are covalently bound to fluorochromes. In rodents, splenocytes are more commonly used than peripheral blood lymphocytes, but the latter may be more sensitive [66]. The use of lymphocyte subset analysis in nonclinical immunotoxicity evaluation largely derives from results obtained in the NTP interlaboratory study in B6C3F1 mice [67]. However, the conclusion of a panel of experts was that immunophenotyping has not been sufficiently validated to be recommended as a routine assay [68]. A major limitation is the current use of a small panel of lymphocyte subsets allowing the enumeration of total B and T lymphocytes, CD4$^+$ T lymphocytes and CD8$^+$ T lymphocytes. An important avenue of research is the use of activation surface markers [69], but no extensive validation studies have so far been conducted to compare changes in the expression of activation surface markers with the results of immune function assays.

Measurement of Humoral Immunity   Besides the measurement of serum immunoglobulin levels, humoral immunity can be assessed by antibody response toward a given antigen injected either a few days before or at the end of drug treatment. In rodents, the duration of treatment should be at least 21–28 days to take into account the half-life of immunoglobulins. The kinetics of antibody production is accelerated and the magnitude of the response is increased in secondary as compared to primary responses. IgM antibodies are initially and predominantly produced in primary responses, whereas IgG of greater affinity are the predominant antibodies in secondary responses. Anyway, primary responses are most often used. Despite obvious differences between primary and secondary responses, no comparative studies on their respective predictive potency have seemingly been performed. Most often, antibody responses are under the control of T lymphocytes because T-dependent antigens are by far the most commonly encountered antigens. Commonly used T-dependent antigens include sheep erythrocytes (SRBCs), bovine serum albumin (BSA), ovalbumin, tetanus toxoid, and keyhole limpet hemocyanin (KLH). SRBCs have long been the preferred antigen. Because they are not standardized and cannot be used in all animal species, they tend to be replaced by KLH. The use of T-independent antigens, such as DNP-Ficoll, TNP-*Escherichia coli* LPS, polyvinylpyrrolidone, and flagellin, is limited to mechanistic studies. Two different approaches can be used to assess humoral immunity, either the enumeration of antigen-specific antibody-producing spleen cells or the measurement of antigen-specific antibody serum levels. Rare comparative studies have been performed [70–72], so that the respective sensitivity of each approach is not known.

PLAQUE-FORMING CELL (PFC) ASSAY   The PFC assay measures the production of specific antibodies by antibody-producing cells following immunization in rodents [73]. SRBCs are the most widely used antigens, but KLH or tetanus toxoid can also be used after coupling to SRBCs using tannic acid, chromic chloride, or carbodiimide. Because of considerable variations depending on the antigen and the experimental protocol, only SRBCs are used in the direct PFC assay for nonclinical immunotoxicity evaluation (Fig. 10.6). Due to variable antigenicity, the same commercial source of SRBCs should be used even though batch-to-batch variability will still exist. SRBCs can be stored at +4 °C for several weeks. Typically, $(1-5) \times 10^8$ SRBCs are injected intravenously. The intraperitoneal route can also be used. The animals are sacrificed after 4–5 days. A suspension of splenocytes is incubated with SRBCs and guinea pig complement for 3 hours over a slide according to Cunningham's technique. At the end of the incubation period, pale areas (plaques) corresponding to the lysis of red blood cells around an antibody-producing cell are counted with the naked eye or at a very small magnification. The number is usually given for 10^5 or 10^6 splenocytes. Based on the results of the NTP interlaboratory validation study [67], the direct PFC assay has long been considered to be the first-line function assay for nonclinical immunotoxicity evaluation. Because SRBCs are not properly standardized antigens, there is marked inter- and intralaboratory variability. In addition, cell counting cannot be automated and results vary depending on the technician's skill. Finally, this is a time-consuming assay that must be

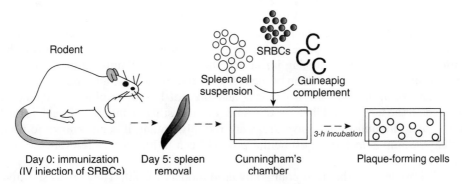

FIGURE 10.6   Plaque-forming cell (PFC) assay.

performed shortly after sacrifice of the animals, which requires appropriate human resources.

ELISA   Enzyme-linked immunoadsorbent assays (ELISA) are increasingly preferred to measure humoral immunity in nonclinical immunotoxicity evaluation. They offer the advantage of measuring a large number of samples in a relatively short period of time using an automated and properly standardized technique. Samples stored at $+4\,^\circ$C or frozen can be measured at a later date, and antibody levels can be measured on several occasions in the same animal. ELISA typically follows a five-step procedure: (1) coating of the microtiter plate wells with antigen; (2) blocking of all unbound sites to prevent false-positive results; (3) addition of the antibody to the wells; (4) addition of anti-IgG conjugated to an enzyme; and (5) reaction of a substrate with the enzyme (e.g., horseradish peroxidase or alkaline phosphatase) to produce a colored product indicative of a positive response. The color intensity is measured by a spectrophotometer. Results are expressed as absorbance values, optical density ratios (by comparing the optical density of the test sample with reference negative samples), or comparison to a standard curve. ELISA consists of relatively complex systems that require careful selection of the technique, adequate reagents and equipment, and technical skill to assure the quality, reproducibility, sensitivity, and accuracy of results. ELISA was first used to measure antibody responses to SRBCs [74], but today KLH is increasingly the most popular antigen [75–77]. As antibody responses vary depending on the antigen, differences in sensitivity can be expected. Decision on the most appropriate antigen as regards sensitivity and predictability can only be made when adequate data are available.

Measurement of Cellular Immunity   *In vivo* animal models or *in vitro* assays can be used to measure cellular immunity in nonclinical immunotoxicity evaluation.

IN VIVO ANIMAL MODELS   *In vivo* models are easy to perform and offer the advantage of taking into account the possible influence of other systems, such as the nervous and endocrine systems that may be negatively affected by the test article, which in turn may result in immune changes. Either the classical delayed-type hypersensitivity (DTH) or contact hypersensitivity model can be used [78]. Whatever the model, the experimental protocol consists of the sensitization (or induction) phase during which the animals receive one or several administrations of the reference immunogen, or contact sensitizer, then a rest period of 7–14 days required for the immune system to mount the expected immune response, and finally the eliciting (or challenge) phase, where the animals are administered the same immunogen, or contact sensitizer as previously. The selection of the immunogen or contact sensitizer, the dose and number of sensitizing injections, the route of administration during the sensitization phase, the duration of the rest period, and the dose and route of administration during the induction phase is actually not based on objective data, but instead on the technical skill and experience of the testing facilities. Although results with potent immunosuppressive drugs are roughly similar, it is not known to what extent variations in the experimental protocol can influence the relevance of the measured effects.

DTH models are the most commonly used models [79, 80]. They are as sensitive as *in vitro* assays. Commonly used T-dependent antigens include SRBCs, KLH, BSA, ovalbumin, and tetanus toxoid. SRBCs are typically preferred in rodents, whereas KLH and tetanus toxoid are preferred in nonrodents. The antigen is injected either subcutaneously or intradermally during the sensitization phase. In rodents, the preferred sites of injection are the back, the basis of the tail, or the footpad for sensitization, and the footpad for elicitation. Hind-footpad thickness is most commonly used to measure the magnitude of the DTH response. The use of a dial caliper is a simple technique and more sophisticated methods, such as ^{125}I diffusion, footpad weight, or footpad dye accumulation, are not more sensitive [81]. Footpad thickness is measured immediately prior to elicitation, and then 24–72 hours later on one or several occasions. The reaction normally peaks at 48 hours. Nonrodents are sensitized either subcutaneously or intradermally in one site and elicited in another site. DTH is assessed after intradermal injection of the antigen, which induces a skin reaction similar to that seen in human skin testing [82]. The magnitude of the reaction is measured semiquantitatively from the size of the erythema and the presence of edema.

Contact hypersensitivity models are primarily used in mice and guinea pigs. The experimental protocol is very close to that of contact sensitization assays [83, 84]. Strong contact sensitizers, such as picryl chloride, oxazolone, and DNFB in mice, and DNCB in guinea pigs, can be used. They are applied topically on the shaved abdomen or interscapular area to sensitize the animals that are elicited topically on the shaved abdomen (guinea pig, mouse) or the ear (mouse) after a short rest period. In guinea pigs, the response (erythema, edema) is measured semiquantitatively. Ear thickness measurement using a dial caliper is the preferred method in mice. Ear thickness is measured immediately prior to elicitation, and again 24–48 hours later. Immunosuppressive drugs decrease ear swelling.

IN VITRO ASSAYS

Lymphocyte Proliferation Lymphocyte proliferation assays are based on the ability of cultured lymphocytes to proliferate. At termination of the drug treatment, animals are killed to collect lymphocytes, either from the peripheral blood, the spleen, or lymph nodes. Lymphocytes are typically cultured for 72 hours. The addition of a mitogen induces the nonspecific proliferation of either T (concanavalin-A, phytohemagglutinin) or B (LPS) lymphocytes, or both (pokeweed mitogen). Proliferation can also be induced by alloantigens. The animals are then sensitized *in vivo* by an antigen, such as tuberculin, and lymphoproliferation is induced *in vitro* by the addition of the mycobacterial extract PPD to lymphocyte cultures. Finally, lymphocyte proliferation can be triggered in a mixed lymphocyte response assay, where a cell suspension derived from the spleen of treated animals is incubated in the presence of pooled stimulator splenocytes from control histoincompatible animals after inactivation by mitomycin C [85]. Whatever the selected assay, tritiated thymidine is added 4–24 hours before culture termination for incorporation into proliferating lymphocytes. The incorporated radioactivity measured using a liquid scintillation counter is a correlate of lymphocyte proliferation and hence of cellular immunity. Colorimetric methods, using MTT or XTT, or BrdU incorporation can also be used to quantitate lymphocyte proliferation [86], but proliferation indices are at least 10 times less than with thymidine so that lower sensitivity or accuracy can be suspected [87].

T Lymphocyte Cytotoxicity   Cytotoxic CD8$^+$ T lymphocytes are specifically cytotoxic to target cells. The *in vitro* induction of T lymphocyte cytotoxicity from splenocytes of treated animals is used to evaluate cellular immunity [87]. Splenocytes of treated and control animals are cocultured for 5 days with histoincompatible target cells, for example, P815 mastocytoma cells in mice and Fu-G1 tumor cells in rats, and inactivated by mitomycin C. Four hours before culture termination, the splenocytes are added to fresh ^{51}Cr-labeled target cells. Cytotoxicity is measured from the radioactivity released into the supernatant. Cell-mediated cytotoxicity can also be measured by flow cytometry [88].

Cytokine Assays   Because cytokines play pivotal roles in the triggering, nature, and control of immune responses, cytokine assays are deemed to become essential components of nonclinical immunotoxicity evaluation [89]. A number of hurdles, however, should be overcome for optimal performance of these assays: (1) very low concentrations of cytokines exert pleiotropic effects on numerous target cells; (2) cytokines can be found under multiple molecular forms with different assay behaviors; (3) a number of endogenous cytokine inhibitors have been described; and (4) the half-life of cytokines is usually less than 10 minutes. The conditions of sampling and storage of biological fluids for cytokine measurements are therefore of crucial importance. Sterile sampling on EDTA, but not heparin, is recommended for immunoassays. Sera must be decanted immediately and frozen at −80 °C. Bioassays measure cytokine levels in a biological system, usually a cell line [90]. Results are calculated by comparing with a standard dose–response curve obtained with known graded concentrations of the cytokine. Bioassays lack specificity and sensitivity and are time consuming. Immunoassays [91], either radioimmunoassays or ELISA, are much more specific and sensitive, but they are based on the binding of antibodies to the cytokine under scrutiny irrespective of its functional role. Many commercial kits are available, but results obtained with one kit may not be reproducible with another kit. Cytokines were initially measured in supernatants of cells stimulated by mitogens or anti-CD3 antibodies in order to achieve measurable levels, but subtle changes in cytokine production may not be detected under these conditions and observed changes may differ from those observed without stimulation. More recent techniques can measure cytokine levels in whole blood [92] or intracellular cytokines [93].

Measurement of Innate Immunity   Although innate immunity plays a major role in the protection of the host against pathogens, measurement of the components and mechanisms involved during nonclinical immunotoxicity evaluation has not been paid as much attention as those involved in adaptive immunity.

PHAGOCYTOSIS   As phagocytosis is a complex process involving different steps, a number of *in vivo* and *in vitro* techniques have been proposed. Most assays have been developed for clinical immunology purposes to investigate primary (hereditary) defects. Overall, they have not been properly standardized and validated from a toxicological point of view. Clearance assays measure the elimination of a substance by phagocytic cells *in vivo*. The standard assay is the *Listeria monocytogenes* clearance assay [94]. Mice or rats are injected intravenously with a suspension of *L.monocytogenes* and then killed at day 1 or 2 postinjection. After spleen removal, serial dilutions are plated to determine the number of colony-forming units. The

L.monocytogenes can also be inoculated intratracheally and the number of viable bacteria in the lungs is counted [95]. Ingestion assays measure the number of pathogens ingested per neutrophil or macrophage *in vitro*. They are not considered to be reliable tools to measure phagocytosis and in addition they are time consuming. The respiratory burst consists of metabolic changes leading to increases in oxygen uptake, oxidation of glucose uptake via the hexose monophosphate shunt, production of hydrogen peroxide and superoxide anion, generation of photons of light, and reduction of tetrazolium dyes. Metabolic assays measure either one of these changes [96]. Superoxide production can be measured from cytochrome-*c* reduction using a spectrophotometer. Chemiluminescence corresponds to light emission by stimulated cells, for example, phagocytes in the early phase of phagocytosis. As the quantity of light emitted is extremely low, amplifying agents, such as luminol, are used. In the presence of hydrogen peroxide or superoxide anion, luminol is converted to aminophthalic acid and photons of light are emitted, which are measured using a chemiluminometer. Chemiluminescence assays are time consuming and require technical skill and dedicated expensive equipment. Interestingly, they can be used *ex vivo* or *in vivo* and comparable results have been obtained in humans, rats, monkeys, and dogs [97]. Flow cytometry is another technique for the evaluation of phagocytosis [98]. The combination of forward-angle light scatter (size) and side-angle light scatter (granularity) allows for the discrimination between lymphocytes and polymorphonuclear leukocytes (PMNLs). Nonlymphocytes are gated to forward-angle light scatter and analyzed for associated fluorescence related to bacteria, fungi, or beads labeled with a fluorescent dye, most often fluorescein isothiocyanate. The oxidative burst can also be measured from the conversion of nonfluorescent substrates into fluorescent products by flow cytometry [99].

CHEMOTAXIS   Infections in patients with congenital disorders of phagocyte motility demonstrate the importance of leukocyte motility and chemotaxis in innate immunity. Several techniques are available [100]. Boyden's technique measures the distance traveled by leukocytes *in vitro* through a polycarbonate or nitrocellulosis filter covered with a chemoattractant substance, such as formyl-methionyl-leucyl-phenylalanine (FMLP). In the agarose technique, migration is measured in wells of 2–3 mm in diameter dug in agarose. Wells contain the leukocyte suspension, the chemoattractant, or a control substance. Chemotaxis is measured by comparing the distance traveled by leukocytes toward the well containing the chemoattractant and the well containing the control substance.

NK CELL ACTIVITY   The gold standard assay to measure NK cell activity is the ^{51}Cr release assay [22]. Target cells, either YAK-1 murine lymphoma cells in rodents or K562 human myeloma cells in monkeys, are labeled with ^{51}Cr. Thereafter, splenocytes or peripheral blood mononuclear cells are incubated with labeled target cells at 37 °C. Different effector:target cell ratios are used, for example, 200:1, 100:1, 50:1, or 25:1, as comparison of the percent lysis at a single effector:target ratio does not provide a quantitative assessment of potency between groups. Radioactivity of the supernatant is measured using a liquid scintillation counter. NK cell activity is calculated by comparing the radioactivity released by target cells in the presence of effector cells with the maximal radioactivity released by target cells in the presence of HCl or Triton X100. Spontaneous release is also taken into account. Flow cytometry is an alternative to the ^{51}Cr release assay. Target cells are labeled with 5-(6)-carboxy-fluorescein succinimidyl ester (CFSE). Subsequent labeling with propidium iodide is used to identify dead target cells. Results are expressed as the percentage of dead targets on a cell-to-cell basis. Flow cytometry has been used in rats and monkeys, and preliminary results suggest sensitivity similar to that of the ^{51}Cr release assay [101]. As compared to the ^{51}Cr release assay, flow cytometry offers the advantage of avoiding the use of radioisotopes, combining the measurement of NK cell activity with NK cell counting in the same animal and measuring NK cell activity on several occasions. The relevance of NK cell activity in nonclinical immunotoxicity evaluation is debatable. Potent immunosuppressive drugs, such as cyclosporine or azathioprine, exerted no effect in most studies. In fact, only a few drugs and chemicals (e.g., some morphine derivatives) were shown to inhibit NK cell activity reproducibly in rodents.

COMPLEMENT   Exploration of the complement system is very rarely included in nonclinical immunotoxicity evaluation and then often is limited to the measurement of CH50 or C3 and C4 component serum levels that are endpoints neither sensitive nor comprehensive enough to provide an in-depth analysis of the effects of medicinal products on the complement system. A comprehensive study performed in a highly specialized laboratory is recommended when the complement system is a suspected target.

Host Resistance Models   As changes in the histology of lymphoid organs and/or immune function may only be mild to moderate, or inconsistent, host resistance models can be helpful to determine whether the observed changes can be associated with impaired resistance to experimental microbial infections or implanted tumors [102]. In the early days of immunotoxicology, host resistance models were considered to be pivotal assays [103]. Their use, however, declined after several studies showed correlations between immune function changes and resistance to infection [104, 105], and also because of the growing concern about animal welfare issues. The use of host resistance models nevertheless is still an open question [106]. In experimental infection models, the pathogenicity of the infectious agent should ideally be as close as can be to that of the spontaneous human disease. It is also essential that the selected infectious agent can be used in conditions ensuring an adequate level of safety and compliance to good laboratory practices. Highly virulent pathogens are a significant biohazard risk and thus require appropriate safety measures. Finally, the immunological mechanisms involved in the infectious model should match with the immunotoxicity profile of the test article. Experimental infections where humoral defense mechanisms are primarily involved (e.g., *Streptococcus pneumoniae* or *Klebsiella pneumoniae* infections) are irrelevant to assess medicinal products that mainly alter cellular immunity. On the other hand, infections involving cellular defense mechanisms, such as *L.monocytogenes* infections, are not helpful to investigate medicinal products that impair humoral immunity. However, most immunotoxic drugs impair more than one aspect of immune functions and several host defense mechanisms are usually involved in fighting pathogens. The selection of an adequate infectious model is therefore difficult.

A variety of viral infection models have been proposed. Two rat models deserve particular attention, namely, infections with cytomegalovirus [104] and influenza virus [107]. NK cell activity was shown to play a major role in the defense against cytomegalovirus, and humoral immunity in the defense against influenza virus. Infection with *L. monocytogenes* is a prototypic bacterial infectious model [108]. In normal animals, most injected *Listeria* are removed by macrophages. Surviving *Listeria* multiply in the liver, but the infection stops within 5–6 days when cell-mediated immunity is not otherwise impaired. Mortality or the number of viable pathogens in the spleen and liver of inoculated animals are the measured endpoints. Infections with *Streptococcus pneumoniae* and *zooepidemicus*, where the complement and humoral immunity play a major role, are also widely used [109]. Parasitic infections offer the advantage of a more consistent virulence and endpoints other than lethality can easily be measured. The *Trichinella spiralis* model, where cellular immunity plays a pivotal role in addition to enhanced parasite elimination by specific antibodies, is the most popular parasitic infection model [110]. An orally administered suspension of larvae induces infection, manifesting after one week with worms in the gut of 50–70% of the animals that are sacrificed on day 14 postinfestation to count adult worms. Immunosuppressed animals have a much higher number of encysted larvae than normal animals. Specific serum IgE levels can also be measured as a correlate to anti-infectious resistance.

Because of their low incidence, spontaneous tumors cannot be used as an indicator of unexpected immunosuppression in nonclinical studies. A number of implanted tumor models have been proposed of which fibrosarcoma PYB6 and melanoma B16F10 were more often used [102]. All tumor models include the injection of a suspension of tumor cells, a rest period to allow for tumor progression, the onset of a palpable tumor, and finally death of the animal. A syngenic tumor must be used to avoid tumor rejection by specific immune mechanisms. A small number of tumor cells to induce tumors in 10–30% of control animals is preferred so that associated drug-induced immunosuppression can be expected to result in increased incidence of tumors in treated animals. Measured endpoints include the incidence of tumors or animals with one or several tumors, the delay between inoculation of tumor cells and the appearance of palpable tumors, the time of tumor growth, the number of nodules, mortality, or the delay to death.

10.5   PRECLINICAL ASSESSMENT OF IMMUNOSTIMULATION

Relatively limited data are available regarding the nonclinical evaluation of (unexpected) immunostimulation as immunotoxicologists have long focused most of their efforts on immunosuppression and potent immunostimulatory drugs have only recently been introduced into the clinical setting.

10.5.1   Histology

Like unexpected immunosuppression, standard histological examination of lymphoid organs in repeated dose toxicity studies can be used to detect unintended immunostimulatory drugs. Technical aspects and the interpretation of results are also globally similar (see Section 10.4). Immunostimulation has been reported to be associated with increased spleen weight, even though no histological changes may be detectable; hyperplasia of the bone marrow, red and white pulps of the spleen, and lymph nodes, with mononuclear cell infiltration and more numerous germinal centers; and mononuclear cell infiltration in the liver, lungs, and adrenal glands [111–113]. Extramedullary hematopoiesis, particularly in the spleen, has been observed in mice [114]. Histology of the thymus does not seem to be affected.

10.5.2   Hematology and Immunology

Mild-to-moderate hyperleukocytosis and lymphocytosis may occur [113, 115]. Depending on the mechanism of action, acute-phase response reflecting immune activation can result in decreased albumin and total protein serum levels [116]. A slight increase in liver weight, liver enzyme serum levels, and bilirubin and fibrinogen levels is possible. Increased serum Ig levels and increased B lymphocyte counts, and decreased CD8+ T lymphocyte counts have rarely been observed.

10.5.3   Immune Function Assays

The immune function assays used to detect unintended immunostimulatory drugs are those used to detect immunosuppressive drugs. Enhanced responses have been reported using the PFC assay [117], antitetanus toxoid antibody levels [118], DTH to SRBCs [119] or *L.monocytogenes* [120], mitogen-stimulated lymphocyte proliferation [121], NK cell activity [122], or resistance to *T.spiralis* experimental infections [123]. Whether the same experimental conditions are appropriate to detect unintended immunostimulatory effects as reliably as immunosuppressive effects has rarely if ever been addressed. Indeed, animal models and assays designed to detect immunosuppression involve the use of optimal doses of the antigen to mount a humoral or cellular response, or optimal mitogen concentration in lymphoproliferation assays. From a theoretical point of view at least, suboptimal antigen doses or mitogen concentrations can be expected to result in improved detection of unintended immunostimulation. *In vitro* screens using various cell lines have been proposed to predict the cytokine-releasing potency of immunostimulatory drugs [124, 125].

10.5.4   Host Resistance Models

Because host resistance models are intended to assess the immunotoxicological relevance of observed immune changes, models applicable for the prediction of adverse consequences related to unexpected immunostimulation differ from those applicable to immunosuppressive drugs. Thus, experimental infection models are intended to detect enhanced resistance and it would be logical to use microbial challenge expected to kill more control animals than in experimental infection models, which are used to predict immunosuppression associated with decreased resistance. However, experimental infection models using the same design as in the evaluation of immunosuppressive drugs have been used [126].

More specific animal resistance models are those intended to predict whether immunostimulatory drugs trigger, accelerate, and/or aggravate autoimmune processes [127]. A variety of genetically prone mouse and rat strains develop frequent autoimmune diseases. NZB × NZW F_1 hybrid female mice develop a syndrome similar to SLE with anti-DNA autoantibodies as early as 2 months of age, and immune complex glomerulonephritis with proteinuria resulting in shorter life expectancy [128]. The IgG and C3 deposits in the mesangium are evidenced by immuno-fluorescence from 5 months of age. Severe cortical thymic atrophy is a consistent finding, whereas spleen and lymph node hyperplasia is of variable intensity. An accelerated time course of the disease in this model reflects the detrimental effects of immunostimulatory drugs [129]. In the MRL-lpr/lpr mouse, the spontaneous disease is characterized by massive generalized lymphadenopathy as early as 8 weeks of age, immune glomerulonephritis, degenerative lesions of the coronary arteries and myocardium, and a high incidence of autoantibodies sometimes associated with polyarthritis, autoantibodies, and circulating immune complexes [130]. Life expectancy is less than 6 months. Clinical features similar to human type-I insulin-dependent diabetes mellitus (IDDM) are noted in nonobese diabetic (NOD) mice with a progressive onset of hyperglycemia, glycosuria, ketonuria, polydipsia, polyuria, and polyphagia [131]. Insulitis consisting of an infiltration of B and T lymphocytes in pancreatic islets resulting in loss of β-cells is evidenced by histological examination. Diabetes is best detected from blood glucose levels, but glycosuria can be used to avoid frequent bleeding. The incidence of diabetes is generally 80–100% in females and 30–50% in males. Female mice are permanently hyperglycemic at 3–6 months of age versus 5–8 months in males. Mice normally die within 5–7 weeks after reaching peak blood glucose levels. The incidence and course of the disease can be altered by immunomodulating drugs [132]. Two autoimmunity-prone rat strains can also be used. Mercuric chloride was shown to induce B lymphocyte polyclonal activation with a massive and rapid increase in IgE levels resulting in immune complex formation and glomerulonephritis in the Brown-Norway (BN) rat [133]. Although mercury has never been convincingly demonstrated to induce autoimmunity in exposed human subjects, the BN rat model is used to investigate the potential of drugs and chemicals for inducing or facilitating autoimmunity [134]. Typically, 60–80% of BB (Bio-Breeding) rats develop IDDM between 60 and 120 days of age, and facilitation of the disease has been reported following treatment with low doses of the interferon inducer poly(I:C) [135]. In addition to genetically autoimmunity-prone animals, a variety of experimental autoimmune diseases can be induced in laboratory animals. Arthritis induced by subcutaneous injections of Freund's complete adjuvant (FCA) or collagen type II in rodents is commonly used [136]. Lesions vary depending on the strain. The progress and severity of the disease are assessed from footpad swelling and joint deformity, histological examination of the joints, and various imaging techniques. Experimental autoimmune encephalomyelitis (EAE) is a model of multiple sclerosis [137]. Following immunization with myelin proteins, rodents develop clinical manifestations, such as loss of tail tonus and forelimb paralysis, which can easily be quantified. Overall, conflicting results have been obtained with genetically prone animal models and extremely few data are available regarding the use of experimental autoimmune disease models for nonclinical immunotoxicity evaluation.

10.6   PRECLINICAL ASSESSMENT OF HYPERSENSITIVITY

In sharp contrast to the growing concern about drug-induced hypersensitivity reactions, only limited aspects can be predicted and most available animal models and assays have at best poor predictability [138, 139].

10.6.1   Models of IgE-Mediated Hypersensitivity Reactions

As most medicinal products are not directly immunogenic because of their small size, they have to bind to carrier macromolecules to induce sensitization. As already mentioned, direct interaction with T lymphocytes bypassing hapten formation has been shown to occur and result in hypersensitivity reactions, but no generally applicable animal models are available to date. Because most medicinal drugs are devoid of the chemical reactivity that is required for covalent binding, reactive metabolites are widely considered to be involved instead of the parent molecule. The site of binding and degree of conjugation are critical factors [140]. Depending on the system used, IgG, IgM, or IgE are raised against the carrier, the hapten, or both. Attempts to reproduce spontaneously occurring haptenization have so far been unsuccessful. The selection of the optimal route of administration is another unsolved issue. The oral route—the most common route of therapeutic administration in humans—typically leads to tolerance instead of sensitization. Sensitization via the intranasal or intratracheal route is possible, but has so far only been documented with highly reactive chemicals [141]. Therefore, caution is required when interpreting positive results with highly reactive chemicals, such as industrial chemicals, intended to support the predictability of models or assays supposedly applicable to medicinal products as well as (false) negative results obtained with nonreactive medicinal products.

Whatever the model used, the induction of drug-specific IgE is a critical step. Although guinea pigs produce more IgG_1 than IgE when sensitized to an allergen, the detection of specific IgE is used for the evaluation of drug allergenicity [142, 143]. Adjuvants can be injected with the test article as a mixture or at different sites in order to increase sensitization. The use of Freund's complete adjuvant (FCA) is illogical as it favors a T_H1 response in contrast to aluminum hydroxide which induces a T_H2 response [144]. Specific IgE levels can be quantitated by passive cutaneous anaphylaxis (PCA) or ELISA. In PCA models, guinea pigs or mice are sensitized by several subcutaneous or intradermal injections of the test article alone or conjugated to a carrier [145]. Serum from sensitized animals is then injected intradermally into nonsensitized (naïve) guinea pigs, mice, or rats, and finally the test article mixed in a dye, such as blue Evans, is injected intravenously. When specific antibodies are present in the dermis, activation of mast cells ensues with subsequent release of vasoacting mediators. Due to increased capillary permeability, extravasation of the dye in tissues surrounding the injection site results in the formation of a blue spot, the size of which reflects the intensity of the reaction. ELISA can detect lower levels of specific IgE than PCA. It is noteworthy that most published results were obtained with penicillins or cephalosporins, and it is unknown to what extent they can be extrapolated to other classes of medicinal products. The induction of systemic anaphylaxis is another approach to evidence the production of specific IgE. During the first phase (elicitation or sensitization), guinea pigs are injected subcutaneously or intradermally on several occasions, and then after a rest phase of variable duration (usually 7–21 days), elicitation or challenge consists of the intravenous or intradermal injection of the test article. Severe acute reactions are characterized by markedly decreased respiratory rate and convulsions, followed by the death of the animal within 10–30 minutes. In mild-to-moderate reactions, clinical signs usually resolve within 30 minutes. Although systemic anaphylaxis guinea pig models have been

widely used, especially by Japanese authors, few validation studies have been conducted. A correlation was found between guinea pig results and the clinical experience with a panel of microbial extracts and vaccines [146]. A major limitation,
however, is that macromolecules of human origin or humanized molecules consistently induce false-positive responses in this model, which may explain why their
use is not recommended by ICH Guideline S6 on the preclinical safety evaluation
of biotechnology-derived pharmaceuticals [147].

10.6.2 Models of Contact Sensitization

Although contact sensitization is an immune-mediated reaction, none of the current
guidelines include contact sensitization in immunotoxicity studies of medicinal
products. Following the pioneer work of Landsteiner and Draize, guinea pig models
were once the most popular methods for the detection of contact sensitizers until
mouse models, particularly the local lymph node assay (LLNA), emerged as alternative models forty years later [148].

Guinea Pig Contact Sensitization Models   At least seven guinea pig models have
been accepted at some time point by regulatory authorities, but a number of other
models have been proposed [14]. No general agreement has ever been reached on
the optimal model or relative sensitivity of available models. Adjuvant-free models
are generally considered to be less sensitive compared to adjuvant models that were
sometimes claimed to be too sensitive and produce false-positive results. Similar
results across guinea pig strains and sex have been reported. The technical skill and
in-house historical data are in fact probably more important than the selected
experimental procedure. All guinea pig contact sensitization models include: (1) an
induction phase during which a mildly to moderately irritating concentration of the
test article is applied epidermally or intradermally (when the test article is absolutely nonirritating, a slightly irritating solvent/vehicle, e.g. sodium lauryl sulfate, can
be used); (2) a rest period of variable duration (e.g., 10–21 days); and (3) an eliciting
(challenge) phase where a nonirritating concentration of the test article is applied
topically on the shaved skin. Concentrations of the test article for the induction and
challenge phases are determined during a preliminary study. The magnitude of the
response is usually assessed by visual scoring including four grades (0 = no visible
change; 1 = discrete or patchy erythema; 2 = moderate and confluent erythema; 3 =
intense erythema and edema). Positive reference contact sensitizers are normally
not included, but the selected assay should be performed at least every 6 months
with positive controls to ensure the consistency of results in the testing facilities.
There is no general consensus regarding the selection of positive controls.

The occlusive patch test was originally proposed by Buehler [149]. It consists of
1 or 3 weekly applications of the test article using induction patches to the same
area of the shaved dorsal surface for 6 hours, and then occlusive patches maintained
for 3–9 hours. After a rest period of 10–14 days, 6 hour challenge patches with a
nonirritating concentration of the test article are applied to a naive clipped skin site.
Reactions are graded for erythema 24 and 48 hours after patch removal. The test
article is considered positive when sensitization is noted in at least 15% of animals.
Validation studies showed a relatively good but inconsistent correlation between
results in the Buehler test and clinical data [150]. One main advantage of the

Buehler test is the possibility to assess the final concentration or the whole formulation to be used commercially. The guinea pig maximization test (GPMT) was initially proposed by Magnusson and Kligman [151]. It consists of paired 0.1 mL intradermal injections of FCA, the test article mixed in a suitable vehicle, and a mixture of the test article dissolved or suspended in FCA into the clipped and shaved shoulders. On day 7, an occlusive patch is applied for 48 hours on the clipped shoulders. On day 21, challenge using a 4 cm² skin site on the left flank of the shaved abdomen is performed by application of a 24 hour occlusive patch with a nonirritating concentration of the test article in a suitable vehicle. The challenge site is observed at 24 and 48 hours after removal of the occlusive patch. The GPMT is a very sensitive test. The ranking of contact sensitizers used to be based on a five-grade scale: grade I (sensitization rate: 0–8%, weak); grade II (sensitization rate: 9–28%, mild); grade III (sensitization rate: 29–64%, moderate); grade IV (sensitization rate: 65–80%, strong); grade V (sensitization rate: 81–100%, extreme). Other guinea pig contact sensitization tests include the Freund's complete adjuvant test, in which the induction phase consists of three intradermal injections of a 1:1 mixture of FCA and the test article at a concentration not exceeding 5% into the suprascapular region, and the challenge phase consists of epicutaneous applications of several concentrations of the test article on 2 cm² areas of the clipped flank skin. The optimization test consists of 10 intracutaneous applications of a 0.1% solution or suspension of the test article every other day. The test article is incorporated in FCA at the same concentration during the second and third weeks. The animals are challenged intradermally 14 days after the last application, and then epicutaneously after a rest period of 10 days. The split adjuvant test was designed to allow assessing formulations following epidermal exposure. A 2 cm² area of shaved suprascapular skin is exposed to dry ice for 5 seconds prior to application of the test article on day 0. Occlusion is maintained for 48 hours until the next application. A total of four applications is used. Two intradermal injections of 0.1 mL of FCA are administered immediately before the fourth application on each side of the application site. The challenge consists of an open or occlusive application of the test article on day 21 and then the reaction is read after 24–72 hours. The open epicutaneous test consists of daily epicutaneous applications of the test article for 5–7 days and then 3:1 progressive dilutions up to a total of 20 applications on the intact skin of the flank. The animals are challenged on the contralateral clipped side of the flank with the test article or a nonirritating concentration on days 21 and 29 and the reactions are read at 24, 48, and 72 hours. Finally, the epicutaneous maximization test was developed to allow for assessing end-use products. The induction consists of topical applications of the test article on days 0, 2, 4, 7, 9, 11, and 14 using a 48 hour occlusive patch on the shaved suprascapular region. On day 0, 0.1 mL of FCA is injected intradermally. The challenge phase consists of the topical application of a nonirritating concentration of the test article on a naive skin site using a 48 hour occlusive patch on day 28.

Mouse Contact Sensitization Models In contrast to guinea pig models, mouse contact sensitization models were developed rather recently after ear swelling had become a popular endpoint to measure murine contact hypersensitivity. The Mouse Ear Swelling Test (MEST) was the first attempt to propose a murine alternative to guinea pig contact sensitization models using a very similar approach [152]. Initially, the MEST design included two intradermal injections of 0.05 mL of FCA into the abdomen immediately prior to the first topical application of the test article. Mice are dosed with 100 μL of a minimally irritating concentration of the test article or the vehicle topically on a previously shaved and tape-stripped abdominal area for 4 consecutive days. Seven days after the last application, 20–40 μL of the test article is applied to the left ear and 20–40 μL of the vehicle to the right ear. The thickness of both ears is measured with a micrometer at 24 and 48 hours postchallenge under light anesthesia. Of 49 known contact sensitizers tested, only vanillin, a mild sensitizer in guinea pigs and humans, was negative in the MEST and all 23 nonsensitizers were negative. Subsequent refinement included a diet supplemented with 250 IU/g vitamin A acetate starting 21 days before and maintained throughout the experiment to enhance ear swelling [153]. Results from several laboratories, however, showed that MEST is not a reliable model to detect weak-to-moderate sensitizers and a poorer predictor of contact sensitizers than the GPMT. MEST is no longer considered to be an alternative to guinea pig models.

Following pioneering work published as early as 1986 [154] and since then extensive interlaboratory validation studies [155, 156], the LLNA is widely accepted by regulatory authorities [157]. In contrast to all other contact sensitization models, the LLNA measures changes in the draining lymph node (i.e., the auricular lymph node) elicited in previously sensitized animals, instead of skin response [158]. Young adult female CBA/Ca or CBA/J mice are recommended as they proved to give more robust results. The test article can be dissolved in a suitable solvent or vehicle, for example, acetone/olive oil (4:1), *N,N*-dimethyl-formamide, methyl ethyl ketone, propylene glycol, or dimethylsulfoxide, and diluted if necessary. Several concentrations of the test article are generally used, but the highest achievable concentration should induce neither overt systemic toxicity nor excessive local irritation. For each mouse, 25 μL/ear of the test article is applied to the dorsum of both ears on days 1, 2, and 3. Then, mice are injected with 250 μL of sterile PBS containing 20 μCi of [^{3}H]-methyl thymidine via the tail vein on day 6. The auricular lymph node of each ear is excised 5 hours later and pooled in PBS for each animal. A single cell suspension of lymph node cells is prepared for each animal (Fig. 10.7). A stimulation index >3 is considered a positive response. Various modifications of the original protocol have been produced and include the measurement of proliferation by immunohistochemistry [159], IL-2 production [160], or BrdU incorporation [161]. Other endpoints including IL-6, IL-12, and IFN-γ production have been used, but none were shown to enhance sensitivity [162, 163]. Overall, the LLNA proved to be a sensitive assay to detect human contact allergens [164]. However, discrimination of primary irritants is a debated issue [165]. The percentage of B220$^+$ B lymphocytes in lymph nodes measured by flow cytometry was increased by contact sensitizers, but not by primary irritants [166].

10.6.3 Other Animal Models of T Lymphocyte-Mediated Hypersensitivity Reactions

Because T lymphocytes are involved in a number of immune-mediated reactions, it is tempting to use DTH or contact sensitization models to assess drug allergenicity. The subcutaneous injection of both benzylpenicillin conjugated to human serum albumin and FCA induced footpad swelling in mice 24 hours after injection of the

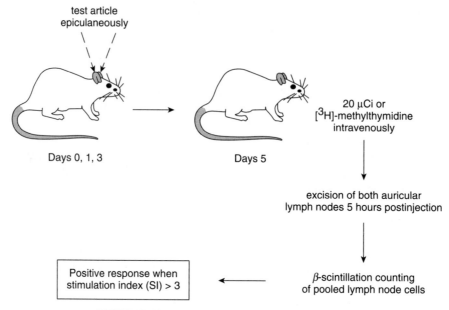

FIGURE 10.7 Local lymph node assay (LLNA).

conjugate into the footpad of previously sensitized mice [167]. Similar findings were obtained with nonconjugated cephalothin. Footpad swelling induced by sulfamethoxazole mixed with S9 mix was obtained in mice previously sensitized by subcutaneous injections in the back, showing the role of metabolites in the induction of DTH by sulfamethoxazole [168]. A comparison of published GPMT results with clinical experience showed a good, or relatively good, correlation for 59 drugs and chemicals and conflicting results for 11 [169]. In contrast, only 14 of 83 drugs reported to the U.S. FDA for inducing systemic hypersensitivity induced a positive guinea pig test [170].

10.6.4 Models of Pseudoallergic Reactions

Only rare animal models are available to predict the risk of drug-induced pseudoallergic reactions. Intravenous administration to dogs that are particularly sensitive to nonspecific degranulation of mast cells and basophils can be helpful to evidence the histamine-releasing properties of a test substance [171, 172]. *In vitro* or *ex vivo* assays, such as histamine release [173], basophil degranulation [174], or complement activation [175] as used for the diagnosis of clinical reactions, may be more valuable.

10.7 PRECLINICAL ASSESSMENT OF AUTOIMMUNITY

Two major hurdles in the preclinical assessment of drug-induced autoimmune reactions are the poor understanding of underlying mechanisms and the role of individual and environmental predisposing factors [176]. As already mentioned, more frequent autoimmune diseases can be associated with immunostimulatory drugs and these should be distinguished from drug-induced autoimmune reactions, which are addressed later. To date, no animal models are available to predict for the risk of drug-induced organ-specific autoimmune reactions. Early studies described autoantibodies in mice, rats, or dogs treated with a variety of drugs, but these findings either were obtained under conditions that did not mimic human treatment or could not be reproduced. Few studies searched for autoantibodies in the course of standard toxicity testing and results were either negative or conflicting [177]. Histological findings suggestive of an autoimmune process have sometimes been described [178]. Inflammation is the hallmark of autoimmunity in laboratory animals. However, mononuclear cell infiltration is not a reliable indicator of autoimmunity as it can be seen in autoimmune diseases as well as other pathological conditions. A predominantly CD4+ T lymphocyte infiltrate and follicular hyperplasia in the spleen and lymph nodes may be more reliable indicators. Because of the key role of genetics in autoimmunity, autoimmunity-prone animal species are often considered for use in nonclinical immunotoxicity evaluation. However, the usefulness of the Brown-Norway (BN) rat model to assess drug-induced autoimmunity is debatable [134] and the same conclusion applies to autoimmunity-prone mouse models [179].

The popliteal lymph node assay (PLNA) may be the only currently available assay that could prove a predictor of systemic autoimmune reactions [180]. The original assay—the direct PLNA—is simple and inexpensive (Fig. 10.8). The test article is injected subcutaneously into one mouse or rat hind footpad, and the same volume of the vehicle (usually 50 μL) into the contralateral footpad. Seven days later, both popliteal lymph nodes are removed and immediately weighed to calculate the treated:control weight ratio (weight index). A weight index >2 is considered to be a positive response; indices >10 are rarely observed. The selection of the vehicle is critical. Saline is the first-choice vehicle, but in case of poor solubility, 20% DMSO or 25% ethanol seems suitable. Acetone, methyl ethyl ketone, and pure

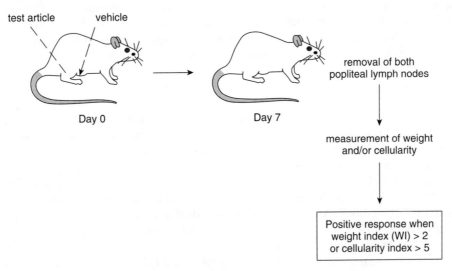

FIGURE 10.8 Popliteal lymph node assay (PLNA).

ethanol because of primary irritancy, and corn oil, paraffin oil, and 1,2-propylene glycol because of excessive viscosity should be avoided as they cause false-positive responses. The dose is selected arbitrarily (usually 1 mg in mice and 5 mg in rats). Similar results have been obtained using various strains of mice and rats. A stronger response has sometimes been observed with PLN removal on days 9–11, instead of day 7. To enhance PLNA sensitivity, additional endpoints have been proposed. The cellularity index (CI) is calculated from the ratio of treated:control cellularity of lymph nodes carefully crushed immediately after weighing. A CI > 5 is considered to be a positive response and indices >50 have been reported. CI has been suggested to enhance PLNA accuracy as well as sensitivity. In contrast, thymidine incorporation 5 hours after the intravenous administration of [^{3}H]methylthymidine or lymphocyte subset analysis did not enhance PLNA sensitivity. Standard histological examination shows changes reminiscent of a graft-versus-host (GvH) reaction with blurring of the lymph node architecture due to an intermingling of the cortical and paracortical areas, numerous immunoblasts in paracortical areas, high-grade maturation of germinal centers, and numerous plasma cells in medullary areas. Results on more than 130 compounds with the direct PLNA have been published and most often there was a parallelism between human and animal data. One interlaboratory study showed consistent blind results with a limited panel of compounds [181]. False-positive responses, however, have been reported. They can be due to sensitization or immunogenicity, but then histological examination shows a conserved architecture of the lymph node and numerous germinal centers. Nonspecific inflammation due to primary irritation is another cause of false-positive responses. Standard histological examination is not helpful in contrast to cytokine production, most notably IL-6 and IFN-γ that are increased by streptozotocin, but not acetone or ethanol [182]. Depletion in CD8$^+$ T lymphocytes by administration of an anti-CD8 monoclonal antibody prior to performing the PLNA is another possibility to rule out false-positive responses due to primary irritants [183]. False-negative responses can also be seen. They are primarily due to the involvement of metabolites. Increasing the dose can positive the response, but systemic toxicity can then occur. *In vitro* preincubation with S9 mix and pretreatment with an enzyme-inducing agent, such as β-naphthoflavone or phenobarbital, are helpful alternatives. As the direct PLNA does not demonstrate whether the reaction is antigen-specific, variations of the original technique have been proposed. The secondary PLNA consists of a first phase where the test article is administered as in the direct PLNA, or by the intranasal, oral, or intravenous route, and then a dose insufficient to induce a primary positive response is injected into one hind footpad of the same animals after a rest period of 4–6 weeks [184]. In the adoptive transfer PLNA, T lymphocytes from a previously exposed donor are injected subcutaneously into the hind footpad of a naive recipient and the next day, a suboptimal dose of the test article is injected subcutaneously at the same site [185]. The modified PLNA was proposed more recently [186]. In this assay, the test article is injected with the reported antigens TNP-Ficoll or TNP-ovalbumin into the footpad and the specific antibody response is measured on day 7 by ELISPOT. Compounds that induce inflammation elicit an IgG response to TNP-ovalbumin, but not to TNP-Ficoll, whereas those inducing a T-lymphocyte-mediated reaction elicit an IgG response to both TNP-ovalbumin and TNP-Ficoll. The measurement of IgG$_1$, and IgG$_{2a}$ and IgE, can differentiate T$_H$2 and T$_H$1 responses, respectively. Even though the available database is still small, the modified PLNA may prove more suitable to identify sensitizing drugs, whereas the direct PLNA seems to be more appropriate to detect drugs with potential for inducing autoimmune reactions [187, 188].

10.8   REGULATORY ASPECTS AND RISK ASSESSMENT

10.8.1   Guidelines

The evolution of concepts and techniques applicable to the nonclinical immunotoxicity evaluation of drugs was accompanied by regulatory documents [189]. The first step was the revision of OECD guideline 407 adopted on 27 July 1995, which requires histological examination of the main lymphoid organs in the control and high dose groups of 28 day rat toxicity studies [190]. The next year, the International Conference on Harmonization (ICH) S6 guideline emphasized the role of immunotoxicity in the safety evaluation of biotechnology-derived products [191]. In 2000, the European Medicines Evaluation Agency (EMEA) issued a note for guidance on repeated dose toxicity including a long annex on immunotoxicity testing [192], and two years later, the U.S. FDA released a guidance on the immunotoxicology evaluation of investigational new drugs [193]. Finally, the ICH S8 guideline on immunotoxicity studies for human pharmaceuticals was adopted on 15 September 2005 [194].

10.8.2   Good Laboratory Practices in Immunotoxicity Evaluation

Nonclinical immunotoxicity evaluation studies should adhere to GLP rules, but this issue has very rarely been addressed [195]. Different commercial sources of animals of the same strain can result in variable immune responsiveness. Transport conditions can also affect immune function, but changes are usually of short duration. Factors of animal environment including light, noise, humidity, temperature, bedding, or cage size can impact on immunocompetence. A critical issue may be the influence of changes in housing conditions. Different immune responses have indeed been described, even though inconsistently, between singly and group-housed animals, or between animals enjoying or not enjoying environmental enrichment. Handling stress is often associated with a certain degree of immunosuppression. The poor standardization of reagents is another issue. Most immunological reagents have not been carefully standardized. SRBCs are a typical example: there is marked variability of results, which is partly due to the use of different animal sources and the time lag between samplings in the same animal. When species-specific reagents are not available, cross-reacting reagents may be used, but careful validation is absolutely required prior to performing the assay. It is also important to bear in mind that similar reagents or kits may generate variable results depending on the commercial source.

10.8.3   Strategy for the Evaluation of Unintended Immunosuppression

The potential for unintended immunosuppression is typically investigated in rodent short-term repeated-dose studies.

Species Selection   General toxicity data should preferably be available in the species selected for nonclinical immunotoxicity assessment to ensure a sound interpretation of histological and/or functional immune changes. Even though the largest interlaboratory study by far was conducted in the B6C3F$_1$ mouse, a hybrid strain bred from C57Bl/6N female and DNA/2N male mice [7], the rat is currently the most commonly used species. It is noteworthy that most current concepts or assays derive from the results of mouse studies and that the available database in rats is much smaller than in mice, and often restricted to a few potent immunosuppressive drugs. The selection of an outbred instead of an inbred strain has been the matter of long debate, but as outbred strains showed no greater interindividual variability, they are currently preferred. It is essential to bear in mind that interindividual variability is a major issue in the interpretation of immunotoxicity studies. Animals as well as human subjects are either good or poor immune responders. As it is absolutely impossible to predict whether a given animal is likely to be a poor or good responder, unexpected difficulties for the interpretation of results may arise when one group of animals (e.g., control animals) obviously includes a greater percentage of poor or good responders. Even though rodents are commonly used, a nonrodent species may be preferred, such as monkeys for the evaluation of biotechnology-derived products with no detectable biological activity in rats. Surprisingly, other nonrodent species, such as dogs or mini-pigs, have so far very rarely been used.

Route and Duration of Administration   The test article is typically administered daily for 28 days using the intended route of administration in human subjects. There is seemingly no evidence that exposure of longer duration can be associated with either exacerbated or delayed immunosuppression. Few data are available for routes other than the oral route, except for the intravenous route.

Dose Selection   Only doses that do not cause overt toxicity should normally be used. It is often recommended that the highest dose should not result in a decrease in weight gain of more than 10% as compared to control animals. Indeed, doses either overtly toxic or associated with exaggerated pharmacodynamic effects can induce stress-related immune changes due to the release of corticosteroid hormones or other mediators, such as increases in circulating neutrophils, decreases in circulating lymphocytes and thymus weight and thymic cortical cellularity, and changes in spleen and lymph node cellularity [194].

Measured Endpoints   Strict tiered protocols [6] are no longer recommended and current strategies to detect unexpectedly immunosuppressive drugs are based primarily on the histological examination of the lymphoid organs as required by the ICH S8 guideline. There is an ongoing debate whether standard histology of the main lymphoid organs is sensitive enough. A number of pathologists claimed that standard histological examination is a reliable tool [196–198], but there was also a wide belief that immune function assays are nevertheless needed [199]. So far, only one study carefully addressed this issue [200]: the critical importance of the pathologist's skill and the criteria selected for scoring histological changes was highlighted, and the conclusion was that histopathology is not as sensitive as immune function assays, even though it may provide a reasonable level of accuracy to identify immunosuppressive chemicals. When an immune function assay is considered to be necessary, for example, because clinical signs or histological changes suggestive of immunosuppression have been noted, or depending on the pharmacological mechanism of action, or the intended therapeutic use (weight of evidence), it is widely agreed that a T-cell-dependent antibody response assay is the first-line immune function assay in additional animals to avoid possible changes caused by antigenic stimulation even though there is no indication that this might happen. Indeed, antibody response assay offers the advantage to assess antigen presentation by APCs, T lymphocyte control, and antibody production by B lymphocytes, simultaneously. As already mentioned, ELISA to measure anti-KLH antibodies is increasingly the preferred method. Second-line assays, such as lymphocyte subset analysis, NK cell activity measurement, delayed-type hypersensitivity or lymphocyte proliferation assays, and macrophage/neutrophil function assays, are only recommended when standard histology and a T-cell-dependent antibody response assay suggest possible immunosuppressive effects. The selection of assays will depend on the type and magnitude of changes observed initially and the weight of evidence.

10.8.4   Strategies for the Nonclinical Evaluation of Other Immunotoxic Effects

No general strategy can be proposed for the prediction of unintended immunostimulation due to the very limited published database. Although medicinal products with unintended immunostimulatory properties have been very infrequently identified, it is not known whether they are actually rare or have been overlooked because of inadequate testing modalities. The prediction of the sensitizing potential of most medicinal products is nearly impossible at the present time, except for contact sensitization. No reliable animal models or assays are available to predict the risk of drug-induced autoimmune reactions.

10.8.5   Immunotoxicity Risk Assessment

Risk assessment is a systematic scientific characterization of adverse health effects potentially resulting from exposure to hazardous agents or situations. No study seemingly ever focused on specific issues related to the immunotoxicity risk assessment of medicinal products. Immunotoxicity risk assessment has often been limited to the extrapolation of animal data for the prediction of unexpected immunosuppression. In the parallelogram concept (Fig. 10.9), results from *in vivo* studies and *in vitro* assays in animals are compared with results from *in vitro* assays using human cells to extrapolate potential *in vivo* changes in human subjects. A major difficulty in immunotoxicity risk assessment is dose response that may follow an atypical pattern. Although dose response is often linear, a hockey cross-type curve reminiscent of the hormesis concept [201] may characterize compounds that exert immunosuppressive properties at high doses, immunoenhancing properties at low doses, and are inactive at mid-doses. In such a situation, totally different health consequences can be expected depending on the level of human exposure. Dose response is also atypical in hypersensitivity reactions. A bell-shaped curve suggests that no reactions may be expected at concentrations below or above an optimal range of concentrations that, in addition, is likely to vary across individuals.

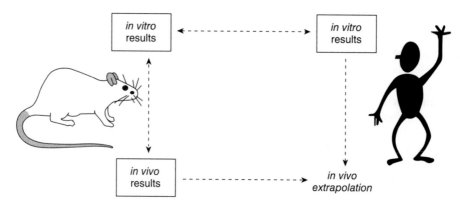

FIGURE 10.9 The parallelogram concept for risk assessment.

10.8.6 Clinical Immunotoxicity Assessment

Clinical immunotoxicology is a neglected area of immunotoxicology and our current ignorance of immunotoxic effects in humans is a hurdle to the development and acceptability of animal models and assays for nonclinical immunotoxicity evaluation. Indeed, so little is known of the impact of most medicinal drugs on the immune system of treated humans that correlation between animal and human results is impossible in the vast majority of cases. The inclusion of immunological endpoints in clinical trials has very rarely been addressed specifically [202]. Immune function assays similar to those used in rodent and nonrodent studies for the identification of unintended immunosuppression or immunostimulation are proposed. However, it is important to bear in mind that such assays are often unable to predict the efficacy of immunosuppressive drugs to prevent organ transplant rejection, or immunoactivating drugs, such as therapeutic cytokines. Therefore, it may be possible that, in the future, modalities to evaluate the immunotoxicity of medicinal products in animal studies as well as clinical trials are based on an entirely different approach. For the time being, recent guidelines emphasize the need for a better prediction of the immunotoxicity of medicinal products, which led to various strategies as briefly reviewed earlier. With nonclinical immunotoxicity evaluation becoming a routine component of safety evaluation, it can be assumed that immunological endpoints will have to be included in clinical trials. For the sake of comparison between animal and human studies, it is logical to recommend that endpoints as close as possible are measured in both situations. Thus, lymphocyte subset analysis, which is not considered to be a first-line assay in nonclinical studies [68], can nevertheless be a helpful endpoint as it is often used in human studies. In contrast, KLH that is increasingly used as a T-cell-dependent antigen in antibody response assays should not be used in humans because of the risk of cross-allergies with seafood.

10.9 CONCLUSION

Current procedures for assessing the immunotoxicological safety of medicinal products are far from perfect because of our poor understanding of most underlying mechanisms, and insufficient standardization and validation. The validation of available animal models and assays has often been restricted to few potent immunosuppressive compounds and there is an urgent need for large interlaboratory validation studies to refine current strategies. In addition, nonclinical immunotoxicity evaluation is currently limited to unintended immunosuppression, even though other immunotoxic effects, in particular, hypersensitivity, are far more critical safety issues in relation to the therapeutic use of medicinal products.

REFERENCES

1. Meylers L. Cytostatic drugs. In Meylers L, Ed. *Side-Effects of Drugs*, 2nd ed. Amsterdam: Excerpta Medica; 1966, pp 472–494.

2. Leibowitz S, Schwartz RS. Malignancy as a complication of immunosuppressive therapy. *Adv Intern Med* 1971;17:95–123.

3. Groupement Lyonnais de Lutte Contre les Intoxications. *L'Immunotoxicologie.* Lyon: Lacassagne; 1975.

4. Abrutyn E. The infancy of immunotoxicology. *Ann Intern Med* 1979;90:118–119.

5. Special issue. *Drug Chem Toxicol* 1979;2:1–89.

6. Dean JH, Padarathsingh ML, Jerrells TR. Assessment of immunobiological effects induced by chemicals, drugs and food additives. I. Tier testing and screening approach. *Drug Chem Toxicol* 1979;2:5–17.

7. Luster MI, Munson AE, Thomas PT, Holsapple MP, Fenters JD, White KL, et al. Development of a testing battery to assess chemical-induced immunotoxicity: National Toxicology Program's guidelines for immunotoxicity evaluation in mice. *Fundam Appl Toxicol* 1988;10:2–19.

8. White KL, Grennings C, Murray MJ, Dean JH. Summary of an international methods validation study, carried out in nine laboratories, on the immunological assessment of cyclosporine A in the Fischer 344 rat. *Toxicol In Vitro* 1994;8:957–961.

9. Richter-Reichhelm HB, Dasenbrock CA, Descotes G, Emmendorffer AC, Ernst HU, Harleman JH, et al. Validation of a modified 28-day rat study to evidence effects of test compounds on the immune system. *Regul Toxicol Pharmacol* 1995;22:54–56.

10. The ICICIS Group Investigators. Report of validation study of assessment of direct immunotoxicity in the rat. *Toxicology* 1998;125:183–201.

11. Behan PO, Behan WMH, Zacharias FJ, Nicholls JT. Immunological abnormalities in patients who had the oculomucocutaneous syndrome associated with practolol therapy. *Lancet* 1976;2:984–987.

12. Posada de la Paz M, Philen RM, Borda AI. Toxic oil syndrome: the perspective after 20 years. *Epidemiol Rev* 2001;23:231–247.

13. Belonga EA, Mayeno AN, Osterholm MT. The eosinophilia-myalgia syndrome and tryptophan. *Annu Rev Med* 1992;12:235–256.

14. Kimber I, Maurer T. *Toxicology of Contact Hypersensitivity*. London: Taylor and Francis; 1996.

15. Ratajczak HV. Drug-induced hypersensitivity: role in drug development. *Toxicol Rev* 2004;23:265–280.

16. Vial T, Choquet-Kastylevsky G, Descotes J. Adverse effects of immunotherapeutics involving the immune system. *Toxicology* 2002;174:3–11.

17. Luster MI, Ackermann MF, Germolec DR, Rosenthal GJ. Perturbations of the immune system by xenobiotics. *Environ Health Perspect* 1989;81:157–162.

18. Metzhitov R, Janeway CA. How does the immune system discriminate self from non-self? *Semin Immunol* 2000;12:185–188.

19. Chaplin DD. Overview of the human immune response. *J Allergy Clin Immunol* 2006;117:S430–S435.

20. Kuper CF, De Heer E, Van Loveren H, Vos JG. Immune system. In Haschek MW, Rousseaux CG, Wallig MA, Eds. *Handbook of Toxicologic Pathology, Volume 2*, 2nd ed. San Diego, CA: Academic Press; 2002, pp 585–646.

21. Alam R, Gorska M. Lymphocytes. *J Allergy Clin Immunol* 2003;111:S476–S485.

22. Descotes J, Ravel G. Role of NK cells in immunotoxicity: an update. *Exp Rev Clin Immunol* 2005;1:605–610.

23. Segal AW. How neutrophils kill microbes. *Annu Rev Immunol* 2005;23:197–223.

24. Gordon S, Taylorn PR. Monocyte and macrophage heterogeneity. *Nat Rev Immunol* 2005;5:953–964.

25. Wallet MA, Sen P, Tisch R. Immunoregulation of dendritic cells. *Clin Med Res* 2005;3:166–175.

26. Prussin C, Metcalfe DD. IgE, mast cells, basophils, and eosinophils. *J Allergy Clin Immunol* 2003;111:S486–S494.

27. Tosi MF. Innate immune responses to infection. *J Allergy Clin Immunol* 2005;116: 241–249.

28. De Smet K, Contreras R. Human antimicrobial peptides: defensins, cathelicidins and histatins. *Biotechnol Lett* 2005;27:1337–1347.

29. Rus H, Cudrici C, Niculescu F. The role of the complement system in innate immunity. *Immunol Res* 2005;33:103–112.

30. Ceciliani F, Giordano A, Spagnolo V. The systemic reaction during inflammation: the acute-phase proteins. *Protein Pept Lett* 2002;9:211–223.

31. Le Y, Zhou Y, Iribarren P, Wang J. Chemokines and chemokine receptors: their manifold roles in homeostasis and disease. *Cell Mol Immunol* 2004;1:95–104.

32. Schnare M, Rollinghoff M, Qureshi S. Toll-like receptors: sentinels of host defence against bacterial infection. *Int Arch Allergy Immunol* 2006;139:75–85.

33. Dustin ML. The immunological synapse. *Arthritis Res* 2002;4:S119–S125.

34. Chatila TA. Role of regulatory T cells in human diseases. *J Allergy Clin Immunol* 2005;116:949–959.

35. http://microvet.arizona.edu/Courses/MIC419/Tutorials/cytokines.html.

36. Fishman JA, Rubin RH. Infection in organ-transplant recipients. *N Engl J Med* 1998;338:1741–1751.

37. Klein NC, Go CH, Cunha BA. Infections associated with steroid use. *Infect Dis Clin North Am* 2001;15:423–32.

38. Giles JT, Bathon JM. Serious infections associated with anticytokine therapies in the rheumatic diseases. *J Intensive Care Med* 2004;19:320–334.

39. Vial T, Descotes J. Immunosuppressive drugs and cancer. *Toxicology* 2003;185:229–240.

40. Georgescu L, Paget SA. Lymphoma in patients treated with rheumatoid patients. What is the evidence of link with methotrexate? *Drug Saf* 1999;20:475–487.

41. Brown SL, Greene MH, Gershon SK, Edwards ET, Braun MM. Tumor necrosis factor antagonist therapy and lymphoma development: twenty-six cases reported to the Food and Drug Administration. *Arthritis Rheum* 2002;46:3151–3158.

42. Descotes J, Vial T. The flu-like syndrome and cytokines. In House RV, Descotes J, Eds. *Cytokines in Human Health: Immunotoxicology, Pathology and Therapeutic Applications.* Totowa, NJ: Humana Press; 2006.

43. Krause I, Valesini G, Scrivo R, Shoenfeld Y. Autoimmune aspects of cytokine and anti-cytokine therapies. *Am J Med* 2003;115:390–397.

44. Shulman KL, Thompson JA, Benyunes MC, Winter TC, Fefer A. Adverse reactions to intravenous contrast media in patients treated with interleukin-2. *J Immunother* 1993; 13:208–212.

45. Renton KW. Hepatic drug metabolism and immunostimulation. *Toxicology* 2000; 142:173–178.

46. Gomes ER, Demoly P. Epidemiology of hypersensitivity drug reactions. *Curr Opin Allergy Clin Immunol* 2005;5:309–316.

47. Choquet-Kastylevsky G, Vial T, Descotes J. Drug allergy diagnosis in humans: possibilities and pitfalls. *Toxicology* 2001;158:1–10.

48. Johansson SG, Hourihane JO, Bousquet J, Bruijnzeel-Koomen C, Dreborg S, Haahtela T, et al. A revised nomenclature for allergy. An EAACI position statement from the EAACI nomenclature task force. *Allergy* 2001;56:813–824.

49. Solensky R. Drug hypersensitivity. *Med Clin North Am* 2006;90:233–260.

50. Descotes J, Choquet-Kastylevsky G. Gell and Coombs classification: is it still valid? *Toxicology* 2001;158:43–49.

51. Naisbitt DJ, Williams DP, Pirmohamed M, Kitteringham NR, Park BK. Reactive metabolites and their role in drug reactions. *Curr Opin Allergy Clin Immunol* 2001; 1:317–325.

52. Britschgi M, Von Greyerz S, Burkhart C, Pichler WJ. Molecular aspects of drug recognition by specific T cells. *Curr Drug Targets* 2003;4:1–11.

53. Descotes J, Payen C, Vial T. Pseudoallergic drug reactions. *Perspect Exp Clin Immunotoxicol* 2006;1:40–49.

54. Vial T, Descotes J. Autoimmunity and toxic exposures. *Perspect Exp Clin Immunotoxicol* 2006;1:2–13.

55. Kuper CF, Harleman JH, Richter-Reichelm HB, Vos JG. Histopathologic approaches to detect changes indicative of immunotoxicity. *Toxicol Pathol* 2000;28:454–466.

56. Haley P, Perry R, Ennulat D, Frame S, Johnson C, Lapointe JM, et al. STP position paper: best practice guideline for the routine pathology evaluation of the immune system. *Toxicol Pathol* 2005;33:404–407.

57. Haley PJ. Species differences in the structure and function of the immune system. *Toxicology* 2003;188:49–71.

58. Haines DM, Westn KH. Immunohistochemistry: forging the links between immunology and pathology. *Vet Immunol Immunopathol* 2005;108:151–156.

59. Kadkol SS, Gage WR, Pasternack GR. *In situ* hybridization—theory and practice. *Mol Diagn* 1999;4:169–183.

60. Hyun BH, Gulati GL, Ashton JK. Bone marrow examination: techniques and interpretation. *Hematol Oncol Clin North Am* 1988;2:513–523.

61. Chadburn A. The spleen: anatomy and anatomical function. *Semin Hematol* 2000;37: S13–S21.

62. MacDonald TT. The mucosal immune system. *Parasite Immunol* 2003;25:235–246.

63. Gergely P. Drug-induced lymphopenia: focus on $CD4^+$ and $CD8^+$ cells. *Drug Saf* 1999;21:91–100.

64. Wierda D, Irons RD. Bone marrow and immunotoxicity. In Smialowicz RJ, Holsapple MP, Eds. *Experimental Immunotoxicity*. Boca Raton, FL: CRC Press; 1996, pp 101–117.

65. Marti GE, Stetler-Stevenson M, Bleesing JJ, Fleisher TA. Introduction to flow cytometry. *Semin Hematol* 2001;38:93–99.

66. Nygaard UC, Lovik M. Blood and spleen lymphocytes as targets for immunotoxic effects in the rat—a comparison. *Toxicology* 2002;174:153–161.

67. Luster MI, Portier C, Pait DG, White KL Jr, Gennings C, Munson AE, et al. Risk assessment in immunotoxicology. I. Sensitivity and predictability of immune tests. *Fundam Appl Toxicol* 1992;18:200–210.

68. Immunotoxicology Technical Committee. Application of flow cytometry to immunotoxicity testing: summary of a workshop. *Toxicology* 2001;163:39–48.

69. Burchiel SW, Lauer FT, Gurule D, Mounho BJ, Salas VM. Uses and future applications of flow cytometry in immunotoxicity testing. *Methods* 1999;19:28–35.

70. Temple L, Kawabata TT, Munson AE, White KL. Comparison of ELISA and plaque-forming cell assays for measuring the humoral response to SRBC in rats and mice treated with benzo[*a*]pyrene or cyclophosphamide. *Fundam Appl Toxicol* 1993;21:412–419.

71. Johnson CW, Williams WC, Copeland CB, DeVito MJ, Smialowicz RJ. Sensitivity of the SRBC PFC assay versus ELISA for detection of immunosuppression by TCDD and TCDD-like congeners. *Toxicology* 2000;156:1–11.

72. Condevaux F, Horand F, Ruat C, Descotes J. Relative sensitivities of the plaque forming cell (PFC) assay and anti-KLH antibody ELISA in the same rats treated with cyclophosphamide. *Toxicol Lett* 2001;123:S58 (abstract).

73. Jerne NK, Henry C, Nordin AA, Fuji H, Koros AM, Lefkovits I. Plaque forming cells: methodology and theory. *Transplant Rev* 1974;18:130–191.

74. Vos JG, Krajnc EI, Beekhof P. Use of the enzyme-linked immunosorbent assay (ELISA) in immunotoxicity testing. *Environ Health Perspect* 1982;43:115–121.

75. Gore ER, Gower J, Kurali E, Sui J-L, Bynum J, Ennulat D, Herzyk D. Primary antibody response to keyhole limpet hemocyanin in rat as a model for immunotoxicity evaluation. *Toxicology* 2004;197:23–35.

76. Ulrich P, Paul G, Perentes E, Mahl A, Roman D. Validation of immune function testing during a 4-week oral toxicity study with FK506. *Toxicol Lett* 2004;149:123–131.

77. Piccotti JR, Alvey JD, Reindel JF, Guzman RE. T-cell-dependent antibody response: assay development in cynomolgus monkeys. *J Immunotoxicol* 2005;2:191–196.

78. Luster MI, Dean JH, Boorman GA. Cell-mediated immunity and its application to toxicology. *Environ Health Perspect* 1982;43:31–36.

79. Descotes J, Tedone R, Evreux JC. Effects of cimetidine and ranitidine on delayed-type hypersensitivity. *Immunopharmacology* 1983;6:31–35.

80. Henningsen GM, Koller LD, Exon JH, Talcott PA, Osborne CA. A sensitive delayed-type hypersensitivity model in the rat for assessing *in vivo* cell-mediated immunity. *J Immunol Methods* 1984;70:153–165.

81. Ponton J, Regulez P, Cisterna R. Comparison of three tests for measuring footpad swelling in the mouse. *J Immunol Methods* 1983;63:139–143.

82. Thilsted JP, Shifrine M. Delayed cutaneous hypersensitivity in the dog: reaction to tuberculin purified protein derivative and coccidioidin. *Am J Vet Res* 1978;39:1702–1705.

83. Descotes J, Tedone R, Evreux JC. Immunotoxicity screening of drugs and chemicals: value of contact hypersensitivity to picryl chloride in the mouse. *Methods Find Exp Clin Pharmacol* 1985;7:303–305.

84. Descotes J, Evreux JC. Effect of chlorpromazine on contact hypersensitivity to DNCB in the guinea-pig. *J Neuroimmunol* 1982;2:21–25.

85. Smialowicz RJ. *In vitro* lymphocyte proliferation assays: the mitogen-stimulated response and the mixed-lymphocyte reaction in immunotoxicity testing. In Burleson GR, Dean JH, Munson AE, Eds. *Methods in Immunotoxicology, Volume 1.* Hoboken, NJ: Wiley-Liss; 1995, pp 197–210.

86. Wemme H, Pfeifer S, Heck R, Muller-Quernheim J. Measurement of lymphocyte proliferation: critical analysis of radioactive and photometric methods. *Immunobiology* 1992;185:78–89.

87. House RD, Dean JH. Studies on structural requirements for suppression of cytotoxic T lymphocyte induction by polycyclic compounds. *Toxicol In Vitro* 1987;1:149–162.

88. Hoppner M, Luhm J, Schlenke P, Koritke P, Frohn C. A flow-cytometry based cytotoxicity assay using stained effector cells in combination with native target cells. *J Immunol Methods* 2002;267:157–163.

89. House RV. Theory and practice of cytokine assessment in immunotoxicology. *Methods* 1999;19:17–27.

90. Meager A. Measurement of cytokines by bioassays: theory and application. *Methods* 2006;38:237–252.

91. De Jager W, Rijkers GT. Solid-phase and bead-based cytokine immunoassay: comparison. *Methods* 2006;38:294–303.

92. Langezaal I, Coecke S, Hartung T. Whole blood cytokine response as a measure of immunotoxicity. *Toxicol In Vitro* 2001;15:313–318.

93. Pala P, Hussell T, Openshaw PJ. Flow cytometric measurement of intracellular cytokines. *J Immunol Methods* 2000;243:107–124.

94. Vos JG, De Klerk A, Krajnc EI, Kruizinga W, Van Ommen B, Rozing J. Toxicity of bis(tri-*n*-butyltin)oxide in the rat. II. Suppression of thymus-dependent immune responses and of parameters of nonspecific resistance after short-term exposure. *Toxicol Appl Pharmacol* 1984;75:387–408.

95. Antonini JM, Roberts JR, Clarke RW, Yang HM, Barger MW, et al. Effect of age on respiratory defense mechanisms: pulmonary bacterial clearance in Fischer 344 rats after intratracheal instillation of *Listeria monocytogenes*. *Chest* 2001;120:240–249.

96. Rodgers K. Measurement of the respiratory burst of leukocytes for immunotoxicologic analysis. In Burleson GR, Dean JH, Munson AE, Eds. *Methods in Immunotoxicology, Volume 2.* Hoboken, NJ: Wiley-Liss; 1995, pp 67–77.

97. Verdier F, Condevaux F, Tedone R, Virat M, Descotes J. *In vitro* assessment of phagocytosis. Interspecies comparison of chemiluminescence response. *Toxicol In Vitro* 1993;7:317–320.

98. Lehmann AK, Sornes S, Halstensen A. Phagocytosis: measurement by flow cytometry. *J Immunol Methods* 2000;243:229–242.

99. Cretinon C, Condevaux F, Horand F, Descotes J. Comparison of the phagocytic activity in rats and monkeys using two commercial kits. *Toxicol Sci* 2003;72:S105 (abstract).

100. Wilkinson PC. Assays of leukocyte locomotion and chemotaxis. *J Immunol Methods* 1998;216:139–153.

101. Cederbrant K, Marcusson-Stahl M, Condevaux F, Descotes J. NK-cell activity in immunotoxicity drug evaluation. *Toxicology* 2003;185:241–250.

102. Thomas PT, Sherwood RL. Host resistance models in immunotoxicology. In Smialowicz RJ, Holsapple MP, Eds. *Experimental Immunotoxicology*. Boca Raton, FL: CRC Press; 1996, pp 29–45.

103. Dean JH, Luster MI, Boorman GA, Luebke RW, Lauer LD. Application of tumor, bacterial, and parasite susceptibility assays to study immune alterations induced by environmental chemicals. *Environ Health Perspect* 1982;43:81–88.

104. Selgrade MK, Daniels MJ, Dean JH. Correlation between chemical suppression of natural killer cell activity in mice and susceptibility to cytomegalovirus: rationale for applying murine cytomegalovirus as a host resistance model and for interpreting immunotoxicity testing in terms of risk of disease. *J Toxicol Environ Health* 1992; 37:123–137.

105. Luster MI, Portier C, Pait DG, Rosenthal GJ, Germolec DR, et al. Risk assessment in immunotoxicology. II. Relationships between immune and host resistance tests. *Fundam Appl Toxicol* 1993;21:71–82.

106. Wierda D. Can host resistance assays be used to evaluate the immunotoxicity of pharmaceuticals? *Hum Exp Toxicol* 2000;19:244–245.

107. Lebrec H, Burleson GR. Influenza virus host resistance models in mice and rats: utilization for immune function assessment and immunotoxicology. *Toxicology* 1994;91: 179–188.

108. Meade BJ, Hayes BB, Klykken PC. Development and validation of a *Listeria monocytogenes* host resistance model in female Fisher 344 rats. *Toxicol Methods* 1998;8:45–57.

109. Bradley SG. Streptococcus host resistance model. In Burleson GR, Dean JH, Munson AE, Eds. *Methods in Immunotoxicology, Volume 2*. Hoboken, NJ: Wiley-Liss; 1995, pp 159–168.

110. De Waal EJ, De Jong WH, Van der Stappen AJ, Verlaan B, Van Der Loveren H. Effects of salmeterol on host resistance to *Trichinella spiralis* in rats. *Int J Immunopharmacol* 1999;21:523–529.

111. Henry SP, Taylor J, Midgley L, Levin AA, Kornbrust DJ. Evaluation of the toxicity of ISIS 2302, a phosphorothioate oligonucleotide, in a 4-week study in CD-1 mice. *Antisense Nucleic Acid Drug Dev* 1997;7:473–481.

112. Anderson TD, Hayes TJ. Toxicity of human recombinant interleukin-2 in rats. Pathologic changes are characterized by marked lymphocytic and eosinophilic proliferation and multisystem involvement. *Lab Invest* 1989;60:331–346.

113. Cesario TC, Vaziri ND, Ulich TR, Khamiseh G, Oveisi F, et al. Functional, biochemical, and histopathologic consequences of high-dose interleukin-2 administration in rats. *J Lab Clin Med* 1991;118:81–88.

114. Sparwasser T, Hultner L, Koch ES, Luz A, Lipford GB, Wagner H. Immunostimulatory CpG-oligodeoxynucleotides cause extramedullary murine hemopoiesis. *J Immunol* 1999;162:2368–2374.

115. Helfand SC, Soergel SA, MacWilliams PS, Hank JA, Sondel PM. Clinical and immunological effects of human recombinant interleukin-2 given by repetitive weekly infusion to normal dogs. *Cancer Immunol Immunother* 1994;39:84–92.

116. Ryffel B, Weber M. Preclinical safety studies with recombinant human interleukin 6 (rhIL-6) in the primate *Callithrix jacchus* marmoset: comparison with studies in rats. *J Appl Toxicol* 1995;15:19–26.

117. Cleveland RP, Kumar A. Enhancement of anti-sheep erythrocyte plaque-forming cell levels by cimetidine *in vivo*. *Immunopharmacology* 1987;14:145–150.

118. Eastcott JW, Holmberg CJ, Dewhirst FE, Esch TR, Smith DJ, Taubman MA. Oligonucleotide containing CpG motifs enhances immune response to mucosally or systemically administered tetanus toxoid. *Vaccine* 2001;19:1636–1642.

119. Descotes J, Tedone R, Evreux JC. Effects of cimetidine and ranitidine on delayed-type hypersensitivity. *Immunopharmacology* 1983;6:31–35.

120. De Waard R, Claassen E, Bokken GC, Buiting B, Garssen J, Vos JG. Enhanced immunological memory responses to *Listeria monocytogenes* in rodents, as measured by delayed-type hypersensitivity (DTH), adoptive transfer of DTH, and protective immunity, following *Lactobacillus casei* Shirota ingestion. *Clin Diagn Lab Immunol* 2003; 10:59–65.

121. Ershler WB, Hacker MP, Burroughs BJ, Moore AL, Myers CF. Cimetidine and the immune response. I. *In vivo* augmentation of nonspecific and specific immune response. *Clin Immunol Immunopathol* 1983;26:10–17.

122. Iho S, Yamamoto T, Takahashi T, Yamamoto S. Oligodeoxynucleotides containing palindrome sequences with internal 5′-CpG-3′ act directly on human NK and activated T cells to induce IFN-gamma production *in vitro*. *J Immunol* 1999;163:3642–3652.

123. Nomoto K, Miake S, Hashimoto S, Yokokura T, Mutai M, et al. Augmentation of host resistance to *Listeria monocytogenes* infection by *Lactobacillus casei*. *J Clin Lab Immunol* 1985;17:91–97.

124. Robinet E, Morel P, Assossou O, Revillard JP. TNF-alpha production as an *in vitro* assay predictive of cytokine-mediated toxic reactions induced by monoclonal antibodies. *Toxicology* 1995;100:213–223.

125. Oshiro Y, Morris DL. TNF-alpha release from human peripheral blood mononuclear cells to predict the proinflammatory activity of cytokines and growth factors. *J Pharmacol Toxicol Methods* 1997;37:55–59.

126. Herzyk DJ, Ruggieri EV, Cunnigham L, Polsky R, Herold C, et al. Single-organism model in host defense against infection: a novel immunotoxicologic approach to evaluate immunomodulatory drugs. *Toxicol Pathol* 1997;25:351–362.

127. Cohen IR, Miller A. *Autoimmune Disease Models. A Guidebook*. San Diego, CA: Academic Press; 1994.

128. Burnett R, Ravel G, Descotes J. Clinical and histopathological progression of lesions in lupus-prone (NZB × NZW) F1 mice. *Exp Toxicol Pathol* 2004;56:37–44.

129. Adam C, Thoua Y, Ronco P, Verroust P, Tovey M, Morel-Maroger L. The effect of exogenous interferon: acceleration of autoimmune and renal diseases in (NZB/W) F1 mice. *Clin Exp Immunol* 1980;40:373–382.

130. Griffin JM, Blossom SJ, Jackson SK, Gilbert KM, Pumford NR. Trichloroethylene accelerates an autoimmune response by Th1 T cell activation in MRL+/+ mice. *Immunopharmacology* 2000;46:123–137.

131. Letter EH, Prochazka M, Coleman DL. The non-obese diabetic (NOD) mouse. *Am J Pathol* 1987;128:380–383.

132. Baxter AG, Healey D, Cooke A. Mycobacteria precipitate autoimmune rheumatic disease in NOD mice via an adjuvant-like activity. *Scand J Immunol* 1994;39:602–606.

133. Pelletier L, Hirsch F, Rossert J, Druet E, Druet P. Experimental mercury-induced glomerulonephritis. *Springer Semin Immunopathol* 1987;9:359–369.

134. White KL, David DW, Butterworth LF, Klykken PC. Assessment of autoimmunity-inducing potential using the Brown-Norway rat challenge model. *Toxicol Lett* 2000; 112–113:443–451.

135. Ewel CH, Sobel DO, Zeligs BJ, Bellanti JA. Poly I:C accelerates development of diabetes mellitus in diabetes-prone BB rat. *Diabetes* 1992;41:1016–1021.

136. Bendele A, McComb J, Gould T, McAbee T, Sennello G, et al. Animal models of arthritis: relevance to human disease. *Toxicol Pathol* 1999;27:134–142.

137. Goverman J, Brabb T. Rodent models of experimental allergic encephalomyelitis applied to the study of multiple sclerosis. *Lab Anim Sci* 1996;46:482–492.

138. Choquet-Kastylevski G, Descotes J. Value of animal models for predicting hypersensitivity reactions to medicinal products. *Toxicology* 1998;129:27–35.

139. Bala S, Weaver J, Hastings KL. Clinical relevance of preclinical testing for allergic side effects. *Toxicology* 2005;209:195–200.

140. Park BK, Kitteringham NR. Drug–protein conjugation and its immunological consequences. *Drug Metab Rev* 1990;22:87–144.

141. Pauluhn J. Predictive testing for respiratory sensitisation. *Toxicol Lett* 1996;86:177–185.

142. Koizumi K, Suzuki S, Fukuba S, Tadokoro K, Hirai K, Muranaka M. Antigenicity of semisynthetic penicillin preparations to evoke systemic anaphylactic reactions in animal models. *Allergy* 1980;35:657–664.

143. Hattori H, Yamaguchi F, Wagai N, Kato M, Nomura M. An assessment of antigenic potential of beta-lactam antibiotics, low molecular weight drugs, using guinea pig models. *Toxicology* 1997;123:149–160.

144. Shibaki A, Katz S. Induction of skewed Th1/Th2 T-cell differentiation via subcutaneous immunization with Freund's adjuvant. *Exp Dermatol* 2002;11:126–134.

145. Verdier F, Chazal I, Descotes J. Anaphylaxis models in the guinea-pig. *Toxicology* 1994;93:55–61.

146. Brutzkus B, Coquet B, Danve B, Descotes J. Systemic anaphylaxis in guinea pigs: intralaboratory validation study. *Fundam Appl Toxicol* 1997;36 (Suppl):192 (abstract).

147. *ICH Guideline S6. Preclinical Safety Evaluation of Biotechnology-Derived Pharmaceuticals.* ICH; 1997. Document available at http://www.ich.org/LOB/media/MEDIA503.pdf.

148. Maurer T. Past, present and future of contact sensitization. *Perspect Exp Clin Immunotoxicol* 2007;1:in press.

149. Buehler EV. Delayed contact hypersensitivity in the guinea pig. *Arch Dermatol* 1965;91:171–177.

150. Basketter DA, Gerberick GF. An interlaboratory evaluation of the Buehler test for the identification and classification of contact sensitizers. *Contact Dermatitis* 1996;35:146–151.

151. Magnusson B, Kligman AM. The identification of contact allergens by animal assay, the guinea pig maximization test method. *J Invest Dermatol* 1969;52:268–276.

152. Gad SC, Dunn BJ, Dobbs DW, Reilly C, Walsh RD. Development and validation of an alternative dermal sensitization test: the Mouse Ear Swelling Test (MEST). *Toxicol Appl Pharmacol* 1986;84:93–114.

153. Gad SC. The Mouse Ear Swelling Test (MEST) in the 1990s. *Toxicology* 1994;93:33–46.

154. Kimber I, Mitchell JA, Griffin AC. Development of a murine local lymph node assay for the determination of sensitization potential. *Fundam Chem Toxicol* 1986;24:585–586.

155. Kimber I, Hilton J, Botham PA, Basketter DA, Scholes EW, Miller K, Robbins MC, Harrison PT, Gray TJ, Waite SJ. The murine local lymph node assay: results of an interlaboratory trial. *Toxicol Lett* 1991;55:203–213.

156. Loveless SE, Ladics GS, Gerberick GF, Ryan CA, Basketter DA, Scholes EW, House RV, Hilton J, Dearman RJ, Kimber I. Further evaluation of the local lymph node assay in the final phase of an international collaborative trial. *Toxicology* 1996;108:141–152.

157. OECD. Skin sensitisation: Local Lymph Node Assay. *OECD Guideline for the Toxicity Testing of Chemicals 429*. Paris: OECD; 2002.

158. Kimber I, Dearman RJ, Basketter DA, Ryan CA, Gerberick GF. The local lymph node assay: past, present and future. *Contact Dermatitis* 2002;47:315–328.

159. Boussiquet-Leroux C, Durand-Cavagna G, Herlin K, Holder D. Evaluation of lymphocyte proliferation by immunohistochemistry in the local lymph node assay. *J Appl Toxicol* 1995;15:465–475.

160. Hatao M, Hariya T, Katsumura Y, Kato S. A modification of the local lymph node assay for contact allergenicity screening: measurement of interleukin-2 as an alternative to radioisotope-dependent proliferation assay. *Toxicology* 1995;98:15–22.

161. Suda A, Yamashita M, Tabei M, Taguchi K, Vohr HW, Tsutsui N, Suzuki R, Kikuchi K, Sakaguchi K, Mochizuki K, Nakamura K. Local lymph node assay with non-radioisotope alternative endpoints. *J Toxicol Sci* 2002;27:205–218.

162. Dearman RJ, Scholes EW, Ramdin LS, Basketter DA, Kimber I. The local lymph node assay: an interlaboratory evaluation of interleukin 6 (IL-6) production by draining lymph node cells. *J Appl Toxicol* 1994;14:287–291.

163. Dearman RJ, Hilton J, Basketter DA, Kimber I. Cytokine endpoints for the local lymph node assay: consideration of interferon-gamma and interleukin 12. *J Appl Toxicol* 1999;19:149–155.

164. Ryan CA, Gerberick GF, Cruse LW, Basketter DA, Lea L, Blaikie L, Dearman RJ, Warbrick EV, Kimber I. Activity of human contact allergens in the murine local lymph node assay. *Contact Dermatitis* 2000;43:95–102.

165. Ulrich P, Streich J, Suter W. Intralaboratory validation of alternative endpoints in the murine local lymph node assay for the identification of contact allergic potential: primary ear skin irritation and ear-draining lymph node hyperplasia induced by topical chemicals. *Arch Toxicol* 2001;74:733–744.

166. Gerberick GF, Cruse LW, Ryan CA, Hulette BC, Chaney JG, Skinner RA, Dearman RJ, Kimber I. Use of a B cell marker (B220) to discriminate between allergens and irritants in the local lymph node assay. *Toxicol Sci* 2002;68:420–428.

167. Shiho O, Nakagawa Y, Kawaji H. Delayed type hypersensitivity for penicillin in mice. I. Induction and characterization of delayed type hypersensitivity for penicillin in mice. *J Antibiot* 1981;34:452–458.

168. Choquet-Kastylevsky G, Santolaria N, Tedone R, Aujoulat M, Descotes J. Induction of delayed-type hypersensitivity to sulfamethoxazole in mice: role of metabolites. *Toxicol Lett* 2001;119:183–192.

169. Vial T, Descotes J. Contact sensitization assays in guinea-pigs: are they predictive of the potential for systemic allergic reactions? *Toxicology* 1994;93:63–75.

170. Weaver JL, Staten D, Swann J, Armstrong G, Bates M, Hastings KL. Detection of systemic hypersensitivity to drugs using standard guinea pig assays. *Toxicology* 2003;193:203–217.

171. Eschalier A, Lavarenne J, Burtin C, Renoux M, Chapuy E, Rodriguez M. Study of histamine release induced by acute administration of antitumor agents in dogs. *Cancer Chemother Pharmacol* 1988;21:246–250.

172. Guedes AG, Rude EP, Rider MA. Evaluation of histamine release during constant rate infusion of morphine in dogs. *Vet Anaesth Analg* 2006;33:28–35.

173. Lorenz W. Histamine release in man. *Agents Actions* 1975;5:402–416.

174. Sanz ML, Maselli JP, Gamboa PM, Oehling A, Dieguez I, De Weck AL. Flow cytometric basophil activation test: a review. J Invest Allergol *Clin Immunol* 2002;12:143–154.

175. Szebeni J, Muggia FM, Alving CR. Complement activation by Cremophor EL as a possible contributor to hypersensitivity to paclitaxel: an *in vitro* study. *J Natl Cancer Inst* 1998;90:300–306.

176. Descotes J. Autoimmunity and toxicity testing. *Toxicol Lett* 2000;112–113:461–465.

177. Verdier F, Patriarca C, Descotes J. Autoantibodies in conventional toxicity testing. *Toxicology* 1997;119:51–58.

178. Kuper CF, Schuurman H, Bos-Kuijpers M, Bloksma N. Predictive testing for pathogenic autoimmunity: the morphological approach. *Toxicol Lett* 2000;112–113:433–442.

179. Pollard KM, Pearson DL, Hultman P, Hildebrandt B, Kono DH. Lupus-prone mice as models to study xenobiotic-induced acceleration of systemic autoimmunity. *Environ Health Perspect* 1999;107 (Suppl 5):729–735.

180. Ravel G, Descotes J. The popliteal lymph node assay: facts and perspectives. *J Appl Toxicol* 2005;25:451–458.

181. Vial T, Carleer J, Legrain B, Verdier F, Descotes J. The popliteal lymph node assay: results of a preliminary interlaboratory validation study. *Toxicology* 1997;122:213–218.

182. Choquet-Kastylevsky G, Descotes J. Popliteal lymph node responses to ethanol and acetone differ from those induced by streptozotocin. *Arch Toxicol* 2004;74:649–654.

183. Choquet-Kastylevsky G, Tedone R, Descotes J. Positive responses to imipramine in the popliteal lymph node assay are due to primary irritation. *Hum Exp Toxicol* 2001;20: 591–596.

184. Nagata N, Hurtenbach U, Gleichmann E. Specific sensitization of Lyt-1$^+$2 T-cells to spleen cells modified by the drug D-penicillamine or a stereoisomer. *J Immunol* 1986;136:136–142.

185. Kubicka-Muryani M, Goebels R, Goebel C, Uetrecht JP, Gleichmann E. T lymphocytes ignore procainamide, but respond to its reactive metabolites in peritoneal cells: demonstration by the adoptive transfer popliteal lymph node assay. *Toxicol Appl Pharmacol* 1993;122:88–94.

186. Albers R, Broeders A, Van Der Pijl A, Seinen W, Pieters R. The use of reporter antigens in the popliteal lymph node assay to assess immunomodulation by chemicals. *Toxicol Appl Pharmacol* 1997;143:102–109.

187. Pieters R, Ezendam J, Bleumink R, Bol M, Nierkens S. Predictive testing for autoimmunity. *Toxicol Lett* 2002;127:83–91.

188. Gutting BW, Updyke LW, Amacher DE. Investigating the TNP-OVA and direct popliteal lymph node assays for the detection of immunostimulation by drugs associated with anaphylaxis in humans. *J Appl Toxicol* 2002;22:177–183.

189. Descotes J. Regulatory aspects of immunotoxicity evaluation. In Descotes J, Ed. *Immunotoxicology of Drugs and Chemicals. An Experimental and Clinical Approach. Vol. 1. Principles and Methods of Immunotoxicology*. Amsterdam: Elsevier Science; 2004, pp 257–268.

190. *OECD Guideline for the Testing of Chemicals. Repeated Dose 28-day Oral Toxicity Study in Rodents OECD*; 1995. Document available at http://www.oecd.org/dataoecd/17/52/1948386.pdf.

191. *Harmonized Tripartite Guideline S6: Preclinical Safety Evaluation of Biotechnology-Derived* Pharmaceuticals. ICH; 1996. Document available at http://www.ich.org/MediaServer.jser?@_ID=503&@_MODE=GLB.

192. *Note for Guidance on Repeated Dose Toxicity*. EMEA; 2000. Document available at http://www.emea.eu.int/pdfs/human/swp/104299en.pdf.

193. *Immunotoxicology Evaluation of Investigational New Drugs*. FDA; 2002. Document available at http://www.fda.gov/cder/guidance/4945fnl.pdf.

194. *Harmonized Tripartite Guideline S8: Immunotoxicity Studies for Human Pharmaceuticals*. ICH; 2005. Document available at http://www.ich.org/MediaServer.jser?@_ID= 1706&@_MODE=GLB.

195. Descotes J. Nonclinical strategies of immunotoxicity evaluation and risk assessment. In Descotes J, Ed. *Immunotoxicology of Drugs and Chemicals. An Experimental and Clinical Approach. Vol. 1. Principles and Methods of Immunotoxicology.* Amsterdam: Elsevier Science; 2004, pp 269–293.

196. Basketter DA, Bremmer JN, Buckley P, Kammuller ME, Kawabata T, Kimber I, et al. Pathology considerations for, and subsequent risk assessment of, chemicals identified as immunosuppressive in routine toxicology. *Food Chem Toxicol* 1995;33:239–243.

197. Gopinath C. Pathology of toxic effects on the immune system. *Inflamm Res* 1996; 2 (Suppl):74–78.

198. Crevel RW, Buckley P, Robinson JA, Sanders IJ. Immunotoxicological assessment of cyclosporin A by conventional pathological techniques and immune function testing in the rat. *Hum Exp Toxicol* 1997;16:79–88.

199. Putman E, Van Loveren H, Bode G, Dean J, Hastings K, Nakamura K, Verdier F, Van Der Laan JW. Assessment of the immunotoxic potential of human pharmaceuticals: a workshop report. *Drug Inf J* 2002;36:417–427.

200. Germolec DR, Kashon M, Nyska A, Kuper CF, Portier C, Kommineni C, Johnson KA, et al. The accuracy of extended histopathology to detect immunotoxic chemicals. *Toxicol Sci* 2004;82:504–514.

201. Calabrese EJ. Hormetic dose–response relationships in immunology: occurrence, quantitative features of the dose response, mechanistic foundations, and clinical implications. *Crit Rev Toxicol* 2005;35:89–295.

202. Buhles WC. Application of immunologic methods in clinical trials. *Toxicology* 1998; 129:73–89.

11

IMMUNOTOXICITY TESTING: ICH GUIDELINE S8 AND RELATED ASPECTS

HANS-GERD PAUELS[1] AND JOHN TAYLOR[2]

[1]*Dr. Pauels–Scientific and Regulatory Consulting, Münster, Germany*
[2]*ProPhase Development Ltd, Harrogate, United Kingdom*

Contents

Preclinical Development Handbook: Toxicology, edited by Shayne Cox Gad
Copyright © 2008 John Wiley & Sons, Inc.

11.1 INTRODUCTION

The physiological role of the immune system is to fight viral, bacterial, and parasitic infections, and perhaps also cancer. The latter, however, is a matter of debate because, with the exception of some rare tumors [1–3], no clear-cut correlation exists between immunosuppression and tumor incidence. Toxicological research over the past decades has indicated that the immune system is a potential target for toxic damage due to xenobiotics, and immunotoxicology has evolved as a discipline concerned with adverse interactions of chemicals and drugs with the immune system.

The immunotoxic effects of chemicals encompass five categories: (1) unintended immunosuppression, (2) unintended immunostimulation, (3) immunogenicity, (4) induction of hypersensitivity, and (5) induction of autoimmunity. The last three categories, however, are variations of the same theme and are discussed together in this chapter.

Immunotoxicology as a discipline has evolved mainly from the 1980s with human health immunotoxicity risk assessments of chemicals, pollutants, and pesticides. Such risk assessments have focused on ensuring that adequate safety factors are applied to dose–response effects such that immunotoxicological risks are negligible for these substances. Various agencies/institutes have been concerned particularly from this period onward in developing immunotoxicity testing strategies and risk assessment processes, as outlined in Section 11.3. Immunotoxicity risk assessment has been integrated in a more general way for pharmaceuticals up until the late 1990s when guidelines were initiated in the ICH regions, culminating in the development of the ICH S8 guideline entitled *Immunotoxicity Studies for Human Pharmaceuticals*, which came into operation in Europe and in the United States in spring 2006. Since immunotoxicity plays a role in some drug-induced adverse effects, resulting in morbidity and mortality, as noted for drugs such as cyclosporine and anticancer cytotoxic agents and more recently for TNF-α antagonists, it is recognized that immunotoxicity risk assessment is an important element of drug safety assessment. The introduction of guidelines including ICH S8 for drugs further supports the clinical risk–benefit assessments that are made for drugs.

Immunotoxicologists have long focused on immunosuppression, but other aspects of immunotoxicity like immunogenicity, induction of autoimmunity, or hypersensitivity have become increasingly important for drugs, especially with the introduction of biotechnology-derived drugs into the pharmaceutical pipeline. A number of well standardized and validated animal models exist for the nonclinical assessment of immunosuppression. Furthermore, some predictive *in vitro* and *in vivo* assays are available for the assessment of unintended immunostimulation. In both cases, many additional techniques can be used to extend the assessment of immunotoxic mechanistic effects on a case-by-case basis. The situation is less satisfactory for the assessment of immunogenicity, allergenicity, and autoimmunity. The main problem, in such cases, is the limited predictive value of animal models for the outcome of a drug treatment in humans.

Over the past decades, several guidelines have been issued by regulatory agencies to integrate immunotoxicity assessment into the risk assessment of chemicals, pollutants, and drugs. To date, these guidelines take a different position whether to make immunotoxicity tests a mandatory step during preclinical safety assessment, or whether the decision on immunotoxicity testing should be based on a weight of evidence basis. Furthermore, different recommendations are given with regard to the kinds of assays that should be employed.

In the pharmaceutical sector, all three ICH regions have made strong efforts to harmonize the immunotoxicity risk assessment for investigational new drugs. These efforts culminated in the release of the ICH S8 guideline, which was adopted by the CHMP in October 2005 and came into operation in April 2006. It was furthermore adopted by the FDA and published in the Federal Register in April 2006, as well as by the MHLW in April 2006. According to this current guideline, initial immunotoxicity assessment should be based on the evaluation of data already available from standard toxicity studies and other characteristics of the drug substance like pharmacological properties, the intended patient population, known drug class effects, clinical data for the drug, and its disposition. The need for additional immunotoxicity testing should be decided on the basis of a weight of evidence assessment, taking into account all available information. Testing should thus be a tiered approach, triggered and determined by concerns from the weight of evidence assessment.

Immunotoxicity is defined in the ICH S8 guideline as unintended immunosuppression or enhancement. It must be noticed that drug-induced hypersensitivity and autoimmunity are not in the scope of ICH S8. Furthermore, the ICH S8 guideline excludes biological and biotechnology-derived products. Nevertheless, these aspects are also addressed in this chapter.

11.2   CATEGORIES OF IMMUNOTOXICITY

11.2.1   Immunosuppression

The immune system is composed of a multitude of cooperating organ systems, cell types, and soluble factors, which are distributed over the entire body, and which normally are in a state of delicate balance. Furthermore, the immune system encompasses a plethora of different signal transduction pathways. As a consequence, multiple entry points exist for unintended noxious actions, and most compounds that interfere with certain signal transduction pathways are likely to find some target structures somewhere in the immune system. Furthermore, since the immune system requires a substantial portion of the body's energy and resources, all metabolic inhibitors are likely to cause an effect on the immune system. In addition, the immune system is closely interrelated with the peripheral and central nervous system [4]. Thus, care must be taken to differentiate noxious toxicological actions on the immune system from secondary effects related to general stress [5].

Immune defense is based on two arms—the evolutionary old arm, called the innate immune system, and the evolutionary younger arm, called the adaptive immune system. In vertebrates, both arms of the immune system are in close interplay, and the adaptive immune system could not work without the sentinel and preparative work of its innate counterpart. A potent innate immune system is found in invertebrates and in vertebrates. Receptors of the innate arm are designed to recognize invariable molecular patterns of microorganisms. A good example of such evolutionary old receptors is the family of toll-like receptors, which have already been identified to be involved in immune defense in *Drosophila*, and which are still in use in humans for the same purposes. In a wider sense, the innate immune system encompasses all physical, chemical, and cellular barriers that protect the individual from microbial infections without the need to learn to discriminate self from nonself. The body protects itself from dangerous actions of the innate immune system by the lack of expression of molecular patterns of microorganisms and by the abundant expression of inhibitors. Most components of the innate immune system can work independently and in parallel to destroy microorganisms (Fig. 11.1). Thus, due to its redundancy, the innate immune system is rather robust regarding its afferent and efferent actions.

The adaptive immune system is only found in vertebrates. Receptors of the adaptive arm are generated by random recombination and mutation processes and sub-

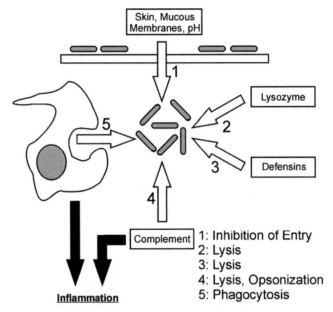

FIGURE 11.1 Parallel actions of the innate immune system during antibacterial defense. Innate defense against bacteria is composed of at least five independent components. (1) Invasion of bacteria from external body surfaces is hampered by keratinized skin, low dermal pH, ciliated epithelia, or mucus layers. (2) Bacterial murein cell walls are digested by the enzymatic activity of the ubiquitous enzyme lysozyme. (3) Bacteria are attacked by antibiotic peptides like defensins (e.g., by pore formation). (4) Bacteria are attacked by the alternative and lectin pathway of the complement cascade, leading to pore formation and 3Cb deposition on the cell wall. (5) Bacteria are recognized by macrophages via receptors for microbial molecular patterns (e.g., LPS receptor, mannose-fucose receptor, scavenger receptor), or via complement receptors detecting deposited C3b. Bacteria are eliminated by macrophages via phagocytosis and intracellular digestion. Both activation of macrophages and activation of the complement system are associated with the release of proinflammatory factors like TNF-α (macrophages) or C3a and C5a (complement).

sequent selection. The adaptive immune system is designed to learn to recognize any foreign antigen that may be expressed by a microorganism. The fact that the adaptive arm of the immune system depends on delicate tolerance mechanisms to shape the repertoire of the randomly produced antigen receptors makes this part of the immune system susceptible for the induction of autoimmunity. In contrast to innate immune responses, induction of an adaptive immune response depends on a well regulated temporal and spatial sequence of activation events, which requires the cooperation of several cell types, and the migration of cells between different organs (Fig. 11.2). As a consequence, activation of adaptive immune responses is a rather slow process, as compared with the activation of innate defense mechanisms. All cellular interactions during the induction of an adaptive immune response are based on differentiated intercellular communications pathways involving a plethora of cytokines and surface receptors. Thus, the four basic types of adaptive immune responses—antigen-specific antibody responses, cytotoxic T cell (CTL) responses, as well as CD4$^+$ inflammatory (T_H1) and helper T cell (T_H2) responses—offer a variety of entry points for immunotoxic actions. A simplified overview of possible entry points for immunotoxic actions, as exemplified by the induction of an antibody response, is given in Table 11.1. As a general rule, the adaptive immune system is more sensitive to the action of immunotoxicants than the innate immune system.

The term immunosuppression refers to the impairment of any component of the immune system resulting in decreased immune function. Immunosuppression may be an intended primary pharmacodynamic action of certain pharmaceuticals (immunosuppressants such as cyclosporine, anti-inflammatory drugs such as corticoids). In such cases, a substantial body of data relating to immunotoxic actions may already be available from basic pharmacodynamic studies. Thus, the need for additional formal immunotoxicity studies may be discussed on a case-by-case basis. The real focus of immunotoxicity assessment is the detection, description, and quantitation of unintended or unforeseen immunotoxic effects.

A critical factor for the risk assessment of potential immunosuppressive compounds is the duration of suppression. The major adverse consequences of long-term immunosuppression are infectious complications and virus-induced malignancies. Short episodes of immunosuppression can be well tolerated by otherwise healthy individuals. However, unless sufficient anti-infective comedication can be provided, even short-term immunosuppression must be avoided in situations of preexisting infectious disease such as parasitoses, systemic mycoses, tuberculosis, and especially viral infections. Therefore, for every drug, the potential to induce unintended immunosuppression should be known, and assessment of potential suppressive effects on the immune system must be regarded as an important component of the overall evaluation of drug safety.

The most robust methods available for practical use in the assessment of adverse drug effects on immune function are those designed to detect and evaluate immunosuppression. For most small molecules, nonclinical assessment of immunosuppression can be performed in small rodent species. Additional general toxicological assessments are also performed using a second (nonrodent) species, and indicators of immunotoxicity are assessed also in the second species. In the case of biotechnology-derived pharmaceuticals like recombinant cytokines or chemokines, however, species specificity of the respective receptors and ligands, as well as immunogenicity

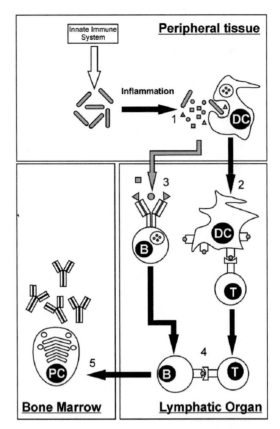

FIGURE 11.2   Temporal and spatial sequence of events leading to the induction of an antibody response. At the first instance, the innate immune system must associate invaded microorganisms with "danger" and cause inflammation. (1) Inflammatory signals instruct immature dendritic cells (DCs) to ingest, process, and finally present external microbial antigens with MHC class I and class II molecules. The immature DCs subsequently differentiate into mature DCs and migrate from the site of antigen exposure to proximal lymphatic organs. (2) In lymphatic organs mature DCs present antigen to resting T cells and stimulate them for proliferation and differentiation into activated T effector cells. (3) B cells have to bind antigens with their membrane immunoglobulins, internalize and process the ingested antigens, and finally present the processed antigens with MHC class II molecules. (4) Inside the lymphatic organ antigen-specific B cells and CD4+ T helper cells (specific for the nominal antigen in processed form) have to enter into direct cellular cross-talk via membrane receptors and cytokines. Depending on the kind of information exchanged between both cells, the B cell gets instructed to proliferate and differentiates into an antibody secreting plasma cell (PC). (5) For long-term antibody production, the PC has to leave the lymphatic organ and find its way to the bone marrow. Note that this picture is still incomplete: antigen presentation to B cells by interdigitating DCs in lymphatic organs is required for affinity maturation of the antibody response; also, antibodies themselves are marker molecules rather than effector molecules. Bound antibodies identify microorganisms for subsequent destruction by the complement cascade via the classical pathway: for antibody-dependent cellular cytotoxicity (ADCC) by NK cells via Fcγ receptors; for phagocytosis by neutrophils or macrophages via Fcγ receptors; or for destruction (e.g., parasitic worms) by eosinophils via Fcε receptors.

TABLE 11.1 Summary of Key Events Required for the Induction of a T-Cell-Dependent Humoral Immune Response and Possible Entry Points for Immunotoxic Actions

Organ	APC	B Cell	CD4+ T Cell	Possible Immunotoxic Entry Point	Possible Immunotoxic Outcome
Bone marrow	Differentiation from pluripotent stem cells	Differentiation from pluripotent stem cells	Differentiation from pluripotent stem cells	• Inhibition of cell proliferation • Interference with signal transduction • Genotoxicity	• Leukopenia • Malignancies
		Rearrangement of antigen receptors Central repertoire selection Homing, antibody production	Rearrangement of antigen receptors	• Interference with gene recombination • Interference with DNA repair • Interference with signal transduction • Interference with apoptosis • Interference with signal transduction • Inhibition of protein synthesis	• Lymphopenia • Selective lymphopenia • Autoimmunity • Impaired adaptive immune response
Thymus			Proliferation and positive/negative repertoire selection	• Interference with signal transduction • Interference with apoptosis	• Selective lymphopenia • Autoimmunity
Peripheral tissue	Antigen uptake and processing			• Inhibition of cell motility • Interference with phagolysosomal degradation • Interference with intracellular transport	• Lack of antigen presentation • Impaired adaptive immune response
	Maturation			• Inhibition of cell motility • Interference with signal transduction	• Lack of antigen presentation • Impaired adaptive immune response
Lymphatic organ	Antigen presentation	Antigen uptake and presentation	Antigen recognition (APC) and activation; proliferation; differentiation	• Inhibition of cell motility • Interference with phagolysosomal degradation or intracellular transport • Interference with signal transduction	• Impaired adaptive immune response
		Cross-communication with T cell Activation, proliferation, differentiation	Cross-communication with B-cell	• Inhibition of cytokine release • Interference with signal transduction	• Impaired adaptive immune response • Autoimmunity; allergy
				• Inhibition of cell proliferation • Interference with signal transduction	• Impaired adaptive immune response

of the compound itself, must be considered when choosing an appropriate test system.

11.2.2 Unintended Immunostimulation

As for immunosuppression, immunostimulation may be an intended primary pharmacodynamic action of drugs. Immunostimulation may be a well justified therapeutic measure in situations of selective impairment of the immune system, or in situations of life-threatening tumor disease, where the potential treatment benefits surpass the risk of unwanted side effects. In general, however, immunostimulation is a double-edged sword. The nonaffected immune system is in a continuous state of homeostatic equilibrium. Disturbing this equilibrium, even by selective activation of single components of the immune system, may lead to severe immunotoxic side effects encompassing hypersensitivity, autoimmunity, or even hematological malignancies.

Some drug substances (or their impurities) may interfere with signal transduction pathways or may be ligands for activating receptors. Such substances may cause a general or selective activation of components of the immune system. Consequences of an unintended activation of the immune system may be fever, influenza-like symptoms, an increased frequency of autoimmune diseases or hypersensitivity reactions, as well as the inhibition of drug-metabolizing cytochrome P450 (CYP) enzymes [6]. Most of these consequences are related to a cytokine burst induced by the activating compound [7]. To make the situation even more complicated, activation of single components of the immune system may cause depression of others, leading to an overall immunosuppression. In general, unintended immunostimulation must be considered as nothing but dysregulation of an otherwise perfectly working immune system. Therefore, for every drug, the potential to induce unintended immunostimulation should be known.

Assessment of unintended immunostimulation *in vivo* is often associated with complex endpoints indicative of lymphoproliferative disorders, inflammation, hypersensitivity, or autoimmunity [8]. Thus, follow-up assessment of immunostimulation should ideally be done *in vitro* using defined cell populations. A number of well established procedures exist to assess immunostimulation *in vitro*, and especially in the case of complex biotechnology-derived pharmaceuticals, species specificity of the respective receptors and ligands can be much better reflected using *in vitro* approaches.

11.2.3 Immunogenicity

Adaptive immune responses fall into four major categories:

1. Antibody responses are based on B cells, which express immunoglobulins as antigen receptors on their cell surfaces, and which differentiate into antibody producing plasma cells after appropriate stimulation. Antibodies bind antigens in their native form.

2. CD4$^+$ inflammatory (T$_H$1) responses are characterized by CD4$^+$ effector T cells secreting the cytokines IL-2 and IFN-γ, but not secreting IL-4, IL-5, and IL-6.

The physiological role of T_H1 cells is to induce inflammation in peripheral tissues and to stimulate macrophages for microbicidal activity [9].

3. CD4+ helper (T_H2) responses are characterized by CD4+ effector T cells secreting the cytokines IL-4, IL-5, and IL-6, but not secreting IL-2 and IFN-γ. The physiological role of T_H2 cells is to activate B cells for antibody production [9]. Both T_H1 and T_H2 cells bind small peptide fragments from extracellular protein antigens, which are processed and presented by professional antigen presenting cells in the context of MHC class II molecules.

4. CD8+ cytotoxic T cell (CTL) responses are characterized by CD8+ effector T cells containing the cytolytic proteins perforin and granzyme. The physiological role of CTLs is to kill virus-infected target cells and tumor cells by direct cell contact. CTLs bind small peptide fragments from intracellular protein antigens, which are processed and presented by all nucleated cells in the context of MHC class I molecules.

There are two major concerns associated with drug immunogenicity: drug allergenicity and the ability of antidrug immune responses to alter the pharmacokinetic and pharmacodynamic profile of a drug substance. Allergy, in this context, is nothing but a special pathological manifestation of immunity, and any drug that induces an allergic reaction must first induce an immune response. Thus, immunogenicity and allergenicity of drugs have to be discussed in the same context.

The immune system is programmed to mount specific immune responses against all kinds of foreign macromolecules like proteins or polysaccharides. Furthermore, even small molecules that may act as "haptens" after binding to carrier proteins can induce immune responses. Good examples of such pharmacologically relevant haptens are penicillin and sulfonamides. When addressing the question of drug immunogenicity, one must keep in mind that almost everything can be made immunogenic, provided the appropriate physical conditions and route of administration are used. Therefore, the question is not whether a drug substance is potentially immunogenic; the question is rather whether a drug substance in its given formulation, dosage, posology, and route of administration can induce an immune response.

Assessment of immunogenicity requires a complete and intact immune system. No *in vitro* procedure is currently in sight to determine the immunogenic potential of a drug, or to replace animal experimentation in this context. However, it must be noted that even the currently available nonclinical *in vivo* immunogenicity tests have only a limited predictive value for the human situation. The ability of a substance to induce an immune response in a given species or even a given individual depends on a variety of factors encompassing the following:

- The chemical nature and dimension of the molecule.
- The ability to form covalent or noncovalent complexes with carrier molecules in the recipient (relevant for small "hapten" molecules).
- The ability to be processed and to be presented with molecules encoded by the recipient's major histocompatibility complex (relevant for proteins and peptides).

- The similarity of the molecule with "self"-antigens of the recipient, and thus the depth of preexisting immunological tolerance of the recipient.
- The site, dose, and frequency of administration.
- The physical form and formulation of the molecule.
- The biological activity of the molecule.
- The genetic background of the recipient.

It is a well known phenomenon that a certain molecule, when administered subcutaneously or intraperitoneally, may cause a vigorous immune response, while the same molecule, when administered via the oral route, causes a state of immunological tolerance. It is furthermore well known to immunologists that mice of a given strain can be good "responders" to a certain antigen, whereas mice of a different strain are "nonresponders" to the same antigen. Thus, when an immunogenicity test in one species gives a negative result, the test should be repeated in at least one further appropriate species to provide a reasonable assessment of immunogenic potential.

As a very rough rule, the predictive value of a nonclinical immunogenicity test increases with increasing "xenogenicity" of the molecule to be assessed. Thus, a molecule that is as foreign to a mouse or guinea pig as it is to humans—for example, an antibiotic or a protein from snake venom—is likely to give predictive results for the human situation in nonclinical immunogenicity investigations. On the other hand, injecting a recombinant human protein into a guinea pig would be a rather senseless approach to assess its potential immunogenicity in humans. The guinea pig is likely to mount an immune response against this foreign protein in such circumstances. Using the recombinant guinea pig homolog to the human protein would be the more informative study design in this case.

11.2.4   Allergenicity

Induction of hypersensitivity resulting in allergic reactions is among the most frequent reasons for terminating a drug treatment. Allergies encompass immune-mediated allergic, as well as non-immune-mediated pseudoallergic, reactions, which can be divided into five categories, depending on the effector molecules and effector mechanisms involved.

> *Type I* (immediate type) hypersensitivity is mediated by antibodies of the IgE isotype, leading to mast cell degranulation after passive adsorption to Fcε receptors on mast cells and cross-linking by allergens. There are two general subtypes of Type I reactions: systemic hypersensitivity (e.g., anaphylaxis, urticaria) and respiratory hypersensitivity (e.g., asthma).
>
> *Type II* hypersensitivity is mediated predominantly by IgG antibodies, which bind to haptenized cell surfaces and elicit cytolytic or inflammatory reactions following binding of natural killer cells or neutrophils via Fcγ receptors.
>
> *Type III* hypersensitivity is mediated by immune complex deposition and subsequent inflammation due to the activation of the complement system.
>
> *Type IV* hypersensitivity (delayed type hypersensitivity, DTH) is mediated by antigen- or hapten-specific T_H1 cells inducing strong inflammatory reactions

after binding antigen on professional antigen presenting cells especially in the skin. A contact allergy, for example against nickel, is a typical manifestation of a Type IV hypersensitivity reaction.

Pseudoallergies are not immunologically mediated, but mediated by active substances that induce or facilitate histamine release from mast cells or basophils. In contrast to real allergies, pseudoallergies show a clear dose–response relationship.

Despite its high clinical relevance, evaluation of drugs for allergenic potential is extremely unreliable in nonclinical toxicology studies. First, a drug that has been proved to be immunogenic in a laboratory animal species may not necessarily be immunogenic in humans, and vice versa. Second, the subtle factors that determine whether an individual responds to an antigen with an IgG or an IgE response can hardly be extrapolated from one species to another. Thus, an immune response that manifests as an allergic response in a laboratory animal may not necessarily manifest as an allergic response in humans, and vice versa.

With regard to antibody-mediated hypersensitivity, three methods have been used extensively to assess the induction of drug-specific (Type I) anaphylactic reactions:

- The passive cutaneous anaphylaxis (PCA) assay.
- The active cutaneous anaphylaxis (ACA) assay.
- The active systemic anaphylaxis (ASA) assay.

All three assays are normally conducted in guinea pigs, which is the only rodent species that actually develops symptoms of severe anaphylactic reactions and even fatal allergic shock. However, the usefulness of these assays for the safety assessment of drugs is considered limited. Since IgE as well as IgG antibodies can cause anaphylactic reactions in guinea pigs, a positive result in any of the three assays can only be weighed as proof of immunogenicity, but not allergenicity of a drug. The PCA, ACA, and ASA assays are therefore not requested or recommended for the routine evaluation of allergenicity of investigational new drugs by any regulatory agency.

The situation is as unsatisfactory for the prediction of a Type II and Type III allergenic potential of drugs. Although there are examples of drugs that are associated with Type II and Type III hypersensitivity reactions, there are no standard nonclinical methods for predicting these effects. Manifestations of both kinds of immunopathies are often indistinguishable from direct, non-immune-mediated drug toxicity. Thus, in some instances of hemolytic anemia, vasculitis, or glomerulonephritis, which may be observed during standard toxicity studies, follow-up studies should be considered to determine if antibody-mediated immune mechanisms are involved.

Since all available nonclinical assays to assess the antibody-based allergenic potential of drugs have a limited predictivity for the human situation [10], detection of drug immunogenicity should already be considered to be a potential safety alert. Whether proven immunogenicity in a nonclinical test does in fact lead to allergic complications in patients can only be convincingly demonstrated (or excluded) in clinical trials or even later still during postmarketing surveillance of the approved drug.

The most robust and predictive procedures available for assessment of allergenicity are those measuring the skin sensitizing potential of topically administered drug substances. In these cases, a drug has to permeate the keratinized skin, bind to MHC molecules of dermal antigen presenting cells, and stimulate CD4$^+$ T cells for proliferation and T$_H$1 differentiation. Any drug that is able to induce the above sequence of events will inevitably induce an inflammatory reaction, a so-called delayed type hypersensitivity reaction, after subsequent challenge exposure to the skin. Thus, in this special situation of dermal sensitization, a proof of immunogenicity is also a proof of allergenicity.

When a drug is intended for topical administration (dermal, ocular, vaginal, rectal), the skin sensitizing potential of the drug should be determined using an appropriate assay based on sensitization and challenge as part of nonclinical safety evaluation. The most common methods for evaluating the dermal sensitizing potential of drugs have been the Buehler assay (BA) and the guinea pig maximization test (GPMT). Both *in vivo* guinea pig based methods are reliable and have demonstrated a high correlation with known human skin sensitizers. Techniques using mice, like the mouse ear swelling test, which uses an induction and challenge pattern similar to the traditional guinea pig tests, or the murine local lymph node assay (LLNA), correlate well with traditional guinea pig tests [11, 12]. Especially the LLNA, which is designed to detect lymphoproliferation in draining lymph nodes of the exposition area instead of inflammation following challenge, gives quantitative results. Furthermore, the assay is now accepted by most regulatory agencies with regard to reduction, refinement, and replacement of animal experimentation.

Pseudoallergic (anaphylactoid) reactions, which are independent of antigen-specific immune responses, result from direct drug-mediated histamine release or complement activation. Anaphylactoid reactions can be differentiated from true IgE-mediated anaphylaxis by *in vitro* testing of drug-induced histamine release from mast cell lines [13], or by the detection of activated complement products in serum of animals showing signs of anaphylaxis [14].

11.2.5 Autoimmunity

Chemical- or drug-induced autoimmune reactions are rather rare events. However, such reactions have been described for heavy metal ions [15] and for vaccines [16]. Drug substances or their impurities may induce autoimmunity by two major mechanisms. Immunogenic drug substances or vaccines may induce autoimmune responses by cross priming for self-antigens. Other drug substances or their impurities may cause an unintended nonspecific activation of the immune system, leading to a break of peripheral self-tolerance. In analogy to allergies, autoimmune reactions may be categorized according to the effector mechanisms involved:

Type II autoimmunity is mediated predominantly by IgG antibodies, which bind to cell surfaces and elicit cytolysis or block cellular functions (e.g., hemolytic anemia, myasthenia gravis).

Type III autoimmunity is mediated by immune complex deposition, activating the complement system (e.g., lupus erythematosus).

Type IV autoimmunity is mediated by self-antigen-specific T cells (e.g., multiple sclerosis, type I diabetes).

There is no Type I (IgE-mediated) autoimmune disease known so far.

An assessment of the potential of a drug (or vaccine) to induce autoimmunity should always be considered when a drug substance, or its impurities, has proved to be immunogenic. The question for autoimmunity should be further addressed when the final formulation of a drug (or vaccine) contains immune response modifiers or adjuvants. However, there are no predictive standard methods for determining the potential of experimental drugs to produce autoimmune reactions [17, 18]. In such situations, special attention should be devoted to signs of glomerulonephritis, lupus-like syndrome, hemolytic anemia, and vasculitis during standard toxicity studies. Furthermore, an assessment of a basic panel of antinuclear or anticytoplasmic auto-antibodies should be considered for inclusion in the study design [19].

11.3   REGULATORY CONSIDERATIONS

11.3.1   History of Regulatory Guidelines

Immunotoxicology regulatory guidelines have evolved from the 1980s. As detailed in Table 11.2, an overview is provided on the chronology of key programs and guidelines that have influenced the development of the science of immunotoxicology and the development of more recent guidelines for pharmaceuticals. It can be seen from this table that the U.S. Environmental Protection Agency and the U.S. National Toxicology Program have been heavily involved in the formative years in the development of tiered immunotoxicology testing guidance. Separate efforts were made in the 1980s in Europe to provide guidance on the prospective assessment of the immunotoxicological potential of chemicals including pharmaceuticals.

The spirit of these immunotoxicology programs and guidelines has been adopted for subsequent testing guidelines issued in the drug-related sector, as detailed later in the text. In particular, tiered approaches to testing have been used for many years, and recent developments for immunotoxicity testing of pharmaceuticals have focused particularly on optimizing tiered testing strategies.

11.3.2   Current Developments for Pharmaceuticals

The developing awareness of the possible unwanted immune-modulating effects of pharmaceuticals has resulted in the release of a number of regulatory guidance documents for immunotoxicity testing in all three ICH regions. Within the various guidelines that have been developed, it is clear that evaluation of the potential adverse effects of human pharmaceuticals on the immune system should be incorporated into standard drug development. Final guidelines for identifying the potential immunotoxicity of new chemical entities have been released by the European Union (EU) Committee for Proprietary Medicinal Products (CPMP) in 2000 [20] and the U.S. Food and Drug Administration Center for Drug Evaluation and Research (CDER) in 2002 [21].

TABLE 11.2   Key Immunotoxicity Programs and Guidelines Prior to Contemporary Immunotoxicity Guidelines for Pharmaceuticals

Key Immunotoxicology Program/Guideline	Main Features of Program/Guideline
U.S. Environmental Protection Agency Office of Pesticide Program guideline for the immunotoxicology evaluation of pesticides (Subdivision M; Pesticide Assessment Guidelines), 1982	New pesticides should be evaluated according to Tier I and Tier II immunotoxicology evaluation.
Council of the European Communities, Official Journal, No. L332/11, 1983 [35]	Recommendation for assessment of immunotoxicity of new medicinal products, with particular emphasis on histopathological assessment of immune system.
National Institute of Public Health and Environmental Protection (RIVM) in The Netherlands [36]	Tiered approach for testing based essentially on OECD Guideline 407 at Tier I. Tier II testing (cell-mediated immunity, humoral immunity, macrophage function, NK function, host resistance) performed where required to further define immunotoxic effects.
U.S. Environmental Protection Agency proposal for first draft revision of 1982 guideline [37]	New pesticides should be evaluated by repeat dose (>30 days) toxicity testing at Tier I (includes functional assays). Tier II would be performed if positive or uninterpretable immunotoxicity results were obtained from Tier I or if other sources indicate immunotoxicity.
U.S. National Toxicology Program [38–40]	Interlaboratory immunotoxicology (repeat dose) validation study in mice of 5 test substances (including diethylstilbestrol and cyclophosphamide). The study later included over 50 test substances. Tier I testing was for general toxicity and pathology and functional endpoints. Tier II testing was performed to further define immunotoxic effects.
Organisation for Economic Development and Cooperation (OECD), Revised Guideline 407, 1995	Repeat dose toxicity guideline, including revised specific guidance on immunotoxicity (pathological) investigations.
U.S. Environmental Protection Agency Toxic Substances Control Act (TSCA) [41]	Update of the pesticides guidelines on immunotoxicity testing covering histopathological and functional endpoints. Tier I testing was for general toxicity and pathology and humoral immunity. Innate immunity (NK assay) may be performed. Tier II testing further defines immunotoxic effects.

The current immunotoxicity guidelines focus on immunosuppression by small chemical entities and exclude biotechnology-derived pharmaceuticals. The latter are presently covered by the ICH S6 guideline, *Preclinical Safety Evaluation of Biotechnology-Derived Pharmaceuticals*, released in 1997 [22]. This guideline considers both the immunogenicity and immunotoxicity of biotechnology-derived pharmaceuticals, many of which are intended to stimulate or suppress the immune system, thus potentially modulating humoral and cell-mediated immunity. The ICH S6 guideline excludes immunotoxicity testing of vaccines, which is covered by a number of specific guidelines focusing on the testing of vaccines or adjuvants released in the three ICH regions. For the United States, the appropriate website is www.fda.gov/cber. For the European Union (EU), the appropriate website is www.emea.europa.eu, and this contains guidance on adjuvants and vaccines. In 2003 the WHO [23] published comprehensive guidelines on the nonclinical evaluation of vaccines, with detailed information on immunotoxicity assessments.

There is still much debate about the best approach for assessing the immunotoxicity potential of new chemical entities. Much of this debate is focused on subtle differences between the FDA and CPMP guidelines with regard to the best approach for determining the risk of immunotoxicity. Efforts to harmonize immunotoxicity testing programs have culminated in development of the ICH S8 guideline, *Immunotoxicity Studies for Human Pharmaceuticals*, which was adopted by the CHMP in October 2005 and came into operation in April 2006. It was furthermore adopted by the FDA and published in the Federal Register in April 2006, as well as by the MHLW in April 2006.

Table 11.3 compares the new as well as the still operating guidelines for immunotoxicity testing issued by the ICH, the FDA CDER (U.S.), and the CPMP (EU).

TABLE 11.3   Comparison of Current ICH, and former EU, and U.S. Immunotoxicity Guidelines

	ICH S8 (In operation in all ICH regions since 2006) [24]	U.S. FDA CDER (Still in operation since 2002) [21]	EU CPMP (Still in operation since 2000) [20]
Specific immunotoxicity guideline	Yes	Yes	No, included in guidance on repeat dose toxicity.
Drug-induced hypersensitivity, immunogenicity, and autoimmunity excluded	Yes	No, these categories are included in the guideline.	Yes. (Note: Skin sensitizing potential addressed in CPMP Note for Guidance on Non-Clinical Local Tolerance Testing, 2001 [42]).
Screening study(ies) required	Yes, the initial screen for potential immunotoxicity involves Standard Toxicity Studies (STSs) from short-term to chronic repeat dose studies in rodents and nonrodents.	Yes, including all standard repeat dose toxicology studies that have been performed.	Yes, screening required for all new active substances in at least one repeat dose toxicity study (duration ideally should be 28 days). Rats or mice are species of choice.

TABLE 11.3   *Continued*

	ICH S8 (In operation in all ICH regions since 2006) [24]	U.S. FDA CDER (Still in operation since 2002) [21]	EU CPMP (Still in operation since 2000) [20]
Screening study(ies) immunotoxicity parameters	Changes in hematology, lymphoid organ weights, histopathology of immune system, and serum globulins and increased incidences of infections and tumors should be evaluated for signs of immunotoxic potential in the STSs.	Changes in hematology, lymphoid organ weights, gross pathology and histopathology of immune system, and serum globulins and increased incidences of infections and tumors should be evaluated for signs of immunotoxic potential.	Hematology, lymphoid organ weights, histopathology of lymphoid tissues, bone marrow cellularity, distribution of lymphocyte subsets, and NK cell activity (if latter two unavailable, primary antibody response to T-cell-dependent antigen).
Other factors to consider in evaluation of potential immunotoxicity and the need for additional immunotoxicity studies	Pharmacological properties of drug; patient population; structural similarities to known immunomodulators; drug disposition; clinical data.	Patient population; known drug class effects (including SARs); drug pharmacokinetics; clinical data. If drug intended for HIV, immune function studies required.	None specifically included in the guideline.
"Follow-on"/ "Additional" immunotoxicity studies	"Additional" studies may be required depending on the "weight of evidence review" of STSs and "Other Factors." "Additional" studies addressed in 3.2, 3.3, and Appendix of guideline.	"Additional" immune function studies (Sections III.B and III.C of guideline) may be required depending on "weight of evidence review" of effects in toxicity studies and "Other Factors."	"Follow-on" functional immunotoxicity studies (Appendix B of guideline) warranted on a case-by-case basis.
Timing of "Follow-on"/"Additional" immunotoxicity testing in relation to clinical studies	"Additional" immunotoxicity testing, if required, should be completed before clinical Phase III, or earlier depending on the effect or the patient population.	Not specified.	Not specified.

The U.S. Food and Drug Administration CDER [21] publication also covers developmental immunotoxicity, which should be addressed where a drug has shown immunosuppressive potential in adult animal studies. More recently, a group of immunotoxicology experts from the United States and European Union has proposed a testing framework for developmental immunotoxicity [25]. The major conclusions are that the rat is the preferred model and that validated developmental immunotoxicity methods should be incorporated into standard developmental and reproductive toxicity protocols where possible.

11.3.3   The Common Spirit of Regulatory Immunotoxicity Guidelines

All current immunotoxicity guidelines for new drug entities are based on a tiered testing approach with a basic set of parameters to be assessed during standard toxicological studies (STSs), and "Additional" or "Follow-up" investigations initiated by alerts from basic toxicological studies. As outlined in the ICH S8 guideline [24] and in the U.S. FDA CDER guideline [21], in addition to the alerts from the STSs, other causes for concern that might prompt additional immunotoxicity studies include the pharmacological properties of the drug, the intended patient population, known drug class effects, the disposition of the drug, and clinical data.

All guidelines from the different ICH regions request that basic immunotoxicity screening should encompass hematology, lymphoid organ weights, and histopathology of the lymphoid organs. All of these parameters are assessed in standard repeat dose toxicity studies. Discrepancy remains in the ICH regions on the need for a functional assay. Currently, only Europe requests functional assays in routine screening. In Europe [20], the routine screening of every compound should include distribution of lymphocyte subsets (by phenotyping) and natural killer cell activity. If these are not available, primary antibody response to a T-cell-dependent antigen may be assessed as an alternative.

The FDA CDER [21] document advocates a case-by-case approach to the need for functional assays. This approach is similar to the position taken by the ICH S8 guideline [24]. Irrespective of whether a functional assay for immunotoxicity was already integrated into the basic toxicological tests (as in Europe), a decision whether additional immunotoxicity follow-up studies are appropriate should be determined by a weight of evidence review of cause(s) for concern. It is generally agreed that a follow-up immunotoxicity testing program must be designed on a case-by-case basis to allow for a sufficient flexibility reflecting the different effects a drug may exert on the immune system. All relevant guidelines only recommend testing methods for follow-up assessment of immunotoxicity. It is at the discretion of the investigator to choose appropriate models, test methods, and protocols for follow-up immunotoxicity studies.

Preclinical programs designed to assess adverse effects of new drugs on the immune system should be based on generally accepted as well as technically and biologically validated methods. The program should furthermore follow the general rules of toxicology by reflecting the following parameters:

- Statistical and biological significance of the changes
- Severity of the effects
- Dose dependency

- Safety factor above the expected clinical dose
- Study duration
- Number of species and endpoints affected
- Changes that may occur secondarily to other factors (e.g., stress)
- Possible cellular targets and/or mechanism of action
- Doses that produce these changes in relation to doses that produce other toxicities
- Reversibility of effect(s)

It must be kept in mind that the availability of biomarkers for evaluating the immune system in clinical trials is limited, and therefore, increased emphasis should be put on preclinical data as is the case for the testing of carcinogenic potential. Preclinical toxicity data support the design of clinical trials and may trigger enhanced screening for certain immune-related effects in clinical trials. The importance of preclinical immunotoxicity risk assessment should not be underestimated, since the findings may affect the indication, patient management, and the labeling of the drug product.

11.4   IMMUNOTOXICITY TESTING STRATEGIES

11.4.1   Initial Considerations

There are some points to consider before collecting data relating to immunotoxicity from standard toxicity studies and before entering into follow-up immunotoxicity testing. The major focus of immunotoxicology is detection and evaluation of undesired effects of substances on the immune system. The prime concern is to assess the importance of these interactions with regard to human health. The basic decision for the selection of assays to be used in evaluating compounds for immunotoxicity must therefore be that the assays are standardized and recognized as validated, meaningful, and predictive for the human situation. Rationales for choosing a certain assay must reflect these criteria. A collection of recommended assays is given in the appendix of the ICH S8 guideline. However, these assays are neither binding nor necessarily suitable to answer all questions related to immunotoxicity.

As stipulated in the ICH S8 guideline, the decision on immunotoxicity testing is driven by alerts from standard toxicity studies, especially from 28 day repeat dose toxicity studies with full assessment of hematology, clinical chemistry, and histopathology. Other causes for concern that might prompt additional immunotoxicity studies include the pharmacological properties of the drug, the intended patient population, known drug class effects, the disposition of the drug, and available clinical data. When no alerts or concerns can be identified during a proper weight of evidence based risk assessment, immunotoxicity testing beyond the parameters already tested during the initial immunotoxicity screening can be omitted. However, the occurrence of immunotoxic potential later in development during clinical trials may require follow-up preclinical investigations.

The immune system is flexible and often able to utilize alternative factors and mechanisms to compensate for deficiencies in a particular immune function. For this reason, tests in appropriate animal models will normally provide a more accurate picture of immune system competence and a more relevant indication of immuno-toxic potential than *in vitro* tests in which compensatory alternative mechanisms may be lacking. However, if a sound scientific rationale can be provided as to why *in vitro* tests will suffice, then their use is encouraged to minimize *in vivo* investigations. Marked differences in the immune system do exist across species. It would therefore be advisable to use more than one species for preclinical immunotoxicity evaluation to confirm that negative as well as positive results in one species are also negative or positive in another species. The use of a rodent and a nonrodent species that are routinely required for standard repeat dose toxicity tests allows for such assessments in two species by assessment of hematology, clinical chemistry, and pathology. However, it must be noted that validated immunotoxicity follow-up testing protocols and methods in nonrodent species are, with a few exceptions, not yet available.

Immunotoxicity studies are expected to be performed in compliance with Good Laboratory Practice (GLP). This is at least binding for the initial immunotoxicity screening during standard toxicology studies, as well as for the assessment of dermal or respiratory sensitization. It is recognized, however, that some specialized assays for follow-up immunotoxicity assessment might not comply fully with GLP. Deviation from GLP rules, or assay performance in a noncertified laboratory, can be justified in such cases. From an analytical point of view, complex biological assays like those used for follow-up immunotoxicity assessment are difficult to validate with regard to accuracy and precision, as well as interassay or interlaboratory reproducibility. Thus, results should ideally not be presented as primary measurements (e.g., optical densities or counts per minute), but rather in terms of more robust derivatives like stimulation indices or percent inhibition data. Furthermore, it is generally recommended to have all necessary positive and negative controls included in the same measurement series. As a matter of course, the weak points and variabilities of an assay should be known and taken into account during the design of a study protocol and final data analysis. Dose comparisons to clinical use should ideally be based on relative body surface areas, as opposed to body weight.

11.4.2 Timing of Immunotoxicity Studies

Some data on the immunotoxic potential of the drug substance or drug product will be known before clinical investigations in humans are initiated, since repeat dose standard toxicity studies are required before human exposure. If required, additional (follow-up) immunotoxicity data should be available before a large number of patients will be treated with an investigational new drug. This means that follow-up immunotoxicity studies, when triggered by an initial weight of evidence risk analysis or by alerts from early clinical trials, are normally performed in parallel with clinical Phase I or Phase II studies. The respective data should be available before entry into clinical Phase III. Nevertheless, a need for additional immunotoxicity studies may also be triggered by unexpected findings during later stages of clinical development or postmarketing pharmacovigilance. An earlier timing of follow-up immunotoxicity studies must be considered when the intended patient group is immunocompromised, suffering from chronic or latent infections, or is affected by allergic or autoimmune disorders.

11.4.3 Choice of Test Species

As a general rule, the same species that gave immunotoxicity alerts during standard toxicity testing should also be employed for follow-up immunotoxicity testing. However, there is only limited availability of validated immunotoxicity test procedures or suitable tools (e.g., monoclonal antibodies, recombinant cytokines, ELISA systems) for otherwise common test species like dogs. In such cases a limitation to rodent tests may be justifiable. The situation is often much better for nonhuman primates. In the latter case, many of the tools designed for human use are also fully compatible with primate material. Thus, nonhuman primates, especially cynomolgus monkeys, may become the "second species" of choice for future nonclinical immunotoxicity assessment. However, in view of the necessary limitations on the use of primates for preclinical testing, primates should only be considered where nonprimate species are not acceptable for human risk assessment.

Assessment of Immunotoxicity of Small Molecules   Given the complexity of the immune system, a species without primary pharmacodynamic activity of the drug (due to different receptors or different drug metabolism) should not be the species of choice for immunotoxicity testing. Concordant with the general rule of drug toxicity assessment, the species should be responsive to the intended primary pharmacodynamic effects of the compound. The same holds for the expected secondary pharmacodynamic effects. For small molecules, the species of choice for immunotoxicity assessment, encompassing immunosuppression and unintended immunostimulation, is mostly the mouse or the rat. In the case of small molecules a good degree of predictivity for the human situation is mostly given. Currently, a preference is given to the rat for mechanistic immunotoxicity testing in Europe, and the mouse in the United States. This, however, has a more historic background and is neither binding nor sustained by a superiority of one system over the other. It should be pointed out, however, that the rat is predominantly used as the rodent species for standard repeat dose toxicity tests and for reproductive toxicity and developmental toxicity testing.

All guidelines in the three ICH regions, as well as the ICH S8 guideline, recommend testing for immunotoxicity in a rodent species in repeat dose toxicity studies. Initial immunotoxicity screening (hematology, clinical chemistry, and pathology) is incorporated into the standard toxicity test(s) also performed in the nonrodent species. The need for additional immunotoxicity testing would be assessed from the results of the standard toxicity tests and other factors as discussed in the ICH S8 guideline. If the preclinical test program is performed in a nonrodent species only (i.e., for a biotechnology drug), additional immunotoxicity testing should then be considered in this species if required based on the initial screen performed in the standard toxicity test(s) using this species.

In contrast to the assessment of immunosuppression and unintended immunostimulation, responsiveness to the pharmacodynamic effects of the drug substance is advisable but not mandatory for immunogenicity or allergenicity testing. However, it must be noted that the kind and strength of an immune response is to a very high degree dependent on the route of antigen administration. Different routes of antigen administration (e.g., oral vs. subcutaneous) may have a totally different outcome with regard to the induced immune response. Thus, the design of an immunogenicity or allergenicity test should always include the intended route of clinical administration.

General humoral immunogenicity of small molecules may be tested in rats and mice, provided a suitable assay system (e.g., ELISA, ELISPOT, PFC assay) is available to detect drug-specific antibodies with sufficient sensitivity. The same holds for immunogenicity assessment with regard to T cells. In this case an *ex vivo* assay for T cell activation following drug administration (e.g., determination of antigen-specific cytokine production or proliferation) may be employed. If such *ex vivo* or *in vitro* assays are not available or technically feasible, the more traditional guinea pig based *in vivo* assays for the determination of Type I and Type IV hypersensitivity (ASA, ACA, PCA, GPMT) may provide a good alternative. Just to reiterate this point, a positive result in any of the above guinea pig assays can be taken as a proof of immunogenicity of a drug but must not be weighed as a proof of allergenicity in humans. In any case, a lack of immunogenicity during nonclinical testing does not necessarily exclude immunogenicity or allergenicity in humans, and vice versa. Thus, preclinical data on immunogenicity or allergenicity of drugs in experimental animals have to be interpreted with the utmost caution.

Assessment of Immunotoxicity and Immunogenicity/Allergenicity of Biotechnology-Derived Drugs The decision on a suitable species for preclinical immunotoxicity assessment of biotechnology-derived drugs must be made on a case-by-case basis. In any case, the limits of predictivity should be clearly stated in the rationales for choosing a certain assay protocol. The biological activity together with species and/or tissue specificity of many biotechnology-derived pharmaceuticals (e.g., recombinant cytokines, therapeutic antibodies) often preclude standard toxicity testing designs in commonly used species (e.g., rats and dogs). The same holds for immunotoxicity testing. The design of immunotoxicity testing programs for biotechnology-derived drugs should include the use of relevant species. A relevant species is one in which the test material is pharmacologically active due to the expression of the receptor or an epitope (in the case of monoclonal antibodies). A variety of techniques (e.g., immunochemical or functional *in vitro* tests) can be used to identify a relevant species. In some cases nonhuman primates may be the only suitable species available. When no relevant species exists, the use of transgenic mice expressing the human receptor or epitope may be accepted by regulatory agencies. The information gained from use of a transgenic mouse model expressing the human receptor is optimized when the interaction of the product and the humanized receptor has similar physiological consequences to those expected in humans.

In other cases, the use of the homologous animal protein instead of the human counterpart may be considered. While useful information may also be gained from the use of homologous proteins, it should be noted that the production process, range of impurities/contaminants, pharmacokinetics, and exact pharmacological mechanism(s) may differ between the homologous form and the product intended for clinical use. Thus, from a formalistic point of view, the test item used in such protocols is not identical to the drug substance to be assessed. Results from such studies can therefore only be weighed as "supportive data." In such situations, it is highly recommended to discuss the testing strategy with the responsible regulatory agency for scientific advice. Where it is not possible to use transgenic animal models or homologous proteins, it may be advisable to assess certain aspects of potential immunotoxicity *in vitro* using human material like PBMCs, monocyte-derived macrophages, or long-term cultivated cell lines of hematopoetic origin.

Most biotechnology-derived pharmaceuticals intended for human use are *per se* immunogenic in animals. The induction of antibody formation in animals is therefore not predictive of a potential for antibody formation in humans. In this regard, the results of, for example, a guinea pig anaphylaxis test, which is usually positive for xenogenic protein products, is not predictive for reactions in humans. Such studies are therefore considered of little value for the routine evaluation of these types of products. It must be kept in mind that even humanized proteins may be immunogenic in humans. In most cases, reliable information on immunogenicity of a biotechnology-derived drug can therefore only be obtained during clinical studies. However, immunogenicity studies in animals using biotechnology-derived drugs may yield valuable information when comparing the immunogenic potential of a test compound with a biosimilar reference compound, or between different production batches.

Even if immunogenicity assessment of biotechnology-derived pharmaceuticals has limited predictivity for the human situation, measurement of antibodies associated with the administration of biotechnology-derived drugs should always be included in the design of a repeat dose toxicity study [26]. Antibody responses should be characterized with regard to titer, number of responding animals, and neutralizing or nonneutralizing antibodies. Furthermore, the detection and quantitation of antibodies should be correlated with any pharmacological and/or toxicological changes. Specifically, the effects of antibody formation on pharmacokinetic/pharmacodynamic parameters, incidence and/or severity of adverse effects, complement activation, or the emergence of new toxic effects should be considered when interpreting the data. Attention should also be paid to the evaluation of possible pathological changes related to immune complex formation and deposition.

11.4.4 Immunotoxicity Alerts

According to the ICH S8 guideline, the decision on "Additional" immunotoxicity studies or a "Follow-up" immunotoxicity program depends on the results of a weight of evidence review of cause(s) for concern of immunotoxicity. This immunotoxicity risk assessment must reflect alerts from basic toxicological studies, pharmacological properties of the drug, the intended patient population, known drug class effects, the disposition of the drug, and clinical data (if available). Results of the entire dataset should be evaluated as to whether sufficient data are available to reasonably determine the risk of immunotoxicity. If the weight of evidence review of cause(s) for concern suggests that the risk of immunotoxicity is acceptable, then no follow-up testing might be called for.

Typical indicators of immunotoxicity, which may be observed during standard short- to long-term repeat dose toxicity studies (STSs), are summarized in Table 11.4. Note that all indicators can also result from non-immune-mediated toxicity of drugs and must not be weighed as a proof of immunotoxicity. Nevertheless, if such indicators are found, additional immunotoxicity studies are needed to identify and assess human risk or exclude immunotoxic mechanisms.

Drug substances encompassing primary pharmacodynamic immunosuppressants, cytostatic and cytotoxic antineoplastic drugs, and steroidal and nonsteroidal anti-inflammatory drugs, as well as primary pharmacodynamic immune response modi-

TABLE 11.4 Typical Indicators of Immunotoxicity, Which May Be Observed During Standard Short- to Long-Term Repeat Dose Toxicity Studies

Findings	Possible Indicator of
During the In-Life Phase	
Increased frequencies of infectious disease	Immunosuppression
Increased frequencies of tumors in long-term studies in the absence of genotoxicity or nongenotoxic indicators of tumorigenicity (e.g., endocrine)	Immunosuppression
Unexpected pathological symptoms or deaths shortly after administration	Hypersensitivity
Strong inflammatory reactions at the site of administration	Hypersensitivity
Gross Necropsy	
Significant increase or decrease of size and weight of lymphatic organs	Unintended immunostimulation or immunosuppression
Hematology	
Changes in total or differential blood counts	Unintended immunostimulation or immunosuppression
Anemia	Type II hypersensitivity
Altered frequencies of lymphocyte subsets (flow cytometry)[a]	Unintended immunostimulation or immunosuppression
Clinical Chemistry	
Altered total globulin levels or albumin : globulin ratio	Unintended immunostimulation or immunosuppression
Changes of immunoglobulin isotype levels[a]	Unintended immunostimulation or immunosuppression
Reduction of hemolytic complement activity[a]	Unintended immunostimulation or Type III hypersensitivity
Antinuclear or anticytoplasmic antibodies[a]	Unintended immunostimulation or autoimmunity
Histopathology	
Changes of cellularity and/or microanatomy of lymphatic organs	Unintended immunostimulation or immunosuppression
Vasculitis, glomerulonephritis	Type III hypersensitivity

[a]This parameter is normally not measured during standard toxicity studies but may be integrated when a focus is drawn on immunotoxicity assessment.

fiers like recombinant cytokines or chemokines, can be assumed to have secondary pharmacodynamic effects on the immune system that might result in immunotoxicity. For all the above drug substances, immunotoxicity studies are mandatory to assess the exact mode of immune interference, as well as the severity, duration, and reversibility of effects. However, in such cases a comprehensive body of data relating to immunotoxic actions may already be available from basic pharmacodynamic studies, and the extent of additional formal immunotoxicity studies may be discussed on a case-by-case basis. It must be reiterated that vaccines and/or adjuvants for vaccines, even if they are not in the scope of immunotoxicity guidelines, may have severe immunotoxic side effects related to hypersensitivity and autoimmunity. Thus, immunotoxicity testing with regard to the latter parameters is stipulated in all vaccine guidelines.

Additional immunotoxicity testing is further mandatory for all drugs intended for the treatment of patients with an increased susceptibility to immunotoxic effects or with an increased risk to be harmed by immunotoxic drugs. These patient populations encompass patients with congenital and acquired immunodeficiency, as well as patients with compromised immune function due to concurrent medical treatment (e.g., antineoplastic chemotherapy, whole body irradiation, or organ/bone marrow transplantation).

Furthermore, additional immunotoxicity studies should be undertaken when drug compounds are structurally similar to compounds with known immunosuppressive properties, with compounds that show strong protein binding properties (testing in this case is required especially with regard to immunogenicity), and with compounds that tend to accumulate in cells or organs of the immune system.

Finally, unexpected clinical findings suggestive of immunotoxicity in patients exposed to the drug should call for additional nonclinical immunotoxicity assessment to identify the degree and mechanisms of immunotoxicity.

11.4.5   Decision Tree

If signs of immunotoxicity are observed in STSs and/or one of the factors relating to pharmacodynamic properties—intended patient population, known drug class effects, pharmacokinetic properties, or clinical findings indicative of immunotoxicity of the drug—apply, it is recommended that the sponsor conducts additional nonclinical studies of drug effects on immune function or provides justification (including clinical risk–benefit analysis) for not performing these evaluations. The decision tree, as recommended by the ICH S8 guideline (Fig. 11.3), starts with a weight of evidence review performed on information from all the factors outlined above. The aim of the review is to determine whether a cause for concern exists. A finding of sufficient magnitude in a single area should trigger additional immunotoxicity studies. Findings from two or more factors, each one of which would not be sufficient on its own, could trigger additional studies. If additional immunotoxicity studies are not performed at the appropriate stage of clinical development, the sponsor will likely be asked by regulatory agencies to provide justification. If this cannot be provided, delays in clinical development and/or regulatory approval for marketing may occur.

11.5   IMMUNOTOXICITY TESTING PROTOCOLS: IMMUNOSUPPRESSION

11.5.1   Basic Testing

The first assessment phase of immunotoxicity testing is the collection and evaluation of toxicological signs indicative of immunotoxicity from standard toxicity studies. These data are regularly generated during 28 day (or similar duration) repeat dose

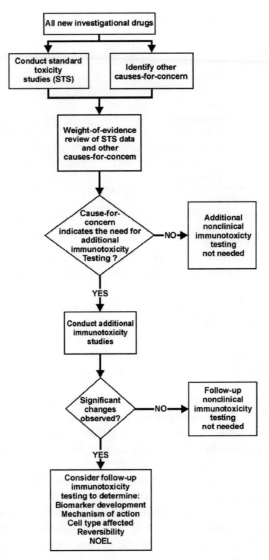

FIGURE 11.3   Decision tree for the conduction of additional and follow-up immunotoxicity studies.

toxicity studies and may be further derived from longer term chronic exposure including carcinogenicity studies. Table 11.5 lists the relevant parameters that must be evaluated in standard toxicity studies for signs of immunotoxicity.

Total and differential leukocyte counts are highly predictive parameters to identify immunotoxicity and to obtain an idea about the involved mechanism. For example, cell loss in peripheral blood resulting from damage to bone marrow cells follows a time course that reflects the half-life of the cell type. Thus, the timing of the onset of any change in blood counts should be carefully evaluated, if possible. In the case of damage to an early stem cell, granulocytopenia is likely to be observed first, followed by thrombocytopenia. Anemia will appear much later, reflecting the

TABLE 11.5   Relevant Parameters that Must Be Evaluated in Standard Toxicity Studies for Signs of Immunotoxicity

Mandatory Parameter	Specific Component
Hematology	Total and differential blood counts
Clinical chemistry	Globulin levels and A/G ratios
Gross pathology	Lymphoid organs/tissues
Organ weights	Thymus, spleen (optional: lymph nodes)
Histology	Thymus, spleen, draining lymph node, and at least one additional lymph node, bone marrow, Peyer's patch[a]; bronchus-associated lymphoid tissue (BALT)[b]; nasal-associated lymphoid tissue (NALT)[b]

[a]In case of oral administration only.
[b]In case of inhalation or nasal route only.

long lifetime (approximately 120 days) of red blood cells. If the loss of a cell type is inconsistent with bone marrow damage, direct attack on mature cells might be indicated.

Changes in serum globulins can be an indication that there are changes in serum immunoglobulins. Thus, when decreased serum globulin level is observed, the protein components affected should be determined using appropriate assays. Although serum immunoglobulins are an insensitive indicator of immunosuppression, changes in immunoglobulin levels can be useful in certain situations in order to better understand target cell populations or mechanism of action.

All lymphoid tissues should be evaluated for gross changes at necropsy. However, this can be difficult for the Peyer's patches of rodents due to their small size. Spleen and thymus weights should be recorded. To minimize variability of spleen weights in dogs and monkeys, bleeding the animals thoroughly at necropsy is recommended. Atrophy of the thymus with aging can preclude obtaining accurate thymus weight.

Histopathological changes of the spleen and thymus should be evaluated as a further highly predictive indicator of systemic immunotoxicity [27]. The lymphoid tissue that drains or contacts the site of drug administration, and therefore is exposed to the highest concentration of the drug, should also be examined. These sites include the Peyer's patches and mesenteric lymph nodes for orally administered drugs, bronchus-associated lymphoid tissue (BALT) for drugs administered by the inhalation route, nasal-associated lymphoid tissue (NALT) for drugs administered by the inhalation or nasal route, and the most proximal regional draining lymph nodes for drugs administered by the dermal, intramuscular, intradermal, or subcutaneous routes. For intravenously administered drugs, the spleen can be considered the draining lymphoid tissue. It is recommended that a "semiquantitative" description of changes in compartments of lymphoid tissues be used in recording changes and reporting treatment-related changes in lymphoid tissues (e.g., –, no changes; +, mild-to-moderate changes; ++, marked changes; +++, severe changes). The parameters that should be evaluated in immunorelevant organs with regard to immunotoxic changes are summarized in Table 11.6.

Other indicators of immunosuppression in nonclinical toxicology studies include treatment-related infections and increased incidences of tumors. Increased treatment-related infections observed in nonclinical toxicology studies, especially infections caused by weakly pathogenic organisms, could be an important indicator

TABLE 11.6   Parameters that Should Be Evaluated in Immunorelevant Organs with Regard to Immunotoxic Changes

Immunorelevant Organ	Parameters
Thymus	• Increased/decreased grade of corticomedullary ratio (related only to area)
	• Increase of starry sky cells
	• Changes of cellular density in the cortex
	• Changes of cellular density in the medulla
Spleen	• Altered cellular composition of follicles
	• Changes of the cellularity of PALS, lymphoid follicles, marginal zone, red pulp
	• Altered number of germinal centers
	• Extramedullary hematopoiesis
	• Congestion
Lymph nodes	• Changes in the cellularity of follicles, interfollicular area, paracortical area, medulla
	• Altered number of germinal centers
	• Changes in the cellularity of sinus
	• Altered cellular composition of paracortex
	• Altered number of germinal centers
	• Hyperplasia of high endothelial venules
Peyer's patches	• Changes of the cellularity of follicles (including mantle zone and germinal centers)
	• Changes of the cellularity of interfollicular area
Bone marrow	• Changes of the cellularity
	• Changes of the myeloid:erythroid ratio

of unintended immunosuppression. It must be noted that no clear-cut correlation exists between the immunosuppressed state and the incidence of common tumors. The relationship between immunosuppression and cancer is controversial, and with the exception of rare lymphoproliferative, reticuloendothelial, or virus-induced tumors, convincing evidence for increased cancer rates due to immunosuppression have not been found. Under most circumstances, when increased incidences of common tumors are observed in standard long-term chronic/carcinogenicity rodent bioassays (or in other nonclinical toxicology studies), the effects are likely to be related to genotoxicity, hormonal effects, or other relatively well understood mechanisms that will require careful analysis and possibly further investigation. However, for some investigational drugs, the cause of tumor findings in nonclinical studies might not be apparent. In those situations, the potential role of immunosuppression should be considered.

It must be kept in mind that, with standard toxicity studies, doses near or at the maximum tolerated dose can result in changes to the immune system related to stress (e.g., by exaggerated pharmacodynamic action). Commonly observed stress-related immune changes include increases in circulating neutrophils, decreases in circulating lymphocytes, decreases in thymus weight, decreases in thymic cortical cellularity and associated histopathologic changes, and changes in spleen and lymph node cellularity. Thymic weight decreases in the presence of clinical signs, such as decreased body weight and physical activity, are too often attributed to stress. These findings on their own should not be considered sufficient evidence of stress-related

TABLE 11.7   Additional Tests that Might Be Technically Integrated into a Standard Repeat Dose Toxicity Study

Parameter	Additional Component
Hematology	• Analysis of lymphocyte subsets by flow cytometry
Clinical chemistry	• Measurement of total hemolytic complement activity
	• Quantitation of immunoglobulin isotypes
	• Detection of antinuclear (ANA) and anticytoplasmic (ACA) autoantibodies
Histology	• Immunohistological or flow cytometric differentiation of lymphocyte subset in lymphatic organs
Functional *ex vivo* tests	• Determination of NK activity in peripheral blood or spleen cells
	• Determination of mitogen responsiveness of peripheral blood or spleen cells
	• Determination of phagocytic activity of peritoneal macrophages
	• Determination of oxidative burst of phagocytes

immunotoxicity. The evidence of stress should be compelling (e.g., by determination of stress-related blood hormone levels [28]), in order to justify not conducting additional immunotoxicity studies.

The minimum parameters that have to be assessed during repeat dose toxicity studies are well defined by regulatory testing guidelines. Nevertheless, the catalog of assays that can be additionally integrated into such studies can be expanded without the need to modify the overall study design. Some additional tests that might give additional valuable information with regard to immunotoxic effects are summarized in Table 11.7. When immunotoxicity assessment is regarded as especially important during preclinical development of certain drug substances, using such additional tests may substantially improve the available database for the weight of evidence review of concern(s) for additional immunotoxicity testing. By the way, such an approach might also help to justify an omission of additional immunotoxicity studies.

Most of the possible additional components that can be integrated into a standard repeat dose toxicity study (Table 11.7) are recommended by regulatory immunotoxicity guidelines as "Additional" or "Follow-up" immunotoxicity assays. Nevertheless, these parameters can already be assessed in a standard repeat dose toxicity study, provided that sufficient amounts of blood can be obtained, and lymphatic organ samples can be obtained under aseptic conditions. Sufficient amounts of blood for the functional assessment of PBMCs can generally not be obtained from mice. For larger animals (including rats, following cardiac puncture), however, obtaining sufficient amounts of blood is not generally a problem.

11.5.2   Additional Testing

If the weight of evidence review of concern(s) indicates that additional immunotoxicity studies are needed, there are a number of animal models that can be used. If there are changes in standard toxicity testing data suggesting immunosuppression, the type of additional immunotoxicity testing that is appropriate will depend on the nature of the immunological changes observed and concerns raised by the class of compound.

To assess drug-induced immunotoxicity, the generally accepted study design is a 28 day study with consecutive daily dosing. Mice or rats are the species of choice (usually the rat since this is routinely used as the rodent toxicity species), but nonrodents should be used if the drug substance to be investigated shows no primary pharmacodynamic activity in rodents. Furthermore, the species, strain, dose, duration, and route of administration used in additional immunotoxicity studies should be consistent, where possible, with the standard toxicity study in which an adverse immune effect was observed. In addition, nonrodents should be used, if possible, to confirm immunotoxicity findings in rodents in a second species. Usually both sexes should be investigated except for studies in nonhuman primates when required. A rationale should be given when only one sex is used in testing. As a central requirement for immunotoxicity studies, the high dose should be above the no observed adverse effect level (NOAEL) but below a level inducing changes secondary to stress. Multiple dose levels are recommended in order to determine dose–response relationships and the dose at which no immunotoxicity is observed.

In concordance with other regional guidelines, the ICH S8 guideline does not stipulate certain tests for additional immunotoxicity testing, but merely gives recommendations. However, due to the dynamic nature of the immune system, immune effects should ideally be demonstrated using a functional immune assay. Where a specific target is not identified, an immune function study such as the T-cell-dependent antibody response (TDAR) is recommended. If specific cell types are affected in STSs or have been identified by immunophenotyping of leukocyte populations, more specific assays that measure function of that specific cell type might be preferable.

In general, the selected immunotoxicity test should be widely accepted and have been demonstrated to be adequately sensitive and specific for known immunosuppressive agents. The limitations of the applied test encompassing intra- and interassay precision, technician-to-technician precision, limit of quantitation, and linear region of quantitation should be known. In addition, assay sensitivity to known immunosuppressive agents should be established. The test should be embedded in an appropriate quality assurance program; for example, the laboratory should conduct a positive control study periodically in order to demonstrate proficiency of performance. However, when extensive validation might have not been completed or the assay might not be widely used, a scientific rationale for use of the assay should be given. Furthermore, a sufficient number of appropriate positive and negative controls should be incorporated.

T-Cell-Dependent Antibody Response (TDAR)   The TDAR should be performed using a recognized T-cell-dependent antigen like sheep red blood cells (SRBCs), bovine serum albumin (BSA), or keyhole limpet hemocyanin (KLH) that result in a robust antibody response. For the SRBC assay, IgM measurement is considered the most appropriate endpoint, whereas IgG measurement is considered to be most appropriate for BSA or KLH. Antibody can be measured by using an ELISA or other immunoassay method. One advantage of ELISA over the traditional plaque forming cell (PFC) assay [29] is that samples can be collected serially during the study, if necessary. Since immunization is likely to have effects on hematology, clinical chemistry, and histology of lymphatic organs, TDAR studies should always be performed as separate studies, or at least in satellite groups of repeat dose toxicity studies.

A protocol for a KLH-based TDAR in mice is depicted in Table 11.8. Brief details of the assay are as follows.

Treatment

1. Use a suitable SPF mouse strain like BALB/c or C57BL/6 × C3H F1 (B6C3F1).
2. Allocate 120 animals in six groups of 10 males and 10 females each according to Table 11.8. The group sizes may be reduced to 5 male and 5 female animals per group, when a substantial immunosuppressive effect can be expected. The larger group size should be chosen when immunosuppression shall be excluded, since otherwise the statistical power of the assay might be insufficient to prove a lack of immunosuppression.
3. Allow acclimatization for 7 days before sampling of pretest serum (day −7) from the test groups, and allow an additional 7 days of rest before first dosing. Pretest serum of recovery groups may be taken on day 35, which is one week postdosing.
4. Administer the test substance and vehicle daily over a period of 28 days (day 1 to day 28) to all animals using an appropriate route of administration.

TABLE 11.8   Design of a Possible Protocol for a KLH-Specific TDAR Study in Mice, Based on a 28 Day Dosing Regimen

Dose Level	Group Size	Start of Acclimatization (day)	Dosing of Vehicle and Test Substance (days)	Immunization with KLH (100 µg IP) Without Adjuvant (day)	Serum Sampling (days)
Test group					
Vehicle	10 male/ 10 female	−14	1–28	14	−7; 29
Low dose	10 male/ 10 female	−14	1–28	14	−7; 29
Intermediate dose	10 male/ 10 female	−14	1–28	14	−7; 29
High dose	10 male/ 10 female	−14	1–28	14	−7; 29
Recovery group					
Vehicle	10 male/ 10 female	−14	1–28	42	35; 57
High dose	10 male/ 10 female	−14	1–28	42	35; 57

5. Use a low, intermediate, and high dose level, whereby the high dose level should be above the NOAEL and below a dose level that causes stress, if possible. The intermediate dose (or low dose) level should ideally represent the intended clinical dose level.

6. Immunize all mice of the test groups on day 14, and mice of the recovery groups on day 42 by intraperitoneal injection of 100 μg KLH per mouse without the use of adjuvant.

7. Sample immune serum from all animals of the test groups on day 29, and from all of the recovery groups on day 57.

8. Store serum at −20 °C until ELISA testing.

ELISA

1. Coat ELISA plates overnight with 10 μg/mL KLH in a carbonate coating buffer, pH 9.6, and block with 1% BSA in PBS or other appropriate blocking agents like casein or dry milk.

2. Distribute pretest and immune serum samples to the ELISA plates in serial or fixed dilutions. The chosen antiserum dilutions should ideally fall into the linear range of the ELISA. Use KLH-specific monoclonal or polyclonal standard antibodies to calculate antibody concentrations, if necessary. Use at least duplicate measurements (triplicates are preferred).

3. Develop the ELISA using biotinylated or enzyme-linked anti-mouse IgG secondary antibodies and appropriate substrate systems.

4. Record direct optical densities or calculate derivatives like antibody concentrations, titers, stimulation indices, percent inhibition, or whatever is found to be appropriate.

The ELISA may be "tuned-up" by using immunoglobulin isotype-specific secondary antibodies to obtain a more detailed picture of the humoral immune response with regard to possible isotype shifts. Such isotype shifts may be indicative of a possible T_H1/T_H2 bias and other cytokine-related modulations of the immune response.

The details of ELISA performance and evaluation are at the discretion of the investigator/sponsor. It must, however, be pointed out that the ELISA, when used in a GLP study, should be thoroughly validated with reference to applicable quality guidelines as, for example, ICH Q2A and Q2B guidelines.

Immunophenotyping   Immunophenotyping is the identification and enumeration of leukocyte subsets using antibodies. Immunophenotyping can be done either by flow cytometric analysis or by immunohistology. With flow cytometry, the percentage and absolute counts of a specific cell type or activation markers can be determined with high precision from large numbers of cells analyzed. When immunophenotyping studies are used to characterize or identify alterations in specific leukocyte populations, the choice of the lymphoid organs to be evaluated should be based on changes observed.

Flow cytometric analysis should at least assess the absolute and relative frequency of the major lymphocyte subsets. No specific recommendations can be made regarding the panel of antibodies to be employed, but at least antibodies specific for T cells (CD3, CD4, CD8), B cells (B220 in mice and CD19 or CD20 or sIg in other species), and NK cells (NK 1.1/CD161 in mice and rats, and CD16 in other species) as well as monocytes/macrophages (Mac-1/CD11b in mice and rats, and CD14 in other species) should be included in the test design. It is at the discretion of the investigator/sponsor to expand the panel by further subset markers for γ, δ-T cells and NK-T cells, by activation markers like CD25, by intracellular cytokine staining, or whatever might make sense to answer special questions with respect to the immunotoxicity assessment. The decision might also be influenced by the capability of the applied flow cytometer with regard to simultaneous multicolor analysis.

Immunophenotyping studies may be designed as separate or satellite studies. As a separate study, the study design should ideally comprise repeated dosing over 28 days; vehicle; low, intermediate, and high dose levels; a sufficient number of animals; and, if possible, both sexes and recovery groups. However, since no immunization or other forms of antigen challenge are required, immunophenotyping can also be easily included in the main groups of a standard repeat dose GLP toxicology study to evaluate changes in lymphocyte subsets. When peripheral blood is used for immunophenotyping, changes can be followed at several time points during the dosing phase and periods without drug exposure (reversal period), if necessary.

Flow cytometry is normally employed to enumerate specific cell populations. It is not a functional assay in this case. However, flow cytometry can be used to measure antigen-specific immune responses of lymphocytes when using fluorescent antigen conjugates for B cells or novel tools like MHC tetramers for T cells. Flow cytometry can also be used for functional endpoints of immune competence like lymphocyte activation, cytokine release, phagocytosis, apoptosis, oxidative burst, and natural killer cell activity [30]. These parameters could be added if the mechanism of action of the drug targets suggests involvement of a particular function of immune cells.

Note that flow cytometry is difficult to validate and hardly meets the criteria of an analytical assay. Thus, to generate an acceptable dataset for immunotoxicity assessment by flow cytometry, a broad set of positive controls (e.g., known marker-positive cells) and negative controls (e.g., isotype-control antibodies) should be included in a test design.

Natural Killer Cell Activity Assays   Natural killer (NK) cell activity assays should be conducted if immunophenotyping studies demonstrate a decrease in NK cell number, or if STSs demonstrate increased viral infection rates, or in response to other causes for concern. In general, all NK cell assays are *ex vivo* assays in which tissues (e.g., spleen) or blood are obtained from animals that have been treated with the test compound. Cell preparations are traditionally coincubated with target cells that have been labeled with chromium. Nevertheless, new methods that involve LDH release from target cells, or labeling of target cells with CFSE and propidium iodide followed by flow cytometry, can be used if adequately validated. Different effector to target cell ratios should be evaluated for each assay to obtain a sufficient picture of the level of cytotoxicity.

As for immunophenotyping, assessment of NK cell activity may be designed as a separate or satellite study. As a separate study, the study design should ideally comprise repeated dosing over 28 days; vehicle; low, intermediate, and high dose levels; a sufficient number of animals; and, if possible, both sexes and recovery groups. However, since no immunization or other forms of antigen challenge are required, assessment of NK cell activity can also be easily included in the main groups of a standard repeat dose GLP toxicology study, provided the technical personnel are able to provide sufficient amounts of blood, and to obtain lymphatic organ samples under aseptic conditions. Sufficient amounts of peripheral blood for the functional assessment of NK cell activity can generally not be obtained from mice. When peripheral blood is used for the assessment of NK cell activity in larger laboratory animals, changes can be followed at several time points during the dosing phase and periods without drug exposure (reversal period), if necessary.

A brief protocol for the assessment of NK cell activity in murine spleen cells during a standard GLP toxicity study could be as follows:

1. Remove spleens under aseptic conditions during necropsy and determine spleen weights (e.g., by using a preweighed tissue culture tube filled with sterile PBS).

2. Remove about one-quarter of the spleen for later histopathology using a sterile scalpel or sterile scissor. Prepare a (sterile) single-cell suspension from the remaining spleen by mechanical disaggregation using surgical pincettes, wire meshes, or whatever method is available.

3. Harvest YAC-1 lymphoma cells (ATCC No. TIB-160) from tissue culture flasks. Label YAC-1 cells in a small volume for 1 h with ^{51}Cr-sodium chromate (~100 μCi per 10^6 cells).

4. Cocultivate 10^4 YAC-1 target cells and spleen cells at effector:target ratios of 100:1, 50:1, 25:1, and 12:1 in 200 μL of cell culture medium containing 10% FCS on round bottomed 96 well microculture plates. Setup of triplicate cultures is recommended. Include at least six 200 μL control cultures, each containing target cells alone (spontaneous ^{51}Cr release) or target cells treated with 1 N NaOH or detergent (maximum ^{51}Cr release).

5. After 6 h of coculture, draw a defined volume (50 or 100 μL) of the culture supernatants and determine radioactivity as counts per minute (cpm) in the samples using a gamma counter.

6. Calculate specific cytotoxicity according to the following formula:

$$\% \text{ Specific release} = \frac{(\text{Mean experimental release} - \text{Mean spontaneous release (cpm)})}{(\text{Mean maximum release} - \text{Mean spontaneous release (cpm)})} \times 100$$

The YAC-1 cells must be harvested from exponentially growing cultures to be in sufficiently good condition. Furthermore, YAC-1 cells must be free from mycoplasms. Since a ^{51}Cr release assay is difficult to validate due to high interassay variability (which is to a high degree related to the actual condition of the YAC-1 cells), all measurements should be conducted in a single measurement series.

Host Resistance Studies   Host resistance studies involve challenging groups of mice or rats treated with different doses of a drug substance with defined doses of a pathogen (bacterial, viral, parasitic) or tumor cells. Infectivity of the pathogens or tumor burden observed in vehicle versus test substance treated animals is used to determine if the test compound is able to alter host resistance [31]. Table 11.9 summarizes the most widely used infectious and tumor models, including endpoints and the defense mechanisms involved. Since the host defense mechanisms in these models are relatively well understood, it is recommended to choose a host resistance assay suitable for a specific target if known.

In conducting host resistance studies, the investigator should carefully consider the direct or indirect (non-immune-mediated) effects of the test compound on the growth and pathogenicity of the organism or tumor cell. For example, compounds that inhibit the proliferation of certain tumor cells can seem to increase host resistance. The same can be expected when using a bacterial challenge model for the immunotoxicity assessment of an antibiotic. In any case, appropriate positive control groups of test animals, dosed with a known immunosuppressive compound, should be included with each host resistance system used.

Listeria Monocytogenes   Resistance to *L. monocytogenes* involves early clearance by neutrophils, followed by the activation of T cells; the latter is required to activate

TABLE 11.9   Widely Used Host Resistance Models, Including Endpoints and Involved Defense Mechanisms

Resistance Model	Endpoints	Defense Mechanisms
Bacterial models		
Listeria monocytogenes	Spleen and lung clearance (rats); mortality (B6C3F1 mice)	Phagocytosis by macrophages and T-cell-dependent lymphokine production
Streptococcus species	Mortality	Complement, neutrophils, antibody
Viral models		
Influenza	Mortality	Cell-mediated immunity, interferon, antibody
Cytomegalovirus	Clearance from salivary gland	Cytotoxic T-cells, NK cells, antibody
Parasite models		
Plasmodium yoelii	Parasitemia	Antibody, macrophages, T cells
Trichinella spiralis	Muscle larvae counts and worm expulsion	T cells (inflammation of the gut), eosinophils, antibodies
Tumor models		
B16F10 melanoma	Lung burden	NK cells, cytotoxic T cells
PYB6 sarcoma	Tumor incidence	NK cells, cytotoxic T cells

macrophages that finally eliminate the remainder of the bacteria. Humoral immunity is not relevant in protection against infection in this model. In rats, clearance of *Listeria* after infection via the intravenous or the intratracheal route can be assessed at various times after infection by determining the numbers of colony forming units in the spleen or lungs, respectively, using serial dilutions of homogenates of the organs. Differences in the numbers of bacteria retrieved from the organs are a measure of the clearance of the bacteria by the host. Histopathology after a *Listeria* infection can also be valuable, since pulmonary infection with *Listeria* induces histopathological lesions characterized by foci of inflammatory cells, such as lymphoid and histiocytic cells, accompanied by local cell degeneration and influx of granulocytes.

When C3H or B6C3F1 mice are challenged with *Listeria*, mortality is the usual endpoint monitored. However, clearance and organ bacterial colony counts can also be determined. In mice the resistance to the organism is genetically regulated, and some strains like C57BL/6 are not useful for assays due to resistance. In studies in susceptible mice, a nonlethal challenge level with *L. monocytogenes* of approximately 10^4 CFU may be given for the enumeration of bacteria in organs, or a 20% lethal challenge level of approximately 5×10^4 CFU for assessment of mortality. Mortality is recorded daily for 14 days. Treatment groups consisting of 12 mice per group have been found to be useful for obtaining statistically meaningful data on host resistance. This assay is extremely reproducible when the organism is administered intravenously. Since *Listeria* is a human pathogen, appropriate precautions are needed in conducting the assay.

Streptococcus Pneumoniae   The first line of defense against *S. pneumoniae* is the complement system. Activation of the complement system can result in direct lysis of certain strains of *S. pneumoniae*. However, due to the nature of their cell wall, some strains may be resistant to lysis by complement. Deposition of complement factor C3b on the surface of the bacteria triggers phagocytosis predominantly by neutrophils. In the later stages of the infection, antigen-specific antibody plays a major role in controlling the infection. Thus, compounds that affect complement, polymorphonuclear leukocytes, B cell maturation and proliferation, or the production of antibody can be evaluated in this system. *Streptococcus pneumoniae* is therefore an excellent model for evaluating immunotoxicity, since it elicits multiple immune components that participate in host resistance, each of which can be a potential target for an adverse effect of an immunotoxic drug.

Routinely, B6C3F1 mice are used. Since the LD_{50} of group B streptococci is approximately 5 living bacteria in this strain, mice are vaccinated twice with 2×10^5 heat inactivated bacteria during the dosing period, the last vaccination given 7 days before the challenge with a lethal dose of living bacteria. Owing to the rapid onset of infection, mortality is recorded twice daily for 7 days during the second half of a 28 day dosing regimen. A nonimmunized control group should be included in each experiment to demonstrate that the challenge dose was lethal to most mice that were not immunized.

B16F10 Melanoma Cells   The B16F10 melanoma line forms tumor metastases almost exclusively in the lungs of C57Bl/6 mice following IV administration, and it is widely used to assess host resistance to nonimmunogenic or minimally immunogenic tumors in mice. NK cells and possibly Tc are involved in resistance to this tumor. Mice are challenged by IV administration of 1×10^5 B16F10 tumor cells on day 12 of a 28 day dosing regime, and lungs are removed for enumeration of experimental metastases using a dissecting microscope 1 day after the last dose.

Mouse and Rat Cytomegalovirus   Cytomegaloviruses are classified as members of the family Herpesviridae. The roles of several arms of the immune system in resistance to cytomegalovirus have been identified, including antibodies, cytotoxic T cells, and NK cells. Antibodies in this case contribute to neutralization and antibody-dependent cell-mediated cytotoxicity. NK cell activity appears to be the most effective during the initial stages of infection [32].

Experimentally, rodents can be inoculated intraperitoneally with a species-specific cytomegalovirus, and the concentration of the virus in tissue can be determined in a plaque-forming assay using susceptible adherent cell lines. Homogenates of different organs (salivary gland, lung, kidney, liver, spleen) may be obtained at various times after infection for this purpose. Plaques are counted under a stereoscopic microscope. In rats, cytomegalovirus is detectable 8 days after infection, although the virus load is much higher on days 15–20.

Macrophage Function   *In vitro* macrophage function assays can be used for several species. These assays assess macrophage function of cells either derived from untreated animals and exposed to the test compound *in vitro* or obtained from animals treated with the test compound as an *ex vivo* assay [33].

Macrophage function assays may be designed as separate or satellite studies. As a separate study, the study design should ideally comprise repeated dosing over 28 days; vehicle; low, intermediate, and high dose levels; a sufficient number of animals; and, if possible, both sexes and recovery groups. However, since no immunization or other forms of antigen challenge are required, macrophage function assays can also be easily included in the main groups of a standard repeat dose GLP toxicology study to evaluate changes in lymphocyte subsets.

An *in vivo* assay could also be used to assess the effects on the reticuloendothelial cells to phagocytize chromium-labeled sheep red blood cells. In this case animals should be treated with the test compound and injected with chromium-labeled sheep red blood cells. Animals should be necropsied and tissues (e.g., liver, spleen, lung, kidney) removed, followed by a quantitation of specific radioactivity incorporated.

A macrophage phagocytosis assay in mice, measuring the ability of peritoneal macrophages to phagocytize latex beads, and assessment by flow cytometry, might by conducted as follows:

1. Collect peritoneal macrophages from mice immediately after euthanasia and before the peritoneal cavity is opened for gross necropsy.
2. Carefully cut the abdominal skin with scissors and pull it back from the abdomen without hurting the abdominal wall.
3. Inject approximately 5 mL of ice cold Ca^{2+} and Mg^{2+} free PBS containing 10 IU/mL sodium heparin intraperitoneally using a thin needle.

4. Gently massage the peritoneum and aspire the peritoneal wash with a separate syringe and a larger needle. Repeat the procedure twice, if possible.

5. Pellet the peritoneal exudate cells by centrifugation and determine cell viability by trypan blue dye exclusion.

6. Adjust cells to 10^6 cells/mL with complete cell culture medium containing 10% FCS, and add carboxyfluorescein modified latex microspheres at a ratio of 100:1 (beads:cells).

7. Incubate aliquots of the cell suspension at either 37 °C or 4 °C for 120 min, subjected to gentle agitation.

8. After 120 min, centrifuge the cells and resuspend in 100 µL PBS containing 0.05% formalin, followed by flow cytometric analysis.

9. Identify and gate macrophages according to forward and side scatter properties, and record data from the fluorescein channel.

10. Analyze recorded histograms with the first fluorescent peak corresponding to a single ingested fluorescent bead, and each successive fluorescent peak corresponding to the phagocytosis of an additional bead.

11. Calculate the frequency of active macrophages with one or more ingested microspheres, and the mean number of microspheres ingested by active macrophages.

12. For each data point subtract the respective measurements at 4 °C to correct for simple adherence of the beads.

This assay may be modified by using antibody-labeled fluorescent erythrocytes instead of latex microbeads or by simple (but time-consuming) microscopic enumeration.

Assays to Measure T-Cell-Mediated Immunity   Three types of assays have been widely used to assess T-cell-mediated immunity. Mostly, delayed type hypersensitivity (DTH) reactions are used, which are based on an immunization with SRBCs, KLH, or BSA, followed by a subsequent challenge with the antigen into the pinna of the ear or the hind footpad, and determination of the degree of inflammation-induced swelling [34]. The above assay may be modified by assessing the *ex vivo* recall response using lymphatic cells derived from spleen or draining lymph nodes. In this case the *in vitro* proliferation of primed T cells in response to the nominal antigen (using [^{3}H]thymidin or BrdU incorporation) or cytokine production is measured. The *ex vivo* modification of the assay is technically more challenging but usually results in less variability of the results.

Instead of vaccination with SRBCs or protein antigens, topical sensitization and challenge with a known contact sensitizer like oxazolone or picrylic acid may be used. The induced contact allergic response is also a T-cell-mediated immune response that may be affected by immunosuppressive drugs.

Alternatively, cytotoxic T cell response can be generated in mice/rats by vaccination with inactivated tumor cells or viruses, followed by an *ex vivo* assessment of the resulting cytotoxic T cell response using a specific ^{51}Cr release assay.

Since immunization is likely to have effects on hematology, clinical chemistry, and histology of lymphatic organs, assays to measure T-cell-mediated immunity should always be performed as separate studies, or at least in satellite groups of repeat dose toxicity studies.

REFERENCES

1. Penn I. Tumors of the immunocompromised patient. *Annu Rev Med* 1988;39:63–73.
2. Penn I. The role of immunosuppression in lymphoma formation. *Springer Semin Immunopathol* 1998;20:343–355.
3. Rygaard J, Povlsen CO. The nude mouse vs. the hypothesis of immunological surveillance. *Transplant Rev* 1976;28:43–61.
4. Ader R, Felten D, Cohen N. Interactions between the brain and the immune system. *Annu Rev Pharmacol Toxicol* 1990;30:561–602.
5. Khansari DN, Murgo AJ, Faith RE. Effects of stress on the immune system. *Immunol Today* 1990;11:170–175.
6. Renton KW, Gray JD, Hall RI. Decreased elimination of theophylline after influenza vaccination. *Can Med Assoc J* 1980;123:288–290.
7. Mannering GJ, Renton KW, el Azhary R, Deloria LB. Effects of interferon-inducing agents on hepatic cytochrome P-450 drug metabolizing systems. *Ann NY Acad Sci* 1980;350:314–331.
8. Farine JC. Animal models in autoimmune disease in immunotoxicity assessment. *Toxicology* 1997;119:29–35.
9. Mosmann TR, Coffman RL. Heterogeneity of cytokine secretion patterns and functions of helper T cells. *Adv Immunol* 1989;46:111–147.
10. Choquet-Kastylevsky G, Descotes J. Value of animal models for predicting hypersensitivity reactions to medicinal products. *Toxicology* 1998;129:27–35.
11. Gad SC, Dunn BJ, Dobbs DW, Reilly C, et al. Development and validation of an alternative dermal sensitization test: the mouse ear swelling test (MEST). *Toxicol Appl Pharmacol* 1986;84:93–114.
12. Kimber I, Hilton J, Botham PA, Basketter DA, et al. The murine local lymph node assay: results of an inter-laboratory trial. *Toxicol Lett* 1991;55:203–213.
13. Baxter AB, Lazarus SC, Brasch RC. *In vitro* histamine release induced by magnetic resonance imaging and iodinated contrast media. *Invest Radiol* 1993;28:308–312.
14. Szebeni J. Complement activation-related pseudoallergy caused by liposomes, micellar carriers of intravenous drugs, and radiocontrast agents. *Crit Rev Ther Drug Carrier Syst* 2001;18:567–606.
15. Bagenstose LM, Salgame P, Monestier M. Cytokine regulation of a rodent model of mercuric chloride-induced autoimmunity. *Environ Health Perspect* 1999;107(Suppl 5):807–810.
16. Ravel G, Christ M, Horand F, Descotes J. Autoimmunity, environmental exposure and vaccination: Is there a link? *Toxicology* 2004;196:211–216.
17. Pieters R, Albers R. Screening tests for autoimmune-related immunotoxicity. *Environ Health Perspect* 1999;107(Suppl 5):673–677.
18. Descotes J. Autoimmunity and toxicity testing. *Toxicol Lett* 2000;112–113:461–465.
19. Verdier F, Patriarca C, Descotes J. Autoantibodies in conventional toxicity testing. *Toxicology* 1997;119:51–58.
20. Committee for Proprietary Medicinal Products (CPMP). *Note for Guidance on Repeated Dose Toxicity* (CPMP/SWP/1042/99 corr.; London, 27 July 2000).

21. US Food and Drug Administration, Center for Drug Evaluation and Research. *Guidance for Industry: Immunotoxicology Evaluation of Investigational New Drugs.* October 2002.

22. *ICH S6 Harmonised Tripartite Guideline. Preclinical Safety Evaluation of Biotechnology-Derived Pharmaceuticals* (Step 4, 1997).

23. *WHO Guidelines on Nonclinical Evaluation of Vaccines. Annex 1.* Adopted by the 54th Meeting of the WHO Expert Committee on Biological Standardization, 17–21 November 2003.

24. *ICH S8 Harmonised Tripartite Guideline. Immunotoxicity Studies for Human Pharmaceuticals.* (Recommended for Adoption at Step 4 of ICH Process on 15 September 2005).

25. Holsapple MP, Burns-Naas LA, Hastings KL, Ladics GS, et al. A proposed testing framework for developmental immunotoxicology (DIT). *Toxicol Sci* 2005;83:18–24.

26. Wierda D, Smith HW, Zwickl CM. Immunogenicity of biopharmaceuticals in laboratory animals. *Toxicology* 2001;158:71–74.

27. Schuurman HJ, Kuper CF, Vos JG. Histopathology of the immune system as a tool to assess immunotoxicity. *Toxicology* 1994;86:187–212.

28. Pruett SB, Ensley DK, Crittenden PL. The role of chemical-induced stress responses in immunosuppression: a review of quantitative associations and cause–effect relationships between chemical-induced stress responses and immunosuppression. *J Toxicol Environ Health* 1993;39:163–192.

29. Jerne NK, Henry C, Nordin AA, Fuji H, et al. Plaque forming cells: methodology and theory. *Transplant Rev* 1974;18:130–191.

30. Burchiel SW, Kerkvliet NL, Gerberick GF, Lawrence DA, et al. Assessment of immunotoxicity by multiparameter flow cytometry. *Fundam Appl Toxicol* 1997;38:38–54.

31. Dean JH, Luster MI, Boorman GA, Leubke RW, et al. Application of tumor, bacterial and parasite susceptibility assays to study immune alterations induced by environmental chemicals. *Environ Health Perspect* 1982;43:81–88.

32. Selgrade MK, Daniels MJ, Dean JH. Correlation between chemical suppression of natural killer cell activity in mice and susceptibility to cytomegalovirus: rationale for applying murine cytomegalovirus as a host resistance model and for interpreting immunotoxicity testing in terms of risk of disease. *J Toxicol Environ Health* 1992;37:123–137.

33. Hubbard AK. Effects of xenobiotics on macrophage function: evaluation *in vitro*. *Methods* 1999;19:8–16.

34. Holsapple MP, Page DG, Bick PH, Shopp GM. Characterization of the delayed hypersensitivity response to a protein antigen in the mouse—I. Kinetics of reactivity and sensitivity to classical immunosuppressants. *Int J Immunopharmacol* 1984;6:399–405.

35. Council of the European Communities. *Official Journal of the European Communities*, No. L332/11, 26 October 1983. Brussels.

36. Vos JG, van Loveren H. Immunotoxicity testing in the rat. In Burger EJ, Tardiff RE, Bellanti JA, Eds. *Environmental Chemical Exposures and Immune System Integrity*. Princeton, NJ: Princeton Scientific Publishing; 1987, pp 167–180.

37. Sjoblad RD. Potential future requirements for immunotoxicology testing of pesticides. *Toxicol Ind Health* 1988;4:391–395.

38. Luster MI, Munson AE, Thomas PT, Holsapple MP, et al. Development of a testing battery to assess chemical-induced immunotoxicity: National Toxicology Program's guidelines for immunotoxicity evaluation in mice. *Fundam Appl Toxicol* 1988;10:2–19.

39. Luster MI, Portier C, Pait DG, White KL Jr, et al. Risk assessment in immunotoxicology. I. Sensitivity and predictability of immune tests. *Fundam Appl Toxicol* 1992;18:200–210.

40. Luster MI, Portier C, Pait DG, Rosenthal GJ, et al. Risk assessment in immunotoxicology. II. Relationships between immune and host resistance tests. *Fundam Appl Toxicol* 1993;21:71–82.

41. Toxic Substances Control Act. Test Guidelines. Final Rule. *Fed Reg* 1997;62: 43819–43864.

42. Committee for Proprietary Medicinal Products (CPMP). *Note for Guidance on Non-Clinical Local Tolerance Testing of Medicinal Products* (CPMP/SWP/2145/00; London, 1 March 2001).

12

REPRODUCTIVE AND DEVELOPMENTAL TOXICOLOGY

RONALD D. HOOD[1,2] AND ROBERT M. PARKER[3]

[1]*Ronald D. Hood & Associates, Toxicology Consultants, Tuscaloosa, Alabama*
[2]*The University of Alabama, Tuscaloosa, Alabama*
[3]*Hoffmann-LaRoche Inc., Nutley, New Jersey*

Contents

Preclinical Development Handbook: Toxicology, edited by Shayne Cox Gad
Copyright © 2008 John Wiley & Sons, Inc.

12.1 REGULATORY AGENCY GUIDANCE

This chapter addresses testing protocols for two general categories of toxicity: (1) reproductive toxicity, which includes effects on fertility, parturition, and lactation; and (2) developmental toxicity, which addresses effects on the developing offspring, namely, mortality, dysmorphogenesis (structural alteration), altered growth, and functional abnormality. It is fortunate that in recent years the United States, the European Community, and Japan have worked together to harmonize their test guidelines via the International Conferences on Harmonization (ICH), thus reducing the regulatory burden inherent in their previously widely differing requirements. According to the ICH S5A document, *Guideline for Industry, Detection of Toxicity to Reproduction for Medicinal Products* [1], a testing regimen should be selected that would "allow exposure of mature adults and all stages of development from conception to sexual maturity. To allow detection of immediate and latent effects of exposure, observations should be continued through one complete life cycle, i.e., from conception in one generation through conception in the following generation." The document further suggests that an integrated test sequence can be subdivided into the following stages:

- *Stage A*. Premating to conception (adult male and female reproductive functions, development and maturation of gametes, mating behavior, fertilization).
- *Stage B*. Conception to implantation (adult female reproductive functions, pre-implantation development, implantation).
- *Stage C*. Implantation to closure of the hard palate (adult female reproductive functions, embryonic development, major organ formation).
- *Stage D*. Closure of the hard palate to the end of pregnancy (adult female reproductive functions, fetal development and growth, organ development and growth).
- *Stage E*. Birth to weaning (adult female reproductive functions, neonate adaptation to extrauterine life, preweaning development and growth).
- *Stage F*. Weaning to sexual maturity (postweaning development and growth, adaptation to independent life, attainment of full sexual function).

Nevertheless, in most cases those six stages are assessed by means of just three studies: (1) the fertility and general reproductive performance study (Segment I, Stages A–B); (2) the prenatal developmental toxicity study (Segment II, Stages C–D); and (3) the perinatal and postnatal study (Segment III, Stages C–F).

In addition, in recent years increased emphasis has been placed on direct toxicity studies in juvenile animals [2, 3]. All of these study types are discussed in some detail later in this chapter. And in some cases, some of the above studies can be omitted. For example, in establishing the safety of veterinary drug residues in human food, a multigeneration study in at least one rodent species is recommended because human exposure may be long term, and the segment studies listed above are not viewed as essential [4].

12.2 FLEXIBILITY IN DEVELOPING A TESTING STRATEGY

The "bad news" about regulatory agency guidelines (i.e., "guidances" according to the FDA) for nonclinical studies is that they are not intended to be specific blueprints that can be followed exactly in every case. That is also the good news regarding such strategies for reproductive and developmental toxicity testing, as they allow for flexibility and use of scientific judgment in those cases in which a "one size fits all" approach would not yield the most useful data. That has led to use of the term "guidance," as opposed to "guideline," by the U.S. FDA, thus implying a less rigid stance. Implementation of flexible test guidelines can be somewhat problematic, however, in that many of the individuals currently designing, implementing, or making regulatory decisions regarding developmental and reproductive toxicology study protocols have had little or no formal education or background knowledge in the disciplines that are especially critical to the field. Of course, a reasonable degree of regulatory guidance flexibility is essential, because no immutable guideline can be designed that would cover all possible eventualities for these complex studies, and guidelines are not typically revised rapidly enough to keep abreast of advances in the relevant testing methodology. It then becomes essential to utilize the training and advice available in relevant references that provide more detail than the current chapter (e.g., Refs. 5 and 6).

Nonclinical testing strategies may require modification to be more predictive of the hazard potential of the particular product under development. Thus, it is important to discuss and consider possible "variations in test strategy according to the state-of-the-art and ethical standards in human and animal experimentation" [7] prior to finalizing study protocols for drug candidates and other products with unique characteristics. For example, the test protocol for new vaccines should be specifically tailored to the particular vaccine under consideration. With regard to reproduction and development, vaccine testing is typically restricted to pre- and postnatal developmental toxicity studies, as no fertility or postweaning studies are conducted for most vaccine products. Such vaccine testing is commonly conducted in only one species, preferably one in which an immune response is elicited, and test agent administration should generally be episodic, rather than by the daily dosing regimen most commonly used for testing other products [8]. As another example of deviation from the usual protocol, for agents typically administered only once, such as diagnostics and medicines used during surgery, dosing repeatedly may be impractical. In such cases, use of high doses for brief treatment periods may be necessary [7]. Also, if an adverse effect is detected, in some cases it can be useful to conduct further studies to more fully characterize the nature of the effect and perhaps provide an explanation for its basis. This can prove valuable if, for example, it is determined that the mechanism for the toxic effect does not apply to humans or would not occur at the likely human equivalent dose.

12.3   FERTILITY AND GENERAL REPRODUCTIVE PERFORMANCE STUDY (SEGMENT I)

12.3.1   Rationale for the Test

Fertility studies (i.e., Segment I studies) test for toxic effects resulting from treatment of both sexes with the test article before mating and during cohabitation and mating, and continuing to treat the females until implantation on gestation day 6 (GD6). This comprises evaluation of ICH Stages A and B of the reproductive process. For females, this should detect effects on the estrous cycle (ovarian and uterine effects), tubal transport, libido, development of preimplantation stages of the embryo, and implantation. For males, it will permit detection of functional effects (e.g., on libido, mating behavior, capacitation, epididymal sperm maturation) that may not be detected by histological examinations of the male reproductive organs.

12.3.2   Male-Only, Female-Only, and Combined Segment I Studies

The fertility study can be performed as male-only [9] (for paternally mediated effects) and female-only [1] (for maternally mediated effects) studies or as a com-

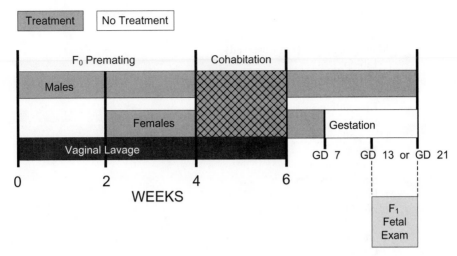

FIGURE 12.1 Fertility study schematic (FDA Segment I and ICH S5 and S5A).

bined male/female study (for couple-mediated effects) (Fig. 12.1). Most regulatory reproduction and fertility guidelines specify cohabitation of treated male rats with treated females, complicating the resolution of gender-specific influences. If male or female reproductive organ toxicity has been observed in subchronic studies, then performance of the male-only and female-only study would allow for greater resolution of gender-based toxicities.

Males are treated with the test article for 2, 4, or 10 weeks (depending on guideline requirements, see later discussion) prior to cohabitation and mating, and continuing until termination. The males are routinely treated until after the female necropsy has been completed; then the males are euthanized and necropsied. Females are treated 2 weeks prior to cohabitation, through cohabitation and mating, and until implantation (usually GD 6). The dam is euthanized on either GD 13 or 21 and necropsied, and the conceptuses are evaluated for viability.

Male-Specific Endpoints and Paternally Mediated Effects Data on the potential male reproductive toxicity of a test article may be collected from subchronic, chronic, and fertility studies. Male-specific endpoints that are determined in these studies are listed in Table 12.1. Several of these parameters are not directly observed (e.g., mating behavior, secretion of hormones), but perturbations to reproductive organs may suggest alterations in these parameters.

Male-only treatment with a variety of agents has been shown to produce adverse effects in offspring, including pre- and postimplantation loss, growth and behavioral deficits, and malformations [10–14]. Many of the chemicals reported to cause paternally mediated effects display genotoxic activity and may cause transmissible genetic alterations. However, other mechanisms of induction of male-mediated effects are also possible, including nongenetic (e.g., presence of drug in seminal fluid) or epigenetic (e.g., an effect on imprinted gene expression from the paternal alleles, resulting in alteration of gene function). Additional studies will be needed to clarify the mechanisms of paternal exposure associated with adverse

TABLE 12.1   Male-Specific Endpoints in Fertility Studies

Body weight
Mating behavior (not observed)
   Libido
   Mounting
   Erection
   Ejaculation
Reproductive organ weights
Histopathology
   Testes
   Epididymides
   Seminal vesicles
   Prostate
   Pituitary
Sperm parameters
   Quality
   Count
   Viability
   Morphology
   Motility
   Transport
   Maturation
   Storage in the epididymis
Production of seminal fluid
Production and secretion of hormones in the pituitary–
   hypothalamus–gonadal axis

effects on offspring. If a test article is identified as causing a paternally mediated adverse effect on offspring in the test species, the effect should be considered an adverse reproductive effect.

Female-Specific Endpoints and Maternally Mediated Effects   The female-specific endpoints in fertility studies are focused on estrous cyclicity, mating, pregnancy, and offspring survival and development. Additional reproductive system endpoints can also be useful in evaluating reproductive toxicity. Adverse alterations in the non-pregnant female reproductive system have been reported at treatment levels below those that result in reduced fertility or produce other effects on pregnancy or pregnancy outcomes. Female-specific endpoints of reproductive toxicity evaluated in the fertility study are listed in Table 12.2. Female mating behavior and tubal transport are not directly observed, but perturbations to reproductive organs may suggest alterations in these parameters.

Unlike the male, the status of the adult female reproductive system fluctuates. In nonpregnant female rats, the ovarian and uterine structures (and other reproductive organs) change throughout the estrous cycle. Although not cyclic, other changes accompany the progression of pregnancy, lactation, and return to cyclicity after lactation. It is important to be aware of the reproductive status of the female at necropsy, including estrous cycle stage. These normal fluctuations may affect or confound the evaluation of female reproductive endpoints. This facilitates interpretation of

TABLE 12.2 Female-Specific Endpoints in Fertility Studies

Body weight
Estrous cycle
   Onset
   Length
   Patterns
Mating behaviors
Reproductive organ weights
Histopathology
   Ovary
   Uterus
   Vagina
Ovulation
Number of corpora lutea
Tubal transport
Implantation
Pre- and postimplantation losses

effects with endpoints such as uterine weight and histopathology of the ovary, uterus, and vagina.

It is well established that female-only treatment can indirectly produce adverse effects in offspring (i.e., maternally mediated effects). If a test article is identified as causing a maternally mediated adverse effect on offspring, the effect should be considered an adverse reproductive effect.

Couple-Mediated Endpoints Couple-mediated endpoints are reproductive endpoints where both parents may have a contributory role. Couple-mediated endpoints from fertility studies include mating behaviors (mating rate, time to mating), pregnancy rate, number of implantation sites, number of conceptuses (total and live), and preimplantation and postimplantation loss. Most regulatory reproduction and fertility guidelines specify cohabitation of treated male rats with treated female rats, complicating the resolution of gender-specific influences.

12.3.3 Animal Species and Strain Selection

Rationale for Species and Strain Selection It is generally desirable to use the same species and strain as in other toxicological studies. Reasons for using rats as the predominant rodent species are practicality, comparability with other results obtained in this species, and the large amount of accumulated background knowledge. The disadvantages of different species are described in Note 5 of the ICH S5A guideline [1].

The animals used must be well defined with respect to their health, fertility, fecundity, prevalence of abnormalities, and embryo–fetal deaths, and their consistency among studies. Within and between studies, animals should be of comparable age, weight, and parity at the start.

When nonhuman primates or other large animal species are used, it is recommended that the protocol design be discussed with the regulatory agencies prior to the conduct of the study to ensure that there is consensus regarding the sensitivity of assay. Because of the normal low pregnancy rate, nonhuman primate fertility studies do not routinely include mating. The treatment effects on menstrual cycle and reproductive hormones are evaluated. Alterations in normal menstrual cycle or reproductive hormone patterns may be considered as adverse.

Number, Sex, and Age of Test Animals   The number of animals per sex per group should be sufficient to allow meaningful interpretation of the data. Routinely, 20 rats per sex per group are evaluated.

12.3.4   Procurement and Acclimation of the Test Animals

The test animals should be young but sexually mature and from the same source and strain, and the females should be nulliparous and as nearly the same age and weight as is practicable. They should be obtained from reputable suppliers that have programs ensuring the genetic integrity of their animals, in addition to their freedom from diseases and parasites. The test animals should be acclimated to the laboratory conditions prior to study start.

12.3.5   Selection of Dosage Groups, Controls, and Route of Administration

Most fertility studies are designed with a vehicle control and at least three dosage groups, all of which should be concurrent and identically housed and handled. Males and females should be assigned by a random procedure to assure that mean body weights are comparable among all test groups. The test compound or vehicle should be administered by the route that most closely approximates the pattern of expected human exposure.

Selection of dosages is one of the most critical issues in design of the reproductive toxicity study. Data from all available studies (pharmacology, acute, subchronic, and chronic toxicity, and kinetic studies) should be used to select the high dose level. A repeated dose toxicity study of about 2–4 weeks' duration provides a close approximation to the duration of treatment in segmental designs of reproductive studies. Using similar doses in the reproductive toxicity studies as in the repeated dose toxicity studies allows interpretation of any potential effects on fertility in context with general systemic toxicity. Some minimal toxicity should be induced in the highest dosage group.

According to the specific compound, factors limiting the high dosage determined from repeated dose toxicity studies could include (1) increased or reduced body weight gain; (2) hematology, clinical chemistry, and histopathology; (3) specific target organ toxicity; (4) exaggerated pharmacological response; (5) physicochemical property limitations in the amount that can be administered; and (6) pharmacokinetic profile.

After deciding on the highest dosage, lower dosages should be selected in a descending sequence, the intervals depending on kinetic and other toxicity factors. The strategy should also result in a no observed adverse effect level (NOAEL) for reproductive aspects.

12.3.6 Treatment Timing and Test Duration

The usual frequency of administration is once daily, but consideration should be given to using either more or less frequent administration, taking kinetics into account.

Males The duration of treatment selected should be adequate for determining effects on spermatogenesis. The duration of spermatogenesis (approximately 63 days in the rat) was the reason that most fertility and reproductive studies require treatment of the males for approximately 10 weeks prior to mating. The premating treatment duration will permit evaluation of functional effects on male fertility that may not be detected by histopathological examination in shorter duration repeated dose toxicity studies.

However, the premating treatment interval may be reduced to 4 weeks in ICH fertility studies if no male reproductive toxicity effects were found in a repeated dose toxicity study (of at least 4 weeks' duration). Validation studies [15, 16] have indicated that a 2 week premating treatment period is adequate to detect male reproductive toxicity. Therefore, treatment of the males for 2 weeks before mating is also acceptable in ICH fertility studies. Justification for the length of the premating treatment period should be stated in the protocol. In fertility studies, treatment should continue throughout the cohabitation period and until termination for males.

Females Provided that no female reproductive toxicity effects were found in a repeated dose toxicity study (of at least 4 weeks' duration), a 2 week premating treatment interval should be used for females in ICH fertility studies. Justification for the length of the premating treatment period should be stated in the protocol. In fertility studies, treatment should continue throughout the cohabitation period and until implantation for females.

12.3.7 Mating Procedures, Detection of Mating, and Housing of Mated Females

Mating Procedure A mating ratio of 1:1 is advisable, and procedures should allow identification of both parents of a litter. This is the safest option for obtaining good pregnancy rates and avoiding incorrect interpretation of results. The female is introduced into the male's cage in the afternoon, and the female is checked for evidence of mating each morning until mating is detected.

Detection of Mating In standard reproductive toxicology studies, the evidence of sexual receptivity and successful mating is based on the presence of copulatory plugs or sperm-positive vaginal lavage. When the male rat ejaculates, the semen quickly coagulates, forming a copulatory plug. Copulatory plugs can remain *in situ* (in the vagina), or they can be dislodged from the vagina and fall into the cage pan (cage plugs). While in cohabitation, the females and their cages should be checked daily for the presence of copulatory plugs. If a copulatory plug is observed *in situ* (in the vagina), a vaginal lavage sample is not necessary. The presence of a copulatory plug in the cage pan is not sufficient evidence that mating has occurred. If only a cage pan plug is observed or no evidence for mating is observed, then a vaginal lavage should be performed and checked for sperm. When sperm are seen, a positive (+) mating is recorded. When no sperm are present in the vaginal smear, a negative (−) mating is recorded.

However, these *post hoc* findings do not demonstrate that male sexual activity resulted in adequate sexual stimulation of the female rat. Failure to provide adequate stimulation to the female has been shown to impair sperm transport in the genital tract of female rats, thereby reducing the probability of successful fertilization [17]. The reduced fertility (as calculated in the Fertility Index) might be erroneously attributed to an effect on the spermatogenic process in the male or on fertility of the female, rather than on altered mating behavior. Effects on sexual behavior should be considered as adverse reproductive effects. However, impairment of sexual behavior that is secondary to more generalized physical debilitation (e.g., intoxication, impaired motor activity, or general lethargy) should not be considered an adverse reproductive effect; such conditions represent adverse systemic effects.

Housing of Mated Females   Once the females have mated, they should be housed individually to allow for monitoring of feed and, if necessary, water consumption. Feed and water should be provided *ad libitum*.

12.3.8   In-Life Observations: Parental Body Weight, Feed Consumption, Estrous Cycles, and Clinical Signs

During study, clinical signs and mortalities should be assessed at least once daily. Body weight should be recorded at least twice weekly. Feed and, if necessary, water intake should be measured at least once weekly (except during cohabitation, when feed consumption is not recorded). Vaginal smears should be collected and evaluated daily for at least 2 weeks during the pretreatment period (baseline), daily during the 2 week treatment period prior to mating, and during the 2 week mating period (for estrous cyclicity and confirmation of mating). Other observations that have proved of value in other toxicity studies may be recorded.

12.3.9   Female Reproductive Evaluation

Assessment of the Dam, Uterine Contents, and Conceptuses at Necropsy   Any mated females that appear moribund should be euthanized appropriately. Any mated females found dead should be necropsied to investigate the cause of death. In all such cases, any evidence of pregnancy and embryonic development should be evaluated and recorded.

Dams are routinely necropsied on GD 13 (early in the second half of gestation). The dam is weighed and euthanized, and the ovary and uterus are examined. Uterine contents (number of implantation sites) are recorded. The dam is subjected to a complete necropsy, and the reproductive organs and other tissues specified in the protocol are weighed and saved for possible histopathological evaluation.

Inspection of Maternal Viscera   The gravid uterus should be removed and weighed. The remaining maternal abdominal and thoracic organs should be inspected grossly for evidence of toxicity, and protocol-specified target organs should be removed and weighed. If gross organ lesions are noted, the affected organs should be preserved for possible histopathologic examination.

The uterus should be examined to determine if the animal was pregnant, and the relative numbers of live and dead conceptuses and their relative positions in the uterus should be recorded. If the uterus shows no signs of implantation, it should be treated with a reagent, such as 10% ammonium sulfide, to reveal any early resorptions (partially autolyzed embryos) that may not have been obvious [18].

Enumeration of Corpora Lutea   Each corpus luteum appears as a round, slightly pink, discrete swelling on the ovarian surface. The corpora lutea can be counted with the naked eye or under a dissecting microscope to determine the number of eggs ovulated. The number of corpora lutea should be recorded for each ovary. In a litter with no obvious signs of resorptions, the number of corpora lutea should be equal to or exceed the number of total implantation sites. Corpora lutea of rats are relatively obvious; however, some corpora lutea may obscure others, making counting difficult. Corpora lutea can be discounted when the count is less than the number of implants, or the number of corpora lutea can be set to correspond to the number of implants to correct for involuting corpora lutea in partially resorbed litters. The corpora lutea count is used in determining preimplantation losses. A reduction in the number of corpora lutea or an increase in the preimplantation loss should be considered an adverse reproductive effect.

Uterine Evaluation   In fertility studies where the pregnant female rodents are necropsied around GD 13, the conceptuses are categorized as live (normal appearance, heart beat, etc.) or dead (discolored, undergoing autolysis). An implanted conceptus that is undergoing autolysis is termed a resorption (see Table 12.3). An early resorption is usually visualized by staining with a 10% aqueous solution of ammonium sulfide by the Salewski method or by observation through pressed glass plates. The number and uterine position of each conceptus is recorded.

In some fertility studies where the necropsy is performed near term, the fetuses are classified as live (fetus exhibits normal appearance, spontaneous movement, heart beat, etc.) or dead (nonliving full size fetus with discernible digits, with a body weight greater than 0.8 g for rats). Resorptions are classified as early or late. An

TABLE 12.3   Categorization Scheme for Offspring from Prenatal Developmental Toxicity Studies

Category	Distinguishing Characteristics
Early resorption	Only dark tissue derived from the placenta remains; if very early, will be visible only with ammonium staining or similar aid to visualize metrial glands and decidual changes in the uterine lining
Mid resorption	Embryonic structures visible but typically show signs of autolysis; may have limb buds but no discernible digits; embryonic remains are generally pale in appearance
Late resorption	Dead fetus that is partially autolyzed
Dead fetus	Dead fetus that shows no signs of autolysis; may be gray in color
Live fetus	Exhibits spontaneous movement, or movement can be elicited by touch; typically pink in color because of circulating blood

early resorption is defined as a conceptus that has implanted but has no recognizable embryonic characteristics evident upon examination. Late resorptions are defined as fetal remains or tissues that have recognizable fetal characteristics (such as limb buds with no discernible digits present) and are undergoing autolysis or maceration.

Vaginal Lavage Methodology   Vaginal lavage is an easy, noninvasive method of collecting vaginal cells for determination of the estrous cycle or to confirm mating (presence of sperm). Vaginal lavage for the determination of the stage of estrus can be performed at any time of the day; however, it is important that the samples be collected at approximately the same time each day over the course of a study. A pre- and postcheck for contamination of the saline should be made. The female rat is removed from the cage, and her identification is verified. One or two drops (approximately 0.25 mL) of physiological (0.9%) saline are withdrawn from the saline aliquot into a new, clean dropping pipette, and the tip of the pipette is gently inserted into the vaginal canal. The pipette bulb is firmly but gently depressed to expel the saline from the pipette into the vagina. The saline is gently drawn back into the dropping pipette, and the pipette is removed from the vaginal canal. If the flush is very clear, the lavage should be repeated. Care must be taken not to insert the tip too far into the vaginal canal, because stimulation of the cervix can result in pseudopregnancy (prolonged diestrus), and the female is returned to her cage. The contents of the pipette are then delivered onto either a clean glass slide or a ring slide containing designated areas for the placement of each sample. Each slide should be numbered, a top and bottom of each slide should be clearly identified, and a corresponding record should be made that indicates the animal number and location for each vaginal smear. All slides should be handled carefully to avoid mixing vaginal lavage samples from different animals. If samples become mixed, they are discarded, and the sampling procedure is repeated for those animals.

The Estrous Cycle   The estrous cycle [19, 20] is separated into distinct phases: metestrus (also called diestrus I), diestrus (also called diestrus II), proestrus, and estrus. The metestrus/diestrus (diestrus I and II) duration is usually 2–3 days, proestrus is usually 1 day, and estrus is also about 1 day.

- Metestrus vaginal smears contain leukocytes, little or few polynucleated epithelial cells, and a variable number of cornified epithelial cells (some of these cells are beginning to roll).
- Diestrus vaginal smears contain a mixture of cell types, mainly leukocytes, a variable number of polynucleated epithelial cells, and few to no cornified epithelial cells. The diestrus period is a time of low serum estradiol, as new follicles mature in the ovary. The transition from diestrus to proestrus is caused by increased estradiol secretion that reaches a peak around the midday of proestrus.
- During the proestrus period, vaginal epithelial cells are proliferating and sloughing off into the vaginal lumen. The proestrus vaginal smear contains numerous round polynucleated epithelial cells (in clumps or strands), a variable number of leukocytes, and few to no cornified epithelial cells. Serum estradiol falls rapidly on the evening of proestrus, as the ovarian follicles leutinize.

- Ovulation occurs early in the morning of vaginal estrus. Proliferation of the vaginal epithelium decreases, and cornified epithelial cells predominate. The estrus vaginal smear contains no leukocytes, few or no polynucleated epithelial cells, and many flat cornified cells.

ESTROUS CYCLE STAGING   Each vaginal lavage sample (fresh or stained) is examined microscopically (low power, 100×). Cellular characteristics of vaginal smears reflect structural changes of vaginal epithelium. The stage of the estrous cycle is determined by recognition of the predominant cell type in the smear. Metestrus smears contain leukocytes and cornified epithelial cells. Diestrus smears contain predominantly leukocytes. The proestrus smears contain predominantly round, polynucleated epithelial cells (in clumps or strands). The estrus smears contain predominantly flat cornified cells. The stage of the estrous cycle is recorded for each female.

ESTROUS CYCLE EVALUATION   Measurement of estrous cycle length is done by selecting a particular stage and counting until the recurrence of the same stage (usually day of first estrus, day of first diestrus, or day of proestrus). The estrous cycle lengths should be calculated for each female. It is often easier to visualize the estrous cycle by plotting the data. The group mean estrous cycle length should be calculated, and the number of females with a cycle length of 6 days or greater should be calculated. A single cycle with a diestrus period of 4 days or longer or an estrus period of 3 days or longer is generally considered aberrant.

Females with two or more days of estrus during most cycles are classified as showing *persistent* estrus. Females with four or more days of diestrus during most cycles are classified as showing *persistent* or prolonged diestrus. Pseudopregnancy is a persistent diestrus (approximately 14 days in duration). Constant estrus and diestrus, if observed, should be reported. Persistent diestrus indicates at least temporary and possibly permanent cessation of follicular development and ovulation, and thus temporary infertility. Persistent diestrus or anestrus may be indicative of interference with follicular development, depletion of the pool of primordial follicles, or perturbation of the gonadotropin support of the ovary.

The presence of regular estrous cycles after treatment does not necessarily indicate that ovulation occurred, because luteal tissue may form in follicles that have not ruptured. However, lack of ovulation should be reflected in reduced fertility parameters. Altered estrous cyclicity or complete cessation of vaginal cycling in response to toxicants should be considered an adverse female reproductive effect. Subtle changes of cyclicity can occur at dosages below those that alter fertility. However, subtle changes in cyclicity without associated changes in reproductive or hormonal endpoints should not be considered adverse.

Oocyte Quantification   Histopathological examination should detect qualitative depletion of the primordial follicle population. However, reproductive study guidelines suggest that a quantitative evaluation of primordial follicles of the F_0 females be performed. Recently, the Society of Toxicologic Pathology [21] has recommended against performing this evaluation. Ovarian histology, oocyte quantification, and differential follicle count methodology have been described in several publications [22–27].

The number of animals, ovarian section selection method, and section sample size should be statistically appropriate for the evaluation procedure used. The guidelines cite ovarian follicular counting methodologies that use a differential count of the primordial follicles, growing follicles, and antral follicles. The current guidelines require evaluation of ovaries from ten randomly selected females from the highest treatment and control groups. Five 6 μm ovarian sections are made from the inner third of each ovary, at least 100 μm apart. The number of primordial follicles (and small growing follicles) is counted, and the presence or absence of growing follicles and corpora lutea is confirmed for comparison of highest dosage group and control ovaries. If statistically significant differences occur, the next lower dosage group is evaluated, and so forth.

12.3.10 Male Reproductive Evaluation

Assessment of the Males at Necropsy In the event of an equivocal mating result, males could be mated with untreated females to ascertain the male's fertility. Males are routinely necropsied after the outcome of mating is known. The males treated as part of the study may also be used for evaluation of toxicity to the male reproductive system if dosing is continued beyond mating and sacrifice is delayed. Any males that are found dead or appear moribund should be necropsied to investigate the cause of death. The male is weighed, euthanized, and subjected to a complete necropsy.

Inspection of Male Viscera The testes and the accessory sex organs are removed and weighed. The remaining abdominal and thoracic organs should be inspected grossly for evidence of toxicity, and target organs should be removed and weighed. If gross organ lesions are noted, the affected organs should be preserved for possible histopathological examination. Although not mandated, evaluation of the histopathology of the testes and epididymides is generally performed, and an evaluation of sperm for motility, count, concentration, and morphology can be performed if that was not done in previous subchronic or chronic studies.

Histopathology

Testis The most sensitive endpoint for the determination of testicular toxicity is histopathology. Testicular histology [28] and sperm parameters are linked, and alterations in testicular structure are usually accompanied by alterations in testicular function. However, some functional changes may occur in the absence of detectable structural changes in the testis. Alterations in the testicular structure and function are also linked to alterations in epididymal structure and function, but changes in epididymal function may occur in the absence of testicular or epididymal structural changes.

Histopathological evaluation of the testis can determine if the germinal epithelium is severely depleted or degenerating, if multinucleated giant cells are present, or if sloughed cells are present in the tubule lumen. The rete testis should be examined for dilation caused by obstruction or disturbances in fluid dynamics and for the presence of proliferative lesions and rete testis tumors. Both spontaneous and chemically induced lesions in the rete testis often appear as germ cell degeneration and depletion. More subtle lesions, such as retained spermatids or missing germ cell types, can significantly affect the number of sperm being released into the tubule lumen.

Several methodologies for qualitative or quantitative assessment of testicular tissues are available that can assist in the identification of less obvious lesions, including use of the technique of "staging spermatogenesis." A detailed morphological description of spermatogenesis and spermiogenesis, with light and electron microscopic photographs of these processes, is available in a book by Russell et al. [29].

Epididymides, Accessory Sex Glands, and Pituitary   Compared with the testes, less is known about structural changes associated with exposure of the epididymides and accessory sex glands to toxicants. Histopathological evaluation should include the caput, corpus, and cauda segments of the epididymis. A longitudinal section of the epididymis that includes all epididymal segments should be obtained for histopathological examination. Presence of debris and sloughed cells in the epididymal lumen indicates damage to the germinal epithelium or to the excurrent ducts. The presence of lesions, such as sperm granulomas, leukocytic infiltration (inflammation), or absence of clear cells in the cauda epididymal epithelium, should be noted. The density of sperm and the presence of germ cells in the lumina reflect time-dependent events in the testis. Sperm in the caput were released from the testis only a few days earlier, while the sperm in the cauda were released approximately 14 days earlier. When decreased copulatory plugs are observed during cohabitation, a careful examination of the accessory sex glands is indicated.

Sperm Evaluation   The sperm quality parameters are sperm number, sperm motility, and sperm morphology [30–32]. Although effects on sperm production can be reflected in other measures, such as testicular spermatid count or cauda epididymis weight, no other measures are adequate to assess effects on sperm motility and velocity. The Computer Assisted Sperm Analysis (CASA) System [33] calculates sperm count, concentration, motility, progressive velocity, track speed, path velocity, straightness, linearity, cross beat frequency, and amplitude of lateral head displacement. For detailed methodologies for epididymal and testicular sample preparations and manual and CASA analysis of epididymal sperm counts and motility and testicular homogenization-resistant spermatid counts, respectively, refer to Parker [34] or the CASA manuals.

While changes in endpoints that measure effects on spermatogenesis and sperm maturation have been related to fertility in several test species, the prediction of infertility from these data (in the absence of actual fertility data) may not be reliable. Fertility is dependent not only on having adequate numbers of sperm, but also on the normality of the sperm. When rat sperm quality is good, rat sperm number must be substantially reduced to affect fertility. Decrements in sperm number or motility may not cause infertility in rats but can be predictive of infertility.

12.3.11   Analysis of Fertility Data

Maternal and paternal toxicity may be evidenced by indicators such as body weight or weight gain, feed and water consumption, organ weights, gross or microscopic

TABLE 12.4   Indices Used in Fertility Study Assessments

$$\text{Male Mating Index} = \frac{\text{Number of males with confirmed matings}}{\text{Number of males cohabitated}} \times 100$$

$$\text{Male Fertility Index} = \frac{\text{Number of males impregnating a female}}{\text{Number of males cohabitated}} \times 100$$

$$\text{Female Mating Index} = \frac{\text{Number of females with confirmed matings}}{\text{Number of females cohabitated}} \times 100$$

$$\text{Female Fertility Index} = \frac{\text{Number of pregnant females}}{\text{Number of females cohabitated}} \times 100$$

$$\text{Fecundity Index} = \frac{\text{Number of pregnant females}}{\text{Number of females with confirmed matings}} \times 100$$

$$\text{Implantation Index} = \frac{\text{Number of implants}}{\text{Number of corpora lutea}} \times 100$$

$$\text{Preimplantation Loss} = \frac{\text{Number of corpora lutea} - \text{Number of implants}}{\text{Number of corpora lutea}} \times 100$$

$$\text{Postimplantation Loss} = \frac{\text{Number of implants} - \text{Number of viable fetuses}}{\text{Number of implants}} \times 100$$

$$\text{Gestation Index} = \frac{\text{Number of females with live born}}{\text{Number of females with evidence of pregnancy}} \times 100$$

Precoital Interval = average number of days after the initiation of cohabitation required for each pair to mate

Mean Gestational Length = Duration from GD 0 to parturition

organ pathology, clinical signs of toxicity, and mortality. Maternal toxicity may be evidenced by indicators such as alterations in the estrous cycle or mating behavior, pre- and postimplantation losses, decreased corpora lutea or ovarian follicle counts, and altered weights and histopathology of the reproductive organs. Paternal toxicity may be evidenced by indicators such as mating behavior, fertility, altered weights and histopathology of the reproductive organs, and abnormal sperm motility and morphology. Fertility data can be analyzed by using the formulas listed in Table 12.4. For further descriptions of each parameter, see Parker [34].

12.3.12   Interpretation of the Data

Importance of Historical Control Data   Of particular concern in reproductive toxicity testing is the development and maintenance of a historical control database [35]. The data should be derived from animals from the same supplier and strain and should be kept current, as animal characteristics can change over time. This database of male and female reproductive information is useful in situations where the data are not otherwise obvious. Published databases are useful for comparison, but they do not take the place of internal historical controls. One must always be aware, however, that even data from animals from a single source may vary unexpectedly or drift over time.

The Need for Expert Judgment and Specialized Technical Training   To assess Segment I studies, the toxicologist must be proficient in reproductive toxicology. To become proficient in reproductive toxicology requires training and experience in a number of different fields, including reproductive anatomy, physiology, endocrinology, pathology, toxicology, and behavior. Fertility is a complex issue encompassing male and female reproductive system function, mating, conception, and implantation.

Reporting the Results of Reproductive Toxicity Studies   Guidelines for reporting the results of reproductive toxicity studies are contained in U.S. FDA *Redbook 2000* [36]. More complete information regarding pathology and statistics can be found in *Redbook* Chapters IVB3c and IVB4a, respectively.

Reproductive toxicity studies are conducted in compliance with Good Laboratory Practice Regulations [37], as specified in Section 21 of the U.S. Code of Federal Regulations (CFR) 58, or, if the study was not conducted in compliance with GLPs, a signed statement including a list of the specific area(s) of noncompliance and the reason(s) for the noncompliance must be included with the study report. Each study report should also include a signed record of periodic inspections conducted by the Quality Assurance Unit (QAU), showing the date of inspection, the phase or segment of the study inspected, and the date the findings were reported to management.

The study report should include all information necessary to provide a complete and accurate description and evaluation of the study procedures and results. The following sections should be included:

- Protocol and Amendments.
- Summary and Conclusions. This section of the study report should contain a brief description of the methods, summary of the data, analysis of the data, and a statement of the conclusions drawn from the analysis.
- Materials. The materials section of the study report should include, but not be limited to, the following information: test substance, storage, animal data, feed and water, diet and availability, facilities, caging, number of animals per cage, bedding material, ambient temperature, humidity, and lighting conditions.
- Methods. The methods section of the study report should include, but not be limited to, the following: deviations from guidelines, specification of test methods, statistical analyses, dosage administration, duration of treatment and study, and method and frequency of observation of the test animals.
- Results. Each study report must include individual animal data and results and tabulation of data must be provided in sufficient detail to permit independent evaluation of the results. The following information should be included for each test animal, where appropriate: time of first observation of each abnormal sign and its subsequent course; time of death during the study; feed consumption data (and water consumption data, if the test compound is administered in the drinking water); body weights and body weight changes; hematology, clinical

chemistry, and other clinical findings; gross necropsy findings including description and incidence of gross lesions; and histopathology findings, including description and incidence of microscopic lesions.

- Data also should be summarized in tabular form, organized by sex and dosage group. When appropriate, data should also be organized by litter. When numerical means are presented, they should be accompanied by an appropriate measure of variability, such as the standard error. For each summarized parameter, the following information should be included: the number of animals at the beginning of the study, the number of animals evaluated for each parameter, the time when animals were evaluated for each parameter, and the number and percentage of animals positive and/or negative for each parameter in comparison to controls.

- All numerical results should be evaluated by an appropriate statistical method. Evaluation of the results should include the following: statements about the nature of relationships, if any, between exposure to the test substance and the incidence and severity of all general and specific toxic effects (such as organ weight effects and mortality effects); statements about the relationships between clinical observations made during the course of a study and postmortem findings; and an indication of the dosage level at which no toxic effects attributable to the test substance were observed.

- References. This section of the study report should include the following information: availability and location of all original data, specimens, and samples of the test substance. The literature or references should include, when appropriate, references for test procedures and statistical and other methods used to analyze the data; compilation and evaluation of results; and the basis on which conclusions were reached.

12.4   PRENATAL DEVELOPMENTAL TOXICITY STUDY (SEGMENT II)

12.4.1   Rationale for the Test

In the developmental toxicity test (i.e., Segment II test, teratology study), pregnant laboratory mammals are exposed to a candidate drug to assess the potential for adverse effects on the developing offspring. This test assesses only prenatal growth, morphological development, and survival, as exposure occurs during gestation and offspring evaluation is carried out prior to the anticipated time of parturition.

12.4.2   Dose Range-Finding Study

A dose range-finding or range-characterization study is a useful preliminary to the developmental toxicity test, and this is especially true for rabbits, as adequate prior toxicity data are seldom available for them. Dosing small groups of dams (generally 5–10 per dosage group) in a pilot study is helpful in selecting appropriate dosages for the definitive study. Although dose selection for this study should be based on any available toxicity and pharmacokinetics data, dosing during gestation in the range-finder controls for physiological differences between pregnant and nonpregnant animals that might cause the choice of inappropriate dosages if selection were based only on findings from the latter. Furthermore, such a study can provide useful preliminary information regarding the test compound's potential for effects on the conceptus. Caution should be used, however, in interpreting the results of a range-finding study, as the small sample size of each treatment group can result in atypical results and inaccurate statistical measures (both Type I and Type II errors), and typically fewer endpoints are examined.

12.4.3 The Definitive Study

Animal Species and Strain Selection   Most commonly, developmental toxicity tests are conducted in two species, rats and rabbits, with mice sometimes used in place of the rat. Other species may be used if they are deemed more relevant in terms of extrapolation of test findings to humans, on the basis of pharmacokinetic or metabolism data or other known attributes of the test compound, or if there are specific toxicity concerns. For example, rabbits are not ideal test animals for antibiotics, as they are dependent on the presence of viable microbial flora in the gut to aid digestion.

Although use of the most relevant species is often said to be desirable, no single animal species has been shown to be an obviously superior model of the human response to developmental toxicants. Thus, rats, rabbits, and mice are used far more often than alternative test species, primarily because of considerations of practicality. They are also used because of regulatory agency recommendations for at least one rodent and one nonrodent species [1]. These animal models offer ready availability, low cost, ease of handling, high fertility, ease of breeding, large litters, short gestation lengths, ease of determination of mating time, low rates of spontaneous deaths and developmental abnormalities, ease with which their fetuses can be examined, and availability of large amounts of information on their reproduction, development, physiology, and response to developmental toxicants [38].

Procurement and Acclimation of the Test Animals   The test animals should be young but fully sexually mature and from the same source and strain, and the females should be nulliparous and as nearly the same age and weight as is practicable. They should be obtained from reputable suppliers that have programs ensuring the genetic integrity of their animals, in addition to their freedom from diseases and parasites. The test animals should be acclimated to the laboratory conditions prior to mating.

Enough females should be used to provide approximately 20 pregnant animals at the time of sacrifice. That is considered to be a minimal number of females to provide adequate data for a developmental toxicity evaluation. Mating 25 rats or mice and 22 rabbits will generally provide at least 20 pregnant dams per test group. Procuring additional female rodents (30–50%) should provide enough matings to result in around 25 mated per test group within a 3–4 day period, whereas an additional two does per group should yield 20 pregnant rabbits at sacrifice [39].

Mating Procedures, Detection of Mating, and Housing of Mated Females   Upon receipt from a supplier, female rodents can be group housed. Once they are mated, females should be housed individually to avoid harassment by dominant individuals and to allow for monitoring of feed consumption. Feed and water should be provided *ad libitum*, except in the case of newly received rabbits, as they may initially benefit from decreased feed availability [39].

It is typical to mate only one or two females to each male, and sibling matings are to be avoided [40]. The number of females to expose to males is limited by the number of litters that can be processed on a given day. As female rodents go through 4–5 day estrous cycles, only a portion will be in estrus and mate on any given day. Thus, it is useful to check female rats for estrous cycle stage by vaginal lavage with physiological (0.9%) saline followed by microscopic examination of the cells thus obtained [34]; only females found to be in estrus or late proestrus should then be placed with males. Care should be taken, however, not to stimulate the cervix when obtaining the cell sample, so as not to induce pseudopregnancy. If estrous cycle stage is not determined, considerably more females must be placed with males than are required to mate on a given day.

Female mice can be influenced by pheromones. If groups of females are housed together, they may cease cycling regularly, but if a male in a wire cage or bedding from a male's cage is placed in a cage housing females, this can synchronize their estrous cycles. A large percentage of female mice can be expected to mate 3 days later if placed with males after such an exposure. Because rabbits are induced ovulators [41], the number mating on a given day is more easily controlled.

Typical ages at mating for rodents and rabbits are shown in Table 12.5, and they differ somewhat among laboratories according to preference. Female rodents to be mated are placed in the male's cage. Rats can be checked each morning by vaginal lavage for the presence of sperm, while mice are examined for the presence of a copulation plug in the vagina as evidence of mating. Alternatively, if rats are kept in wire bottom cages the pan below each cage can be inspected for a copulation plug, as the plug falls out intact by about 6–8 h after mating. Copulation plugs in mice remain in the vagina and are often readily visible. However, in some cases it is necessary to use a small probe to expand the vaginal opening to facilitate detection of the plug, and even with experienced examiners, a few matings can go unrecognized. It is also possible to purchase timed-mated rats and mice, but this practice does not allow for an acclimation/quarantine period, and shipping stress can cause implantation failure. The day on which mating is detected in rodents is, by convention, most commonly referred to as gestation day 0 (GD 0).

Ovulation in rabbits can be induced by natural mating or by injection of luteinizing hormone. Hormone injection is used in conjunction with artificial insemination, employing semen collected via an artificial vagina. Semen can be collected by enticing the buck with an infertile "teaser" doe or by means of a rabbit skin sleeve on the collecting technician's arm. Artificial insemination allows examination of the

TABLE 12.5 Typical Ages and Weights of Laboratory Animals at Time of Mating for Use in Developmental Toxicity Tests

Test Species	Age at Mating (weeks)		Weight of Females at Mating
	Females	Males	
Rat	8–12	10–25	200 g
Mouse	8–12	10–25	25 g
Rabbit	5–6	29–104	2.5–5 kg

semen prior to use, and more than one female can be inseminated with a single ejaculate. However, care must be taken to eliminate any bucks that produce abnormal offspring from untreated females [39]. It is also possible to purchase timed-pregnant rabbits if the vendor is based in close proximity to the test facility. The day on which mating is observed or the day on which the doe is inseminated is designated as GD 0. GD 0 body weights provided by vendor are often used for randomization.

Selection of Dosage Groups and Route of Administration   Typically, developmental toxicity studies are designed with a vehicle control and at least three dosage groups, all of which should be concurrent and housed and handled identically. Mated females should be assigned by a random procedure in a manner that assures that mean maternal body weights are comparable among all test groups and that mating days are similarly represented across dosage groups. The test compound or vehicle must be administered by the route that most closely approximates the pattern of expected human exposure. The highest dosage group should be selected to induce observable maternal toxicity, but without an excessive incidence of maternal mortality (often defined as no more than 10% maternal deaths) [42] or of complete litter loss.

For a given route of administration, the physicochemical characteristics of the test article or dosage formulation may impose practical limitations on the amount that can be successfully administered. In the absence of observable maternal toxicity, a high dose of 1000 mg/kg, a so-called limit dose, is generally acceptable [7]. Alternatively, a high dose that is at least 1000 times the highest expected human dose may be adequate. Ideally, the low dose should be selected so as to provide an NOAEL and to provide a margin of safety [42]. The intermediate dose should be a threshold dose, and the high dose should approximate the maximum tolerated dose (MTD). In practice, this ideal is difficult to achieve with only three dosage levels, making the added information from a well-conducted preliminary dose-characterization study of considerable value. Also, it must be kept in mind that developmental toxicity dose–response curves are often relatively steep, and thus wide separation of dosages above the threshold dose should generally be avoided [43]. Moreover, the dosage intervals should be close enough so as to reveal possible dose-related trends [7].

Treatment Timing and Test Duration   The originally recommended developmental toxicity test (Segment II) study design called for dosing to extend from the time of embryonic implantation until closure of the hard palate of the specific test species (Figs. 12.2 and 12.3), thereby encompassing the period of major organogenesis. Thus, treatments were administered as shown in Table 12.6. However, recently the FDA has recommended extending the dosing period until the day before the scheduled necropsy and fetal examination [40]. The FDA also considers treatment beginning on GD 0, rather than after implantation, an acceptable alternative. Starting the treatment period prior to implantation is particularly desirable for drug candidates that require prolonged exposure to achieve a steady-state concentration in the maternal system [43]. The test compound is usually administered once daily, but pharmacokinetic considerations may suggest an alternative schedule. Dosing should take place at approximately the same time each day for all dosage

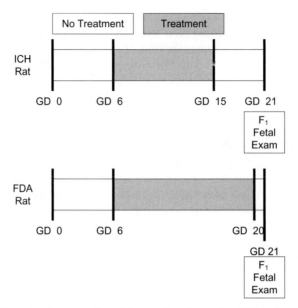

FIGURE 12.2   Rat developmental toxicity study schematics (FDA Segment II and ICH OPPTS 870.3700 and OECD 414).

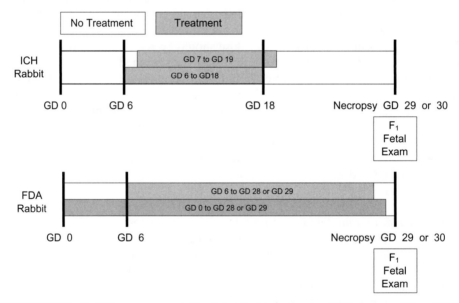

FIGURE 12.3   Rabbit developmental toxicity study schematics (FDA Segment II and ICH S5A).

groups. Aside from considerations of diurnal maternal physiological differences that may influence toxicity response in the dam, development of the offspring is rapid and exact stage of development at the time of toxic insult can influence any prenatal effects.

TABLE 12.6   Timing of Maternal Treatment and Necropsy in Developmental Toxicity Tests

Test Species	ICH[a]	FDA[b]	Necropsy Day
		Guideline and Dosing Period	
Rat	6–15	6 (or 0)–19 or 20	20 or 21
Mouse	6–15	6 (or 0)–17 or 18	17 or 18
Rabbit	6–18	6 (or 0)–28 or 29	29 or 30

[a]From Ref. 1.
[b]From Ref. 40.

TABLE 12.7   Typical Endpoints for Assessment of Maternal Toxicity in Developmental Toxicity Studies

Mortality
Mating index [(Number with seminal plugs or sperm/Number mated) × 100]
Fertility index [(Number with implants/Number of matings) × 100]
Gestation length (useful when animals are allowed to deliver pups)
Body weight
  Gestation day 0
  During gestation
  On day of necropsy
Body weight change
  Throughout gestation
  During treatment (including increments of time within treatment period)
  Posttreatment to sacrifice
  Corrected (body weight change throughout gestation minus gravid uterine weight or litter weight at sacrifice)
Organ weights (in cases of suspected target organ toxicity and especially when supported by adverse histopathology findings)
  Absolute
  Relative to body weight
  Relative to brain weight
Food and water consumption (where relevant)
Clinical evaluations
  Type, incidence, degree, and duration of clinical signs
  Clinical chemistries
Gross necropsy and histopathology

Source: Adapted from Ref. 62.

Maternal and Fetal Endpoints Measured   Typical maternal and fetal endpoints are shown in Tables 12.7 and 12.8, and selected aspects of the test protocols are discussed in the following sections.

Clinical Signs, Maternal Body Weight, and Feed Consumption   The FDA suggests that mated females be observed at least twice daily for clinical signs of toxicity and mortality and advises that the first examination be a thorough examination, while the second can be limited to observing the animals in their cages [40]. If possible, the second observation should be timed appropriately after dosing to allow for detection of the onset and progression of any toxic or pharmacologic effects, and

TABLE 12.8   Typical Endpoints for Assessment of Developmental Toxicity

Litters with Implants

Number of implantation sites/dam
Number of corpora lutea (CL)/dam
Percent preimplantation loss: (CL − Implantations) × 100/CL
Number and percent live fetuses/litter
Number and percent resorptions/litter
Number and percent litters with resorptions
Number and percent late fetal deaths/litter
Number and percent nonlive (late fetal deaths + resorptions) implants/litter
Number and percent litters with nonlive implants
Number and percent affected (nonlive + malformed) implants/litter
Number and percent litters with affected implants
Number and percent litters with total resorptions
Number and percent stillbirths/litter
Number and percent litters with live fetuses

Litters with Live Fetuses

Sex ratio/litter
Mean fetal body weight/litter
Mean male or female fetal body weight/litter
Number and percent fetuses with malformations/litter
   External
   Visceral
   Skeletal
Number and percent malformed fetuses/litter
Number and percent litters with malformed fetuses
Number and percent fetuses with variations/litter
   External
   Visceral
   Skeletal
Number and percent fetuses with variations/litter
Number and percent litters having fetuses with variations
Types and incidence of individual fetal malformations
Types and incidence of individual fetal variations
Individual fetuses with malformations or variations (grouped by litter and dose)

Source: Adapted from Ref. 62.

to permit moribund or dead animals to be removed and preserved prior to excessive tissue deterioration.

All dams should be weighed on GD 0 and daily or at least every 3 days during the dosing period and at necropsy. If dosing does not commence until GD 6, the dams should also be weighed on GD 3. Gains and losses of body weight are often comparatively sensitive indicators of maternal toxicity. Body weight changes are more sensitive than body weights as indicators of effects, and at times they may be the only means of demonstrating toxicity at the high dose. Such body weight changes should be calculated during any preexposure period, for each interval for which weights were recorded, and for the entire period of exposure. This allows detection of temporary effects and compensatory weight gains.

Regulatory guidelines [8, 40] suggest measuring feed consumption weekly as a minimum, but taking such measurements on the same days as body weights are obtained will give more useful data in those instances in which maternal toxicity alters test diet intake. Feed consumption can be calculated as grams/animal/day or as grams/kg/day to adjust for relative maternal size. Water consumption should be measured if suggested by prior test results on the current or similar test compounds.

Maternal Toxicity and Its Significance   Maternal toxicity may be evidenced by indicators such as body weight or weight gain, feed and water consumption, organ weights, gross or microscopic organ pathology, clinical signs of toxicity, and mortality. Of course, interpretation of putative signs of toxicity should consider the timing of their onset or disappearance in relation to the period of dosing in cases where treatment does not span the entire time between mating and necropsy.

In addition to fulfilling the requirement for evidence of maternal toxicity at the high dose, signs of such toxicity have a special significance in developmental toxicity testing. That is because these tests involve two organisms concurrently, the dam and the conceptus (the products of conception, i.e., the embryo or fetus and its membranes), and the conceptus is dependent on the dam for its survival and well-being. Deleterious effects on the embryo/fetus in the absence of discernible maternal toxicity are viewed as especially troublesome, as they suggest that the developing organism is especially sensitive to the test compound. However, if adverse effects on the offspring are observed only at maternally toxic dosages, their interpretation can be confounded by the presence of said maternal toxicity. The default position of the U.S. FDA [40] is that developmental effects occurring in the presence of minimal maternal toxicity are considered to be evidence of developmental toxicity unless it can be shown that those effects are clearly maternally mediated. If developmental effects are seen only at substantially maternally toxic dose levels, then the possibility that said effects were maternally mediated should be investigated before a valid assessment can be made regarding the hazard potential of the test compound. The FDA's position appears to be valid, in that numerous examples of relatively severe maternal toxicity without concomitant developmental effects have been reported, although other instances have been noted in which mechanisms have been found to support the presumption of maternally related causation of embryo–fetal toxicity or teratogenicity [44]. An example of the latter was the finding that diflunisal-associated skeletal defects in rabbits were apparently caused by maternal hemolytic anemia [45]. Additional discussion of the relationship between maternal and developmental toxicity can be found in the review by Hood and Miller [46].

Assessment of the Dam, Uterine Contents, and Fetuses at Necropsy   Any mated females that appear moribund or that appear to have aborted or prematurely delivered should be euthanized appropriately and necropsied to investigate the cause of death. Animals found dead should also be necropsied. In all such cases any evidence of pregnancy and of embryonic or fetal development [47] should be evaluated as well. All surviving females should be humanely euthanized prior to term (see Table 12.6 for timing), laparohysterectomized, and examined as described in the following.

INSPECTION OF MATERNAL VISCERA, ENUMERATION OF CORPORA LUTEA, AND ASSESSMENT OF PRENATAL MORTALITY   The gravid uterus should be removed and weighed, and the female's carcass should be weighed to allow determination of the net maternal weight at sacrifice (the maternal body weight without the uterine weight). The remaining maternal abdominal and thoracic organs should be inspected grossly for evidence of toxicity, and the liver and any known target organs should be removed and weighed. If gross organ pathology is noted or anticipated, the affected organs should be preserved for possible histopathologic examination. The numbers of corpora lutea should be counted and recorded. Corpora lutea of rats and rabbits are relatively obvious, but those of mice must be counted with the aid of a dissecting microscope. Such counts aid in assessing preimplantation mortality, keeping in mind that evidence of preimplantation mortality is only treatment related if dosing began prior to implantation.

The uterus should be examined to determine if the animal was pregnant, and the relative numbers of live, dead, and resorbed offspring and their relative positions in the uterus should be recorded. If the uterus shows no signs of implantation, it should be treated with a reagent, such as 10% ammonium sulfide, to reveal any early resorptions (partially autolyzed embryos) that may not have been obvious [18]. Each remaining uterus should be cut open so that the contents can be examined and characterized. Different characterization schemes can be used, but all bear similarity to the classification scheme shown in Table 12.9. Once fetuses are removed from the uterus and determined to be alive, they should be anesthetized or euthanized prior to weighing or any further examination.

ASSESSMENT OF FETAL GROSS MORPHOLOGY AND BODY WEIGHT   Generally, fetuses from the control and all dosage groups are weighed and examined grossly for developmental defects. In some cases inspection of the low dose and mid-dose fetuses for visceral or skeletal anomalies can be omitted if no differences are found between the control and high dose groups, but in such cases, fixation and storage of the unexamined fetuses is advisable.

Once each fetus is removed from the uterus, its umbilical cord should be cut, and the fetus should be blotted on absorbent paper to remove blood and amniotic fluid. Especially in the case of mouse fetuses, the paper should be slightly damp lest the fetal skin adhere to it and become torn. Then each fetus is carefully inspected for externally visible anatomical abnormalities. This examination should be conducted in a standardized, repeatable manner for each fetus, and the results recorded as either normal or abnormal, with any deviations from normal specifically described. In addition, the sex of each rat or mouse fetus should be assessed by careful measurement of the anogenital distance, which is roughly twice as great in males as in females. Rabbit fetuses must be sexed internally. Fetal inspections of rats, and especially of mice, should be carried out under magnification. Additional endpoints, such as fetal crown-to-rump distance, can also be measured if desired.

The placenta should also be grossly evaluated. Some laboratories weigh the placentas or preserve them in fixative for possible histopathological evaluation. Although not required by regulatory guidelines, placental weights can be useful in cases in which the test chemical may have estrogenic properties.

Each fetus should be numbered individually, weighed, and placed initially in a multi compartmented container, so that all fetuses can be individually identifiable

TABLE 12.9   Comparison of Advantages and Disadvantages of the Major Visceral Examination Methods Used in Developmental Toxicity Studies

Fresh Dissection (Staples' Method)	Free-Hand Sectioning (Wilson's Method)
The same fetus can be examined for both soft tissue and skeletal changes, if desired, increasing the reliability of the study findings and statistical analyses.	Fetuses cannot be examined for skeletal defects once they have been sectioned, so only half of the total available fetuses can be examined for either endpoint.
Training of technicians is simpler, as the viscera are examined *in situ*; that is, structures are visualized as they are learned in anatomy courses.	Technicians must be trained in the normal appearance of two-dimensional serial cross sections and in visualizing anatomical alterations in each such section.
Allows the use of the same general technique for rodents and nonrodents.	Wilson's method cannot be used for nonrodents.
Decreases the likelihood of overlooking clefts, breaches, or absence of a structure (e.g., a heart valve).	Certain anomalies are more likely to be missed.
Avoids the difficulty of sectioning every fetus in exactly the same way, as is needed to ensure comparability of views among fetuses.	Requires relatively precise and consistent sectioning of each fetus, including fetuses of different sizes.
Allows viewing fresh coloration of organs, vessels, and tissues; detection of color changes; and evaluation of vascular tissue perfusion by coloration.	All structures may be colored more or less alike.
The probability of creating artifacts is relatively low.	Artifacts may be created by improper sectioning or fixation.
No chemicals are required except for fixing fetal heads, although a method is now available that uses quick freezing of the heads with dry ice [53].	Has traditionally required use of picric acid, which is a strong irritant, an allergen, and explosive, although other fixation methods have now been described [52].
Organs can be saved for histopathology if desired, although this is rarely done.	Organs can't be saved intact, but all sections can be saved for future re-inspection if needed.
Allows shorter study turnaround.	Requires extra time for fixation and decalcification of fetuses (approximately 1 week).
Requires that more technicians are available to process the fetuses in a timely manner.	Fetuses can be stored until technicians are available to examine them.

throughout the assessment process. Individual identification is then assured by means such as use of chemical-resistant tags. Rabbits can be tagged or numbered on top of the head with a permanent marker (assuming that the area is normally intact). Individual fetal identification is important so that all findings, such as body weight and gross, visceral, and skeletal examinations, can be related to a specific individual.

FETAL VISCERAL EVALUATION   Many fetal abnormalities are only detectable internally, so it is imperative that both the soft tissues and the skeleton are examined.

All nonrodent fetuses, being larger, are examined for visceral defects by fresh dissection, with only the heads subjected to sectioning. Typically half of each litter of rodent fetuses is randomly selected and examined by either a fresh dissection (Staples') method [39, 48] or the free-hand sectioning (Wilson's) method [49, 50]. There are positive and negative attributes of both methods (Table 12.9) but there are more positives for the fresh dissection method if enough technicians are available to examine all fetuses in a reasonable amount of time. Even if availability of technical staff is limiting, rodent fetuses can be refrigerated for a day or so prior to visceral examination if necessary. Visceral examination is often best carried out under magnification, and detailed instructions for visceral exams can be found in the references listed above, and in other sources, such as Christian [51].

Whole fetuses and fetal heads to be examined by Wilson's method must be preserved with an appropriate decalcifying fixative prior to sectioning. It should be noted that alternate fixatives, such as Davidson's [52], may be preferable to Bouin's fixative for that method. They avoid the use of picric acid, and they may produce superior contrast and enhanced definition of organs and vessels, as well as allowing the sections to remain moist for a greater length of time. Another method for preparing fetal heads for sectioning has been described for rat fetuses by Astroff et al. [53]. This method employs freezing with dry ice, avoids the use of fixative chemicals entirely, and avoids the delay of several days necessitated by use of chemical fixatives.

FETAL SKELETAL EVALUATION   All rabbit fetuses and at least half of each litter of rodent fetuses should be processed and examined for skeletal defects. There are two general skeletal staining techniques, with several published variations of each. For staining only the ossified structures, rodent fetuses are first fixed in 70% ethanol. Then each fetus is cut open along the ventral midline, and the viscera are removed. The soft tissues are macerated with a strong alkaline solution and simultaneously stained with alizarin red S, and then the soft tissues are "cleared" (i.e., made transparent), by use of glycerin-containing solutions. Rabbit fetuses are processed similarly, following their visceral examination, but should be skinned first. Alternatively, the cartilage is stained blue with alcian blue, and the mineralized bone is stained red with alizarin red S. To facilitate penetration of the alcian blue dye, rats and rabbits should be skinned prior to this "double-staining" process. Moreover, although the original double-staining technique called for use of glacial acetic acid, hazards posed by exposure to that substance make its use problematic. According to Webb and Byrd [54], "replacement of the glacial acetic acid with potassium hydrogen phthalate eliminates these hazards without compromising the quality of the stained specimen."

Although there is disagreement on the matter [51], there have been published comparisons claiming that double-staining was to be preferred [55]. Detailed instructions for macerating and staining fetuses can be found in a number of sources [54, 56–60]. Such methods can generally be adapted for use with automated staining systems designed for the purpose, and use of such systems can decrease processing time and labor. However, it must be kept in mind that unusually small fetuses, especially those of mice, can disintegrate if kept too long in strong alkali solutions. Maceration times may have to be adjusted in such cases, and this is especially of concern when automatic processors are employed.

Analysis of Maternal and Fetal Data   Obviously, both the maternal and fetal data must be subjected to appropriate statistical analysis. The FDA [40] has suggested that maternal body weights be compared by analysis of covariance, with adjustment for initial body weight, followed by analysis by protected least significant difference tests. The FDA also suggested comparison of fetal weight by nested ANOVA, fetal abnormalities by Fisher's exact test, and fetal mortality and litter incidence of anomalies by arcsine transformation followed by ANOVA. There has been considerable interest in exactly how fetal data should be analyzed; as the data may not be "normally distributed," they tend to be interrelated in various ways, and their endpoints range from relatively continuously distributed to the highly categorical. Fetal findings are commonly influenced by the so-called "litter effect" (i.e., fetuses within a litter tend to be affected more similarly), giving rise to the admonition that the litter, rather than the fetus or neonate, should be the experimental unit [61]. Moreover, inappropriately calculating fetal malformation data is a common error. The percentage of affected fetuses should be determined for each litter, allowing calculation of an overall mean of the litter means [43]. Complexities such as the foregoing make it imperative to consult with an experienced statistician, beginning at the study design stage.

12.4.4 Interpretation of the Data

Importance of Historical Control Data   Of particular concern in developmental toxicity testing is the development and maintenance of a historical control database for each test species. The data should be derived from animals from the same supplier and strain and should be kept current, as animal characteristics can change over time. This database of litter and fetal characteristics is invaluable in situations in which it is not otherwise obvious whether a finding, such as an apparent increase in resorptions (evidence of prenatal demise) or of specific malformations or developmental variations, is treatment related. Although comparisons with data from the same species and strain from other suppliers or collected by other laboratories may be of some value for comparison purposes, *such data cannot take the place of data collected in-house and from the same source.* One must always be aware, however, that even animals from a single source may vary unexpectedly over time.

Possible Adverse Effects on the Offspring   There are four major categories of toxicity effects on the conceptus: mortality, structural alteration, altered growth, and functional deficit. Prenatal mortality can be revealed as pre- or peri-implantation loss (which may be treatment related if dosing was initiated prior to implantation), early or late resorption, abortion, or fetal death. Manifestations of abnormal fetal anatomical development (dysmorphology) are often categorized as malformations or variations. Malformations can be defined as permanent structural changes that may adversely affect survival, development, or function, whereas variations may be regarded as deviations beyond the usual range of structural constitution that may not adversely affect survival or health [62]. However, the division between variations and malformations is somewhat artificial, as there is a continuum of responses from the normal to the extremely abnormal, and there are numerous classification schemes for malformations and variations [63]. Growth alteration is almost always seen as diminished growth, although there can be other possibilities, such as localized overgrowth or altered anogenital distance, and increased fetal weight can be secondary to generalized edema. Functional deficits can be manifested as abnormal physiological or biochemical parameters, although these are not routinely measured. Behavioral parameters are sometimes affected, but they can only be assessed postnatally.

Evaluation of Low Incidence Effects   The U.S. FDA [64] has defined "rare event" as "an endpoint that occurs in less than 1% of the control animals in a study and in historical control animals." When such small numbers of adverse fetal findings, such as malformations, are observed, it is often difficult to ascertain whether they are spontaneous background events or the result of test article toxicity. The incidences of malformations in typical guideline studies are generally too low to be considered statistically significantly elevated above the control incidence, thus increasing the difficulty in separating such events from normal biological variation. Nevertheless, appearance of two or three malformed fetuses in a test group, especially if they occur in different litters, is cause for concern that they may be treatment related.

Detailed guidance for evaluation of the biological significance of low incidence adverse events can be found in the discussion of the issue by Holson et al. [43]. They advise that careful examination of the test facility's historical control database is the logical initial step in assessing whether a small, statistically nonsignificant alteration in an endpoint should be considered a possible treatment effect. They further advise that reliable estimation of the incidence of a low incidence developmental defect in the test population requires approximately 100 control datasets, thus rendering the concurrent controls relatively unhelpful for discerning treatment-related versus spontaneous occurrences for low incidence developmental toxicity endpoints.

Distinguishing between spontaneous adverse findings and those caused with low frequency by a test compound is a daunting task for developmental toxicologists, because the usual insights provided by statistical analyses are generally unavailable. Thus, Holson et al. [43] suggest reliance on additional tools, such as "probabilistic theory, intuition for developmental processes and patterns, and arrays and timing of effects."

The Need for Expert Judgment and Specialized Technical Training   It may perhaps be appreciated from the foregoing that developmental toxicology is a complex subject. It requires knowledge of a number of different fields, including embryology, anatomy, physiology, reproductive biology, endocrinology, laboratory animal science, biochemistry, cell biology, statistics, and, of course, toxicology. Such knowledge is important because development of the embryo and fetus encompasses a highly complex series of many events occurring concurrently at the organ, tissue, cellular, and molecular levels, and these events are also continually changing over time. An additional level of complexity is added by the relationship of the embryo/fetus to the mother via the placenta and the extraembryonic membranes. That relationship is further influenced by the mother's physiology, which is changing throughout pregnancy. If postnatal survival and development are assessed, maternal behaviors and lactation are also influential.

Unfortunately, as affirmed by Kimmel et al. [65], "many of the current graduate programs have an academic/basic science focus that gives the student neither an understanding of the complex interplay of anatomy with physiological and bio-chemical processes, nor a perspective of more applied areas of toxicology." Relatively few students are currently being exposed to relevant courses, such as developmental anatomy, or even to basic anatomy and physiology, and they may have never even worked with live animals [66]. In-depth principles of developmental toxicology are not often taught in college or graduate school, even in toxicology programs, and few graduate students are engaged in research that prepares them to conduct or interpret guideline compliant studies, such as the prenatal developmental toxicity study. New entrants to the field are often life sciences majors. They are intelligent, but when they have not been exposed to the relevant disciplines much of their training must be on-the-job training. And then they are asked to design, perform, and interpret some of the most technically and numerically complex studies in the entire discipline of toxicology!

To make matters even more challenging, a large number of endpoints are examined in developmental toxicity assessments, and it is not unusual for at least a few of the findings to be problematic to interpret. In part, that is because some of these findings may be differences from the controls that are deemed statistically significant merely because of the combination of biological variability and the large number of comparisons that must be made. Others may fall into the category of "rare events," as described earlier. All of these factors make expert judgment of considerable importance in interpreting developmental toxicity test findings, and especially in evaluating potential human risk. They also highlight the relevance of organized approaches to interpretation of the data, as detailed in Holson et al. [43].

12.4.5   Reporting the Results of Developmental Toxicity Studies

Study reports should include complete tabulated data on the dams and individual fetuses, as well as tables summarized by litters. The data should be calculated by litter incidence and by the number and percent of litters with a specific endpoint. The dosages employed should be reported as mg/kg/day, that is, milligrams of test compound per kilogram of body weight per day [40]. It is also extremely important to report all relevant historical control data, as this is critical in allowing reviewers to evaluate the biological significance of findings, such as malformations, variations, resorptions, and the like. The historical control data should include all significant factors, such as the dates when they were obtained, the strain of animals used (which should preferably be the strain that was used in the current study), the group sizes, and the range as well as the mean of the values for specific parameters.

The most common problems seen when developmental toxicity studies are reviewed by the FDA are failure to use adequate numbers of pregnant dams in each test group, not using random selection procedures for allocating dams to test groups, and use of the individual fetus rather than the litter as the experimental unit for statistical analysis [40]. It is also all too common to see errors in test protocol descriptions, and these often arise whenever "boilerplate" text is taken from previous reports and put together in new combinations.

12.5   PERINATAL AND POSTNATAL STUDY (SEGMENT III)

The Segment III study or perinatal/postnatal evaluation was designed to evaluate the effects of a test article on gestation, parturition, and lactation. The perinatal/postnatal study is generally performed with treatment of pregnant female rats beginning on GD 7 and continuing through gestation, parturition, and through a 21 day lactation period. This combines embryo, fetal, and perinatal/postnatal exposures in one study. Postnatal changes may be induced by insult at any time during treatment. Parturition and pup survival and development are monitored with observations for prolonged gestation, dystocia, impaired maternal nesting or nursing behavior, and postnatal mortality. If indicated by the results of this study or other studies, a cross-fostering procedure may be included to demonstrate whether findings in the pups are direct effects of exposure during gestation and/or lactation or if they are associated with abnormalities in maternal reproductive behavior or health. The peri/postnatal evaluation is not required by the FDA *Redbook*, OECD, or U.S. EPA guidelines. Rather, these evaluations are part of the multigeneration studies performed to meet the needs of these regulatory bodies, which consider this design an appropriate overall evaluation of reproductive capacity. The ICH guideline acknowledges the overlap in the methods used to test chemicals and pharmaceuticals for adverse effects on the reproductive process, but recommends that segmented study designs generally be used because humans usually take a pharmaceutical product for limited intervals, rather than an entire lifetime. However, the ICH document [2] also notes that lifetime exposure to a drug sometimes occurs, and that there may be drugs that can be more appropriately tested by exposure throughout the entire reproductive life (i.e., through use of a multigeneration study design) (see later discussion).

Rather than a standard "checklist" approach, the ICH guideline [1] emphasizes flexibility in developing the testing strategy. Although the most probable options are identified in the guideline, the development of the testing strategy is to be based on the following points:

1. Anticipated drug use, especially in relation to reproduction.
2. Form of the test article and route(s) of administration intended for humans.
3. Use of any existing data on toxicity, pharmacodynamics, kinetics, and similarity to other compounds in structure/activity.

The notes in the ICH guideline describe some methods appropriate for use in specific portions of the tests; however, it emphasizes that the individual investigator is at liberty to identify the tests used, and that the ICH guideline is truly a guideline and not a set of rules. The overall aim of the described reproductive toxicity studies is to identify any effect of an active substance on mammalian reproduction, with subsequent comparison of this effect with all other pharmacologic and toxicologic data. The objective is to determine whether human risk of effects on the reproductive process is the same as, increased, or reduced in comparison with the risks of other toxic effects of the agent. The document clearly states that, for extrapolation of results of the animal studies, other pertinent information should be used, including human exposure considerations, comparative kinetics, and the mechanism of the toxic effect.

12.5.1   Rationale for the Test

The Segment III study or perinatal/postnatal evaluation was designed to detect adverse effects following exposure of the female from implantation through weaning (Fig. 12.4). Since manifestations of effect induced during this period may be delayed, observations should be continued through sexual maturity (i.e., Stages C–F). The adverse effects assessed in a perinatal/postnatal study include enhanced toxicity relative to that in nonpregnant females, maternal nursing behavior (including milk production), pre- and postnatal death of offspring, altered growth and development, and functional deficits in offspring, including behavior, maturation (puberty), and reproduction.

12.5.2   Animal Species and Strain Selection

It is generally desirable to use the same species and strain as in other toxicological studies. Reasons for using rats as the predominant rodent species are practicality, comparability with other results obtained in this species, and the large amount of background knowledge accumulated. Within and between studies, animals should be of comparable age, weight, and parity at the start of the study.

Number of Test Animals   The number of animals per group should be sufficient to allow meaningful interpretation of the data. Routinely, 20–25 pregnant female

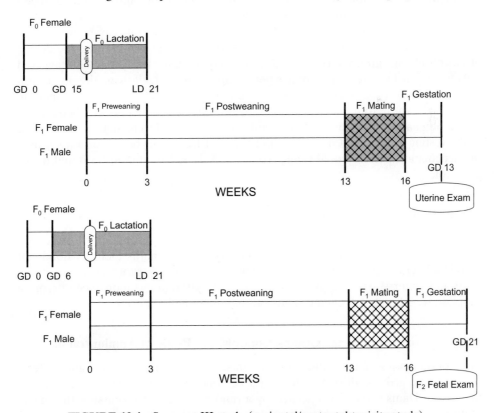

FIGURE 12.4   Segment III study (perinatal/postnatal toxicity study).

rats per group are used. If lethality is expected, then an increased number of animals should be mated. Usually 16–20 litters per group are required for evaluation. With less than 16 litters per group, the study results can become inconsistent, while greater than 20–24 litters per group does not greatly enhance the group consistency.

Statistical Considerations   When using statistical procedures, the experimental units of comparison should be the dam and the litter, not the individual offspring.

The endpoints observed in reproductive tests are usually nonnormal and extend from the continuous to the categorical. The interpretation of the data *must* be based on biological plausibility. To assume that a difference from control values is not biologically relevant simply because it is not "statistically significant" is unfounded, while the assumption that a "statistically significant" difference must be biologically relevant is also unwise. Statistical tests should be used only as a support for the interpretation of results. The statistical tests and statistical programs used should be stated in the protocol and their use justified.

12.5.3   Procurement and Acclimation of the Test Animals

The test animals should be young but sexually mature and from the same source and strain, and the females should be nulliparous and as nearly the same age and weight as is practicable when mated. However, the availability of timed-mated pregnant rats from vendors has reduced the need to maintain a breeding colony to deliver the requisite number of pregnant rats. The pregnant rats can be ordered to arrive at the testing facility with staggered days of conception, allowing the dosing of subsets of each group to begin on different days (usually four). A 4 day staggered start will allow five pregnant females per group as a subset, allowing the pup evaluation workload to be distributed over several days for each task. The acclimation period may vary from the usual laboratory acclimatization period when timed-mated pregnant rats are used. If pregnant rats are ordered to be delivered to arrive at the testing facility on GD 2, 3, 4, and 5, and if treatment begins on GD 7, then the acclimation period would range from 2 to 5 days. This should be stated in the protocol.

12.5.4   Housing of Female Rats

Upon receipt from a supplier, nonpregnant females can be group housed. Once they are mated, dams should be housed individually to avoid harassment by dominant individuals and to allow for monitoring of feed and, if necessary, water consumption. Feed and water should be provided *ad libitum*. Alternately, upon receipt from a supplier, timed-mated pregnant dams can be individually housed.

12.5.5   Selection of Dosage Groups, Controls, and Route of Administration

Most perinatal/postnatal studies are designed with a vehicle control and at least three dosage groups, all of which should be concurrent and housed and handled identically. Dams should be assigned by a random procedure to assure that mean body weights are comparable for all test groups. The test compound or vehicle should be administered by the route that most closely approximates the pattern of expected human exposure.

12.5.6   Treatment Timing and Test Duration

Females are exposed to the test article daily from implantation (GD 7) to the end of lactation (LD 21). Dosing should take place at approximately the same time each day for all dosage groups. F_1 generation pups are not directly given the test article and/or vehicle, but may possibly be exposed to the test article during gestation (*in utero* exposure) or via milk during the lactation period.

12.5.7 F_0 Generation

Maternal Endpoints Measured

Maternal Body Weight, Feed Consumption, Behavior, and Clinical Signs   Clinical signs and mortalities should be recorded at least once daily. Body weight values should be recorded at least twice weekly but are routinely collected daily or at protocol-specified intervals (e.g., GD 0, 7, 9, 12, 15, 18, and 20, and LD 0, 7, 14, and 21). Food consumption should be measured at least once weekly up to LD 14 at the same interval as the body weight collection. Pups begin feeding on their own at this time, so food consumption measurement on LD 21 would not be reliable. Duration of pregnancy, parturition, and nursing behaviors, and any additional observations that have proved of value in other toxicity studies are also recorded.

Assessment of the Dam at Necropsy   Dams are routinely necropsied on LD 21. The dam is weighed and euthanized, and the ovary and uterus are examined. Any mated females that appear moribund should be euthanized appropriately, and mated females that are found dead should be necropsied to investigate the cause of death. Any evidence of pregnancy and of embryonic development should be recorded.

Inspection of Maternal Viscera   If necropsy occurs prior to parturition, then the gravid uterus should be removed and weighed. The uterus should be examined to determine if the animal was pregnant, and the relative numbers of live and dead conceptuses and their relative positions in the uterus should be recorded. If the uterus shows no signs of implantation, it should be treated with a reagent, such as 10% ammonium sulfide, to reveal any early resorptions [18]. The remaining maternal abdominal and thoracic organs should be inspected grossly for evidence of toxicity, and target organs should be removed and weighed. If gross organ lesions are noted, the affected organs should be preserved for possible histopathologic examination.

If necropsy occurs as scheduled or after parturition, then the uterus should be removed and weighed. The remaining maternal abdominal and thoracic organs should be inspected grossly for evidence of toxicity, and target organs should be removed and weighed. If gross organ lesions are noted, the affected organs should be preserved for possible histopathologic examination.

Enumeration of Corpora Lutea   The number of corpora lutea should be recorded for each ovary as described earlier.

Parturition   Dams should be housed in litter boxes with bedding material no later than GD 20 (two days prior to expected parturition, earlier if required by protocol). The dams are observed periodically throughout the day for stretching, visual uterine contractions, vaginal bleeding, and/or placentas in the nesting box. These signs are strong indicators of parturition onset and indicate that dams should be closely monitored for the delivery of the first pup. As soon as the first pup is found, parturition is considered initiated. Once delivery has begun, the dams should be checked periodically for evidence of difficulty of labor or delivery (e.g., dam cold to touch or pale, partially delivered pup). Dams should not be treated during delivery.

The calendar date when delivery is completed is designated as LD 0, PND 0 (postnatal day 0), and day 0 of age. The following maternal behaviors are indicators that parturition is complete: removal of the amniotic sacs, placentas, and umbilical cords, and grooming of the pups by the dam; self-grooming; nesting behavior; and nursing. However, parturition may be complete without all of these behaviors present. Individual pup observations should not be made until delivery is completed. Apparently dead pups should be removed from the nesting box to preclude cannibalization by the dam.

Milk Collection (if Required)   Prior to milk collection, the pups are withheld from the dam for approximately 4 hours. At least 5 minutes prior to milk collection, 0.05 mL of oxytocin (20 units/mL) is administered intravenously to the dam. The time that the oxytocin is administered should be documented on the appropriate form. The dam is then held in a position that facilitates access to the teats. Milk is expressed from one teat at a time by applying gentle digital pressure. Initially the pressure is applied at the base of the teat and then is directed distally. The milk is collected into a microtainer or other suitable container (labeled with the protocol and animal number, date, identification of sample and test system, i.e., rat milk). The time of collection and volume of milk collected are documented, and the dam is returned to her litter.

12.5.8   F₁ Generation

Litter Evaluations   The general appearance of the entire litter and maternal and pup nesting behavior are observed. The following items should be checked: (1) that there is evidence of a nest, (2) that the pups are grouped together, (3) that the pups are warm and clean, and (4) that the pups are nursing or have milk present in their stomachs (milk spot).

After the litter observations, the bedding in the nesting box can be replaced with clean bedding or a new box with clean bedding can be obtained. The dam is weighed and observed for clinical signs, the feed jar is weighed (if appropriate), and the dam and pups are placed into the clean box.

Gender Determination   The pups are removed from the nesting box, and the gender of each pup is determined. Anogenital distance (the length between the anus and the genital tubercle) is used to determine gender. Beginning on DG 17 and continuing through PND 21, anogenital distances are greater for male than for female rodents. The increased growth of this region occurs in response to testosterone.

Anogenital distances for rat fetuses (DG 20 or 21) or pups on PND 0 to 3 are measured with a micrometer and a stereomicroscope [43]. Pups that have been cannibalized to the extent that their gender cannot be determined are recorded as "sex unable to be determined because of cannibalization." If a malformation precludes sex determination, this is recorded (e.g., "tail absent, no apparent anus, sex could not be determined"). If the malformed pup is dead, the sex is determined internally.

Viability   The viability of each pup is determined, and dead pups are removed from the nesting box to prevent cannibalization. The dead pup is necropsied, the trachea is tied off with string, and the lungs are removed and placed in a container of water. If the dead pup's lungs float, the pup is assumed to have breathed, and the viability is recorded as "born alive, but found dead." If the lungs sink, the pup is assumed to have never taken a breath, and the viability is recorded as "stillborn." Dead pups can be cannibalized to the point where viability cannot be determined. The sex and viability status are recorded for each pup (including dead, cannibalized, and malformed pups) in all litters.

External Alterations   Each pup in the litter is evaluated for external alterations. The following items are evaluated for each pup: the general shape of the head; presence/completeness of features; trunk continuity; presence of bruises, lesions, or depressions; length and shape of limbs (digits are counted); length and diameter of the tail; presence of an anus; milk in the stomach; and whether partial cannibalization has occurred. All live pups are weighed.

Missing Pups   If a pup cannot be found during the daily litter count, the pups are sorted by gender in order to determine the sex of the missing pup(s) by process of elimination. The missing pup is recorded as "missing, presumed cannibalized." If the pups have been tattooed or otherwise identified, the actual identification number of the missing pup(s) should be recorded.

Pups Found Dead   All found dead pups are necropsied. Stomach contents of all dead pups should be recorded (i.e., "stomach contains/does not contain milk"). Unless otherwise dictated by the protocol, dead pups with gross lesions found on LD 0 to 4 should be fixed in Bouin's fixative. Gross lesions from pups found dead on LD 5 through weaning are fixed in 10% neutral buffered formalin. Because of postmortem autolysis, dead pups are not routinely weighed.

Dam Dies Before Scheduled Sacrifice or All Pups in a Litter Die   If a dam with a litter dies before her scheduled sacrifice, the pups are sacrificed and necropsied. If all the pups in a litter die, the dam may remain on study until her scheduled sacrifice date, or the dam may be sacrificed at the discretion of the study director. The sacrifice and necropsy observations are recorded.

Pup Evaluations

Pup Body Weights   Individual pup weights should always be measured on the day of parturition. The statistical unit is the litter; therefore, data from the individual pups are reported as the entire litter weight and as weight by sex per litter. Birth weights are influenced by maternal nutritional status, intrauterine growth rates, litter size, and gestation length. Individual pups in small litters tend to be larger than pups in larger litters; conversely, individual pups in large litters tend to be smaller. Therefore, reduced birth weights that can be related to large litter size or increased birth weights that can be related to small litter size should not be considered an adverse effect unless the altered litter size is considered treatment related and survivability and/or development of the offspring have been compromised.

Postnatal Pup Body Weights   Postnatal weights are dependent on litter size and on pup gender, birth weight, suckling ability of the offspring, and normality of the individual, as well as on maternal milk production. With large litters, small or weak offspring may not thrive and may show further impairments in growth or development. Because one cannot determine whether growth retardation or decreased survival rate was due solely to the increased litter size, these effects are usually considered adverse developmental effects. Conversely, pup weights in very small litters may appear comparable to or greater than control weights and therefore may mask decreased postnatal weights in other litters.

Crown–Rump Length   Crown–rump lengths for fetuses are measured with a caliper. Fetuses may be euthanized before measuring the crown–rump length. Place each fetus on its side on a flat surface, and place the caliper with one prong touching the top of the head and the opposite prong touching the base of the tail. Do not stretch or compress the fetus. Record the measurements in millimeters.

Standardization of Litter Sizes   Animals should be allowed to litter normally and rear their offspring to weaning. Standardization of litter sizes is optional. If standardization is performed, the procedure should be described in detail in the protocol or Standard Operating Procedure. On PND 4, the size of each litter may be adjusted by eliminating extra pups by random selection to yield, as nearly as possible, four males and four females per litter or five males and five females per litter. Selective elimination of pups based on body weight, size, and/or activity is not appropriate. Whenever the number of male or female pups prevents having four (or five) of each sex per litter, partial adjustment (e.g., five males and three females, or four males and six females) is acceptable. Adjustments are not appropriate for litters of eight pups or less.

Survival Indices   The following survival indices should be calculated and reported: Live Birth Index and Survival Index on PND 4, 7, 14, and 21. These indices are primary endpoints in a reproduction study, reflecting the offspring's ability to survive postnatally to weaning. If litter standardization or culling of the litter is performed on PND 4, then the PND 4 *Survival Index* should be based on the preculling number of offspring. All subsequent *Survivability Index* calculations will use the number of offspring remaining after standardization as the denominator in the equation. If litter standardization was performed, the PND 21 survival index is known as the *Lactation Index*. If litter standardization was not performed, the PND 21 survival index is known as the *Weaning Index*. Pup survival endpoints can be affected by the toxicity of the test article, either by direct effects on the offspring (e.g., low birth weight, impaired suckling ability, structural or functional developmental defects), indirectly through effects on the dam (e.g., neglect, poor milk production, acute intoxication), or by a combination of maternal and offspring effects. Pup survival may also be impaired by nontreatment-related factors, such as litter size or improper husbandry. The methods of calculation of the survival indices are as follows:

$$\text{Live Birth Index} = \frac{\text{Number of pups born alive}}{\text{Total number of pups born}} \times 100$$

$$\text{Survival Index} = \frac{\text{Total number of live pups (at designated timepoint)}}{\text{Number of pups born}} \times 100$$

Sex Ratio   Offspring gender in mammals is determined at fertilization of an ovum by sperm with an X or a Y chromosome. Altered sex ratios may be related to several factors, including selective loss of male or female offspring, sex-linked lethality (genetic germ cell abnormalities), abnormal production of X- or Y-chromosome-bearing sperm, or hormonal alterations that result in intersex conditions. The calculations should include both live and dead pups, because sex can easily be determined (except in the case of cannibalized pups or in some sexually ambiguous offspring). Treatment effects on sex ratio can indicate an adverse reproductive effect, especially if embryonic or fetal loss is observed. Because of the altered anogenital distance, visual determination of sex is often incorrect when the pups have an intersex condition (masculinized females or feminized males). The correct diagnosis is usually determined later during lactation when the condition becomes obvious or at the postmortem evaluation, when the reproductive organs are examined. The data are usually presented as a ratio, using the following formula:

$$\text{Sex ratio} = \frac{\text{Number of male offspring}}{\text{Number of female offspring}}$$

Data are often presented as a percentage of male offspring, using the following formula:

$$\text{Percentage of male offspring} = \frac{\text{Number of male offspring}}{\text{Total number of offspring}} \times 100$$

Weaning   Weaning is usually performed at LD 21. At weaning, one male and one female offspring per litter are selected for rearing to adulthood and for mating with a non-littermate from the same dosage group to assess reproductive competence.

Assessment of F_1 Weanlings Not Selected for Continuation   At the time of termination or death during the study, when the litter size permits, pups should be examined macroscopically for any structural abnormalities or pathological changes. Special attention should be paid to the reproductive organs. Dead pups or pups that are terminated in a moribund condition should be examined for possible defects and/or cause of death.

Developmental Landmarks The onset of various developmental landmarks can be used to assess postnatal development. Sexual maturation landmarks (balanopreputial separation and vaginal patency) are required in perinatal/postnatal studies, where the offspring are raised to adulthood. Additional developmental landmarks can be assessed, including pinna detachment, hair growth, incisor eruption, eye opening, nipple development, and testes descent. The development of the following reflexes can also be evaluated: surface righting reflex, cliff avoidance, forelimb placing, negative geotaxis, pinna reflex, auditory startle reflex, hindlimb placing, air righting reflex, forelimb grip test, and pupillary constriction reflex. For a description of these developmental landmarks and reflexes, see Parker [34]. The examinations must begin prior to the landmark's historical day of onset and continue daily until each animal in the litter meets the criterion [67]. Data for each day's testing should be expressed as the number of pups that have achieved the criterion for each developmental landmark, divided by the total number of pups tested in the litter. Forelimb grip test and pupillary constriction tests are conducted on PND 21 only. Data for the forelimb grip test and pupillary constriction tests should be expressed as the number of pups that have achieved the criterion, divided by the total number of pups tested in the litter.

Balanopreputial Separation In rats, balanopreputial separation is considered to result from membrane cornification, which leads to the detachment of the prepuce from the glans penis in the rat. Preputial separation occurs dorsolaterally and then ventrally on the penis and down the shaft of the penis. The prepuce remains attached to the glans penis on its ventral surface by the frenulum of the prepuce of the penis. Male rats are examined for balanopreputial separation beginning on PND 35 to 40. Published preputial separation age ranges from PND 32 to 42 in Japanese studies [68–70] to PND 41 to 46 in American studies, depending on the observation criterion.

Because manipulation of the prepuce can accelerate the process of preputial separation, the males must be examined gently. Each male is removed from its cage and held in a supine position. Gentle digital pressure is applied to the sides of the rodent's prepuce, and the criterion is met when the prepuce completely retracts from the head of the penis. The foreskin can be attached along the shaft of the penis, but it cannot be attached to the opening of the urethra. Each male is examined daily until acquisition or until PND 55, whichever is earliest. Body weight should be recorded on the day the criterion is met.

Vaginal Patency After vagina canalization occurs in rats, the vaginal opening remains covered by a septum or membrane. The age of vaginal patency (when the septum is no longer evident) occurs around the time of puberty in rats, and it is their most readily determined marker for puberty. Female rats are examined beginning a few days prior to the expected age of maturation (e.g., PND 25 to 28) and examinations are continued until the criterion for patency has been achieved or until PND 43, whichever comes first.

The female is removed from the cage and held in a supine position, exposing the genital area. Gentle pressure is applied to the side of the vaginal opening to determine if it is patent. When the membrane is present, the area has a slight "puckered" appearance; however, when the membrane has broken, the vaginal opening is about the size of a pinhead. The criterion has been met when the vaginal opening is observed. Body weight should be recorded on the day the criterion is met.

F_1 Mating Procedure   At approximately 90 days of age, the F_1 rats are cohabitated for a period of 21 days. A mating ratio of 1:1 from the same dosage group but from different litters allows identification of both parents of a litter. Females with sperm observed in the vaginal lavage and/or having a copulatory plug will be presumed pregnant and at day 0 of gestation and will be housed individually. Females that do not mate within 14 days will be cohabitated with an alternate male animal from the same dosage group that has mated.

F_1 Female Observations

F_1 Female Body Weight, Feed Consumption, Behavior, and Clinical Signs   Clinical signs and mortalities should be recorded at least once daily. Body weight values should be recorded on first day of dosing and at least weekly thereafter. Food consumption should be measured at least once weekly, at the same interval as the body weight collection. Water consumption should be measured weekly if the test article is administered in the drinking water.

F_1 Maternal Observations

Maternal Body Weight, Feed Consumption, Behavior, and Clinical Signs   Maternal body weight, feed consumption, behavior, and clinical signs should be recorded at the same intervals as for the F_0 maternal observations.

Laparohysterectomy   Female F_1 rats will be laparohysterectomized on GD 21. The dams should be examined for numbers and distribution of corpora lutea, implantation sites, placentas, live and dead fetuses, and early and late resorptions. The location of each fetus should be recorded. Each fetus will be examined for gender and gross external alterations (representative photographs of alterations may be taken). Fetuses will be tagged with individual identification number, litter number, uterine distribution, and fixative. Approximately one-half of the fetuses in each litter should be retained in Bouin's solution; the remaining fetuses should be retained in alcohol. If a Segment II study has already been performed, then the fetuses do not require further evaluation but should be retained for possible future evaluation. If a Segment II or other supplementary study has not been performed, then evaluation of the viscera and skeleton should be performed as described earlier (Section 12.4.3).

F_1 Paternal Observations

Paternal Body Weight, Feed Consumption, Behavior, and Clinical Signs   Clinical signs, mortalities, and body weight values should be recorded at the same intervals and in the same manner as for the F_1 females.

Assessment of the F_1 Males at Necropsy

Unscheduled Deaths   Any males that are found dead or appear moribund are subjected to a complete necropsy, and the viscera are examined to investigate the cause of death.

Scheduled Deaths   Males are routinely euthanized and necropsied after the outcome of mating is known. In the event of an equivocal mating result, males can be mated with untreated females to ascertain their fertility or infertility. The males treated as part of the study may also be used for evaluation of toxicity to the male reproductive system if dosing is continued beyond mating and sacrifice is delayed. Routinely, after day 21 of cohabitation, the male is weighed, euthanized, and subjected to a complete necropsy.

Inspection of F_1 Male Viscera   The thoracic, abdominal, and pelvic organs should be inspected grossly for evidence of toxicity. If gross organ lesions are noted, the affected organs should be preserved for possible histopathological examination. The testes and epididymides should be excised and their weights recorded (total weights paired and individual organ weights). The epididymides should be stored in neutral buffered 10% formalin. The testes should be fixed in Bouin's solution for 48–96 hours and then retained in 10% neutral buffered formalin.

12.5.9   Analysis of Maternal and Litter/Pup Data

Interpretation of the Data   Values from control and test groups of animals should be compared statistically. The following techniques may be used, but others may be substituted if they are appropriate. The fertility and gestation indices may be analyzed by a one-tailed Fisher exact test. For the sex ratio index, a two-tailed Fisher exact test may be used. Data for the viability and weaning indices may be transformed by the Freeman–Tukey arcsine transformation for binomial proportions. The transformed data may then be analyzed by an analysis of variance (ANOVA) followed by a one-tailed protected least significant difference (LSD) test to compare the control with the treated groups if the ANOVA yields $p < 0.10$. The average litter size and the number of viable pups throughout the reproduction phase may be analyzed by ANOVA followed by a protected LSD test (one-tailed). For the growth (weight gain) and organ weight analyses, an analysis of covariance may be used, followed by a protected LSD test (two-tailed) to compare the control and treated groups.

Importance of Historical Control Data   Historical control data should be used to enhance interpretation of study results. Historical control data, when used, should be compiled, presented, and evaluated in an appropriate and relevant manner. In order to justify its use as an analytical tool, information such as the dates of study conduct, the strain and source of animals, and the vehicle and route of administration should be included.

12.6   TWO-GENERATION REPRODUCTIVE TOXICITY STUDIES

12.6.1   Rationale for the Test

The multigeneration study (two-generation reproduction testing guideline, OPPTS 870.3800 [71] and OECD 416 [72]) was designed to detect adverse effects on the integrity and performance of the male and female reproductive systems, including

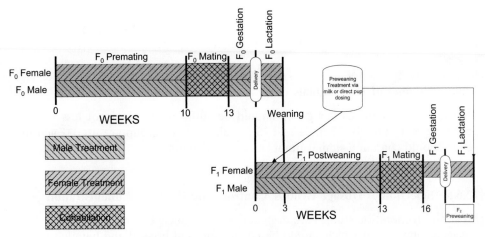

FIGURE 12.5 Multigeneration study.

gonadal function, estrous cycle, mating behavior, conception, gestation, parturition, lactation, and weaning, and on the growth and development of the offspring (Fig. 12.5). The adverse effects assessed in a multigeneration study also include neonatal mortality, mortality, target organs in offspring, and functional deficits in offspring, including behavior, maturation (puberty), and reproduction.

12.6.2 Principle of the Test Method

The test article is administered to the parental animals (F_0) prior to and during mating, during gestation, parturition, and lactation, and through weaning of the F_1 offspring. The test article is administered to selected F_1 offspring from weaning through adulthood, during cohabitation and mating, and through gestation, parturition, and lactation until the F_2 generation is weaned (PND 21).

12.6.3 Animal Species and Strain Selection and Rationale

The rat is the commonly used species for multigeneration studies. It is generally desirable to use the same species and strain as in other toxicological studies. If another mammalian species is used, then justification for its use should be provided in the protocol. Within and between studies, animals should be of comparable age, weight, and parity at the start of the study. In OECD 416, the weight variation at the commencement of study should be minimal and not exceed 20% of the mean weight of each sex.

12.6.4 Procurement and Acclimation of the Test Animals

The test animals should be young (4–8 weeks of age) upon arrival. The test animals should be from the same source and strain, and the females should be nulliparous, nonpregnant, and approximately the same age and weight. The test animals should be acclimated to the laboratory conditions at least 5 days prior to study start. Each animal should be assigned a unique identification number. This is done just prior to initiation of dosing for the F_0 generation and just after weaning for the F_1 generation.

12.6.5 Number of Test Animals

The number of animals per group should be sufficient to yield not less than 20 pregnancies. Routinely, 25 male and 25 female rats per group are used. Each test group should contain a similar number of mating pairs.

12.6.6 Selection of Dosage Groups, Controls, and Route of Administration

Most multigeneration studies are designed with a vehicle control and at least three dosage groups, all of which should be concurrent and housed and handled identically. Males and females should be assigned by a randomization procedure that assures that mean body weights are comparable among all test groups. The test compound and vehicle should be administered by the route that most closely approximates the pattern of expected human exposure. If the route of administration differs from the expected human exposure, a justification will be required in the protocol.

12.6.7 Selection of Dosage Levels

The dosage levels should be spaced to produce a gradation of toxic effects. Unless limited by physiochemical or biological properties, the highest dose should be chosen to produce reproductive and/or systemic toxicity. For the F_0 generation, the highest dose selected should not have caused greater than 10% mortality in previous toxicity studies. The intermediate dose should only produce minimal observable toxic effects. The low dose should not produce any evidence of either systemic or reproductive toxicity (NOAEL). Two- or fourfold intervals are often used for spacing of the dosage levels. For dietary studies, the dosage interval should not exceed threefold (OECD 416). Metabolism and pharmacokinetics of the test article should be available from previously conducted studies to demonstrate the adequacy of the dosing regimen.

A concurrent control group (either untreated, sham treated, or vehicle treated) should always be used. If a vehicle control group is used, then the dosing volume should be equal to the highest volume used. If the test article is administered in the diet and causes reduced dietary intake, then the use of a pair-fed control group may be necessary.

12.6.8 Treatment Timing and Test Duration

The F_0 animals are dosed daily beginning at 5–9 weeks of age. Daily dosing of the selected F_1 generation offspring commences at weaning. For both generations (F_0 and F_1) dosing should be continued for at least 10 weeks prior to mating. Daily dosing of the F_0 and F_1 animals should continue until termination.

12.6.9 Mating Procedures, Detection of Mating, and Housing of Mated Females

A mating ratio of 1:1 from the same dosage group allows identification of both parents of a litter. The mating pair is cohoused until evidence of copulation is observed or either three estrous periods or 2 weeks have elapsed. Animals should be separated as soon as evidence of copulation is observed (as described earlier). Once they are pregnant, females should be housed individually to allow for monitoring of feed and, if necessary, water consumption. Feed and water should be provided *ad libitum*. Pregnant animals should be provided with nesting materials near the end of gestation.

12.6.10 F_0 Generation

F_0 Maternal Observations

Maternal Body Weight, Feed Consumption, Behavior, and Clinical Signs   Clinical signs and mortalities should be recorded at least once daily throughout the test period. Body weight values should be recorded on the first day of dosing and at least weekly, but during gestation and lactation body weights are routinely collected at protocol-specified intervals (e.g., GD 0, 7, 14, and 21, and LD 0, 4, 7, 14, and 21). Food consumption should be measured at least once weekly and at the same interval as the body weight collection through LD 14. Water consumption should be measured weekly if the test article is administered in the drinking water. Estrous cycle length and pattern should be determined from vaginal smears (see earlier discussion) during a minimum of 3 weeks prior to mating and throughout cohabitation.

F_0 Parturition   Dams should be housed in litter boxes with bedding material no later than DG 20 (2 days prior to expected parturition, earlier if required by protocol). The dams are observed periodically for signs of parturition onset. Individual pup observations should not be made until delivery is completed. Dead pups should be removed from the nesting box to preclude cannibalization by the dam.

Assessment of the F_0 Dam at Necropsy

Unscheduled Deaths   Any mated females that appear moribund should be euthanized appropriately. Any mated females that are found dead should be necropsied to investigate the cause of death. Any evidence of pregnancy and of embryonic development should be evaluated. A vaginal smear should be taken and the stage of estrus determined.

Scheduled Deaths   All F_0 females Should be terminated when they are no longer needed for assessment of reproductive effects. Dams are routinely necropsied on LD 21. A vaginal smear should be taken and the stage of estrus determined. The dam is weighed and euthanized, her ovaries and uterus are examined, and she is subjected to a complete necropsy.

Inspection of F_0 Maternal Viscera

Unscheduled Deaths   If necropsy occurs prior to parturition, then the gravid uterus should be removed and weighed. The uterus should be examined to determine if the animal was pregnant, and the relative numbers of live and dead conceptuses and their relative positions in the uterus should be recorded. If the uterus shows no signs of implantation, it should be treated with a reagent, such as 10% ammonium sulfide, to reveal any early resorptions. The number of corpora lutea should be recorded for each ovary, as described earlier. The remaining maternal abdominal and thoracic organs should be inspected grossly for evidence of toxicity. The following organs should be weighed from all F_0 females: uterus with oviducts, ovaries, brain, pituitary, liver, kidneys, adrenal glands, spleen, and any known target organs. The vagina, uterus with oviducts, cervix, ovaries, pituitary, and adrenal glands should be removed, fixed, and stored in appropriate medium for histopathological examination. If gross organ lesions are noted, the affected organs should be preserved for possible histopathological examination.

Scheduled Deaths   If necropsy occurs as scheduled, then the uterus should be removed and weighed. The number of corpora lutea should be recorded for each ovary as described earlier. The remaining maternal abdominal and thoracic organs should be inspected grossly for evidence of toxicity. The organs for organ weight collection and possible histopathological examination are listed below. If gross organ lesions are noted, the affected organs should be preserved for possible histopathological examination.

Histopathology for F_0 Females   The vagina, uterus with oviducts, cervix, ovaries, pituitary and adrenal glands, and any target organs and gross lesions should be fixed and stored in a suitable medium for histopathological examination. Complete histological evaluation is performed on the listed organs from ten randomly selected control and high dose F_0 females. Organs demonstrating treatment-related changes should be examined from the remainder of the high dose and control animals, and for all F_0 females in the low and mid-dose groups. Additionally, reproductive organs of the low and mid-dose females suspected of reduced fertility (those that failed to mate, conceive, or deliver healthy offspring, or for which estrous cyclicity was affected) should be subjected to histopathological evaluation as described previously (Segment I). Histopathological examination should detect qualitative depletion of the primordial follicle population; however, reproductive study guidelines require a quantitative evaluation of primordial follicles of the F_0 females (see Segment I).

F_0 Paternal Observations

Paternal Body Weight, Feed Consumption, Behavior, and Clinical Signs   Clinical signs and mortalities should be recorded at least once daily. Body weight values should be recorded on first day of dosing and at least weekly thereafter. Food consumption should be measured at least once weekly at the same interval as the body weight collection. Water consumption should be measured weekly if the test article is administered in the drinking water.

Assessment of the F_0 Males at Necropsy

Unscheduled Deaths   Any males that are found dead or appear moribund are subjected to a complete necropsy, and their visceral contents are examined to investigate the cause of death.

Scheduled Deaths Males are routinely euthanized and necropsied after the outcome of mating is known. In the event of an equivocal mating result, males can be mated with untreated females to ascertain their fertility or infertility. The males treated as part of the study may also be used for evaluation of toxicity to the male reproductive system if dosing is continued beyond mating and sacrifice is delayed. The male is weighed, euthanized, and subjected to a complete necropsy.

Inspection of F_0 Male Viscera The testes, epididymides (paired and individually), seminal vesicles (with coagulating glands and their fluids), prostate, brain, pituitary, liver, kidneys, adrenal glands, spleen, and any known target organs are removed and weighed. For all F_0 males, sperm from one testis and one epididymis should be collected for enumeration of homogenization-resistant sperm and caudal epididymal sperm reserves, respectively. In addition, sperm from one cauda epididymis (or vas deferens) should be collected for evaluation of sperm motility and morphology. The remaining abdominal and thoracic organs should be inspected grossly for evidence of toxicity. If gross organ lesions are noted, the affected organs should be preserved for possible histopathological examination.

Histopathology for F_0 Males One testis (preserved in Bouin's fixative or a comparable preservative), one epididymis, seminal vesicles, prostate, coagulating, pituitary, and adrenal glands, and any target organs and gross lesions should be fixed and stored in a suitable medium for histopathological examination. Complete histological evaluation is performed on the listed organs from ten randomly selected control and high dose F_0 males. Organs demonstrating treatment-related changes should be examined from the remainder of the high dose and control animals, and from all F_0 males in the low and mid-dose groups. Additionally, reproductive organs of the low and mid-dose males suspected of reduced fertility (those that failed to mate or impregnate or had abnormal sperm number, motility, or morphology) should be subjected to histopathological evaluation as described earlier (Segment I).

F_0 Sperm Evaluation The sperm quality parameters are sperm number, sperm motility, and sperm morphology. Sperm evaluation will be performed on all control and high dose group F_0 males unless treatment-related effects have been observed; in that case, the lower dosage groups should be evaluated. The sperm evaluation methodologies were described earlier (Section 12.3.10). A morphological evaluation of epididymal (or vas deferens) sperm sample should be performed. If sperm evaluation parameters have already been evaluated as part of a systemic toxicity study of at least 90 days' duration, the evaluations need not be repeated in this study.

12.6.11 F_1 Generation

F_1 Litter Evaluations The general appearance of the entire F_1 litter and maternal and pup nesting behavior is observed as described earlier for Segment III.

F_1 Pup Evaluations The litter is evaluated as soon as possible after delivery to establish the number and sex of pups, stillbirths, live births, and the presence of gross anomalies. Pups that are found dead should be examined for possible defects and

cause of death. Pups that have been cannibalized to the extent that their gender cannot be determined are recorded as "sex unable to be determined due to degree of cannibalization" (see earlier discussion).

Live pups should be counted, sexed, and weighed individually at birth, and on LD 4, 7, 14, and 21. If a pup cannot be found during the daily litter count, the pups are sorted by gender in order to determine the sex of the missing pup(s) by process of elimination. The missing pup is recorded as "missing, presumed cannibalized." If the pups have been tattooed or otherwise identified, the actual identification number of the missing pup(s) should be recorded.

The pup survival indices (e.g., Live Birth Index, Survival Index, and Sex Ratio) should be calculated as described previously (Section 12.5.8).

Standardization of F_1 Litter Sizes   Animals should be allowed to litter normally and rear their offspring to weaning. Standardization of litter sizes at LD 4 is optional (see Section 12.5.8).

Weaning   Weaning is usually performed on LD 21. At weaning, one male and one female offspring per litter are selected for rearing to adulthood and mating to assess reproductive competence.

Test Article Administration   The test article is administered to selected F_1 offspring from weaning through adulthood, during cohabitation and mating, and through gestation, parturition, and lactation until the F_2 generation is weaned.

F_1 Postweaning Developmental Landmarks   Sexual maturation landmarks (balanopreputial separation and vaginal patency) are required in multigeneration studies where the selected offspring are raised to adulthood. The OECD 416 guideline recommends that additional developmental parameters be evaluated for supplementary information (e.g., eye and ear opening, tooth eruption, hair growth). Other functional investigations are also recommended before and/or after weaning, such as motor activity, sensory function, and reflex ontogeny. These observations should not be performed on the pups selected for mating. These landmarks are described in Parker [34].

F_1 Mating Procedure   A mating ratio of 1:1 from the same dosage group but from different litters allows identification of both parents of a litter. The mating pair is cohoused as described above. Pregnant animals should be provided with nesting materials near the end of gestation. In instances of poor reproductive performance in the controls or in the event of a treatment-related alteration in the litter size, the adults of that generation may be remated to produce an F_{1b} litter. The dams should not be remated until approximately 1–2 weeks following weaning of the F_{1a} litter.

F_1 Maternal Observations

Maternal Body Weight, Feed Consumption, Behavior, and Clinical Signs   Maternal body weight, feed consumption, behavior, and clinical signs should be recorded at the same intervals as the F_0 maternal observations. Estrous cycle length and pattern should be determined from vaginal smears during a minimum of 3 weeks prior to mating and throughout cohabitation. Observations that have proved of value in other toxicity studies, as well as duration of pregnancy, parturition, and nursing behaviors, are recorded.

F_1 *Parturition* Dams should be housed in litter boxes with bedding material no later than DG 20 (2 days prior to expected parturition, earlier if required by protocol). The dams are observed periodically throughout the day for signs of parturition onset. As soon as the first pup is found, parturition is considered initiated and should be observed as described earlier (Section 12.5.7).

Assessment of F_1 Weanlings Not Selected for Continuation At the time of termination or death during the study, when the litter size permits, at least three pups per sex per litter should be examined macroscopically for structural abnormalities or gross lesions, paying special attention to the reproductive organs. Dead pups or pups that are terminated in a moribund condition should be examined for possible defects and cause of death. The following organs should be weighed from one randomly selected pup per sex per litter: brain, spleen, and thymus. The following organs should be fixed and stored for histopathological examination: gross lesions and any target organs.

Assessment of the Parental F_1 Female at Necropsy Same as assessment of the parental f_0 female at necropsy, as described in Section 12.5.7.

F_1 Male Observations Same as F_0 male observations, as described in Section 12.5.8.

12.6.12 F_2 Generation

F_2 Litter and Pup Evaluations The general appearance of the entire F_2 litter and maternal and pup nesting behavior should be observed as described earlier for the F_1 pups. The litter is evaluated as soon as possible after delivery to establish the number and sex of pups, stillbirths, live births, and the presence of gross anomalies as described earlier for the F_1 pups. Live F_2 pups should be counted, sexed, and weighed individually at birth, and on LD 4, 7, 14, and 21 as described for F_1 pups. Pup survival indices should be calculated and reported as described earlier (Section 12.5.8).

Assessment of F_2 Pups at Weaning At weaning or death during the study, when the litter size permits, at least three pups per sex per litter should be examined macroscopically for any structural abnormalities or pathological changes, paying special attention to the reproductive organs. Dead pups or pups that are terminated in a moribund condition should be examined for possible defects and/or cause of death. The following organs should be weighed from one randomly selected pup per sex per litter: brain, spleen, and thymus. The following organs should be fixed and stored for histopathological examination: any gross lesions and target organs.

12.6.13   Analysis of Maternal and Litter/Pup Data

Values from control and test groups of animals should be compared statistically as described in Section 12.5.9. Historical control data should be used to enhance interpretation of study results, as described in Section 12.5.9.

12.7   JUVENILE TOXICITY TESTING

12.7.1   Rationale for the Test

Drug development programs have used safety data from preclinical and clinical studies in adults to support the use of a drug in pediatric patients. This method assumes that the pediatric population has a similar disease progression and responds to the therapy in a similar fashion as the adult. Unfortunately, adult clinical trials and supportive preclinical animal studies may not always assess drug effects on developmental processes that are pediatric age-group specific. Pharmacological and pharmacodynamic processes in the pediatric population may differ from those of the adult population, resulting in adverse effects that may not be detected in adult preclinical or clinical studies. Juvenile animal studies can be designed to characterize postnatal developmental toxicities that would not be detected by use of the routine perinatal/postnatal toxicity study design. See Brent [73] for a review of the utilization of juvenile animal studies to determine human effects.

In 1997, the FDA [75] stated that the lack of pediatric labeling information posed a significant risk for children. The lack of pediatric safety information in product labeling exposes pediatric patients to the risk of age-specific adverse reactions unexpected from adult experience. These reactions could be avoided by development of appropriate pediatric dosage information. In addition to adverse effects due to overexposure, the absence of pediatric testing and labeling may also expose pediatric patients to ineffective treatment through underdosing, or may deny pediatric patients therapeutic advances because physicians choose to prescribe existing, less effective medications in the face of insufficient pediatric information about a new medication. Failure to develop a pediatric formulation of a drug or biological product, where younger pediatric populations cannot take the adult formulation, may also deny pediatric patients access to important new therapies, or may require pediatric patients to take the drug in formulations that may be poorly or inconsistently bioavailable. Also in 1997, the ICH M3 guidance, *Nonclinical Safety Studies for the Conduct of Human Clinical Trails for Pharmaceuticals* [74], states that juvenile animal studies should be considered on an individual basis when previous animal data and human safety data are insufficient.

In February 2006, the U.S. FDA Center for Drug Evaluation and Research (CDER) issued a *Guidance for Industry: Nonclinical Safety Evaluation of Pediatric Drug Products* [75]. It discusses the conditions when a juvenile animal study should be conducted, describes the design of juvenile animal studies, and makes recommendations on nonclinical testing (e.g., the timing and utility of juvenile animal studies in relation to phases of clinical development). This guidance is available on the FDA website (http://www.fda.gov/cder/guidance/5671fnl.htm).

12.7.2   Study Justification

Before performing a juvenile animal toxicity study, several questions should be addressed. The first question to address is the justification of the juvenile animal study. To answer this question, several additional questions must be answered.

- What is the age of the targeted pediatric population?

  Consideration should be given to the age of the intended population and its stage of postnatal development. The endpoints assessed in the nonclinical juvenile studies should be tailored to address concerns for a particular pediatric population. In addition, the disease indication may influence the type, duration, and timing of the testing.

- Is the target organ or system developing during the juvenile period in the species of choice?

  The toxic effects of drugs on postnatal development are believed most likely to occur in those organs and tissues that are undergoing significant postnatal development. The nervous, reproductive, pulmonary, renal, skeletal, and immune systems undergo considerable postnatal growth and development. Exposure to the drug must occur during the appropriate periods of growth and development in the animal species. A comparison of the times of target organ or system development between the species of choice and humans should be reviewed, usually by literature mining. Anatomical development as well as physiological development must be considered. For example, the timing of the presence of functional metabolic enzymes varies among species, as well as during the developmental period for each species. The FDA guidance has tables that give basic information; however, a series of articles on comparative organ system development are also available that provides more in-depth information (many of these are collected in Hood [38, Appendix C]): male and female reproductive system [76, 77], lung [78, 79], renal [80, 81], heart [82], skeletal system [83], behavioral aspects of the central nervous system [84], immune system [85, 86], brain [87], and gastrointestinal system [88].

- Is there enough preexisting data from juvenile animal studies with a compound that is structurally similar (e.g., same class of chemicals) or pharmacologically similar (same mechanism of action) that this study may not be required?

  Many potential pediatric drugs have established adult efficacy and safety profiles and there may be limited data available from pediatric patients 12 years or older. For marketed drugs that have already undergone extensive adult clinical trials, nonclinical pharmacology and toxicology data are available, including studies of general, reproductive, and genetic toxicity, as well as carcinogenicity and other special toxicology studies. Studies in juvenile animals such as perinatal/postnatal studies may be available. Target organs of toxicity in animals and adult humans have already been identified in these studies. A careful evaluation of these data should enable the toxicologist to (1) identify potential safety concerns for the intended pediatric population, (2) judge the adequacy of the nonclinical studies, and (3) identify gaps in the data that could be addressed by juvenile animal testing. Based on this assessment, a juvenile animal study might not be warranted.

- Are the metabolic profiles similar during the juvenile period between the animal species and humans?

  Metabolic profiles should be considered in determining the selection of an appropriate species. The adult human metabolic pathways are not necessarily the same as the pediatric metabolic pathways, and the pediatric metabolic pathways may differ from juvenile animal metabolic pathways. The presence or absence of functional metabolic enzymes in the juvenile animal species may alter the pharmacokinetics and toxicology of the therapeutic agent. By altering drug metabolism, increased drug accumulation or elimination can occur that affects exposure and duration. In addition, new reactive metabolites can be created or fail to be metabolized.
- Is the pediatric formulation different from the adult formulation?

  If, after pharmacokinetic bridging studies, it is determined that the pediatric formulation is pharmacokinetically (e.g., altered absorption, clearance, C_{max}, T_{max}, AUC) sufficiently different from the adult formulation, a juvenile animal study should be performed using the pediatric formulation.
- If the juvenile animal study is justified, what are the key experimental design issues—for example, species, age at start and end of treatment, route of administration (maternal and fetal/neonatal through adulthood), duration of exposure, endpoints, and general or specific histopathology?

  When determining the appropriate species, the following factors should be considered: (1) pharmacology, pharmacokinetics, and toxicology of the compound; (2) comparative developmental stage of major target organs; and (3) sensitivity of the selected species to a particular toxicity.

12.7.3   Species of Choice

The rat is generally the species of choice, even though the rat may not be most sensitive or the most relevant species. This preference is based on the fact that appropriate developmental windows in the rat cover all postnatal developing target organs and because of the large rat postnatal database. There will be cases where the rat is not an appropriate species (e.g., when the target organ toxicity is not observed in the rat but is observed in the second species) and another species should be considered. The usual second species of choice is the dog (although nonhuman primates, pigs, and minipigs may be appropriate when drug metabolism in the rat differs significantly from that of the human).

12.7.4   Age at Start and End of Treatment

Age at start and end of treatment may vary depending on the target pediatric population and the timing of the corresponding developmental stage in the animal model. The specific age ranges for pediatric populations are presented in the ICH E11 guideline, *Clinical Investigation of Medicinal Products in the Pediatric Population* [89].

12.7.5   Route of Administration

The route of administration is usually the route in human adults. However, pharmacologic/pharmacodynamic differences in the juvenile animal model may require an alternate route. If multiple routes of administration are planned for the different pediatric populations and/or indications, then multiple routes of exposure should also be tested. Assessment of differential drug pharmacokinetics should be made prior to the study according to established guidelines (ICH S3A guideline, *Note for Guidance on Toxicokinetics: Assessment of Systemic Exposure in Toxicity Studies* [90].

12.7.6   Frequency of Administration and Duration of Treatment

The frequency of administration should be relevant to the intended use of the drug. However, sometimes this is not feasible because of technical considerations or metabolic or pharmacokinetic differences. The duration of treatment should include the relevant period of postnatal development for the selected species and may be expanded to cover a longer duration, based on chronic pediatric administration. The assessment of delayed toxicity may require continuation of exposure through organ maturity or until adulthood, based on the safety concern. Addition of a treatment-free period should also be considered to assess potential reversibility of adverse effects, thereby distinguishing short-term pharmacodynamic effects from frank organ developmental toxicity.

12.7.7   Range-Finding Studies

Range-finding studies (including toxicokinetic/pharmacokinetic parameters) are highly recommended for establishment of a maximum tolerated dose, tolerability, target organs, and subsequent dose level selection. These studies can also be used to address specific questions and develop methodologies. For the definitive juvenile animal study, the highest dosage should cause toxicity (developmental or general), while the lowest dosage should produce little to no toxicity and should establish a NOAEL.

12.7.8   Juvenile Animal Study Design

There are two options for juvenile animal study design. The study can be (1) designed to address a specific safety concern (i.e., known or anticipated effects based on adult studies or drug class effects), or (2) a modified perinatal/postnatal developmental toxicity study designed to evaluate most potential outcomes. The target organ toxicity directed specific study design can be developed using a modified repeat dose toxicity study design. The design is modified for species considerations, age of the animal at initiation of exposure, duration of treatment, and endpoints evaluated. Routinely, both sexes are evaluated. When the magnitude of the biological effect is small, greater numbers of animals per group may be required.

The second design is a modified Segment III study (as described earlier) that assures adequate exposure during the target organ(s) development and assessment of specific organ requirements (e.g., additional developmental landmarks or reflex ontogeny). The routine Segment III design consists of maternal dosing from GD 6 through PND 20, with weaning on PND 21. If the drug or active metabolite is not transferred through the milk, then direct dosing of the pup throughout the preweaning phase may be necessary. Selected pups are raised to adulthood and mated after 80 days of age, and their offspring are evaluated. Developmental and behavioral assessments (e.g., reflex ontogeny, vaginal patency, preputial separation, reactivity, sensorimotor function, motor activity, and learning and memory assessments) are performed. Additional developmental and behavioral landmarks may need to be assessed, based on target organs. Additional measurements of overall growth are required (growth velocity over time and tibial length). Additional endpoints should be considered on a case-by-case basis. Juvenile animal studies are conducted on a case-by-case basis, and the study design should be discussed with the regulatory agency.

12.7.9   Timing of the Juvenile Animal Study

If a juvenile animal study is justified, when will the study be conducted relative to clinical trial? The timing of the juvenile animal study used to support the pediatric clinical trials depends on the duration of the juvenile animal study and the subsequent timing of the pediatric clinical trial. A juvenile animal study using the Segment III design will require approximately 5 months for in-life data collection and up to six additional months for data analysis and reporting. Therefore, the juvenile animal study should be initiated at least 1 year prior to the pediatric clinical study. If toxicities identified in the juvenile animal studies are likely to occur in pediatric patients, cannot be clinically monitored, and do not have adequate safety margins, then, after risk–benefit analysis for the therapeutic indication, it may not be possible to safely conduct pediatric clinical trials.

12.8   CONCLUSION

The design and conduct of developmental and reproductive toxicity (DART) studies and juvenile animal studies for pediatric drugs are among the most difficult in toxicology. These studies are run under FDA/ICH Good Laboratory Practice and Good Automated Laboratory Practice regulations, which also require computer database validation and validation of behavioral testing paradigms. These are monumental tasks requiring significant expenditures of personnel and money. Behavioral testing requires that the apparatus and data collection system has been validated and the conduct of positive control studies using drugs that achieve both ceiling and floor effects. Apparatuses or methods used in adult animal behavioral assessments may not be sensitive enough or small enough to test pups. DART studies require highly trained and skilled technicians to properly evaluate the reproductive and developmental aspects, and now many such studies require behavioral evaluations calling for behaviorally trained technicians and scientists. Interobserver variations must be minimized, which requires significantly more training and evaluation than routine clinical observations. In order to evaluate the data and report the results, trained reproductive and behavioral toxicologists are needed. Furthermore, while Segment I, II, and III protocols do not routinely need review by regulatory agencies prior to conduct, it is recommended that regulatory review be carried out prior to commencing juvenile animal studies to support pediatric clinical trials.

REFERENCES

1. US Food and Drug Administration. International Conference On Harmonisation; Guideline on Detection of Toxicity to Reproduction for Medicinal Products. *Fed Reg Part IX* 1994;59(183):48746–48752.

2. Hurtt ME, Daston G, Davis-Bruno K, Feuston M, Silva Lima B, Makris S, McNerney ME, Sandler JD, Whitby K, Wier P, Cappon GD. Workshop summary: juvenile animal studies: testing strategies and design. *Birth Defects Res (Part B)* 2004;71:281–288.

3. US Food Drug Administration. *Guideline for Industry. Nonclinical Safety Evaluation of Pediatric Drug Products.* CDER; 2006. http://www.fda.gov/cder/guidance/5671fnl.pdf.

4. US Food and Drug Administration. *Guidance for Industry. Safety Studies for Veterinary Drug Residues in Human Food: Reproduction Studies.* VICH GL22. Rockville, MD: US Department of Health and Human Services; 2000.

5. Slikker W, Chang LW, Eds. *Handbook of Developmental Neurotoxicology.* San Diego: Academic Press; 1998.

6. Hood RD, Ed. *Developmental and Reproductive Toxicology, A Practical Approach.* Boca Raton, FL: CRC Press; 2006.

7. US Food Drug Administration. Guideline for industry, detection of toxicity to reproduction for medicinal products. *Fed Reg* 1994;59(183). (Same as ICH Guideline for Industry S5A.)

8. US Food and Drug Administration. *Guidance for Industry. Considerations for Reproductive toxicity Studies for Preventive Vaccines for Infectious Disease Indications.* Rockville, MD: US Department of Health and Human Services; 2000.

9. International Conference on Harmonisation. ICH harmonized tripartite guideline: Maintenance of the ICH guideline on toxicity to male fertility, An addendum to the ICH tripartite guideline on detection of toxicity to reproduction for medicinal products, S5B(M). (Amended 9 November, 2000).

10. Davis DL, Friedler G, Mattison D, Morris R. Male-mediated teratogenesis and other reproductive effects: biologic and epidemiologic findings and a plea for clinical research. *Reprod Toxicol* 1992;6:289–292.

11. Colie CF. Male mediated teratogenesis. *Reprod Toxicol* 1993;7:3–9.

12. Savitz DA, Sonnenfeld NL, Olshan AF. Review of epidemiologic studies of paternal occupational exposure and spontaneous abortion. *Am J Ind Med* 1994;25:361–383.

13. Trasler JM, Doerksen T. Teratogen update: paternal exposures—reproductive risks. *Teratology* 1999;60:161–172.

14. Ulbrich B, Palmer AK. Detection of effects on male reproduction—a literature survey. *J Am Coll Toxicol* 1995;14:293–327.

15. Takayama S, Akaike M, Kawashima K, Takahashi M, Kurokawa Y. Collaborative study in Japan on optimal treatment period and parameters for detection of male fertility disorders in rats induced by medicinal drugs. *J Am Coll Toxicol* 1995;14:66–292.

16. Sakai T, Takahashi M, Mitsumori K, Yasuhara K, Kawashima K, Mayahare H, Ohno Y. Collaborative work to evaluate toxicity on male reproductive organs by 2-week repeated dose toxicity studies in rats. Overview of the studies. *J Toxicol Sci* 2000;25:1–21.

17. Adler NT, Toner JP. The effect of copulatory behavior on sperm transport and fertility in rats. In Komisaruk BR, Siegel HI, Chang MF, Feder HH, Eds. *Reproduction: Behavioral and Neuroendocrine Perspective.* New York: New York Academy of Science; 1986, pp 21–32.

18. Salewski E. Färbemethode zum makroskopischen nachweis von implantationsstellen am uterus der ratte. *Naunyn-Schmiedebergs Arch Exp Pathol Pharmakol* 1964;247:367.

19. Long JA, Evans HM. The oestrous cycle in the rat and its associated phenomena. *Mem Univ Calif* 1922;6:1–111.

20. Cooper RL, Goldman JM, Vandenbergh JG. Monitoring of the estrous cycle in the laboratory rodent by vaginal lavage. In Heindel JJ, Chapin RE, Eds. *Methods in Toxicology: Female Reproductive Toxicology*. San Diego: Academic Press; 1993, pp 45–56.

21. STP Working Group. STP Position Paper: ovarian follicular counting in the assessment of rodent reproductive toxicity. *Toxicol Pathol* 2005;33:409–412.

22. Plowchalk DR, Smith BJ, Mattison DR. Assessment of toxicity to the ovary using follicle quantitation and morphometrics. In Heindel JJ, Chapin RE, Eds. *Methods in Toxicology: Female Reproductive Toxicology*. San Diego: Academic Press; 1993, pp 57–68.

23. Pedersen T, Peters HJ. Proposal for the classification of oocytes and follicles in the mouse ovary. *Reprod Fertil* 1968;17:555–557.

24. Bolon B, Bucci TJ, Warbritton AR, Chen JJ, Mattison DR, Heindel JJ. Differential follicle counts as a screen for chemically induced ovarian toxicity in mice: results from continuous breeding bioassays. *Fundam Appl Toxicol* 1997;39:1–10.

25. Bucci TJ, Bolon B, Warbritton AR, Chen JJ, Heindel JJ. Influence of sampling on the reproducibility of ovarian follicle counts in mouse toxicity studies. *Reprod Toxicol* 1997;11:689–696.

26. Heindel JJ, Thomford PJ, Mattison DR. Histological assessment of ovarian follicle number in mice as a screen of ovarian toxicity. In Hirshfield AN, Ed. *Growth Factors and the Ovary*. New York: Plenum; 1989, pp 421–426.

27. Christian MS, Brown WR. Control primordial follicle counts in multigeneration studies in Sprague–Dawley ("gold standard") rats. *Toxicologist* 2002;66(No. 1-S).

28. Russell LD, Ettlin R, Sinha Hikim AP, Clegg ED. The classification and timing of spermatogenesis. In Russell LD, Ettlin R, Sinha Hikim AP, Clegg ED, Eds. *Histological and Histopathological Evaluation of the Testis*. Clearwater, FL: Cache River Press; 1990, Chap 2.

29. Russell LD, Ettlin R, Sinha-Hikim AP, Clegg ED, Eds. *Histological and Histopathological Evaluation of the Testis*. Clearwater, FL: Cache River Press; 1990.

30. Chapin RE, Filler RS, Gulati D, Heindel JJ, Katz DF, Mebus CA, Obasaju F, Perreault SD, Russell SR, Schrader S, Slott V, Sokol RZ, Toth G. Methods for assessing rat sperm motility. *Reprod Toxicol* 1992;6:267–273.

31. Toth GP, Stober JA, Zenick H, Read EJ, Christ SA, Smith MK. Correlation of sperm motion parameters with fertility in rats treated subchronically with epichlorohydrin. *J Androl* 1991;12:54–61.

32. Toth GP, Read EJ, Smith MK. Utilizing Cryo Resources CellSoft computer-assisted sperm analysis system for rat sperm motility studies. In Chapin RE, Heindel JJ, Eds. *Methods in Toxicology: Male Reproductive Toxicology*. San Diego: Academic Press; 1993, pp 303–318.

33. UK Industrial Reproductive Toxicology Discussion Group (IRDG). Computer-Assisted Sperm Analysis (CASA) Group, rat sperm morphological assessment, guideline document, edition 1, October 2000. http://www.irdg.co.uk/IRDG_spermmorphology.doc.

34. Parker RM. Testing for reproductive toxicity. In Hood RD, Ed. *Developmental and Reproductive Toxicology, A Practical Approach*. Boca Raton, FL: CRC Press; 2006, pp 425–487.

35. MARTA and MTA. Historical Control Data (1992–1994) for developmental and reproductive toxicity studies using the Crl:CD®(SD)BR Rat. 1996. http://www.criver.com/flex_content_area/documents/rm_rm_r_tox_studies_crlcd_sd_br_rat.pdf.

36. US Food Drug Administration. *Redbook 2000*. Toxicological principles for the safety assessment of food ingredients, section IV.B.2. Guidelines for reporting the results of toxicity studies. CFSAN; 2000. http://www.cfsan.fda.gov/~redbook/red2ivb2.html.

37. US Food Drug Administration. Good Laboratory Practice Regulations, Final Rule. 21 CFR 58, 33768. 1987.

38. Hood RD. Animal models of effects of prenatal insult. In Hood RD, Ed. *Developmental Toxicology—Risk Assessment and the Future*. New York: Van Nostrand Reinhold; 1990, pp 183–188.

39. Tyl RW, Marr MC. Developmental toxicity testing—methodology. In Hood RD, Ed. *Developmental and Reproductive Toxicology, A Practical Approach*. Boca Raton, FL: CRC Press; 2006, pp 201–261.

40. US Food and Drug Administration. *Redbook 2000*. Toxicological principles for the safety assessment of food ingredients. Rockville, MD: US Department of Health and Human Services, Food and Drug Administration, Center for Food Safety and Applied Nutrition; 2000.

41. Johnson M, Everitt B. *Essential Reproduction*. Oxford: Blackwell Scientific Publications; 1984.

42. Collins TFX, Sprando RL, Shackelford ME, Hansen DK, Welsh JJ. Food and Drug Administration proposed testing guidelines for developmental toxicity studies. *Regul Toxicol Pharmacol* 1999;30:39–44.

43. Holson JF, Nemec MD, Stump DG, Kaufman LE, Lindstrom P, Varsho BJ. Significance, reliability, and interpretation of developmental and reproductive toxicity study findings. In Hood RD, Ed. *Developmental and Reproductive Toxicology, A Practical Approach*. Boca Raton, FL: CRC Press; 2006, pp 3–14.

44. Hood RD. Maternal vs. developmental toxicity. In Hood RD, Ed. *Developmental Toxicology—Risk Assessment and the Future*. New York: Van Nostrand Reinhold; 1990, pp 67–75.

45. Clark RL, Robertson RT, Minsker DH, Cohen SM, Tocco DJ, Allen HL, James ML, Bokelman DL. Diflunisal-induced maternal anemia as a cause of teratogenicity in rabbits. *Teratology* 1984;30:319–332.

46. Hood RD, Miller DB. Maternally mediated effects on development. In Hood RD, Ed. *Developmental and Reproductive Toxicology, A Practical Approach*. Boca Raton, FL: CRC Press; 2006, pp 93–124.

47. Solecki R, Bergmann B, Burgin H, Buschmann J, Clark R, Druga A, Van Duijnhoven EA, Duverger M, Edwards J, Freudenberger H, Guittin P, Hakaite P, Heinrich-Hirsch B, Hellwig J, Hofmann T, Hubel U, Khalil S, Klaus A, Kudicke S, Lingk W, Meredith T, Moxon M, Muller S, Paul M, Paumgartten F, Rohrdanz E, Pfeil R, Rauch-Ernst M, Seed J, Spezia F, Vickers C, Woelffel B, Chahoud I. Harmonization of rat fetal external and visceral terminology and classification. Report of the Fourth Workshop on the Terminology in Developmental Toxicology, Berlin, 18–20 April 2002. *Reprod Toxicol* 2003;17:625–637.

48. Stuckhardt JL, Poppe SM. Fresh visceral examination of rat and rabbit fetuses used in teratogenicity testing. *Teratog Carcinog Mutagen* 1984;4:181–188.

49. Wilson JG, Warkany J. *Teratology: Principles and Techniques* (Lectures and demonstrations Given at the first workshop in teratology, University of Florida, 2–8 February, 1964). Chicago: University of Chicago Press; 1965.

50. Wilson JG. *Environment and Birth Defects*. New York: Academic Press; 1973, Appendix III, pp 228–232.

51. Christian MS. Test methods for assessing female reproductive and developmental toxicology. In Hayes AW, Ed. *Principles and Methods of Toxicology*, 4th ed. Philadelphia: Taylor & Francis; 2001, pp 1301–1381.

52. Jonassen H, Lucacel C, Agajanov T, Gondek H, Schoenfeld HA. Comparison of modified Davidson's fixative and Bouin's solution in fixation of fetal soft tissue for evaluation using the Wilson's technique. *Teratology* 2002;65:332.

53. Astroff AB, Ray SE, Rowe LM, Hilbish KG, Linville AL, Stutz JP, Breslin WJ. Frozen-sectioning yields similar results as traditional methods for fetal cephalic examination in the rat. *Teratology* 2002;66:77–84.

54. Webb GN, Byrd RA. Simultaneous differential staining of cartilage and bone in rodent fetuses: an alcian blue and alizarin red S procedure without glacial acetic acid. *Biotech Histochem* 1994;69:181–185.

55. Menegola E, Broccia ML, Di Renzo F, Giavina E. Comparative study of sodium valproate-induced skeletal malformations using single or double staining methods. *Reprod Toxicol* 2002;16:815–823.

56. Crary DD. Modified benzyl alcohol clearing of alizarin stained specimens without loss of flexibility. *Stain Technol* 1962;37:124–125.

57. Kimmel CA, Trammel C. A rapid procedure for routine double staining of cartilage and bone in fetal and adult animals. *Stain Technol* 1981;56:271–273.

58. Narotsky MG, Rogers JM. Examination of the axial skeleton of fetal rodents. In Taun RS, Lo CW, Eds. *Methods in Molecular Biology. Developmental Biology Protocols, Volume 1*. Totowa, NJ: Humana Press; 2000, pp 139–150.

59. Young AD, Phipps DE, Astroff AB. Large-scale double-staining of rat fetal skeletons using alizarin red S and alcian blue. *Teratology* 2000;61:273–276.

60. Tyl RW, Marr MC. Developmental toxicity testing—methodology. In Hood RD, Ed. *Developmental and Reproductive Toxicology, A Practical Approach*. Boca Raton, FL: CRC Press; 2006, pp 201–261.

61. Chen JJ. Statistical analysis for developmental and reproductive toxicologists. In Hood RD, Ed. *Developmental and Reproductive Toxicology, A Practical Approach*. Boca Raton, FL: CRC Press; 2006, pp 697–711.

62. US Environmental Protection Agency. Guidelines for developmental toxicity risk assessment; notice. *Fed Reg* 1991;56(234):63798–63826.

63. Hood RD. Malformations vs. variations and "minor defects." In Hood RD, Ed. *Developmental Toxicology—Risk Assessment and the Future*. New York: Van Nostrand Reinhold; 1990, pp 178–182.

64. US Food Drug Administration. *Reviewer Guidance: Integration of Study Results to Assess Concerns About Human Reproductive and Developmental Toxicities* (draft). Rockville, MD: US Department of Health and Human Services, Food and Drug Administration, Center for Drug Evaluation and Research; 2001.

65. Kimmel G, Harris S, Tassinari M, Knudsen T, Cunny H, Tyl R, Carlton B, Holson J, Slikker W. Concern over decreased training in embryology and developmental/reproductive toxicology. *Birth Defects Res (Part B)* 2004;71:191–192.

66. Hood RD. Principles of developmental toxicology revisited. In Hood RD, Ed. *Developmental and Reproductive Toxicology, A Practical Approach*. Boca Raton, FL: CRC Press; 2006, pp 3–14.

67. Bates HK, Cunny HC, Kebede GA. Developmental neurotoxicity testing methodology. In Hood RD, Ed. *Handbook of Developmental Toxicology*. Boca Raton, FL: CRC Press; 1997, pp 291–324.

68. Kai S, Kohmura H. Comparison of developmental indices between Crj:CD(SD)IGS rats and Crj:CD(SD) rats. In Matsuzawa T, Inoue H, Eds. *Biological Reference Data on CD(SD)IGS-1999*. Yokohama: CD(SD)IGS Study Group; 1999, pp 157–167.

69. Ohkubo Y, Furuya K, Yamada M, Akamatsu H, Moritomo A, Ishida S, Watanabe K, Hayashi Y. Reproductive and developmental data on Crj:CD(SD)IGS rats. In Matsuzawa T, Inoue H, Eds. *Biological Reference Data on CD(SD)IGS-1999*. Yokohama: CD(SD)IGS Study Group; 1999, pp 153–156.

70. Ema M, Fujii S, Furukawa M, Kiguchi M, Ikka T, Harazano A. Rat two-generation reproductive toxicity study of bisphenol A. *Reprod Toxicol* 2001;15:505–523.

71. US Environmental Protection Agency. *Health Effects Test Guidelines OPPTS 870.3800, Reproduction and Fertility Effects*. Washington, DC: EPA 712-C-96-208; 1996, pp 1–11.

72. Organization for Economic Cooperation and Development. *OECD 416: Two-Generation Reproduction Toxicity Study* (updated guideline, adopted 22 January 2001). Paris: OECD; 2001.

73. Brent R. Utilization of juvenile animal studies to determine the human effects and risks of environmental toxicants during postnatal developmental stages. *Birth Defects Res (Part B)* 2004;71:303–320.

74. US Food and Drug Administration, Center for Drug Evaluation Research (CDER), Center for Biologics Evaluation and Research (CBER). *Guidance for Industry: M3 Nonclinical Safety Studies for the Conduct of Human Clinical Trials for Pharmaceuticals*. 1997.

75. US Food and Drug Administration, Center for Drug Evaluation and Research (CDER). *Pharmacology and Toxicology, Guidance for Industry: Nonclinical Safety Evaluation of Pediatric Drug Products*. 2006. http://www.fda.gov/cder/guidance/5671fnl.pdf.

76. Beckman DA, Feuston M. Landmarks in the development of the female reproductive system. *Birth Defects Res (Part B)* 2003;68P:137–143.

77. Marty MS, Chapin R, Parks L, Thorsrud B. Development and maturation of the male reproductive system. *Birth Defects Res (Part B)* 2003;68:125–136.

78. Zoetis T, Hurtt ME. Species comparison of lung development. *Birth Defects Res (Part B)* 2003;68:121–124.

79. Burri PH. Structural aspects of prenatal and postnatal development and growth of the lung, lung growth and development. In McDonald JA, Ed. *Lung Growth and Development*. New York: Marcel Dekker; 1997, pp 1–35.

80. Zoetis T. Species comparison of anatomical and functional renal development. *Birth Defects Res (Part B)* 2003;68:111–120.

81. Radde IC. Mechanism of drug absorption and their development. In Macleod SM, Radde IC, Eds. *Textbook of Pediatric Clinical Pharmacology*. Littleton, MA: PSG Publishing Co; 1985, pp 17–43.

82. Hew KW, Keller KA. Postnatal anatomical and functional development of the heart: a species comparison. *Birth Defects Res (Part B)* 2003;68:309–320.

83. Zoetis T, Tassinari MS, Bagi C, Walthall K, Hurtt ME. Species comparison of postnatal bone growth and development. *Birth Defects Res (Part B)* 2003;68:86–110.

84. Wood SL, Beyer BK, Cappon GD. Species comparison of postnatal CNS development: functional measures. *Birth Defects Res (Part B)* 2003;68:391–407.

85. Holsapple MP, West LJ, Landreth KS. Species comparison of anatomical and functional immune system development. *Birth Defects Res (Part B)* 2003;68:321–334.

86. Miyawaki T, Moriya N, Nagaoki T, Taniguchi N. Maturation of B-cell differentiation and T-cell regulatory function in infancy and childhood. *Immunol Rev* 1981;57:61–87.

87. Rice D, Barone S Jr. Critical periods of vulnerability for the developing nervous system: evidence from human and animal models. *Environ Health Perspect* 2000;108(Suppl 3):511–533.

88. Walthall K, Cappon GD, Hurtt ME, Zoetus T. Postnatal development of the gastrointestinal system: a species comparison. *Birth Defects Res (Part B)* 2005;74:132–156.

89. US Food Drug Administration, Center for Drug Evaluation and Research (CDER), Center for Biologics Evaluation and Research (CBER). ICH, Guidance for Industry: E11. *Clinical* investigation of medicinal products in the pediatric population. *Fed Reg* 2000;65:19777–19781. Docket No. 00D-1223.

90. ICH Harmonised Tripartite Guideline. *Guideline for Industry S3A, Note for Guidance on Toxicokinetics: Assessment of Systemic Exposure in Toxicity Studies.* ICH; 1994. http://www.ich.org/LOB/media/MEDIA495.pdf.

13

CARCINOGENICITY STUDIES

Shayne Cox Gad

Gad Consulting Services, Cary, North Carolina

Contents

Preclinical Development Handbook: Toxicology, edited by Shayne Cox Gad
Copyright © 2008 John Wiley & Sons, Inc.

13.1   INTRODUCTION

In the experimental evaluation of substances for carcinogenesis based on experimental results of studies in a nonhuman species at some relatively high dose or exposure level, an attempt is made to predict the occurrence and level of tumorigenesis in humans at much lower levels. Examined here are the assumptions involved in this undertaking and a review of the aspects of design and interpretation of traditional long-term (lifetime) animal carcinogenicity studies as well as some of the alternative short-term models.

When are carcinogenicity studies required?

- Studies should be performed for pharmaceuticals with continuous clinical use for at least 6 months. (Most compounds indicated for 3 months of treatment would likely be used for 6 months and longer.)
- Studies are needed for pharmaceuticals used frequently in an intermittent manner. For example, carinogenicity studies would be needed for drugs used to treat allergic rhinitis, depression, and anxiety; while no carcinogenicity studies would be needed for anesthetics and radiolabeled imaging compounds.
- Additional criteria for defining cases of concern include:

    Previous demonstration of a carcinogenic potential in the product class.

    Structure–activity relationship suggesting carcinogenic risk.

    Evidence of preneoplastic lesions in repeat-dose toxicity studies.

    Long-term tissue retention of compound or metabolites resulting in local tissue reactions.

- Unequivocally genotoxic compounds do not need carcinogenicity studies.
- Carcinogenicity studies have the following timing considerations:

    Carcinogenicity studies should be completed before application for marketing approval (i.e., upon NDA filing).

    In the case of certain serious (life-threatening or limiting) diseases, studies may (should) be conducted postapproval.

    Complete rodent carcinogenicity studies are not needed in advance of the conduct of large scale clinical trials, unless there is a special concern.

    Where patient life expectancy is short (i.e., less than 2–3 years), no carcinogenicity studies are required.

    Pharmaceuticals in tumor *adjuvant* therapy usually do need studies.

At least in a general way, we now understand what appear to be most of the mechanisms underlying chemical- and radiation-induced carcinogenesis. The most recent regulatory summary on identified carcinogens [1] lists 44 agents classified as "Known to be Human Carcinogens." Several hundred other compounds are also described as having lesser degrees of proof. A review of these mechanisms is not germane to this chapter (readers are referred to Miller and Miller [2] for a good short review), but it is now clear that cancer as seen in humans is the result of a multifocal set of causes.

Mechanisms and theories of chemical carcinogenesis include (1) *genetic* (all due to some mutagenic event), (2) *epigenetic* (no mutagenic event), (3) *oncogene activation*, (4) *two-step* (induction/promotion), and (5) *multistep* (combination of 1–4) [3].

Considered in another way, the four major carcinogenic mechanisms are DNA damage, cell toxicity, cell proliferation, and oncogene activation. Any effective program to identify those drugs that have the potential to cause or increase the incidence of neoplasia in humans must effectively screen for these mechanisms [4].

The single most important statistical consideration in the design of bioassays in the past was based on the point of view that what was being observed and evaluated was a simple quantal response (cancer occurred or it didn't), and that a sufficient number of animals needed to be used to have reasonable expectations of detecting any meaningful risks of such an effect. Although the single fact of whether or not the simple incidence of neoplastic tumors is increased due to an agent of concern is of interest, a much more complex model must now be considered. The time-to-tumor, patterns of tumor incidence, effects on survival rate, and age of first tumor all must now be captured in a bioassay and included in an evaluation of the relevant risk to humans [5].

The task of interpreting the results of any of the animal-based bioassays must be considered from three different potential perspectives as to organ responsiveness:

Group I. Those organs with high animal and low human neoplasia rates.

Group II. Those organs with high neoplasia rates in both animals and humans.

Group III. Those organs with low animal but high human neoplasia rates.

Note that not considered is the potential other case—where the neoplasia rates are low for both animals and humans. This is a very rare case and one for which our current bioassay designs probably lack sufficient power to be effective.

In group I, the use of animal cancer data obtained in the liver, kidney, forestomach, and thyroid gland are perceived by some as being hyperresponsive, too sensitive, and of limited value and utility in the animal cancer data obtained in group I organs. The liver is such a responsive and important organ in the interpretation of cancinogenesis data that the discussion of this subject area has been broken up into three sections for human, rat, and mouse data. Peroxisome proliferation in the liver, particularly in mice, is an area of interpretive battle as in many cases the metabolism and mechanisms involved are not relevant to humans.

Group II organs (mammary gland, hematopoietic, urinary bladder, oral cavity, and skin) are less of an interpretive battleground than group I organs. For group II organs, all four major mechanisms of carcinogenesis (electrophile generation, oxidation of DNA, receptor–protein interactions, and cell proliferation) are known to be important. The high cancer rates for group II organs in both experimental animals and humans may at first give us a false sense of security about how well the experimental animal models are working. As we are better able to understand the probable carcinogenic mechanism(s) in the same organ in the three species, we may find that the important differences between the three species are more numerous than we suspect. This is particularly true for receptor-based and for cell-proliferation-based carcinogenic mechanisms.

Animal cancer data for group III organs are the opposite of group I organs. Group III organs have low animal cancer rates and high human cancer rates. In contrast to the continuing clamor and interpretive battleground associated with group I organs, there is little debate over group III organs. Few voices have questioned the adequacy of the present-day animal bioassay to protect the public health from possible cancer risks in these group III organs. Improved efforts must be made toward the development of cancer-predictive systems or short-term tests for cancer of the prostate gland, pancreas, colon/rectum, and cervix/uterus.

Carcinogenicity bioassays are the longest and most expensive of the extensive battery of toxicology studies required for the registration of pharmaceutical products in the United States and in other major countries. In addition, they are often the most controversial with respect to interpretation of their results. These studies are important because, as noted by the International Agency for Research on Cancer [6], "in the absence of adequate data on humans, it is biologically plausible and prudent to regard agents for which there is sufficient evidence of carcinogenicity in experimental animals as if they presented a carcinogenic risk to humans."

In this chapter, we consider the major factors involved in the design, conduct, analysis, and interpretation of carcinogenicity studies as they are performed in the pharmaceutical industry.

13.2   REGULATORY REQUIREMENTS AND TIMING

The prior FDA guidance on the need for carcinogenicity testing of pharmaceuticals presented a dual criteria: such studies were required to support registration of a drug that was to be administered for a period of 3 months or more (in Japan and Europe this was stated to be 6 months or more); and such testing had to be completed before filing for registration in such cases. ICH guidelines [5] now fix this human exposure period that triggers the need for testing at 6 months, excluding agents given infrequently through a lifetime or for shorter periods of exposure unless there is reason for concern (such as positive findings in genotoxicity studies, structure–activity relationships suggesting such risk, evidence of preneoplastic lesions in repeat dose studies, or previous demonstration of carcinogenic potential in the product class that is considered relevant to humans). Such studies are still only required to be completed before filing for registration. Most developers conduct carcinogenicity studies in parallel with Phase III clinical studies.

Endogenous peptides, protein substances, and their analogues are generally not required to be evaluated for carcinogenicity. There are three conditions that call the need into question, however:

- Products where there are significant differences in biological effects to the natural counterparts.
- Products where modifications lead to significant changes in structure compared to the natural substance.
- Products resulting in humans having a significant increase over the existing local or systemic concentration.

The ICH and EMEA have also given guidance on design, dose selection, statistical analysis, and interpretation for such studies [7–11]. The FDA has also offered guidance; the most recent form is a 44 page document available online [12].

There has been extensive debate and consideration on the relevance and value of the traditional long-term rodent bioassays. The FDA looked at rat and mouse studies for 282 human pharmaceuticals, resulting in the conclusion that "sufficient evidence is now available for some alternative *in vivo* carcinogenicity models to support their application as complimentary studies *in combination with a single 2-year carcinogenicity study* [italics added] to identify trans-species tumorigens" [13].

The Europeans, meanwhile, have focused on the need for better care in study design, conduct, and interpretation [14], aiming to incorporate these in the revision of the Center for Proprietary Medicinal Products (CPMP) carcinogenicity guidelines.

13.3 SPECIES AND STRAIN

Two rodent species are routinely used for carcinogenicity testing in the pharmaceutical industry—the mouse and the rat. Sprague–Dawley derived rats are most commonly used in American pharmaceutical toxicology laboratories. However, the Wistar and Fischer 344 strains are favored by some companies, while the Long Evans and CFE (Carworth) strains are also used but rarely [15].

With respect to mice, the CD-1 is by far the most commonly used strain in the pharmaceutical industry. Other strains used less frequently are the B6C3F1, CF-1, NMRI, C57B1, BALB/c, and Swiss [15, 16]. "Swiss" is the generic term since most currently used inbred and outbred strains were originally derived from the "Swiss" mouse.

If either the mouse or the rat is considered to be an inappropriate species for a carcinogenicity study, the hamster is usually chosen as the second species.

The use of two species in carcinogenicity studies is based on the traditional wisdom that no single species can be considered an adequate predictor of carcinogenic effects in humans. Absence of carcinogenic activity in two different species is thought to provide a greater level of confidence that a compound is "safe" for humans than data derived from a single species.

One may question this reasoning on the basis that data from two "poor predictors" may not be significantly better than data from a single species. It is also reasonable to expect that the ability of one rodent species to predict a carcinogenic effect in a second rodent species should be at least equal to, if not better than, its ability to predict carcinogenicity in humans. The concordance between mouse and rat carcinogenicity data has been investigated and a summary of the results is presented in the next paragraph.

A review of data from 250 chemicals found an 82% concordance between results of carcinogenicity testing in the mouse and the rat [17]. Haseman et al. [18] reported a concordance of 73% for 60 compounds studied in both species. However, 30–40% of 186 National Cancer Institute (NCI) chemicals were found to be positive in one species and negative in the other [19]. It is reasonable to conclude that neither rodent species will always predict the results in the other rodent species or in humans, and that the use of two species will continue until we have a much better understanding of the mechanisms of carcinogenesis.

The choice of species and strain to be used in a carcinogenicity study is based on various criteria including susceptibility to tumor induction, incidence of spontaneous tumors, survival, existence of an adequate historical database, and availability.

Susceptibility to tumor induction is an important criterion. There would be little justification for doing carcinogenicity studies in an animal model that did not respond when treated with a "true" carcinogen. Ideally, the perfect species/strain would have the same susceptibility to tumor induction as the human. Unfortunately, this information is usually unavailable, and the tendency has been to choose animal models that are highly sensitive to tumor induction to minimize the probability of false negatives.

The incidence of spontaneous tumors is also an important issue. Rodent species and strains differ greatly in the incidence of various types of spontaneous tumors. The Sprague–Dawley strain, although preferred by most pharmaceutical companies, has a very high incidence of mammary tumors in aging females, which results in substantial morbidity during the second year of a carcinogenicity study. If one chooses the Fischer 344 (F344) strain, the female mammary tumor incidence will be lower, but the incidence of testicular tumors will be higher (close to 100%) than that in Sprague–Dawley rats.

A high spontaneous tumor incidence can compromise the results of a carcinogenicity study in two ways. If a compound induces tumors at a site that already has a high spontaneous tumor incidence, it may be impossible to detect an increase above the high background "noise." Conversely, if a significant increase above control levels is demonstrated, one may question the relevance of this finding to humans on the basis that the species is "highly susceptible" to tumors of this type.

The ability of a species/strain to survive for an adequate period is essential for a valid assessment of carcinogenicity. Poor survival has caused regulatory problems for pharmaceutical companies and is therefore an important issue [15]. The underlying concept is that animals should be exposed to the drug for the greater part of their normal life span to make a valid assessment of carcinogenicity. If animals on study die from causes other than drug-induced tumors, they may not have been at risk long enough for tumors to have developed. The sensitivity of the bioassay would be reduced and the probability of a false-negative result would be increased.

The availability of an adequate historical database is often cited as an important criterion for species/strain selection. Historical control data can sometimes be useful in evaluating the results of a study. Although such data are not considered equal in value to concurrent control data, they can be helpful if there is reason to believe that the concurrent control data are "atypical" for the species/strain.

Although outbred stocks (e.g., Sprague–Dawley rats and CD-1 mice) are generally favored in the pharmaceutical industry, inbred strains are also used (e.g., Fischer 344 rats and B6C3F1 mice). Inbred strains may offer greater uniformity of response, more predictable tumor incidence, and better reproducibility than outbred strains. However, their genetic homogeneity may also result in a narrower range of sensitivity to potential carcinogens than exists in random-bred animals. In addition, extrapolation of animal data to humans is the ultimate goal of carcinogenicity studies, and the human population is anything but genetically homogeneous.

The ideal species for carcinogenicity bioassays should absorb, metabolize, and excrete the compound under study exactly as humans do. Unfortunately, because of the small number of species that meet the other criteria for selection, there is limited practical utility to this important scientific concept, as applied to carcinogenicity studies.

Before concluding this discussion of species/strain selection, it may be worthwhile to take a closer look at the animals preferred by pharmaceutical companies to determine to what extent they meet the conditions described earlier. Advantages of the CD-1 mouse are (1) a good historical database including various routes of exposure, (2) demonstrated susceptibility to induction of tumors, and (3) relatively low spontaneous incidence of certain tumors to which other strains are highly susceptible, especially mammary and hepatic tumors. Disadvantages are (1) lack of homogeneity, (2) relatively low survival, (3) moderate to high incidence of spontaneous pulmonary tumors and leukemias, and (4) high incidence of amyloidosis in important organs, including the liver, kidney, spleen, thyroid, and adrenals [20].

There was a reduction in survival of Sprague–Dawley rats and rats of other strains during the 1990s [21]. This reduction may have been the result of *ad libitum* feeding, as preliminary results suggest that caloric restriction may improve survival. Leukemia appears to be the major cause of decreasing survival in the F344 rat. While this reduced survival trend has flattened out, a resumption of the problem of reduced survival may necessitate a reevaluation of the survival requirements for carcinogenicity studies by regulatory agencies.

13.4 ANIMAL HUSBANDRY

Because of the long duration and expense of carcinogenicity studies, the care of animals used in these studies is of paramount importance. Various physical and biological factors can affect the outcome of these studies. Some important physical factors include light, temperature, relative humidity, ventilation, atmospheric conditions, noise, diet, housing, and bedding [22]. Biological factors include bacteria and viruses that may cause infections and diseases.

The duration, intensity, and quality of light can influence many physiological responses, including tumor incidence [23, 24]. High light intensity may cause eye lesions, including retinal atrophy and opacities [25, 26]. Rats housed in the top row and the side columns of a rack may be the most severely affected.

The influence of light on the health of animals may be managed in several ways. The animals may be randomly assigned to their cages on a rack such that each column contains animals of a single dose group. The location of the columns on the rack may also be randomized so that the effect of light is approximately equal for all dose groups. In addition, the cages of each column of the rack may be rotated from top to bottom when the racks are changed.

Room temperature has been shown to influence the incidence of skin tumors in mice [27]. Changes in relative humidity may alter food and water intake [28]. Low humidity may cause "ringtail," especially if animals are housed in wire mesh cages [29].

Diets for rodents in carcinogenesis studies should ideally be nutritionally adequate while avoiding excesses of nutrients that may have adverse effects.

Types of caging and bedding have been shown to affect the incidence and latency of skin tumors in mice. In a study by DePass et al. [30], benzo[a]pyrene-treated mice were housed either in stainless steel cages or polycarbonate shoebox cages with hardwood bedding. The mice housed in shoebox cages developed tumors earlier and with higher frequency than those housed in steel cages.

Housing of rats in stainless steel cages with wire mesh floors may result in decubitous ulcers on the plantar surfaces. This condition may be a significant problem associated with high morbidity and may affect survival of the animals if euthanasia is performed for humane reasons. Ulcers are particularly frequent and severe in older male Sprague–Dawley rats, perhaps because of their large size and weight compared with females and rats of other strains.

Common viral infections may affect the outcome of carcinogenicity studies by altering survival or tumor incidence. Nevertheless, viral infections did not cause consistent adverse effects on survival or tumor prevalence in control F344 rats from 28 NCI-NTP studies, although body weights were reduced by Sendai and pneumonia viruses of mice [31]. The probability of such infections can be minimized by using viral-antibody-free animals, which are readily available.

13.5   DOSE SELECTION

13.5.1   Number of Dose Levels

For pharmaceuticals, most carcinogenicity studies employ at least three dose levels in addition to the controls, but four levels have occasionally been used [15]. The use of three or four dose levels satisfies regulatory requirements [32] as well as scientific and practical considerations. If a carcinogenic response is observed, information on the nature of the dose–response relationship will be available. If excessive mortality occurs at the highest dose level, a valid assessment of carcinogenicity is still possible when there is adequate survival at the lower dose levels.

13.5.2   Number of Control Groups

Pharmaceutical companies have frequently favored the use of two control groups of equal size [15]. A single control group of the same size as the treated groups is also used and, less frequently, one double-sized control group may be used. The diversity of study designs reflects the breadth of opinion among toxicologists and statisticians on this issue.

Use of two control groups has the advantage of providing an estimate of the variation in tumor incidence between two groups of animals in the absence of a drug effect. If there are no significant differences between the control groups, the data can be pooled, and the analysis is identical to that using a single, double-sized group. When significant differences occur between the control groups, one must compare the data from the drug-treated groups separately with each control group.

There will be situations in which the incidence of a tumor in one or more drug-treated groups is significantly higher than that of one control group but similar to that of the other control group. In such a situation, it is often helpful to compare the tumor incidences in the control groups to appropriate historical control data. One may often conclude that, for this tumor, one of the control groups is more "typical" than the other and should therefore be given more weight in interpreting the differences in tumor incidence.

In spite of its popularity in the pharmaceutical industry, the use of two control groups is opposed by some statisticians on the grounds that a significant difference between the two groups may indicate that the study was compromised by excessive, uncontrolled variation. Haseman et al. [33], however, analyzed tumor incidence data from 18 color additives tested in rats and mice and found that the frequency of significant pairwise differences between the two concurrent control groups did not exceed that which would be expected by chance alone.

The use of one double-sized group is sometimes preferred because it may provide a better estimate of the true control tumor incidence than that provided by a smaller group. Nevertheless, more statistical power would be obtained by assigning the additional animals equally to all dose groups rather than to the control group only, if power is a primary consideration.

13.5.3   Criteria for Dose Selection

Dose selection is one of the most important and difficult activities in the design of a toxicology study. It is especially critical in carcinogenicity studies because of their long duration. Whereas faulty dose selection in an acute or subchronic toxicity study can easily be corrected by repeating the study, this situation is much less desirable in a carcinogenicity study, especially since such problems may not become evident until the last stages of the study.

The information used for dose selection usually comes from subchronic toxicity studies, but other information about the pharmacological effects of a drug and its metabolism and pharmacokinetics may also be considered. The maximum recommended human dose (MRHD) of the drug may be an additional criterion, if this is known when the carcinogenicity studies are being designed. An additional consideration is that for U.S. FDA submissions, protocols must be reviewed and dose selections justified (prior to study start) by the Carcinogenicity Advising Committee (CAC) [34].

For most pharmaceutical companies, the doses selected are as follows. The highest dose is selected to be the estimated maximum tolerated dose (MTD). The lowest dose is usually a small multiple (one to five times) of the MRHD, and the mid-dose approximates the geometric mean of the other two doses [15, 35].

The MTD is commonly estimated to be the maximum dose that can be administered for the duration of the study that will not compromise the survival of the animals by causes other than carcinogenicity. It should be defined separately for males and females. ICH [6] states that the MTD is "that dose which is predicted to produce a minimum toxic effect over the course of the carcinogenicity study, usually predicted from the results of a 90-day study." Factors used to define minimum toxicity include no more than a 10% decrease in body weight gain relative to controls, target organ toxicity, and/or significant alterations in clinical pathology parameters. If the MTD has been chosen appropriately, there should be no adverse effect on survival, only a modest decrement in body weight gain and minimal overt signs of toxicity. The procedures for dose selection described above are generally consistent with major regulatory guidelines for carcinogenicity studies[1] [21, 32]. There are,

---

[1]Note that the FDA *Redbook 2000* applies, strictly speaking, only to food additives. It is cited here because it is a well-known toxicology guideline routinely applied to animal pharmaceuticals to which humans may be exposed. The *Redbook* has recently been updated by the FDA [16].

however, exceptions to the general approach described above. For example, for nontoxic drugs, the difference between the high and the low doses may be many orders of magnitude, if the high dose is set at the estimated MTD and the low dose is a small multiple of the clinical dose. Some guidelines suggest that the low dose be no less than 10% of the high dose [32]. In this situation, it may be acceptable to set the high dose at 100 times the MRHD, even if the MTD is not achieved [32]. Similarly, when a drug is administered in the diet, the highest concentration should not exceed 5% of the total diet, whether or not the MTD is achieved [36].

MTD (Maximum Tolerated Dose) Concept

- Criteria of MTD
    Dose to elicit signs of minimum toxicity without altering the animal's normal life span due to effects other than carcinogenicity.
    No more than 10% decrease in body weight gain.
    Target organ toxicity and/or alterations in clinical pathological parameters.
- Criticism: For compounds with low toxicity, extremely high unrealistic doses may result.
- Threshold concept for nongenotoxic compounds: alterations of normal physiology.
- The high dose should allow an adequate safety margin over the human therapeutic exposure and should be tolerated without significant physiological dysfunction or increased mortality.

High Dose Selection

- Toxicity endpoints
    Traditionally, carcinogenicity studies have relied on the MTD (maximum tolerated dose) concept; no other toxicological endpoints are agreed upon.
    Pharmacokinetic endpoints may determine the high dose (you reach a saturation of absorption plateau, where additional dosing does not achieve any higher plasma levels (systemic exposure).
    Systemic exposure represents a large multiple of the human dose (minimum 25×) on a basis of mg/m^2 body surface.
- Pharmacodynamic endpoints: receptor selectivity, specific argumentation.
- Maximally feasible or practicable dose (i.e., you cannot give any more): 5% of the diet or 1500 mg/kg/day (only for human doses up to 500 mg/day).
- Additional endpoints: must be scientifically justified.

Metabolism and/or pharmacokinetic data, when available, should also be considered in the dose selection process. It is desirable that a drug not be administered at such a high dose that it is excreted in a different manner than at lower doses, such as the MRHD. Similarly, the high dose should not lead to the formation of metabolites other than those formed at lower (clinical) doses. If data show that a given dosage produces maximum plasma levels, administration of higher doses should be unnecessary. These considerations may be very useful when interpreting the results of the study or attempting to extrapolate the results to humans.

13.6 GROUP SIZE

The minimum number of animals assigned to each dose group in pharmaceutical carcinogenicity studies is 50 of each sex [15]. Most companies, however, use more than the minimum number, and some use up to 80 animals per sex per group. The most important factor in determining group size is the need to have an adequate number of animals for a valid assessment of carcinogenic activity at the end of the study. For this reason, larger group sizes are used when the drug is administered by daily gavage because this procedure may result in accidental deaths by perforation of the esophagus or aspiration into the lungs. Larger group sizes are also used when the carcinogenicity study is combined with a chronic toxicity study in the rat. In this case, serial sacrifices are performed at 6 and 12 months to evaluate potential toxic effects of the drug.

In the final analysis, the sensitivity of the bioassay for detecting carcinogens is directly related to the sample size. Use of the MTD has often been justified based on the small number of animals at risk compared to the potential human population, in spite of the difficulties inherent in extrapolating effects at high doses to those expected at much lower clinical doses. A reasonable compromise may be the use of doses lower than the MTD combined with a larger group size than the 50 per sex minimum accepted by regulatory agencies.

13.7 ROUTE OF ADMINISTRATION

In the pharmaceutical industry, the two most common routes of administration are via diet and gavage [15]. Some compounds are given by drinking water, topical (dermal) application, or injection, depending on the expected clinical exposure route, which is the primary criterion for determining the route of administration in carcinogenicity studies. When more than one clinical route is anticipated for a drug, the dietary route is often chosen for practical reasons.

Dietary administration is often preferred over gavage because it is far less labor intensive. Another advantage is that the MTD has rarely been overestimated in dietary studies, whereas it has often been overestimated in gavage studies, according to data from the NTP [37]. The dietary route is unsuitable for drugs that are unstable in rodent chow or unpalatable. The dietary route is also disadvantaged by the fact that dosage can only be estimated based on body weight and food intake data, in contrast with gavage by which an exact dose can be given. Disadvantages of gavage testing are the likelihood of gavage-related trauma, such as puncture of the trachea or esophagus, and possible vehicle (e.g., corn oil) effects.

When doing studies by the dietary route, the drug may be administered as a constant concentration at each dose level, or the concentration may be increased as body weight increases to maintain a constant dose on a milligram per kilogram basis. The latter method allows greater control of the administered dose and avoids age- and sex-related variations in the dose received, which occur with the former method. Both methods are acceptable to regulatory agencies.

13.8   STUDY DURATION

The duration of carcinogenicity studies for both rats and mice is 2 years in most pharmaceutical laboratories [15]. Occasionally, rat studies are extended to 30 months, while come companies terminate mouse studies at 18 months. The difference in duration between mouse and rat studies is based on the belief that rats have a longer natural life span than mice. Recent data indicate, however, that this is not the case. The most commonly used strains, the Sprague–Dawley rat and the CD-1 mouse, have approximately equal survival at 2 years, based on industry data [15]. The same is true for the most popular inbred strains, the Fischer 344 rat and the B6C3F1 mouse [15]. Data from NCI studies confirm that the 2 year survival of the B6C3F1 mouse is at least equal to, if not greater than, that of the Fischer 344 rat [38].

13.9   SURVIVAL

As stated earlier, adequate survival is of primary importance in carcinogenicity studies because animals must be exposed to a drug for the greater part of their life span to increase the probability that late-occurring tumors can be detected. Early mortality, resulting from causes other than tumors, can jeopardize the validity of a study because dead animals cannot get tumors.

In general, the sensitivity of a carcinogenicity bioassay is increased when animals survive to the end of their natural life span, because weak carcinogens may induce late-occurring tumors. The potency of a carcinogen is often inversely related to the time to tumor development. By analogy, as the dose of a carcinogen is reduced, the time to tumor occurrence is increased [30, 39].

Why do we not allow all animals in a carcinogenicity study to live until they die a natural death if by so doing we could identify more drugs as carcinogens? In fact, the sensitivity of a bioassay may not be improved by allowing the animals to live out their natural life span because the incidence of spontaneous tumors tends to increase with age. Thus, depending on the tumor type, the ability of the bioassay to detect a drug-related increase in tumor incidence may actually decrease, rather than increase, with time. Therefore, the optimum duration of a carcinogenicity study is that which allows late-occurring tumors to be detected but does not allow the incidence of spontaneous tumors to become excessive.

Reduced survival in a carcinogenicity study may or may not be drug related. Sometimes, the MTD is exceeded and increased mortality occurs at the highest dose level and occasionally at the mid-dose level as well. This situation may not necessarily invalidate a study; in fact, the protocol may be amended to minimize the impact of the drug-induced mortality. For example, cessation of drug treatment may enhance the survival of the animals in the affected groups and allow previously initiated tumors to develop. As shown by Littlefield et al. [39] in the CNTR ED01 study, liver tumors induced by 2-acetylaminofluorene, which appeared very late in the study, were shown to have been induced much earlier and not to require the continuous presence of the carcinogen to develop. By contrast, bladder tumors that occurred in the same study were dependent on the continued presence of the carcinogen.

Whether drug treatment is terminated or not, drug-related toxicity may also be managed by performing complete histopathology on animals in the lower dose groups rather than on high dose and control animals only. If there is no increase in tumor incidence at a lower dose level that is not compromised by reduced survival, the study may still be considered valid as an assessment of carcinogenicity.

When reduced survival is related to factors other than excessive toxicity, the number of animals at risk for tumor development may be inadequate, and the validity of the study may be compromised even in the absence of a drug effect on survival. Obviously, the adjustments described above for excessive, drug-related toxicity are not relevant to this situation.

There is no unanimity of opinion among regulatory agencies as to the minimum survival required to produce a valid carcinogenicity study or as to the best approach for dealing with survival problems. Even within a single agency such as the FDA, different opinions exist on these issues. For example, the recently issued FDA *Redbook II Draft Guideline* [21] requires that rats, mice, or hamsters be treated for 24 months. Early termination due to decreased survival is not recommended. The EEC guidelines differ in that they suggest termination of the study when survival in the control group reaches 20%, while Japanese guidelines suggest termination at 25% survival in the control or low dose groups [32]. These provisions make good sense in that they do not request termination of the study when drug-related mortality may be present only at the highest dose.

13.10   ENDPOINTS MEASURED

A carcinogenicity study is more focused than a chronic toxicity study—fewer endpoints are evaluated and as such it is a simpler study. The key endpoints are actually few:

Pathology (limited to neoplastic and preneoplastic tissue transformations).

Body weight (to ensure that toxicity is not so great as to invalidate the assays— and also that it is just sufficient to validate the assay).

Survival (key to determining when to terminate the study).

Clinical pathology (limited to evaluating the morphology of white blood cells, and usually this is actually deferred until there are indications that such data is needed).

Food consumption (actually measured to ensure that dietary administration doses are accurate).

Only pathology will be considered in detail.

The primary information for carcinogenicity evaluation is generated by pathologists. Table 13.1 lists the tissues normally collected, processed, and evaluated (see also Table 13.2). These professionals, like any other group of professionals, vary in

TABLE 13.1   Standard Tissue List

Kidney	Urinary bladder	Aorta
Heart	Trachea	Lungs
Liver	Gallbladder	Pancreas
Fat	Salivary gland	Spleen
Cervical lymph node	Mesenteric lymph node	Thymus
Tongue	Esophagus	Stomach
Duodenum	Jejunum	Ileum
Cecum	Colon	Mammary gland
Skin	Skeletal muscle	Sciatic nerve
Parathyroid	Thyroid	Adrenal gland
Pituitary	Prostate	Seminal vesicles
Testes	Epididymides	Ovaries
Oviducts	Uterine horns	Uterine body
Cervix	Vagina	Brain
Spinal cord	Sternum	Rib/bone
Eyes	Harderian glands	BM smear
Nares	Clitoral/preputial gland	Zymbal's gland
Gross lesions		

TABLE 13.2   Current Global Carcinogenicity Study Requirements

Guide	Eye	Blood Smear	RBC	WBC	Differential	Clinical Chemistry	Urine	Organ	Histopathology
EPA 1998	–	+	–	–	+ C+H	–	–	+	C+H
Redbook 1993; 2000	–	–	+	+	+	+	+	+	All?
Japan 1999	–	+	+	+	–	–	–	–	C+H
CHMP 2003	+	–	+	+	+	+	+	+	All
CDER 1993	–	+	+	+	–	–	–	–	C+H

their training and experience, and these are characteristics that may influence the evaluation in a number of ways.

1. Differences in terminology may be important when considering controversial lesions.
2. Lack of consistency throughout a study is likely when a pathologist has only recently become involved with rodent carcinogenicity. Training is often in a clinical situation (especially in Europe), where each animal or person is unique, and a rodent carcinogenicity study can consist of 500 animals.
3. Unfamiliarity with the observed lesion in a particular species may cause problems in interpretation.

Possible bias introduced by knowledge of treatment can be corrected in several ways, but the use of a two-stage process would seem to be most efficient:

1. An initial evaluation is performed with full knowledge of the animal's history, including treatment.
2. A second evaluation of specific lesions is then carried out. This should be done blind, either by the same pathologist or, preferably, by the same and a second pathologist.

Differences in evaluation between pathologists should always be discussed by them to resolve the differences; they may be due to subtle differences in diagnosis and do not indicate incompetence in one of the pathologists. It is unacceptable for a study sponsor to shop around until a pathologist is found who gives (for whatever reason) the result the sponsor is looking for without giving an opportunity for interaction with all of the other evaluators. Sometimes these diagnoses are given years apart, during which time understanding of the pathogenesis of lesions may change, and even the first pathologist may not arrive at the same conclusion as he/she did some years ago.

Evaluation of the data is not purely a statistical exercise. A number of important factors should be considered: (1) dose–effect relationship, (2) a shift toward more anaplastic tumors in organs where tumors are common, (3) earlier appearance of tumors, and (4) presence of preneoplastic lesions.

The language used to describe the carcinogenic response has masked its complexity and presents a stumbling block to its understanding among nonhistopathologists. Benign or malignant neoplasms do not arise without some precursor change within normal tissue. An important concept in carcinogenicity evaluation is that of neoplastic progression, which was derived from studies on skin tumors and expanded to a number of other tissues. There is, on many occasions, a far from clear distinction between hyperplastic and "benign" neoplasia and between benign and malignant neoplasia.

Hyperplasia and benign and malignant neoplasia are convenient medical terms with prognostic significance. Hyperplasia can occur either as a regenerative response to injury, with no neoplastic connotations, or as a sustained response to a carcinogenic agent. It is an increase in the number of normal cells retaining normal intercellular relationships within a tissue. This normally may break down, resulting in altered growth patterns and altered cellular differentiation—a condition that may be described as atypical hyperplasia or presumptively as preneoplastic lesions. Possible sequelae to hyperplasia are (1) persistence without qualitative change in either structure or behavior, (2) permanent regression, (3) regression with later reappearance, and (4) progression to develop new characteristics indicating increased probability of malignancy. The last of these in the least likely to occur in experimental multistage models, such as in mouse skin or rat liver, where large numbers of hyperplastic lesions may occur, but notably fewer carcinomas develop from them.

Benign neoplasms in most rodent tissues apparently arise in hyperplastic foci, for example, squamous cell papillomas of the skin and forestomach. Furthermore, these papillomas seldom demonstrate autonomous growth and even fewer progress to squamous cell carcinomas. This decisive progression to carcinoma, when it occurs, provides powerful evidence for the multistage theory of carcinogenesis: the new, malignant cells arising as a focus within the papilloma or even in an area of hyperplasia, since the papilloma is not a necessary intermediate stage. In other organs, benign neoplasia is usually characterized by well differentiated cell morphology, a fairly uniform growth pattern, clear demarcation from surrounding tissues, and no evidence of invasion. The progression toward malignancy involves anaplasia (loss of differentiation) and pleomorphism (variety of phenotypic characteristics within the neoplasm). These changes may be focal in an otherwise benign neoplasm and may vary in degree and extent. Evidence of invasion into surrounding tissues or of metastasis is not an essential characteristic of malignancy, although it strengthens the diagnosis.

The grouping together of certain tumor types can aid statistical analysis, but it must be done carefully, with full appreciation of the biology and whatever is known of the pathogenesis of the lesions. Grouping for analysis of all animals showing neoplasia, irrespective of the tumor type, is inappropriate because the incidence in most treatment control groups can be very high and, in U.S. National Toxicology Program studies, approaches 100% in rats and 50–70% in mice (Table 13.3).

There may be similar incidences of tumors in aging people, but the real prevalence of tumors in human populations is uncertain. In the United States, where autopsies are uncommon, over one-third reveal previously undiagnosed cancers when they are conducted. A single type of neoplasm, renal adenoma, is present in 15–20% of all adult kidneys, although it is unclear whether these 2–6 mm foci of proliferating tubular and papillary epithelium represent small carcinomas or benign precursors of renal cell carcinomas. Irrespective of the significance of these lesions in human pathology, the presence of similar foci in a rodent carcinogenicity experiment would trigger the recording of renal tumor-bearing animals and hence their consideration in the statistical and pathological evaluation processes. Evaluation is further complicated by the increased background incidences of tumors as animals get older.

TABLE 13.3   Tumor-Bearing Animals in Control Groups from Rodent Studies

Control Animals for 2 year NTP Bioassay	Number of Animals	Those (%) with Tumors		
		Malignant	Benign	Total
B6C3F1 mice				
Male	1692	42	35	64
Female	1689	45	33	64
F344 rats				
Male	1596	55	95	98
Female	1643	38	76	88
Osborne–Mendel rats				
Male	50	26	68	78
Female	50	12	80	88
Sprague–Dawley rats				
Male	56	9	36	39
Female	56	30	68	79

Source: J. K. Haseman (unpublished summary of U.S. NTP data).

The independent analysis of every different diagnosis in rodent studies would also mask significant effects in many cases, while enhancing them in others. Benign and malignant neoplasms of a particular histogenesis are often grouped because the one is seen as a progression from the other. However, this grouping may result in a nonsignificant difference from the controls because there has been an acceleration of progression toward malignancy, the incidence of benign neoplasms decreasing while the malignant neoplasms increase. Guidelines are available for "lumping" or "splitting" tumor types, but in using them, the basis for the classification of neoplastic lesions should be clarified, especially when data generated over several or many years are coupled, since diagnostic criteria and ideas regarding tumor histogenesis may have changed. Reliance on tabulated results alone can lead to serious misinterpretation by those not closely connected with a particular study. For this very important reason, the pathology and toxicology narrative should be full and clear. If it is not, then there will always be doubts about future interpretations, even if these doubts are not, in reality, justified.

13.11 STATISTICAL ANALYSIS

Irrespective of the specific protocols used, all carcinogenicity studies end with a statistical comparison of tumor proportions between treated and control groups. This analysis is necessary because the control incidence of most tumor types is rarely zero. In the unlikely case that a type of tumor is found in treated animals but not in concurrent or appropriate historical controls, it is reasonable to conclude that the tumor is drug-related without statistical analysis.

Most pharmaceutical companies analyze tumor data using mortality-adjusted methods [15, 40]. The Peto/International Agency for Research on Cancer (IRC) methodology is most commonly used, perhaps because this method is currently favored by the FDA [41]. The use of life-table methods is most appropriate for "lethal" tumors, that is, those that cause the death of the animals. Various statistical methods are available for analyzing the incidence of the lethal and nonlethal tumors [42–45]. These methods are especially useful when there are drug-related differences in mortality rates. When there is no drug effect on survival, unadjusted methods will generally give the same results.

As a general approach, most pharmaceutical statisticians begin by testing for the presence of a dose-related trend in tumor proportions. If the trend test is significant, that is, the p value is less than or equal to 0.05, pairwise comparisons are performed between the treated and control groups. Trend and pairwise analyses may be adjusted for mortality as stated earlier, or performed without mortality adjustment using such simple methods as chi-square or Fisher's exact tests.

Although in most cases the use of trend tests is appropriate since most biological responses are dose related, there are exceptions to this rule. Certain drugs, especially those with hormonal activity, may not produce classical dose responses and may even induce inverse dose–response phenomena. In these cases, a pairwise comparison may be appropriate in the absence of a significant positive trend.

Most (70%) pharmaceutical companies use one-tailed comparisons, and a substantial number use two-tailed methods [15]. Since regulatory agencies are primarily interested in identifying carcinogenic drugs, as opposed to those that inhibit carcinogenesis, the use of one-tailed tests is generally considered more appropriate. Some companies prefer two-tailed comparisons because, in the absence of a true carcinogenic effect, there is an equal probability of seeing significant decreases as well as significant increases by chance alone.

One of the most important statistical issues in the analysis of carcinogenicity data is the frequency of "false positives" or Type I errors. Because of the multiplicity of tumor sites examined and the number of tests employed, there is concern that non-carcinogenic drugs may be erroneously declared carcinogens. If a $p < 0.05$ increase in tumor incidence is automatically regarded as a biologically meaningful result, then the false-positive rate may be as high as 47–50% [33].

Several statistical procedures designed to correct for the multiplicity of significance tests have been published (and reviewed by Haseman [46]). One approach to the problem of multiple tumor site/type testing is a procedure attributed to Tukey by Mantel [47]. This method is used to adjust a calculated p value based on the number of tumor types/sites for which there are a minimum number of tumors in the particular study. The reasoning here is that, for tumor sites, the number of tumors found is so small that it is impossible to obtain a significant result for that tumor site no matter how the tumors might have been distributed among the dose groups. Only those sites for which a minimum number of tumors are present can contribute to the false-positive rate for a particular study.

A method proposed by Schweder and Spjotvoll [48] is based on a plot of the cumulative distribution of observed p values. Farrar and Crump [49] have published a statistical procedure designed not only to control the probability of false-positive findings but also to combine the probabilities of a carcinogenic effect across tumor sites, sexes, and species.

Another approach to controlling the false-positive rate in carcinogenicity studies was proposed by Haseman [50]. Under this "rule," a compound would be declared a carcinogen if it produced an increase that was significant at the 1% level in a common tumor or an increase that was significant at the 5% level in a rare tumor. A rare neoplasm was defined as a neoplasm that occurred with a frequency of less than 1% in control animals. The overall false-positive rate associated with this decision rule was found to be not more that 7–8%, based on control tumor incidences from NTP studies in rats and mice. This false-positive rate compares favorably with the expected rate of 5%, which is the probability at which one would erroneously conclude that a compound was a carcinogen. The method is notable for its simplicity and deserves serious consideration by pharmaceutical statisticians and toxicologists. Without resorting to sophisticated mathematics, this method recognizes the fact that tumors differ in their spontaneous frequencies and therefore in their contribution to the overall false-positive rates in the carcinogenicity studies. False-positive results are much less likely to occur at tissue sites with low spontaneous tumor incidences than at sites with high frequencies.

As a final point that has special relevance to pharmaceutical carcinogenicity studies, one may question whether the corrections for multiple comparisons and their effect on the overall false-positive rate are appropriate for all tumor types. For example, if a compound is known to bind to receptors and produce pharmacological effects in a certain organ, is it justified to arbitrarily correct the calculated p value for the incidence of tumors in that organ, using the methods described above? It is difficult to justify such a correction considering that the basis for correcting the calculated p value is that the true probability of observing an increased incidence of tumors at any site by chance alone may be much higher than the nominal alpha level (usually 0.05). It is reasonable to expect that, when a drug has known pharmacological effects on a given organ, the probability of observing an increased tumor incidence in that organ by chance alone is unlikely to be higher than the nominal 5% alpha level.

Although most pharmaceutical statisticians and toxicologists agree on the need to control the probability of false-positive results, there is no consensus as to which method is most appropriate or most acceptable to regulatory agencies. The FDA and other such agencies will accept a variety of statistical procedures but will often reanalyze the data and draw their own conclusions based on their analyses.

13.12   TRANSGENIC MOUSE MODELS

Sine the early 1970s, the standard for adequate evaluation of the carcinogenic potential of a candidate pharmaceutical has been the conduct of lifetime, high dose assays in two species—almost always the rat and the mouse.

The relevance (and return on investment) for the bioassays preformed in mice has been questioned for some time. In 1997, the ICH opened the possibility for the substitution of some form of short- or medium-term mouse test as an alternative for the traditional lifetime mouse bioassay. The FDA has subsequently stated that it would accept "validated" forms of a set of medium-term mouse studies based on transgenic models, and significant effort has since gone into such validation.

The huge advances made in molecular biology since the late 1980s have provided the possibility of evaluating chemicals and potential drugs for carcinogenic potential by approaches that are different, less expensive, and take a shorter period of time than traditional long-term bioassays. This work has also been stimulated by dissatisfaction with the performance of traditional test systems.

The traditional long-term bioassays use highly inbred animals, developed with the goal of reducing the variability in background tumor incidences as a means of increasing the statistical sensitivity of the bioassays. This inbreeding has led to narrowing of the allelic pool in the strains of animals that are currently used for testing, as opposed to the wild-type populations (of humans) that the tests are intended to protect [51]. Transgenic models should serve to improve the identification of carcinogens by providing the gene-specific mechanistic data, minimizing the influence of spontaneous tumors and strain-specific effects, and reducing time required and cost and animal usage [52].

As it has become possible to transfer new or engineered genes to the germlines of mammals, the results have been transgenic mice that can be used in shorter term *in vivo* assays for carcinogenicity and that are also useful for research into the characterization of genotoxic events and mechanisms in carcinogenesis. By coupling reporter phenotypes (such as papillomas in the Tg·AC mouse), the task of "reading" results in test animals is made much less complex.

There are four transgenic mouse models that have been broadly evaluated—the Tg·AC, the Tg.rasH2, the TSP p53$^{+/-}$ and the XPA$^{-/-}$. Each of these has its own characteristics, and each of these merits some consideration. They are each made by either zygote injection or specific gene targeting in embryonic cells [53, 54].

13.12.1   The Tg·AC Mouse Model

This was the earliest of the models to be developed, and its use in mouse skin carcinogenicity studies was first reported in 1990. The mice have four copies of the v-H-ras oncogene in tandem on chromosome 11, and the transgene is fused with a fetal ζ-globin gene that acts as a promoter. The transgene codes for a switch protein, which is permanently "on," and this results in the mice having genetically initiated skin cancer. The application of tumor promoters to the surface of the skin causes the rapid induction of pedunculate papillomas that arise from the follicular epithelium. This is despite the fact that the transgene is not expressed in the skin, although it is present in the papillomas that form, and also in the focal follicular hyperplastic areas that are the precursors to the papillomas. In about 40% of the mice, the papillomas become malignant skin tumors—mainly squamous cell carcinomas and sarcomas.

The first assessments of this model as an alternative to traditional carcinogenicity studies were performed by the U.S. NIEHS and NTP, and the results with over 40 chemicals have been published. The majority of studies were performed by skin painting, regardless of whether the product was a dermal or systemic carcinogen. However, a good correlation was found with the known carcinogenicity of the test compounds, and both mutagenic and nonmutagenic were identified. It was found that great care had to be taken with the skin, because damage could also induce papillomas, which means that these animals cannot be identified using transponder chips. This sensitivity may also explain some of the false-positive results that have occurred with resorcinol and rotenone. Of more concern is that there have been false negatives with known carcinogens, namely, ethyl acrylate and *N*-methyl-*o*-acrylamide. The model was designed for use in the context of the two-stage model of carcinogenesis with the underlying mechanistic pathway involving specific transcription factors, hypomethylation, and cell-specific expression of the results. Along with the p53 model, this model has seen the widest use and evaluation (in terms of number of agents evaluated) so far. The carrier mouse strain employed, the FVB/N, is not commonly employed in toxicology and is prone to sound-induced seizures. It may be that the dermal route is not suitable for all systemic carcinogens, and this is the reason that in the ILSI program, both the dermal and systemic routes are being investigated in this model.

Another problem with this model was the occurrence of a nonresponder genotype to positive control agents. This was found to be attributable to a rearrangement of the ζ-globin promoter region, but it is claimed that this problem has been resolved. However, this has considerably delayed the ILSI studies with this model [52, 53]. It is already clear that the model gives a robust response to the positive control agent, 12-*o*-tetradecanoylphorbol 13-acetate (TPA).

13.12.2   The Tg.rasH2 Mouse Model

This model was developed at CIEA in Japan, and the first information about the mouse was published in 1990. The mice have five or six copies of the human H-ras proto-oncogene inserted in tandem into their genome surrounded by their own promoter and enhancer regions. This transgene has been very stabile, with no loss of responsiveness since the model was developed. The transgene codes for a molecular switch protein in the same way as the previous model, but the transgene is expressed in all organs and tissues. Thus, the response endpoint is not primarily dermal.

The initial studies with this model revealed a rapid appearance of forestomach papillomas with *N*-methyl-*N*-nitrosourea (MNU), and this compound has already been used as the positive control agent in subsequent studies with this strain. A study duration of 6 months is sufficient to obtain a positive response, and longer periods should be avoided because the mice start to develop various spontaneous tumors, such as splenic hemangiosarcomas, forestomach and skin papillomas, lung and Harderian gland adenocarcinomas, and lymphomas. The model has a high level of constitutive expression and some spontaneous tumors even when the animals are younger. It is, however, very responsive to carcinogens—one gets a rapid onset after exposure and a higher response incidence than with the other models. The underlying mechanism is still not certain.

A large number of studies have been run in this strain in Japan in advance of the ILSI program. The model is sensitive to both mutagenic and nonmutagenic carcinogens, although cyclophosphamide and furfural have given equivocal results in each category, respectively. The majority of noncarcinogens have also been identified correctly, although again, there are a small number of compounds that have given equivocal results.

13.12.3 The TSP *p53*$^{+/-}$ Mouse Model

The TSP *p53*$^{+/-}$ (hereafter referred to as the *p53*—the designation of the tumor suppressor gene involved) is a heterozygous knockout with (up to seven or so months of age) a low spontaneous tumor incidence. It is responsive to the genotoxic carcinogens by a mechanism based on the fact that many (but not all) tumors show a loss of the wild-type allele. The *p53* has been extensively worked on by Tennant's group at NIEHS [55, 56]. This model was developed in the United States and carries a hemizygous knockout of the *p53* gene, which was developed by integrating a mutated copy of the gene into the genome of mice. The *p53* gene is known as a tumor-suppressor gene, and it is the most commonly mutated gene in human malignancies. It searches for a protein transcription factor, which activates multiple genes when damage to DNA strands occurs, and this in turn leads to either the arrest of the cell cycle while DNA repair occurs, or to apoptosis (programmed cell death), which removes the damaged cell. The heterozygote is used because homozygotes show a very high incidence of spontaneous tumors within a few months of birth. The heterozygotes have a low background incidence of tumors up to 12 months, but during this time there is a high chance of a second mutagenic event occurring—following exposure to a carcinogen, for example—and this would result in a loss of suppressor function or an increase in transforming activity.

The initial studies with this model as an alternative in traditional carcinogenicity testing were performed at the U.S. NIEHS, and these suggested that it was sensitive to mutagenic carcinogens such as benzene and *p*-cresidine within 6 months. Nonmutagenic carcinogens were negative in the assay, as were mutagenic noncarcinogens. However, subsequent studies and some parts of the ILSI program have shown clear indications that a 6 month duration may be insufficient. In particular, benzene has given negative or equivocal results within 6 months, although positive results have been obtained by extending the study to 9 months. It will be very important to assess the results of the ILSI program when deciding the best study duration for this model. This is the most popular model in the United States.

13.12.4   The XPA$^{-/-}$ Mouse Model

This was the last of the models to be developed and was created using a knockout technique after the *XPA* gene had been cloned. The first data were published by RIVM in The Netherlands in 1995. Both alleles of the *XPA* gene have been inactivated by a homologous recombination in ES cells, resulting in a homozygous deletion of the gene spanning exons 3 and 4. The protein coded by this gene is essential for the detection and repair of DNA damage, using the nucleotide excision repair (*NER*) pathway. This model only has between 2% and 5% of residual *NER* activity.

The initial studies at RIVM demonstrated that exposure of these mice to IV-B radiation or 7,12-dimethylbenz[*a*]anthracene resulted in the rapid induction of skin tumors. It was also shown that various internal tumors could be induced following oral administration of mutagenic carcinogens such as benzo[*a*]pyrene (B[*a*]P) and 2-acetylaminofluorene (2-AAF). The early studies suggested that this response could occur within 6 months, but further experience has indicated that a 9 month treatment period is essential in order to obtain a response with positive control agents such as B[*a*]P,2-AAF, and *p*-cresidine.

It is generally proposed that while such models can improve the identification of carcinogens in three ways (providing gene-specific mechanistic data, minimizing the influence of spontaneous tumors and strain-specific effects, and reducing the time, cost, and animal usage involved), they have two potential uses in pharmaceutical development. These are either in lieu of the mouse 2 year cancer bioassay or in subchronic toxicity assessments prior to making a decision to commit to a pair of 2 year carcinogenicity bioassays.

As performance data has become available on these strains, the ICH [8] has incorporated their use into pharmaceutical testing guidelines in lieu of the second rodent species tests (i.e., to replace the long-term mouse bioassay when the traditional rat study has been performed). The FDA has stated that it would accept such studies when "performed in a validated mode." In fact, the CBER has accepted such studies as a sole carcinogenicity bioassay in some cases where there was negative traditional genotoxicity data and strong evidence of a lack of a mechanistic basis for concern.

A joint ILSI and HESI validation program has been completed, looking at the results of the four prime candidate models in identifying carcinogens as compared to the results of traditional long-term rodent bioassays. This validation program involved 51 different laboratories and imposed protocol standards to allow comparison of results. Three dose levels were studied per chemical, with 15 males and 15 females being used for each dose group. A vehicle and high dose control in wild-type animals was also included, with information from NTP bioassays and 4 week range-finding assays being used to help set doses. Animals were dosed for 26 weeks. The issues in and coming out of these validation programs bear consideration [56].

- Is human or rodent bioassay data the proper comparator data for evaluating performance? It should be kept in mind that there are sets of rodent bioassay data (particularly those involving liver tumors in mice) that are widely accepted as irrelevant in the prediction of human risk.
- How will the data from these assays be incorporated into any weight-of-evidence approach to assessing human health risk?
- What additional mechanistic research needs to be undertaken to improve our understanding of the proper incorporation and best use of the data from these assays?
- How can the results of current validation efforts be best utilized in the timely evaluation of the next generation of assays?
- Given that, at least under some conditions, assays using these models tend to "blow up" (have high spontaneous tumor rates) once the animals are more than 8 or 9 months of age, how critical are age and other not currently apprehended factors to optimizing both sensitivity and specificity?
- How wide and unconditional will FDA (and other regulatory bodies) acceptance be of these models in lieu of the traditional 2 year mouse bioassay?

13.13 INTERPRETATION OF RESULTS

13.13.1 Criteria for a Positive Result

There are three generally accepted criteria for a positive result in a carcinogenicity study. The first two are derived directly from the results of the statistical analysis: (1) a statistically significant increase in the incidence of a common tumor and (2) a statistically significant reduction in the time to tumor development. The third criterion is the occurrence of very rare tumors, that is, those not normally seen in control animals, even if the incidence is not statistically significant.

13.13.2 Statistical Analysis

The actual statistical techniques used to evaluate the results of carcinogenicity bioassays basically utilize four sets of techniques, three of which have been presented earlier in this book. These methods are *exact tests, trend tests, life tables* (such as log rank techniques), and *Peto analysis*. These are then integrated into the decision-making schemes discussed earlier in this chapter. The methods themselves and alternatives are discussed elsewhere in detail [11, 57].

Exact Tests   The basic forms of these (the Fisher exact test and chi-squared) have previously been presented, and the reader should review these. Carcinogenicity assays are, of course, conducted at doses that are at least near those that will compromise mortality. As a consequence, one generally encounters competing toxicity producing differential mortality during such a study. Often, particularly with certain agricultural chemicals, latency of spontaneous tumors in rodents may shorten as a confounded effect of treatment with toxicity. Because of such happenings, simple tests on proportions, such as χ^2 and Fisher–Irwin exact tests on contingency tables,

TABLE 13.4 Trend Versus Heterogeneity

Number at Risk	Number with Tumor	Dose Level
50	2	0
50	4	1
50	6	2
50	7	3

may not produce optimal evaluation of the incidence data. In many cases, however, statisticians still use some of these tests as methods of preliminary evaluation. These are unadjusted methods without regard for the mortality patterns in a study. Failure to take into account mortality patterns in a study sometimes causes serious flaws in interpretation of the results. The numbers at risk are generally the numbers of animals histopathologically examined for specific tissues.

Some gross adjustments on the numbers at risk can be made by eliminating early deaths or sacrifices by justifying that those animals were not at risk to have developed the particular tumor in question. Unless there is dramatic change in tumor prevalence distribution over time, the gross adjusted method provides fairly reliable evidence of treatment effect, at least for nonpalpable tissue masses.

Trend Tests   Basic forms of the trend tests (such as that of Tarone [58]) have previously been presented in this text.

Group comparison tests for proportions notoriously lack power. Trend tests, because of their use of prior information (dose levels), are much more powerful. These are illustrated in Table 13.4. Also, it is generally believed that the nature of true carcinogenicity (or toxicity for that matter) manifests itself as dose response. Because of these facts, evaluation of trend takes precedence over group comparisons. In order to achieve optimal test statistics, many people use ordinal dose levels $(0, 1, 2, \ldots)$ instead of the true arithmetic dose levels to test for trend. However, such a decision should be made *a priori*. The following example demonstrates the weakness of homogeneity tests.

COCHRAN–ARMITAGE TEST FOR TREND

	Calculated χ^2 Subgroup	DF	Alpha	Two-Tail Probability
Trend	3.3446	1	0.0500	0.0674
Departure	0.0694	2	0.0500	0.9659
Homogeneity	3.4141	3	0.0500	0.3321

ONE-TAIL TESTS FOR TREND

Type	Probability
Uncorrected	0.0337 (direction = +)
Continuity corrected	0.0426 (direction = +)
Exact	0.0423 (direction = +)

MULTIPLE PAIRWISE GROUP COMPARISONS BY FISHER–IRWIN EXACT TEST

Groups compared	Alpha	One-Tail Probability
1 vs. 2	0.0500	0.33887
2 vs. 3	0.0500	0.13433
1 vs. 4	0.0500	0.07975

As is evident from this example, often group comparison tests will fail to identify significant treatment but a trend test will. The same arguments apply to survival adjusted tests on proportions as well. In an experiment with more than one dose group ($K > 1$), the most convincing evidence for carcinogenicity is given by tumor incidence rates that increase with increasing dose. A test designed specifically to detect such dose-related trends is Tarone's [52] trend test.

Letting $\mathbf{d} = (O, d_1, d_2, \dots, d_k)^T$ be the vetor of dose levels in *all $K + 1$ groups* and letting

$$(\mathbf{O} - \mathbf{E}) = (O_0 - E_0, \dots, O_k - E_k)^T \quad \text{and} \quad \mathbf{V} = \begin{pmatrix} \mathbf{V}_{00} & \cdots & \mathbf{V}_{0K} \\ \vdots & & \vdots \\ \mathbf{V}_{K0} & \cdots & \mathbf{V}_{KK} \end{pmatrix}$$

contain elements as described in the previous section but for *all $K + 1$ groups*, the trend statistic is given by

$$\mathbf{X}_T^2 = \frac{[d^T(\mathbf{O} - \mathbf{E})]^2}{d^T \mathbf{V} \mathbf{d}}$$

The statistic $\mathbf{X}_T^2$ will be large when there is evidence of a dose-related increase or decrease in the tumor incidence rates, and small when there is little difference in the tumor incidence between groups or when group differences are not dose related. Under the null hypothesis of no differences between groups, $\mathbf{X}_T^2$ has approximately a chi-squared distribution with one degree of freedom.

Tarone's trend test is most powerful at detecting dose-related trends when tumor onset hazard functions are proportional to each other. For more power against other dose-related group differences, weighted versions of the statistic are also available; see Breslow [59] or Crowley and Breslow [60] for details.

These tests are based on the generalized logistic function [61]. Specifically, one can use the Cochran–Armitage test (or its parallel, the Mantel–Haenszel version) for monotonic trend as the heterogeneity test.

Life-Table and Survival Analysis   These methods are essential when there is any significant degree of mortality in a bioassay. They seek to adjust for the differences in periods of risk that individual animals undergo. Life-table techniques can be used for those data where there are observable or palpable tumors. Specifically, one should use Kaplan–Meier product limit estimates from censored data graphically,

Cox–Tarone binary regression (log-rank test), and Gehan–Breslow modification of Kruskal–Wallis tests [62] on censored data.

The Kaplan–Meier estimates produce a step function for each group and are plotted over the lifetimes of the animals. Planned, accidentally killed, and lost animals are censored. Moribund deaths are considered to be treatment related. A graphical representation of Kaplan–Meier estimates provide excellent interpretation of survival adjusted data except in the cases where the curves cross between two or more groups. When the curves cross and change direction, no meaningful interpretation of the data can be made by any statistical method because the proportional odds characteristic is totally lost over time. This would be a rare case where treatment initially produces more tumor or death and then, due to repair or other mechanisms, becomes beneficial.

For Cox–Tarone binary regression [58, 62], censored survival and tumor incidence data are expressed in a logistic model as dose over time. The log-rank test [63] is based on the Weibull distribution, and the Mantel–Haenszel test [64] is very similar to this test when there are no covariates or stratifying variables in the design. The logistic regression based Cox–Tarone test is preferable because one can easily incorporate covariates and stratifying variables, which one cannot do in the IARC methods.

Gehan–Breslow modification of the Kruskal–Wallis test is a nonparametric test on censored observations. It assigns more weight to early incidences compared to the Cox–Tarone test.

For survival adjusted tests on proportions, as mentioned earlier, instead of having a single $2 \times k$ table, one has a series of such $2 \times k$ tables across the entire lifetime of the study. The numbers at risk for such analyses will depend on the type of tumor one is dealing with:

1. *Palpable or Lethal Tumors.* Number at risk at time t = number of animals surviving at the end of time $t - 1$.
2. *Incidental Tumors.* Number at risk at time t = number of animals that either died or were sacrificed whose particular tissue was examined histopathologically.

The methods of analyzing the incidences, once the appropriate numbers at risk are assigned for these tumors, are rather similar, either binary regression based or by pooling evidence from individual tables [43].

Peto Analysis   The Peto method of analysis of bioassay tumor data is based on careful classification of tumors into five different categories, as defined by the IARC.

1. Definitely Incidental.
2. Probably Incidental.
   Comment: Combine (1) and (2).
3. Probably Lethal.
4. Definitely Lethal.
   Comment: These categories may be combined into one (otherwise it requires a careful cause of death determination).

5. Mortality Independent (such as mammary, skin, and other observable or superficial tumors).

Interval Selection for Occult (Internal Organ) Tumors

1. FDA: 0–50, 51–80, 81–104 Weeks, Interim Sacrifice, Terminal Sacrifice.
2. NTP: 0–52, 53–78, 79–92, 93–104 Weeks, Interim Sacrifice, Terminal Sacrifice.
3. IARC: *Ad hoc* Selection Method [41].
   Comment: Any of the above may be used. There are problems with the IARC selection method, however, Two sexes or two or more strains will have different intervals for the same compound. Different interval selection methods will produce different statistical significance levels. This may produce bias and requires an isotonic tumor prevalence for ready analysis.

Logistic Regression Method for Occult (Internal Organ) Tumors [65]

Tumor prevalence is modeled as a logistic function of dose and polynomial in age.
Comment: The logistic tumor prevalence method is unbiased, requires maximum likelihood estimation, and allows for covariates and stratifying variables. It may be time consuming and have convergence problem with sparse tables (low tumor incidences) and clustering of tumors.

13.13.3   Methods to Be Avoided

The following methods and practices should be avoided in evaluation of carcinogenicity:

1. Use of only the animals surviving after 1 year in the study.
2. Use of a two-strata approach—separate analyses for animals killed during the first year of the study and the ones thereafter.
3. Exclusion of all animals in the study that died on test and analysis of only the animals that are sacrificed at the end of the study.
4. Exclusion of interim sacrifice animals from statistical analyses.
5. Evaluation of number of tumors of all sites as opposed to the number of animals with tumors for specific sites of specific organs.

Another issue is subjectivity in slide reading by most pathologists who do not want to read them in a coded fashion, whereby they will not know the dose group an animal is coming from. This is not under statisticians' control but they should be aware of that in any case.

Often a chemical being tested is both toxic as well as potentially carcinogenic. When competing toxicity causes extreme differences in mortality or there is a clustering effect in tumor prevalence in a very short interval of time, none of the adjusted methods works. One then must use biological intuition to evaluate the tumor data.

Use of historical control incidence data for statistical evaluation is controversial. There are too many sources of variation in these data. For example, different pathologists use different criteria for categorizing tumors (in fact, the same pathologist may change opinion over time); there is laboratory-to-laboratory variation; there may be genetic drift over time; location of suppliers may make a difference; and finally, these data are not part of the randomized concurrent control. Regulatory agencies and pathologists generally use these data for qualitative evaluation. My personal view is that that is where they belong.

13.13.4   Use of Historical Controls

When the study is over, the data analyzed, and the p values corrected, as appropriate, one may find that one or more tumor types increased in drug-treated groups relative to concurrent controls. Although the FDA and other regulatory agencies play down the importance of historical control data, it is common practice in the pharmaceutical industry to use historical data in the interpretation of tumor findings. The first and most appropriate comparison of a treated group is with concurrent control group(s), but it is of interest to see how tumor incidences in the treated groups compare with the historical incidence, and such a comparison is an accepted practice in toxicology and biostatistics [42, 66, 67]. A treated group may have a tumor incidence significantly higher than that of the concurrent control groups, but comparable to or lower than the historical incidence. Occasionally, a small number of tumors may be found in a treated group and the incidence may be significant because of the absence of this tumor in the concurrent controls. Review of appropriate historical control data may reveal that the low tumor incidence in the treated group is within the "expected" range for this tumor.

The role of historical control data in interpreting carcinogenicity findings depends on the "quality" of the historical data. Ideally, the data should be derived from animals of the same age, sex, strain, and supplier, housed in the same facility, and the pathology examinations should have been performed by the same pathologist or using the same pathological criteria for diagnosis. Since genetic drift occurs even in animals of a given strain and supplier, recent data are more useful than older data. The value of historical control data is directly proportional to the extent to which these conditions are fulfilled.

Although methods are available for including historical control data in the formal statistical analysis [68, 69], this is usually not done and for good reason. The heterogeneity of historical data requires that they be used qualitatively and selectively to aid in the final interpretation of the data, after completion of the formal statistical analysis. Table 13.5 presents a summary of background tumor incidences for the most commonly employed rodent strains.

13.13.5   Relevance to Humans

After statistical analyses have been performed and historical data consulted, the final interpretation may be that a drug appears to cause tumors at one or more tissue sites in the mouse or the rat. But what does this mean for the species to which the drug will be administered, namely, the human? Extrapolation of rodent carcinogenicity data to humans remains one of the greatest challenges of modern toxicol-

TABLE 13.5 Comparative Percent Incidence of Pertinent Neoplasia in Different Strains of Rats and Mice (104 Weeks Old)

Types of Neoplasia	F344 Rats		S-D Rats		Wistar Rats		B6C3F₁ Mice		CD-1 Mice	
	Males	Females	Males	Females	Males	Females	Males	Females	Males	Females
Hepatocellular adenoma	4	<1	5	<1	1	2	29	30	26	5
Hepatocellular carcinoma	2	0	2	0	<1	<1	26	16	10	1
Pancreas islet adenoma	12	2	8	9	4	2	2	0	<1	<1
Pancreas islet carcinoma	3	0	<1	5	<1	<1	0	0	0	0
Pancreas acinar adenoma	6	0	1	0	13	<1	2	0	<1	0
Pheochromocytoma	21	4	23	5	10	2	0	2	<1	<1
Adrenocortical adenoma	0	2	3	0	8	9	<1	0	1	<1
Pituitary adenoma	49	42	62	85	34	55	2	8	0	5
Thyroid C-cell adenoma	17	8	7	6	6	8	0	0	0	0
Thyroid follicular adenoma	0	0	4	2	2	1	2	6	1	<1
Mammary gland fibroadenoma	4	57	2	54	3	36	0	0	<1	1
Mammary gland carcinoma	0	4	<1	26	1	13	0	0	0	6
Skin fibroma	10	2	2	<1	5	1	1	2	<1	<1
Skin papilloma	6	0	2	0	2	<1	0	0	<1	0
Pulmonary adenoma	4	4	<1	<1	<1	0	22	6	15	15
Preputial gland neoplasia	10	NA	>1	NA	<1	NA	<1	NA	<1	NA
Leydig cell neoplasia	89	NA	7	NA	11	NA	0	NA	1	NA
Clitoral gland neoplasia	NA	14	NA	<1	NA	<1	NA	<1	NA	0
Uterine polyps	NA	14	NA	6	NA	16	NA	1	NA	<1
Ovarian neoplasia	NA	6	NA	1	NA	8	NA	6	NA	1
Mononuclear cell leukemia	62	42	0	0	<1	<1	0	0	2	2
Lymphoma	0	0	2	1	3	5	14	24	8	22
Forestomach papilloma	0	2	<1	<1	0	<1	4	2	<1	<1
Scrotal mesothelioma	5	NA	1	NA	2	NA	0	NA	0	NA

Note: F344, Fischer 244 rats; S-D, Sprague–Dawley rats; B6C3F1, mice, (C57BL/6N+C3H/HeN)F1; CD-1, 1CRCr: CD-1 mice; NA, nonapplicable; the average number used by species/strain/gender was in excess of 750 animals.

451

ogy. There is no simple formula, and each case must be evaluated on its own merits. Very generally speaking, the FDA and other major regulatory agencies consider compounds that are tumorigenic in one or more animal species to be "suspect" tumorigens in humans. The actual impact of this conclusion on the approval of a drug depends on the target population and the indication. For example, even a suspicion of carcinogenic activity may be fatal for a potential contraceptive drug intended for use in a very large population of healthy people. By contrast, clear evidence of carcinogenic activity may be overlooked in a drug being considered for use in a restricted population with a life-threatening disease.

Regardless of the target population and indication, the FDA and other agencies have, in recent years, attempted to consider the mechanism of tumor induction in rodents and its relevance for humans. If a drug is known to cause tumors in a rodent via a mechanism that does not exist in humans, the importance of the tumor findings may be markedly reduced. For example, drugs that cause tumors by a secondary hormonal mechanism shown to be inapplicable to humans may be given special consideration. It is the sponsor's responsibility to provide pertinent data on the mechanism of tumor induction and its relevance, or irrelevance, for humans. If the sponsor can show that an apparently drug-related tumor is species specific, the importance of the tumor in the overall evaluation of the drug will be greatly minimized. Table 13.5 presents a list of neoplastic /tumorigenic responses seen in rodents, which have limited relevance to human safety. Part of the consideration must also be a recognition of the main characteristics of nongenotoxic carcinogens. These are recognized to be dose-dependent responses with operative thresholds. The major characteristics [14] are:

- Specificity (of species, sex, and organ).
- A threshold is operative and must be exceeded for cell proliferation and tumor development to occur.
- There is a step wise dose–response curve/relationship between exposure, cell proliferation, and tumor development.
- The response is reversible with a cessation of dosing unless a point of no return has been passed.

Not all tumors seen in animals are revelant to predicting human risk, particularly these in rodents. Table 13.6 summarizes such situations.
Interpretation of the data and results from a carcinogenicity study is generally not simply a yes or no (or counting turnovers) matter. Rather, one must also consider effects on survival. An approach to this is shown in Table 13.7.

13.14   CONCLUSION

The design, conduct, and interpretation of carcinogenicity studies is one of the major challenges for the pharmaceutical toxicologist, pathologist, biostatistician, and regulator. This is a rapidly changing field generating more questions than answers. The biggest question continues to be the extrapolation of rodent data to humans,

TABLE 13.6   Examples of Neoplastic Effects in Rodents with Limited Significance for Human Safety

Neoplastic Effect	Pathogenesis (Agents)
Renal tubular neoplasia in male rats	$\alpha_2\mu$-Globulin nephropathy/hydrocarbons (*d*-limonene, *p*-dichlorobenzene)
Hepatocellular neoplasia in rats and mice	Peroxisome proliferation (clofibrate, phthalate esters, phenoxy agents) Phenobarbital-like promotion
Urinary bladder neoplasia in rats	Crystalluria, carbonic anhydrase inhibition, urine pH extremes, melamine, saccharine, carbonic anhydrase inhibitors, dietary phosphates
Hepatocellular neoplasia in mice	Enzymatic-metabolic activation (in part unknown)/phenobarbital-like promotion
Thyroid follicular cell neoplasia in rats	Hepatic enzyme induction, thyroid enzyme inhibition/axazepam, amobarbital, sulfonamides, thioureas
Gastric neuroendocrine cell neoplasia mainly in rats	Gastric secretory suppression, gastric atrophy induction (climetidine, omeprazole, butachlor)
Adenohypophysis neoplasia in rats	Feedback interference/neuroleptics (dopamine inhibitors)
Mammary gland neoplasia in female rats	Feedback interference/neuroleptics, antiemetics, antihypertensives (calcium channel blockers), serotonin agonists, anticholinergics, exogenous estrogens
Pancreatic islet cell neoplasia in rats	Feedback interference/neuroleptics
Harderian gland neoplasia in mice	Feedback interference/misoprostol (PGE_1), nalidixic acid, aniline dyes
Adrenal medullary neoplasia in rats	Feedback interference (lactose, sugar alcohols)
Forestomach neoplasia in rats and mice	Stimulation of proliferation/butylated hydroxyanisole, phthalate esters, proprionic acid
Lymphomas in mice	Immunosuppression/cyclosporine
Mononuclear cell leukemia in rats (mainly F344)	Immunosuppression (in part unknown)/furan, iodinated glycerol
Splenic sarcomas in rats	Methemoglobinemia (in part unknown)/dapsone
Osteomas in mice	Feedback interference/lactose, sugar alcohols, H2 antagonists, carbamazepine, vidarabine, isradipine, dopaminergics, finasteride
Leydig cell testicular neoplasia in mice	Feedback interference (proestrogens, finasteride, methoxychlor, cadmium)
Endometrial neoplasia in rats	Feedback interference (proestrogens, dopamine agonists)
Uterine leiomyoma in mice	Feedback interference (β_1-antagonists)
Mesovarial leiomyoma in rats (occasionally in mice)	Feedback interference (β_2-agonists)

TABLE 13.7   Interpretation of the Analysis of Tumor Incidence and Survival Analysis (Life Table)

Outcome Type	Tumor Association with Treatment[a]	Mortality Association with Treatment	Interpretation[b]
A	−	+	Unadjusted test may underestimate tumorigenicity of treatment.
B	+	+	Unadjusted test gives valid picture of tumorigenicity of treatment.
C	+	−	Tumors found in treated groups may reflect longer survival of treated groups. Time adjusted analysis is indicated.
D	−	+	Apparent negative findings on tumors may be due to the shorter survival in treated groups. Time adjusted analysis and/or a retest at lower doses is indicated.
E	−	0	Unadjusted test gives a valid picture of the possible tumor-preventive capacity of the treatment.
F	−	−	Unadjusted test may underestimate the possible tumor-preventive capacity of the treatment.
G	0	+	High mortality in treated groups may lead to unadjusted test missing a possible tumorigen. Adjusted analysis and/or retest at lower doses is indicated
H	0	0	Unadjusted test gives a valid picture of lack of association with treatment.
I	0	−	Longer survival in treated groups may mask tumor-preventive capacity of treatment.

[a]+, Yes; −, No; and 0, No bearing on discussion.
[b]The unadjusted test referred to here is a contingency table type of analysis of incidence, such as Fisher's exact test.

especially when data on mechanisms of tumor induction are unavailable or controversial. Much has been written on the difficulties inherent in extrapolating results from rodents treated with MTDs of a compound to humans who will be exposed to much lower doses and often for shorter periods. A discussion of these and other aspects of carcinogenic risk assessment is beyond the scope of this chapter.

Regulatory agencies are very aware of these challenges and deserve credit for attempting to respond to changes in the state of knowledge, while still discharging their responsibility to protect the public health. For example, the latest version of the Japanese guidelines [27] acknowledges that the highest dose in a carcinogenicity study may be set at 100 times the clinical dose, instead of requiring that the MTD be achieved. It is also noteworthy that the FDA Center for Drug Evaluation has announced the formation of a Carcinogenicity Assessment Committee representing all drug review divisions. This group will advise all the divisions on issues related to carcinogenicity. Creation of such a group reflects the importance that the FDA places on carcinogenicity data in evaluating the safety of new drug candidates.

REFERENCES

1. NIH *9th Report on Carcinogens.* Washington, DC: US Department of Health and Human Services; 2000.
2. Miller EC, Miller JA. Mechanisms of chemical carcinogenesis. *Cancer* 1981;47:1055–1064.
3. Powell CJ, Berry CL. Non-genotoxic or epigenetic carcinogenesis. In Ballantyne B, Marrs T, Syversen T, Eds. *General and Applied Toxicology*, 2nd ed. London: MacMillan; 2000.
4. Kitchin KT. *Carcinogenicity.* New York: Marcel Dekker; 1999.
5. Williams GM, Iatropoulos MJ. and Enzhmann HG. Principles of testing for carcinogenic activity. In Hayes AW, Ed. *Principles and Methods of Toxicology*, 5th ed. Philadelphia: Taylor and Francis; 2007.
6. International Agency for Research on Cancer. IARC Monographs on the Evaluation of Carcinogenic Risks to Humans—Preamble. *IARC Internal Technical Report 87/001.* Lyon: IARC; 1987.
7. *The Need for Long-Term Rodent Carcinogenicity Studies of Pharmaceuticals.* ICH; 1996.
8. *Testing for Carcinogenicity of Pharmaceuticals.* ICH; 1997.
9. *Dose Selection for Carcinogenicity Studies of Pharmaceuticals.* ICH; 1997.
10. *CPMP Note for Guidance on Carcinogenic Potential.* EMEA; July 2002.
11. Weaver RJ, Brunden MN. The design of long-term carcinogenicity studies. In Chow S, Lide J, Eds. *Design and Analysis of Animal Studies in Pharmaceutical Development.* New York: Marcel Dekker; 1998.
12. FDA. *Guidance for Industry: Statistical Aspects of the Design, Analysis and Interpretation of Chronic Rodent Carcinogenicity Studies of Pharmaceuticals.* Washington, DC: USDHEW; 2001.
13. Contrera JF, Jacobs AC, DeGeorge JJ. Carcinogenicity testing and the evaluation of regulatory requirements for pharmaceuticals. *Regul Toxicol Pharmacol* 1997;25:130–145.
14. Spindler P, Loan J, Ceuppens P, Harling R, Eittlin R, Lima BS. Carcinogenicity testing of pharmaceuticals in the European Union: a workshop report. *Drug Inf J* 2000; 34:821–828.
15. Pharmaceutical Manufacturers Association. *Results of a Questionnaire Involving the Design of and Experience with Carcinogenicity Studies.* PMA; 1988. This document has not been published in the open literature but is widely available within the pharmaceutical industry. It may be obtained by writing to the Pharmaceutical Manufacturers Association.

16. Rao GN, Birnbaum LS, Collins JJ, Tennant RW, Skow LC. Mouse strains for chemical carcinogenicity studies: overview of a workshop. *Fundam Appl Toxicol* 1988;10:385–394.

17. Purchase IFH. Interspecies comparisons of carcinogenicity. *Br J Cancer* 1980;41:454–468.

18. Haseman JK, Crawford DD, Huff JE, Boorman GA, McConnell EE. Results for 86 two-year carcinogenicity studies conducted by the National Toxicology Program. *J Toxicol Environ Health* 1984;14:621–639.

19. Gold LS, Sawyer CB, Magaw R, Blackman G, deVeciana M, Levenson R, Hooper NK, Havender WR, Bernstein L, Peto R, Pike MC, Ames BN. A carcinogenic potency data base of the standardized results of animal bioassays. *Environ Health Perspect* 1984;58:9–319.

20. Sher SP, Jensen RD, Bokelman DL. Spontaneous tumors in control F344 and Charles River CD rats and Charles River CD-1 and B6C3F1 mice. *Toxicol Lett* 1982;11:103–110.

21. Food and Drug Administration (FDA). Toxicological principles for the safety assessment of direct food additives and color additives used in food. In *Redbook II (draft)*. Washington, DC: Food and Drug Administration; 1993, pp 111–115.

22. Rao GN, Huff J. Refinement of long-term toxicity and carcinogenesis studies. *Fundam Appl Toxicol* 1990;15:33–43.

23. Greenman DL, Kodell RL, Sheldon WG. Association between cage shelf level and spontaneous induced neoplasms in mice. *J Natl Cancer Inst* 1984;73:107–113.

24. Wiskemann A, Sturm E, Klehr NW. Fluorescent lighting enhances chemically induced papilloma formation and increases susceptibility to tumor challenge in mice. *J Cancer Res Clin Oncol* 1986;112:141–143.

25. Bellhorn RW. Lighting in the animal environment. *Lab Anim Sci* 1980;30:440–450.

26. Greenman DL, Bryant P, Kodell RL, Sheldon W. Influence of cage shelf level on retinal atrophy in mice. *Lab Anim Sci* 1982;32:353–356.

27. Weisbrode SE, Weiss HS. Effect of temperature on benzo[*a*]pyrene induced hyperplastic and neoplastic skin lesions in mice. *J Natl Cancer Inst* 1981;66:978–981.

28. Fox JG. Clinical assessment of laboratory rodents on long term bioassay studies. *J Environ Pathol Toxicol* 1977;1:199–226.

29. Flynn RJ. Studies on the aetiology of ringtail in rats. *Proc Anim Care Panel* 1960;9:155–160.

30. DePass LR, Weil CS, Ballantyne B, Lewis SC, Losco PE, Reid JB, Simon GS. Influence of housing conditions for mice on the results of a dermal oncogenicity bioassay. *Fundam Appl Toxicol* 1986;7:601–608.

31. Rao GN, Haseman JK, Edmondson J. Influence of viral infections on body weight, survival, and tumor prevalence in Fisher 344 rats on two-year studies. *Lab Anim Sci* 1989;39:389–393.

32. Speid LH, Lumley CE, Walker SR. Harmonization of guidelines for toxicity testing of pharmaceuticals by 1992. *Regul Toxicol Pharmacol* 1990;12:179–211.

33. Haseman JK, Winbush JS, O'Donnell MW. Use of dual control groups to estimate false positive rates in laboratory animal carcinogenicity studies. *Fundam Appl Toxicol* 1986;7:573–584.

34. *Guidance for Industry: Carcinogenicity Study Protocol Submissions*. CDER; May 2002.

35. McGregor D. Carcinogenicity and genotoxic carcinogens. In Ballantyne B, Marrs T, Syversen T, Eds. *General and Applied Toxicology*, 2nd ed. London: MacMillan; 2000.

36. Japanese Ministry of Health and Welfare (MHW). *Revised Guidelines for Toxicity Studies Required for Application for Approval of Manufacturing/Importing Drugs.* Tokyo: Ministry of Health and Welfare; 1989, pp 37–48.

37. Haseman JK. Issues in carcinogenicity testing: dose selection. *Fundam Appl Toxicol* 1985;5:66–78.

38. Cameron TP, Hickman RL, Kornreich MR, Tarone RE. History, survival, and growth patterns of B6C3F1 mice and F344 rats in the National Cancer Institute Carcinogenesis Testing Program. *Fundam Appl Toxicol* 1985;5:526–538.

39. Littlefield NA, Farmer JH, Gaylor DW, Sheldon WG. Effects of dose and time in a long-term, low-dose carcinogenic study. In Staffa JA, Mehlman MA, Eds. *Innovations in Cancer Risk Assessment (ED01Study).* Chicago, Illinois: Pathotox Publishers; 1979, pp 17–34.

40. Gaylor DW, Kodell RL. Dose–response trend tests for tumorigenesis adjusted For differences in survival and body weight across doses. *Toxicol Sci* 2001;59:219–225.

41. Peto R, Pike MC, Day NE, Gray RG, Lee PN, Parish S, Peto J, Richards S, Wahrendorf J. Guidelines for simple, sensitive significance tests for carcinogenic effects in long-term animal experiments. In *IARC Monographs on the Evaluation of the Carcinogenic Risk of Chemicals to Humans.* Lyon: International Agency for Research on Cancer; 1980.

42. Gart JJ, Chu KC, Tarone RE. Statistical issues in interpretation of chronic bioassay tests for carcinogenicity. *J Natl Cancer Inst* 1979;62:957–974.

43. Gart JJ, Krewski D, Lee PN, Tarone RE, Wahrendorf J. The design and analysis of long-term animal experiment. In *Statistical Methods in Cancer Research, Volume III.* IARC Scientific Publication No. 79. Lyon: International Agency for Research on Cancer; 1986.

44. Dinse GE, Lagakos SW. Regression analysis of tumor prevalence data. *Appl Stat* 1983;32:236–248.

45. Portier CJ, Bailer AJ. Testing for increased carcinogenicity using a survival-adjusted quantal response test. *Fundam Appl Toxicol* 1989;12:731–737.

46. Haseman JK. Use of statistical decision rules for evaluating laboratory animal carcinogenicity studies. *Fundam Appl Toxicol* 1990;14:637–648.

47. Mantel N. Assessing laboratory evidence for neoplastic activity. *Biometrics* 1980; 36:381–399.

48. Schweder T, Spjotvoll E. Plots of *p*-values to evaluate many tests simultaneously. *Biometrika* 1982;69:493–502.

49. Farrar DB, Crump KS. Exact statistical tests for any carcinogenic effect in animal bioassays. *Fundam Appl Toxicol* 1988;11:652–663.

50. Haseman JK. A reexamination of false-positive rates for carcinogenicity studies. *Fundam Appl Toxicol* 1983;3:334–339.

51. Festing MW. Properties of inbreed strains and outbreed stocks, with special reference to toxicity testing. *J Toxicol Environ Health* 1979;5:53–68.

52. Eastin WC, Haseman JK, Mahler JF, Bucher JR. The National Toxicology Program evaluation of genetically altered mice predictive models for identifying carcinogens. *Toxicol Pathol* 1998;26:461–584.

53. McAnulty PA. Transgenic mouse models in carcinogenicity testing. *European Pharmaceutical Contractor*; 2000.

54. French JE, Spalding JW, Dunnick JK, Tice RR, Furedi-Marchacck M, Tennant RW. The use of transgenic animals in cancer testing. *Inhalation Toxicol* 1999;11:541–544.

55. Tennant RW, French JE, Spalding JW. Identification of chemical carcinogens and assessing potential risks in short-term bioassays using transgenic mouse models. *Environ Health Perspect* 1995;103:942–950.

56. Tennant RW, Stasiewicz S, Mennear J, French JE, Spalding JW. Genetically altered mouse models for identifying carcinogens. In McGregor DB, Rice JM, Venith S, Eds. *The Use of Short and Medium-Term Tests for Carcinogens and Data on Genetic Effects in Carcinogenic Hazard Evaluation.* IARC Science Publication No. 146. Lyon, France: IARC; 1999, pp 23–148.

57. Gad SC. *Statistics and Experimental Design for Toxicologists,* 4th ed. Boca Raton, FL: CRC Press; 2007.

58. Tarone RE. Tests for trend in life table analysis, *Biometrika* 1975;62:679–682.

59. Breslow N. Comparison of survival curves. In Buyse ME, Staquet MJ, Sylvester RJ, Eds. *Cancer Clinical Trials: Methods and Practice.* Oxford, UK: Oxford University Press; 1984, pp 381–406.

60. Crowley J, Breslow N. Statistical analysis of survival data. *Annu Rev Public Health* 1984;5:385–411.

61. Cox DR. Regression models and life-tables. *J R Stat Soc* 1972;34B:187–220.

62. Thomas DG, Breslow N, Gart JJ. Trend and homogeneity analyses of proportions and life table data. *Comput Biomed Res* 1977;10:373–381.

63. Peto R. Guidelines on the analysis of tumor rates and death rates in experimental animals. *Br J Cancer* 1974;29:101–105.

64. Mantel N, Haenszel W. Statistical aspects of the analysis of data from the retrospective studies of disease. *J Natl Cancer Inst* 1952;22:719–748.

65. Dinse GE. Estimating tumor prevalence, lethality and mortality. Presented at the Symposium on Long-Term Animal Carcinogenicity Studies: A Statistical Perspective, 4–6 March 1985, Bethesda.

66. Hajian G. Statistical issues in the design and analysis of carcinogenicity bioassays. *Toxicol Pathol* 1983;11:83–89.

67. Haseman JK, Huff J, Boorman GA. Use of historical control data in carcinogenicity studies in rodents. *Toxicol Pathol* 1984;12:126–135.

68. Tarone RE. The use of historical control information in testing for a trend in proportions. *Biometrics* 1982;38:215–220.

69. Dempster AP, Selivyn MR, Weeks BJ. Combining historical and randomized controls for assessing trends in proportions. *J Am Stat Assoc* 1983;78:221–227.

14

TOXICOKINETICS: AN INTEGRAL COMPONENT OF PRECLINICAL TOXICITY STUDIES

SONU SUNDD SINGH

Nektar Therapeutics India Private Limited, Secunderabad, India

Contents

Preclinical Development Handbook: Toxicology, edited by Shayne Cox Gad
Copyright © 2008 John Wiley & Sons, Inc.

14.1   INTRODUCTION

The establishment of preclinical safety data for an investigational new drug (IND) is a global regulatory requirement. Recently, it has been universally recognized that efficacy and safety of a drug can be better correlated with systemic drug exposure rather than directly with dose [1]. Drug discovery scientists now believe that toxicological experiments should include the assessment of the concentration–time course of the investigated agent for proper interpretation of the toxicological data. Several regulatory guidelines recommend toxicokinetic evaluation of an investigational drug. Toxicokinetics has emerged as an area distinct from pharmacokinetics, where kinetic data for a new compound are generated at subtherapeutic dose levels. The Toxicokinetics guideline of the International Conference on Harmonization (ICH S3A) defines toxicokinetics [1, 2] as "the generation of pharmacokinetic data, either as an integral component of non-clinical toxicity studies or in specially designed supportive studies, to assess systemic exposure." In other words, kinetics and tissue distribution studies performed on the same animals (large animals) or a satellite group of animals (small animals such as rodents) during a nonclinical toxicity study to augment the interpretation of toxicological findings are known as *toxicokinetics*. Here the term "satellite group of animals" refers to a group of animals included in the design and conduct of a toxicity study, which are treated and housed under similar conditions as those of the main toxicity study but used for generating toxicokinetic data.

Toxicokinetics is a relatively small but important component of preclinical animal toxicology studies, which form the foundation of a preclinical program leading to the filing of an IND application. Therefore, the sole purpose of conducting toxico-kinetic studies is to add value to the existing toxicological data. Incorporation of toxicokinetics in the design of conventional toxicity studies helps in ratifying the design of the study with respect to pharmacokinetic and metabolic principles by providing a proof of concept that the animals were really exposed to appropriate systemic levels of administered test compound and/or its metabolites. Toxicokinetics brings in better understanding of toxicity data and better extrapolation of nonclini-cal data for clinical use. Most importantly, toxicokinetic evaluation makes for good science [2]. The term "pharmacokinetics" should not be confused with "toxicokine-tics" as the parameters obtained from the former are used for the characterization of the drug, whereas "toxicokinetics" serves as a fundamental tool for assessing the safety profile of a drug at toxic dose levels. The toxicokinetic data thus obtained are utilized in co-relating the plasma/tissue levels to toxicological findings and their relevance to clinical safety. Toxicokinetic profiling of toxicity studies should estab-lish the level of exposure that has been achieved during the course of the study and may also serve as an alert to toxicologists toward nonlinear, dose-related changes in exposure that may have occurred. Toxicokinetics allows better interspecies com-parisons than simple dose/body weight (or surface area) comparisons. The extrapo-lation of data between animals and humans for the purpose of establishing safety margin, when solely based on doses (mg/kg), can give very misleading results due to vast pharmacokinetic differences between species and gender. Invariably, there appears to be much greater safety margin when plasma concentration data, which represent actual drug exposure, are used [2].

Toxicokinetic (TK) evaluation can be performed during safety pharmacology, single dose and dose escalation studies, repeated dose toxicity studies, reproductive toxicity, genotoxicity, and carcinogenicity studies. TK data at "no observed toxic effect dose" provide a suitable safe starting and upper dose for the clinical investiga-tor in designing a Phase I clinical trial. Since new drug development is a dynamic process and continuous feedback between clinical and nonclinical studies is required for proper safety assessment, flexible procedures based solely on pure scientific judgments are recommended [1]. TK evaluation should conform to Good Labora-tory Practice (GLP) as described in 21 CFR Part 58 [3] and OECD GLP guidelines 1997 (F) [4]. Meaningful TK data should be based on reliable and well validated analytical methods [5].

14.2   OBJECTIVES OF TOXICOKINETIC STUDY

The prime objective of a toxicokinetic study is to estimate the systemic exposure of a drug achieved at different dose levels in a toxicity study and to establish a dose versus exposure relationship. The secondary objectives may be to correlate the expo-sure achieved with the toxicological findings and to contribute to the assessment of the relevance of these findings to clinical safety. The toxicokinetic data in conjugation with toxicity findings also help in identifying the right toxicity species and in design-ing the subsequent nonclinical toxicity studies. The measurement of various toxico-kinetic parameters results in meeting all the above objectives. The parameters usually measured are maximum plasma concentration (C_{max}), time point of maximum plasma concentration (T_{max}), area under the plasma concentration–time curve

(AUC), and half-life of drug elimination during the terminal phase ($T_{1/2}$). These parameters are usually calculated from the concentration/time data, using a curve prediction package (e.g., Win Nonlin from Pharsight: http://www.pharsight.com).

14.3 TOXICOKINETICS IN VARIOUS TOXICITY STUDIES FOR PHARMACEUTICALS

14.3.1 Safety Pharmacology

These studies comprise a battery of tests for assessing the CNS, cardiovascular, and respiratory functions. The ICH guideline for safety pharmacology [6] does not specifically mention the requirement of toxicokinetic measurement during these studies. Nevertheless, the estimation of systemic exposure helps immensely in correlating any adverse effects to plasma concentrations.

14.3.2 Single Dose-Ranging Toxicity Studies

These studies are carried out primarily in rodents, generally at early stages of development. As a common practice, toxicokinetics is not routinely incorporated due to nonavailability of validated bioanalytical methods. However, some samples are taken and stored for future analysis without any insight into the stability of the samples. Ideally, the kinetic data for the single dose studies should be generated initially for the intended broad dose range as a separate study on the same animal models. This would give a fairly good idea of dose linearity range, that is, the dose versus exposure (AUC) relationship. In addition, it would also provide information about the presence of metabolites, the highest possible dose with no mortality, the exhibition of some toxic effects, the dose administration constraints due to absorption saturation, and formulation-related problems (at very high concentrations the permissible volumes may not be possible). Single dose-ranging studies designed and conducted with the background of this data would certainly provide meaningful results.

14.3.3 Rising Dose Toxicity Studies

These studies are carried out in nonrodents or higher animal models (e.g., dogs, monkeys). Here toxicokinetics can easily be incorporated into the main study, as there is no constraint on the number of sampling points due to the large blood volume. Moreover, these studies are usually carried out after the rodent single dose studies. Thus, by that time, the bioanalytical methods are usually available. Here toxicokinetics is performed on the same animal at various time points for each new dose level. Such an evaluation gives very good information about the dose linearity range and clinical symptoms can be readily co-related with plasma concentration of the parent compound or the metabolites.

14.3.4 Repeated Dose Toxicity Studies (4 Weeks)

Single/rising dose toxicity studies are followed by repeated dose studies in both rodent and nonrodent species. These studies are carried out at three dose levels—low, intermediate, and high—along with a vehicle control group. The low dose lies near the efficacy dose, whereas the high dose falls near the end of the dose response–linearity curve and this dose is expected to exhibit some signs of toxicity. The control samples should be analyzed along with the treated samples [1]. The selection of dose levels and the treatment regimen (dosage, formulation, route of administration, and dosing frequency) are based on the results of previous single dose and rising dose toxicity studies. Usually a duration of 4 weeks is recommended for supporting Phase I clinical trials. A satellite group of animals is generally used for rodent studies due to the sampling constraint of low blood volumes, as only 10% of the total blood volume can be withdrawn [7]. Samples are withdrawn on day 1, day 14, and day 28. Sampling times are based on earlier pharmacokinetic data or on the toxicokinetic data obtained for single dose/rising dose studies. Typically, three or more animals are used for each dose level. An average of drug concentrations at each time point is taken and toxicokinetic parameters are also presented as the mean ± SD. In some instances, pooling of equal volumes of plasma samples for each time point is also done prior to sample analysis. Tissue distribution is also incorporated in the design of the study and organs of interest are removed after sacrifice and analyzed for the drug and metabolites. A typical design of a 4 week toxicokinetic study is shown in Table 14.1. A comparison of systemic exposure in terms of plasma and tissue concentrations and AUC is done in order to interpret the outcome of the study. Proper designing of a toxicokinetic study would provide valuable information about the accumulation of drug and/or metabolites in body fluids or organs/tissues. There is also a possibility of reduction in the overall exposure after repeated dose administration, which may be attributed to autoinduction of drug metabolizing enzymes, saturated absorption, or increased clearance [2]. At low doses, blood levels may indicate nonaccumulation but tissue distribution could reveal accumulation of drug in specific organs.

14.3.5 Repeated Dose Toxicity Studies (6 and 12 Months)

In order to assess longer exposure, repeated dose studies are conducted for 6 and 12 months in rodents and nonrodents, respectively. Toxicokinetics can be incorporated in a similar manner as 4 week studies, covering the entire span of the study.

TABLE 14.1 Animal Grouping for a 4 Week Toxicokinetic Study

		Day of Sampling					
		Day 1[a]		Day 14[b]		Day 28	
		Animal Numbers					
Group	Dose (mg/kg)	Male	Female	Male	Female	Male	Female
I	10.0	1–3	19–21	4–6	22–24	7–9	25–27
II	30.0	10–12	28–30	13–15	31–33	16–18	34–36

[a]Animals were bled on day 1 for toxicokinetics data and dosing of these animals was continued for 28 days and on day 29 the animals were sacrificed for tissue distribution after 24 hours from the last dosing.
[b]These animals would be sacrificed after day 14 for toxicokinetics data.

14.3.6   Genotoxicity Studies

Generally, two *in vitro* tests and one *in vivo* tests are recommended for genotoxicity testing [8, 9]. A rodent micronucleus (bone marrow or peripheral erythrocytes) test or chromosomal aberration test is carried out for *in vivo* investigation of genotoxicity. The ICH toxicokinetics guideline [1] recommends that for "negative results of *in vivo* geno toxicity studies, it may be appropriate to have demonstrated systemic exposure in the species used or to have characterized exposure in indicator organs."

14.3.7   Carcinogenicity Studies

Carcinogenicity studies are generally conducted to identify a tumorigenic potential of a drug in animals and to assess the relevant risk in humans. Pharmaceuticals that are proposed for continuous use for at least 6 months of clinical use should be considered for carcinogenicity testing. Pharmaceuticals administered for a short duration of exposure, such as anesthetics, critical care medications, and radiolabeled imaging agents, do not need carcinogenic assessment. Certain formulations or delivery systems that prolong the exposure of the test compound need carcinogenicity studies. Carcinogenicity studies are not needed for endogenous substances like peptides, proteins, and their analogues. Carcinogenicity studies should be completed before filing an NDA (New Drug Application). Complete rodent carcinogenicity studies are not needed in advance for conducting clinical trials. The following ICH guidelines address the various issues concerning nonclinical carcinogenicity studies:

S1A: Guidance on the Need for Carcinogenicity Studies of Pharmaceuticals, March 1996 [10].

This guideline defines the need and conditions under which carcinogenicity studies should be conducted in order to avoid unnecessary usage of animals.

S1B: Testing for Carcinogenicity of Pharmaceuticals, July 1997 [11].

This guideline describes the experimental approaches for the evaluation of carcinogenic potential of pharmaceuticals. This also outlines the necessity of two routine long-term rodent studies in rats and mice.

S1C: Dose Selection for Carcinogenicity Studies of Pharmaceuticals, March 1995 [12].

S1C (R): Addendum to Dose Selection for Carcinogenicity Studies of Pharmaceuticals: Addition of a Limit Dose and Related Notes, July 1997.

These guidelines address the issues of dose selection for long-term carcinogenicity studies.

Additionally the Center for Drug Evaluation and Research of the U.S. FDA in May 2002 issued the guidance *Carcinogenicity Protocol Submission*.

The basic scheme consists of a dose range-finding study, generally of 90 days' duration. Dose selection requires an in-depth knowledge of the pharmacology, repeated dose toxicology, toxicokinetics, and human pharmacokinetics of the test compound. All regulatory authorities recommend that a high dose be set with no mortality for the study period. There are six different methods for selection of high dose for range–finding studies: (1) toxicity based endpoints, (2) pharmacokinetic endpoints, (3) saturation of absorption, (4) pharmacodynamic endpoints, (5) maximum feasible dose, and (6) additional endpoints.

This is followed by two main studies—(a) long-term (2 year) study in rats and another long-term or short-term study that provides additional information that is not readily available from the first long-term study. This is either a long-term study in a second rodent species (e.g., mouse) or a short- or medium-term study in alternative models of carcinogenicity. There are four short- or medium-term transgenic models in common use: (1) activated oncogene (Tg.AC model), (2) activated oncogene (rasH2 model), (3) inactivated tumor suppressor gene ($p53^{+/-}$ model), and (4) inactivated DNA repair gene ($XPA^{-/-}$ model). The short-term studies can provide better answers for differences in the range of susceptible target tissues, in which tumors develop, and knowledge of a compounds' ADME profile for human risk assessment. There is a regulatory requirement for information on the assessment of systemic exposure to the parent compound and its metabolites [1]. For the toxicokinetic study, blood samples are collected from the caudal vein in the unanesthetized state from satellite animals (~5–10 per sex/group) at various time intervals such as 4, 12, 26, 52, and 103 weeks (morning and afternoon). These satellite animals are sacrificed after final sampling without any further investigation.

14.3.8 Reproductive Toxicity Studies

Although no specific guidance [1, 13] is available, regulatory authorities still expect toxicokinetic studies to be conducted on pregnant animals. The toxicokinetic data are generated for fertility studies in rats—embryo and fetal development. Reproductive toxicity studies became very important after the tragic thalidomide story, where the drug caused rare birth defects in pregnant women. The tragedy led to the passage of the Harris–Kefauver Amendment to the Federal Pure Food and Drug Act in the United States in 1962 to ensure that approved drugs have proof of safety and efficacy [14]. Data from nonpregnant animals is used to set the dose levels for the reproductive toxicity study. The toxicokinetic evaluation should be carried out in embryo–fetal studies at the beginning and end of gestation in the animal study. However, it can also be conducted in preliminary studies or in the main study with a satellite group of animals.

14.4 TOXICOKINETIC EVALUATION OF BIOPHARMACEUTICALS

The toxicokinetic assessment of biotechnology products is a difficult exercise. However, some information on the absorption, disposition, and clearance in relevant models is essential in order to predict safety prior to clinical investigation. Therefore, wherever possible, systemic exposure should be monitored during toxicity studies [1, 15]. The species difference in pharmacokinetics would help in assigning dose–response relationships in toxicity studies. Single- and multiple-dose pharmacokinetic, toxicokinetic, and tissue distribution studies have proved useful in the interpretation of safety data. However, mass balance studies may not yield useful results. A common problem encountered during the measurement of biotechnology products is the presence of neutralizing antibodies raised in animals against human proteins. The neutralizing antibodies alter the pharmacokinetic profile due to immune-mediated clearance and affect the interpretation of toxicity data. Some biotechnology products may exhibit a significant delay or prolongation in the expression of pharmacodynamic effect relative to pharmacokinetic profile/plasma levels. While measuring radioactivity it is important that the radiolabeled linkage is stable. The assessment of radioactivity becomes difficult due to rapid *in vivo* metabolism of radiolabel. Care should be taken in the interpretation of studies using radioactive tracers incorporated into specific amino acids because of recycling of amino acids into non-drug-related proteins/peptides. The biotech products are metabolized into small peptides and individual amino acids. Since the metabolic pathways are generally understood, classical biotransformation studies are not required. Selection of assay methods should be based on a proper understanding of the behavior of the biopharmaceutical in the biological matrix such as plasma, serum, whole blood, and cerebrospinal fluid. Protein binding is an important factor that can affect the assay. One quantitative assay should be sufficient, provided it is specific for the analyte, and the effect of plasma protein binding and antibodies on the assay should be predetermined.

14.5 FACTORS THAT AFFECT THE MEASUREMENT AND INTERPRETATION OF TOXICOKINETIC DATA

14.5.1 Measuring Unbound Versus Bound Drug

Plasma protein binding of a drug influences its pharmacokinetic parameters [16–23] (i.e., distribution, clearance, and elimination half-life) and pharmacodynamic parameters (i.e., efficacy and toxicity) [24]. A drug may bind to several components/macromolecules, for example, albumin, α1-acid glycoprotein (AGP), lipoproteins, immunoglobulins (IgG), and erythrocytes within the blood. The formation of a drug–protein complex is termed drug–protein binding. Most drugs bind to proteins in a reversible manner by means of weak chemical bonds such as ionic, van der Waals, hydrogen, and hydrophobic bonds with the hydroxyl, carboxyl, or other reversible sites available in the amino acids that constitute the protein chain. The major contribution to drug binding in the plasma is made by albumin [25], which is synthesized in the liver and constitutes about half of total plasma proteins. The molecular weight of albumin ranges between 65,000 and 69,000 daltons. Acidic drugs are known to bind strongly [25] to human serum albumin (HSA), which has two ligand-specific binding sites [26, 27], namely, site I and site II. The ligand selectivity is comparatively broader for these two sites, allowing a range of drug molecules to bind at these sites. This broad selectivity is considered to be a consequence of the significant allosteric effects in HSA [28] and drug molecules can also interact non-specifically with HSA. HSA is responsible for maintaining the osmotic pressure of the blood and is a carrier of many molecules [29], such as free fatty acids, bilirubin, and various hormones (e.g., cortisone, aldosterone, thyroxin).

α1-Acid glycoprotein (AGP) is a relatively low molecular weight (approximately 40,000 daltons) protein. Its concentration in plasma is about 40–100 mg/100 mL and primarily binds to basic (such as lidocaine, propranolol, imipramine, and quinidine) and neutral drugs [25] in addition to some acidic drugs [30]. In general, gyrase inhibitors [31] and NSAID (nonsteroidal anti-inflammatory drugs) [32] bind to albumin and antiretroviral compounds [33] bind to AGP. Binding of drugs to lipoproteins, red blood cells, and other membranes is not a true binding reaction but is similar to dissolving of the drugs in the lipids of the membrane. Very lipophilic drugs partition preferentially into the membrane lipids rather than the plasma water. Some drugs bind strongly to particular tissue components such as DNA (e.g., some anti-cancer drugs) and melanin-rich tissues (e.g., chloroquine, amiodarone).

Free drug concentration in plasma is responsible for the observed pharmacological effect or therapeutic response [34–36]. The drug bound to plasma protein is not available for distribution, hepatic metabolism, and renal elimination. The drug–protein complex does not permeate phospholipid bilayers, including capillary membranes, glomerular membranes in the nephrons, and the blood–brain barrier. Bound drugs are also less available to the cytochrome P450 and other enzymes involved in first-pass metabolism. The driving force for drug excretion in the kidney is the free drug concentration in the plasma. The glomerular capillaries permit the passage of free drug molecules but restrict the passage of plasma proteins and drug–protein complexes and, as a consequence, only free or unbound drug is filtered. After the metabolic and excretory processes have cleared much of the free drug, the reversible drug–protein complex serves as a depot to replenish the concentration *in vivo* [35]. Drugs with high protein binding tend to have a greater elimination half-life compared to those with low binding. The prolonged pharmacological activity resulting from these factors may be desirable or may promote the emergence of undesirable side effects. Therefore, estimation of the extent of drug–protein binding is crucial for clinical drug development. Ideally, determination of both total and unbound plasma drug concentrations is necessary to obtain an understanding of drug available for pharmacological effect.

In the past, several techniques have been explored for quantitative determination of drug–protein binding *in vitro*. Among those, equilibrium dialysis, gel filtration, ultrafiltration, and ultracentrifugation [31, 37–41] have been conventionally and most commonly used. These conventional methods suffer from long analysis time. Different *in vitro* methods yield different results; for example, equilibrium dialysis indicated 23% plasma protein binding for fleroxacin whereas ultrafiltration indicated 47% plasma protein binding [31]. A lot of interlaboratory variation in plasma protein binding data obtained via the same technique leading to a broad range for ciprofloxacin (20–40%), ofloxacin and norfloxacin (8–30%), and enoxacin (30–50%) [31] has been reported. Although the ultrafiltration method is believed to be comparable to *in vivo* processes, such as ultrafiltration of drug in the kidney [31], it still suffers from the limitation of nonspecific binding of the drug to the membrane and leakage of drug from the membrane.

In comparison to conventional methods, chromatography-based methods [37, 42–46] employing columns immobilized with plasma proteins have gained popularity over the years because of their simplicity, specificity, and speed.

14.5.2   Racemic Compound Versus Enantiomer

Enantiomers must be considered as essentially different chemical compounds, as they usually differ in their pharmacokinetic and pharmacodynamic properties due to stereoselective interaction with biological macromolecules. Early evaluation of stereoselective pharmacokinetics, pharmacodynamics, and toxicity of individual enantiomers is essential to decide whether to develop the racemate or an individual enantiomer. Absorption from the gastrointestinal tract, tissue distribution, and renal excretion are passive processes for most drugs, where the extent and rate are mainly governed by physiological properties of the drug. Since the physiological properties of stereoisomers are the same, stereoselectivity is not expected for these processes unless active transport is involved. On the contrary, stereoselective plasma protein binding and metabolism are common and well documented [47, 48]. In addition, both plasma protein binding and metabolism of different enantiomers are species specific due to structural differences in plasma proteins and drug metabolizing enzymes across species. The plasma protein binding of MK-571 [49] is extensive, stereoselective, and species dependent. The R enantiomer was bound to rat plasma to a greater extent as compared to the S enantiomer, whereas in dog and monkey the reverse was true [50]. The elimination of the enantiomers was directly related to plasma protein binding in a particular species and the unbound enantiomer was more rapidly cleared. Mephenytoin exhibits stereoselective metabolism, which is also species specific. In *in vitro* studies using liver microsomes [51], it was observed that the rate of 4-hydroxylation was twofold to sixfold higher for R enantiomer as compared to S enantiomer in rabbit, dog, and rat, whereas 4′-hydroxylation of S enantiomer was 5–15 times higher as compared to R enantiomer in human and monkeys. Similarly, the S enantiomer of propranolol had a higher intrinsic clearance in liver microsomes of dog as compared to R enantiomer. On the contrary, human microsomes exhibited higher clearance for R enantiomer [52]. Flurbiprofen, an aryl propionic acid NSAID, is marketed as a racemic compound. Its anti-inflammatory activity is believed to reside with the S enantiomer [53, 54]. *In vivo*, the R enantiomer gets irreversibly converted to the S enantiomer. The extent of this unidirectional conversion is 100% in guinea pigs, 40% in dog, and ~5% in rat, gerbil, and human [55, 56]. Ketoprofen, another 2-aryl propionic acid NSAID, also exhibits *in vivo* chiral inversion. The extent of inversion was high in rat [57], low in rabbit [58], and insignificant in human [48].

The large differences in pharmacokinetic profile of enantiomers result in stereoselective safety and efficacy. Thalidomide, the hypnotic that caused birth defects called phocomelia, was administered as a racemic compound, where both the enantiomers had equal sedating effect. After its withdrawal, studies in pregnant mice and rats revealed that the S enantiomer of thalidomide was teratogenic, whereas the R enantiomer was devoid of any such symptoms [59, 60]. Following intraperitoneal administration of S enantiomer (200 mg/kg/day) to pregnant animals, 30% of mice and 50% of rats had deformed fetuses; however, there was no deformity reported after the administration of R enantiomer. On the other hand, both R and S enantiomers were equally teratogenic in rabbit: 40% of deformed fetuses were recorded from pregnant rabbits that were administered racemic thalidomide, whereas 16–17% when R or S enantiomer was administered individually [61, 62]. Thalidomide is a stark example of stereoselective toxicity.

After the administration of a racemic drug, it becomes important to monitor the respective enantiomers *in vivo*. Development of a more potent and safer enantiomer instead of the racemic compound not only reduces the dose but also addresses the concerns of toxicity. For the racemic drug, it becomes important to demonstrate that the administered enantiomer is stable *in vivo* and does not get converted into the undesired enantiomer. In other words, a sensitive bioanalytical method for monitoring the *in vivo* chiral conversion of such a drug candidate during toxicokinetic analysis is desirable.

14.5.3   Nonlinear Dose Kinetics

When the dose of a drug is increased, we expect that the concentration at steady state will increase proportionately: that is, if the dose rate is increased or decreased, say, twofold, the plasma drug concentration will also increase or decrease twofold. This is known as linear dose kinetics or first-order kinetics. The rate constants of such models do not change with concentration in the body. However, for some drugs, the plasma drug concentration changes either more or less than would be expected from a change in dose rate. Such drugs do not obey first-order kinetics. In such cases, the first-order kinetics get transformed into a mixture of first-order and zero-order rate processes. This is known as nonlinear pharmacokinetic behavior and can cause problems when adjusting doses. For such drugs that behave nonlinearly within the therapeutic range (e.g., ascorbic acid and naproxen), it is difficult to predict the plasma concentrations achieved. Nonlinear kinetic behavior may occur due to various reasons, such as saturation of first-pass metabolism causing an increase in bioavailability; saturation of protein binding sites causing a change in fraction of drug unbound in plasma; saturation of elimination mechanisms causing a change in intrinsic clearance; and absorption being rate limited.

14.5.4   Measurement of Metabolites

Although the primary concern of toxicokinetics is to determine the plasma and tissue levels of the parent compound in the toxicology species, there are instances when measurement of metabolite concentrations in plasma or other body fluids may become essential for the conduct of toxicokinetic studies. For a "prodrug," the primary active metabolite is monitored. If the administered compound undergoes extensive metabolism, the measurement of plasma or tissue concentrations of a major metabolite is the only practical means of estimating exposure. The metabolites are also monitored in addition to the parent compound when the compound is metabolized to one or more pharmacologically or toxicologically active metabolites that could significantly contribute to pharmacological responses. Measurement of metabolites, however, cannot account for toxic reactive intermediate metabolites, which are known to cause idiosyncratic reactions.

14.5.5   Measurement of Produgs in Biological Fluids and Tissues

The term prodrug was first introduced by Albert in 1958 [63] to describe compounds that undergo *in vivo* biotransformation before exhibiting their pharmacological effect. Prodrugs are precursors of active principles that can be used to modify the pharmacokinetics of a drug. This may lead to improvement in bioavailability, increased drug stability, enhancement of patient acceptance, and compliance by minimizing taste and odor problems or elimination of pain on injection. Prodrugs do not possess any pharmacological effect, but their metabolite is pharmacologically active. Piva ampicillin, tala ampicillin, and baca ampicillin are ester prodrugs of ampicillin. The absorption of these prodrugs is complete as compared to 50% absorption of ampicillin [64, 65]. Enalapril, a prodrug of enaprilate, is a popular ACE inhibitor with an oral absorption of 100%, whereas the parent compound is poorly absorbed (~10%) [66, 67]. Acyclovir, a potent antiherpes drug, is poorly absorbed after oral administration. Deoxyacyclovir is the prodrug of acyclovir, which provides superior delivery of acyclovir [68–70]. γ-Glutamyldopa is a kidney-specific prodrug of levodopa [71], responsible for receptor-mediated vasodilation in the kidney. It is a precursor of the neurotransmitter dopamine, which plays an important role in the CNS. During the toxicokinetic evaluation of a prodrug, the analytical method should be sensitive enough to distinguish between the prodrug and the active metabolite in biological matrices of interest.

14.5.6   Measurement of Labile Reactive Metabolites

Following an oral administration in humans, the plasma levels of clopidogrel are extremely low due to extensive metabolism and are difficult to quantify. The active metabolite (thiol) is highly labile and remains undetected in plasma. The main circulating metabolite (carboxylic acid derivative) is pharmacologically inactive. Since the parent compound and the active metabolite cannot be detected, the estimation of the major inactive metabolite is the only way of assessing systemic exposure [72, 73]. The half-life of acetaminophen is two- to threefold longer in rat than in mouse, it is toxic in mice at a low dose of 200–300 mg/kg but well tolerated in rats up to a dose of 1500 mg/kg. The hepatotoxicity caused by acetaminophen is due to a reactive toxic metabolite, which is labile and too small in quantity to be detected in plasma [74]. Therefore, the parent compound and its sulfate conjugate are monitored *in vivo*, which is of little relevance in predicting hepatotoxicity.

14.5.7   Human Metabolites that Are Absent in Animal Models

Major metabolic differences between the animal and human studies reduce the confidence in toxicity studies as predictors of safety. A method of comparing *in vitro* metabolic profiles of various animal models with that of humans using recombinant liver microsomes and/or recombinant drug metabolizing enzymes [75] has recently come to the rescue of toxicologists. An early *in vitro* comparison of the metabolic profile of test species with humans helps in selecting the relevant animal models for the assessment of potential human risk.

14.5.8   Species Differences in Pharmacokinetics

Due to ethical reasons, the safety of all pharmaceutical drugs cannot be directly evaluated on humans but should be tested on rodents and nonrodents prior to approval for clinical investigation. The extrapolation of risk assessment from animal to human is a challenge, as it is far from straightforward to extrapolate animal toxicity to human toxicity. This is because the drug-induced toxicity is often species dependent and to date no single animal model resembles humans completely. Among rodents, there are vast differences in response to the same drug. Most common antibiotics are lethal in guinea pigs and hamsters but may be tolerated by mice, rats, and gerbils. Fleming had used the rat as the animal model for penicillin; had he used guinea pigs or hamsters in his research, the wonder drug would have been dropped at an early stage. When there is so much difference among various rodent species, one can imagine the amount of variability that could be expected between rodents and humans. Aspirin causes birth defects in most rodents but not in humans. Cortisone causes birth defects in mice but not in rats and humans. Aspartame, an artificial sweetener, has been shown to cause lymphoid cancer in rats, whereas there is no clear evidence of its toxicity in humans, and has been in use for a long time. A drug may cause cancer in development in certain animal species but not in humans and vice versa.

Acetaminophen caused hepatotoxicity [74] in mice at the low dose of 200–300 mg/kg but was tolerated in rats up to a high dose of 1500 mg/kg. In humans, it is well tolerated within the therapeutic range but is toxic at a high dose of 10–15 g (150–200 mg/kg). Dichloromethane, a common industrial chemical, causes lung and liver cancer in mice after chronic inhalation exposure but not in rats and hamsters under similar exposure [76]. Treatment with perfluoro decanoic acid, a potent peroxisome proliferator, led to the development of pronounced hepatomegaly in rats but not in guinea pigs [77]. The sulfonamide, sulfomethoxazole, produced thyroid nodules in rats at 50 mg/kg/day dose for 1 year, whereas rhesus monkeys treated with a higher dose (300 mg/kg/day) for the same time period exhibited no increase in thyroid weight and no morphological alterations [78].

Indomethacin, an anti-inflammatory agent used widely for the treatment of rheumatoid arthritis, caused ulcers in rats and dogs but not in humans [79].

Species differences in toxicity of a drug can be interpreted and explained in terms of species differences in the pharmacokinetics or ADME of a drug. Species differences in metabolism, which is the major cause of diversity, arise due to structural differences in drug metabolizing enzymes. Since drug-induced toxicity is directly related to systemic exposure to drug and its metabolites, the species differences in metabolism of the drug are perhaps the most important factor in explaining the observed differences in toxicity. The nucleotide and amino acid sequence of CYP450 varies in different species. Even small changes in the amino acid sequence can give rise to a large difference in substrate specificity [80]. Similarly, uridine diphosphoglucuronyl transferases (UDPGTs), responsible for glucuronidation, also exhibit species differences in structure. Comparison of 10 rat UDPGTs and 8 human UDPGTs showed that they have a common C terminal domain but the N terminal is quite variable. As a result, their substrate specificities are different, although they still have overlapping substrate specificities [81]. Carboxyl esterases hydrolyze drugs containing ester bonds and amide linkages. They exist as multiple isoforms and exhibit significant species differences in their activities. The carboxyl esterases across various species (i.e., mouse, hamster, rat, guinea pig, rabbit, and monkey) exhibit high homology in amino acid sequence but have different N terminal amino acids, resulting in different substrate specificity [82, 83].

A comparison of the *in vitro* metabolic profile of losartan, a potent nonpeptide angiotensin II receptor antagonist, in hepatic slices obtained from rat, monkey, and human provides clear evidence of species differences in metabolism [84]. Rat liver slices primarily oxidize losartan to monohydroxylated and carboxylic metabolites. Glucuronidation of tetrazole moiety predominated in monkey, whereas in human both the oxidized and glucuronidated metabolites were equally present.

The metabolic clearance of dihydropyridine calcium channel blockers amlodipine, felodipine, nicardine, nisoldipine, nitrendipine, and nilvadipine was compared in rat, dog, and human. For all the compounds, the metabolism in humans was quantitatively similar to dogs, whereas rats show a much higher capacity of metabolism [85]. Azidothymidine (AZT), an HIV reverse transcriptase inhibitor, is extensively metabolized in humans, but not in rats [86, 87]. Acetaminophen is primarily sulfated in rats but glucuronidation is more prominent in humans [88, 89]. There is a marked species difference in enzyme induction. For example, the gastric acid-suppressing drug omeprazole is a CYP1A2 enzyme inducer in humans but has no such inductive effect in mice or rabbits [90, 91]. Furthermore, members of the CYP3A subfamily in rats are inducible by the steroidal agent pregnenolone-16α-carbonitrile, but not by the antibiotic rifampin. The opposite is true in rabbits and humans [92, 93]. Therefore, the assumption that xenobiotics that do not induce drug-metabolizing enzymes in animal models would not induce human enzymes as well and vice versa is totally baseless. To overcome this drawback, both *in vitro* (human hepatocytes) and *in vivo* (probe drugs for certain human cytochrome P450s) techniques have become available and have increasingly been used by investigators to evaluate the potential induction of human cytochrome P450s by a variety of therapeutic agents. The above examples demonstrate that extrapolation of drug metabolism from animals to human is difficult, if not impossible.

14.5.9   Gender Differences in Pharmacokinetics

Sex-related differences in metabolism have been known for more than sixty years. Recent studies have shown that gender differences in xenobiotic metabolism are more pronounced in rat than any other species. Early studies designed to examine the mechanism of sex-dependent differences in response to specific barbiturates [94] demonstrated that female rats had higher and more prolonged serum concentration of parent compound due to lower rate of metabolism as compared with male rats. Female rats have 10–30% less total cytochrome P450 (CYP450) as compared to male rats. This explains why female rats in general metabolize many drugs and compounds more slowly than male rats. Cocaine, diazepam, hexobarbital, indinavir, morphine, phenobarbital, and tolbutamide are some of the drugs and chemicals that have a higher rate of metabolism in male rats as compared to female rats [95]. Although male rats generally have a higher rate of metabolism, there are instances where female rats exhibit a higher metabolic rate than males. There are sex-dependent differences in the expression of microsomal CYP isoforms, which could be attributed to the fact that the CYP isoforms are very different in male and female rats. Immunological data have shown that CYP2C11 is expressed only in male rats, whereas CYP2C12 expression is specific to female rats. CYP2A2 and CYP3A2 are male dominant whereas CYP2A1 and CYP2C7 are female dominant enzymes [96–99]. Sprague–Dawley rats treated with phenobarbital (1,3, or 20 mg/kg) for 6 days showed an increase in hexobarbital hydroxylase activity and aminopyrine N demethylation in hepatic microsomes prepared from male rats but not in those prepared from female rats [100]. Sex-dependent differences have also been observed in the expression of conjugative enzymes such as sulfotransferase, glutathione S transferases, and glucuronyl transferases [95]. In general, male rats have higher drug metabolizing enzyme activities than female rats. Sex-related differences in metabolism are not unique to rats but have been observed in mice [101], ferrets [102], dogs [103], and humans [104]. However, the magnitude of differences in these species is less pronounced as compared to rats.

After rat, xenobiotic metabolism has been best characterized in mouse. Sex-related differences in mice are often strain dependent [101]. Males have a high rate of metabolism in some strains while females have a high rate in other strains. In general, female mice more commonly have a higher rate of metabolism than males [101]. The magnitude of sex-dependent differences in metabolism is subtle compared to rats. For example, a male rat can have enzyme activities as much as fivefold greater than a female rat, whereas the greatest degree of difference in mice is twofold. Sex-dependent differences in the xenobiotic metabolism of rabbit has been reported in the flavine containing monooxygenase flavo proteins that oxidize nitrogen and sulfur containing compounds [105].

Indinavir, a potent HIV protease inhibitor, exhibits sex-related differences in clearance in rats and dogs but not in monkeys and humans. Rats exhibited a clearance of 89 mL/min/kg for male and 41 mL/min/kg for female. Dogs exhibited just the opposite trend, with higher rate of clearance in female dogs (26 mL/min/kg) as compared to male dogs (15 mL/min/kg) [106]. The *in vitro* liver microsome data was consistent with the *in vivo* data, where male rats had substantially higher metabolizing activity toward indinavir as compared to female rats. Hepatic microsomes from female dogs exhibited a higher metabolic rate than male dogs. Monkey and human liver microsomes exhibited no differences in the metabolism of indinavir. The functional activity of CYP3A when measured in liver microsomes exhibited significant gender differences in rat and dog [106].

In general, when sex-dependent differences in pharmacokinetics of xenobiotics are observed in humans, females have higher plasma concentrations compared to males. This difference has been reported with drugs like acetaminophen, aspirin, chlorophenicol, diazepam, lidocaine, mephobarbital, nortriptyline, oxazepam, propranolol, rifampicin, and tetracycline [95]. Unlike the rat, the sex-related differences in the pharmacokinetics in humans are not related to differences in CYP isoforms. This lack of sex-dependent isoform in humans indicates that the rat, the most popular animal model so far, is not an accurate model for prediction of sex-dependent pharmacokinetic differences in humans. Furthermore, these differences in humans are not as significant as those in rodents. In humans, interindividual differences in metabolism due to genetic polymorphism outweigh any differences regulated by sex-related factors [104]. Therefore, metabolism is not the sole factor for the gender differences in humans: the basic differences in physiology and body composition are responsible for it.

Absorption of certain drugs from the gastrointestinal tract may be affected by the fact that both gastric acid secretion and gastric emptying are lower in women as compared to men [107]. The difference in rates of gastric absorption cause men to achieve peak sodium salicylate plasma concentration more quickly than women. Moreover, the volume of distribution of certain drugs can be affected by the fact that lean body mass is greater in men while adipose tissue content is greater in women [107]. For example, intramuscular injection of drugs is handled differently between men and women because of sex differences in the differences of gluteal fat. Because of this, lipophilic chemicals can have a greater volume of distribution in woman as compared to men. Hormonal regulation also plays a role in metabolism in humans and the manipulation of normal levels of circulating steroid hormones can alter the way men and women metabolize xenobiotics. There is evidence that the phase of a woman's menstrual cycle can affect the pharmacokinetics of a number of xenobiotics by altering their distribution and clearance. There are changes in gastric emptying rate and acidity of stomach contents at about day 14 of a 28 day menstrual cycle. As progesterone rises, ovulation increases the gastric emptying rate and the secretion of acid in the stomach. Therefore, the bioavailability of a compound may change depending on the phase of a woman's menstrual cycle. The phase of the menstrual cycle has also been shown to affect the volume of distribution and half-life of various drugs, including diazepam and acetaminophen [108].

14.5.10   Interpretation of Drug Plasma Concentrations

Higher plasma concentration in the later stage of a repeated dose toxicokinetic study is caused by the accumulation of drug. The accumulation of drug occurs due to long plasma half-life, reduced clearance, inhibition of drug metabolizing enzymes, or enterohepatic recirculation. Clearance can be affected by impaired hepatic function or capacity-limited elimination. Lower plasma concentrations at a later stage of a study as compared to initial levels could be related to high first-pass metabolism or autoinduction of drug metabolizing enzymes. At times low plasma concentrations may be interpreted as no accumulation but exceptionally high drug levels may be present in the tissues. Therefore, toxicokinetic evaluation should be carried out after careful comparison of both plasma and tissue levels. Lack of dose proportionality occurs due to either autoinduction of drug metabolizing enzymes or saturation of mechanisms such as intestinal absorption, enzyme metabolizing systems, and tubular reabsorption.

14.5.11   Choice of Biological Fluid

Plasma is the most common matrix of choice. The less common ones are serum, whole blood, or cerebrospinal fluid. Whole blood estimation is generally carried out for compounds that tend to accumulate in blood cells. CNS drugs are monitored in cerebrospinal fluid.

14.5.12   Combination Drugs May Cause Drug–Drug Interactions

Marketed drugs that are intended for combination therapy need special toxicokinetic evaluation for possible drug–drug interactions. Pharmacokinetic drug interactions are consequences of altered levels of exposure to the drugs or its metabolites through one or more of the following mechanisms: altered absorption by chelation or complex formation, altered distribution due to the competition of two coadministered drugs for the same plasma protein binding site, altered transport inhibition of transporter proteins, induction and/or inhibition of CYP450, altered drug excretion because of competition for renal anion or cation transport systems, changes in urinary pH, or inhibition of renal metabolism. Among these, "inhibition" and 'induction' of cytochrome P450 is of prime importance and should be extensively explored in the preclinical stage, as they have been known to be notoriously associated with the withdrawal of several drugs (suruvidine, terfinadine, mibefradil, astemizole, cisapride, levacetylmethadol, cerivastatin, and repaglinide) in the past.

When administered in combination, the drug metabolizing enzymes, especially cytochrome P450, may be transcriptionally activated or induced by one of the drugs, resulting in increased production of the enzyme. The pharmacological consequences of enzyme induction could lead to faster metabolism, reduced efficacy, and/or formation of toxic metabolites, resulting in treatment failure and/or toxicity of drugs, which is the basis of undesirable drug–drug interactions. Evaluation of drug–drug interactions in animal models is less relevant due to the structural differences in the drug metabolizing enzymes across species. For instance, omeprazole induces CYP1A2 in humans but not in mice and rabbits [90, 91]. Rifampicin induces CYP3A in human and rabbit but not in rat. Pregnenolone-16-α-carbonitrile induces rat CYP3A but not human [92, 93].

When the enzyme responsible for metabolizing a drug is inhibited by the coadministered drug, there is usually an increased plasma concentration of the former, which may lead to toxicity—another major reason of drug–drug interaction. The enzyme inhibition potential of drugs also differs across species. For instance, furafylline is a more potent inhibitor of phenacetin O-deethylation catalyzed by CYP1A2 in humans as compared to rats [109]. Quinidine is a more potent inhibitor of debrisoquine 4-hydroxylation in humans than in rats [110]. To overcome these obstacles, the enzyme inductive or inhibitory potential of combination drugs should first be evaluated *in vitro* on recombinant enzymes from human and relevant animal species [75]. If the *in vitro* enzyme inductive or inhibitory effect of the animal model is comparable to humans, only then should an *in vivo* study be designed. *In vitro* drug interaction studies should be conducted at concentrations similar to those attained *in vivo*.

Drugs that are metabolized by more than one drug metabolizing enzyme generally have a decreased likelihood of clinically significant drug interactions due to the availability of compensatory metabolic pathways if one is inhibited. Drug interactions are likely to be particularly important when the elimination of a drug occurs primarily through a single metabolic pathway, the drug is a potent inhibitor or inducer of a drug metabolizing enzyme, one or both of the interacting drugs have a steep dose–response curve, one or both of the interacting drugs have a narrow therapeutic range, inhibition of the primary metabolic enzyme or induction of a secondary metabolic enzyme results in diversion of the drug into an alternative pathway that generates a metabolite having toxic or modified pharmacodynamic activity, the drug has nonlinear pharmacokinetics, or the interaction results in conversion from linear to nonlinear pharmacokinetics.

14.6 TOXICOKINETICS AND GOOD LABORATORY PRACTICE (GLP)

There are two main guidelines of GLP.

14.6.1 Overview of Federal Register (21 CFR Part 58)

In 1976, the FDA proposed GLP guidelines; they were finalized in 1978 and became effective in 1979. The GLP guidelines continue to evolve with additional changes made in September 1987 and updates in April 2006.

The FDA GLP guidelines are divided into nine subparts, dealing with general provisions, organization and personnel, facilities, equipment, testing facility operations, test and control articles, protocol for and conduct of a nonclinical laboratory study, records and reports, and disqualification of testing facilities.

21 CFR PART 58
Subpart A—General Provisions
        58.1 Scope
        58.3 Definitions
        58.10 Applicability to studies performed under grants and contracts
        58.15 Inspection of a testing facility
Subpart B—Organization and Personnel
        58.29 Personnel
        58.31 Testing facility management
        58.33 Study director
        58.35 Quality assurance unit
Subpart C—Facilities
        58.41 General
        58.43 Animal care facilities
        58.45 Animal supply facilities
        58.47 Facilities for handling test and control articles
        58.49 Laboratory operation areas
        58.51 Specimen and data storage facilities
Subpart D—Equipment
        58.61 Equipment design
        58.63 Maintenance and calibration of equipment
Subpart E—Testing Facilities Operation
        58.81 Standard operating procedures
        58.83 Reagents and solutions
        58.90 Animal care
Subpart F—Test and Control Articles
        58.105 Test and control article characterization
        58.107 Test and control article handling
        58.113 Mixture of articles with carriers
Subpart G—Protocol for and Conduct of a Nonclinical Laboratory Study
        58.120 Protocol
        58.130 Conduct of a nonclinical laboratory study
Subparts H, I—[Reserved]
Subpart J—Records and Reports
        58.185 Reporting of nonclinical laboratory study results
        58.190 Storage and retrieval of records and data
        58.195 Retention of records

Subpart K—Disqualification of Testing Facilities

Subpart A—General Provisions   This part prescribes the scope of good laboratory practices for conducting nonclinical laboratory studies that support or are intended to support applications for research or marketing permits for products regulated by the Food and Drug Administration, including food and color additives, animal food additives, human and animal drugs, medical devices for human use, biological products, and electronic products. The Definitions describe the meaning of certain terms used in the regulation such as Act, Test Article, Control Article, Nonclinical Laboratory Study, Sponsor, Testing Facility, Application for Research or Marketing Permit, Person, Test System, Specimen, Raw Data, Quality Assurance Unit, Study Director, Batch, Study Initiation Date, and Study Completion Date.

Applicability to studies performed under grants and contract fall under the provision of this regulation. An authorized FDA employee can inspect a laboratory's facility, records, and specimens at any time and without warning.

Subpart B—Organization and Personnel   Each personnel engaged in the conduct of or responsible for supervision of a study must possess appropriate education, training, and experience to perform the assigned tasks; the education, training and experience must be documented. Job descriptions must be available and current for each individual. The laboratory must have available the appropriate number of personnel required to perform each task as stated in the standard operating procedures (SOPs). Personnel must take all necessary precautions to avoid contamination of any testing materials.

The management of the laboratory testing facility must designate a study director; create a quality assurance unit; assure that test materials are assayed as required; make available personnel, resources, facilities, equipment, materials, and methodologies as scheduled; assure that the testing personnel clearly understand their duties; and assure that any deviations from protocols and SOPs are communicated, corrected, and documented.

The study director has the overall responsibility for the conduct of the study and is the single point of study control. The responsibilities of the study director include assuring that the protocol is approved and followed, all data are recorded and verified, unforeseen circumstances are noted and corrective action is taken and documented, test systems are specified in the protocol, GLP is followed, and documentation is archived.

GLP regulations mandate that the testing facility has a QA (Quality Assurance) unit that is separate from and independent of the personnel engaged in the conduct and direction of each study. The duties of the QA unit are extensive and include monitoring each study; assuring that the facility, equipment, personnel, methods, practices, records, and controls conform to GLP; maintaining a master schedule of duties being performed; maintaining copies of all protocols; periodically completing internal audits and submitting status reports, which include descriptions of problems noted and any corrective actions; submitting written status reports to management and the study director; ensuring no deviations occur from the approved protocols or SOPs without appropriate authorization and documentation; reviewing the final study reports; enclosing the QA report in the final study report; and preparing and maintaining QA SOPs and making documentation available for regulatory inspections.

Subpart C—Facilities   Each testing facility should be of suitable size and construction to facilitate the proper conduct of nonclinical laboratory studies. A separate laboratory operations area is needed. Storage space to archive specimens and data must be adequate. To avoid contamination and mix-ups between test and control articles, separate areas are needed for receipt, storage, and preparation of materials and the storage of products.

Subpart D—Equipment   GLP regulation mandates that equipment used in the generation, measurement, or assessment of data and equipment used for facility environmental control should be of appropriate design and adequate capacity to function according to the protocol and should be suitably located for operation, inspection, cleaning, and maintenance. Detailed written SOPs are needed for each instrument. All instrumentation must be adequately operated, inspected, cleaned, maintained, tested, calibrated, and standardized. Equipment performance, use, and maintenance are documented.

Subpart E—Testing Facilities Operation   A testing facility should have standard operating procedures in writing setting forth nonclinical laboratory study methods that management is satisfied are adequate to ensure the quality and integrity of the data generated in the course of a study. All deviations in a study from standard operating procedures should be authorized by the study director and should be documented in the raw data. Significant changes in established standard operating procedures should be properly authorized in writing by management. The GLP SOP states exactly how the procedure is to be done each time, every time. The SOPs must be current, clearly written, and immediately available to the staff, adhered to and authorized. A historical file of SOPs is maintained. The regulations list those procedures requiring SOPs.

All reagents and solutions in the laboratory areas should be labeled to indicate identity, titer or concentration, storage requirements, and expiration date. Deteriorated or outdated reagents and solutions should not be used.

There should be standard operating procedures for the housing, feeding, handling, and care of animals. Detailed guidelines governing animal care are mentioned in the regulation.

Subpart F—Test and Control Articles   Test and control materials are handled in such a way as to ensure receipt documentation, proper identification, appropriate storage, and adequate distribution processes to avoid contamination, deterioration, or damage. For each batch of test and control materials, the identity, strength, purity, composition, and stability must be determined and documented. Methods of synthesis for the materials are documented. Each batch is labeled with the material name, CAS number, batch number, and expiration date and storage conditions. If test or control articles are mixed with carriers, the uniformity, concentration, stability, and expiration date of the mixture must be determined.

Subpart G—Protocol for and Conduct of a Nonclinical Laboratory Study   Each study should have an approved written protocol that clearly indicates the objectives and all methods for the conduct of the study. A minimum applicable requirement of study protocol is described in the regulation. All changes in or revisions of an approved protocol and the reasons thereof should be documented, signed by the study director, dated, and maintained with the protocol.

The nonclinical laboratory study should be conducted in accordance with the protocol and documented accordingly. All data generated during the conduct of a nonclinical laboratory study, except those that are generated by automated data collection systems, should be recorded directly, promptly, and legibly in ink. All data entries should be dated on the date of entry and signed or initialed by the person entering the data. Any change in entries should be made so as not to obscure the original entry, should indicate the reason for such change, and should be dated and signed or identified at the time of the change.

Subpart H and I—[Reserved]

Subpart J—Records and Reports   The testing laboratory's final report must state the laboratory's name and address, the start and end dates of the study, the objectives and procedures of the protocol, statistical methods used, and the identification of test and control articles.

The final report should be signed and dated by the study director. Corrections or additions to a final report should be in the form of an amendment by the study director. The amendment should clearly identify that part of the final report that is being added to or corrected and the reasons for the correction or addition, and should be signed and dated by the person responsible.

Archiving is an assigned responsibility because access to the archives is restricted to authorized personnel only. Archiving must be timely and all archived data are indexed to permit expedient retrieval.

Subpart K—Disqualification of Testing Facilities   This part of the regulation describes the purpose and grounds for disqualification of a nonclinical testing facility. An opportunity for hearing on disqualification should be provided, followed by a final order for disqualification. Once a testing facility has been disqualified, each application for a research or marketing permit, whether approved or not, containing or relying on any nonclinical laboratory study conducted by the disqualified testing facility may be examined to determine whether such study was or would be essential to a decision.

A testing facility that has been disqualified may be reinstated as an acceptable source of nonclinical laboratory studies, to be submitted to the Food and Drug Administration if the Commissioner determines, upon an evaluation of the submission of the testing facility, that the facility can adequately assure that it will conduct future nonclinical laboratory studies in compliance with the good laboratory practice regulations set forth in this part and, if any studies are currently being conducted, that the quality and integrity of such studies have not been seriously compromised.

14.6.2 Overview of OECD Principles of GLP

The OECD published GLP principles in 1981. These were readily accepted by 30 member industrial countries including the European Union, the United States, and Japan. As a result, it became popular internationally. The OECD guidelines are on the same lines of 21 CFR Part 58. The document has been divided into two sections. Section I gives the introduction to GLP principles. It consists of a preface, scope, and definitions of important terms. Section II describes GLP principles.

Section I

Scope   The principles of GLP are applicable to the testing of chemicals for characterizing their properties and assessing their safety with respect to human safety.

Definition of Terms   This section defines important terms concerning the organization of the test facility, the study, and test substances. The term "GLP is concerned with the organizational process and the conditions under which laboratory studies are planned performed, monitored, recorded and reported." The "test facility" means persons, premises, and operational units that are necessary for conducting the study. Study director, quality assurance program, standard operating procedures, and sponsor are some of the important terms concerning the organization of a facility.

The term "study" has been defined as an experiment or a set of experiments in which a test substance is examined to obtain data on its properties and/or its safety with respect to human health and the environment. The other important terms related to the study are study plan, OECD test guidelines, test system, specimen, and raw data. "Raw data" means all original laboratory records and documentation or verified copies thereof, which are the result of original observations and activities in a study. As per the OECD definition, "test substance" is a chemical substance or a mixture that is under investigation. The other important terms concerning the test system are reference standard, batch, vehicle, and sample.

Section II   Section II has been further subdivided into 10 subsections: (1) test facility organization and personnel, (2) quality assurance program, (3) facilities, (4) apparatus, material, and reagents, (5) test systems, (6) test and reference substances, (7) standard operating procedures, (8) performance of the study, (9) reporting of study results, and (10) storage and retention of records and material.

Test Facility Organization and Personnel   This section of OECD principles of GLP describes the responsibilities of management, the study director, and personnel. It is the responsibility of management to ensure that the principles of GLP are complied with in a test facility.

The management must designate a study director, establish a quality assurance unit, and assign personnel responsible for managing the archives. It should appoint a sufficient number of qualified personnel and provide appropriate facilities, equipment, and material. The management should ensure that the persons involved in the study are properly trained and the records of their qualification, training experience, and job description are maintained. It should ensure that all safety and health precautions are taken as per national regulations. It should also ensure that appropriate SOPs are established and followed, and amendments to the study plan are agreed upon and documented. It is also the responsibility of management to maintain copies of the study plan and historical files of SOPs.

The study director is an individual responsible for the overall technical conduct of the study, including interpretation, analysis, documentation, report generation, archiving of documents/reports, and GLP compliance. The study director should ensure that the study is conducted in accordance with the study plan. The study plan is a document that defines the entire scope of the study. It is the director's responsibility to see that any amendment/modification is done after proper authorization and is documented, stating the reason for the change. The study director is supposed to sign the final report in order to certify the validity of data and GLP compliance.

The personnel conducting the study are expected to follow safety precautions in the laboratory and handle hazardous chemicals cautiously. They should ensure health precautions as well to minimize risk to themselves and integrity of the study. Diseased and sick personnel likely to have an adverse effect on the study should be excluded from the study or a particular sensitive operation.

Quality Assurance (QA) Program   The QA program is an internal control system designed to ascertain that the study is in compliance with the principles of GLP. This subsection deals with the general description of a quality program and the responsibilities of QA personnel. The QA program ensures that the studies performed conform to the principles of GLP. QA personnel are independent entities designated directly by the management and are expected to be familiar with the test procedures. They are supposed to report their observations directly to the management and the study director.

QA personnel should ensure that the study plan and standard operating procedures (SOPs) are accessible to the study personnel and should conduct frequent inspections of the facility and audit the study in progress to ensure that the study plan and SOPs are being adhered to. Proper documentation and records of the inspections and/or audits should be maintained by the QA unit. Any unauthorized deviation from the final plan or SOPs should be immediately brought to the attention of the study director. The QA unit should review the final report to assure that the methods, procedures, and observations are correct and that the reported results are in agreement with the raw data generated during the study. The final report should contain a statement prepared and signed by the QA unit, specifying the dates of inspection and dates of findings reported to the management and study director.

Facilities   In general, it is required that the test facility should be of a suitable size, construction, and location to meet the study requirements. The design of the study should allow separation of different activities to avoid cross contamination and mix-ups and in turn preserve the integrity of the study. The facilities can be categorized into test system facilities, facilities for handling test and reference substances, archive facilities, and waste disposal facilities. The test system facilities should have enough rooms or separate areas to allow isolation of various test systems based on species, strain, and individual projects involving biohazardous substances. The health of the test system is an important aspect that can affect the outcome of the study, and therefore it is mandatory for the test facility to have separate areas for diagnosis, treatment, and control of disease in test systems.

There should be separate storage areas for supplies and equipment. Perishable materials should be kept under refrigeration. The storage areas should be distinctly separated from animal housing areas to prevent contamination and infestation.

It has been recommended that the test and reference substance should be isolated from the test system housing area and should be such that their identity, purity, concentration, and stability are maintained. There should be a provision for safe storage of hazardous substances. The facility should have a separate archival area for the purpose of retrieval of raw data, reports, and specimens.

The waste should be handled and disposed of in such a manner that the ongoing studies are not affected in any way. The waste disposal procedures should be consistent and meet regulatory requirements. This would include provision for collection, storage, and disposal facilities and decontamination and transportation procedures. The waste disposal/ handling activities should be properly documented and records maintained.

Apparatus, Material, and Reagents   The apparatus used for analysis and data generation should be of suitable design and capacity and appropriately located. There should be a system of periodic calibrations, maintenance, and performance checks of all the apparatus and proper records should be maintained. These procedures should be written down in the form of SOPs. All reagents should be properly labeled indicating the source, identity, concentration, date of preparation, expiration date, and storage conditions.

Test Systems   Any animal, plant, microbial, or other cellular, subcellular, chemical, or physical system or a combination used in the study is referred to as the test system. Test systems have broadly been categorized into physical/chemical and biological test systems. The physical or chemical data generation should be performed using well calibrated apparatus of appropriate design and capacity. The integrity of physical and chemical test systems should be verified against a highly pure reference substance. Biological systems should be housed and cared for under appropriate conditions in accordance with national regulatory requirements for the import, collection, care, and use of animals. There should be a systematic health checkup program for newly arrived systems, until which time they should be kept in isolation. If the newly arrived animals are diseased or exhibit unusual mortality or morbidity, they should be destroyed as per regulatory guidelines. Upon new arrival of animals, the source, date of arrival, and health condition upon arrival should be documented and records maintained. For obtaining reliable data, the test system should be properly acclimatized prior to study initiation. The containers housing the test systems should bear all information related to the identity of the test systems. The diagnosis and treatment of any disease before or during the study should be properly documented.

Test and Reference Substances   A test substance is a chemical substance or a mixture under investigation. A reference substance is any well defined chemical substance or any mixture other than the test substance used to provide a basis for comparison with the test substance. Proper records of characterization, date of receipt, quantity received, and consumption should be maintained after the receipt of the substance. The procedures for handling, sampling, and storage of these substances should be laid down in relevant SOPs so as to maintain the homogeneity and stability of the substances and avoid possible contamination and mix-ups. The storage container should be labeled with the information on identity, expiration date, and storage conditions. The characterization of each substance should be done with respect to code, name, and chemical abstract number (CAS). The reference substance used in each study should also have a known identity, batch number, purity, composition, and concentration. The stability of both the test and reference substances along with the storage conditions should be known. The stability and homogeneity of the formulation in the vehicle should be established before the initiation of a study. Here the vehicle is an agent that serves as a carrier used to mix, disperse, or solubilize the test or reference substance to facilitate the administration to the test system.

Standard Operating Procedures   Standard operating procedures (SOPs) are written procedures that describe how to perform certain routine laboratory tests or activities normally not specified in detail in study plans or guidelines. In order to ensure the quality and integrity of data, each test facility should have written SOPs approved by management. The SOPs should be immediately available in each laboratory. Published textbooks, articles, and journals may be used as supplements to these SOPs. In general, the written approved SOPs are required in the following areas:

a. Receipt, identification, labeling, handling, sampling, and storage of test and reference substances.
b. Use, maintenance, cleaning, calibration of measuring apparatus, and preparation of reagents.
c. Coding of studies, data collection, report preparation, indexing systems, handling of data including computerized data systems are some important SOPs in the area of record keeping, reporting, storage, and retrieval of data.
d. Test systems should have SOPs on (1) room preparation and environmental room conditions for the test system; (2) procedures for receipt, transfer, proper placement, characterization, identification, and care of test system; (3) test system preparation, observations, and examinations, before, during, and at termination of the study; (4) handling of test system individuals found moribund or dead during the study; (5) collection, identification, and handling of specimens including necropsy and histopathology.
e. Operation of quality assurance personnel in performing and reporting study audits, inspections, and final study report reviews.

    f. SOPs on health and safety precautions as required by national and/or international legislation or guidelines.

Performance of the Study   This section has been divided into study plan, content of study plan, and conduct of study.

The study plan is a document that defines the entire scope of the study. It should be written before the initiation of a study and retained as raw data. It should contain all changes, modifications, and revisions including justifications as agreed to, signed and dated by the study director.

The study plan should consist of the following minimum information:

    a. The study should be identified by a descriptive title and a statement that reveals the nature and purpose of the study and the test substance and reference substance should be identified by code or name (IUPAC, CAS number, etc.).

    b. Name and address of the sponsor, test facility, and study director.

    c. The date of agreement to the study plan by signature of the study director and, when appropriate, of the sponsor and/or the test facility management along with the proposed starting and completion dates.

    d. Test methods should have reference to OECD test guidelines or other test guidelines to be used.

    e. Study plan should address issues (where applicable) such as the justification for selection of the test system, characterization of the test system, such as the species, strain, substrain, source of supply, number, body weight range, sex, age, and other pertinent information.

    f. It should also contain the method of administration, and the reason for its choice, the dose levels and/or concentration(s), frequency, duration of administration, detailed information on the experimental design, including a description of the chronological procedure of the study, all methods, materials, and conditions, type and frequency of analysis, measurements, observations, and examinations to be performed.

    g. A list of records to be retained.

Each study should be identified by a separate identification number and all study items should bear this number. The study should be conducted as per the previously compiled and approved study plan. The raw data should be entered directly, promptly, and accurately and legibly signed or initialed and dated by study personnel. The changes or corrections in the raw data should be made in such a way that the previous entry is not obscured. A reason for the change must be indicated along with the date and signature of the person making the change. The data generated directly into the computer should also indicate the person responsible for data input. Corrections in such case should be entered separately with the reason for change and the date and identity of the individual making the change.

Reporting of Study Results   The study results should be compiled in the form of a final report, which is signed and dated by the study director. If reports from principal scientists from various disciplines are included in the final report, they should be signed and dated by them. Corrections can be made in the final report in the form of amendments clearly specifying the reason for the change and signed and dated by the study director and principal scientists.

The final report should contain the following minimum information:

1. Identification of the Study and the Test and Reference Substances
   (a) A descriptive title
   (b) Identification of the test substance by code or name (IUPAC, CAS number, etc.)
   (c) Identification of the reference substance by chemical name
   (d) Characterization of the test substance including purity, stability, and homogeneity
2. Information Concerning the Test Facility
   (a) Name and address
   (b) Name of the study director
   (c) Name of other principal personnel having contributed reports to the final report
3. Dates
   (a) Dates on which the study was initiated and completed
4. Statement
   (a) A quality assurance statement certifying the dates inspections were made and any findings were reported to management and to the study director
5. Description of Materials and Test Methods
   (a) Description of methods and materials used
   (b) Reference to OECD test guidelines or other test guidelines
6. Results
   (a) A summary of results
   (b) All information and data required in the study plan
   (c) A presentation of the results, including calculations and statistical methods
   (d) An evaluation and discussion of the results and, where appropriate, conclusions
7. Storage
   (a) The location where all samples, specimens, raw data, and the final report are to be stored

Storage and Retention of Records and Material   The archive should be equipped to securely store the study plan, raw data, final report, records of laboratory inspection and study audits, samples, and specimens. All archived materials should be indexed to ensure orderly storage and rapid retrieval. Movement of material into and out of the archive should be properly recorded and only persons authorized by management should have access to the archive.

14.7   SELECTION AND EXTRAPOLATION OF DOSE

14.7.1   Dose Levels

Dose levels for repeated dose studies are largely governed by toxicological findings in dose range-finding studies. Toxicokinetics is generally conducted at three dose levels [1]—low dose, intermediate dose, and high dose.

> *Low Dose Level.* This is preferably the "no toxic effect" dose or "no observed adverse effect" dose level. At this dose pharmacological response is observed but no adverse effect is observed. Here the exposure in animal models should ideally be equal to or just exceed the maximum exposure in human patients.
>
> *Intermediate Dose Level.* Exposure at the intermediate dose level should normally represent an appropriate multiple or fraction of exposure of lower or higher dose level.
>
> *High Dose Level.* This is the highest dose that is chosen with the aim of inducing toxic effects but no mortality or severe suffering. There may be certain dose-related constraints in choosing the high dose. The toxicokinetic data may indicate that the absorption of the compound limits exposure. Under these circumstances, it should be ensured that absorption is the rate-limiting step and not increased clearance. Hence, the lowest dose producing maximum exposure should be considered as the highest dose. The limits for acceptable volumes [7] that can be administered to animals at times constrain the dose levels for solutions and suspensions.

14.7.2   Interspecies Scaling: Extrapolation of Dose

The ultimate aim of interspecies scaling of dose is to derive the maximum recommended starting dose (MRSD) for "first in human" studies. The U.S. FDA guidance [111] for "estimating safe starting dose in clinical trials for therapeutics in adult healthy volunteers" describe sit as a five step process:

> *Step 1.* No observed adverse effect level (NOAEL) determination.
> *Step 2.* Human equivalent dose (HED) calculation.
> *Step 3.* Most appropriate species selection.
> *Step 4.* Application of safety factor.
> *Step 5.* Consideration of the pharmacologically active dose (PAD).

NOAEL is the highest dose level achieved in an animal toxicity study that dose not produce a significant increase in adverse effect. The NOAEL is generally the accepted benchmark for safety and serves as a starting point for the calculation of a safe starting human dose, which is subsequently converted to HED. It is a usual assumption that after systemic administration of therapeutics to animals, toxic endpoints such as maximum tolerated dose (MTD) and NOAEL scale well between various species when doses are normalized to body surface area (mg/m^2). The following equation is applied for interspecies scaling:

$$HED = \text{Animal NOAEL} \times (W_{\text{animal}}/W_{\text{human}})^{1-b}$$

The derivation of the above equation is not within the scope of this chapter and is reported elsewhere [111]. Conventionally, for body surface area (mg/m²), normalization of the value of the allometric exponent b would be 0.67 as originally derived by Freireich et al. [112] and Schein et al. [113]. Although subsequent analysis showed that $W^{0.75}$ was a better normalization factor, the use of body surface area ($W^{0.67}$) and normalization to body surface area has remained a widespread practice for extrapolation of animal dose to humans. The guidance document recommends the conversion of NOAEL dose to HED based on the body surface area correction factor $W^{0.67}$ for selection of a starting dose in initial studies on healthy human volunteers. An analysis conducted to address the effect of body weight on actual body surface area correction factor (BSA CF) demonstrated that it provides a reasonable estimate of HED over a broad range of human and animal weights. Table 14.2 shows the standard interspecies conversion factors as recommended by the CDER and CBER. Any deviation from the body surface area approach needs a proper justification. An alternative approach for determining initial clinical dose would be the use of animal pharmacokinetics and modeling rather than body surface area. However, in the initial stages of an IND study, animal data are not sufficient to construct a scientifically valid model. There are occasions when scaling based on body weight (mg/kg)

TABLE 14.2 Conversion of Animal Doses to Human Equivalent Doses (HEDs) Based on Body Surface Area

Species	To Convert Animal Dose in mg/kg to Dose in mg/m², Multiply by	To Convert Animal Dose in mg/kg to HED[a] in mg/kg, either:	
		Divide Animal Dose by	Multiply Animal Dose by
Human	37	—	—
Mouse	3	12.3	0.08
Hamster	5	7.4	0.13
Rat	6	6.2	0.16
Ferret	7	5.3	0.19
Guinea pig	8	4.6	0.22
Rabbit	12	3.1	0.32
Dog	20	1.8	0.54
Primates			
Monkeys[b]	12	3.1	0.32
Marmoset	6	6.2	0.16
Squirrel monkey	7	5.3	0.19
Baboon	20	1.8	0.54
Micro-pig	27	1.4	0.73
Mini-pig	35	1.1	0.95

[a]Assumes 60 kg human. For species not listed or for weights outside the standard ranges, human equivalent dose can be calculated from the formula:

$$HED = (\text{Animal dose in mg/kg}) \times (\text{Animal weight in kg/human weight in kg})^{0.33}.$$

[b]For example, cynomolgus, rhesus, and stumptail.

instead of body surface area may be appropriate. In order to consider mg/kg scaling, the available data should show that NOAEL occurs at a similar dose across species. If only two NOAELs from toxicity studies in separate species are available, one of the following criteria should be met:

1. After oral dose administration, the dose is limited by local toxicity.
2. The toxicity in humans is dependent on the exposure parameter (i.e., C_{max}) that is highly correlated with dose across species.
3. Other pharmacological and toxicological endpoints such as MTD and lowest lethal dose also scale between species by mg/kg.

However, mg/kg scaling gives a 12-, 6-, and 2-fold higher HED than the default mg/m^2 approach for mouse, rat, and dog, respectively. Therefore, if the above stated factors are not complied with, the body surface area scaling would be a safer approach.

There are other exceptions to the body surface area approach such as:

1. Therapeutics administered by alternative routes, such as topical, intranasal, subcutaneous, and intramuscular, for which dose is limited by local toxicity, should be normalized to concentration (mg/area of application) or amount (mg) of drug at application site.
2. Administration of drugs into anatomical compartments such as intrathecal, intranasal, intraocular, intrapleural, and intraperitoneal, with little distribution outside the compartment, should be normalized according to the volume of the compartment and the concentration of the drug.
3. Intravenously administered biological products with molecular weight >100,000 daltons should be mg/kg.

When there is no knowledge on the relevant species, by default the most sensitive species with the lowest HED should be chosen for MRSD calculation. Following are factors that influence the choice of appropriate species instead of using the most sensitive species.

1. Differences in ADME between species. While determining MRSD for the Phase I clinical trial, the ADME for humans is not known. But comparative *in vitro* data might be available. These data are relevant when there are marked differences in both the *in vivo* metabolic profiles and HEDs in animals.
2. Class experience may indicate a particular model is predictive of human toxicity.
3. There is limited biological cross-species pharmacologic reactivity of the therapeutics.
4. If a species is most sensitive but is different in terms of physiology as compared to humans, the species may not be the most appropriate one for MRSD calculations.

The application of a safety factor provides a margin of safety for protection of human subjects receiving the initial clinical dose. It protects from uncertainties due to enhanced sensitivity to therapeutic activity in humans versus animals, difficulties in detecting certain toxicities in animals (e.g., headache, myalgias, mental disturbances), differences in receptor densities or affinities, unexpected toxicities, and interspecies differences in absorption, distribution, metabolism, and excretion of the therapeutic. These differences may be accommodated by lowering the human starting dose from the HED of the selected species NOAEL.

A default safety factor of 10 is generally recommended for adequate protection of human volunteers. The safety factor can be raised in case of increased safety concerns such as:

Steep Dose–Response Curve. Steep dose–response curves for significant toxicities in the most appropriate species or in multiple species may indicate a greater risk to humans.

Severe Toxicities. Qualitatively severe toxicities or damage to an organ system (e.g., central nervous system (CNS)) indicate increased risk to humans.

Nonmonitorable Toxicity. Nonmonitorable toxicities may include histopathologic changes in animals that are not readily monitored by clinical pathology markers.

Toxicities Without Prodromal Indicators. If the onset of significant toxicities is not reliably associated with premonitory signs in animals, it may be difficult to know when toxic doses are approached in human trials.

Variable Bioavailability. Widely divergent bioavailability in several species, with poor bioavailability in the test species used to derive the HED, suggests a greater possibility for underestimating the toxicity in humans.

Irreversible Toxicity. Irreversible toxicities in animals suggest the possibility of permanent injury in human trial participants.

Unexplained Mortality. Mortality that is not predicted by other parameters raises the level of concern.

Large Variability in Doses or AUC Levels Eliciting Effect. When doses or exposure levels that produce a toxic effect differ greatly across species, the ability to predict a toxic level in humans is reduced and a greater safety factor may be called for.

Questionable Study Design or Conduct. Poor study design or conduct casts doubt on the accuracy of the conclusions drawn from the data. For instance, few dose levels, wide dosing intervals, or large differences in responses between animals within dosing groups may make it difficult to characterize the dose–response curve.

Novel Therapeutic Targets. Therapeutic targets that have not been previously clinically evaluated may increase the uncertainty of relying on the nonclinical data to support a safe starting dose in humans.

Animal Models with Limited Utility. Some classes of therapeutic biologics may have very limited interspecies cross reactivity or pronounced immunogenicity, or may work by mechanisms that are not known to be conserved between (nonhuman) animals and humans; in these cases, safety data from any animal studies may be very limited in scope and interpretability.

A safety factor lower than 10 can be used for drugs of well characterized class, same route of administration, same schedule and duration of administration, similar metabolic profile and bioavailability, and similar toxicity across species including human. A smaller safety factor might also be used when toxicities of drugs are easily monitored, reversible, and predictable and exhibit a moderate to shallow dose–response relationship with toxicities that are qualitatively and quantitatively consistent across the tested species. When NAOEL is based on safety studies of longer duration than proposed clinical schedule, a greater margin of safety is built into NOAEL and hence a factor lower than 10 is justified.

14.8   ROUTE OF DOSE ADMINISTRATION

The route of administration in animals should be similar to the intended clinical route [1]. Adoption of an alternative route should be based on pharmacokinetic considerations. A comparison of systemic exposure and metabolic profile of the investigational compound should be made by both routes of administration. If there is a significant change in pharmacokinetic parameters, a rigorous safety evaluation is required. When similar metabolism and exposure can be demonstrated by the alternative route, then nonclinical toxicity studies may focus only on local toxicity.

14.9   SAMPLING APPROACHES

The number of sampling time points should be frequent enough to estimate exposure but not so frequent as to cause physiological stress to animals. The justification of sampling time points should be based on kinetic data obtained from previous pilot studies or dose range-finding studies in similar animal models. Usually three or more animals are used to assess the concentration at each time point. The time points can be analyzed individually or after pooling.

14.9.1   Serial Sampling Approach

Systemic exposure is generally determined in terms of area under plasma/serum concentration versus time curve (AUC) [114] and C_{max}. This requires withdrawal of 10–20 samples [115] from the animal at different time points. Withdrawal of multiple samples from the same experimental animal at different time points for drug exposure assessment is reffered to as serial sampling. Withdrawal of multiple samples from the same animal is feasible in large animals such as dog and monkey. However, blood sampling in rodents is restricted due to low blood volume [116]. Moreover, the trauma and stress caused by frequent venipuncture and blood loss could cause adverse changes in the animal physiology and ultimately the pharmacokinetics of the drug. A satellite group of animals (4–5 animals/dose) is recommended for rodent toxicokinetics [1], and these animals undergo exactly the same treatment as those in the main study. The approach requires more animals, greater amount of drug, and increased personnel for dose administration and veterinary care. In addition, there may be lack of correlation in plasma drug concentration and toxicity findings.

14.9.2   Sparse Sampling Approach

To overcome these problems, several investigators [116–118] suggested the use of the sparse sampling approach (SSA) within the toxicity study itself. The basic characteristic of the SSA is that a complete profile is not sampled in every animal; that is, serial sampling is not done. Rather, each animal contributes to the profile with just one or two samples. Hence, blood samples can be generated directly from animals in toxicity studies as one or two samples will not effect the toxicity findings [116, 119], thereby precluding the need for separate toxicokinetic studies. This also enables direct correlation of plasma drug concentrations and toxicity findings within the same study and hence leads to a more efficient preclinical drug development program.

14.10   ANALYTICAL METHODOLOGY

All analytical methods should be developed and validated before the initiation of a toxicokinetic study. The methods should possess the desired sensitivity, precision, and accuracy and should be selective for the analyte with no interference from the endogenous components of the matrix. It is also important to study the stability of the analyte in the matrix.

14.10.1   Bioanalytical Method

The choice of biological should be continuously reviewed and methods should be developed in the adequate matrices—blood, plasma, serum, urine, and so on. If tissue distribution is also incorporated in the study, then it is required to develop methods in all organs of interest—for example, brain, heart, liver, kidney, adipose tissue, and skeletal muscles—and properly validate them. There should be clarity about the type of analyte to be analyzed—be it the parent compound, the active or inactive metabolites, or the enantiomers. Generally, the administered dose range in a toxicity study is broad, ranging from a lower dose to a higher toxic dose level. Therefore, the linearity curve should be capable of covering all the doses, or there can be two linearity curves—one for the low dose levels and another for the higher dose levels. For higher dose levels for which the concentrations falls beyond the upper limit of quantitation, a dilution integrity test should be done and, if convenient, the samples should be diluted appropriately to bring them within the linearity range. Later, these concentrations can be back calculated based on the dilution factor.

14.10.2   Bioanalytical Method Development

This general strategy is applicable to high-pressure liquid chromatography bioanalytical methods performed on drugs and metabolites present in biological matrices, such as blood, serum, plasma, or urine.

Formula Goals to Be Achieved

1. LLOQ. Minimum quantifiable concentration of drug and/or metabolites in biological fluid (approximately 20-fold less than reported C_{max} values).

2. Concentration range. Linearity is preferred: a concentration range from LLOQ to a value greater than C_{max} is expected in the study (preferably 10-fold more than the value of C_{max} in reported values). Calibration standards in the 1, 2, 5, 10, 20, 50, ... pattern of concentration are preferable. The shape of the calibration curve should be defined in mathematical terms.

3. Number of samples for calibration curve. At least seven or eight nonzero standards.

4. Strategy.

    a. Collect information on physicochemical properties of the drug and/or metabolites—structure, solubility, and stability in solution (including photostability).

    b. Check literature for information on sample preparation and chromatographic methods of compounds with closely related chemical structure.

    c. Select appropriate internal standard that is structurally similar.

    d. Select an appropriate detector—variable wavelength detector, photodiode array detector, fluorescence detector, and or electrochemical detector, depending on the sensitivity and selectivity required.

    e. Chromatography.

    Select suitable detecting wavelengths (the most sensitive wavelength of the drug is preferable—more than 250 nm in the case of UV—and the most sensitive excitation and emission wavelengths in the case of fluorescence).

    Check columns with different physical properties and/or from different suppliers (preferably with C_{18} or C_8).

    Check for pH effects (pH range 2–7).

    Optimize flow rate.

    Optimize mobile phase composition to obtain optimal retention (5–14 min) and peak shape.

    Select appropriate injection volume (20–100 μL).

    f. Sample preparation. Select an appropriate method—dilution, protein precipitation, liquid–liquid extraction, or solid phase extraction.

    Protein precipitation. Suitable for highly water-soluble drugs. Precipitating agents used are perchloric Acid (5–28% solutions), trichloroacetic acid (5–25% solutions), and acetonitrile (two- to fivefold of sample volume).

    Liquid–liquid extraction. Based on distribution coefficient of analytes, the preferable organic solvents employed are methanol, acetonitrile, diethyl ether, dichloromethane, chloroform, hexane, *t*-butyl methyl ether, and toluene, and/or their appropriate mixtures.

    Solid phase extraction. Based on the partition coefficient of analytes, a cartridge having suitable sorbent is selected (C_{18}, C_8, etc.). A typical solid phase extraction (SPE) procedure consists of the following steps: (i) condition and equilibrate the cartridge bed, (ii) load the sample, (iii) wash off interferences, (iv) elute analyte(s) of interest, and (v) dry the elution solvent in a hot water bath under a stream of nitrogen air.

g. Prepare a spiked sample. Elution or reconstitution solvent must be compatible with HPLC mobile phase.

h. Check recovery and optimize sample preparation procedure.

i. Reoptimize chromatography, if necessary.

j. Assay performance.

Analyze a solution of analyte(s) and internal standard in the mobile phase, $n \geq 5$, to determine the robustness of the spectrometric detection. Prepare one spike sample and analyze at least three times to determine the robustness of the chromatographic method. Prepare at least five spike samples of the same concentration and analyze to determine the robustness of the total method. Partly validate the method for linearity of spiked and nonspiked standards and their recovery.

14.10.3   Bioanalytical Method Validation

In order to define the various prestudy validation parameters for a validating bioanalytical [5] method for toxicokinetic studies, the following parameters should be assessed during prestudy validation:

- Specificity,
- Calibration curve
- Accuracy and precision
- Recovery (of analyte and the internal standard)
- Stability

This procedure is applicable to high-pressure liquid chromatography analytical methods performed on drugs and/or metabolites obtained from biological matrices such as blood, serum, plasma, or urine.

Specificity   At least six randomly selected control blank biological matrix samples should be chromatographed to determine the extent to which endogenous biological matrix components may contribute to interference at the retention time of analyte and internal standard. Any interference should be compared with the response of the LLOQ and internal standard. Chromatograms should be evaluated to make sure that there is no interference at the retention times of analyte and internal standard. Any interference is compared with the analyte response of the LLOQ. For hyphenated mass spectrometry based methods, testing six independent matrices for interference may not be important. Any significant interference peak corresponding to analyte and internal standard peak should not be present. The significance of the interference peak should be considered if it meets the following criteria:

- The retention time of the interference peak corresponds to the analyte peak and the internal standard peak.

- The response of interference peak is greater than or equal to 20% of the response of LLOQ.
- The response of the interference peak is greater than or equal to 5% of the response of the internal standard.

Linearity   For the establishment of linearity, a series of calibration samples should be prepared, by spiking a known concentration of drug with a working standard solution. The calibration curve should consist of a blank sample (matrix sample processed without IS and analyte), a zero sample (matrix sample processed only with IS), and six to eight nonzero samples covering the range of expected concentrations.

A minimum of four linearity curves containing not less than six nonzero concentrations should be analyzed.

The factors calculated from the calibration curve should match the following acceptance criteria:

- The deviation of the LLOQ from nominal concentration should not be more than 20%.
- The deviation of the standards, other than LLOQ, from nominal concentration should not be more than 15%.
- A minimum of six nonzero standards should meet the above criteria, including the LLOQ and the calibration standard at the highest concentration.
- The correlation coefficient should be more than 0.95.

Accuracy and Precision   The precision of an analytical method describes the closeness of individual measures of an analyte when the procedure is applied repeatedly to multiple aliquots of a single homogeneous volume of biological matrix.

- The accuracy of an analytical method describes the closeness of test results obtained by the method to the true value of the analyte.
- Within-batch accuracy and precision evaluations should be performed by replicate analysis of the same concentration of drug in biological matrix. The run should consist of a calibration curve and six replicates of each LLOQ, low, medium, and high quality control samples, that is, precision and accuracy (PA) batches.
- The between-batch accuracy and precision are assessed by analysis of a minimum of four precision and accuracy batches.
- For the evaluation of precision, the %CV of each concentration level should not be more than 15%, except for the LLOQ, for which it should not be more than 20%. The same is true for accuracy: the mean value should not deviate by more than ±15% of the actual concentration, except for the LLOQ, where it should not deviate by more than ±20% of the actual concentration. At least 67% of QC samples should be within 15% of their respective nominal (theoretical) values; 33% of the QC samples (not all replicates at the same concentration) can be outside ±15% of the nominal value.

Recovery   The recovery of an analyte in an assay is the detector response obtained from an amount of the analyte added to and recovered from the biological matrix, compared to the detector response obtained for the pure authentic standard. Recovery pertains to the extraction efficiency of an analytical method within the limits of variability.

Recovery of drug in biological matrix should be evaluated by comparing the mean peak responses of a minimum of three samples of low, medium, and high quality control samples, prepared in biological matrix, to mean peak responses of a minimum of three samples prepared in diluent. Recovery of internal standard in the biological matrix should be evaluated by comparing the mean peak responses of a minimum of three quality control samples, prepared in biological matrix, to mean peak responses of a minimum of three samples of the same quality control samples prepared in diluent. Recovery of the analyte need not be 100%, but the extent of recovery of an analyte and of the internal standard should be consistent, precise, and reproducible.

Dilution Integrity   A minimum of three replicates of each low and high QC sample should be used to prepare the required concentration by multiple aliquoting of their actual concentration. Then the samples should be diluted with biological matrix to meet their actual concentration. The samples should be analyzed and the results should be compared against the theoretical values. The percent change in concentration of the prepared samples from the theoretical value should not be more than ±15%.

Interaction with Anticoagulant   Interaction of anticoagulant with the drug is established as the vacutainers are coated with anticoagulant. A minimum of three replicates of each low and high QC sample should be prepared in the subject sample collection culture tube having an anticoagulant coating and be kept in a deep freezer at −70°C until completion of the stability testing period. After completion of the stability testing period, the samples should be processed along with a precision and accuracy batch and compared against the theoretical values. The percent change in concentration of the prepared samples from the theoretical value should not be more than ±15%.

Stability   Drug stability in a biological fluid is a function of the storage conditions, the chemical properties of the drug, the matrix, and the container system.

Freeze and Thaw Stability   Testing for freeze and thaw cycles on stability should be determined after three freeze and thaw cycles. At least three aliquots of each of the low and high concentrations should be stored at the same storage conditions as the study samples for 24 hours and thawed unassisted at room temperature. When completely thawed, the samples should be refrozen for 12–24 hours under the same conditions. The freeze–thaw cycle should be repeated two more times and then analyzed on the third cycle, and results should be compared against the theoretical value of QC sets. If there is a remarkable instability, the test should be repeated with one or two cycles. The percent change in concentration of the stability samples should not be more than ±15% from the theoretical value.

Short-Term Stability of Samples   A minimum of three aliquots each of the low and high QC samples should be kept at room temperature (25 ± 5 °C) for 4–24 hours after spiking into biological matrix. After completion of the stability testing period, the samples should be analyzed and compared against the theoretical value of QC sets. If there is a remarkable instability, the test should be performed for a suitably shorter duration. The percent change in concentration of the stability samples should not be more than ±15% from the theoretical value.

Long-Term Stability   The storage time in long-term stability evaluation should exceed the time difference between the date of first sample collection and the date of the last sample analysis. Long-term stability should be determined by storing at least three aliquots of each of the low and high concentrations or near to them under the same conditions as the study samples. The samples should be analyzed and compared to the theoretical value of QC sets. The test should be performed periodically to establish long-term stability from suitable duration to optimum duration. The percent change in concentration of the stability samples should not be more than ±15% from the theoretical value.

Autosampler Stability   The stability of processed samples in the autosampler should be determined at the autosampler temperature over the anticipated run time for the batch size to be used in studies. The minimum of three QC sets of low and high concentrations should be kept in the autosampler for the expected duration and analyzed. The drug concentrations obtained should be compared against their theoretical value. The percent change in concentration of the stability samples should not be more than ±15% from the theoretical value.

Stock Solution Stability   The stock solutions of drug and the internal standard stability under suitable conditions such as ambient temperature (20–30 °C), or refrigerated (2–8 °C) should be established by comparing the response or ratio of drug and internal standard from the system suitability chromatogram area of the first day of preparation of the solution and the system suitability chromatogram area of the last day of validation or any other relevant analysis. The duration of stock solution stability can be established, if required, by periodic analysis of system suitability. The percent change in area or the area ratio of the drug and internal standard of the stability samples should not be more than ±15% from the theoretical value.

Dry Extract Stability   Dry extract stability should be determined by storing at least three aliquots of each of the low and high concentrations, after processing without reconstitution under the same conditions as the study samples (at about −70 °C in a deep freezer). After completion of the anticipated stability testing period, the samples should be reconstituted and analyzed and results should be compared against the theoretical value of the QC set. The percent change in concentration of the stability samples should not be more than ±15% from the theoretical value.

Partial Validation   Partial validations are modifications of already validated bioanalytical methods. Partial validation should be performed after analyzing a minimum of one precision and accuracy batch. Partial validation can range from as little as one PA batch to nearly full validation based on requirement. Some typical bioanalytical method changes that require partial validation are:

- Bioanalytical method transfers between laboratories or analysts.
- Change in analytical methodology (e.g., change in detection systems).
- Change in anticoagulant in harvesting biological fluid.
- Change in matrix within species (e.g., human plasma to human urine).
- Change in sample processing procedures.
- Change in species within matrix (e.g., rat plasma to mouse plasma).
- Change in relevant concentration range.
- Changes in instruments and/or software platforms.
- Limited sample volume (e.g., pediatric study).
- Rare matrices.
- Selectivity demonstration of an analyte in the presence of concomitant medications.
- Selectivity demonstration of an analyte in the presence of specific metabolites.

Data Handling   The regression equation and the correlation coefficient should be calculated by performing a linear regression analysis according to the least squares method of the peak area response versus analyte concentration.

14.10.4   Method for the Formulation

In order to ensure proper dose administration, it is very important to establish the stability data for the formulation used in the study. At the preclinical stage, the formulation is generally very simple with minimum excipients. Several strengths are required to cover the broad range of dose levels. Therefore, scientists prefer to prepare them more frequently depending on the requirement. The minimum stability period should cover the time required for dosing all the animals on one particular day. In the case where a longer stability period is achieved, the formulation can be prepared accordingly. The formulation cannot be used beyond the established stability period, or if stored in conditions (temperature, humidity, and packing/container) other than established during stability studies. The formulation should be assayed on the first and last day of the study with some intermediate points in order to ascertain that the right dose was administered during the study. Therefore, it is mandatory to develop and validate a sensitive stability indicating method for the formulation.

14.10.5   Method Validation for the Formulation

Validation [120, 121] should be performed for each chemical species to be measured in the placebo/vehicle. Typical performance parameters that should be assessed during method validation include: accuracy, linearity range, limit of quantitation, precision, ruggedness, and specificity.

Accuracy Accuracy is the measure of how close the experimental value is to the true value. Accuracy studies for drug substance and drug product are performed at the 80%, 100%, and 120% levels of label claim. For the drug product, this is performed frequently by the addition of known amounts of drug by weight or volume (dissolved in diluent) to the placebo formulation working in the linear range of detection of the analyte. This would be a true recovery for liquid formulations. This test evaluates the specificity of the method in the presence of the excipients under the chromatographic conditions used for the analysis of the drug product. It will pick up recovery problems that could be encountered during the sample preparation and the chromatographic procedures. Recovery data should be assayed at least in triplicate, at each level (80%, 100% and 120% of label claim). The RSD of the replicates will provide the analysis variation or how precise the test method is. The mean of the replicates (expressed as % label claim) indicates how accurate the test method is.

Linearity Range The linear range of detectability that obeys Beer's law is dependent on the compound analyzed and the detector used. The working sample concentration and samples tested for accuracy should be in the linear range. The linearity range for an assay method will be evaluated by spiking the test compound to placebo formulation with 40%, 60%, 100%, 120%, and 140% of label claim. The regression coefficient (r) should be about 0.999. Intercept and slope should be indicated.

Limit of Quantitation (LOQ) Quantitation limit is the lowest concentration of analyte in a sample that can be determined with acceptable precision and accuracy under the stated experimental conditions. The limit of quantitation is expressed as the concentration of the analyte in the sample. LOQ is the concentration at which the signal-to-noise ratio is 10:1.

Precision Precision is the measure of how close the data values are to each other for a number of measurements under the same analytical conditions.

- *Injection Repeatability.* The precision as measured by multiple injections or a system suitability test of a homogeneous sample (prepared solution) indicates the performance of the HPLC instrument under the chromatographic conditions and day tested. An RSD of 1% RSD for precision of the system suitability tests for at least five injections ($n = 5$) for the active drug product is desirable.
- *Analysis Repeatability.* Determination, expressed as the RSD, consists of multiple measurements of a sample by the same analyst under the same analytical conditions on the same day (intraday). An RSD of 2% RSD for precision of the system suitability tests for 80%, 100%, and 120% levels of label claim for at least two determinations is desirable. For practical purposes, it is often combined with accuracy and carried out as a single study.

Ruggedness This attribute evaluates the reliability of the method in a different environment other than that used during development of the method. The objective is to ensure that the method will provide the same results when similar samples are analyzed once the method development phase is over. Depending on time and resources, the method will be tested by conducting the same assay on multiple days, with multiple analysts and instruments. Intermediate precision in the test method can be partly assured by good system suitability specifications.

Robustness   Robustness is a measure of the method's capability to remain unaffected by small but deliberate variations in method parameters. Robustness can be partly assured by good system suitability specifications. Thus, it is important to set tight, but realistic, system suitability specifications. Robustness of the method will be evaluated by varying some or all conditions, for example, columns, flow rate, slight change in mobile phase composition, pH of buffer in mobile phase, and reagents.

Specificity   The analyte should have no interference from other extraneous components and should be well resolved from them. A representative HPL chromatogram or profile should be generated to show that the extraneous peaks from either addition of known compounds or samples from stress testing (thermal degradation at 55 °C for 3 hours) are baseline resolved from the parent analyte. The photodiode array detector will determine peak purity.

Acceptance Criteria   An analytical method can be considered fully validated when it meets the following criteria:

- Accuracy: RSD should not be more than 2% at all three concentrations.
- Linearity: The regression coefficient (r) should be about 0.999 for the linearity range.
- Limit of quantitation (LOQ) : Signal-to-noise ratio should be 10:1.
- Precision: Injection repeatability—RSD of 5 replicate injections should not be more than 1%. Analysis repeatability—RSD for two determinations on the same day at 80%, 100%, and 120% levels of label claim should be no more than 2%.
- Ruggedness: RSD for two determinations on two different days at 80%, 100%, and 120% levels of label claim by different analysts and on two different instruments should be no more than 2%.
- Robustness: Changes in column, flow rate, or a slight change in mobile phase should not significantly affect the % Assay of the same formulation.
- Specificity: There should be no interfering peak below the main peak for stressed and nonstressed samples. Peak purity should not be less than 0.99.

14.10.6   Method Development Issues for Biotech Products

Many bioanalytical validation parameters are also applicable to microbiological and ligand-binding assays for biotech products also. However, these assays possess some selectivity and quantitation issues that need to be considered along with method development and validation.

Selectivity Issues   Similar to chromatographic methods, selectivity is important for microbiological and ligand-binding assays also. Here selectivity needs to be shown in terms of (1) interference from substances physicochemically similar to the analyte and (2) interference from matrix components that are unrelated to the analyte.

1. Interference from Substances Physicochemically Similar to the Analyte
    (a) Cross-reactivity of metabolites, concomitant medications, or endogenous compounds should be evaluated individually and in combination with the analyte of interest.
    (b) When possible, the immunoassay should be compared with a validated reference method (such as LC-MS) using already analyzed samples and predetermined criteria for agreement of accuracy of the immunoassay and the reference method.
    (c) The dilution linearity to the reference standard should be assessed using study (incurred) samples.
    (d) Separation steps can be incorporated prior to the immunoassay in order to improve selectivity.

2. Matrix Effects Unrelated to the Analyte

    (a) The standard curve should be prepared in biological fluids and should be compared with standard in buffer to rule out matrix effects.
    (b) Parallelism of diluted study samples should be evaluated with diluted standards to rule out any matrix effects.
    (c) Nonspecific binding should be determined.

Quantification Issues   Microbiological and imunoassay standard curves are inherently nonlinear and, in general, more concentration points may be required to define the standard curve [5]. In addition, the response–error relationship for immunoassay standard curves is a nonconstant function of the mean response. Therefore, a minimum of six nonzero calibrator concentrations, run in duplicate, is recommended. The concentration–response relationship is most often fitted to a four- or five-parameter logistic model, although others may be used with suitable validation. The overall curve fit can be improved by employing anchoring points in the asymptotic high- and low-concentration ends of the standard curve. Generally, these anchoring points will be at concentrations that are below the established LLOQ and above the established ULOQ. Calibrators should be prepared in the same matrix as the study samples or in an alternate matrix of equivalent performance. Both ULOQ and LLOQ should be defined by acceptable accuracy, precision, or confidence interval criteria based on the study requirements. The accuracy can be improved by the use of replicate samples. In the case where replicate samples should be measured during the validation to improve accuracy, the same procedure should be followed as for unknown samples.

The following recommendations apply to quantification issues:

• If separation is used prior to assay for study samples but not for standards, it is important to establish recovery and use it in determining results. Efficiency and reproducibility of recovery can be achieved by (1) the use of radiolabeled tracer analyte (quantity too small to affect the assay), (2) the advance establishment of reproducible recovery, and (3) the use of an internal standard that is not recognized by the antibody but can be measured by another technique.

- Key reagents, such as antibody, tracer, reference standard, and matrix, should be characterized appropriately and stored under defined conditions.
- Assessments of analyte stability should be conducted in true study matrix and not in a matrix from which endogenous interference has been removed.
- Acceptance criteria: At least 67% (4 out of 6) of QC samples should be within 15% of their respective nominal value; 33% of the QC samples (not all replicates at the same concentration) may be outside 15% of nominal value. In certain situations, wider acceptance criteria may be justified.
- Assay reoptimization or revalidation may be important when there are changes in key reagents, as follows:

  Labeled Analyte (Tracer). Binding should be reoptimized and performance should be verified with standard curve and QCs.

  Antibody. Key cross-reactivities should be checked and tracer experiments above should be repeated.

  Matrix. Tracer experiments above should be repeated and method development experiments should include a minimum of six runs conducted over several days,with at least four concentrations (LLOQ, low, medium, and high) analyzed in duplicate in each run.

14.11   CONCLUSION

Toxicokinetic evaluation is a small but vital part of the drug development process and plays a crucial role in deciding the fate of a drug candidate. Reliable toxicokinetic evaluation should consist of a correct study design, adequate sampling, sensitive and robust analytical methodology, accurate raw data, proper interpretation of toxic response versus exposure of drug and/or metabolites, and overall GLP compliance.Toxicokinetics provides a proof of concept for animal exposure to appropriate concentrations of administered drug or its metabolites. It brings in better understanding of toxicity data in terms of pharmacokinetic and metabolic principles and facilitates better extrapolation of preclinical data for clinical use. It is important to generate toxicokinetic data in safety pharmacology, repeated dose toxicity studies, genotoxicity studies, carcinogenicity studies, and reproductive toxicity studies. The primary concern of generating toxicokinetic data is to determine the plasma and tissue levels of the parent compound in the toxicology species; however, measurement of metabolite concentrations in plasma or other body fluids may be required for "prodrug," extensively metabolized drugs, or when one or more pharmacologically or toxicologically active metabolites are formed. The drug bound to plasma proteins is not available for distribution, hepatic metabolism, and renal elimination and is therefore pharmacologically inactive. Drug-induced toxicity is often species dependent due to species differences in pharmacokinetics, which can reduce the confidence in preclinical toxicity data. Other factors to be considered are sex differences in kinetics. Prolonged plasma half-life, reduced clearance, inhibition of drug metabolizing enzymes, or enterohepatic recirculation cause accumulation of drug after repeated administration. On the other hand, first-pass metabolism or autoinduction of drug metabolizing enzymes may cause reduced drug levels. Lack of dose proportionality also has clinical relevance and may occur either due to autoinduction of drug metabolizing enzymes or because of saturation of mechanisms such as intestinal absorption, enzyme metabolizing systems, and tubular reabsorption.

ACKNOWLEDGMENT

The authors is thankful to Shriprakash Singh, group leader at Ranbaxy Laboratories, Gurgaon, India, for his valuable contribution in compiling the GLP guidelines and in editing of manuscript for this chapter.

REFERENCES

1. ICH Topic S3A, CPMP/ICH/384/95: Operational June 1995. *Toxicokinetics: A Guidance for Assessing Systemic Exposure in Toxicology Studies.* (See http://www.emea.eu.int.)
2. Baldrich P. Toxicokinetics in preclinical evaluation. *Drug Discov Today* 2003;8(3): 127–133.
3. *Federal Register—FDA 21 CFR Part 58.*
4. OECD GLP guidelines 1997.
5. *Guidance for Industry: Bioanalytical Method Validation.* US Department of Health and Human Services, Food and Drug Administration, Center for Drug Evaluation and Research (CDER), Center for Veterinary Medicine (CVM), May 2001. www.fda.gov/cder/guidance/4252fnl.htm.
6. ICH Topic S7A, CPMP/ICH/539/00: Operational June 2001. *Safety Pharmacology Studies for Human Pharmaceuticals.* (See http://www.emea.eu.int.)
7. Diehl KH, Hull R, Morton D, Pfister R, Rabemampianina Y, Smith D, Vidal JM, van de Vorstenbosch C. A good practice guide To the administration of substances and removal of blood, including routes and volumes. *J Appl Toxicol* 2001;21:15–23.
8. ICH Topic S2B, CPMP/ICH/174/95: Operational March 1998. *Genotoxicity: A Standard Battery of Genotoxicity Testing of Pharmaceuticals.* (See http://www.emea.eu.int.)
9. ICH Topic S2A, CPMP/ICH/141/95: Operational April 1996. *Genotoxicity: Guidance on Specific Aspects of Regulatory Genotoxicity Tests for Pharmaceuticals.* (See http://www.emea.eu.int.)
10. ICH Topic S1A. *Guideline on the Need for Carcinogenicity Studies of Pharmaceuticals.* International Conference on Harmonization on Technical Requirements for Registration of Pharmaceuticals for Human Use. Harmonized Tripartite Guideline; 1995.
11. ICH Topic S1B: *Testing for Carcinogenicity of Pharmaceuticals.* International Conference on Harmonization on Technical Requirements for Registration of Pharmaceuticals for Human Use. Harmonized Tripartite Guideline; 1996.
12. ICH S1C: *Dose Selection for Carcinogenicity Studies of Pharmaceuticals.* International Conference on Harmonization on Technical Requirements for Registration of Pharmaceuticals for Human Use. Harmonized Tripartite Guideline; 1994.
13. ICH Topic S5A: CPMP/ICH/386/95, Operational March 1994. *Reproductive Toxicology: Detection of Toxicity to Reproduction for Medicinal Products.* (See http://www.emea.eu.int.)

14. Blaschke TF, Nies AS, Mamelok RD. Principles of therapeutics. In Gilman AF, Goodman LS, Rall TW, Murad F, Eds. *The Pharmacological Basis of Therapeutics*, 7th ed. New York: Macmillan Publishing; 1985, pp 49–65.

15. ICH Topic S6: CPMP/ICH/302/95, Operational March 1998. *Preclinical Safety Evaluation of Biotechnology Products Derived Pharmaceuticals.* (See http://www.emea.eu.int.)

16. van de Waterbeemd H. *Curr Opin Drug Discov Dev* 2002;5:33.

17. Viswanathan VN, Balan C, Hulme C, Cheetham JC, Yaxiong Sun Y. *Curr Opin Drug Discov Dev* 2002;5:400.

18. Chaturvedi PR, Decker CJ, Odinecs A. *Curr Opin Chem Biol* 2001;5:452.

19. Banik GM. *Curr Drug Discov* 2004;31.

20. Segall MD. *Future Drug Discov* 2004;81.

21. van de Waterbeemd H, Gifford E. *Nat Rev in Drug Discov* 2003;2:192.

22. Clark DE, Grootenhuis PD. *Curr Opin Drug Discov Dev* 2002;5:382.

23. Fichtl B, Nieciecki A, Walter K. *Adv Drug Res* 1991;20:117.

24. Olson RE, Christ DD. *Annu Rep Med Chem* 1996;31:327.

25. Naranjo CA, Sellers EM. *Drug–Protein Binding.* New York: Praeger; 1986, pp 233–251.

26. Carter DC, He XM, Munson SH, Twigg PD, Gernert KM, Broom MB, Miller TY. *Science* 1994;244:1195.

27. Curry S, Mandelkow H, Brick P, Franks N. *Nat Struct Biol* 1998;5:827.

28. Diaz N, Suarez D, Sordo TL Jr, Merz KM. *J Med Chem* 2001;44:250.

29. Herve F, Urien S, Albengres E, Duche JC, Tillement JP. *J Clin Pharmacokinet* 1994;26:44–58.

30. Kremer JM, Wilting J, Janssen LH. *Pharmacol Rev* 1988;40:1.

31. Zlotos G, Bucker A, Kinzig-Schippers M, Sorgel F, Holzgrabe U. *J Pharm Sci* 1998;87:215.

32. Borga O, Borga B. *J Pharmacokinet Biopharm* 1997;25:63.

33. Hoggard PG, Owen A. *J Antimicrob Chemother* 2003;51:493.

34. Goodman A, Gilman AG. *The Pharmacological Basis of Therapeutics*, 9th ed. New York: McGraw-Hill; 1996, pp 1712–1792.

35. Kratochwil NA, Huber W, Muller F, Kansy M, Gerber PR. *Biochem Pharmacol* 2002;64(9):1355.

36. Ebert SC. *Pharm Ther* 2004;29(4):244.

37. Cheng Y, Ho E, Subramanyam B, Tseng JL. *J Chromatogr B* 2004;809:67.

38. Kwong TC. *Clin Chim Acta* 1985;151:17.

39. Melten JW, Witterbrood AJ, Willems HJJ, Faber GH, Wemer J, Faber DB. *J Pharm Sci* 1985;74:692.

40. Machinist JM, Kukulka MJ, Bopp BA. *Clin Pharmacokinet* 1995;29:34.

41. Fung EN, Chen Y-H, Lau YY. *J Chromatogr B* 2003;795:187.

42. Beaudry F, Coutu M, Brown NK. *Biomed Chromatogr* 1999;13:401.

43. Bertucci C, Bartolini M, Gotti R, Andrisano V. *J Chromatogr B* 2003;797:111.

44. Kim HS, Hage DS. *J Chromatogr B* 2005;816:57.

45. Chen J, Ohnmacht C, Hage DS. *J Chromatogr B* 2004;809:137.

46. Bertucci C, Andrisano V, Gotti R, Cavrini V. *J Chromatogr B* 2002;768:147.

47. Lee EJD, Williams KM. Chirality: clinical pharmacokinetic and pharmacodynamic considerations. *Clin Pharmacokinet* 1990;18:339–345.

48. Jamali F, Mehvar R, Pasutto FM. Enantioselective aspects of drug action and disposition: therapeutic pitfalls. *J Pharm Sci* 1989;78:695–715.

49. Lin JH, deLuna FA, Ulm EH, Tocco DJ. Species-dependent enantioselective plasma protein binding of MK-571, a potent leukotriene D4 antagonist. *Drug Metab Dispos* 1990;18:484–487.

50. Tocco DJ, deLuna FA, Duncan AEW, Hsieh JH, Lin JH. Interspecies differences in stereoselective protein binding and clearance of MK-571. *Drug Metab Dispos* 1990;18:388–392.

51. Yasumori T, Chen L, Nagata K, Yamazoe Y, Kato R. Species differences in stereoselective metabolism of mephenytoin by cytochrome P-450 (CYP 2C and CYP 3A). *J Pharmacol Exp Ther* 1993;264:89–94.

52. Silber B, Holford NHG, Riegelman S. Stereoselective disposition and glucuronidation of propranolol in humans. *J Pharm Sci* 1982;71:699–704.

53. Wechter WJ, Loughead DG, Reischer RJ, Van Giessen GJ, Kaiser DG. Enzymatic inversion at saturated carbon: nature and mechanism of the inversion of R(−)-p-isobutyl-hydratropic acid. *Biochem Biophys Res Commun* 1974;61:833–837.

54. Hutt AJ, Caldwell J. The metabolic chiral inversion of 2-arylpropionic acids: a novel route with pharmacological consequences. *J Pharm Pharmacol* 1983;35:693–704.

55. Manzel-Soglowek S, Geisslinger G, Beck WS, Brune K. Variability of inversion of (R)-flurbiprofen in different species. *J Pharm Sci* 1992;81:888–891.

56. Jamali F, Berry BW, Tehrani MR, Russell SA. Stereoselective pharmacokinetics of flurbiprofen in humans and rats. *J Pharm Sci* 1988;77:666–669.

57. Foster RT, Jamali F. Stereoselective pharmacokinetics of ketoprofen in the rat: influence of route of administration. *Drug Metab Dispos* 1988;16:623–626.

58. Abas A, Meffin PJ. Enantioselective disposition of 2-arylpropionic acid nonsteroidal anti-inflammatory drugs: IV—ketoprofen disposition. *J Pharmacol Exp Ther* 1987;240:637–641.

59. Blaschke TF. Chromatographic resolution of racemates. *Angew Chem Int Ed Engl* 1980;19:13–24.

60. Blaschke TF, Kraft HP, Fickentscher K, Köhler F. Chromatographische racemattrennung von thalidomid und teratogene wirkung der enantiomere. *Drug Res* 1979;29:1640–1642.

61. Fabro S, Smith RL, Williams RT. Toxicity and teratogenicity of optical isomers of thalidomide (Comment). *Nature (London)* 1967;215:296.

62. Simonyi M. On chiral drug action. *Med Res Rev* 1984;4:359–413.

63. Albert A. Chemical aspects of selective toxicity. *Nature (London)* 1958;182:421–426.

64. Loo JCK, Foltz EL, Wallick H, Kwan KC. Pharmacokinetics of pivampicillin and ampicillin in man. *Clin Pharmacol Ther* 1974;16:35–43.

65. Clayton JP, Cole M, Elson SW, Ferres H. BRL 8988 (talampicillin): a well absorbed oral form of apicillin. *Antimicrob Agents Chemother* 1975;5:670–671. Bodin NO, Ekström B, Forsgren U, Jular LP, Magni L, Ramsey CH, Sjöberg B. An orally well-absorbed derivative of ampicillin. *Antimicrob Agents Chemother* 1978;8:518–525.

66. Ulm EH, Hichens M, Gomez HJ, Till AE, Hand E, Vassil TC, Biollaz J, Brunner HR, Schelling JL. Enalapril maleate and a lysine analogue (MK-521) disposition in man. *Br J Clin Pharmacol* 1982;14:357–362.

67. Tocco DJ, deLuna FA, Duncan AEW, Vassil TC, Ulm EH. The physiological disposition and metabolism of enalapril maleate in laboratory animals. *Drug Metab Dispos* 1982;10:15–19.

68. Rees PJ, Selby P, Prentice HG, Whiteman PD, Grant DM. A prodrug of acyclovir with increased bioavailability. *J Antimicrob Chemother* 1986;18(Suppl B):215–222.

69. Krasny HC, Petty BG. Metabolism of desciclovir, a prodrug of acyclovir, in humans after multiple oral dosing. *J Clin Pharmacol* 1987;27:74–77.

70. Krenitsky TA, Hall WW, de Miranda P, Beauchamp LM, Schaeffer MJ, Whiteman PD. 6-Deoxyacyclovir: a xanthine oxidase-activated prodrug of acyclovir. *Proc Natl Acad Sci USA* 1984;81:3209–3213.

71. Wilk S, Mizoguchi H, Orlowski M. γ-Glutamyl dopa: a kidney-specific dopamine precursor. *J Pharmacol Exp Ther* 1978;206:227–232.

72. Clarke TA, Waskell LA. *Drug Metab Dispos* 2003;31(1):53.

73. Pereillo JM, Maftouh M, Andrieu A, Uzabiaga MF, Fedeli O, Savi P, Pascal M, Herbert JM, Mafford JP, Picard C. *Drug Metab Dispos* 2002;30:1288–1295.

74. Gillette JR. Problems in extrapolations from animals to man. In Kato R, Estabrook RW, Cayen MN, Eds. *Xenobiotic Metabolism and Disposition*. London: Taylor & Francis; 1989, pp 209–216.

75. *Guidance for Industry: Drug Metabolism/Drug Interaction Studies in the Drug Development Process: Studies In Vitro*. Department of Health and Human Services, US Food and Drug Administraion, Center for Drug Evaluation and Research, Center For Biologics Evaluation and Research; April 1997. http://www.fda.gov/cder/guidance.htm.

76. Burek DJ, Nitschke KD, Bell TJ, Wackerle DL, Childs RC, Beyer JE, Dittenber DA, Rampy LW, McKenna MJ. Methylene chloride: a two year inhalation toxicity and oncogenicity study in rats and hamsters. *Fundam Appl Toxicol* 1984;4:30–47.

77. Chinje E, Kentish P, Jarnot B, George M, Gibson G. Induction of the CYP 4A subfamily by perfluorodecanoic acid: the rat and the guinea pig as susceptible and non-susceptible species. *Toxicol Lett* 1994;71:69–75.

78. Swarm RL, Roberts GKS, Levy AC, Hines LR. Observations on the thyroid gland in rats following the administration of sulfamethoxazole and trimethoprim. *Toxicol Appl Pharmacol* 1973;24:351–363.

79. Duggan DE, Hooke KF, Noll RM, Kwan KC. Enterohepatic circulation of indomethacin and its role in intestinal irritation. *Biochem Pharmacol* 1975;24:1749–1754.

80. Lindberg LP, Negishi M. Alternation of mouse cytochrome P450 substrate specificity by mutation of a single amino-acid residue. *Nature (London)* 1989;339:632–634.

81. Clarke DJ, Burchell B. The uridine diphosphate glucuronosyltransferase multigene family: function and regulation. In Kauffman FC, Ed. *Conjugation–Deconjugation Reactions in Drug Metabolism and Toxicity*. Berlin: Springer-Verlag; 1994, pp 3–43.

82. Satoh T. Role of carboxylesterases in xenobiotic metabolism. In Hodgson E, Bend JR, Philot RM, Eds. *Review in Biochemical Toxicology*, Vol 8. Amsterdam: Elsevier; 1987, pp 155–181.

83. Hosokawa M, Maki T, Satoh T. Characterization of molecular species of liver microsomal carboxylesterases of several animal species and human. *Arch Biochem Biophys* 1990;277:219–227.

84. Stearns RA, Miller RR, Doss GA, Chakravarty PK, Rosegay A, Gatto GJ, Chiu S-HL. The metabolism of Dup 753, a nonpeptide angiotensin II receptor antagonist by rat, monkey and human liver slices. *Drug Metab Dispos* 1992;20:281–287.

85. Smith DA. Species differences in metabolism and pharmacokinetics: are we close to an understanding? *Drug Metab Rev* 1993;23:355–373.

86. Blum MR, Liao SHT, Good SS, deMiranda P. Pharmacokinetics and bioavailability of zidovudine in man. *Am J Med* 1988;85:189–196.

87. Resetar A, Spector T. Glucuronidation of 3'-azido-3'-deoxythymidine: human and rat enzyme specificity. *Biochem Pharmacol* 1989;38:1389–1393.

88. Lin JH, Levy G. Effect of prevention of inorganic sulfate depletion on the pharmacokinetics of acetaminophen in rats. *J Pharmacol Exp Ther* 1986;239:94–98.

89. Slattery JT, Levy G. Acetaminophen kinetics in acutely poisoned patients. *Clin Pharmacol Ther* 1979;25:185–195.

90. McDonnell WM, Scheiman JM, Traber PG. Induction of cytochrome P450 IA genes (CYP 1A) by omeprazole in the human alimentary tract. *Gastroenterology* 1992;103:1509–1516.

91. Diaz D, Fabre I, Daujat M, Saint Aubert B, Bories P, Michel H, Maurel P. Omeprazole is an aryl hydrocarbon-like inducer of human hepatic cytochrome P-450. *Gastroenterology* 1990;99:737–747.

92. Strolin Benedetti M, Dostert P. Induction and autoinduction properties of rifamycin derivatives: a review of animal and human studies. *Environ Health Perspect* 1994;102(Suppl 9):101–105.

93. Nebert DW, Gonzalez FJ. The P450 gene superfamily. In Ruckpaul K, Rein H, Eds. *Principles, Mechanisms and Biological Consequences of Induction*. London: Taylor & Francis; 1990, pp 35–61.

94. Holk HGO, Munir AK, Mills LM, Smith EL. Studies upon the sex differences in rats in tolerance to certain barbiturates and to nicotine. *J Pharmacol Exp Ther* 1973;60:323–346.

95. Gregory L, Kedderis GL, Mugford CA. Sex dependent metabolism of xenobiotics. *Drug Metab Rev* 1998;30:441–498.

96. Kobliakov V, Popova N, Rossi L. Regulation of the expression of the sex-specific isoforms of cytochrome P-450 in rat liver. *Eur J Biochem* 1991;195:585–591.

97. Bandiera S. Expression and catalysis of sex-specific cytochrome P-450 isozymes in rat liver. *Can J Physiol Pharmacol* 1990;68:762–768.

98. Legraverend C, Mode A, Wells T, Robinson I, Gustafsson J-A. Hepatic steroid hydroxylating enzymes are controlled by the sexually dimorphic pattern of growth hormone secretion in normal and dwarf rats. *FASEB J* 1992;6:711–718.

99. Waxman DJ, Dannan GA, Guengerich FP. Regulation of rat hepatic cytochrome P450: age-dependent expression, hormonal imprinting and xenobiotic inducibility of sex-specific isoenzymes. *Biochemistry* 1985;24:4409–4417.

100. Shapiro BH. Sexually dimorphic response of rat hepatic monooxygenases to low dose phenobarbital. *Biochem Pharmacol* 1986;35:1766–1768.

101. Macleod JN, Sorensen MP, Shapiro BH. Strain independent elevation of hepatic monooxygenase enzyme in female mice. *Xenobiotics* 1987;17:1095–1102.

102. Ioannides C, Sweatman B, Richards R, Parke DV. Drug metabolism in the ferret: effects of age, sex and strain. *Gen Pharmacol* 1977;8:243–249.

103. Dogterom P, Rothuizen J. A species comparison of tolbutamide metabolism in precision-cut liver slices from rats and dogs: qualitative and quantitative sex differences. *Drug Metab Dispos* 1993;21:705–709.

104. Hunt CM, Westerkam WR, Stave GM. Effect of age and gender on the activity of human hepatic CYP3A. *Biochem Pharmacol* 1992;44:275–283.

105. Tynes RE, Philpot RM. Tissue and species dependent expression of multiple forms of flavine monooxygenases. *Mol Pharmacol* 1987;31:569–574.

106. Lin JH, Chiba M, Balani SK, Chen I-W, Kwei GY-S, Vastag KJ, Nishime JA. Species differences in the pharmacokinetics and metabolism of indinavir, a potent HIV protease inhibitor. *Drug Metab Dispos* 1996;24:1111–1120.

107. Gludicelli JF, Tillement JP. Influence of sex on drug kinetics in man. *Clin Pharmacokinet* 1977;2:157–166.

108. Macleod SM, Giles HG, Bengeret B, Lui FF, Sellers EM. Age and gender related differences in diazepam pharmacokinetics. *J Clin Pharmacol* 1979;19:15–19.

109. Sesardic D, Boobis AR, Murray P, Murray S, Segura J, de la Torre R, Davies DS. Furafylline is a potent and selective inhibitor of cytochrome P450 IA2 in man. *Br J Clin Pharmacol* 1990;29:651–663.

110. Kobayashi S, Murray S, Watson D, Sesardic D, Davies DS, Boobis AR. The specificity of inhibition of debrisoquine 4-hydroxylase activity in quinidine and quinine in the rat is the reverse of that in man. *Biochem Pharmacol* 1989;38:2795–2799.

111. *Guidance for Industry and Reviewers: Estimating the Safe Starting Dose in Clinical Trials for Therapeutics in Adult Healthy Volunteers.* US Department of Health and Human Services, Food and Drug Administration, Center for Drug Evaluation and Research (CDER), Center for Biologics Evaluation and Research (CBER); December 2002. Pharmacology and Toxicology, http://www.fda.gov/cber/guidelines.htm.

112. Freireich EJ, Gehan EA, Rall DP, Schmidt LH, Skipper HE. Quantitative comparison of toxicity of anticancer agents in mouse, rat, hamster, dog, monkey, and man. *Cancer Chemother Rep* 1966;50:219–244.

113. Schein PS, Davis RD, Carter S, Newman J, Schein DR, Rall DP. The evaluation of anti-cancer drugs in dogs and monkeys for the prediction of qualitative toxicities in man. *Clin Pharmacol Ther* 1970;11:3–40.

114. Cayen MN. Consideration in the design of toxicokinetic studies. *Toxicol Pathol* 1995;23:148–157.

115. Gibaldi M, Perrier D, Eds. *Pharmacokinetics*, 2nd ed. New York: Marcel Dekker; 1982.

116. Dahlem AM, Allerheiligen SR, Vodicnik MJ. Concomitant toxicokinetics techniques for interpretation of exposure data obtained during the conduct of toxicology studies. *Toxicol Pathol* 1995;2:170–178.

117. Bree JV, Nedelman J, Steimer JL, Tse F, Robinson W, Niederberger W. Application of sparse sampling approaches in rodent toxicokinetics: a prospective view. *Drug Inf J* 1994;28:263–279.

118. Campbell DB, Jochemsen R. Nonclinical pharmacokinetics and toxicokinetics. In Cartwright AC, Mathews BR, Eds. *International Pharmaceutical Product Registration, Aspects of Quality, Safety, and Efficacy—Chemistry, Pharmacy and Manufacturing.* Chichester: Ellis Horwood; 1994, pp 560–627.

119. Tse F, Nedelman J. Serial versus sparse sampling in toxicokinetic studies. *Pharm Res* 1996;13:1105–1108.

120. *Reviewer Guidance: Validation of Chromatographic Methods.* Center for Drug Evaluation and Research (CDER), November 1994.

121. *United States Pharmacopoeia* 2000;24:⟨1225⟩.

15

IN VITRO TOXICOKINETICS AND DYNAMICS: MODELING AND INTERPRETATION OF TOXICITY DATA

ARIE BRUININK

Materials–Biology Interactions, Materials Science & Technology (EMPA), St. Gallen, Switzerland

Contents

15.1 INTRODUCTION

If the dose of a bioactive test compound (drug, chemical, protein, etc.) exceeds a certain concentration and/or if the exposure duration at subtoxic doses is lengthened, adverse effects may develop in organisms. Knowledge about toxicokinetics and toxicodynamics is of crucial importance for various areas of research: this ranges from risk assessment of compounds, to the development of new drugs and new biomedical materials. Toxicokinetics is generally regarded as an area of science dealing with kinetics of exposure, absorption, distribution, metabolism, and excretion of test compounds and metabolites. Toxicodynamics, however, focuses on studying dose–response relationships. Depending on the application of test compound, the *no adverse effect level* (NOAEL)—the dose or dose/concentration at which the parameter of interest is reduced by 50% (e.g., *lethal dose* 50 (LD$_{50}$))—is of importance. Whereas numerous publications have described approximations of the fate of test compounds in the intact body and dose–effect relationships, no such information is currently available for *in vitro* systems.

This chapter describes *in vitro* concentration–effect relationships, taking variations in toxic compound concentration into account. For this, a set of equations are presented that are based on known first-order equations describing uptake and elimination-based fluctuations in compound blood levels [1] and equations describing receptor–ligand interaction relationships [2]. Furthermore, special attention is paid to determine inhibitory concentrations reducing the parameter of interest by 50% (IC$_{50}$) or 5% (IC$_5$; benchmark dose 5%).

15.2 BENCHMARK DOSE

All compounds are toxic under certain exposure conditions. The change of the occurrence of these adverse effects can be minimized by limiting the dose or exposure period. A basis for hazard assessment of chemicals is the no observed adverse effect level (NOAEL). For assessment of the NOAEL, only animal toxicity data are used. It represents the highest dose at and below which no significant adverse effects are seen. In reality, it is defined by the *lowest adverse effect level* (LOAEL)—the dose at which a significant effect is seen [3]. Instead of NOAEL, recent alternative approach is to use the *benchmark dose* [4]. In contrast to the NOAEL, in this approach all data obtained are taken into account. A line is fitted through the data using a mathematical model for the dose–response relationship. With the help of this fitted relationship, we can calculate the dose at which the incidence or frequency of a toxic adverse effect is increased (in the case of the benchmark dose by 5%). In addition, the statistical confidence limits of this dose are estimated. Both values are dependent on the mathematical model for the dose–response relationship used. Still, no general model for the dose–response relationship exists against which the line should be fitted. In most cases, a log-probit extrapolation of concentration–response data to the 95% lower confidence limit on the toxic concentration is employed. The practical use of the benchmark dose has been evaluated by applying dose–response models to an extensive historical database [5]. It was found that the lower confidence limit on the 5% benchmark dose is comparable to the NOAEL for most datasets. In this chapter a mathematical base is given to calculate the effective concentration of a test compound that reduces the parameter of interest by 5% and 50%.

15.3 TOXICOKINETICS *IN VIVO*

One simplified model that has gained wide acceptance in toxicokinetics is that of describing the system in terms of a single compartment in which the test compound is homogeneously distributed after administration. This is the case if (1) the distribution equilibrium between test compound in blood and tissues is reached before a significant amount of test compound has been eliminated, and (2) the equilibrium constant is such that the concentration ratio between blood and tissues remains stable during the period of elimination. The one-compartment model is a strong simplification of the *in vivo* situation but, to a large extent, is applicable for several types of test compound.

After intravenous (IV) application, the serum level exponentially decreases due to elimination processes. In the intact animal, the administered compounds are eliminated from the circulation by various routes. By assuming one homogeneous compartment, the serum level of the compound can be described mathematically [1] by

$$y_i = y_0 e^{-k_{el}t_i} \tag{15.1}$$

where y_i is the blood concentration of the compound at time t_i after addition at t_0, y_0 is the blood concentration of the compound just after administration at t_0, and k_{el} is the elimination constant.

The elimination velocity is characterized by the elimination half-life ($t_{1/2}$). The elimination half-life is defined as the period that is needed to reduce the serum level by a factor of 2 ($y_i = 0.5 y_0 = y_0 e^{-k_{el}t_{1/2}}$). Thus,

$$t_{1/2} = \frac{\ln 2}{k_{el}} \tag{15.2}$$

After an extravascular administration, the compound first has to enter the circulation before it is eliminated from this compartment. The delay and magnitude of the peak plasma concentration following extravascular administration are a function of the kinetics of absorption as well as, in the case of inhalation and oral administration, the fraction (f) of the absorbed unchanged compound (Fig. 15.1). The value of f normally equals 1 for an extravascular injection of the compound (IM, SC, IP) but is lower than 1 after an oral intake or after inhalation. The volume of distribution V is strongly compound dependent and may generally vary between 0.1 and 10 L/kg body weight.

The equation for the concentration of the test compound y_i in the blood serum assuming one compartment corresponds to the Bateman equation [1]:

$$y_i = \left(\frac{Df}{V}\right) k_{abs} \left(\frac{e^{-k_{el}t_i} - e^{-k_{abs}t_i}}{k_{abs} - k_{el}}\right) \tag{15.3}$$

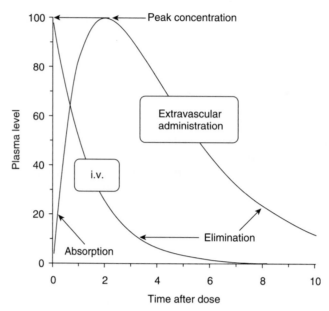

FIGURE 15.1   Simulated plasma concentration–time curve assuming the one-compartment model. These relationships are characterized by an elimination and, in the case of extravascular administration, an absorption phase. The AUC is the area below each curve.

in which k_{abs} is the absorption constant, D is the dose, f is the fraction of the test compound dose taken up (extent of absorption), and V is the distribution volume.

Independent of the route of administration, a similar plasma concentration–time curve is obtained for the metabolite(s) of the test compound.

One assumption in toxicology is that the cumulative dose at the sensitive site determines the reaction. A simplification can be made: the extent of adverse effects is correlated to the *area under the curve* (AUC) of the concentration–time relationship of the active form of the compound at the site of action (Fig. 15.1). Based on the latter yet unproven assumption, other theories (e.g., linear systems theory) have been hypothesized to characterize toxicokinetics and toxicodynamics [6]. Later on, it will be shown that, based on the premises made in this chapter, this assumption is only correct in some selected cases.

15.4   BASICS OF *IN VITRO* TOXICODYNAMICS

In the *in vivo* situation, multiple relatively large compartments are present in which the administered compounds can be distributed, metabolized, and redistributed. Various physiologically based toxicokinetic models have been developed as tools to describe blood levels after exposure [7–9]. Normally, the various compartments of the *in vitro* systems are composed of large (the medium part of the culture) and negligibly small (the cells) parts. Models to be developed can assume one compartment, that is, the sensitive target cell component is directly accessible, or two compartments, that is, the culture medium and the compartment within the cell that the toxic compound first has to reach and develop a certain concentration before adverse effects are seen.

In *in vivo* studies, benchmark dose, NOAEL, LOAEL, as well as cumulative dose are generally used to describe the concentration–effect relationships of a test compound; equivalent expressions for describing *in vitro* effects do not exist in the case of the benchmark dose or are only rarely used. *In vitro*, the potency of a test compound in affecting cell functions is defined by the *effective culture medium concentration* (EC) or *inhibiting culture medium concentration* (IC). In general, the expressions EC_{50} and IC_{50} are used. They represent the concentrations of a test compound that modify or diminish, respectively, the value of a given measured parameter (cell function, concentration of certain proteins, etc.) by 50% relative to control. In analogy to the NOAEL, its *in vitro* equivalent, the *no observed effect medium concentration* (NOEC), is strongly dependent on the choice of the test compound concentration and reproducibility of the measurements of the given parameter. In contrast, like the *in vivo* benchmark dose approach, all results are taken into account for the estimation of EC_{50} and IC_{50} values. Thus, taking a certain additional safety factor into account, the use of EC_{50} and IC_{50} values for risk analysis seem to be justified. However, the appearance of biphasic effects makes it very difficult to assess these EC_{50} and IC_{50} values correctly. Furthermore, the differences between medium concentrations of the test compound, which only negligibly affect the parameter of interest, and EC_{50} or IC_{50} levels are determined by the shape of the medium concentration–effect relationships and are cell culture, compound, and parameter dependent. This means that an approach equivalent to *in vivo* benchmark dose 5% would be more adequate for defining *in vitro* threshold medium concentrations. For the estimation of both the benchmark dose 5% in *in vivo* studies and the *benchmark culture medium concentration 5%* (BMC_5) in *in vitro* studies, a mathematical model for the dose–response relationship is needed, according to which the lines are fitted.

The description of the dose–response curves obtained from *in vivo* and *in vitro* experiments is generally based on a linear regression analysis of a near linear portion of the concentration–response curve, plotting the logarithm of the dose on the horizontal axis and the response on the vertical axis. This method permits the calculation of an effective dose. However, the latter value can be manipulated by the choice of data points. Complex dose–response curves, such as those showing stimulation at low concentrations but inhibition at high concentrations, cannot be described. Moreover, the slope of the curve, another important index characterizing the effects of a compound, also depends on the data points chosen and is nearly always neglected.

In 1992, I proposed a new mathematical approach to analyze *in vitro* toxicity data [3]. Since the book in which this approach is described is no longer available and because the present paper is built on this, the approach is briefly described here. The statistical method is based on models of enzyme kinetics and the law of mass action. This method allows both the effective concentration and the slope of the dose–response curve to be reliably estimated, as well as the IC_5 and the benchmark dose 5% [10–13]. The values of the various parameters in the following formulas can be calculated using available spreadsheet programs with macro possibilities; the contribution from each data point is weighted according to the standard error of the mean. Based on this model, the toxic effects of several neurotoxic compounds have been evaluated [14–18]. Recently, other very similar approaches have been suggested [19].

The description of the test compound concentration/dose–effect relationship is based on the primary toxic event. The exposure of cells to a test compound or its toxic metabolite generally first results in the test compound binding to one or more of the proteins in the outer membrane of the cells, where it may intercalate into the membrane or diffuse (transported) into the cell and bind to one or more intracellular proteins (Fig. 15.2). Binding of the test compound induces a range of effects, such as stimulation or inhibition of synthesis or degradation of various cellular molecules directly or mediated indirectly by secondary processes. It is reasonable to assume that the effect on the various cell functions will be directly related to the first event, by the fraction of target protein sites occupied by the test substance. The measurement of binding is amenable to mathematical analysis and therefore also its evoked effects. The effects on the measured cell function(s) can be positive or negative depending on the compound and the compound concentration.

15.4.1   Test Substance Binds Predominantly to One Important Effectual Cell Protein

Generally, duration of exposure to the test compound is sufficient to ensure that, within the most sensitive cell compartment, binding to cell effectual protein involved in cell function reaches equilibrium. If equilibrium is established and degradation of the test compound is negligible, the law of mass action is valid as described by

$$\frac{[SB]}{[B_{max}]} = \frac{[S]}{K_d + [S]} \tag{15.4}$$

where S is the test compound, B is the unbound effectual protein, and SB is the test compound–effectual protein complex. In this equilibrium state, only the complex SB induces, directly or indirectly, the changes in cell function. K_d represents the

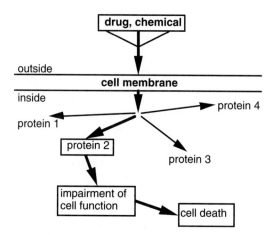

FIGURE 15.2   Exposure of a cell with a test compound or chemical: schematic representation.

equilibrium dissociation constant. The total amount of protein $[B_{max}]$ is the sum of $[B]$ and $[SB]$. $[SB]/[B_{max}]$ is the fraction of effectual protein sites to which the test compound is bound. If the relationship between the fraction of bound sites and the changes in the cell function(s) being measured is linear, then Eq. 15.4 can be rewritten to incorporate the cell function:

$$\frac{E_i}{E_u} = \frac{[S]}{K_r + [S]} \tag{15.5}$$

where E_u is the experimental value of the cell function in untreated cells, E_i is the reduction in E_u caused by the test substance, and K_r is the response constant of the cell for the test substance.

The value of cell function of interest in the presence of the test substance as a fraction of the value of the cell function in untreated cells (E_t/E_u) is, therefore

$$\frac{E_t}{E_u} = \frac{K_r}{K_r + [S]} \tag{15.6}$$

where E_t is the measured value of the cell function in treated cells and $E_u = E_t + E_i$.

Generally, the toxic effects are expressed by IC_{50} or BMC_5. With this equation, IC_{50} and BMC_5 can be calculated. As defined previously, IC_{50} is the concentration of the test substance when the measured value of cell function is reduced to half its maximum value: $E_t/E_u = 0.5$ (see Fig. 15.3: $N_c = 1$). Thus,

$$0.5 = \frac{K_r}{K_r + IC_{50}} \quad \text{or} \quad IC_{50} = K_r \tag{15.7}$$

The BMC_5 is defined as the concentrations where $E_t/E_u = 0.95$. Thus,

$$BMC_5 = \frac{K_r}{19} \tag{15.8}$$

If in Eq. 15.8 K_r is replaced by IC_{50}, then according to Eq. 15.7 BMC_5 can be related to IC_{50} as follows:

$$BMC_5 = \frac{IC_{50}}{19} \tag{15.9}$$

In most cases, however, the effect on the cell function(s) of the binding of the test substance to the relevant effectual protein is not linearly related to the fraction of bound effectual protein sites $([SB]/[B_{max}])$. Generally, as the number of occupied sites increases, the effect on the measured cell function will be enhanced with every additional occupied site. Thus, as $[S]$ increases, K_r decreases. In other words, a positive cooperativity analogous to the binding of oxygen to hemoglobin as described by Hill [2] is observed. Therefore,

$$\frac{E_t}{E_u} = \frac{1}{i}\left(\frac{K_{r1}}{K_{r1}+[S]} + \frac{K_{r2}}{K_{r2}+[S]} + \cdots + \frac{K_{ri}}{K_{ri}+[S]}\right)$$

in which i is the number of effectual protein molecules or, more generally,

$$\frac{E_t}{E_u} = \frac{K_c}{K_c + [S]^{N_c}} \tag{15.10}$$

where K_c is the response constant under cooperativity conditions, and N_c is the cooperativity constant. Examples of concentration–effect relationships with varying N_c values are shown in Fig. 15.3.

Equation 15.6 is a special case of Eq. 15.10, where $N_c = 1$, and because of that, $K_c = K_r$. The concentration of the substance where the measured value of the cell parameter is half the maximum value is

$$0.5 = \frac{K_c}{K_c + (IC_{50})^{N_c}} \Rightarrow$$

$$IC_{50} = K_c^{1/N_c} \quad (\text{or } K_c = (IC_{50})^{N_c}) \tag{15.11}$$

In analogy, the BMC_5 can be calculated:

$$0.95 = \frac{K_c}{K_c + (BMC_5)^{N_c}} \Rightarrow$$

$$BMC_5 = \left(\frac{K_c}{19}\right)^{1/N_c} \tag{15.12}$$

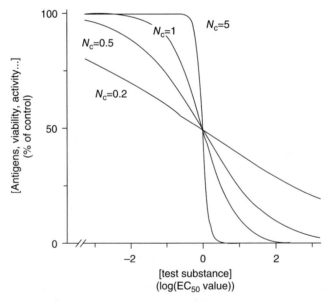

FIGURE 15.3   Relationship between the cell parameter and the concentration of the test substance calculated from Eq. 15.10 for various values of the cooperativity constant N_c, assuming that $K_c = IC_{50}$ and $E_u = 100$ (arbitrary units).

Small variations of N_c strongly affect the BMC_5 value. In analogy to Eq. 15.9, by combining Eqs. 15.11 and 15.12, the BMC_5 in relation to N_c and IC_{50} can be described by the following equation:

$$BMC_5 = \frac{IC_{50}}{19^{1/N_c}} \tag{15.13}$$

By reducing N_c values, the ratio IC_{50}/BMC_5 increases exponentially. Thus, small variations of N_c value affect the BMC_5 value maximally at very small N_c.

The distribution of the logarithm of the IC_{50} and BMC_5 values found under experimental conditions is (as stated for the *in vivo* situation [20]) log-normal Gaussian around the mean of the logarithm of the IC_{50} and BMC_5 values, respectively, for each experiment and not (as suggested by others [19]) normal at the nonlogarithmic linear scale. The same appears to be true for the N_c values.

15.4.2 Test Substance Binds to Two Important Effectual Proteins with Different Affinities

After application of a compound under the present assumption, two different main effects on cells can be discriminated depending on the applied concentration. In this case, E_t/E_u represents a combination of the effects induced by effectual protein 1 with parameters E_{u1}, K_{c1}, and N_{c1} and by effectual protein 2 with parameters E_{u2}, K_{c2}, and N_{c2}. Thus,

$$\frac{E_t}{E_u} = \frac{\dfrac{E_{u1}K_{c1}}{K_{c1}+[S]^{N_{c1}}} + \dfrac{E_{u2}K_{c2}}{K_{c2}+[S]^{N_{c2}}}}{E_{u1}+E_{u2}} \tag{15.14}$$

where

$$E_u = E_{u1} + E_{u2} \tag{15.15}$$

For both phases of the medium concentration–effect relationship, BMC_5 values can be calculated. Binding of the test substance to the effectual proteins can stimulate or inhibit cell function. In case that binding to effectual protein 1 stimulates cell function and binding to effectual protein 2 inhibits cell function, the value of E_{u2} will represent the sum of the control value and the increase induced by binding to effectual protein 1 (Fig. 15.4) where E_{u1} has a negative value. Instead of IC_{50}, the more general term *effective concentration 50%* (EC_{50}) is used to describe the concentration resulting in a 50% stimulation or inhibition. Examples of both situations, namely, where both E_u values are positive or one is positive and one is negative, are shown in Figs. 15.4 and 15.5 (line D in Fig. 15.5 is the sum of B and C, and line E is the sum of A and C). Equation 15.14 also applies if a test substance in the concentration range investigated only affects a fraction of the measured functional parameter (Fig. 15.4 in the concentration range 0–$1000EC_{50,1}$, and Fig. 15.5 lines A and B). In this case, the IC_{50} value for binding to the second protein is outside the tested concentration range and the cooperativity constant N_c must be set to $10^{-\infty}$.

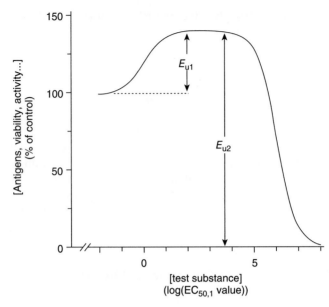

FIGURE 15.4   Relationship between the cell parameter and the concentration of the test substance calculated from Eq. 15.14 where the test substance binds to two of the effectual proteins involved in the measured cell function (E_{u1} = –40, K_{c1}=EC$_{50,1}$, N_{c1} = 1; E_{u2} = 140, K_{c2} = 100,000EC$_{50,1}$, and N_{c2} = 1) (arbitrary units).

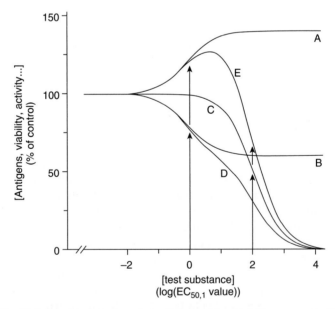

FIGURE 15.5   Relationship between the cell parameter and the concentration of the test substance calculated from Eq. 15.10 (line C: K_c = 100EC$_{50,1}$, E_u = 100, N_c = 1) and Eq. 15.14 (line A: K_{c1} = EC$_{50,1}$, E_{u1} = –40, N_{c1} = 1, K_{c2} = ∞, E_{u2} = 140, N_{c2} = 10$^{-∞}$; line B: K_{c1} = EC$_{50,1}$, E_{u1} = 40, N_{c1} = 1, K_{c2} = ∞, E_{u2} = 60, N_c = 10$^{-∞}$; line D: K_{c1} = EC$_{50,1}$, E_{u1} = 40, N_{c1} = 1, K_{c2} = 100EC$_{50,1}$, E_{u2} = 60, N_{c2} = 1; line E: K_{c1} = EC$_{50,1}$, E_{u1} = –40, N_{c1} = 1, K_{c2} = 100EC$_{50,1}$, E_{u2} = 140, N_{c2} = 1) (arbitrary units).

For certain indices of *in vivo* response, animals react to test compound treatment mainly by stimulation/increase at low doses and inhibition at high doses (e.g., behavioral response to benzodiazepine receptor ligands [21]). Using Eq. 15.14, the BMC_5 and EC_{50} for the low concentration effect and the BMC_5 and IC_{50} of the inhibitory effect observed at the high compound concentration range may be determined correctly.

15.4.3 Test Substance Binds to Many Important Effectual Proteins with Approximately Equal Affinity

In this case, the effect on the cell function induced by binding of the test substance to various effectual proteins involved in cell function is cumulative. If the relationship between the change in the cell function and the fraction of bound sites is linear for each of the proteins (no cooperativity), the value of the cell function in the presence of the test substance as a fraction of the control value (E_t/E_u) is

$$\frac{E_t}{E_u} = \frac{\dfrac{E_{u1}K_{c1}}{K_{c1}+[S]^{N_{c1}}} + \dfrac{E_{u2}K_{c2}}{K_{c2}+[S]^{N_{c2}}} + \cdots + \dfrac{E_{ui}K_{ci}}{K_{ci}+[S]^{N_{ci}}}}{E_{u1}+E_{u2}+\cdots+E_{ui}} \tag{15.16}$$

As the number of different proteins (i) increases and assuming that the distribution of the logarithm of the affinities to the various proteins is Gaussian, the generalized form of Eq. 15.16 will approach the situation described by Eq. 15.10. If, as described for the one effector site model, there is a cooperative effect for each single effector protein, this equation will still hold, but the values of N_c and K_c will change. Thus, if there is a cooperative effect or the test substance binds to many proteins that are involved in the measured cell functions, the results are similar. Depending on the precise values of EC_{50}, N_c, and the standard deviations of the values of the measured cell function, the phenomenon can even take place for the two effector site model (compare Fig. 15.5 line D and Fig. 15.3).

15.5 RATIONALE DESCRIBING *IN VITRO* TOXICOKINETICS AND DYNAMICS AND AIM OF THE PRESENT STUDY

As in *in vivo*, the *in vitro* toxicity of compounds and test compounds is determined by toxicokinetic parameters in addition to the sensitivity of the cells. Although the concentrations of the test compounds are in most cases not or relatively slowly modified in *in vitro* systems, medium has to be partly replaced from time to time, especially in long-term cultures. The medium replacement may affect the medium test compound concentration. Furthermore, the compound may need an accumulation within the target compartment (e.g., cytoplasm, lysosomes) before toxic effects are induced. As a result, the toxicity for two different situations can be discriminated: toxicity of a compound and/or of its metabolite(s) is determined by peak concentrations or by the treatment period times concentration. It depends on the compound tested which of the two possibilities is crucial for the toxicity. So far, no mathematical approach exists for the data analysis of *in vitro* pharmaco/toxicokinetic data. In Sections 15.6.1 and 15.6.2 eight different hypothetical extreme *in vitro* scenarios are discussed. In Models 1–4, toxicity is solely determined by the C_{max} (Section 15.6.1) and in Models 5–8 toxicity is determined by the treatment period (Section 15.6.2). Concerning the stability of the compound, in Models 1 and 5 the compound is stable; in Models 2 and 6 the toxic test compound is inactivated, similar to the *in vivo* situation after IV administration; in Models 3 and 7 the nontoxic test compound is modified into a toxic compound; and in Models 4 and 8 the toxic metabolite formed (Models 3 and 7) is thereafter inactivated (Fig. 15.6). This latter case is similar to an *in vivo* extravascular administration of a test compound. It must be noted that Models 4 and 8 are only mentioned for the sake of completeness and will only be discussed briefly. Furthermore, a scheme is presented that may help select the model according to how the given test compound behaves (Section 15.7). In this chapter, it is assumed that test compound concentration–effect relationship characteristics can be described using the equations in Section 15.4. Furthermore, in this chapter the equations are simplified: it is assumed that the effects are induced according to the single effector site model (Section 15.4.1). One must be aware that Models 1–8, as mathematical models for describing *in vivo* serum concentrations, simplify the real existing situation found in the culture dish and are based on the premises made. However, the discussed models may be of help to optimize experiments, to provide additional data from the obtained results, and to understand the collected results.

The outcome of experiments, in which concentration–effect relationships are investigated, is generally expressed in calculated compound concentrations, taking the known concentrations of the test compound in the stock solution just after dissolving in the culture medium as a starting point; however, concentration during the experiment may vary and the modified form of the test compound is responsible

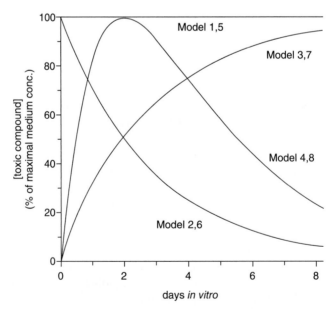

FIGURE 15.6   Concentration of the toxic compound in the culture medium in the eight hypothetical models after various periods of time.

for the observed adverse effects. Because of these reasons, instead of concentration–effect relationship, the term *initial outer compartment (cell culture medium) test compound concentration–effect relationship* (OCER) is used. Furthermore, the calculated *initial (starting) concentration* of the compound causing certain effects is based on the compound concentration in the stock solution and is called the *effective initial concentration* (EIC). In EIC_z, z stands for the observed effect relative to control. Here, z is 50 if at the end of the treatment period, the value of the parameter of interest is exactly between the value of (untreated) controls and the maximal possible change. EIC_{50} is thereby the starting (initial) concentration at which, at the end of the treatment period, this 50% reduction (or stimulation) occurs. In analogy, in BMC_5 z is 5 and represents a 5% change relative to control values. One possibility to determine the velocity of activation or inactivation of a test compound in the cell cultures is to modify the treatment schedules in such a way that the C_{max} (Models 1–4) and AUC (Models 5–8) of the toxic compound or of its toxic metabolite are changed. These modifications in the treatment schedule include **(a)** a partial replacement of the culture medium by fresh culture medium not containing any compound (*compound dilution*) during the treatment period; **(b)** a partial replacement of the culture medium during the treatment period by fresh culture medium *containing* the compound at the initial concentration (*compound replacement*); and **(c)** a preincubation of the compound of interest at nearly the final concentration before adding to the cell cultures (*compound preincubation*).

As mentioned above, schedules (a) and (b) normally occur if cultures are treated or kept for prolonged periods of time. In some labs, stock solutions of test compounds are made and kept until use. In that case, treatment schedule (c) takes place even if the person involved is unaware of it. This chapter takes these situations into account and even makes use of it. Models 1–4 are based on the assumption that the test compound does not penetrate into the cells (or, in the case where it is taken up, the test compound does not interact with intracellular components) and exerts its influence by interacting with components of the cell membrane: that is, a change in C_{max} will result in a change in EIC_z values (one-compartment models). In contrast, Models 5–8 are based on the assumption that the test compound first has to penetrate into the cells and exert its influence by interacting with an intracellular component; that is, the AUC and/or shape of the AUC will result in a change in EIC_z values (two-compartment models). The observed differences in EIC_z values in relation to experiments in which no compound dilution, replacement, and preincubation are performed (termed *control experiments*) are used as a base for the assessment of the test compound activation (k_{met}) and/or inactivation (k_{el}) constants. In this case test compound activation means modification of the test compound in a way that the resulting modified test compound is toxic. The opposite is meant with inactivation.

15.6 *IN VITRO* TOXICOKINETICS AND DYNAMICS

15.6.1 Effects Based on Peak Concentrations (One-Compartment Models)

Certain classes of compound either cannot overcome the cell membrane or they specifically interact with components of the outer cell membrane like receptors and ion channels. In this case, the reaction occurs if enough test compound binds to the receptive membrane component. The threshold treatment period is assumed to be the time needed to reach equilibrium. The presumption is made that the latter period is negligible and is therefore not taken into account in Models 1–4.

Model 1: The Compound Is Stable   In this model the concentration of the test compound does not vary during the treatment period. The medium compound concentration at the end of the treatment period corresponds to the initial concentration at the beginning of the treatment period. Since the maximum medium concentration is assumed to be the effective compound concentration, a compound dilution, such as occurs as a result of feeding the cultures by replacing old medium with fresh culture medium without test compound during the treatment period, or a compound preincubation before addition will not affect or shift the effective initial medium compound concentration (EIC)–response curves (OCERs).

Model 2: The Toxic Compound Is Inactivated   *In vitro*, compounds are inactivated (eliminated) on the one hand by the cultured cells, or on the other hand extracellularly by decomposition, by reducing the cellular accessibility, such as binding to released products of the cultured cells or by interaction with medium constituents (mainly proteins). The half-life of the compound due to intracellular inactivation and extracellular inactivation as a result of the interaction with released products is determined by the cell density and the cellular activity. Since the volume of the culture medium relative to the number of cells is extremely large, of the three inactivation pathways, the effect of inactivation by cells or their products is mainly negligible. The inactivation due to decomposition is exponential with a constant half-life. The half-life of the test compound that is inactivated by interaction with medium constituents depends on the medium concentrations of these constituents. A nearly constant half-life will only be found at small test compound concentrations relative to the concentration of these constituents; otherwise the half-life will increase exponentially with time.

Due to the inactivation of the test compound, its maximum concentration is present at the moment of addition of the test compound to the cultures. Therefore, a dilution of the culture medium after addition will not affect the OCERs. The maximum medium concentration will only be reduced in the case of compound preincubation, but only if the test compound is inactivated by decomposition or by interaction with medium constituents and not by cell-related processes.

Assuming one compartment and a single treatment of the cultures, the culture medium concentration of the toxic compound (y_i) follows the OCER as the one described for blood concentrations after an IV administration *in vivo* under the same assumptions. Thus, Eqs. 15.1 and 15.2 are also applicable for the present model for describing the culture medium concentration and the inactivation half-life, respectively.

After preincubation, less toxic compound will be present, resulting in an apparent shift in the OCER in which the effect is related to the test compound at the moment before preincubation was started (initial or starting concentration, EIC). Comparing EIC_{50} values as calculated by Eq. 15.11, an inactivation of 50% of the compound implies that, before preincubation, twice the concentration had to be present to give the same concentrations at the moment that the dilutions are added to the cultures and thus in concentrations giving the same effect. The presence of equal effects implies that at the beginning of the treatment period equal toxic compound concentrations were present in the cell cultures. An increase in EICz as result of preincubation can be explained by a partial conversion of the toxic compound into a non-toxic substance. For example if 50% is inactivated during the preincubation period twice the concentration is needed to have at start of the treatment the same concentration of toxic compound. This can be described by the following equation,

$$EIC_{z1} = EIC_{z2} \cdot e^{-k_{el}t_p} \tag{15.17}$$

where k_{el} is the elimination constant in the culture medium, t_p is the preincubation duration (difference between the time point at which the preincubation was started and t_0), EIC_{z1} is the obtained EIC_z in experiments without compound preincubation, and EIC_{z2} is the EIC_z in experiments with compound preincubation.

The k_{el} can be calculated with the following equation, which is obtained by rearranging Eq. 15.17:

$$k_{el} = \left(\frac{-1}{t_p}\right)\ln\left(\frac{EIC_{z1}}{EIC_{z2}}\right) \tag{15.18}$$

Model 3: The Nontoxic Compound Is Modified into a Toxic Compound   This model describes the concentration and effects of those test compounds that are bioactivated as a result of an interaction with components of the culture medium. Effects of biotransformation by a rate-limiting process inside the cells or at the cell surface are not described by this model but are by Model 5 (Section 15.6.2). Although a nontoxic test compound may give rise to a range of products, each of them having different toxic effects, generally one product dominates in its toxic effects on the cell culture. The formation of this main important toxic product is subjected to the same kind of processes as described for inactivation of the test compound (Model 2). The only difference is that in Model 3 the product is the toxic compound and in Model 2 the product is the original test compound. If one molecule of test compound gives rise to one toxic molecule, the concentration of the toxic product can be calculated by subtracting the concentration of the test compound at time t_i from the initial test compound concentration at time t_0. Otherwise, the test compound concentrations need to be multiplied by a factor representing the largest number of toxic molecules that are obtained from one molecule of test compound. The concentration of toxic product (A_i) increases with treatment period (t_i) (see Eq. 15.1) and is

$$A_i = A_0(1 - e^{-k_{met}t_i}) \tag{15.19}$$

where A_0 is the final concentration of the toxic product when all test compound is bioactivated, A_i is the concentration of the toxic product at t_i, and k_{met} is the rate constant of activation (*met*abolism) [1].

Like the elimination half-life, the rate of bioactivation can also be expressed in a "half-life period" defined as the time needed to activate half of the test compound. Thus, $A_i = 0.5A_0 = A_0(1 - e^{-k_{met}t_{1/2}})$ and, in analogy to Eq. 15.2,

$$t_{1/2} = \frac{\ln(2)}{k_{met}} \tag{15.20}$$

Although the nontoxic test compound only evokes toxic effects by its toxic product(s), the extent of toxic effects is related to the concentration of the nontoxic compound added to the culture medium. This characteristic can be used to assess k_{met} experimentally without measuring the concentrations in the culture medium. The k_{met} can be calculated if results from the control experiment are compared with data from experiments using compound dilution, compound replacement, or compound preincubation.

COMPOUND DILUTION   According to Eq. 15.19, the concentration of the toxic product at the time point just before medium dilution (t_1) corresponds to

$$A_1 = A_0(1 - e^{-k_{met}t_1})$$ (15.21)

and at the end of the treatment period after dilution of the medium by a factor x to

$$A_i = \frac{A_0(1 - e^{-k_{met}t_i})}{x}$$ (15.22)

By comparing data obtained from dilution and control experiments, the following scenarios may occur:

1. The medium is diluted by test compound-free medium after full activation of the test compound in the cell cultures. Under these circumstances, the concentration–response curve will not be affected by the dilution.
2. The medium is diluted by test compound-free medium before the test compound is fully activated in the cell cultures.
   (a) The dilution factor and/or t_1 is large enough that $A_1 > A_i$. Under these conditions, identical maximum concentrations and thus effects are obtained if

$$A_{01}(1 - e^{-k_{met}t_i}) = A_{02}(1 - e^{-k_{met}t_1})$$

where

A_{01} is the initial, starting concentration of the test compound in experiments without dilution and A_{02} is the initial, starting concentration of the test compound in experiments with dilution.

If the maximum concentrations that are reached in culture medium during cell treatment are directly correlated with the resulting cellular effects,

$$\frac{A_{01}}{A_{02}} = \frac{EIC_{z1}}{EIC_{z2}}$$ (15.23)

Thus,

$$\frac{EIC_{z1}}{EIC_{z2}} = \frac{1 - e^{-k_{met}t_1}}{1 - e^{-k_{met}t_i}}$$ (15.24)

k_{met} can be calculated after filling in EIC_{z1}, EIC_{z2}, t_1, and t_i.

(b) The most common situation is that x is large and so $A_1 < A_i$. Under these circumstances, identical maximum concentrations are obtained if

$$A_{01}(1-e^{-k_{met}t_i}) = \frac{A_{02}(1-e^{-k_{met}t_i})}{x}$$

where again x is the dilution factor (see Eqs. 15.21 and 15.22). Also, in combination with Eq. 15.23 and after some rearrangement,

$$\frac{EIC_{z1}}{EIC_{z2}} = \frac{1}{x}$$

This implies that under these circumstances k_{met} *cannot* be assessed.

COMPOUND REPLACEMENT   An analogue situation as described earlier occurs if the replacing medium contains the test compound at an identical concentration as present at t_0. The EIC_z in experiments with compound replacement will increase in comparison to control experiments. This will occur because at t_1 not only is the test compound replaced but the toxic product formed in the cultures is diluted by a factor x. No change or only a negligible change in EIC_z will occur if the activation half-life is very small and at t_1 or t_i the maximum concentration of the toxic metabolite is already present. A similar situation occurs if both x and t_1 are very large ($t_1 \gg 0.5t_i$). The increase in EIC_z value is maximum in the case where the concentrations of the toxic product at t_1 and t_i are the same (i.e., after complete replacement $t_1 = 0.5t_i$). In the latter situations, the maximum concentration of the toxic product is reached in the culture just before the compound replacement and Eq. 15.24 can be used for calculating k_{met}. Otherwise, the following correlation between A_{01} (Eq. 15.21) and A_{02} (see Eq. 15.22) exists:

$$A_{01}(1-e^{-k_{met}t_1}) = \frac{A_{02}(1-e^{-k_{met}t_i})}{x} + \frac{(x-1)A_{02}(1-e^{-k_{met}(t_i-t_1)})}{x}$$

or in combination with Eq. 15.23

$$\frac{EIC_{z1}}{EIC_{z2}} = \frac{x - e^{-k_{met}t_i} + (1-x)e^{-k_{met}(t_i-t_1)}}{x(1-e^{-k_{met}t_1})}$$

Again, k_{met} can be calculated after filling in EIC_{z1}, EIC_{z2}, x, t_1, and t_i.

COMPOUND PREINCUBATION   If no full activation is achieved, the final concentration A_i of the activated compound is $A_0(1-e^{-k_{met}(t_i+t_p)})$ instead of $A_0(1-e^{-k_{met}t_i})$ after inclusion of a preincubation period. To obtain identical concentrations at the end of the treatment period, the starting concentration must be comparably higher to the extent that

$$A_{01}(1-e^{-k_{met}t_i}) = A_{02}(1-e^{-k_{met}(t_i+t_p)})$$

By assuming that the effects seen are directly dependent on the final concentration of the bioactivated compound, we find

$$\frac{\text{EIC}_{z1}}{\text{EIC}_{z2}} = \frac{1 - e^{-k_{\text{met}}(t_p + t_i)}}{1 - e^{-k_{\text{met}}t_i}}$$

in which EIC_{z1} and EIC_{z2} are the concentrations needed to obtain similar effects (EIC_{z1} (controls) and EIC_{z2} (experiment with compound preincubation) according to Eq. 15.19 and in combination with Eq. 15.23).

Model 4: The Nontoxic Test Compound Is Transformed into a Toxic Product that Afterwards Is Inactivated   This model finds its analogue in the *in vivo* situation after extravascular administration of a toxic compound, when absorption and elimination are first-order processes as described in Section 15.3. This means that the pattern of the toxic product A_i in the culture medium can be described by the Bateman equation (Eq. 15.3, also like *in vivo*). For the *in vitro* situation, the absorption constant (k_{abs}) has to be replaced by the metabolization constant (k_{met}) and the ratio (Df/V) by A_0, representing the maximum concentration of toxic product in the case $k_{\text{el}} = 10^{-\infty}$, or

$$A_i = A_0 k_{\text{met}} \left(\frac{e^{-k_{\text{el}}t_i} - e^{-k_{\text{met}}t_i}}{k_{\text{met}} - k_{\text{el}}} \right) \tag{15.25}$$

where k_{met} is the activation constant and k_{el} is the inactivation (elimination) constant.

Although the nontoxic test compound only evokes toxic effects by its toxic products(s), the extent of toxic effects is directly related to and can be expressed in the concentration of the nontoxic compound like in Model 3. Therefore, k_{met} and k_{el} can also be expressed in nontoxic test compound concentrations. Important for the observed effects in Models 1–4 are the peak concentration of the toxic product and the time at which this peak concentration is present in the medium. The time point (t_{max}) in this model at which the peak concentration is reached is

$$t_{\text{max}} = \frac{\ln(k_{\text{met}}/k_{\text{el}})}{k_{\text{met}} - k_{\text{el}}} \tag{15.26}$$

and the peak concentration (A_{max}) is [1]

$$A_{\text{max}} = A_0 \left(\frac{k_{\text{met}}}{k_{\text{el}}} \right)^{k_{\text{el}}/(k_{\text{el}} - k_{\text{met}})} \tag{15.27}$$

Up to the time point t_{max} a direct relationship exists between EIC_z and y_i of Eq. 15.25. After t_{max} the EIC_z is constant and directly related to A_{max} (Eq. 15.27).

COMPOUND DILUTION   If the culture medium is replaced by medium without a compound (compound dilution) at a time point after t_{max}, then the EIC_z value is not affected. A dilution before t_{max} is similar to the situation described by Model 3: the maximum concentration of toxic product is present in the culture medium at the end of the treatment period. Comparing data obtained from dilution and control experiments, the same scenarios may occur as in Model 3. However, EIC_z correlates with Eq. 15.25 and not with Eq. 15.19. Since before t_{max} A_i can nearly be mimicked by Eq. 15.19, in practice it will not be possible to discriminate between Model 3 and 4 under these circumstances using compound dilution experiments.

COMPOUND PREINCUBATION   In analogy to compound dilution, the value of t_{max} is decisive as to which effect a compound preincubation has on the EIC_z value. Of the four different scenarios that can be discriminated, three are possible in practice: (1) The t_{max} in both cases (with and without preincubation) has a value between $t0$ and t_i. In this scenario a compound preincubation has no effect on EIC_z. (2). The t_{max} is reached during the preincubation period. In this case a preincubation of the compound dilutions results in an increase in the EIC_z value. The compound behaves very similarly to that described in Model 2. (3) The t_{max} is greater than t_i, irrespective of the value of t_p, or occurs only after preincubation. Under these circumstances, a compound preincubation results in a decrease in the EIC_z value. The compound behaves as described in Model 3. Since under possibilities (2) and (3) the OCER can be mimicked fairly well by the equations describing Models 2 and 3, respectively, it is not possible to discriminate between these models and Model 4 under experimental conditions.

15.6.2   Effects Based on Accumulation (Two-Compartment Models)

Several compounds of different compound classes seem not to have an acute effect or only after extreme doses. Their toxicity seems to be dependent on the total cumulative dose received and not merely on the treatment schedule. Therefore, their effects seem to be related with the *in vivo* area under the serum concentration–time curve (AUC) (Fig. 15.1) and not by a single dose or by the maximum serum concentration.

The reason why one toxic compound at a given blood concentration is effective at a short exposure time while other compounds require a prolonged period of time to be effective is assumed to be the difference in the accessibility of the target protein(s) for the toxic test compound. Whereas some compounds introduced into a test system are obviously able to interact directly and freely with the target protein(s) resulting in acute effects, others are not. These latter compounds first have to overcome some kind of "barrier," which is not only determined by diffusion velocity. This barrier consists of saturable processes that limit transfer into the target compartment, such as carrier dependent transport, or saturable processes in which certain enzymes play a key role (formation of toxic product S*; Fig. 15.7). In the latter case, a complex or a metabolite may be formed. In these kinds of barrier, accumulation is restricted by the number of interaction sites (binding sites). Binding site-limited processes can be described by the Michaelis–Menten relationship [22]:

$$\frac{v_0}{V_{max}} = \frac{[S]}{K_m + [S]}$$

(15.28)

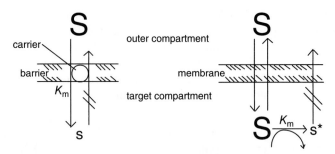

FIGURE 15.7 Entry of a toxic compound into the target compartment: example of a carrier-mediated inward transport and of an enzyme-dependent accumulation.

where [S] is the external concentration of the test compound (termed the outer compartment test compound concentration), v_0 is the compound transfer velocity per time unit at [S], V_{max} is the maximum compound transfer velocity per time unit, and K_m is the Michaelis–Menten constant representing the [S] at which $v_0 = 0.5V_{max}$.

Besides K_m, the stability of the test compound plays an important role in how much of the toxic product finally reaches the target compartment. Previously, we described what occurs if the compound is **(a)** stable (Model 5), **(b)** modified into a nontoxic compound (Model 6), **(c)** modified into a toxic product, the test compound being nontoxic (Model 7), and **(d)** in addition to (c) the resulting toxic product is thereafter modified into a nontoxic compound (Model 8). For these four models, it is assumed that the toxic test compound, test compound complex, or product (termed toxic compound in the target compartment) cannot be released from the target compartment. In other words, the process of accumulation is assumed to be unidirectional. Furthermore, it is assumed that the effects are induced according to the single effector site model (see Section 15.4.1). For model 5, we discuss the possibility that the effects are due to an interaction with two different effector sites. The compound concentration outside the target compartment is assumed to be homogeneous and is termed the outer compartment. The following models are simplified with the restriction that the delay, which may occur between reaching the toxic compartment concentration and the onset of effects, is not taken into account.

Model 5: The Test Compound Concentration Is Stable   Assuming that [S] is constant, the concentration s of the toxic compound within the target compartment equals

$$s = t_i S_f \left(\frac{v_0}{V_{max}} \right) \tag{15.29}$$

where t_i is the period between the addition and the time of interest, S_f is the maximum concentration increase per time unit of the toxic compound within the target compartment, and V_0/V_{max} is the fraction of compound transferred relative to the maximum.

The relationship between the outer compartment and target compartment concentrations can be obtained by replacing the ratio v_0/V_{max} in Eq. 15.29 by Eq. 15.28:

$$s = t_i S_f \left(\frac{[S]}{K_m + [S]} \right)$$

(15.30)

Thus, at a given outer compartment concentration, the maximum target compartment concentration is determined by only t_i, K_m (Fig. 15.8a), and S_f. The transfer of the compound into the target compartment may be altered under certain circumstances, such as modified culture conditions. Effects on S_f can be mimicked by changes in t_i (doubling of S_f has the same effect as doubling t_i (see Eq. 15.30). In contrast, a change in K_m value does not affect the maximum compound concentration within the target compartment after a given treatment period but only affects the concentration at which the transfer into the target compartment reaches maximum values (Fig. 15.8b). The slope of the outer compartment–target compartment compound concentration relationship remains unchanged under these conditions. By testing different compound concentrations, it is possible to discriminate between effects on S_f and K_m on the target compartment concentration.

After a certain period of time, the concentration of toxic compound/product within the target compartment reaches a critical level: the compound/product starts to noticeably interfere with cell functions (Fig. 15.9a). It is reasonable to assume that these interferences are directly related with binding of the toxic compound to effector molecules within the target compartment. If the induced effects are concentration dependent according to the one effector site model (Section 15.4.1), [S] of Eq. 15.10 has to be changed to s (or s^*). The variables s and s^* represent the concentrations of the toxic test compound/product within the target compartment. In the next step, s (or s^*) is replaced by Eq. 15.30, or

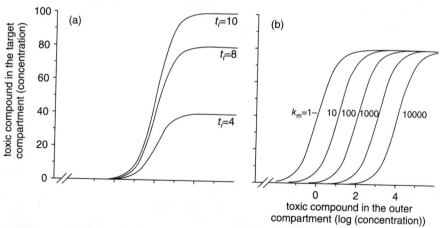

FIGURE 15.8   Correlation between the concentration of the toxic compound in the outer compartment and the concentration in the target compartment according to Eq. 15.30: effects of variations in (a) the treatment period t_i ($S_f = 10$, $K_m = 100$) and (b) the Michaelis–Menten constant K_m ($t_i = 8$; $S_f = 10$) (arbitrary units).

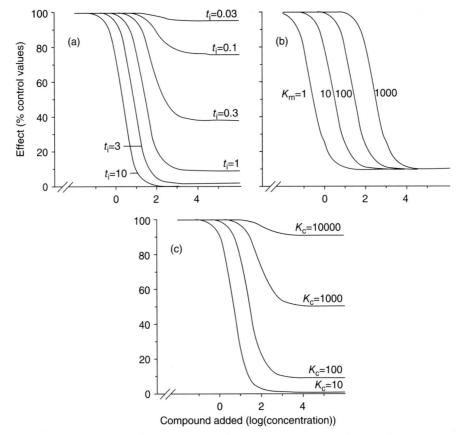

FIGURE 15.9 Outer compartment compound concentration–effect relationships (OCERs) according to Eq. 15.31. $N_c = 1.5$, $K_c = 100$, $t_i = 1$, $S_f = 100$, and $K_m = 100$ (arbitrary units) or as mentioned in the figure. Effects on the outcome are shown for variations in (a) the treatment period t_i, (b) the Michaelis–Menten constant K_m, and (c) the cooperativity constant K_c.

$$\frac{E_t}{E_u} = \frac{K_c}{K_c + \left(t_i S_f \left(\dfrac{[S]}{K_m + [S]}\right)\right)^{N_c}} \tag{15.31}$$

or

$$\frac{E_t}{E_u} = \frac{1}{1 + \dfrac{(t_i S_f)^{N_c}}{K_c}\left(\dfrac{[S]}{K_m + [S]}\right)^{N_c}} \tag{15.32}$$

Thus, *the response constant K_c and the slope N_c in Eq. 15.31 and 15.32 are characterized by the target compartment and not by the outer compartment concentration! In addition, the shape of the present relationship is not the same as the one described by Eq. 15.10, although the obtained relationships are apparently very similar.*

In Eq. 15.32, $(t_i S_f)^{N_c}/K_c$ behaves like a single constant. This implies that modifications in the K_c, t_i, or S_f value can be mimicked by changes in one of the other parameters. At a given test compound outer compartment concentration, the parameters K_c, t_i, and S_f determine the maximum effect level. The maximum effect level is reached when [S] is large, and therefore when the ratio $[S]/(K_m + [S])$ reaches the value 1. Thus, under the assumptions of Model 5, the maximum effect level is *independent* of K_m. As clearly demonstrated by Eq. 15.33, a decrease in K_m value by a factor of x can be mimicked by an increase in test compound in the outer compartment by the same factor.

$$\frac{x[S]}{K_m + x[S]} = \frac{[S]}{(K_m/x)+[S]} \qquad (15.33)$$

Thus, modifications in K_m, in contrast to t_i, S_f, and K_c, shift the OCER (Fig. 15.9b) without effect on its shape. It must be noted that a change in the K_m, K_c, or S_f value influences the shape but not the slope of the OCER. In analogy to s (or s^*), modifications of the compound toxicity due to changes in culture conditions can be based on modifications of S_f, K_m, and/or K_c values. By measuring the effect of various compound concentrations under different culture conditions and assessing the effects on the maximum effect level and location of the OCER, it is possible to discriminate between effects on S_f or K_c and K_m but not between S_f and K_c. To discriminate between the effect on S_f and K_c, the concentration of the compound in the target compartment has to be measured and related to the observed effects. The latter, however, will in most cases not be possible.

For calculation of the EIC_{50} value, two reference levels are needed: control values and a reference value for maximum effects. For maximum effects, two different reference lines can be considered: (1) the 0% activity line, corresponding to the effect of the compound at maximum concentration and treatment duration, and (2) the activity percentage reached at large [S] values at t_i.

The 0% activity is taken as the reference for maximum effects. Under this assumption, the EIC_{50} is defined as the outer compartment compound concentration at which at the chosen treatment period $E_t = 0.5E_u$. In Eq. 15.31, if we replace E_t/E_u by 0.5 and [S] by EIC_{50}, the following equation can be obtained after some rearrangements:

$$EIC_{50} = \frac{K_m\{(K_c)^{1/N_c}/S_f\}}{t_i - \{(K_c)^{1/N_c}/S_f\}}$$

or

$$EIC_{50} = \frac{K_m}{t_i S_f (K_c)^{-1/N_c} - 1} \qquad (15.34)$$

For calculation of BMC_5, where $E_t/E_u = 0.95$, K_c must be replaced by $K_c/19$, or

$$BMC_5 = \frac{K_m}{t_i S_f (K_c/19)^{-1/N_c} - 1} \qquad (15.35)$$

Using this equation, N_c, K_m, and S_f must be calculated by taking into account the activity percentage reached at large [S] values *at the given* t_i. An example of such a relationship between EIC_{50} and t_i according to Eq. 15.34 is shown in Fig. 15.10. A positive, fictitious value for EIC_{50} is only obtained if $t_i S_f (K_c)^{-1/N_c} > 1$. In this equation, $(K_c)^{-1/N_c}$ represents the target compartment EIC_{50} (see Eq. 15.11). Only if this target compartment concentration is reached, can measurement of a 50% reduction be possible.

At short t_i values, when $t_i S_f$ values are near $(K_c)^{1/N_c}$, a doubling of t_i will reduce EIC_{50} much *more* than 50% due to the subtraction of 1 from $t_i S_f (K_c)^{-1/N_c}$. *Thus, the toxicity is not directly related to the AUC.* If the compound concentration in the outer compartment is stable, the AUC after the treatment period t_i is defined by

$$AUC_{t_i} = (AUC_{t_0 \Rightarrow t_i}) = [S]t_i$$

where t_i is the difference between the time at the end of the treatment period and the time at the beginning of the treatment period (t_0).

At large t_i the subtraction of 1 from $t_i S_f (K_c)^{-1/N_c}$ will only marginally influence the outcome. Only under these circumstances does a doubling of t_i bisect the EIC_{50} value or, in other words, EIC_{50}/t_i is constant. This implies that only *at large t_i can an inverse linear relationship exist between toxicity expressed by EIC_{50} value and AUC.*

If the results of two experiments are compared in which only t_i was varied, an estimate of K_m can be made if an inhibition of the parameter of interest of at least

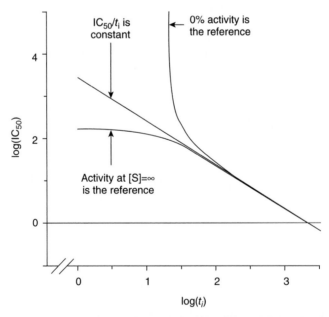

FIGURE 15.10   Correlation between EIC_{50} defined by 0% activity or by the activity percentage reached if $[S] = \infty$ and treatment period t_i. The effects are simulated according to the one effector site model (Eq. 15.34 and 15.39, respectively) ($S_f = 100$, $K_c = 100{,}000$, $K_m = 100$, $N_c = 1.5$) (arbitrary units).

$z\%$ at maximum [S] is reached. The two different treatment periods are termed t_{i1} and t_{i2}. As a new variable, r is introduced representing the ratio $r = (t_{i1} - t_{i2})/t_{i2}$, or $t_{i1} = t_{i2}(1 + r)$. In Models 5–8, the effects after t_{i1} and t_{i2} are the same if $s_1 = s_2$, or

$$(1+r)t_{i2}S_f\left\{\frac{\text{EIC}_{z1}}{K_m + \text{EIC}_{z1}}\right\} = t_{i2}S_f\left\{\frac{\text{EIC}_{z2}}{K_m + \text{EIC}_{z2}}\right\}$$

where EIC_{z1} and EIC_{z2} are the initial outer compartment concentration after t_{i1} and t_{i2}, respectively, resulting in a reduction of the parameter of interest by $z\%$. Or after rearrangement,

$$K_m = \frac{r \cdot \text{EIC}_{z1} \cdot \text{EIC}_{z2}}{\text{EIC}_{z2} - (r+1) \cdot \text{EIC}_{z1}} \tag{15.36}$$

Besides the possibility of calculating K_m, this equation also indicates that a relation between treatment period and EIC_{z1} and EIC_{z2} exists, independent of S_f, K_c, and N_c.

The reference for maximum effects is defined by the activity percentage reached at large [S] values. As mentioned before, at large [S] values the ratio $[S]/(Km + [S])$ in Eq. 15.31 reaches the value 1. Thus, the maximum possible effect level (E_{tmax}/E_u) after the given treatment period t_i equals

$$\frac{E_{tmax}}{E_u} = \frac{K_c}{K_c + (t_iS_f)^{N_c}} \tag{15.37}$$

The EIC_{50} at the treatment period chosen under the present assumptions is defined as the outer compartment concentration at which

$$1 - \frac{E_t}{E_u} = 0.5\left(1 - \frac{E_{tmax}}{E_u}\right) \tag{15.38}$$

In Eq. 15.38, (E_t/E_u) can be replaced by Eq. 15.31 and (E_{tmax}/E_u) by Eq. 15.37. After some rearrangements, the following is obtained:

$$\text{EIC}_{50} = \frac{K_m}{\{2 + (t_iS_f)^{N_c}/K_c\}^{1/N_c} - 1} \tag{15.39}$$

In analogy, the BMC_5 can be calculated:

$$1 - \frac{E_t}{E_u} = 0.05\left(1 - \frac{E_{tmax}}{E_u}\right)$$

or

$$\text{BMC}_5 = \frac{K_m}{\{20 + 19(t_iS_f)^{N_c}/K_c\}^{1/N_c} - 1} \tag{15.40}$$

As in the previous case, in which the 0% activity is taken as a reference, only at large t_i can doubling of t_i bisect the EIC_{50} value. However, in contrast to the previous case, at very small t_i a doubling of t_i will reduce the EIC_{50} value by *less* than 50%. This is due to the presence of the constant with a value of 2 in the denominator. Thus, again toxicity is inversely linearly correlated with the AUC *only* at large treatment periods (Fig. 15.10). Roughly, one can say that a linear relationship between AUC and EIC_{50} exists as far as Eqs. 15.34 and 15.39 give similar EIC_{50} values.

COMPOUND DILUTION   If during the treatment period at a time t_1 the medium of the cultures is partially replaced by fresh medium without the test compound, the remaining compound is diluted, corresponding to the ratio of remaining old medium divided by total medium volume (factor x). As a result, the increase in s per time unit is reduced after t_1. Mathematically, the obtained OCER can be described by Eq. 15.32, including an adaptation for the dilution of [S] at t_1:

$$\frac{E_{\text{tdil}}}{E_{\text{u}}} = \frac{K_{\text{c}}}{K_{\text{c}} + \left(t_1 S_{\text{f}} \left\{ \dfrac{[S]}{K_{\text{m}} + [S]} \right\} + (t_i - t_1) S_{\text{f}} \left\{ \dfrac{x[S]}{K_{\text{m}} + x[S]} \right\} \right)^{N_{\text{c}}}} \tag{15.41}$$

where E_{tdil} and E_{u} are values of the parameter of interest at the end of the treatment period, in which a dilution or no dilution step was carried out, respectively; $t_1 S_{\text{f}}\{[S]/(K_{\text{m}} + [S])\}$ is the concentration of the test compound in the target compartment at the moment of dilution (t_1), and $(t_i - t_1)S_{\text{f}}\{x[S]/(K_{\text{m}} + x[S])\}$ is the increase of test compound in the target compartment from t_1 to the end of the treatment period (t_i).

At large [S], however, the ratio $x[S]/(K_{\text{m}} + x[S])$ is still near 1 except if x is extremely small (see Fig. 15.8 and Eq. 15.30). This implies that the *same* maximum effect level is obtained with or without compound dilution. Depending on the location of the maximum effect level at t_1, two different situations can be discriminated after a compound dilution.

(a) *The parameter of interest is completely inhibited at t_1 at maximum [S] values.* With decreasing x values, the OCER found at t_i will shift asymptotically toward the OCER measured at t_1. No swallowed OCER will be obtained (Fig. 15.11). Independent of the value of t_i, if $x[S]$ is relatively small in comparison to K_{m}, then in $(t_i - t_1)S_{\text{f}}\{x[S]/(K_{\text{m}} + x[S])\}$, a decrease in the x value can be mimicked by an increase in t_i and by that of $t_i - t_1$.

(b) *Even at very large [S], s (or s^*) at t_1 is still too low to inhibit completely the parameter of interest.* Only the part of the curve that represents the effect due to the treatment period to t_1 will behave in a similar way as described under (a). The other part will be shifted corresponding to the dilution. A dilution of 0.1 will shift the latter part of the relationship by a factor of 10, a dilution of 0.01 will result in a shift of a factor 100, and soon (see Fig. 15.11). At relatively large x values (0.01–1), only a change in the apparent N_{c} will be observed and a swallowed OCER cannot be recognized. A complete removal of the compound at t_1 ($x = 10^{-\infty}$) will result in an OCER corresponding to the effect of a treatment to t_1. Thus, only under these extreme situations (complete removal) can a dilution of the compound be mimicked by a reduction in the total treatment period without dilution!!

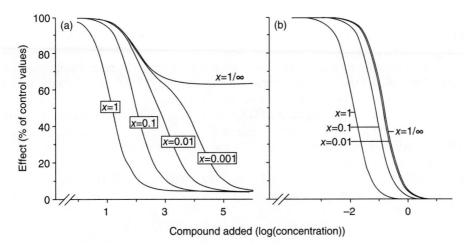

FIGURE 15.11 Simulation of initial outer compartment concentration–effect relationship (OCER) according to Eq. 15.41: effects on the outcome due to variations of dilution factor x ($K_m = 100$, $K_c = 100$, $N_c = 1.5$ (arbitrary units)). (a) $t_1 = 0.15$ and $t_i = 1.65$, (b) $t_1 = 150$ and $t_i = 1650$.

The K_m value can be estimated if an inhibition of the parameter of interest is present by more than z%, at least at maximum [S]. The reference for maximum effects is 0% (complete inhibition or absence of the parameter of interest). Comparing the effective outer compartment concentrations giving the same effect z in experiments with and without compound dilution: E_i/E_u (Eq. 15.31) = E_{tdil}/E_u (Eq. 15.41), or

$$
\frac{K_c}{K_c + \left((1+r)t_1 S_f \left\{ \dfrac{\mathrm{EIC}_{z1}}{K_m + \mathrm{EIC}_{z1}} \right\} \right)^{N_c}}
$$
$$
= \frac{K_c}{K_c + \left(t_1 S_f \left\{ \dfrac{\mathrm{EIC}_{z2}}{K_m + \mathrm{EIC}_{z2}} \right\} + r t_1 S_f \left\{ \dfrac{x\mathrm{EIC}_{z2}}{K_m + x\mathrm{EIC}_{z2}} \right\} \right)^{N_c}}
$$

where EIC_{z1} and EIC_{z2} are the EIC_z values measured in experiments without and with compound dilution, respectively, at t_1, and r is the ratio $(t_i - t_1)/t_1$.

After some rearrangements, the following equation can be obtained:

$$
K_m = \frac{\mathrm{EIC}_{z2}\{x\mathrm{EIC}_{z2}(1+r) - \mathrm{EIC}_{z1}(x+r)\}}{\mathrm{EIC}_{z1}(1+r) - \mathrm{EIC}_{z2}(1+rx)} \tag{15.42}
$$

At extremely small x values ($x \Rightarrow 10^{-\infty}$), Eq. 15.42 resembles Eq. 15.36.

COMPOUND REPLACEMENT AND PREINCUBATION   Compound replacement and compound preincubation have no effect, since the concentration of the test compound in the cultures and within the outer compartment will not be modified due to these treatments.

Special Cases: Two or More Effector Sites Are Present   If two or more effector sites are present, these various sites may be located in the same or in different target compartments.

(a) *Both sites are located within the target compartment.* The interaction between test compound and the main effector site need not always result in cell death. When numerous effector sites play a role in the observed effects, the resulting OCER can be described by Eq. 15.16, replacing [S] by the *s* of Eq. 15.30. The resulting equation is indistinguishable from Eq. 15.31. Interactions of the test compound with two effector sites (the main and another effector site causing cell death) will result in swallowed or at least a less steep OCER. Mathematically, this OCER can be described by Eq. 15.14, replacing [S] by the *s* (or *s**) of Eq. 15.30. The latter substitution results in the following equation:

$$\frac{E_t}{E_u} = \frac{\dfrac{K_{c1} E_{u1}}{K_{c1} + \left(t_i S_f \left\{ \dfrac{[S]}{K_m + [S]} \right\} \right)^{N_{c1}}} + \dfrac{K_{c2} E_{u2}}{K_{c2} + \left(t_i S_f \left\{ \dfrac{[S]}{K_m + [S]} \right\} \right)^{N_{c2}}}}{E_{u1} + E_{u2}} \qquad (15.43)$$

After a short treatment period, the maximum test compound concentration in the target compartment will be low. After reaching a certain concentration, the compound will interact with the high-affinity, in the present example (Fig. 15.12) stimulatory, effector site. Parallel with a prolongation of the treatment period, the maximum compound concentration within the target compartment will increase.

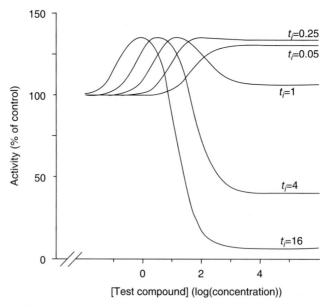

FIGURE 15.12   Simulation of outer compartment compound concentration–effect relationships according to Eq. 15.43 in relation to the treatment period t_i. ($E_{u1} = -40$, $N_{c1} = 1.5$, $K_{c1} = 0.1$, $E_{u2} = 140$, $N_{c2} = 1.5$, $K_{c2} = 100$, $S_f = 10$, and $K_m = 100$ (arbitrary units)).

The OCER of the first effector site will shift to the left. In addition, other cell functions will be affected due to the interaction with the second effector site. With further prolongation of the treatment period, both OCERs will shift to the left. Since only the combined effects can be detected, this shift will be reflected in a change in the overall shape of the outer culture medium concentration–response curve (Fig. 15.12).

(b) *The two effector sites are located in different compartments.* One of these compartments may represent a directly and freely accessible compartment, that is, the compartment to which the compound is added, and is termed the "outer" compartment. The second compartment represents a compartment outside the latter compartment. The compound first has to be transferred to this compartment and it is termed the "target" compartment. This implies that, as a result of an increase of the treatment period, only that part of the OCER will be shifted which is the result of the effector site being located within the target compartment. The other part of the OCER remains unaffected by a variation of the treatment period. If the various effector sites induce the *same* effect(s), their contributions for the observed effect(s) will change with the increase in treatment period. Otherwise, if the effector sites affect *different* functional parameters, the characteristics of the altered functional state of the cell will depend on the treatment period. *With prolonged treatment periods, the effect induced by the effector site located in the outer compartment will be totally overshadowed by the effect induced by the other effector site(s) inside the target compartment.* Often, two effects are characterized by different N_c values. In this case, a treatment-period-dependent change in N_c values will be observed. The sum of both effects can be characterized mathematically by multiplying Eq. 15.10, which describes the treatment-period-independent effects, by Eq. 15.31 or 15.43, which describes the transfer-dependent effects. Since transfer-dependent and acute effects can be described according to the one site effector model, the OCER can be characterized by the following equation:

$$
\frac{E_t}{E_u} = \left\{ \frac{K_{c1}}{K_{c1} + \left(t_i S_f \left[\dfrac{[S]}{K_m + [S]} \right] \right)^{N_{c1}}} \right\} \left\{ \frac{K_{c2}}{K_{c2} + [S]^{N_{c2}}} \right\}
\tag{15.44}
$$

in which effector site 1 (characterized by K_{c1} and N_{c1}) is responsible for the transfer-dependent effects and effector site 2 (characterized by K_{c2} and N_{c2}) is responsible for transfer-independent effects. In analogy, the same transition can be made if the transfer-dependent effects can be described according to the two effector site model (not shown).

The presence of such a mixture of effects, in which one effector site is located in the outer compartment and the other(s) is not, is typical for toxic compounds, with different EIC_{50} values for acute and long-term exposure (Fig. 15.13). For acute effects, no transfer into a certain target compartment is needed. Mainly the effective concentration is high and the OCER is steep (N_c is large) relative to the transfer-dependent effects. To avoid intermediate effects, representing a mixture of transfer-dependent and transfer-independent effects, prolonged treatment periods are preferred.

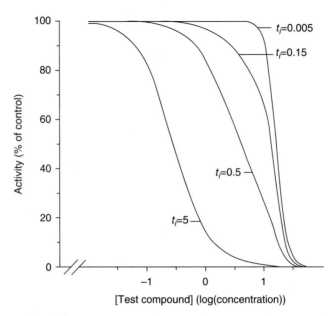

FIGURE 15.13   Simulation of an outer compartment compound concentration–effect relationship (OCER) according to Eq. 15.44 in relation to the treatment period t_i ($E_u = 100$). Target compartment effector site: $N_{c1} = 1.5$, $K_{c1} = 0.1$, $S_f = 10$ and $K_m = 10$. Outer compartment effector site: $N_{c2} = 5$, $K_{c2} = 100{,}000$; (all in arbitrary units).

Special Cases: The Accumulation Is Limited   In some cases accumulation of the test compound in the target compartment seems to be limited. Apparently only during the first part of the treatment period does a correlation between toxic effects and treatment period exist at a constant outer compartment test compound concentration.

An explanation for this phenomenon is the presence of a retro transport of the test compound (or its metabolite) out of the target compartment (Fig. 15.14). As a result, the accumulation in the target compartment is limited. The retrotransport may be due to diffusion or may be the result of a carrier-dependent retrotransport of the test compound. The increase of the target compartment concentration is maximum at small s_i (Fig. 15.14). A maximum concentration is reached the moment that the outward flux is equivalent to the inward flux. It must be noted that test compounds that are metabolized or activated inside the target compartment and the metabolite or activated test compounds that are able to leave the target compartment in one way or another behave identically.

The target compartment concentration s is dependent on the rat of influx (Fig. 15.14 left) or conversion rate (Fig. 15.14 right) and efflux rate. This influx/conversion is constant due to a constant outer compartment concentration (Eq. 15.30). The efflux, however, is dependent on the target compartment concentration and thus changes during the treatment period. If the efflux is carrier dependent, this may be described, in analogy to Eq. 15.4, as follows:

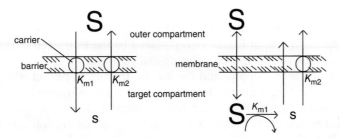

FIGURE 15.14 Entry of a toxic compound into the target compartment: example of a carrier mediated inward and outward transport (left) and of an enzyme-dependent accumulation with diffusion or carrier-mediated outward flux (right).

$$s_{\text{out},i} = S_{\text{f}} \left(\frac{s_i}{K_{\text{m}} + s_i} \right) \tag{15.45}$$

where $s_{\text{out},i}$ is the quantity of compound transported to the outer compartment expressed in concentration units of the target compartment, S_{f} is the maximum concentration decrease per time unit of the toxic compound within the target compartment, s_i is the target compound concentration at t_i, and K_{m} is the Michaelis–Menten constant representing the s_i at which efflux velocity $v_0 = 0.5V_{\text{max}}$.

The concentration s_i can be described as the difference between the quantity that is transported into the target compartment (Eq. 15.30) and the quantity that is transported out of the target compartment during the treatment period (see Eq. 15.45), or

$$s_i = t_i S_{\text{f1}} \left(\frac{[\text{S}]}{K_{\text{m1}} + [\text{S}]} \right) - S_{\text{f2}} \int_{\tau=0}^{\tau=t_i} \left(\frac{s_\tau}{K_{\text{m2}} + s_\tau} \right) d\tau \tag{15.46}$$

in which s_τ is the target compound concentration at $t = \tau$, S_{f1} and S_{f2} are the maximum concentration increase and decrease, respectively, per time unit of the toxic compound within the target compartment, and K_{m1} and K_{m2} are the Michaelis–Menten constants representing s_i at which, respectively, inward and outward flux velocity $v_0 = 0.5V_{\text{max}}$.

Since the target compartment concentration is present on the left and right sides of Eq. 15.46, this equation can be simplified not toward t_i but only toward s_i. After differentiation of Eq. 15.46 the following can be obtained:

$$S_{\text{f1}} \left(\frac{[\text{S}]}{K_{\text{m1}} + [\text{S}]} \right) - S_{\text{f2}} \left(\frac{s}{K_{\text{m2}} + s} \right) = \frac{ds}{dt} \tag{15.47}$$

or after some rearrangements

$$t_i = \frac{s_i}{a - S_{\text{f2}}} + \left(\frac{K_{\text{m2}}}{a - S_{\text{f2}}} \right) \left(1 - \frac{a}{a - S_{\text{f2}}} \right) \log \left(1 + \frac{s_i(a - S_{\text{f2}})}{aK_{\text{m2}}} \right) \tag{15.48}$$

in which a stands for $S_{\text{f1}}[\text{S}]/(k_{\text{m1}} + [\text{S}])$

For describing the OCER, for each S and t_i the s_i must be estimated using a numerical approach. An example of a relationship between s_i and t_i is presented in Fig. 15.15. Thereafter, [S] of Eq. 15.10 is replaced by the estimated s_i. The characteristics of the OCER can be estimated as described above.

A dilution of the test compound during the treatment period will result in an adjustment of the target compartment concentration asymptotically to the new equilibrium according the new outer compartment concentration. A dilution will have no effect on the OCER if the maximum target concentration is reached at the time of dilution. Thus, it appears that the treatment period is unimportant for the toxicity and important only for the peak concentration (Model 1). Therefore, the system has characteristics in-between Model 1 and Model 5 without outward transport. Compound replacement and compound pretreatment will have no effects on toxicity, as mentioned for Model 5 in the absence of outward transport.

Model 6: The Toxic Compound Is Inactivated   In analogy to Model 2, it is assumed that the compound is inactivated within the outer compartment during the treatment period. The concentration just after the addition of the compound (S_0) is reduced with increase of the treatment period according to Eq. 15.1. [S] at time point t_i (S_i) is equal to $S_0 e^{-k_{el}t_i}$. Not only the concentration in the outer compartment, per time unit ($t - t_{-1}$), but also the ratio $[S_i]/(K_m + [S_i])$ is slowly reduced during the treatment period. Therefore, the quantity of the test compound that is transferred from the outer compartment into the target compartment is continuously reduced. No compound is transferred at the moment that no compound is left in the outer compartment. The final concentration within the target compartment represents the

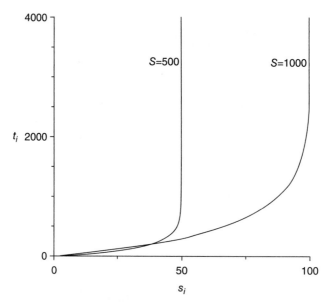

FIGURE 15.15   Correlation between the concentration of the toxic compound in the target compartment and the treatment period according to Eq. 15.48: effects of variations in the outer compartment concentration S ($S_{f1} = 10$, $S_{f2} = 10$, $K_{m1} = 100$, $K_{m2} = 100$ (arbitrary units)).

quantity of compound that is transferred into the target compartment over the whole treatment period. Thus, the concentration within the target compartment is

$$s_i = \sum_{t=0}^{i} (t - t_{-1}) S_f \left\{ \frac{S_0 e^{-k_{el}t}}{S_0 e^{-k_{el}t} + K_m} \right\}$$

or

$$s_i = S_f \int_{t=0}^{i} \left\{ \frac{S_0 e^{-k_{el}t}}{S_0 e^{-k_{el}t} + K_m} \right\} dt$$

Thus,

$$s_i = \left(\frac{S_f}{k_{el}} \right) \ln \left\{ \frac{K_m + S_0}{K_m + S_0 e^{-k_{el}t_i}} \right\} \qquad (15.49)$$

At large S_0 the ratio $(K_m + S_0)/(K_m + S_0 e^{-k_{el}t_i})$ has the value $e^{k_{el}t_i}$. After introducing this factor into Eq. 15.49, the following equation is obtained: $s_i = S_f t_i$. This equation is identical to Eq. 15.30. This means that *at large S_0 the maximum concentration level is time dependent and not dependent on K_m and k_{el} (see also Fig. 15.16). Furthermore, this implies that at large S_0 the same maximum s level is found within the target compartment independent of the stability of the toxic test compound!!*

$S_0 e^{-k_{el}t_i}$ will be 0 at the moment that all compound is inactivated. At this time point, the maximum target compartment concentration (s_{max}) is reached.

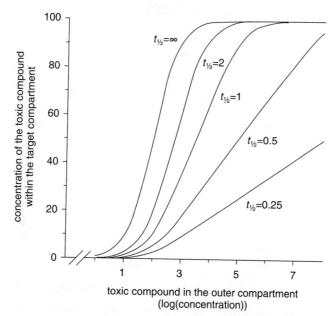

FIGURE 15.16 Correlation between the concentration of the toxic compound in the outer compartment and the concentration in the target compartment according to Eq. 15.49: effects of variations in the elimination half-life ($t_i = 10$; $S_f = 10$; $K_m = 100$ (arbitrary units)).

$$s_{max} = \left(\frac{S_f}{k_{el}}\right) \ln\left\{\frac{K_m + S_0}{K_m}\right\} \qquad (15.50)$$

If the induced effects are target compartment concentration-dependent, the OCER can be simulated in analogy to Model 5. Since the effects can be described according to the one effector site model, [S] of Eq. 15.10 can be replaced by Eq. 15.49, or

$$\frac{E_t}{E_u} = \frac{K_c}{K_c + \left(\left(\frac{S_f}{k_{el}}\right)\ln\left\{\frac{K_m + S_0}{K_m + S_0 e^{-k_{el}t_i}}\right\}\right)^{N_c}} \qquad (15.51)$$

An example of such a relationship is shown in Fig. 15.17. Please note that *the maximum effect level is only dependent on t_i (Fig. 15.17a) and not dependent on k_{el} (Fig. 15.17b)*.

Taking the 0% activity as a reference for maximum effects, the EIC_{50} value at the given treatment period can be calculated in analogy to Eq. 15.34 by $E_t = 0.5E_u$. By replacing S_0 by EIC_{50} and E_t/E_u by Eq. 15.51, the following equation can be obtained after some rearrangements:

$$EIC_{50} = \frac{K_m(v-1)}{1 - ve^{-k_{el}t_i}} \qquad (15.52)$$

in which v stands for

$$v = \exp\left(\frac{k_{el}(K_c)^{1/N_c}}{S_f}\right) \qquad (15.53)$$

For calculation of BMC_5, K_c must be replaced by $K_c/19$.

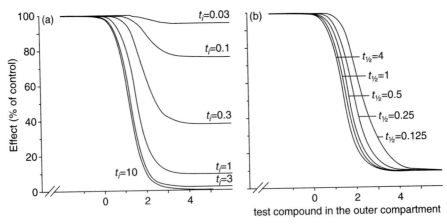

FIGURE 15.17 Simulation of outer compartment compound concentration–effect relationships (OCERs) according to Eq. 15.51 ($N_c = 1.5$, $K_c = 100$, $t_i = 1$, $S_f = 100$, and $K_m = 100$ (arbitrary units) or as mentioned in the figure): effects of variations in (a) the treatment period t_i and (b) the elimination half-life ($t_{1/2}$).

The reference value for maximum effects can also be defined as the activity percentage reached at large [S] values. In analogy to Eq. 15.39, Eq. 15.38 is used for the calculation of the EIC$_{50}$. In this case, the EIC$_{50}$ equals Eq. 15.52; however, in this case v stands for

$$v = \exp\left\{ \left(\frac{k_{el}}{S_f}\right)\left(\frac{2K_c}{1 + K_c/(t_iS_f)^{N_c}} - K_c\right)^{1/N_c} \right\}$$

(15.54)

At short treatment periods, the relationship between EIC$_{50}$ and the duration of the treatment period is similar to the one described for Model 5 (compare Figs 15.10 and 15.18). Because no test compound is present in the outer compartment at large t_i, no change in EIC$_{50}$ value is observed with increasing t_i (Figs. 15.17 and 15.18). *As a result, only during a short time period does a nearly linear relationship between t_i and EIC$_{50}$ exist!* In contrast to Model 5, a linear relationship between AUC and EIC$_{50}$ may not automatically be assumed if Eq. 15.52 in combination with Eq. 15.54 and Eq. 15.52 in combination with Eq. 15.53 give similar EIC$_{50}$ values!

COMPOUND DILUTION   A dilution of the compound during the treatment period will have less effect on the OCER as in the previous case (Model 5), since during the period before the dilution some test compound is already inactivated. To measure identical effects in cultures with or without compound dilution, the concentrations within the target compartment(s) need to be the same at t_i. Thus, s_1(without compound dilution) $= s_2$(with compound dilution). If in the cultures without compound dilution at t_i no compound is present, then

$$\left(\frac{S_f}{k_{el}}\right)\ln\left\{\frac{K_m + EIC_{z1}}{K_m}\right\} = \left(\frac{S_f}{k_{el}}\right)\ln\left\{\frac{K_m + EIC_{z2}}{K_m + EIC_{z2}e^{-k_{el}t_1}}\right\}$$

(15.55)

$$+ \left(\frac{S_f}{k_{el}}\right)\ln\left\{\frac{K_m + xEIC_{z2}e^{-k_{el}t_1}}{K_m}\right\}$$

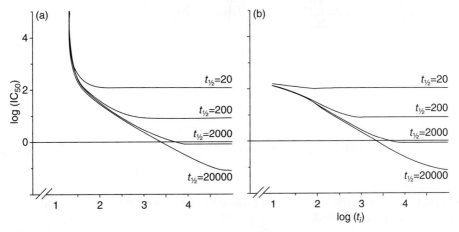

FIGURE 15.18 Correlation between EIC$_{50}$ defined by 0% activity (a) or by the activity percentage reached if [S] $= \infty$ and treatment period t_i (b). The effects are simulated according to the one effector site model (Eq. 15.52 and with v defined by Eqs. 15.53 and 15.54, respectively) ($S_f = 100$, $K_c = 100{,}000$, $K_m = 100$, $N_c = 1.5$ (arbitrary units)).

in which EIC_{z1} is the obtained EIC_z in experiments without dilution, EIC_{z2} is the EIC_z in experiments in which the compound was diluted during the treatment period, $(S_f/k_{el})\ln\{(k_m + EIC_{z1})/k_m\}$ is the test compound concentration in the target compartment at t_i in experiments without dilution according to Eq. 15.48, $(S_f/k_{el})\ln\{(K_m + EIC_{z2})/(K_m + EIC_{z2}e^{-k_{el}t_1})\}$ is the test compound concentration in the target compartment at $t1$ according to Eq. 15.47, and $(S_f/k_{el})\ln\{(K_m + xEIC_{z2}e^{-k_{el}t_1})/K_m\}$ is the increase of target compartment concentration after dilution by a factor x over the period t_1 to t_i (according to Eq. 15.50).

After a rearrangement of Eq. 15.55, we find

$$k_{el} = \left(\frac{-1}{t_1}\right)\ln\left(\frac{K_m(EIC_{z2} - EIC_{z1})}{EIC_{z2}\{K_m(1-x) + EIC_{z1} - EIC_{z2}x\}}\right) \tag{15.56}$$

or

$$K_m = \frac{(xEIC_{z2} - EIC_{z1})EIC_{z2}e^{-k_{el}t_1}}{(1-x)EIC_{z2}e^{-k_{el}t_1} + EIC_{z1} - EIC_{z2}} \tag{15.57}$$

The same equations can also be used if experiments with different treatment periods are compared. In this case, $x = 0$ and t_1 and t_i represent the different treatment periods. The disadvantage of Eq. 15.56 and 15.57 is that K_m has to be known in order to calculate k_{el}. It may be possible to estimate k_{el} and K_m by including within the same experiment the effects of a dilution at different time points to obtain Eq. 15.57 with other values for EIC_{z2} and t_1. Since in both obtained equations the value for K_m is the same, k_{el} can theoretically be resolved.

A more complex situation exists if at the end of the treatment period not all test compound is inactivated. In this case, a correction needs to be included for the remaining compound. Therefore, Eq. 15.50 may not be used. Under the present assumptions, Eq. 15.55 is adapted to

$$\left(\frac{S_f}{k_{el}}\right)\ln\left\{\frac{K_m + EIC_{z1}}{K_m + EIC_{z1}e^{-k_{el}t_i}}\right\} = \left(\frac{S_f}{k_{el}}\right)\ln\left\{\frac{K_m + EIC_{z2}}{K_m + EIC_{z2}e^{-k_{el}t_1}}\right\}$$
$$+ \left(\frac{S_f}{k_{el}}\right)\ln\left\{\frac{K_m + xEIC_{z2}e^{-k_{el}t_i}}{K_m + xEIC_{z2}e^{-k_{el}t_1}e^{-k_{el}(t_i - t_1)}}\right\}$$

or after rearrangement,

$$K_m = \{(1-x)EIC_{z1}EIC_{z2}e^{-k_{el}(t_i - t_1)} + (xEIC_{z2} - EIC_{z1})EIC_{z2} +$$
$$(EIC_{z2} - EIC_{z1})EIC_{z2}e^{-k_{el}(t_i - t_1)}\}/ \tag{15.58}$$
$$\{(1-x)EIC_{z2} + (xEIC_{z2} - EIC_{z1})e^{-k_{el}(t_i - t_1)}\}$$

Again, by changing the time point of dilution as mentioned before, k_{el} and K_m can theoretically be calculated.

COMPOUND REPLACEMENT Compound replacement during treatment maximally results in a doubling of the target compartment concentration if all compound is inactivated at the moment of replacement and in addition at the moment that the measurement is done again all compound is inactivated. If not all compound is inactivated at t_1 or at t_i, the change will be much less. Because of this, an effect on EIC_{50} will hardly be measurable under experimental conditions. Thus, the description of models 6–8 for the effect of compound replacement is only briefly discussed.

COMPOUND PREINCUBATION   During the preincubation period (t_p), the toxic compound is inactivated as described by Eq. 15.1. Thus, at t_0 only $S_0\exp(-k_{el}t_p)$ is left of the test compound. The presence of identical effects in cultures with and without compound preincubation implies that at the time of measurement the concentrations within the target compartment are the same (s_1 (without) = s_2 (with)). Thus,

$$\left(\frac{S_f}{k_{el}}\right)\ln\left\{\frac{K_m+EIC_{z1}}{K_m+EIC_{z1}e^{-k_{el}t_i}}\right\}=\left(\frac{S_f}{k_{el}}\right)\ln\left\{\frac{K_m+EIC_{z2}e^{-k_{el}t_p}}{K_m+EIC_{z2}e^{-k_{el}t_p}e^{-k_{el}t_i}}\right\} \qquad (15.59)$$

where EIC_{z1} is the obtained EIC_z in experiments without compound preincubation, and EIC_{z2} is the EIC_z in experiments with compound preincubation.

After rearrangement of Eq. 15.59, Eq. 15.18 is obtained! Thus, from preincubation experiments, Models 2 and 6 cannot be discriminated! Furthermore, k_{el} can be calculated without knowing K_m and t_i. This implies that the outcome is not affected by the transfer velocity into the target compartment. *Moreover, the outcome is not influenced by the remaining unchanged test compound at time t_i at which the effects are measured!*

Model 7: The Nontoxic Compound Is Modified into a Toxic Compound   In analogy to Model 3, in the present model the test compound in the outer compartment is modified into a toxic compound by interaction with the culture medium or by cells at a constant rate. The target compartment concentration can be described in analogy to Model 6 by

$$a_i = \sum_{t=0}^{i}(t-t_{-1})S_f\left(\frac{A_0(1-\exp(-k_{met}t))}{A_0(1-\exp(-k_{met}t))+K_m}\right)$$

or

$$a_i = S_ft_i - S_f\int_{t=0}^{i}\left\{\frac{1}{1+(A_0/K_m)-(A_0/K_m)e^{-k_{met}t}}\right\}dt$$

resulting in

$$a_i = \left(\frac{S_f}{A_0+K_m}\right)\left\{A_0t_i-\left(\frac{K_m}{k_{met}}\right)\ln\left[1+\left(\frac{A_0}{K_m}\right)(1-e^{-k_{met}t_i})\right]\right\} \qquad (15.60)$$

If, as assumed, the induced effects are only dependent on s, the OCER can be simulated in analogy to Models 5 and 6. Since the effects may be described according to the one effector site model, [S] of Eq. 15.10 can be replaced by Eq. 15.60, or

$$\frac{E_t}{E_u} = \frac{K_c}{K_c + \left(\left(\frac{S_f}{A_0 + K_m}\right)\left\{A_0 t_i - \left(\frac{K_m}{k_{met}}\right)\ln\left\{1 + \left(\frac{A_0}{K_m}\right)(1 - e^{-k_{met}t_i})\right\}\right\}\right)^{N_c}} \tag{15.61}$$

Since the transfer from the outer compartment into the target compartment (or the enzymatic modification of S to s^*; see Fig. 15.7) is a rate-limiting process, only at low concentrations does the rate of transfer parallel the outer compartment concentration of the toxic product (Fig. 15.19). At large concentrations, this transfer is constant and is not or only negligibly changed by an increase in the outer compartment concentration. If the treatment period is increased, a disproportionate increase in target compartment concentration is seen if the $t_{1/2}$ value relative to the treatment period is large (slow activation; Fig. 15.20). Under testing conditions, the shift in OCER of the toxic product is larger than expected if erroneously Model 5 is assumed. Thus a compound dilution affects the EIC_z value more, as expected if we assume Model 5. At small $t_{1/2}$ values, no difference between the present model and Model 5 can be detected in dilution and preincubation experiments under experimental conditions. The equations describing the effects of compound dilution, compound replacement, and compound preincubation are extremely complex. Since a suspicion of compound activation implies retesting with the toxic product, a more detailed description is not needed. However, if under some circumstances such a description is necessary, the equations can easily be derived from Eq. 15.60.

Model 8: The Nontoxic Test Compound Is Transformed into a Toxic Product that Afterwards Is Inactivated   For the sake of completeness, Model 8 is mentioned in

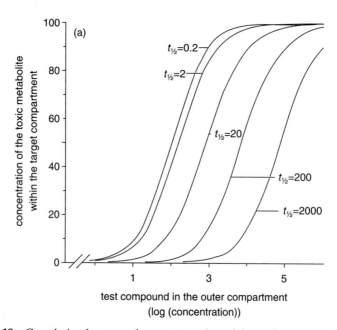

FIGURE 15.19   Correlation between the concentration of the toxic compound in the outer compartment and the concentration in the target compartment according to Eq. 15.60: effects of variations in the elimination half-life ($t_i = 10$; $S_f = 10$; $K_m = 100$ (arbitrary units)).

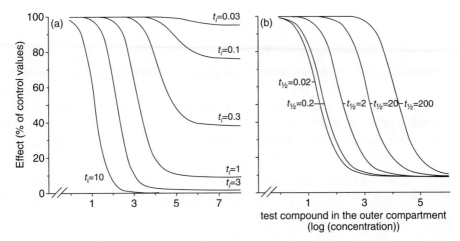

FIGURE 15.20   Outer compartment compound concentration–effect relationships (OCERs) according to Eq. 15.61. (a) Effects of variations in the treatment period t_i. (b) Effects of variations in the elimination half-life ($t_{1/2}$). In the present example, $N_c = 1.5$, $K_c = 100$, $t_i = 1$, $S_f = 100$ and $K_m = 100$ (arbitrary units) or as mentioned in the figure.

which, like Model 4, a nontoxic test compound is added to the cultures. Due to an interaction with components of the outer compartment, this test compound is activated into a toxic product, which is inactivated afterwards. The concentration of the toxic product inside the target compartment can be described by the following equation:

$$s_i = S_f \int_{t_0}^{t_i} \left(\frac{S_0 * k_{met}\left(\dfrac{e^{-k_{el}*t} - e^{-k_{met}*t}}{k_{met} - k_{el}} \right)}{S_0 * k_{met} * \left(\dfrac{e^{-k_{el}*t} - e^{-k_{met}*t}}{k_{met} - k_{el}} \right) + K_m} \right) dt$$

The target compartment concentration can only be calculated using a numerical approach by employing computer programs such as MatLab or MAPLE.

Variations in treatment period, inclusion of dilution, or inclusion of preincubation steps will result in a mixture of the effects observed in Models 6 and 7. Which of these effects dominate depends on the location of t_{max} (see Eq. 15.26) in relation to t_i (see also Model 4). Under experimental conditions, only having knowledge of the fate of the test compound in the culture medium (k_{el} and k_{met} are known), an estimate can be made for compound is probably the most toxic component: the test compound itself (behavior like Model 6), an active intermediate of the test compound (behavior like Model 8), or a stable product or complex of the test compound (behavior like Model 7).

15.7   CONCLUDING REMARKS REGARDING THE EIGHT MODELS OF TOXICITY AND THE DISCRIMINATION BETWEEN THEM

The OCERs that are defined by multiple data points, each with very small standard deviations, can be used to distinguish Models 1–8. Mostly, the behavior of the test compound in the medium and the location and number of target proteins are unknown before experiments are started. Generally, OCERs can roughly be described by Eq. 15.15–15.26. The following series of experiments should be performed to distinguish roughly among the eight models:

- Standard experiments (no dilution, no preincubation of the test compound).
- Experiments in which the dilutions of the test compound before addition to the cells are preincubated for a certain period (e.g., 24 hours) under the same conditions as the cell cultures.
- Experiments in which the treatment period is reduced due to nearly complete dilution of the test compound shortly after addition (e.g., after a few hours).

If the results of these experiments are compared as described in Fig. 15.21, the most probable model may be assessed according to which toxicity is induced. Fur-

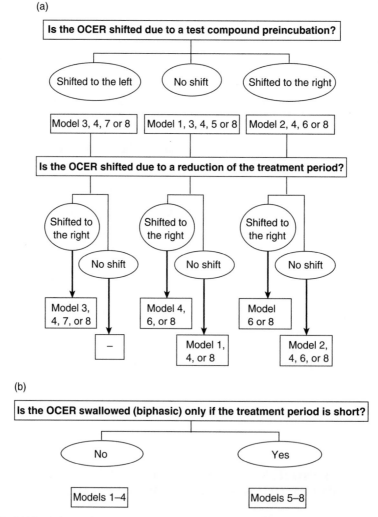

FIGURE 15.21 Schematic representation to discriminate Models 1–8. (a) Comparison of the location of the OCERs. (b) Comparsion of the course of the OCERs.

thermore, the data may help to decide which further experiments, like measurement of the test compound concentration and/or its metabolite(s) at the end of the treatment period, are needed to further specify the obtained characteristics.

In summary, the present chapter describes tools to elucidate the toxicomechanisms under *in vitro* conditions. For this, equations were developed to describe *in vitro* toxicokinetics and toxicodynamics under various conditions and assumptions.

ACKNOWLEDGMENT

The present study was supported by the European Commission through the specific targeted research project CellForce (Contract No. NMP4-CT-2005-016626).

REFERENCES

1. Dost FH. *Grundlagen der Pharmakokinetik*. Stuttgart: Thieme; 1968, p 450.
2. Hill AV. The possible effects of the aggregation of the molecules of haemoglobin on its oxygen dissociation curve. *J Physiol (London)* 1913;40:IV–VII.
3. Bruinink A. Serum-free monolayer cultures of fetal chick brain and retina: immunoassays of developmental markers, mathematical data analysis, and establishment of optimal culture conditions. In Zbinden G, Ed. *The Brain in Bits and Pieces*. Zollikon: MTC Verlag; 1992, pp 23–50.
4. Filipsson AF, Sand S, Nilsson J, Victorin K. The benchmark dose method—review of available models, and recommendations for application in health risk assessment. *Crit Rev Toxicol* 2003;33:505–542.
5. Auton TR. Calculation of benchmark doses from teratology data. *Regul Toxicol Pharmacol* 1994;19:152–167.
6. Links JM, Schwartz BS, Simon D, Bandeen-Roche K, Stewart WF. Characterization of toxicokinetics and toxicodynamics with linear systems theory: application to lead-associated cognitive decline. *Environ Health Perspect* 2001;109:361–368.
7. Nakayama Y, Kishida F, Nakatsuka I, Matsuo M. Simulation of the toxicokinetics of trichloroethylene, methylene chloride, styrene and *n*-hexane by a toxicokinetics/toxicodynamics model using experimental data. *Environ Sci* 2005;12:21–32.
8. Bois FY, Gelman A, Jiang J, Maszle DR, Zeise L, Alexeef G. Population toxicokinetics of tetrachloroethylene. *Arch Toxicol* 1996;70:347–355.
9. Haddad S, Krishnan K. Physiological modeling of toxicokinetic interactions: implications for mixture risk assessment. *Environ Health Perspect* 1998;106(Suppl 6):1377–1384.
10. Bruinink A, Rasonyi T, Sidler C. Reduction of ochratoxin A toxicity by heat-induced epimerization. *In vitro* effects of ochratoxins on embryonic chick meningeal and other cell cultures. *Toxicology* 1997;118:205–210.
11. Bruinink A, Sidler C. The neurotoxic effects of ochratoxin-A are reduced by protein binding but are not affected by l-phenylalanine. *Toxicol Appl Pharmacol* 1997;146: 173–179.
12. Bruinink A, Rasonyi T, Sidler C. Differences in neurotoxic effects of ochratoxin A, ochracin and ochratoxin-alpha *in vitro*. *Natural Toxins* 1998;6:173–177.
13. Bruinink A, Faller P, Sidler C, Bogumil R, Vasak M. Growth inhibitory factor and zinc affect neural cell cultures in a tissue specific manner. *Chemi-Biol Interact* 1998;115: 167–174.

14. Müller JP, Bruinink A. Neurotoxic effects of aluminium on embryonic chick brain cultures. *Acta Neuropathol* 1994;88:359–366.

15. Bruinink A, Birchler F. Effects of cisplatin and ORG.2766 in chick embryonic brain cell cultures. *Arch Toxicol* 1993;67:325–329.

16. Bruinink A, Reiser P, Müller M, Gähwiler BH, Zbinden G. Neurotoxic effects of bismuth *in vitro*. *Toxicol In Vitro* 1992;6:285–293.

17. Bruinink A, Zimmermann G, Riesen F. Neurotoxic effects of chloroquine *in vitro*. *Arch Toxicol* 1991;65:480–484.

18. Bruinink A, Sidler C, Birchler F. Neurotrophic effects of transferrin on embryonic chick brain and neural retina cell cultures. *Int J Dev Neurosci* 1996;14:785–795.

19. Goldoni M, Vettori MV, Alinovi R, Caglieri A, Ceccatelli S, Mutti A. Models of neurotoxicity: extrapolation of benchmark doses in vitro. *Risk Anal* 2003;23:505–514.

20. *Progress Report of the Ecological Committee on FIFRA Risk Assessment Methods: V. Terrestrial Effects Assessment*. US EPA; 2005.

21. Stephens DN, Voet B. Differential effects of anxiolytic and non-anxiolytic benzodiazepine receptor ligands on performance of a differential reinforcement of low rate (DRL) schedule. *Behav Pharmacol* 1994;5:4–14.

22. Michaelis L, Menten ML. Die Kinetik der Invertinwirkung. *Biochem Z* 1913;49: 333–369.

16

TOXICOLOGIC PATHOLOGY

PAUL B. TCHOUNWOU[1] AND JOSÉ A. CENTENO[2]

[1]*Jackson State University, Jackson, Mississippi*
[2]*Armed Forces Institute of Pathology, Washington, DC*

Contents

16.1 INTRODUCTION

Toxicologic pathology is defined as a scientific discipline that integrates two important areas of scientific endeavors: toxicology and pathology. Toxicology is the study of the deleterious effects of chemical compounds on biologic systems and the evaluation of the probability of their occurrence. Pathology, on the other hand, is the study of the nature and magnitude of diseases and the evaluation of structural and functional changes in cells, tissues, and organs in response to the exposure to physical, chemical, and/or biological agents. Hence, the new discipline of toxicologic pathology requires knowledge of toxicology and pathology, as well as other related disciplines, such as molecular and cellular biology, biochemistry, histology, chemistry, microbiology, bioengineering, anatomy, and homeostasis, to provide a scientific understanding of the biologic significance of the biochemical, functional, cellular, and morphological changes arising from various environmental exposures. Understanding the biologic significance of health-related conditions at the cellular, molecular, and morphological levels is critical to assessing the health risk associated with environmental exposures, for developing safety standards, and for developing cost-effective management strategies. This chapter discusses important aspects of toxicologic pathology at the molecular and cellular levels and uses arsenic and radiation as model toxicants to provide relevant information on chemically induced toxicologic pathology at the cellular and target organ levels.

16.2 TOXICOLOGIC PATHOLOGY OF THE CELL

16.2.1 Introduction

Toxicologic pathology has been defined as the study of the molecular, cellular, tissue, and/or organ responses of the living organism when exposed to injurious agents or deprivations. These responses represent a spectrum of cellular changes ranging from cell death to malignant transformations; tissue and organ responses, including regeneration, inflammation, and organization; and the overall response as identified by clinical changes and alterations in body fluids [1]. The cell constitutes the basic unit of life. Hence, morphologic changes in organs and tissues as a result of injury begin with the responses of underlying cells to the toxic insult. A thorough evaluation and understanding of related pathology must logically begin at the cellular level. Several cellular components whose alterations have been reported to be critically associated with cell injury include the plasma membrane, site of osmotic, electrolyte, and water regulation, as well as signal transduction; the mitochondrion, site of energy storage and aerobic respiration; the endoplasmic reticulum, site of much protein synthesis, as well as calcium storage in some cases; and the nucleus, which contains the genetic material and where transcription of the genetic code takes place [2].

Biochemical changes such as enzyme induction and gene expression occur at the earlier stages of the exposure–disease continuum. The degree of cellular injury depends on the metabolic rate. Cells with high metabolic rates such as neurons, myocardial cells, and renal proximal convoluted tubule epithelial cells (PTCs) may suffer from injury more quickly than low metabolizing ones. These high metabolism cells depend on a continuous flow of oxygen to perform aerobic metabolism necessary to provide required energy in the form of ATP for the maintenance of membrane polarity and membrane integrity (neurons), for the continual muscular contraction/relaxation and calcium transport (myocardium), and for the transport of fluids, electrolytes, and metabolites (renal PTCs). Hence, any depletion in oxygen supply is likely to have a significant impact on their survival. In contrast, cells with low metabolic activity such as fibroblasts and adenocytes are less affected by the low supply of oxygen, and hence their prominent role in regeneration and scarring [2].

16.2.2   Cellular Responses to Insult

Homeostasis is one of the most remarkable and most typical properties of highly complex biologic systems. It defines the ultimate environment under which cells maintain the physio- chemical conditions (intracellular pH, cytosolic osmolarity, ion gradients) necessary to perform their biologic functions. In biologic systems, homeostasis is maintained by means of a multiplicity of dynamic equilibriums rigorously controlled by interdependent regulation mechanisms. Hence, the homeostatic system reacts to changes or disturbances in response to various insults by exerting a series of modifications or adjustments to maintain the internal balances and conditions within tolerable limits.

In recent years, the hypothalamus has been identified as one of the critical sites involved in energy homeostasis. Earlier experimental studies with rodents have pointed out that food intake and body weight are under the control of specific hypothalamic subregions. A recent review on the hormonal regulation of the neuronal circuits of the arcuate nucleus of the hypothalamus also reported that the central nervous system (CNS) and the hypothalamus in particular are key players in the regulation of food intake and energy expenditure by peripheral signals such as hormones [3]. Accumulating evidence indicates that the melanocortin (MC) system plays a key role in the regulation of food intake and energy balance. This evidence includes findings that either spontaneous genetic mutations or targeted gene deletions that impair melanocortin signaling cause disrupted food intake and body-weight control. In addition, expression of the mRNA that encodes the endogenous agonists and antagonists for CNS melanocortin receptors is regulated by changes in energy balance and body-adiposity signals [4]. Regulation of signaling by melanocortin 3 and melanocortin 4 receptors in the CNS is controlled via neuronal cell bodies in the arcuate nucleus of the hypothalamus that synthesize melanocortin receptor agonists such as alpha-melanocyte-stimulating hormone (alpha-MSH) or antagonists such as Agouti-related protein (AgRP). The activity of these two populations of neurons is reciprocally regulated by a number of peripheral and central systems that influence energy balance [5].

Deviations from homeostasis may lead to cell injury and eventually cell death, depending on the degree of alterations. Biologic systems must be able to sense and respond rapidly to changes in their environment in order to maintain homeostasis and survive. The induction of heat shock proteins (Hsps) is a common cellular defense mechanism for promoting survival in response to various stress stimuli. Heat shock factors (HSFs) are transcriptional regulators of Hsps, which function as molecular chaperones in protecting cells against proteotoxic damage. Mammals have three different HSFs, which have been considered functionally distinct; HSF1 is essential for the heat shock response and is also required for developmental processes, whereas HSF2 and HSF3 are important for differentiation and development. Recent evidence, however, suggests a functional interplay between HSF1 and HSF2 in the regulation of Hsp expression under stress conditions [6]. Given the broad cytoprotective properties of the heat shock response, there has been a strong interest in discovering and developing pharmacological agents capable of inducing the heat shock response [7].

Cellular adaptation defines the mechanisms by which cells attempt to regulate their internal environment. Two types of adaptation have been reported: atrophy and hypertrophy. Atrophy is an adaptation in which there is a reduction in cell, organ, or tissue mass. At the cellular level, atrophy is often a response to decreased demand for the specialized functions of a particular cell. At the most basic level, atrophied cells undergo a catabolism, often reflected ultrastructurally by an overt breakdown of cellular organelles, including mitochondria, endoplasmic reticulum, microfilaments, and microfilaments [2]. Hypertrophy, on the other hand, is an adaptation in which there is an increase in cell, tissue, or organ mass without cellular proliferation. In general, it is a response to increased metabolic activity/demand for the particular cell. At the ultrastructural and histological levels, this translates into an increase in volume of the cytoplasm and an increase in the number of cell organelles, microfilaments, microtubules, and other specialized structures [2].

In a review of recent experimental insights into the molecular mechanisms underlying organellar protein quality control processes, Leidhold and Voos [8] reported that organellar protein homeostasis is maintained by a combination of specific protein biogenesis processes and protein quality control mechanisms that together guarantee the functional state of the organelle. Organelles like mitochondria, chloroplasts, or the endoplasmic reticulum (ER) are essential subcompartments of eukaryotic cells that fulfill important metabolic tasks. Based on their endosymbiotic origin, mitochondria and chloroplasts contain internal protein quality control systems that consist of a cooperative network of molecular chaperones and proteases. In contrast, the ER employs the main cytosolic degradation machinery, the proteasome, for the removal of damaged or misfolded proteins [8]. In all eukaryotic cells, the ER is the site where folding and assembly occurs for proteins destined to the extracellular space, plasma membrane, and the exo/endocytic compartments. The ER is exquisitely sensitive to alterations in homeostasis and provides stringent quality control systems to ensure that only correctly folded proteins transit to the Golgi and unfolded or misfolded proteins are retained and ultimately degraded. A number of biochemical and physiologic stimuli, such as perturbation in calcium homeostasis or redox status, elevated secretory protein synthesis, expression of misfolded proteins, sugar/glucose deprivation, altered glycosylation, and overloading of cholesterol, can disrupt ER homeostasis, impose stress on the ER, and subsequently lead to accumulation of unfolded or misfolded proteins in the ER lumen [9].

In a study of metabolic homeostasis and tissue renewal, Cheung et al. [10] reported that Golgi beta1,6N-acetylglucosaminyltransferase V (Mgat5) produces beta1,6GlcNAc-branched N-glycans on glycoproteins, which increases their affinity for galectins and opposes loss from the cell surface to constitutive endocytosis. Oncogenic transformation increases Mgat5 expression, beta1,6GlcNAc-branched N-glycans on EGF, and TGF-beta receptors, and enhances sensitivities to ligands, cell motility, and tumor metastasis [10]. From another recent study, Wellen et al. [11] pointed out that metabolic and inflammatory pathways crosstalk at many levels, and, while required for homeostasis, interaction between these pathways can also lead to metabolic dysregulation under conditions of chronic stress. This study also demonstrated that the six-transmembrane protein STAMP2 is a critical modulator of this integrated response system of inflammation and metabolism in adipocytes. Lack of STAMP2 in adipocytes resulted in aberrant inflammatory responses to both nutrients and acute inflammatory stimuli; indicating that STAMP2 plays a key role in systemic metabolic homeostasis [11].

There is accumulating evidence that reactive oxygen species (ROSs) are not only toxic but play an important role in cellular signaling and in the regulation of gene expression. Biochemical and physiologic stimuli, such as perturbation in redox status, expression of misfolded proteins, altered glyc(osyl)ation and glucose deprivation, overloading of products of polyunsaturated fatty acid peroxidation (hydroxynonenals, HNE), or cholesterol oxidation and decomposition, can disrupt redox homeostasis, have been found to impose stress, and subsequently lead to accumulation of unfolded or misfolded proteins in brain cells. Alzheimer disease (AD), Parkinson disease (PD), Huntington disease (HD), amyotrophic lateral sclerosis (ALS), and Friedreich ataxia (FRDA) are major neurological disorders associated with production of abnormal proteins and, as such, belong to the "protein conformational diseases." The brain response to detect and control metabolic or oxidative stress is accomplished by a complex network of "longevity assurance processes" integrated to the expression of genes termed vitagenes [12]. Nitric oxide and other reactive nitrogen species appear to play crucial roles in the brain such as neuromodulation, neurotransmission, and synaptic plasticity but are also involved in pathological processes such as neurodegeneration and neuroinflammation. Acute and chronic inflammation result in increased nitrogen monoxide formation and nitrosative stress. It has been well documented that NO and its toxic metabolite, peroxynitrite, can inhibit components of the mitochondrial respiratory chain leading to cellular energy deficiency and, eventually, to cell death [13]. Gestational diabetes mellitus (GDM) and type 2 diabetes mellitus (DM2) have been suggested to be caused by the same metabolic disorder, and defects in gut hormone-dependent regulation of beta-cell function (enteroinsular axis) have been proposed to contribute to the pathogenesis of DM2 [14].

16.2.3 Cell Death

Severe disruption in homeostasis can lead to an irreversible injury to the cell, resulting in cell death in which the normal cell function can no longer be restored. Two distinct types of cell death have been reported: oncotic or accidental necrosis, and apoptotic/programmed cell death.

Oncotic/Accidental Necrosis   Necrotic cell death is characterized by several ultrastructural changes including cell swelling with rarefaction of the cytosol due to the influx of water, loss of plasma membrane integrity, dilation of the cisternae of the endoplasmic reticulum, loss or deformation of other specialized surface features, and subsequent loss of cellular integrity resulting in recruitment of cells that cause inflammation and phagocytes and cellular fragments. Hence, necrotic death has been described as a toxic process in which the cell is not a targeted cell but a passive victim that does not sustain the energy level for an orderly process of cell destruction and assassination [2, 15]. Changes in plasma membrane characterized by the loss of surface specialization including the disappearance of microvilli and swelling of cilia are among the first necrotic changes. Other changes include intercellular attachment breakdown leading to neighboring cell detachment because of separation of gap junctions, dissolution of the terminal web, and degradation of maculae densae and zonulae adherentes. Cytoplasmic blebs or outpocketing may form on the surface of injured cells. Mitochondria are the most dramatically affected organelles from the depletion of ATP, leading to necrotic cell death [2]. Morphological changes in the nucleus are associated with changes in the structure of chromatin. Gross changes associated with oncotic necrosis are variable and very much dependent on the tissue in which the injury has occurred and the etiology of the injury in the response of surrounding tissues [2].

Apoptotic Cell Death   Apoptosis plays a critical role in maintaining tissue homeostasis and represents a normal function to eliminate excess or dysfunctional cells. Cell death typically follows one of two patterns: oncotic necrosis and apoptosis. Necrosis is typically the consequence of acute metabolic perturbation with ATP depletion, as occurs in ischemia/reperfusion and acute drug-induced hepatotoxicity. Apoptosis, in contrast, represents the execution of an ATP-dependent death program often initiated by death ligand/death receptor interactions, such as Fas ligand with Fas, which leads to a caspase activation cascade. A common event leading to both apoptosis and necrosis is mitochondrial permeabilization and dysfunction, although the mechanistic basis of mitochondrial injury may vary in different settings [16].

For many years cell death was considered to be an uncontrolled, degenerative, and catastrophic failure of homeostasis in response to cellular injury, and thus of little scientific interest. However, scientific discovery over the past two and a half decades has pointed out that cells within multicellular organisms have the ability to undergo a programmed cell death termed "apoptosis." From a toxicological point of view, it is believed that cells can be killed by exposure to various toxicants and hazardous conditions, and especially if the chemical dose is high enough to induce lethality through oncotic necrosis or cell "murder." However, it is now recognized that it is more common for chemically exposed cells to be destroyed by apoptosis or cell "suicide" [17]. Apoptosis is now believed to be a pathophysiological cell death that is much more common than necrosis and is a desirable mechanism by which biologic systems dispose or get rid of cells that have been damaged by mutagenic chemicals or irradiation without perturbing the homeostatic balance of its environment.

Apoptosis has been reported to play a role in the pathogenesis of several health conditions. This process of programmed cell death has been implicated in diseases such as cancer and AIDS [18], neurologic disorders including ischemic brain injury, Alzheimer disease, amyotrophic lateral sclerosis or Lou Gehrig disease, Huntington disease, and Parkinson disease [19], renal diseases including congenital dysplastic kidneys, diabetic nephropathy, glomerulonephritis, glomerulous sclerosis hemolytic uremic syndrome, HIV nephropathy, obstructive uropathy and hydronephrosis polycystic kidney disease, and renal cancer, reproduction abnormalities including the disruption of spermatogenesis and male infertility by toxicants and hormone exposure [20] and the induction of ovarian toxicity in females [21].

Apoptotic cell death has been described as occurring in three phases: first, a receptor-mediated commitment to the cell death, which is termed induction phase, followed by an effector phase characterized by distinct morphological changes in cell structure with modification of mitochondrial functions including change in the status of ATP and other intracellular constituents, and finally a degradation phase with extensive break up of the targeted cell. Figure 16.1 presents the morphological features of necrosis and apoptosis [22].

Utrastructurally, apoptotic cell death has unique features that are quite distinct from necrotic cell death (Table 16.1). Its execution phase has striking morphological characteristics including the loss of cell contact with neighboring viable cells, chromatin condensation to form dense compact masses, and breakdown of the cytoskeletal scaffolding. The cell surface membrane, which is already contracted, begins to bleb. This is followed by breakdown of the cell into membrane-bound fragments or "apoptotic bodies" [17]. In contrast to necrosis, the plasma membrane and cytoplas-

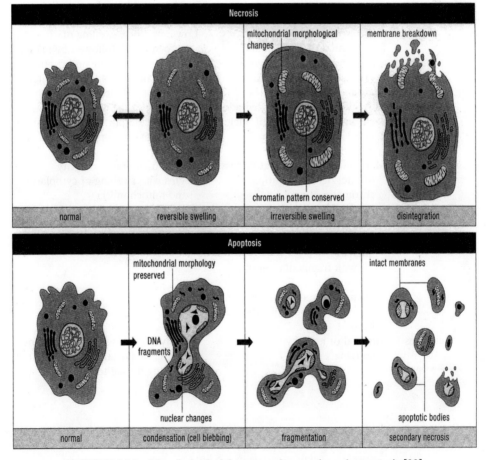

FIGURE 16.1   Morphological features of necrosis and apoptosis [22].

TABLE 16.1   Differential Characteristics of Apoptotic and Necrotic Cell Death[a]

Characteristic	Apoptosis	Necrosis
Histological changes	Individual cells scattered throughout the affected tissue Heperbasophilia or hyperiosinophilia Formation of round bodies, often within a "halo" Chromatin condensation into "caps" or "crescents," with round nuclear bodies; preservation of nuclear envelope	Whole fields of cells affected Hyperiosinophilia Loss of cell border with irregular fragmentation Irregular chromatin clumping, pyknosis, karyorhesis, and/or karyolysis; rupture of nuclear envelope
Ultrastructural changes	Condensation followed by rapid "zeoisis" (budding) Condensation of cytoplasm followed by rarefaction after ingestion by phagocytes Preservation of organellar integrity Preservation of mitochondrial ultrastructure Preservation of internal and external membranes with preservation of membranes around apoptotic bodies Migration of uniformly degraded chromatin to margin of nuclear envelope; preservation of nuclear envelope	Swelling and loss of surface structures with "blebbing" and loss of apical portions of cytoplasm Rarefaction of cytoplasm followed by condensation after death Swelling and loss of organellar integrity Low amplitude swelling of mitochondria followed by high amplitude swelling and rupture Rupture and degradation of internal and external membranes with bursting of the cell Irregular clumping and degradation of chromatin; rupture of nuclear envelope
Morphological changes	Membrane blebbing, but no loss of integrity; aggregation of chromatin at nuclear membrane Begins with shrinking of cytoplasm and condensation of nucleus Ends with fragmentation of cell into smaller bodies Formation of membrane-bound apoptotic bodies; mitochondria become leaky	Loss of membrane integrity Begins with swelling of cytoplasm and mitochondria Ends with total cell lysis Disintegration/swelling of organelles
Gross changes	Minimal or atrophy without scarring	Grossly evident with disruption of normal tissue structure and detail, scarring if long term

TABLE 16.1 *Continued*

Characteristic	Apoptosis	Necrosis
Biochemical features	Tightly regulated process involving activation and enzymatic steps Energy (ATP) dependent; active process Nonrandom mono- and oligonucleosomal length fragmentation of DNA (ladder pattern after agarose gel electrophoresis) Prelytic DNA fragmentation Release of cytochrome-*c*, AIF from the mitochondria into the cytoplasm Activation of caspase cascade Alteration in membrane asymmetry; phosphatidylserine translocation	Loss of regulation of ion homeostasis No energy requirement; passive process Random digestion of DNA (smear of DNA after agarose gel electrophoresis) Postlytic DNA fragmentation (late event of death)
Sequelae	Retention of intracellular enzymes within the apoptotic bodies No release of proinflammatory products Ingestion by adjacent cells or by tissue macrophages Atrophy with stromal collapse but no scarring	Release of intracellular enzymes into extracellular milieu Release of proinflammatory cell breakdown products Ingress of neutrophils followed by macrophages Active inflammation with scarring

[a]See Refs. 2 and 22.

mic organelles of the apoptotic cells remain intact. The biochemical effect most commonly associated with apoptosis is the cleavage of chromosomal DNA, resulting in nucleosomal fragments recognizable as a DNA ladder on agarose gel electrophoresis. This DNA fragmentation induced preferentially in the linker region between nucleosomes is generally believed to be catalyzed by an apoptotic specific Ca^{2+}/Mg^{2+}-dependent endonuclease [23]. An increase in intracellular Ca^{2+} has been reported in early apoptosis to occur in many cell types. This process may activate a nucleolus apoptotic specific endonuclease that cleaves genomic DNA to nucleosomal oligomers [23]. It has been reported that the apoptotic process requires energy from ATP and sometimes depends on new gene expression for completion.

The molecular mechanisms of apoptosis involve a signal transduction in plasma membranes, during which second messengers including CAMP, inositol-1,4,5 triphosphate (IP_3), diacyl glycerol, and CGMP are produced through the signal transduction systems, such as adenylase cyclase, phospholipase C, guanylate cyclase, and ion channel systems, which are essential in living systems. Although it is unclear what happens downstream of the apoptosis-specific Fas/APO-1 (CD 95) and tumor necrosis factor (TNF), the crosstalk of the second messengers produced results in the expression of apoptosis-regulator genes, the activation of preexisting apoptotic gene products, and/or suppression of the expression of survival genes [23].

Several oncogenes such as c-myc, p53, bcl2, c-fos, c-gun, and Rb, have been shown to modulate apoptosis. Changes in these gene products can be responsible for initiation of apoptosis that is dependent on induction of the *de novo* synthesis of either RNA or protein or on suppression. The tumor suppressor oncogene p53 has been shown to have dramatic effect on apoptosis. Several studies have shown that DNA damaging agents such as alkylating agents and UV radiation require p53 for apoptosis induction. Mutations of p53 have been observed in many human cancers [23]. On the other hand, overexpression of bcl2 has been linked to oncogenic activation and the prevention of apoptosis induced by irradiation, glucocorticoid or c-myc. The c-myc protooncogene, known to be important for cell proliferation control, plays a part in the regulation of apoptosis. Its ability to regulate apoptosis results from the coordinated activation of c-myc and several protein partners (such as Max) that facilitate DNA binding and activate transcription. C-myc can regulate apoptosis induced by a variety of insults such as hypoxia, glucose deprivation, cancer chemotherapeutics, and DNA damage [24].

Programmed cell death is essential for the development and maintenance of cellular homeostasis of the immune system. B-cell lymphoma-2 (Bcl2) family members have been demonstrated to play a crucial role in the regulation of apoptosis as mediators between the apical stimuli sensing steps and the executory mechanisms of apoptosis. Deregulation of their role may subvert the homeostasis of a given tissue and collaborate in the genesis of a myriad of diseases characterized by exacerbated or insufficient apoptosis, including neurodegenerative diseases and cancer [25]. The Bcl2 family of proteins comprises both proapoptotic and antiapoptotic members. They are characterized by the presence of conserved sequence motifs, known as Bcl2 homology (BH) domains. Antiapoptotic members share all four BH domains, designated as BH1–4; the multidomain proapoptotic members contain BH1–3 domains, whereas another subgroup of proapoptotic members only have a BH3 domain. The BH3-only proteins act as sensors for distinct apoptosis pathways, whereas multidomain proapoptotic Bax and Bak are executioners of death orders relayed by the BH3-only proteins. Antiapoptotic Bcl2 family members appear to function, at least in part, by interacting with and antagonizing proapoptotic family members [26]. The functional balance of proapoptotic versus antiapoptotic influences, which operates at organelles, determines whether cells will live or undergo apoptosis [27]. BH3-only molecules, often working in concert, compete for downstream multidomain pro- and antiapoptotic Bcl2 members to control serial stages of lymphocyte development and homeostasis [28]. In a study of the modulation of proapoptotic (Bax) and antiapoptotic (Bcl2) gene expression in isolated porcine hepatocytes perfused within a radial-flow bioreactor after low-temperature storing, Mischiati et al. [29] demonstrated that the loss in Bax expression was paralleled with the increase in Bcl2 expression, indicating that the proapoptotic activity seems to balance the antiapoptotic activity. Accumulated evidence suggests that apoptosis helps to maintain cellular homeostasis during the menstrual cycle by eliminating senescent cells from the functional layer of the uterine endometrium during the late secretory and menstrual phase of the cycle. The Bcl2 family and the Fas/FasL system have been extensively studied in human endometrium and endometriotic tissues [30].

The family of nuclear factor kB (NF-kB) nuclear transcription factors also regulates cell survival by inhibiting or promoting apoptosis in several cell types. The antiapoptotic role of NF-kB has been demonstrated in several models of apoptosis including Ras-induced apoptosis of NIH 3T3 cells, nitric-oxide induced apoptosis, and anti-IgM-induced apoptosis of lymphoma cells [24].

Cell cycle regulation is essential for proper cellular homeostasis. In hematopoietic cells, cycling dependent kinase-2 (Cdk2), a major regulator of S phase entry, is activated by mitogenic cytokines and has been suggested to be involved in antigen-induced apoptosis of T lymphocytes. However, a recent report indicates that Cdk2 is not required for proliferation and differentiation of hematopoietic cells *in vivo*, although *in vitro* analyses consider Cdk2 a main player for the proliferation and apoptosis in these cells, and a potential target for therapy [31].

16.2.4   Carcinogenesis

It is estimated that cancer causes at least one million deaths worldwide each year, and exposure to carcinogenic compounds constitutes a major risk factor. Cancer is not a single disease but a large group of diseases, all of which can be characterized by the uncontrolled growth of an abnormal cell to produce a population of cells that have acquired the ability to multiply and invade surrounding and distant tissues [32].

Stages of Carcinogenesis   Carcinogenesis is a complex multistep process that involves epigenetic events such as the inappropriate expression of certain cellular genes, and genetic events that include the mutational activation of oncogenes and the inactivation of tumor suppressor genes. Multistep models of carcinogenesis have been useful for defining events in the neoplastic process and form the cornerstone of current hypotheses of the biological mechanisms of carcinogenesis [33]. This process has been divided into at least three stages known as initiation, promotion, and progression. Table 16.2 presents its morphological and biological features [34].

During the initiation phase, a normal cell undergoes an irreversible change characterized by an intrinsic capacity for autonomous growth. However, this capacity remains latent for a period of time during which the initiated cell is morphologically similar to the normal cell. Initiation involves alteration of cellular DNA, and this effect may be triggered by exposure to a known carcinogen or to an ultimate carcinogen generated by metabolic activation of a procarcinogen. Initiators interact with host cellular macromolecules and nucleic acids in a specific pattern typically involving the generation of reactive oxygen species (electrophiles) esters or free radicals that bind covalently to nucleophilic sites in critical cellular molecules [13]. Initiation is hence a genotoxic or DNA-damaging event, one in which an alteration in the DNA sequence is produced.

In the promotion stage of carcinogenesis, specific agents known as promoters enhance the development of neoplasm in initiated cells. Promoters do not cause cancer by themselves. The temporal sequence of exposure is important in characterizing promotion, a process that is considered as a nongenotoxic or epigenetic event. If the agent potentiates carcinogenesis from coexposure with an initiation, it is called a cocarcinogen rather than a promoter. Tumor promotion has been found to be modulated by various factors including age, gender, and hormonal status [32, 33].

TABLE 16.2   Morphological and Biological Features of the Stages of Carcinogenesis[a]

Initiation	Promotion	Progression
Irreversible	Operationally reversible, both at the level of gene expression and at the cellular level	Irreversible
Initiated stem cell not morphologically identifiable		Morphologically discernible alteration in cellular genomic structure resulting from karyotypic instability
Efficiency is sensitive to xenobiotic and other chemical factors	Promoted cell population existence dependent on continued administration of promoting agent	
Spontaneous (endogenous) occurrence of initiated cells	Efficiency is sensitive to aging and dietary and hormonal factors	Growth of altered cells sensitive to environmental factors during early phase
Requirement for cell division for fixation	Endogenous promoting agents may effect spontaneous promotion	Benign or malignant neoplasms observed at this stage
Dose–response not exhibiting a readily measurable threshold	Dose–response exhibits measurable threshold and maximum effect	Progressor agents advance promoted cells into this stage
Relative potency of initiators dependent on quantitation of preneoplastic lesions after defined period of promotion	Relative potency of promoters measured by their effectiveness in causing an expansion of the initiated cell population	

[a]See Ref. 14.

The third stage of carcinogenesis progression involves additional genetic damage and enhances the development of malignant tumors from benign tumors [32, 33]. Associated with progression is the development of an increased degree of karyotypic instability and of aneuploidy leading to chromosomal rearrangements, especially in leukemia. Table 16.3 presents a comparison of specific features of benign and malignant neoplasms [34].

Regulation of Carcinogenesis   Both oncogenes and tumor-suppressor genes have been involved in the regulation of carcinogenesis. Oncogenes are dominant-acting structural genes that encode for protein products capable of transforming the phenotype of a cell. They are known to encode for growth factors, growth factor receptors, regulatory proteins in signal transduction, nuclear regulatory proteins, and protein kinases. The activation of these gene products including c-onc, c-myc, c-abl, N-myc, K-ras, C-H-ras, C-U-ras, C-K-ras, myc, myb, erb B, mos, Ink1, Ink2, and Jun contributes to the neoplastic process. Tumor suppressor genes, on the other hand, are regulatory genes that function to suppress or limit growth by inhibiting the activity of structural genes that are responsible for cellular growth. While proto-oncogenes have to be activated to influence carcinogenesis, tumor suppressor genes have to be inactivated for the transformed phenotype to be expressed. Hence, several human cancers have been associated with mutations in various tumor suppressor genes including p53, RB1, APC, WT-1, NF-1, p16INK4, BRCA1, BRCA2, TSC2, MSH2, MLH1, VHL, and PTC [32].

TABLE 16.3   Comparative Features of Benign and Malignant Neoplasms[a]

Characteristic	Benign Neoplasms	Malignant Neoplasms
General effect on the host	Little, usually do not cause death	Will always kill the host if untreated
Rate of growth	Slow; may stop or regress	More rapid, but slower than repair tissue; autonomous; never stop or regress
Histological features	Encapsulated; remain localized at primary site	Infiltrate or invade; metastasize
Mode of growth	Usually grow by extension, displacing surrounding normal tissue	Invade, destroy, and replace surrounding normal tissue
Metastasis	Do not metastasize	Most can metastasize
Architecture	Encapsulated; have complex stroma and adequate blood supply	Not encapsulated; usually have poorly developed stroma; may become necrotic at center
Danger to host	Most are without lethal signature	Always ultimately lethal unless removed or destroyed *in situ*
Injury to host	Usually negligible but may become very large and compress or obstruct vital tissue	Can kill host directly by destruction of vital tissue
Radiation sensitivity	Sensitivity near that of half of normal parent cell; rarely treated with radiation	Sensitivity increases in rough proportion to malignancy; often treated with radiation
Behavior in tissue	Cells are cohesive and inhibited by mutual contact	Cells do not cohere; frequently not inhibited by mutual contact
Resemblance to tissue	Cells and architecture resemble tissue of origin	Cells are atypical and pleomorphic; disorganized bizarre architecture
Mitotic figures	Mitotic figures are rare and normal	Mitotic figures may be numerous and abnormal in polarity and configuration
Shape of nucleus	Normal and regular; show usual stain affinity	Irregular; nucleus frequently hyperchromatic
Size of nucleus	Normal; ratio of nucleus to cytoplasm near normal	Frequently large; nucleus to cytoplasm ratio increased
Nucleolus	Not conspicuous	Hyperchromatic and larger than normal

[a]See Ref. 34.

The ubiquitin-proteasome system (UPS) has been reported to play a significant role in cell fate and carcinogenesis. It is comprised of a multiunit cellular protease system that controls several of the proteins that regulate the cell cycle, apoptosis, angiogenesis, adhesion, and cell signaling. Inhibition of this UPS has been found to be a prerequisite for apoptosis and is already clinically exploited with the proteasome inhibitor bortezomib in multiple myeloma [35].

The cyclooxygenase (COX) enzymatic system has also been implicated in carcinogenesis and apoptosis. It includes two isoenzymes, COX1 and COX2, that convert arachidonic acid to prostaglandins. COX1 is constitutively expressed and considered to be a housekeeping gene, while COX2 is not usually detectable in normal tissues but can readily be induced in processes like inflammation, reproduction, and carcinogenesis [36]. The mechanisms by which COX2 is thought to be involved in carcinogenesis include resisting apoptosis, increasing cell proliferation, stimulating angiogenesis, and modulating the invasive properties of cancer cells [36]. Buskens et al. [37] reviewed the mechanisms by which COX2 contributes to carcinogenesis, its role in prognosis, and the possible place of selective COX2 inhibitors in the prevention and treatment of gastrointestinal malignancies, focusing particularly on esophageal cancer. Inhibition of COX2 by aspirin and other nonsteroidal anti-inflammatory drugs (NSAIDs) has been found to inhibit proliferation of colorectal cancer cells and in epidemiologic studies has been shown to reduce colon polyp formation in genetically predisposed populations and in the general population [35]. Epidemiological studies have also reported that long-term use of NSAIDs is associated with a reduced incidence of breast, colorectal, gastric, and esophageal cancers, while experimental and clinical studies have demonstrated that treatment with NSAIDs causes a statistically significant reduction in both the number and the size of polyps in familial adenomatous polyposis patients [36, 37].

Disruptions of the control mechanisms of the cell cycle can initiate carcinogenesis and play a role in progression to cancer. A recent study by Horree et al. [38] has shown that the increase in cell proliferation during endometrial carcinogenesis paralleled the progressive derailment of cyclin B1, cyclin D1, cyclin E, p16, p21, p27, p53, and cdk2, indicating the importance of these cell cycle regulators in endometrial carcinogenesis.

Inactivation of the p53 tumor suppressor gene through a point mutation and/or loss of heterozygosity is one of the most common genetic changes found in various types of human tumors. Mitsudomi et al. [39] investigated the relationship between the presence of p53 gene mutations and survival of patients with non-small-cell lung cancer (NSCLC) of all stages who underwent surgery with preoperative curative intent as a routine therapeutic intervention. The prognostic significance of parameters like sex, age, tumor histology, and the stage of the disease was also evaluated. Overall, the p53 mutations did not correlate with sex, age, or the clinical stage of the disease but showed frequent association with tumors of squamous cell histology. It was concluded that the occurrence of p53 mutations in some NSCLC tumors may be independently associated with a shortened overall survival and may be of somewhat more prognostic significance in patients with advanced stage than in those with early stage of the disease [39].

16.3 CHEMICAL–INDUCED TOXICOLOGIC PATHOLOGY AND ORGAN–SPECIFIC RESPONSES

Understanding the mechanisms of chemical-induced toxicologic pathology is pivotal to evaluating the health-related risks of drugs and other chemical compounds. A high degree of toxicologic pathology has been associated with exposure to many types of chemical substances including heavy metals, pesticides, pharmaceuticals, and various industrial compounds. The toxicologic pathology of these compounds, and especially their impact on human health, has received a great deal of attention. This attention is mostly due to the availability of new data indicating the need to reevaluate the health effects, and to revise the existing criteria and standards. The following discussion focuses on arsenic as an example to illustrate the toxicologic pathology associated with chemical exposure on various organ systems.

16.3.1   Arsenic-Induced Health Effects

A review of biological properties and toxic effects of arsenic indicates that this chemical is a systemic toxicant capable of causing a significant number of health effects, including cardiovascular disease, peripheral vascular disease, developmental effects, neurologic and neurobehavioral effects, diabetes, hearing loss, portal fibrosis of the liver, lung fibrosis, hematologic effects (anemia, leukopenia, and eosinophilia), and carcinogenic effects [40–42]. Table 16.4 presents a summary of health effects associated with arsenic exposure [43].

Research has also pointed to significantly higher standardized mortality rates for cancers of the bladder, kidney, skin, and liver in many areas of arsenic pollution. The severity of adverse health effects is related to the chemical form of arsenic and is also time and dose dependent [44, 45]. Although the evidence of carcinogenicity of arsenic in humans seems strong, the mechanism by which it produces tumors in humans is not completely understood [43].

16.3.2   Mechanisms of Arsenic-Induced Toxicologic Pathology

One of the major mechanisms by which arsenic exerts its toxic effect is through impairment of cellular respiration by the inhibition of various mitochondrial enzymes, and the uncoupling of oxidative phosphorylation. Most toxicity of arsenic results from its ability to interact with sulfhydryl groups of proteins and enzymes, and to substitute phosphorus in a variety of biochemical reactions [46]. Arsenic *in vitro* reacts with protein sulfhydryl groups to inactivate enzymes, such as dihydrolipoyl dehydrogenase and thiolase, thereby producing inhibited oxidation of pyruvate and betaoxidation of fatty acids [47]. Although the evidence of carcinogenicity of arsenic in humans seems strong, the mechanism by which it produces tumors in humans is not completely understood. In contrast to most other human carcinogens, it has been difficult to confirm the carcinogenicity of arsenic in experimental animals. Research evaluating the chronic effects in laboratory animals exposed to inorganic and organic arsenic compounds by the oral route or skin contact has not shown any potential for initiation or promotion of carcinogenicity [48].

In the absence of animal models, *in vitro* studies become particularly important in providing information on the carcinogenic mechanisms of arsenic toxicity. Arsenic and arsenical compounds are toxic and induce morphological changes in cultured cells [49]. Studies in our laboratory have indicated that arsenic is cytotoxic and able to transcriptionally activate a significant number of stress genes in transformed human liver cells [50, 51]. Recently, we have also demonstrated that the toxicity of arsenic depends on its chemical form, the inorganic form being more toxic than the organic one [45]. Arsenic and arsenic containing compounds have also been shown to be potent clastogens both *in vivo* and *in vitro*. They have been reported to induce sister chromatid exchanges and chromosome aberrations in both human and rodent cells in culture [52, 53] and in cells of exposed humans [54]. Arsenical compounds have also been shown to induce gene amplification, arrest cells in mitosis, inhibit DNA repair, and induce expression of the *c-fos* gene and the oxidative stress protein

TABLE 16.4   Clinical and Pathological Manifestations of Acute and Chronic Arsenic Poisoning[a]

Organ/Tissue Level	Acute Effects	Chronic Effects
Dermatologic	• Capillary flush • Contact dermatitis • Folliculitis • Hair loss	• Melanosis • Bowen disease • Facial edema • Palmoplantar hyperkeratosis • Cutaneous malignancies • Hyperpigmentation • Desquamation
Neurologic	• Hyperpyrexia • Convulsions • Tremor/coma • Disorientation	• Encephalopathy • Headache • Peripheral neuropathy • Axonal degeneration
Gastrointestinal/ hepatic	• Abdominal pain • Dysphagia • Vomiting • Blood/rice water diarrhea • Garlicky odor to breath • Mucosal erosions • Fatty liver • Cholangitis • Cholecystitis	• Nausea • Vomiting • Diarrhea • Anorexia • Weight loss • Hepatomegaly • Jaundice • Pancreatitis • Cirrhosis • Liver cancer
Renal	• Tubular damage • Glomerular damage • Oliguria • Uremia	• Nephritis • Proteinuria
Hematologic	• Anemia • Thrombocytopenia	• Bone marrow hypoplasia • Anemia • Thrombocytopenia • Basophilic stippling • Karyorrhexis
Cardiovascular	• Ventricular fibrillation • Tachycardia	• Arrhythmias • Pericarditis • Acrocyanosis • Raynaud's gangrene
Respiratory	• Pulmonary edema • Bronchial pneumonia • Tracheobronchitis	• Cough • Pulmonary fibrosis • Lung cancer

[a]See Ref. 44.

heme oxygenase in mammalian cells [55], and have been implicated as promoters and comutagens for a variety of agents [56].

Various hypotheses have been proposed to explain the carcinogenicity of inorganic arsenic [57]. Nevertheless, molecular mechanisms by which this arsenical induces cancer are still poorly understood. Results of previous studies have indicated that inorganic arsenic does not act through classic genotoxic and mutagenic mechanisms, but rather may be a tumor promoter that modifies signal transduction pathways involved in cell growth and proliferation [58]. Inorganic arsenic has been shown to modulate expression and/or DNA-binding activities of several key transcription factors, including nuclear factor kappa B, tumor suppressor protein (p53), and activating protein-1 (AP-1) [59, 60]. Mechanisms of AP-1 activation by trivalent arsenic include stimulation of the mitogen-activated protein kinase (MAPK) cascade with a consequent increase in the expression and/or phosphorylation of the two major AP-1 constituents, *c-jun* and *c-fos* [60].

Although much progress has recently been made in the area of arsenic's possible mode(s) of carcinogenic action, a scientific consensus has not yet been reached. A recent review discusses nine different possible modes of action of arsenic carcinogenesis: induced chromosomal abnormalities, oxidative stress, altered DNA repair, altered DNA methylation patterns, altered growth factors, enhanced cell proliferation, promotion/progression, suppression of p53, and gene amplification [57]. Presently, three modes (chromosomal abnormality, oxidative stress, and altered growth factors) of arsenic carcinogenesis have shown a degree of positive evidence, both in experimental systems (animal and human cells) and in human tissues. The remaining possible modes of carcinogenic action (progression of carcinogenesis, altered DNA repair, p53 suppression, altered DNA methylation patterns, and gene amplification) do not have as much evidence, particularly from *in vivo* studies with laboratory animals, *in vitro* studies with cultured human cells, or human data from case or population studies. Thus, the mode-of-action studies suggest that arsenic might be acting as a cocarcinogen, a promoter, or a progressor of carcinogenesis.

16.3.3 Arsenic-Induced Keratosis

Arsenical keratosis is often regarded as premalignant and the clinical syndrome comprises several pathological features including hyperkeratosis, parakeratosis, arsenical pigmentation, and squamous cell carcinoma *in situ* (Bowen disease). There are two gross variations; the first being multiple, punctate, hard, yellow, corn-like papules arising in areas of friction such as on the soles and palms, and the second being slightly elevated, scaly, erythematous or pigmented patches appearing on non-sun-exposed areas.

Arsenical bowenoid lesions are noninvasive squamous cell carcinomas (*in situ*) that can be found in both sun-exposed and nonexposed areas of the skin. Atypical epithelial cells occupy the full thickness of the surface epithelium. Arsenical keratosis and Bowen disease tend to persist for many years before becoming invasive squamous cell carcinoma. Gross pigmentary changes in chronic arseniasis include hyperpigmentation (darker color) and hypopigmented (lighter color) raindrop-like macules ranging in size from 1 to 2 millimeters. Figure 16.2 presents three examples of arsenic-induced keratotic lesions [61].

16.3.4 Arsenic-Induced Skin Cancer

The skin manifestations are most diagnostic for chronic arsenic toxicity as internal organ cancers have no characteristic histologic features suggestive of arsenical etiology. Some studies of arsenic toxicity suggest that internal cancers behave differently and may have a different mechanism from skin cancers as related to concentration and length of exposure [62].

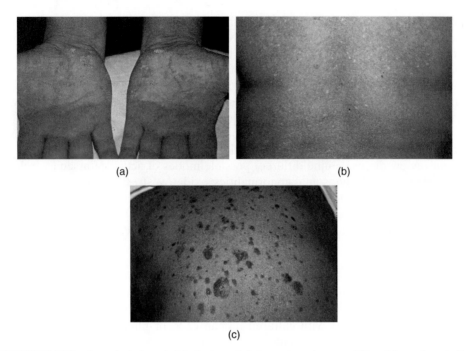

FIGURE 16.2 Arsenic-induced skin lesions: (a) the palms show multifocal hyperkeratotic lesions; (b) skin of back with "rain-drop" like hyperpigmented and hypopigmented macules; and (c) skin of back with chronic arsenical keratotic lesions.

Squamous cell carcinomas (SCCs) are invasive skin tumors that arise from the surface epidermal layer. Histologically, they resemble normal surface squamous cells but with atypical features and growth patterns. SCCs typically arise in sun-exposed areas of the body, but in chronic arsenic ingestion, they are usually found in sun-protected areas.

Basal cell carcinomas (BCCs) that are arsenic-induced most often arise from normal tissue, are almost always multiple, and frequently occur on the trunk. Malignant cells in the lower part of the epidermis show a variety of growth patterns including adenoid, reticulated, trichoepitheliomatous, and hyperpigmented. In one study, arsenical BCC was associated with multinucleated giant cells, some of which had a bizarre appearance and atypical mitoses [63]. Figure 16.3 illustrates two cases of arsenic-induced basal cell carcinoma [61].

Malignant melanomas arise from pigment making cells, melanocytes, that are scattered along the base of the squamous epithelium. Several conflicting reports tying arsenic exposure to the development of malignant melanoma are found in the literature. One report on art glassware workers exposed to arsenic in Italy found one adenocarcinoma, one melanoma, and one squamocellular carcinoma in the sinonasal tract [64]. However, the National Cancer Registry Program in Taiwan contained information on cell types of arsenic-related skin cancers in 2369 patients, and all were either associated with squamous cell carcinoma or basal cell carcinoma, but none with malignant melanoma [65].

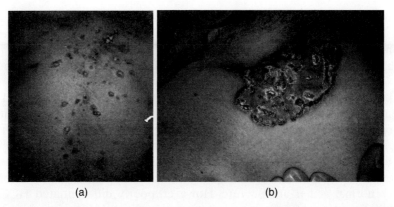

(a)   (b)

FIGURE 16.3   Photograph demonstrating patients with basal cell carcinoma: (a) multifocal basal cell carcinoma of the back; and (b) patient with a single lesion of the left groin.

16.3.5   Arsenic-Induced Liver Cancer

The liver is the main organ for detoxification of substances entering the body. Exposure to toxic agents may result in a variety of hepatic lesions that may resolve when the toxin is removed, or evolve to hepatic failure, malignancy, or death. Chronic arsenic exposure causes liver injury when it accumulates and damages the cells' organelles: these include macrovesicular steatosis, phospholipidosis, cholestatic lesions, steatohepatitis, granulomatous reactions, fibrosis, cirrhosis, vascular lesions, and neoplasms. Arsenic has been reported to enhance hepatic morphological and biochemical changes in phenobarbital-pretreated rats. Hydrophic degeneration, total loss of glycogen, necrosis in some centrolobular zones, and an increase in lipid vacuoles around the periportal area have been observed [66]. Subchronic exposure to arsenic has also been associated with hepatic histopathological changes in rats including the disruption of hepatic cord, sinusoidal dilation, fatty infiltration, and altered expression of cyclin D1, p27, JLK, PTEN, and beta-catenin in the liver [67]. In a study evaluating the combined effect of a mixture of chemicals (arsenic, benzene, chloroform, chromium, lead, phenol, and tetrachloroethylene) on Fischer-344 rats, Constan et al. [68] reported a direct correlation between apoptosis and changes in cell proliferation associated with low level exposure.

Liver angiosarcomas have been associated through medical treatment with inorganic trivalent arsenic compounds, particularly Fowler's solution. Angiosarcoma of the liver is the malignant transformation of the sinusoidal endothelial cells and is linked to exposure to inorganic arsenic as well as vinyl chloride, anabolic steroids, and Thorotrast [69]. Histologically, angiosarcomas exhibit two growth patterns—cavernous and solid. The cavernous areas contain plump, atypical endothelial cells that line the dilated sinusoids, while solid areas show sheets of anaplastic-spindled tumor cells and often have areas with hemorrhage and necrosis. The cells are immunopositive for the endothelial markers CD31, CD34, and Factor VIII-related antigen [70].

Hepatocellular carcinoma (HCC) constitutes a malignant transformation of hepatocytes. Recent studies have documented its association with ingested inorganic arsenic [42]. Large populations exposed to elevated levels of arsenic in drinking water have been studied in Japan, Mexico, Chile, Germany, Argentina, Taiwan, China, India, and Bangladesh. In Taiwan, Japan, and Germany, a dose–response relationship between inorganic arsenic and HCC has been reported. This has also been linked to the interaction of arsenic with other risk factors, including hepatitis B and C infection, aflatoxin exposure, alcohol abuse, and genetic hemochromatosis [71, 72]. Histologically, hepatocellular carcinoma resembles normal liver, and a well-differentiated HCC requires close examination for lack of acinar architecture, growth pattern, and positivity for sinusoidal staining with CD34 (Q-Bend-10) immunostain, which will be increased in neoplastic liver [73]. Moderately differentiated HCCs are easier to diagnose, as they still resemble liver but have increased nuclear pleomorphism, mitoses, and growth pattern abnormalities (thickened trabeculae) and lack normal acinar architecture. However, poorly differentiated HCCs need clinical investigations to exclude metastatic disease. Figure 16.4 shows the histological sections of a normal liver (A), and neoplasia associated with chronic exposure to arsenic, including hepatocellular carcinoma (B) and liver angiosarcoma (C).

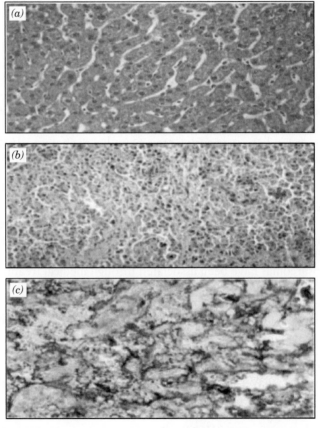

FIGURE 16.4 Histological sections of (a) normal liver, and neoplasia associated with chronic exposure to arsenic, including (b) hepatocellular carcinoma and (c) liver angiosarcoma.

16.3.6 Arsenic-Induced Kidney Cancer

Chronic arsenic exposure has been associated with kidney cancer. A 30% increased incidence of renal carcinoma has been reported in smelter workers in Tacoma, Washington (USA), who were chronically exposed to arsenic as a by-product of smelting nonferrous metal ores [43]. Mining workers and copper smelters not only develop renal carcinoma but also have increased rates of lung cancer, gastrointestinal cancer, and hematolymphatic malignancies. The development of carcinoma appears to be a clear dose-related response. Histologically, the renal tumor is not renal cell carcinoma, but a malignancy of the lining epithelium of the renal pelvis, or transitional cell carcinoma, similar to that of the urinary bladder (see Section 16.3.7).

16.3.7 Arsenic-Induced Urinary Bladder Cancer

Transitional cell carcinoma (TCC) from arsenic exposure in drinking water has been reported in Argentina, Chile, and Taiwan [71, 74, 75]. It has an 8–20 year latent period and appears to be dose related. This tumor develops in the lining of the renal pelvis, ureters, and urinary bladder. Urothelial carcinomas comprise two distinct diseases, both biologically and molecularly: a low-grade papillary tumor, which frequently recurs; and a high-grade malignancy, which can present as dysplasia or carcinoma *in situ* but frequently presents as invasive disease. Histologically, more than seven layers of urothelium cover the papillae. The cells vary from almost normal in appearance to highly atypical. The cytoplasm is pale eosinophilic and usually moderate in amount but can vary and be more abundant, densely eosinophilic, or clear. There are three grades using cytologic criteria that correlate with prognostic significance. Grades 1 through 3 increase with the number of layers of urothelial cells, cytologic atypia, and mitotic figures present. Invasive TCC can arise from both papillary and sessile precursors. The histologic appearance is variable and there are several specific variants. The tumor frequently grows in nests, small clusters, and single cells, dispersed in the lamina propria or invading into the muscularis propria. The tumor cells are usually medium in size with modest eosinophilic cytoplasm, but in some cases the cytoplasm is abundant, densely eosinophilic, or clear. The urothelial characteristics of the tumor cells are usually appreciable, except in cases of high-grade tumors [76].

16.3.8 Arsenic-Induced Lung Cancer

Recent evidence from both epidemiological and experimental studies have indicated that arsenic and cigarette smoking exposure act synergistically to increase the incidence of lung cancer, through induction of oxidative stress leading to an increase in DNA oxidation and reduction of glutathione levels in the lung [77]. Arsenic-related lung cancers reported in smelter workers tend to be adenocarcinomas, followed by small cell carcinoma [78]. Bronchogenic "non-small-cell" carcinoma is the most common type of primary lung cancer. The incidence is clearly higher in smokers and is increased with the number of "pack-years" of smoking. Other etiologic factors include exposure to radiation, asbestos, radon, and inhaled substances, such as nickel, chromates, and arsenic, and genetic factors [79]. It is estimated that

1.5 million workers in the United States are occupationally exposed to arsenic in industries that manufacture glass, pigments, pesticides, and paints. Studies have shown a dose-related association between arsenic in drinking water with both kidney and lung cancers [71].

Primary pulmonary adenocarcinoma is a malignant epithelial neoplasm with features of glandular differentiation. It tends to arise in the periphery of the lung and is more common in women. The tumor histology may vary from well-differentiated glands, to poorly differentiated single cells that are only recognized as adenocarcinoma based on the demonstration of intracellular mucin production. In well-differentiated adenocarcinoma, the glands are lined by tall columnar or mucinous epithelium with ample cytoplasm, basal nuclei, prominent nucleoli, and frequent mitoses. As differentiation decreases, there is increased nuclear atypia and mitosis [80].

Squamous cell carcinoma (SCC) is a malignant epithelial neoplasm with features of squamous differentiation. It arises in the bronchus, close to the hilum. Grading depends on the presence of intercellular bridges and keratinization, and higher grades have more pronounced cytologic atypia, increased mitoses, and frequent foci of necrosis and hemorrhage. *In situ* lesions are recognized in this type of tumor, but there is no *in situ* counterpart for adenocarcinoma. Histologically, the cells show a plate-like growth pattern, have ample eosinophilic cytoplasm, round to oval nuclei, prominent nucleoli, and well-defined cell borders with intercellular bridges [80]. Occasionally, the cytoplasm appears water-clear due to glycogen accumulation, but the tumor still behaves like conventional SCC. Other variants include spindle cell squamous carcinoma, basaloid carcinoma, and lymphoepithelioma-like carcinoma [81].

Small cell carcinoma is one of the least differentiated neuroendocrine neoplasms of the lung and is often centrally located. Patients typically present with symptoms of airway obstruction or may have signs of one of the paraneoplastic syndromes, that is, Cushing syndrome, inappropriate antidiuretic hormone secretion, and Eaton–Lambert syndrome. Histologically, the tumor is composed of small, round to oval, primitive appearing cells, growing in haphazard sheets and nests with scant cytoplasm, round to oval nuclei, dense granular chromatin, and inconspicuous nucleoli. There is brisk mitotic activity and cellular "molding." Distortion "crush" artifact is commonly seen in biopsy material, as well as basophilic deposition of DNA around blood vessels (Azzopardi phenomenon). In Nakajo, Japan, small cell carcinoma was reported in patients exposed to arsenic in well-water with an exposure of five years [82]. Neuroendocrine differentiation may be difficult to demonstrate immunohistochemically, but sometimes positive reactions can be seen using chromogranin A or synaptophysin [81].

16.3.9 Arsenic-Induced Gastrointestinal Cancer

Conflicting reports linking carcinoma of the gastrointestinal tract and arsenic ingestion are scattered in the literature [83]. Most cases are of multiple cancers developing many years after initial exposure. A Japanese study of 839 copper smelters showed significantly increased mortalities from lung and colon cancers [84], while gold miners in Ontario, Canada had excess mortality from *stomach cancer* [85]. Swedish glass-blowers exposed to high levels of lead, arsenic, antimony, and manganese had increased risk of dying from cancer of the stomach, lung, and colon [86]. Although histologic types are not listed, adenocarcinoma would be the most common in the gastrointestinal tract.

16.3.10   Arsenic-Induced Brain Cancer

A Swedish study of occupational exposure to chemicals including arsenic, mercury, and petroleum products found an increased incidence of gliomas in men and an increased incidence of both gliomas and meningiomas in women [87]. About half of all primary brain tumors and about one-fifth of all primary spinal cord tumors are gliomas. Gliomas grow from glial cells within the brain and usually occur in the cerebral hemispheres but may also strike other areas, especially the optic nerve, the brain stem, and, particularly among children, the cerebellum. Gliomas are classified into several groups because there are different kinds of glial cells.

Astrocytomas, the most common type of glioma, are also the most common type of primary brain tumor. They develop from star-shaped glial cells called astrocytes. Well-differentiated or low-grade (grade I or II) astrocytomas contain cells that are relatively normal and are less malignant than the other two. They grow relatively slowly and may sometimes be completely removed through surgery. In some cases these tumors can also progress or recur as higher grade tumors. Anaplastic (or high-grade) astrocytomas (grade III) grow more rapidly than lower grade astrocytomas and contain cells with malignant traits.

16.4   RADIATION-INDUCED TOXICOLOGIC PATHOLOGY

16.4.1   Ionizing Radiation and Ultraviolet Radiation

Both ionizing radiation and ultraviolet radiation appear to be important in the evaluation of radiation effects on humans. Human exposure to ionizing radiation involves external exposures from radioactive materials in the environment, and internal exposures from naturally occurring radionuclides deposited in the body. Diagnostic X-rays used for medical purposes are the second largest source of human exposure for ionizing radiation. The sun is the most common source of ultraviolet radiation (UV) exposure for humans and other animals [88]. UV exposure from the sun is also considered as the most important cause of skin cancer. It has been reported that sunburns and excessive exposures cause cumulative damage, which induces immunosuppression and skin cancers [89]. Although the relationship for melanoma and basal cell carcinoma (BCC) is complex, there exists strong evidence implicating the sun as a potent inducer of squamous cell carcinoma (SCC) [85].

It has been reported that intermittent sun exposure is important in the pathogenesis of BCC, whereas cumulative exposure is important for both BCC and SCC [90, 91]. Other studies have pointed out that sunlight and psoralen and UV-A are risk factors for the development of SCC and, to a lesser extent, BCC. UV-A irradiation has been associated with free radical formation, including peroxides, superoxide anion, and hydroxyl radical, and macromolecule damage, including DNA, RNA, proteins, and lipids. Adverse cellular effects include apoptotic cell death, cell cycle arrest, mutation, and altered gene expression [88]. Most target organs of toxicity include the skin, with skin cancer being the most critical effect, the eyes, and the immune system. UV-B used in the treatment of psorasis might also increase the risk of these tumors [92].

The biologic effect of ionizing radiation has been attributed to its direct interaction with macromolecules or its indirect effect associated with free radical generation and subsequent induction of oxidative stress. Most of the significant effects of ionizing radiation from cell killing to carcinogenesis appear to be related to DNA damage. Ionizing radiation has been implicated in the induction of large scale structural DNA damage, resulting in the loss of entire genes or groups of genes from aberrations such as deletions, rearrangements, and recombination. Radiation-induced genomic instability is characterized by alterations in the mammalian genome and is recognized as a hallmark of cancer cells and carcinogenesis [88]. Studies of childhood thyroid cancers in the territories affected by the Chernobyl nuclear accident have demonstrated a significant increase in these cancers associated with the presence of I-131 and other short-lived isotopes of idione released into the environment. Also, the mutational spectrum of these cancers demonstrates that gene rearrangements that lead to the activation of protein kinase signaling seem to have a pivotal role; point mutations are rare [93].

Alteration in cell cycle progression and chromosome damage has also been reported in radiation pathology. Ionizing radiation is considered as being a complete carcinogen because it has been fully implicated in all three stages of carcinogenesis including initiation, promotion, and progression. It is also considered to be a systemic toxicant capable of causing injury to various organ systems/tissues including the hematopoietic and lymphoid systems, the respiratory system, the dermatologic system, the gastrointestinal system, the skeletal system, the ocular system, the cardiovascular system, the urogenital/reproductive system, and the integumentary system [87].

16.4.2 Nonionizing Radiation

Nonionizing radiation (NIR) includes electromagnetic energy distributed as near-ultraviolet and visible light, infrared radiation, microwaves, radio frequencies, and very low frequency and extremely low frequency alternating electric and magnetic fields. Almost every member of modern society is exposed to it in some form. Usually the intensity of exposure is low in the general population but can be greatly increased in the workplace [94]. However, the biological effects of NIR remain to be elucidated [95]. Although sunlight contains all UV wavelengths, only the UV-A and a portion of the UV-B are of biologic significance because the Earth's atmosphere screens out UV wavelengths shorter than 280 nm [88].

16.5   CONCLUSION

The science of toxicologic pathology has been critical for the evaluation and understanding of adverse effects of physical, chemical, and biologic agents on biologic systems. This emerging science is very important in health risk assessment and management as it provides public health officials with a strong scientific basis for informed decision making. It serves as a tool for the diagnosis of disease status and the evaluation of the toxicity induced by various environmental exposures. The examination of tissues at the molecular, cellular, target organ, and organismal levels provides an excellent opportunity to describe the adverse effects that are associated with environmental exposure, and to understand the pathological manifestations of toxicity. This includes the description of adaptive changes in response to perturbations of homeostasis, and degenerative lesions and alterations induced by toxic exposures.

ACKNOWLEDGMENTS

This work has been supported in part by the NIH-RCMI Center for Environmental Health (Grant No. 1G12RR13459) and the United States Department of the Army Chemical Materials and Computational Modeling Cooperative Agreement No. W912H2-04-2-0002 to Jackson State University (Jackson, Mississippi, USA), and in part by the Armed Forces Institute of Pathology (Washington DC, USA).

REFERENCES

1. Rousseaux CG, Haschek WM, Wallig MA. Toxicologic pathology: an introduction. In Haschek WM, Rousseaux CG, Wallig MA, Eds. *Handbook of Toxicologic Pathology*. New York: Academic Press; 2002, pp 31–114.

2. Wallig MA. Morphologic manifestations of toxic cell Injury. In Haschek WM, Rousseaux CG, Wallig MA, Eds. *Handbook of Toxicologic Pathology*. New York: Academic Press; 2002, pp 39–65.

3. Coppola A, Diano S. Hormonal regulation of the arcuate nucleus melanocortin system. *Front Biosci* 2007;12:3519–3530.

4. Seeley RJ, Drazen DL, Clegg DJ. The critical role of the melanocortin system in the control of energy balance. *Annu Rev Nutr* 2004;24:133–149.

5. Benoit S, Schwartz M, Baskin D, Woods SC, Seeley RJ. CNS melanocortin system involvement in the regulation of food intake. *Horm Behav* 2000;37(4):299–305.

6. Akerfelt M, Trouillet D, Mezger V, Sistonen L. Heat shock factors at a crossroad between stress and development. *Ann NY Acad Sci* 2007 (in press).

7. Calabrese V, Lodi R, Tonon C, D'Agata V, Sapienza M, Scapagnini G, Mangiameli A, Pennisi G, Stella AM, Butterfield DA. Oxidative stress, mitochondrial dysfunction and cellular stress response in Friedreich's ataxia. *J Neurol Sci* 2005;233(1–2):145–162.

8. Leidhold C, Voos W. Chaperones and proteases: guardians of protein integrity in eukaryotic organelles. *Ann NY Acad Sci* 2007 (in press).

9. Zhang K, Kaufman RJ. The unfolded protein response: a stress signaling pathway critical for health and disease. *Neurology* 2006;66(2):S102–S109.

10. Cheung P, Pawling J, Partridge EA, Sukhu B, Grynpas M, Dennis JW. Metabolic homeostasis and tissue renewal are dependent on {beta}1,6GlcNAc-branched N-glycans. *Glycobiology* 2007;17(8):828–837.

11. Wellen KE, Fucho R, Gregor MF, Furuhashi M, Morgan C, Lindstad T, Vaillancourt E, Gorgun CZ, Saatcioglu F, Hotamisligil GS. Coordinated regulation of nutrient and inflammatory responses by STAMP2 is essential for metabolic homeostasis. *Cell* 2007;129(3):537–548.

12. Calabrese V, Guagliano E, Sapienza M, Mancuso C, Butterfield DA, Stella AM. Redox regulation of cellular stress response in neurodegenerative disorders. *Ital J Biochem* 2006;55(3–4):263–282.

13. Calabrese V, Boyd-Kimball D, Scapagnini G, Butterfield DA. Nitric oxide and cellular stress response in brain aging and neurodegenerative disorders: the role of vitagenes. *In Vivo* 2004;18(3):245–267.

14. Cypryk K, Vilsboll T, Nadel I, Smyczynska J, Holst JJ, Lewinski A. Normal secretion of the incretin hormones glucose-dependent insulinotropic polypeptide and glucagon-like peptide-1 during gestational diabetes mellitus. *Gynecol Endocrinol* 2007;23(1):58–62.

15. Reed DJ. Mechanisms of chemically induced cell injury and cellular protection mechanisms. In Hodgson E, Smart RC, Eds. *Introduction to Biochemical Toxicology*, 3rd ed. Hoboken NJ: Wiley; 2001, Chap 10, pp 221–253.

16. Malhi H, Gores GJ, Lemasters JJ. Apoptosis and necrosis in the liver: a tale of two deaths? *Hepatology* 2006;43(2):S31–S44.

17. Gill JH, Dive C. Apoptosis: basic mechanisms and relevance to toxicology. In Roberts R, Ed. *Apoptosis in Toxicology*. New York: Taylor & Francis; 2000, Chap 1, pp 1–19.

18. Cosulich SC, Roberts RA. Perturbation of apoptosis as a mechanism of action of non genotoxic carcinogens. In Roberts R, Ed. *Apoptosis in Toxicology*. New York: Taylor & Francis, 2000, pp 169–185.

19. Gibson RM. Role of apoptosis in neuronal toxicology. In Roberts R, Ed. *Apoptosis in Toxicology*. New York: Taylor & Francis; 2000, pp 145–167.

20. Woolveridge I, Morris I. Apoptosis in male reproductive toxicology. In Roberts R, Ed. *Apoptosis in Toxicology*. New York: Taylor & Francis; 2000, pp 71–93.

21. Tilly JL. Apoptosis in female reproductive toxicology. In Roberts R, Ed. *Apoptosis in Toxicology*. New York: Taylor & Francis; 2000, pp 95–115.

22. Wyllie A. Cell death–apoptosis and necrosis. In *Apoptosis and Cell Proliferation*, 2nd ed. Mannheim, Germany: Boehringer Mannheim Gmbh; 1998, pp 1–61.

23. Tanuma SI. Molecular mechanisms of apoptosis. In Sluyser M, Ed. *Apoptosis in Normal Development and Cancer*. New York: Taylor & Francis; 1996, pp 39–59.

24. Davis MA, Jeffery EH. Organelle biochemistry and regulation of cell death. In Haschek WM, Rousseaux CG, Wallig MA, Eds. *Handbook of Toxicologic Pathology*, 2nd ed. New York: Academic Press; 2002, pp 67–81.

25. Roset R, Ortet L, Gil-Gomez G. Role of Bcl-2 family members on apoptosis: what we have learned from knock-out mice. *Front Biosci* 2007;1(12):4722–4730.

26. Chan SL, Yu VC. Proteins of the bcl-2 family in apoptosis signaling: from mechanistic insights to therapeutic opportunities. *Clin Exp Pharmacol Physiol* 2004;31(3):119–128.

27. Lanave C, Santamaria M, Saccone C. Comparative genomics: the evolutionary history of the Bcl-2 family. *Gene* 2004;333:71–79.

28. Opferman JT, Korsmeyer SJ. Apoptosis in the development and maintenance of the immune system. *Nat Immunol* 2003;4(5):410–415.

29. Mischiati C, Puviani AC, Brogli M, Guarniero S, Sereni A, Breda L, Ricci D, Galavotti D, Morsiani E, Gambari R. Modulation of pro-apoptotic (Bax) and anti-apoptotic (Bcl-2) gene expression in isolated porcine hepatocytes perfused within a radial-flow bioreactor after low-temperature storing. *Int J Artif Organs* 2003;26(2):139–148.

30. Harada T, Taniguchi F, Izawa M, Ohama Y, Takenaka Y, Tagashira Y, Ikeda A, Watanabe A, Iwabe T, Terakawa N. Apoptosis and endometriosis. *Front Biosci* 2007;12:3140–3151.

31. Berthet C, Rodriguez-Galan MC, Hodge DL, Gooya J, Pascal V, Young HA, Keller J, Bosselut R, Kaldis P. Hematopoiesis and thymic apoptosis are not affected by the loss of Cdk2. *Mol Cell Biol* 2007;2714:5079–5089.

32. Smart RC, Akunda JK. Carcinogenesis. In Hodgson E, Smart RC, Eds. *Introduction to Biochemical Toxicology*, 3rd ed. Hoboken, NJ: Wiley; 2001, pp 343–395.

33. Mostorides S, Maronpot RR. Carcinogenesis. In Haschek WM, Rousseaux CG, Wallig MA, Eds. *Handbook of Toxicologic Pathology*. New York: Academic Press; 2002, pp 3–122.

34. Pilot HC, Dragan YP. Chemical carcinogenesis. In Klaassen CD, Ed. *Cassarett & Doull's Toxicology: The Basic Science of Poisons*. New-York: McGraw-Hill; 1996, pp 201–267.

35. Voutsadakis IA. Pathogenesis of colorectal carcinoma and therapeutic implications: the roles of the ubiquitin-proteasome system and Cox-2. *J Cell Mol Med* 2007; 11(2):252–285.

36. Moran EM. Epidemiological and clinical aspects of nonsteroidal anti-inflammatory drugs and cancer risks. *Environ Pathol Toxicol Oncol* 2002;21(2):193–201.

37. Buskens CJ, Ristimaki A, Offerhaus GJ, Richel DJ, van Lanschot JJ. Role of cyclooxygenase-2 in the development and treatment of oesophageal adenocarcinoma. *Scand J Gastroenterol* Suppl 2003;239:87–93.

38. Horree N, van Diest PJ, van der Groep P, Sie-Go DM, Heintz AP. Progressive derailment of cell cycle regulators in endometrial carcinogenesis. *J Clin Pathol* 2007 (in press).

39. Mitsudomi T, Oyama T, Kusano T, Osaki T, Nakanishi R, Shirakusa T. Mutations of the p53 gene as a predictor of poor prognosis in patients with non-small-cell lung cancer. *J Natl Cancer Inst* 1993;85(24):2018–2023.

40. NAS (National Academy of Science). *Arsenic in Drinking Water*. Washington, DC: National Academies Press; 1999, pp 299–301.

41. NRC (National Research Council). *Arsenic in Drinking Water: Update*. Washington, DC: National Academies Press; 2001.

42. Tchounwou PB, Wilson B, Ishaque A. Important considerations in the development of public health advisories for arsenic and arsenic-containing compounds in drinking water. *Rev Environ Health* 1999;14(4):211–229.

43. Tchounwou PB, Centeno JA, Patlolla AK. Arsenic toxicity, mutagenesis, and carcinogenesis—a health risk assessment and management approach. *Mol Cell Biochem* 2004; 255(1-2):47–55.

44. Tchounwou PB, Patlolla AK, Centeno JA. Carcinogenic and systemic health effects associated with arsenic exposure—a critical review. *Toxicol Pathol* 2003;31(6):575–588.

45. Tchounwou PB, Wilson BA, Abdelgnani AA, Ishaque AB, Patlolla AK. Differential cytotoxicity and gene expression in human liver carcinoma (HepG2) cells exposed to arsenic trioxide and monosodium acid methanearsonate (MSMA). *Int J Mol Sci* 2002;3:1117–1132.

46. Li JH, Rossman TC. Inhibition of DNA ligase activity by arsenite: a possible mechanism of its comutagenesis. *Mol Toxicol* 1989;2:1–9.

47. Belton JC, Benson NC, Hanna ML, Taylor RT. Growth inhibition and cytotoxic effects of three arsenic compounds on cultured Chinese hamster ovary cells. *J Environ Sci Health* 1985;20A:37–72.

48. Goyer RA. Toxic effects of metals. In Klaassen CD, Ed. *Cassarett & Doull's Toxicology: The Basic Science of Poisons*. New York: McGraw-Hill; 1996, pp 691–736.

49. Lee TC, Oshimura M, Barrett JC. Comparison of arsenic-induced cell transformation, cytotoxicity, mutation and cytogenetic effects in Syrian hamster embryo cells in culture. *Carcinogenesis* 1985;6(10):1421–1426.

50. Tchounwou PB, Wilson BA, Ishaque A, Schneider J. Atrazine potentiation of arsenic trioxide-induced cytotoxicity and gene expression in human liver carcinoma cells (HepG2). *Mol Cell Biochem* 2001;222:49–59.

51. Tchounwou PB, Wilson BA, Schneider J, Ishaque A. Cytogenetic assessment of arsenic trioxide toxicity in the Mutatox, Ames II, and CAT-Tox assays. *Metal Ions Biol Med* 2000;6:89–91.

52. Vega L, Gonsebatt ME, Ostrosky-Wegman P. Aneugenic effect of sodium arsenite on human lymphocytes *in vitro*: an individual susceptibility effect detected. *Mutat Res* 1995;334(3):365–373.

53. Patlolla A, Tchounwou PB. Cytogenetic evaluation of arsenic trioxide toxicity in Sprague–Dawley rats. *Mutat Res Genet Toxicol Environ Mutagen* 2005;587(1–2):126–133.

54. Gonsebatt ME, Vega L, Salazar AM, Montero R, Guzman P, Blas J, Del Razo LM, Garcai-Vargas G, Albores A, Cebrian ME, Kelsh M, Ostrosky-Wegman P. Cytogenetic effects in human exposure to arsenic. *Mutat Res* 1997;386:219–228.

55. Jingbo Pi, Hiroshi Y, Yoshito K, Guifan S, Takahiko Y, Hiroyuki A, Claudia HR, Nobuhiro S. Evidence for induction of oxidative stress caused by chronic exposure of Chinese residents to arsenic contained in drinking water. *Environ Health Perspect* 2002;110(4): 331–336.

56. Cavigelli M, Li WW, Lin A, Su B, Yushioka K, Karin M. The tumor promoter arsenite stimulates AP-1 activity by inhibiting a JNK phosphatase. *EMBO J* 1996;15:6269–6279.

57. Kitchin K. Recent advances in arsenic carcinogenesis: modes of action, animal model systems, and methylated arsenic metabolites. *Toxicol Appl Pharmacol* 2001;172: 249–261.

58. Simeonova PP, Luster MI. Mechanisms of arsenic carcinogenicity: genetic or epigenetic mechanisms? *J Environ Pathol Toxicol Oncol* 2000;19:281–286.

59. Barchowsky A, Dudek EJ, Treadwell MD, Wetterhahn KE. Arsenic induces oxidant stress and NF-kB activation in cultured aortic endothelial cells. *Free Radic Biol Med* 1996;21:783–790.

60. Simeonova PP, Wang S, Toriumi W, Kommineni C, Matheson J, Unimye N, Kayama F, Harki D, Ding M, Vallyathan V. Arsenic mediates cell proliferation and gene expression in the bladder epithelium: association with AP-1 transactivation. *Cancer Res* 2000;60: 3445–3453.

61. Centeno JA, Tchounwou PB, Patlolla AK, Mullick FG, Murakat L, Meza E, Gibb H, Longfellow D, Yedjou CG. Environmental pathology and health effects of arsenic poisoning: a critical review. In Naidu R, Smith E, Smith J, Bhattacharya P, Eds. *Managing Arsenic In the Environment: From Soil to Human Health*. Adelaide, Australia: CSIRO Publishing Corp; 2006.

62. Centeno JA, Martinez L, Ladich ER, Page NP, Mullick FG, Ishak KG, Zheng B, Gibb H, Thompson C, Longfellow D. *Arsenic-Induced Lesions*. Washington, DC: Armed Forces Institute of Pathology, American Registry of Pathology; 2000.

63. Schwartz RA. Arsenic and the skin. *Int J Dermatol* 1997;36:241–250.

64. Battista G, Bartoli D, Iaia TE, Dini F, Fiumalbi C, Giglioli S, Valiani M. Art glassware and sinonasal cancer: report of three cases. *Am J Ind Med* 1996;30(1):31–35.

65. Guo HR, Yu HS, Hu H, Monson RR. Arsenic in drinking water and skin cancers: cell-type specificity. *Cancer Causes Control* 2001;12(10):909–916.

66. Albores A, Cebrian ME, Garcia-Vargas GC, Connelly JC, Price SC, Hinton RH, Bach PH, Bridges JW. Enhanced arsenite-induced hepatic morphological and biochemical changes in phenobarbital-pretreated rats. *Toxicol Pathol* 1996;24(20):172–180.

67. Cui X, Li S, Shraim A, Kobayashi T, Hayakawa T, Kanno S, Yamamoto M, Hirano S. Subchronic exposure to arsenic through drinking water alters expression of cancer-related genes in rat liver. *Toxicol Pathol* 2004;32(1):64–72.

68. Constan AA, Benjamin SA, Tessari JD, Baker DC, Yang RS. Increased rate of apoptosis correlates with hepatocellular proliferation in Fischer-344 rats following long-term exposure to a mixture of groundwater contaminants. *Toxicol Pathol* 1996;24(3):315–322.

69. Tsai S, Wang T, Ko Y. Mortality for certain diseases in areas with high levels of arsenic in drinking water. *Arch Environ Health* 1999;54:186–193.

70. Centeno JA, Mullick FG, Martinez L, Page NP, Gibb H, Longfellow D, Thompson C, Ladish ER. Pathology related to chronic arsenic exposure. *Environ Health Perspect* 2002;110(5):883–886.

71. Hopenhayn-Rich C, Biggs ML, Smith AH. Lung and kidney cancer mortality associated with arsenic in drinking water in Cordoba, Argentina. *Int J Epidemiol* 1998;27:561–569.

72. Chen CJ, Yu MW, Liaw YF. Epidemiological characteristics and risk factors of hepatocellular carcinoma. *J Gastroenterol Hepatol* 1997;12(9–10):S294–S308.

73. Di Carlo I, Fraggetta F, Lombardo R, Azzarello G, Vasquez E, Puleo S. CD 34 expression in chronic and neoplastic liver diseases. *Panminerva Med* 2002;44(4):365–367.

74. Johansson SL, Cohen SM. Epidemiology and etiology of bladder cancer. *Semin Surg Oncol* 1997;13(5):291–298.

75. Chiou HY, Chiou ST, Hsu YH, Chou YL, Tseng CH, Wei ML, Chen CJ. Incidence of transitional cell carcinoma and arsenic in drinking water: a follow-up study of 8,102 residents in an arseniasis-endemic area in northeastern Taiwan. *Am J Epidemiol* 2001;153(5):411–418.

76. Royce RK, Ackerman LV. Carcinoma of the bladder: therapeutic and pathologic aspects of 135 cases. *J Urol* 1951;65:66–86.

77. Hays AM, Srinivasan D, Witten ML, Carter DE, Lantz RC. Arsenic and cigarette smoke synergistically increase DNA oxidation in the lung. *Toxicol Pathol* 2006;34(4):396–404.

78. Wicks MJ. Arsenic exposure in a copper smelter as related to histological type of lung cancer. *Am J Ind Med* 1981;2:25–31.

79. Reger RB, Morgan WK. Respiratory cancers in mining. *Occup Med* 1993;8(1):185–204.

80. Travis WD, Travis LB, Deveesa SS. Lung cancer. *Cancer* 1995;75:191–202.

81. Travis WD. Pathology of lung cancer. *Clin Chest Med* 2002;23(1):65–81.

82. Nakadaira H, Endoh K, Katagiri M, Yamamoto M. Elevated mortality from lung cancer associated with arsenic exposure for a limited duration. *J Occup Environ Med* 2002;44(3):291–299.

83. Murata K, Iwazawa T, Takayama T, Yamashita K, Okagawa K. Quadruple cancer including Bowen's disease after arsenic injections 40 years earlier: report of a case. *Surg Today* 1994;24(12):1115–1118.

84. Tokudome S, Kuratsune M. A cohort study on mortality from cancer and other causes among workers at a metal refinery. *Int J Cancer* 1976;17(3):310–317.

85. Kusiak RA, Ritchie AC, Springer J, Muller J. Mortality from stomach cancer in Ontario miners. *Br J Ind Med* 1993;50(2):117–126.

86. Wingren G, Axelson O. Mortality in the Swedish glassworks industry. *Scand J Work Environ Health* 1987;13(5):412–416.

87. Navas-Acien A, Pollan M, Gustavsson P, Plato N. Occupation, exposure to chemicals and risk of gliomas and meningiomas in Sweden. *Am J Ind Med* 2002;42(3):214–227.

88. Benjamin SA, Powers BE, Haln FF, Kusewitt DF. Radiation and heat. In Haschek WM, Rousseaux CG, Wallig MA, Eds. *Handbook of Toxicologic Pathology*, 2nd eds. New York: Academic Press; 2002, pp 529–594.

89. Saladi RN, Persaud AN. The cause of skin cancer: a comprehensive review. *Drugs Today* 2005;41(1):37–53.

90. English DR, Armstrong BK, Kricker A, Fleming C. Sunlight and cancer. *Cancer Causes Control* 1997;8(3):271–283.

91. Almahroos M, Kurban AK. Ultraviolet carcinogenesis in nonmelanoma skin cancer, part II: review and update on epidemiologic correlations. *SkinMed* 2004;3(3):132–139.

92. Lim JL, Stern RS. High levels of ultraviolet B exposure increase the risk of non-melanoma skin cancer in psoralen and ultraviolet A-treated patients. *J Invest Dermatol* 2005;124(3):505–513.

93. Yamashita S, Saenko V. Mechanisms of disease: molecular genetics of childhood thyroid cancers. *Nat Clin Pract Endocrinol Metab* 2007;3(5):422–429.

94. Yost MG. Occupational health effects of nonionizing radiation. *Occup Med* 1992;7(3):543–566.

95. Hietanen M. Health risks of exposure to non-ionizing radiation—myths or science-based evidence. *Med Lav* 2006;97(2):184–188.

17

SECONDARY PHARMACODYNAMIC STUDIES AND *IN VITRO* PHARMACOLOGICAL PROFILING

DUNCAN ARMSTRONG,[1] JACQUES MIGEON,[2] MICHAEL G. ROLF,[1] JOANNE BOWES,[1] MARK CRAWFORD,[2] AND JEAN-PIERRE VALENTIN[1]

[1]*AstraZeneca R&D, Alderley Park, Macclesfield, Cheshire, United Kingdom*
[2]*Cerep, Redmond, Washington*

Contents

Preclinical Development Handbook: Toxicology, edited by Shayne Cox Gad
Copyright © 2008 John Wiley & Sons, Inc.

17.1   INTRODUCTION

17.1.1   Definitions

Pharmacological investigations during the drug discovery process may be divided into three distinct categories: primary pharmacodynamic, secondary pharmacodynamic, and safety pharmacological studies. Primary pharmacodynamic studies are those in which the mode of action of a substance is investigated in relation to its desired (therapeutic) effect. In contrast, secondary pharmacodynamic studies are defined as those that "investigate the mode of action and/or effects of a substance not related to its desired therapeutic target" [1]. Finally, safety pharmacological studies are those that "investigate the potential undesirable pharmacodynamic effects of a substance on physiological functions in relation to exposure in the therapeutic range and above" [1].

This chapter discusses drivers for secondary pharmacodynamic studies and different strategic approaches to such studies, focusing specifically on *in vitro* pharmacological profiling techniques, data analysis, and interpretation. Some examples of the impact of pharmacological profiling on the drug discovery and development process are provided.

17.1.2   Historical and Regulatory Perspectives

In Japan, the Ministry of Health and Welfare (MHW), now referred to as the Ministry of Health, Labour, and Welfare, promulgated comprehensive guidance for organ function testing as early as 1975 (see Table 17.1). These guidelines describe which organ systems should be included in a first tier evaluation (Category A studies) and make specific recommendations regarding study design (including description of models, criteria for dose selection, and which endpoints would be included in the investigation). These guidelines also describe a second phase of studies (Category B) to be conducted, as necessary, in the light of the results of the Category A studies (Table 17.1 [2]). As the Japanese guidelines were the most comprehensive of their time, they became the *de facto* foundation for organ function testing throughout the pharmaceutical industry [3–5]. The organ function studies included in Categories A and B were intertwined with studies whose aim was to identify functions and activities in addition to the primary pharmacological function/activity. Kinter et al. [6] distinguished two subgroups of objectives embedded in the Japanese studies as safety pharmacology and pharmacological profiling. This concept was enlarged upon by the International Conference on Harmonization (ICH) safety pharmacology Expert Working Group (EWG) to define three categories of pharmacology studies: primary and secondary pharmacodynamic studies, and safety pharmacology studies [1, 5, 7] (Table 17.1).

The origin of the term secondary pharmacodynamic studies is obscure. It first appeared in the draft guidelines of the ICH M3 and S6 (see Table 17.1 [8, 9]). ICH S6 stated that secondary pharmacodynamic studies aimed to "investigate the mode of action and/or effects of a substance not related to its desired therapeutic target." The ICH S7 EWG began its work in the first quarter of 1999 and a harmonized safety pharmacology guidance was finalized and adopted by the regional regulatory authorities over 2000–2001 (ICH S7A [1]). The ICH S7A guidance defines the objectives and general principles of secondary pharmacodynamic studies, including the timing of these investigations in relation to the clinical development program and the requirement for Good Laboratory Practice (GLP), where applicable [1, 10].

17.2   DRIVERS FOR SECONDARY PHARMACODYNAMIC STUDIES

17.2.1   Regulatory Requirements

The ICH S7A guideline [1] provides a definition for secondary pharmacodynamic studies (see Section 17.1.1); however, unlike safety pharmacological studies, secondary pharmacodynamic studies are not required as part of the core assessment of the safety of a new drug substance. The guidance suggests that secondary pharmacodynamic studies performed early in the drug discovery process may contribute to the design of safety pharmacological studies, providing information relevant to, for example, dose selection.

The ICH S7A guidance suggests that in some cases secondary pharmacodynamic findings may contribute to the safety evaluation of a substance and may be considered along with the findings of safety pharmacology studies. In cases where the secondary pharmacodynamic findings are pivotal to the safety evaluation, it may be necessary to conduct secondary pharmacodynamic studies to the Good Laboratory Practice standard [1, 10].

The ICH M4(R3) [14] guideline describes an acceptable format and content for a Common Technical Document (CTD) suitable for submission to regulatory agencies in all three ICH regions. Secondary pharmacodynamic studies should be submitted as part of the pharmacology section of the CTD.

17.2.2   Economic Environment

Drug development is a high-risk venture. Estimates for the full cost of bringing a new drug to market are U.S. $800M for compounds approved in the late 1990s, U.S. $1.1B in 2001, and expected to rise to U.S. $1.9B in 2013 [15]. It is estimated that 70% of this figure supports projects that do not lead to a marketed product [16]. Adding to the development risk is the fact that some compounds succeed in clinical development, reach the market, and, only after widespread use, are found to have unexpected adverse effects. The consequences of these postapproval failures are

TABLE 17.1 Regulatory Guidance Documents Referring to Secondary Pharmacodynamic Studies for Pharmacological Profiling[a]

Document and Source	Comments	Reference
Japanese Guidelines for Non-clinical Studies of Drugs Manual 1995—Guidelines for General Pharmacology Studies	Defines a list of studies to be conducted on all NCE (Category A) and a list of studies to be conducted on a case-by-case basis (Category B). Recommends the use of *in vitro* assays such as isolated organs and tissues. Indicates that ligand-binding methods should be positively adopted. Guidance to be superseded by ICH S7A and S7B.	1, 2, 11
Committee for Proprietary Medicinal Products—*Points to Consider: The Assessment of QT Interval Prolongation by Non-cardiovascular Medicinal Products*	Recommends a set of nonclinical (including *in vitro* assays) and clinical studies to address the risk for a noncardiovascular drug to slow cardiac repolarization and prolong the QT/QTc interval. Considers *in vitro* assays aimed at assessing activity at cardiac ion channels.	12
ICH M3—Timing of Non-clinical Safety Studies for the Conduct of Human Clinical Trials for Pharmaceuticals	Provides guidance on the timing of safety pharmacology studies in relation to clinical development. Establishes that safety pharmacology studies should be conducted prior to first administration to humans.	8
ICH S7A—Note for Guidance on Safety Pharmacology Studies for Human Pharmaceuticals	Provides clear definitions for primary, secondary, and safety pharmacology studies. Provides the general framework for *in vitro* and *in vivo* safety pharmacology studies. Ligand-binding or enzyme assays data suggesting a potential for adverse effects should be considered in selecting and designing safety pharmacology studies.	1
ICH S7B—Note for Guidance on the Non-clinical Evaluation for Delayed Ventricular Repolarization (QT Interval Prolongation) by Human Pharmaceuticals	Describes a nonclinical testing strategy for assessing the potential of a test substance to slow ventricular repolarization. Includes information concerning nonclinical assays and integrated risk assessment. Effects on I_{Kr} current and other cardiac ion channels should be considered as part of "core battery" and "follow-up" studies, respectively.	3
Draft Guideline on the Non-clinical Investigation of the Dependence Potential of Medicinal Products	Provides guidance on the need for testing of dependence potential in animals during the development of medicinal products and indicates what type of information is expected as part of a MAA. Receptor-binding studies of parent drug and metabolites should be considered to reveal signals pointing toward dependence potential.	13
ICH M4—Common Technical Document	Describes an acceptable format and content for submission to regulatory agencies. Secondary pharmacodynamics studies should be submitted as part of the pharmacology section.	14

[a]ICH, International Conference on Harmonization; IND, investigational new drug; MAA, Marketing Authorization Application; NCE, new chemical entity.

enormous from the perspective of individual patients, public health, and the pharmaceutical industry. Thus, there is a high value in all technologies that can identify potential clinical liabilities at an early stage.

At this time technologies are not available to accurately predict, through preclinical experiments, the many factors related to clinical safety and efficacy. To understand the full scope of this problem, it must be recognized that:

1. The patient population is heterogeneous [17]. Patients differ at the genetic level with regard to drug transport, drug metabolism, expression of disease, and many other factors not yet understood. Humans change with age [18] and are changed by disease [19].
2. Early testing using tissues, cells, and subcellular components is only modestly predictive; it is not yet possible to reduce human physiology to an array of *in vitro* tests.
3. Preclinical testing using animal models is only modestly predictive of effects in humans.

The pharmaceutical industry has long recognized the magnitude of this problem and made significant investments to address it. As one example of success [20], in 1991 ~40% of attrition was due to poor pharmacokinetics/bioavailability. By 2000, attrition due to these factors was reduced to ~10%. During this time period, most pharmaceutical companies had implemented sophisticated panels of early *in vitro* absorption, distribution, metabolism, and excretion (ADME) assays in the discovery/development process. These included intestinal permeability assays, hepatic metabolism assays, and physicochemical characterization. Many in the industry believe that the use of this early testing strategy is the basis for the profound reduction in attrition due to poor pharmacokinetics.

At this time the major factors leading to clinical attrition are safety/toxicology issues and lack of efficacy that is only apparent at the clinical level. Unanticipated safety and efficacy issues each account for approximately 30% of current attrition [20]. This chapter focuses on some of the key *in vitro* technologies that can improve early prediction of clinical safety and efficacy. It is anticipated that, over time, these methods will have a profound impact on clinical attrition and on the economics of drug development.

17.3   APPROACHES TO PHARMACOLOGICAL PROFILING

17.3.1   Factors Influencing the Approach to Secondary Pharmacodynamics

In addition to regulatory requirements, several factors will influence the strategy for secondary pharmacology in any given pharmaceutical organization. The main factors are presented in Table 17.2. Thus, the pharmaceutical industry is beset with a number of significant challenges to achieve high quality, high throughput, and predictive secondary pharmacological studies, during the early stages of the drug discovery process. As well as satisfying project demands, scientific efficacy, selectivity and safety questions, international regulatory guidelines, and increased patient awareness, secondary pharmacology is increasingly being used to enable informed

TABLE 17.2   Factors Influencing the Approach to Secondary Pharmacodynamic Studies

Increasing	Decreasing
Number, complexity, and stringency of regulatory requirements	Supply of compound during the early discovery stages
Number and novelty of new chemical entities	Availability of scientific and technical expertise in key areas (e.g., Integrative Physiology and Pharmacology)
Number, diversity, and novelty of molecular targets and approaches	Late stage attrition
Throughput of *in vitro* versus *in vivo* assays	Discovery and development time
Risk identification initiatives during early discovery stages (e.g., "front loading" initiatives)	Numbers of animals used in the pharmaceutical industry
Patient awareness and expectations	
Predictive value of *in vivo* and *in vitro* nonclinical assays with respect to human safety	

decision making. One of the key factors influencing the approach to secondary pharmacology is the rapidly evolving scientific and technological knowledge. A recent example is the evolution from conventional labor-intensive patch-clamp electrophysiology to medium throughput electrophysiology-based platforms to assess activities at ion channels [21].

17.3.2   *In Vivo* and *In Vitro* Approaches to Secondary Pharmacodynamics

Two complementary approaches to secondary pharmacodynamic studies may be considered: *in vivo* observational methods and *in vitro* pharmacological profiling.

An *in vivo* strategy may be employed to measure the integrated response to drug challenge in the whole animal, where a variety of factors such as genetics, biochemistry, metabolism, and environment combine to influence the observed effect. The advantage of such an approach is that the effect of the test substance is determined in an intact physiological system; of course, this offers its own challenge in interpretation and translating the results to other species.

The complexity of study design, numbers of animals, and quantity of compound required to conduct *in vivo* studies require a rationally designed, hypothesis-driven approach. Prior knowledge of adverse events associated with a related target class or chemical structure is invaluable in designing effective studies. Selection of the most appropriate animal model is also important: studies may be conducted in specific disease models, or in knock-out animals in order to increase the predictive power of the chosen model.

Interpretation of data from *in vivo* studies is complex as the molecular target or targets responsible for mediating a given response are unknown and it may be difficult to distinguish the effects of the drug due to action at the primary target from effects mediated through secondary targets.

In vivo secondary pharmacodynamic studies are clearly not suited to a high throughput approach, which would make it difficult to apply an *in vivo* approach to a feedback system in early drug discovery. However, this approach may be more applicable in later stages of compound development, where refinement of predictions from *in vitro* studies on small numbers of compounds becomes important.

A complementary approach to *in vivo* studies is the more recent and now more common *in vitro* method of pharmacological profiling in which the compound of interest is screened in a battery of *in vitro* assays to determine its affinity at a range of receptors, ion channels, transporters, and enzymes. Determination of the potency and efficacy of the drug in functional assays may generate useful information in defining whether it is an agonist or antagonist at a given target. The technologies available for these kinds of analyses are discussed in detail in Section 17.4.1.

In vitro approaches offer a high throughput method for studying secondary pharmacodynamics; integration of *in vitro* secondary pharmacodynamic analyses into early drug discovery is therefore relatively simple as capacity and turnaround time are likely to be equivalent to primary pharmacologic assays. No prior knowledge of target class or chemical structure is required in the experimental design, although such knowledge can be used to enhance the power of the design. Assay panel design is discussed further in Section 17.4.2.

The key limitation of the pharmacological profile approach is in the translation of simple quantitative pharmacological data (affinity or efficacy values) from *in vitro* systems to whole organism physiology, although one method to address this is discussed in Section 17.4.4.

It should be noted that the *in vitro* and *in vivo* approaches discussed are not mutually exclusive and may indeed be complementary: *in vivo* experiments may be carefully designed around the results of *in vitro* panel screening to investigate the effect of any significant activity in an intact physiological system; *in vitro* panels may be employed to deconvolute an observed physiological response in order to identify the underlying molecular target(s) involved.

17.3.3   Strategies for *In Vitro* Pharmacological Profiling

Stepwise Approach   Pharmacological profiling may be applied in a stepwise, or tiered, process, where compounds are assayed for activity at an increasing number of molecular targets as the chemical series progresses through the drug discovery and development process (Fig. 17.1). The screens applied in the early stages of discovery consist of a small panel of key targets that mediate functional effects of the vital physiological systems: cardiovascular, central nervous, and respiratory systems. This early screening may aid selection between multiple lead series. During the optimization phases of discovery, the profile is expanded to a greater number of assays, adding targets that mediate effects on other organs systems such as the gastrointestinal system, enabling refinement of compound selectivity alongside primary target affinity/efficacy. As the drug evolves into a candidate for the development phase, a greater number of targets covering all organ systems are screened. The result is the generation of a comprehensive pharmacological profile of the drug before it is first administered to humans.

The assay methodologies applied are firstly to perform *in vitro* radioligand binding assays and enzyme activity assays, where possible using recombinant human targets. The drug is initially screened at an appropriate single concentration and any

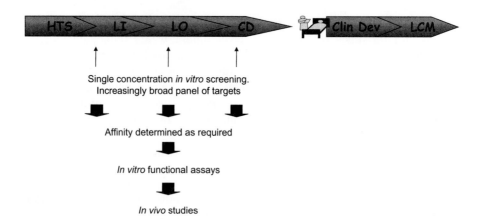

FIGURE 17.1   Stepwise pharmacological profiling in drug discovery. Compounds are assayed in single concentration screens for activity at an increasing number of molecular targets as the chemical series progresses through the drug discovery and development process. In the early stages of discovery, the profiling panel may be small and focussed toward those targets of greatest impact, allowing fast and efficient generation of data, perhaps to select between lead series. As compounds progress, the number of secondary targets screened increases to broaden the biological space searched for potential undesirable effects. At any stage, identification of significant activity at a secondary target may trigger determination of affinity in order to estimate selectivity compared with the primary target. Further investigation for targets of concern may be determination of functional activity: agonism or antagonism, which may dictate the likely effect of the compound *in vivo*. Finally, specific *in vivo* studies may be necessary to fully explore the activity of the compound at secondary targets. (HTS = high throughput screening; LI = lead identification; LO = lead optimization; CD = candidate drug; Clin Dev = clinical development; LCM = life cycle management)

targets that show significant activity are retested in concentration–response studies to provide a quantitative analysis of the activity (Fig. 17.1). The test concentration selected may be based on the affinity of the drug at the therapeutic target, and it is recommended that the test concentration should be a multiple of the primary therapeutic target affinity or efficacy value, in order to use the data to assess the selectivity of the compound for the primary target. Alternatively, a therapeutic margin (the ratio of the dose at which desired therapeutic activity occurs to the dose at which unacceptable adverse events occur) may be considered by comparing the affinity of the compound for secondary targets with the measured (or predicted) maximum exposure *in vivo*. For example, a compound in the early phases of discovery may be tested at concentration 10-fold higher than its affinity for the primary target, but for compounds in later phases it may be appropriate to test at 100-fold higher than the primary target potency or affinity.

Once the activity of the drug at the secondary molecular target has been quantified in a radioligand binding assay or enzyme activity assay, the mode of action may be explored in *in vitro* functional assays to determine whether the drug is an agonist or antagonist at that target. Functional effects in relation to dose and plasma exposure of the drug may then be explored in specifically designed *in vivo* studies (Fig. 17.1).

Reverse Sequential Approach Some pharmaceutical companies have initiated intensive profiling programs to define chemical space that is most suitable for the use of discovering lead compounds against important target classes [22, 23]. This approach requires the ability to test large series of molecules in large panels of assays at low cost in order to build a dataset correlating diverse areas of chemical space with pharmacological profiles. This database will form the foundation for new drug discovery programs, allowing focused libraries of compounds likely to have affinity for the target of interest, and limited secondary target affinity, to be designed *in silico*. These libraries may be screened by traditional high throughput methods, resulting in high quality lead compounds. Lead optimization, screening compounds for both primary target efficacy and secondary profile, will cycle until a suitable candidate drug can be selected, but this process should not operate in isolation: data generated should be added to the database, and analysis and predictions from alignment of lead compounds with data already in the database should allow rapid optimization of the compound. This reverse sequential drug discovery process is described in Fig. 17.2.

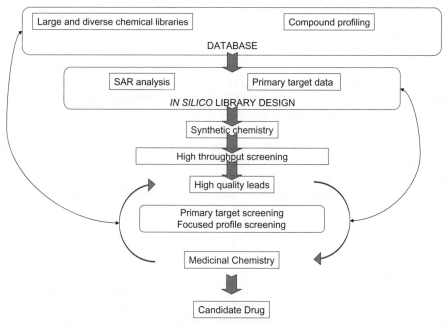

FIGURE 17.2 Reverse sequential drug discovery. A database containing pharmacological profiles for large and diverse chemical libraries is generated. *In silico* analysis of these data allow prediction of structures likely to have affinity at the primary target of interest, and limited off-target affinities. Small, focused libraries based on these analyses may be synthesized and screened to generate high quality leads. Optimization of these leads for primary target efficacy and lack of secondary target effects along with other key properties, including ADME and PK, will cycle until a suitable candidate drug may be selected. Data generated in this process should be captured in the original database to enhance its power for future use.

Problem Solving   *In vitro* profiles of compounds may be generated in an attempt to find the molecular mechanism behind observed *in vivo* effects of a new drug substance. These observations may come from animal models used in early efficacy testing, toxicological studies, or core battery safety pharmacology studies; or they may be observations from clinical trials of a candidate drug. A broad spectrum profile may be generated in order to attempt to find a molecular target responsible for some physiological effect, or perhaps more focused screening of key molecular targets involved in specific physiological systems may be employed to determine rapidly whether a particular pathway is involved in the observed physiology. An example of this approach is given in Section 17.5.2.

17.4   TECHNICAL CONSIDERATIONS FOR *IN VITRO* PROFILING

17.4.1   Assay Technologies

A wide variety of assay technologies are available for compound profiling. These range from assays using highly purified single protein reagents, to subcellular fractions, to whole cells, to tissues, and finally to animals. Within each level there are a variety of detection techniques available. Here we focus on the underlying assay parameters rather than the chemistry, physics, and engineering behind various signal detection systems.

Most profiling is done in a tiered fashion with the first tier consisting primarily of assays using highly purified protein targets or subcellular fractions. Compounds with activity in these primary assays are then progressed to more physiologically relevant functional assays. Primary assays generally measure competition between the test compound and either a receptor–ligand or enzyme–substrate interaction. These types of assays have the advantage of using reagents that can be well characterized and easily produced. For this reason, these biochemical assays generally give consistent results over time and are suitable for the rapid testing of large numbers of compounds.

It is important to recognize that the interaction of test compounds with the assay method and technology will have a profound effect on the results. Compounds must be soluble in the assay buffer at all test concentrations. Test compounds that either fluoresce or have strong absorbance can interfere with optical detection systems. Compounds with high protein binding will give variable results depending on the assay protein content. Many test compounds show nonspecific binding to plastics used in pipette tips, assay plates, and filtration media; thus, the actual concentration available to interact with the target may be substantially lower than the theoretical test concentration. Changing consumables or taking steps to block nonspecific binding will impact assay results. Test results for lipophilic compounds will vary with amount of membrane fraction in receptor binding and cytochrome P450 assays. These types of physicochemical interactions can generally be anticipated based on a prior understanding of the nature of the test compounds (solubility, optical properties, protein binding, lipophilicity).

Some assay technologies are optimized for throughput, good signal-to-noise ratio, and signal stability in ways that severely constrain the concentration or type of key assay components. To optimize assay robustness and signal-to-noise ratio, high affinity antagonists will often be chosen as the radioligand in receptor binding assays. In some cases, these ligands are not effective for detecting agonists and important interactions may be missed. There are many kinase assay technologies that require substrate or cofactor concentrations well above K_m and/or require the use of substrates with no physiological relevance. Many assays are run using receptors expressed at high density, which may exist in abnormal states and thus exhibit aberrant pharmacology. Many assays use the active site fragment of an enzyme or receptor, which may yield results different from those obtained using the entire protein. In many pharmacology profiles, ion channel targets are tested in binding rather than functional assays; these binding assays are known to miss some channel-blocking compounds. There are a number of cases of assay format variations leading to significant and consistent changes in test results that are more difficult to anticipate.

In many cases, both human and animal forms of important targets are available. Not surprisingly, there are examples of species-specific differences in the affinities for some compounds [24]. For this reason, there has been a great effort to introduce human forms of the target of interest into all profiles. There are, however, good reasons to retain assays based on relevant animal-derived targets, as most models for *in vivo* safety and efficacy are in animals. It is important to anticipate these differential results in animal models and expected clinical outcome. There are also several examples of important targets, where the human form is not yet cloned or is unavailable due to blocking patents. Over time, most early pharmacology profiles have incorporated, whenever available, the human form of important targets with animal targets primarily used in focused studies to support a full understanding of *in vivo* animal models.

The difficulties outlined in the preceding paragraphs highlight the importance of informed assay design and a full understanding of the relationship between an *in vitro* assay result and the *in vivo* outcome that it is designed to predict. This understanding can come only from full characterization of each assay using as many known effectors as possible. For example, if a cardiovascular safety profile contains a group of adrenergic receptor subtype assays, it is important to know how all reference compounds with well characterized *in vivo* outcomes perform across the panel. These reference compounds would include marketed drugs, compounds that have been characterized in animal studies, and include a selection of agonists and antagonists. Only with this data as context can there be an informed interpretation of data from new test compounds.

Once a compound has been shown to have significant activity in an *in vitro* assay, the next step or tier of assays is designed to define the likely functional outcome of the compound–target interaction. For enzyme targets, this would normally be definition of the mechanism (competitive, noncompetitive, uncompetitive). For receptor targets, this would normally be differentiation between agonists, partial agonists, antagonists, and inverse agonists. For transporters, this could be differentiation between substrates and inhibitors. In some cases, these assays can be run using the same target reagent as the initial screening assay. However, in many cases (primarily receptors, ion channels, and transporters), the relevant experiments can only be done in living cells or isolated organs. These more biologically complex assays open up a new area of difficulty in assay design and data interpretation. Some of these difficulties can be addressed by a good understanding of the physicochemical properties of each test compound: Is it likely to reach an intracellular target? Is it soluble at the highest test concentration? Will results be influenced by serum proteins? Some of the difficulties must be addressed by having a good understanding of the additional factors in cells and tissues that will influence assay results. For example, is the signal transduction between a highly expressed receptor and the measured signal a good representation of normal physiology? Can interactions between the test compound and endogenous nontarget proteins in the cell line or tissue influence the assay results? Thus, once again, it is essential to fully characterize each assay by having tested all known effectors. This reference dataset is the context in which data on new compounds can be fully understood.

The third tier of testing often involves animal experiments to explore fully the functional effect of an activity discovered in the early tiers of profiling. These models are based on specific organ functions known to be associated with the earlier observed *in vitro* assay results. Testing at this level may be the first time a compound has been used *in vivo* and brings up questions of formulation, dosage, route of administration, and pharmacokinetics. Consideration of these factors is beyond the scope of this chapter; however, once again, it is key to have a strong set of reference compound data in each model, which can be used as the context in which to interpret data on new compounds.

In conclusion, regardless of the particular assay technology chosen, profiling assays should meet two basic requirements. First, the relationship between the assay result and one or more clinical outcomes should be well understood; and second, the assay should produce consistent results over time.

17.4.2 *In Vitro* Panel Design

Introduction *In vitro* assay panels can be designed using two major strategies. Assays can be selected one-by-one based on known safety issues associated with those assays [25] or the assay panel can be chosen on the basis of assay diversity as determined by a variety of different methods [22]. In reality, most assay panels are designed using a combination of these two strategies. With greater technological advancement, a large number of cell lines and expression systems have been engineered to allow development of assays using human targets. As a result, a wide range of *in vitro* pharmacology assays have been developed to act as models for predicting *in vivo* effects. With such a great diversity of assays available to choose from, efforts have been made to determine the most clinically important side effects and to link those side effects with assays [26].

Growing experience with profiling has facilitated the selection of assay panels. As pharmaceutical companies screen an increasing number of drug candidates, this experience, in the form of data, can be applied to better understand the assays and to fine-tune the assay selections. In-house, public, and commercial profiling databases offer unique opportunities to analyze the relationships between targets as well as to access the profiles of drugs and drug-like molecules (e.g., see Refs. 22 and 23). Standard statistical methods such as clustering and correlation can be applied to these datasets to elucidate the sometimes counterintuitive relationships between assays. In this section, the application of the knowledge from long-running screening programs to assay panel design is discussed.

Assay-by-Assay Choice: Beyond Known Pharmacology   The most intuitive methods of assay selection are based on known pharmacology and clinical experience. Experience from long-running screening programs and commercial drug information databases can be applied to enhance these methods of selection. For example, associations between assays and adverse drug reactions (ADRs) can be generated using a database of *in vitro* pharmacology data for drugs and the accompanying *in vivo* ADR data. In this example, uniformly generated *in vitro* pharmacology data is coupled with *in vivo* ADR data gathered from drug labels and mined for significant correlations between the *in vitro* pharmacology and *in vivo* clinical effects [26]. In this analysis, the natural language of drug label ADRs were translated into COSTART (Coding Symbols for Thesaurus of Adverse Reaction Terms, U.S. Food and Drug Administration) ADR terms and loaded into a database. Each COSTART ADR term was compared with each pharmacology assay to identify significant correlations. The hits in a given assay were binned by strength, and among the drugs in a given bin, the percentage of those drugs that report each of the 800 ADR terms was determined. Assay bin/ADR pairs were flagged when the percentage of compounds in that bin that list the ADR on the label was significantly higher than the baseline level for that ADR across all the drugs in the dataset. Further analysis looked for an *in vitro* activity–ADR dose response across the hit strength bins for a given assay or target. In other words, as the *in vitro* potency against a target goes up, the ADR should be increasingly present on the labels of the drugs in those bins.

An example of the results of this analysis can be seen in Fig. 17.3. This figure illustrates the association of mydriasis with the M_3 muscarinic receptor. The baseline frequency of this ADR is 5.99%, while nearly half of the drugs with M_3 hits in the <100 nM IC_{50} bin list this ADR on the drug label.

Over 5000 significant *in vitro* assay–ADR associations were found covering over 100 assays/targets. Close examination of this set of associations yields many results

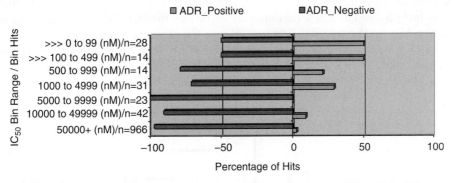

FIGURE 17.3   Significant statistical association between in vitro binding to the M_3 muscarinic receptor and clinical mydriasis. Seven IC_{50} activity bins are found on the y-axis ranging from the 0-99 nM bin to the greater-than-50000 nM bin which is the default bin for the non-hits. The number of compounds in each bin is indicated. The bars shown with each bin represent the percentage of compounds in that bin that are positive (light bars on the right) or negative (dark bars on the left) respectively for the ADR in question. The baseline percentage for that ADR is 5.99%. The result of a Spearman rank correlation of this association is a robust 0.82. Data from BioPrint (Cerep SA).

that are consistent with known pharmacology and many others that appear to be novel. Another useful feature of these associations is that they aid in interpretation of *in vitro* data because one can identify the hit strength bins where the association becomes significant. For instance, in the case of M_3 and mydriasis, the association only becomes of concern in the 1000–4999 nM bin.

Diversity: Beyond Phylogenetics Phylogenetic or pharmacological diversity can be applied to the selection of assays for profiles. Phylogenetic and pharmacological descriptions of how the members of a receptor or enzyme family are related are not necessarily in agreement. Here too, the availability of large *in vitro* datasets is useful, allowing analysis of interassay overlap, correlation, and clustering.

The muscarinic acetylcholine receptor can act as an interesting test case for assay selection. Among the five different muscarinic receptor subtypes, which and how many of these receptors should be included in a profile? While all five may eventually be tested, which ones might prove most informative for the earliest testing? Several different kinds of information can be brought to bear in making this evaluation. While clustering compounds by an *in vitro* profile is now a common practice, there is less recognition of the utility of using those same datasets to cluster the assays. In the case of compound clustering, the assay data is used to probe the relationships of the compounds to one another. Similarly, the compounds can be used as probes to define how the *in vitro* assays relate to one another. From the clustering of receptors by pharmacological activity, it can be seen that the M_1 and M_2 are most closely related to one another followed by the pair of M_3 and M_4 with M_5 most distantly related to both pairs (Fig. 17.4).

Assuming that it is desirable to cover muscarinic pharmacology as completely as possible without having to run all five assays, it would follow that one might choose to run three assays, one chosen from each pair of related assays and M_5. To help choose between these pairs, the overlap of hits on each of these assays can be examined (Fig. 17.5) as well as the number of ADR associations that have been found for each of these targets (Table 17.3). The overlap matrix shows what proportion of the hits (defined as >30% inhibition at 10 μM) on the target defining each column are also hits on the target defining each row. For instance, looking at the first row in Fig. 17.5, 88% of the hits at M_2 are also hits at M_1, 96% of the hits on M_3 are also hits at M_1, 85% of hits at M_4 are also hits at M_1, and 86% of hits at M_5 are also hits at M_1.

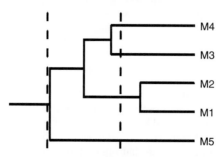

FIGURE 17.4   Clustering by Pearson correlation using the complete linkage. A dataset of nearly 2500 molecules tested on all five subtypes was used to define the relationship between muscarinic acetylcholine receptor targets. Data from BioPrint (Cerep SA).

	M1	M2	M3	M4	M5
M1	1	0.88	0.96	0.85	0.86
M2	0.88	1	0.96	0.85	0.84
M3	0.96	0.96	1	0.71	0.77
M4	0.85	0.85	0.71	1	0.78
M5	0.86	0.84	0.77	0.78	1

FIGURE 17.5 Overlap matrix for the five muscarinic acetylcholine receptors. The matrix shows the overlap frequency between hits on the individual mAChRs. For example, 62% of hits on M_1 are also hits on M_3. Conversely, 96% of hits on M_3 are also hits on M_1. Data from BioPrint (Cerep SA).

TABLE 17.3   Distribution of ADR Association Across the mAChRs[a]

Assays	Number of ADR Associations that Are Unique to the Assay or Group of Assays
M_1 alone	24
M_5 alone	20
M_4 alone	4
M_1 and M_4	9
M_1 and M_2	4
M_1, M_2, and M_3	2
M_1, M_2, M_3, and M_4	36
M_1, M_2, and M_4	1
M_1, M_3, and M_4	1

[a]For example, there are 24 ADR associations unique to M_1 and 9 associations shared by M_1 and M_4. Data from BioPrint (Cerep SA).

Table 17.3 shows the number of ADR associations found for each receptor subtype. As the five subtypes are highly correlated, they share many of the same ADR associations; for example, there are 36 ADR associations common to M_1, M_2, M_3, and M_4. Based on the information presented in the table, M_1 should be chosen over M_2 because although the two are highly correlated, M_1 has the greater overlap with other subtypes and has many unique ADR associations while M_2 has no unique associations. M_3 and M_4 cluster together even though M_3 is more highly correlated with M_1. Most of the hits at M_3 (96%) are also hits at M_1. M_4 is the better choice here because it is less correlated and has less overlap with M_1 and M_2. M_4 also has more unique ADR associations than M_3. M_5 should be included because it differs most from the other family members by correlation, clustering, and overlap and has a large number of ADR associations uniquely associated with it. Based on this analysis, the best assays to include would be M_1, M_4, and M_5.

It is important to recognize that this kind of analysis is limited by the dataset used to generate associations. For example, there are currently very few muscarinic receptor subtype-selective compounds on the market, which may explain some of the overlap and correlations described here. It is important, therefore, that the analyses used to define profiling panels are reviewed regularly, especially as novel compounds are profiled, in order to ensure that the relationships still hold. Likewise, new scientific knowledge of targets and effects should be incorporated in order to maximize the value of the profiling panel.

17.4.3 ADME/PK Profiling

Introduction   While the pharmacological screening of development compounds has been widely accepted by the pharmaceutical industry, *in vitro* ADME/PK screening has been adopted more slowly. Nevertheless, ADME/PK profiling is now widely performed at early stages in lead development. Selection of leads with favorable *in vitro* ADME properties is important because it is much harder to design them in after a compound with the appropriate pharmacology has been identified. *In vitro* ADME assay panels are chosen for their potential to predict *in vivo* pharmacokinetics. Some of the *in vitro* assays measure properties that contribute to the *in vivo* bioavailability of the new drug candidate. These include aqueous solubility, log D, and physicochemical properties known to play a role in drug absorption. More direct assays such as immobilized artificial membrane (IAM) columns and parallel artificial membrane permeation assay (PAMPA) are also gaining popularity as measures of passive permeability. Results from these types of assay are useful by themselves but interpretation of these data is enhanced by the use of large *in vitro* and *in vivo* datasets that act as a context in which to understand these *in vitro* results.

In Fig. 17.6, a histogram shows the distribution of the log D values for compounds with poor (<20%) and good (>80%) oral absorption. The distributions are overlapping but offset and as such log D alone cannot be used to make a clear determination of potential permeability. Nevertheless, information like this can be taken into

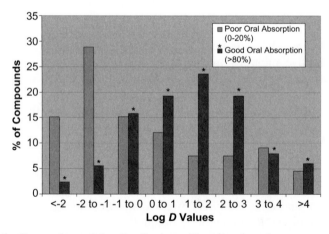

FIGURE 17.6   Comparison of the distribution of log D values for compounds with good (>80%, bars with asterisk) and poor (<20%, plain bars) oral absorption. Data from BioPrint (Cerep SA).

account for library design by trying to target compound libraries to have log D values that fall into the range preferred for good oral absorption. In-house or commercially available software can be used for *in silico* log D or log P predictions for potential libraries. Early screening of drug candidates can allow selection of those with the best possible *in vitro* ADME properties.

Permeability assays using cell lines like Caco-2, MDCK, or HT-29 may be employed to make permeability determinations that are able to take into account the diverse transporters and efflux pumps that play a significant role in drug permeability *in vivo*. In the case of the Caco-2 assay, it is most informative to run the assay in both the apical (A) to basolateral (B) and the basolateral to apical directions in order to identify compounds that might be differentially transported in one direction versus another. The P-glycoprotein (P-gp) inhibition (of the B-to-A flux of P-gp transporter substrate digoxin) and P-gp ATPase assays are used further to identify whether a compound is likely to be effluxed *in vivo*. Figure 17.7 plots percent oral absorption versus Caco-2 cell permeability data. This view of the data shows that while the general trends are as expected—drugs with low permeability are poorly absorbed and drugs with high permeability are well absorbed—this is not the complete answer. As a rule of thumb, an apparent permeability value (P_{app}) of 5 or greater indicates that a compound is not likely to be permeability-limited; however, there are clearly many exceptions.

In vitro metabolic stability assays using liver microsome preparations and isolated cytochrome P450s allow a qualitative assessment of the likely metabolic fate of the test compound. Figure 17.8 shows that there is no direct correlation between *in vitro* metabolic stability and oral bioavailability. However, it is worth noting that there are very few compounds having both poor metabolic stability (<20% remaining) and high oral bioavailability (>80).

Drug Interactions at Cytochrome P450   Panels of cytochrome P450 inhibition assays can aid in identifying compounds that might be susceptible to P450-mediated

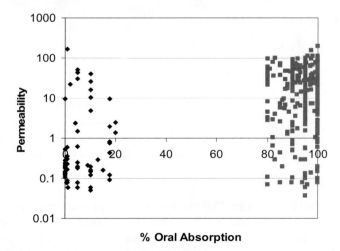

FIGURE 17.7   Comparison of the distribution of apical to basolateral apparent permeability values (P_{app} 1×10^{-6} cm/s) for compounds with good (>80%) and poor (<20%) oral absorption. Data from BioPrint (Cerep SA).

Oral Bioavailability
120
100
80
60
40
20
0
0
20
40
60
80
100
120
140
HLM Metabolic Stability (% Remaining)

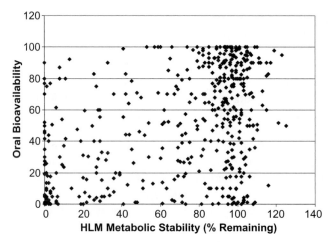

FIGURE 17.8 Plot of human liver microsome metabolic stability (% remaining) versus human oral bioavailability (%); $n = 468$ compounds. Data from BioPrint (Cerep SA).

Compound Name
CYP1A2
CYP2B6
CYP2C19
CYP2C8
CYP2C9 (MFC)
CYP2C9 (Tolbutamide)
CYP2D6
CYP2E1
CYP3A4 (BFC)
CYP3A4 (Benzoxyresorufin)
CYP3A4 (Midazolam)
CYP3A4 (Testosterone)
CYP3A5
Cimetidine
Clarithromycin
Ketoconazole
Terfenadine
Omeprazole
Lovastatin
Ritonavir

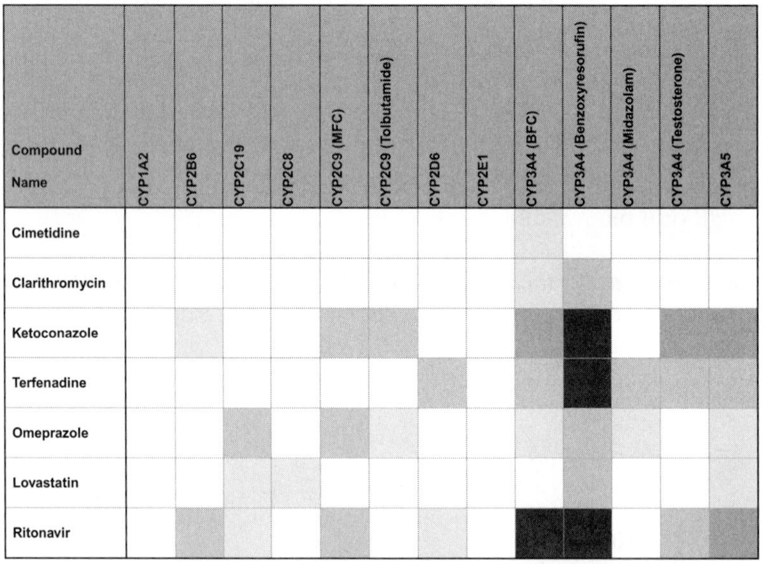

FIGURE 17.9 Heat map of P450 profiles of a selection of compounds known to be involved in clinically relevant drug–drug interactions: individual drug data is shown in the rows, while the assays are named at the top of the columns. Data from BioPrint (Cerep SA).

drug–drug interactions. Figure 17.9 shows the P450 interactions of a selection of drugs known to be vulnerable to drug–drug interactions as either substrates or inhibitors. For instance, lovastatin is a CYP3A4 substrate susceptible to interactions with potent CYP3A4 inhibitors such as ketoconazole [27]. Terfenadine is metabolized by CYP3A4 [28] and has been involved in adverse interactions with inhibitors such as ritonavir.

Use of an ADME Profile   All together, these assays can be used to create an ADME profile that is useful both as individual results and as a collective ADME profile. The use of the collective profile may help to overcome the limitations of the individual assays. Very low solubility as determined in the solubility assay might explain why compounds like albendazole or niclosamide that have good *in vitro* permeability characteristics are poorly absorbed. Standard statistical methods can be used to identify which marketed drugs have ADME profiles similar to that of a test compound of interest. The well understood clinical PK properties of these known compounds can be used to help predict the *in vivo* properties of the clinical candidate. Figure 17.10 shows the *in vitro* ADME profiles for two sets of drugs and some corresponding pharmacokinetic data. Both sets of drugs share similar results in the four permeability assays, but differ in metabolic stability and log *D* values. Both sets of compounds are generally well absorbed orally, but the set with low metabolic stability understandably has low oral bioavailability. When comparing the *in vitro* ADME profile of a drug candidate to those of known drugs, one can have greater confidence in extrapolating from the neighbors (compounds with similar *in vitro* ADME profiles) when most of the neighbors have homogeneous *in vivo* ADME properties. If the neighbors have very diverse properties, there is little basis for extrapolation.

17.4.4   Data Analysis and Interpretation

Introduction   Can *in vitro* pharmacological profiling capture information relevant to drug biology and drug development? The heat map in Fig. 17.11 shows the profiles of tricyclic antidepressants versus the newer second and third generation antidepressants. The antidepressants are divided into three tiers in the figure. In the upper tier are the older tricyclic antidepressants, the second tier are the popular second generation antidepressants, and some of the newer antidepressants are found in the

Compound Name	Permeability A to B pH 7.4/7.4 (Papp 10e-6 cm/s)	Permeability B to A pH 7.4/7.4 (Papp 10e-6 cm/s)	Permeability A to B pH 6.5/7.4 (Papp 10e-6 cm/s)	Permeability B to A pH 7.4/6.5 (Papp 10e-6 cm/s)	Aqueous Solubility (10e-6 M)	HLM Metabolic Stability (% Remaining)	LogD (octanol)	LogD (Cyclohexane)	Oral Bioavailibility (%)	Oral Absorption (%)
Nefazodone	96	19	36	15	72	0	3.53	1.68	19	100
Lovastatin	14	7	26	10	13	0	4.08	1.28	5	10
Ergotamine l-Tartrate	20	17	26	23	41	1	3.57	0.71	4	55
Astemizole	14	9	26	16	42	3	4.05	2.1	7	90
Benzarone	38	8	36	8	31	6	4.04	1.1	1	73
Sildenafil	42	23	35	41	32	19	2.8	0.65	40	92
Quinidine	43	18	25	51	200	69	1.96	-1.5	74	80
Yohimbine	43	21	31	47	196	69	1.98	na	28	
Clozapine	32	14	26	31	203	78	2.98	1.23	53	93
Amitriptyline	25	78	26	51	175	79	2.77	1.7	48	100
Tramadol	56	19	38	44	200	90	1.24	1.12	77	75
Pantoprazole	31	28	35	23	166	91	1.93	-1.1	79	

FIGURE 17.10   Compounds with similar *in vitro* ADME profiles and corresponding *in vivo* pharmacokinetics. Data from BioPrint (Cerep SA).

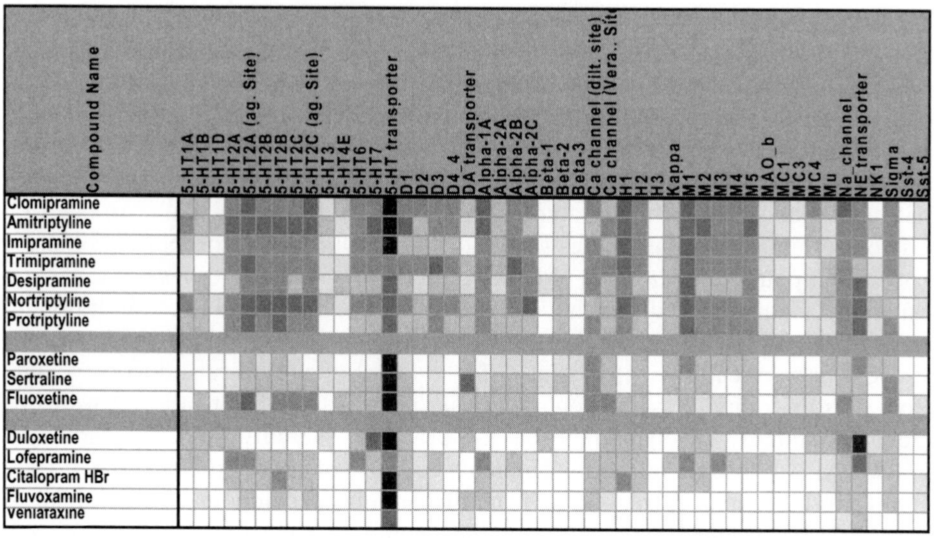

FIGURE 17.11   Heat map of antidepressant profiles. In this heat map, the individual drugs are shown in the rows, while the assays are named at the top of the columns. Data from BioPrint (Cerep SA).

third tier. Nearly all the drugs share strong interactions with the 5-HT transporter. Further visual inspection shows that the tricyclics also share hits on the muscarinic, histamine, and adrenergic targets, all of which are known to be associated with the commonly reported side effects of these drugs. Each succeeding generation of drugs has fewer and weaker hits on these targets. Thus, in this case, profiling clearly captures the differences between these generations of drugs.

The profile similarities shared by the many antidepressants make great sense both from the standpoints of shared therapeutic targets such as the serotonin and norepinephrine transporters and of the shared muscarinic and histaminic adverse effects. Nevertheless, it is not necessary that a drug's target class be included in the profile for that class to cluster together. An example of this is shown in Fig. 17.12, where a large group of the "conazole" family of antifungals are found to cluster together despite the absence of the therapeutic target in the assay panel used to cluster the compounds. These drugs are clustering together based on rich profiles of weak hits.

Profile Interpretation on a Hit-by-Hit Basis   The most obvious way to interpret profile data is on a hit-by-hit basis. When following up on hits, the first consideration is the strength of the off-target effect relative to the therapeutic target. The hit strength and agonist/antagonist status can be determined by IC_{50} or K_i and functional assay follow-up. Having obtained an IC_{50} for a hit in question, the value may be compared with available plasma exposure data or with the projected therapeutic concentration of the drug candidate. If there is good (>100-fold) separation between these values, the hit may be of little concern.

Another line of investigation involves exploring the ADR associations discussed previously in Section 17.4.2. ADR associations for the assay of interest can be

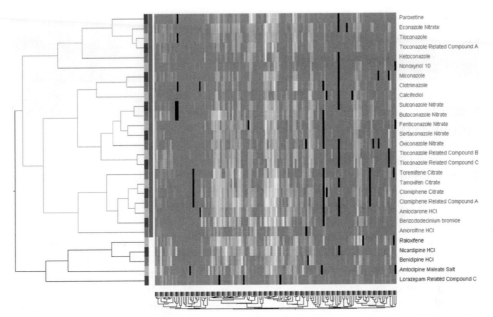

Paroxetine
Econazole Nitrate
Tioconazole
Tioconazole Related Compound A
Ketoconazole
Nonoxynol 10
Miconazole
Clotrimazole
Calcifediol
Sulconazole Nitrate
Butoconazole Nitrate
Fenticonazole Nitrate
Sertaconazole Nitrate
Oxiconazole Nitrate
Tioconazole Related Compound B
Tioconazole Related Compound C
Toremifene Citrate
Tamoxifen Citrate
Clomiphene Citrate
Clomiphene Related Compound A
Amiodarone HCl
Benzododecinium bromide
Amorolfine HCl
Raloxifene
Nicardipine HCl
Benidipine HCl
Amlodipine Maleate Salt
Lorazepam Related Compound C

FIGURE 17.12   Clustered heat map. Individual drugs are clustered on the *y*-axis while the pharmacology assays are clustered on the *x*-axis. Clustering of both the compounds and the assays is performed using the conventional Pearson correlation and complete linkage. This figure only shows a subcluster of an original clustering of over 2000 compounds. Data from BioPrint (Cerep SA).

retrieved and examined. The ADR associations only become significant at a certain hit level (IC_{50} bin). This information can be used to estimate a hit strength threshold at which the risk of a given ADR becomes significant from the clinical point of view. These data can be considered in the context of other compounds, in particular, marketed pharmaceuticals that have similar levels of activity at the target of interest. It can be considered whether or not the ADRs associated with the target of interest proved to be a liability for these marketed drugs.

While binding assays make up a large part of a pharmacology safety profile, it is also important to be aware of the limitations of these assays. First, radioligands can be either agonist or antagonist and the choice can influence the ability to detect agonists. For instance, the neurotransmitters serotonin, dopamine, and norepinephrine have broad ranges of potency on the diverse members of their own and related receptor families (see Fig. 17.13). Second, binding assays for ion channels and enzymes using a single ligand are not able to assess fully the many ways a test compound might interact with the normal functioning of the native protein. These binding assays only monitor drug interactions at a specific site.

Using the Entire Profile   The previous section discussed profile analysis based on individual assay results. Using standard statistical clustering techniques, compounds with profiles similar to the compound of interest can be identified. Examples of this have been provided, where even profiles of weak hits not including the therapeutic target cause a group of antifungal drugs to cluster together (Fig. 17.12). The group-

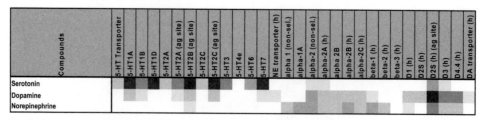

FIGURE 17.13   Binding assay data for serotonin, dopamine, and norepinephrine across a panel of aminergic targets. In the case of serotonin, the potency of the endogenous ligand varies greatly ranging from no hit on 5-HT$_{4E}$ to a nM hit on the 5-HT$_{2C}$ agonist site assay. Data from BioPrint (Cerep SA)

ing of the *in vitro* pharmacological profiles of the antidepressants also makes the point that compounds with similar profiles have similar side effects (Fig. 17.11). The *in vivo* properties (ADRs) of the compounds with similar profiles can be tabulated. Investigation of the ADRs common to the group of similar compounds may help in predicting the potential of ADRs for the profiled compound. It is also worth noting that this technique allows identification of ADRs that might be associated with the drug class but which are not captured by the individual assay pharmacology.

Thus, the profile data can be interpreted at a variety of levels and interpretation is greatly aided by access to large datasets of *in vitro* and *in vivo* data on compounds with well documented *in vivo* history. Interpretation of individual hits is facilitated by comparison to drugs or benchmark compounds with similar activities. Assay/ADR associations mined from these large datasets can help to assess the risk associated with the off-target hits of a drug candidate. Analysis of the profile as a whole allows one to identify compounds or drugs with similar profiles with the added benefit of introducing drug class ADRs that are not captured by the profile assays or our understanding of the *in vivo* biology from those assays.

17.5   IMPACT OF SECONDARY PHARMACODYNAMIC PROFILING: CASE STUDIES

In this section, three case studies are presented to offer a context for the application of secondary pharmacodynamic studies and *in vitro* pharmacological profiling.

17.5.1   Case Study 1. Ranolazine: Secondary Pharmacodynamic and Nonclinical Safety Pharmacology Studies Supporting Regulatory Approval

Ranolazine (Raxena™) is a new anti-anginal agent approved in the United States for use as combination therapy when chronic stable angina is not adequately controlled with other anti-anginal agents (for review, see Ref. 29). While the exact mechanism of action of ranolazine is not known, its anti-anginal and anti-ischemic effects do not appear to depend on changes in blood pressure or heart rate. Purported primary mechanisms of action include inhibition of the late sodium (I_{Na}) current and partial inhibition of fatty acid oxidation. In patients, ranolazine has been associated with a slight but dose-dependent prolongation of the rate corrected QT interval of the surface electrocardiogram (QTc; mean increases of 4–12 ms at 500–1500 mg dose, which equates to plasma exposures of ~2–6 μM).

It is recognized that some drug-induced sudden deaths are secondary to the development of an arrhythmia called torsades de pointes (TdP). Recent advances in the understanding of this issue indicate that the primary event is likely to be inhibition of the rapid component of the delayed rectifier potassium current (I_{Kr}) by such drugs. Since I_{Kr} plays a key role in repolarization of the cardiac action potential, its inhibition slows repolarization and this is manifested on the electrocardiogram as a prolongation of the QT interval. While QT interval prolongation is not a safety concern *per se*, in a small percentage of people it is associated with TdP and degeneration into ventricular fibrillation (for review see Refs. 30 and 31).

Since the cardiac action potential is generated by a complex interplay between several voltage-gated ion channel types and also involves transporters, a series of experiments were carried out to assess the effects of ranolazine on cardiac electrophysiology using electrophysiology-based techniques. In dog myocytes, ranolazine inhibits I_{Kr}, late I_{Na}, and I_{Ca} at clinically relevant therapeutic concentration (IC_{50} of 12, 6, and 50 μM, respectively) [32]. Ranolazine also blocks the peak I_{Ca} and $I_{Na/Ca}$ exchange although with lower potencies (296 and 91 μM, respectively) [32]. Subsequently, the effects of ranolazine in *in vitro* and *in vivo* repolarization assays were evaluated. In the canine wedge preparation, ranolazine caused a slight prolongation of action potential duration (APD) in epicardial cells [33]. Furthermore, in an atrioventricular block dog model, ranolazine produced modest, nonsignificant prolongation of QT interval [34]. Since ranolazine has the ability to block I_{Kr} and to prolong, although minimally, the APD and the QT interval, its proarrhythmogenic potential was evaluated to refine further its cardiac safety profile. In the canine wedge preparation, ranolazine, in contrast to selective I_{Kr} blockers, causes a shortening of the APD in M cells but a slight prolongation of APD in epicardial cells [33]. This leads to a rate-independent reduction in transmural dispersion of repolarization, a key arrhythmogenic factor. In an atrioventricular block dog model, ranolazine, in contrast to D-sotalol, produces modest, nonsignificant prolongation of QT interval that was not associated with reverse use dependency [33]. Furthermore, ranolazine abolishes sea anemone toxin-induced early after depolarization (EADs) in guinea pig ventricular myocytes and suppresses sotalol-induced EADs in Purkinje fiber preparations; ranolazine *per se* failed to induce EADs in these preparations [35]. Furthermore, in the isolated female rabbit Langendorff heart, ranolazine *per se* did not induce TdP but suppressed TdP-induced by I_{Kr} blockers and I_{Na} activators [33]. Finally, in a dog in an atrioventricular block dog model, ranolazine, in contrast to D-sotalol or epinephrine, failed to induce TdP [34]. Overall, ranolazine failed to demonstrate a proarrhythmic profile and showed some antiarrhythmic properties in nonclinical models.

The overall polypharmacology of ranolazine may explain in part its overall modest ability to prolong the QT interval and its lack of arrhythmogenic potential. The nonclinical experiments described above were instrumental in supporting the approvability by regulatory agencies of ranolazine.

17.5.2   Case Study 2. Muscarinic M_3 Receptors and Mydriasis: Linking a Molecular Target to a Physiological Effect

Compound AZ123 was profiled in a panel of 150 *in vitro* radioligand binding and enzyme assays at a single concentration of $10\,\mu M$ as a routine part of the drug discovery process. Significant activity, defined as greater than 50% inhibition at $10\,\mu M$, was detected in one radioligand binding assay, the human recombinant muscarinic M_3 receptor, where 75% inhibition of the binding of $[^3H]$-*N*-methylscopolamine to the human muscarinic M_3 receptor was detected. No significant activity was detected in any of the other muscarinic receptor radioligand binding assays (human recombinant M_1, M_2, M_4, or M_5). A concentration–effect curve was constructed in the human M_3 receptor binding assay and the affinity (K_i) was determined to be $0.3\,\mu M$.

The compound was subsequently tested in the core battery of safety pharmacology studies to explore its effects on physiological functions. The doses selected achieved free plasma levels greater than that predicted to drive efficacy at the primary molecular target. In the rat functional observational battery (FOB) test, used to assess effects on nervous system function, AZ123 caused a dose-dependent increase in pupil diameter (mydriasis) under ambient lighting, an impairment of the pupillary light reflex and a reduction in body weight gain over 24 h. The free plasma level at which the effect was observed was greater than $1\,\mu M$. Literature investigations indicated these effects could be linked to antagonist action at the muscarinic M_3 receptor, as there is good evidence that reflex contraction of the iris in response to light is under parasympathetic nervous system control [36]. The muscarinic M_3 receptor is expressed on the iris sphincter pupillae and parasympathetic innervation of this sphincter regulates pupil diameter to constrict and reduce pupil diameter in response to light [37]. In addition, parasympathetic innervation of the gastrointestinal tract causes contraction of the gastrointestinal tract and this is mediated by acetylcholine action at muscarinic M_3 receptors expressed on smooth muscle. Antagonists of the muscarinic M_3 receptor inhibit the contraction of gastrointestinal tract smooth muscle and reduce spontaneous gastrointestinal motility and gastric emptying [38]. Muscarinic M_3 receptor antagonists are used in the clinic to prevent the gastrointestinal tract peristalsis when performing radiological diagnosis of gastrointestinal disorders [39].

AZ123 was subsequently tested in an *in vitro* functional assay using the guinea pig isolated ileum preparation to explore its functional effects at muscarinic M_3 receptors. AZ123 alone had no effect on the guinea pig ileum preparation but inhibited the contraction caused by methacholine in a concentration-dependent manner with an IC_{50} of $9.5\,\mu M$ suggesting that AZ123 was a functional antagonist of the muscarinic M_3 receptor. It can therefore be concluded that the effects of AZ123 observed in the rat are likely to be mediated by antagonist activity at the muscarinic M_3 receptor. These data can be used to make predictions of the potential effects in the clinic. AZ123 has the potential to cause the classical side effects caused by other drugs that have antagonist activity at the muscarinic M_3 receptor, such as dry mouth, effects on pupil diameter, and subsequent effects on vision as well as effects on gastrointestinal motility (constipation) [40] if free plasma levels are achieved that exceed the K_i for AZ123 at the human muscarinic M_3 receptor. Pharmacological profiling has enabled explanation of *in vivo* observations from an animal model and allowed predictions to be made of potential effects in the clinic.

17.5.3 Case Study 3. Chlorpromazine and Reprofiling: The Application of Pharmacological Profiling Beyond Secondary Pharmacodynamics

The development of novel uses for known compounds, called "drug repurposing" or "drug repositioning," is becoming increasingly important in the pharmaceutical industry. Although life-cycle management of compounds by large companies to extend the use of a current drug into new indications is nothing new, a number of recent publications [41–44] and the emergence of biotechnology companies focused on drug repurposing highlight the increasing interest in finding new therapeutic indications for existing compounds.

Although there are several examples of repurposed drugs, where a new indication is to be treated using the same primary mechanism of action, there are fewer examples of drugs that have been reused with an entirely different primary target for a new indication. However, there may be one historical lesson worthy of consideration.

In the late 1940s and early 1950s, Rhône-Poulenc synthesized a series of antihistaminergic compounds, including the successfully marketed promethazine. These compounds had high affinity for, and were antagonists at, histamine receptors. However, effects of promethazine were also observed in the central nervous system [45].

Chlorpromazine, a derivative of promethazine, was found to have a wide range of pharmacological actions, including cardiovascular effects, antiemetic action, and antagonism of alpha adrenoceptors [46]. However, it had a lower potency than promethazine as an antihistamine and so was perhaps of little interest to Rhône-Poulenc.

Smith, Kline and French subsequently negotiated an agreement with Rhône-Poulenc to study the efficacy of chlorpromazine as an antiemetic but found that although it prevented apomorphine-induced vomiting in the dog, side effects included sedation and hypotension, and so chlorpromazine was dismissed as unsuitable as an antiemetic [47].

The value of chlorpromazine began to be realized when it was used in a "lytic cocktail" to enhance surgical anesthesia [48, 49] and later suggested that chlorpromazine alone be used in psychiatry [50]. Subsequently, the successful use of chlorpromazine in the treatment of psychiatric patients was described [51, 52], marking the beginning of the era of antipsychotic drugs.

Chlorpromazine is an example of a compound for which (by modern standards) a limited pharmacological profile was developed. Clearly, the compound was of little use as an antihistamine due to low affinity, while undesired side effects limited its use as an antiemetic. However, in retrospect, it is easy to see that a high affinity for dopamine D_2 receptors may explain its undesirable side effects as an antihistamine or antiemetic and its subsequent use as an antipsychotic [53]. In the modern era with the ability to develop rapidly detailed profiles for compounds at the molecular level, pharmacological profiling may have a key role to play in drug repurposing by identifying new targets for which old compounds have high affinity.

17.6 CONCLUSION

The study of secondary pharmacodynamics for candidate drugs is now essential, as embodied in the International Committee for Harmonisation guidelines for drug development (ICH S7A [1]). Both *in vivo* and *in vitro* approaches to secondary pharmacodynamic studies have been discussed, but it is clear that, at the present time, *in vitro* pharmacological profiling is becoming the method of choice for many of the large pharmaceutical companies. The ability to interpret such profile data is rapidly being enhanced with the advent of databases containing pharmacological profiles linked to *in vivo* observations and adverse drug reactions.

In the short term, the application of *in vitro* pharmacological profiling to both secondary pharmacodynamics and to other areas in the pharmaceutical industry is likely to expand. The ability to interpret *in vitro* data to predict *in vivo* effects is likely to increase and be refined. In the medium term, it is likely that the generation of very large datasets linking chemical structures to *in vitro* profiles will enable *in silico* prediction of a chemical's likely profile, and thus its potential physiological effects, without ever having to synthesize or to test the compound.

REFERENCES

1. Anon. ICH S7A: *Note for Guidance on Safety Pharmacology Studies for Human Pharmaceuticals*. CPMP/ICH/539/00. 2000.
2. Anon. *Guidelines for General Pharmacology Studies—Japanese Guidelines for Nonclinical Studies of Drugs Manual*. Tokyo, Japan: Nippo Yakuji; 1995, pp 71–80, pp 125–129.
3. Kinter LB, Valentin JP. Safety pharmacology and risk assessment. *Fundam Clin Pharmacol* 2002;16:175–182.
4. Redfern WS, Wakefield ID, Prior H, Hammond TG, Valentin JP. Safety pharmacology—a progressive approach. *Fundam Clin Pharmacol* 2002; 16:161–173.
5. Bass AS, Kinter LB, Williams P. Origins, practices and future of safety pharmacology. *J Pharmacol Toxicol Methods* 2004;49:145–151.
6. Kinter LB, Gossett KA, Kerns WD. Status of safety pharmacology in the pharmaceutical industry—1993. *Drug Dev Res* 1994;32:208–216.
7. Bass AS, Williams PD. Status of international regulatory guidelines on safety pharmacology. In Williams PD, Bass AS, Eds. *Safety Pharmacology A Practical Guide*. TherImmune Research Corporation, USA; 2003, pp 9–20.
8. Anon. ICH M3: *Timing of Non-clinical Safety Studies for the Conduct of Human Clinical Trials for Pharmaceuticals*. CPMP/ICH/286/95. 1997.
9. Anon. ICH S6: *Preclinical Safety Evaluation of Biotechnology-Derived Pharmaceuticals*. CPMP/ICH/302/95. 1997.
10. Anon. *The GLP Pocket Book: The Good Laboratory Practice Regulations 1999 and Guide to UK GLP Regulations*. London: MCA Publications; 1999, pp 1–75.
11. Anon. ICH S7B: *The Non-clinical Evaluation of the Potential for Delayed Ventricular Repolarization (QT Interval Prolongation) by Human Pharmaceuticals*. CPMP/ICH/423/02. 2005.
12. Anon. Committee for Proprietary Medicinal Products. *Points to Consider: The Assessment of QT Interval Prolongation by Non-cardiovascular Medicinal Products*. CPMP/986/96. 1997.

13. Anon. *Draft Guideline on the Non-clinical Investigation of the Dependence Potential of Medicinal Products*. EMEA/CHMP/SWP/94227/2004. 2005.

14. Anon. ICH M4: *Organization of the Common Technical Document for the Registration of Pharmaceuticals for Human Use*. CPMP/ICH/2887/99 rev.2. 1999.

15. DiMasi JA, Hansen RW, Grabowski HG. The price of innovation: new estimates of drug development costs. *J Health Econ* 2003;22:151.

16. Kola I, Rafferty M. Oral communication: new technologies that may impact drug discovery in the 5–10 year time frame workshop. Presented at Biomed Expo, Ann Arbor, Michigan, USA, 2002. Data derived from Prous Science, Drug News Prospect.

17. Shastry BS. Pharmacogenetics and the concept of individualized medicine. *Pharmacogenetics J* 2006;6:16–21.

18. Mangoni AA. Cardiovascular drug therapy in elderly patients: specific age-related pharmacokinetic, pharmacodynamic, and therapeutic considerations. *Drugs Aging* 2005; 22:913–941.

19. Feldman DS, Carnes CA, Abraham WT, Bristow MR. Mechanisms of disease: β-adrenergic receptors—alterations in signal transduction and pharmacogenomics in heart failure. *Nat Clin Practice Cardiovasc Med* 2005;2:475–483.

20. Kola I, Landis J. Can the pharmaceutical industry reduce attrition rates? *Nat Rev Drug Discov* 2004;3:711.

21. Bridgland-Taylor MH, Hargreaves AC, Easter A, Orme A, Henthorn DC, Ding M, Davis AM, Small BG, Heapy CG, Abi-Gerges N, Persson F, Jacobson I, Sullivan M, Albertson N, Hammond TG, Sullivan E, Valentin JP, Pollard CE. Optimisation and validation of a medium-throughput electrophysiology-based hERG assay using IonWorks HT. *J Pharmacol Toxicol Methods* 2006;54:189–199.

22. Fliri AF, Loging WT, Thadeio PF, Volkmann RA. Biological spectra analysis: linking biological activity profiles to molecular structure. *Proc Nat Acad Sci USA* 2005; 102:261–266.

23. Fliri AF, Loging WT, Thadeio PF, Volkmann RA. Analysis of drug-induced effect patterns to link structure and side effects of medicines. *Nat Chem Biol* 2005;1:389–391.

24. Maemoto T, Finlayson K, Olverman HJ, Akahane A, Horton RW, Butcher SP. Species differences in brain adenosine A1 receptor pharmacology revealed by use of xanthine and pyrazolopyridine based antagonists. *Br J Pharmacol* 1997;122:1202–1208.

25. Whitebread S, Hamon J, Bojanic D, Urban L. Keynote review: *in vitro* safety pharmacology profiling: an essential tool for successful drug development. *Drug Discov Today* 2005;10:1421–1433.

26. Krejsa CM, Horvath D, Rogalski SL, Penzotti JE, Mao B, Barbosa F, Migeon JC. Predicting ADME properties and side effects: the BioPrint approach. *Curr Opin Drug Discov Dev* 2003;6:470–480.

27. Law M, Rudnicka AR. Statin safety: a systematic review. *Am J Cardiol* 2006;17: S52–S60.

28. Zhou S, Yung Chan S, Cher Goh B, Chan E, Duan W, Huang M, McLeod HL. Mechanism-based inhibition of cytochrome P-450 3A4 by therapeutic drugs. *Clin Pharmacokinet* 2005;44:279–304.

29. Siddiqui MAA, Keam SJ. Ranolazine: a review of its use in chronic stable angina pectoris. *Drugs* 2006;66:693–710.

30. Antzelevitch C. Arrhythmogenic mechanisms of QT prolonging drugs: is QT prolongation really the problem? *J Electrocardiol* 2004;37(Suppl):15–24.

31. Belardinelli L, Antzelevitch C, Vos MA. Assessing predictors of drug-induced torsades de pointes. *Trends Pharmacol Sci* 2003;24:619–625.

32. Antzelevitch C, Belardinelli L, Zygmunt AC, Burashnikov A, Di Diego JM, Fish JM, Cordeiro JM, Thomas G. Electrophysiological effects of ranolazine, a novel anti-anginal agent with anti-arrhythmic properties. *Circulation* 2004;110:904–910.

33. Antzelevitch C, Belardinelli L, Wu L, Fraser H, Zygmut AC, Burashnikov A, Diego JM, Fish JM, Cordeiro JM, Goodrow RJ Jr , Scornik F, Perez G. Electrophysiologic properties and anti-arrhythmic actions of a novel anti-anginal agent. *J Cardiovasc Pharmacol Ther* 2004;9(Suppl 1):S65–S83.

34. Schram G, Zhang L, Derakhchan K, Ehrlich JR, Belardinelli L, Nattel S. Ranolazine: ion-channel blocking actions and in vivo electrophysiological effects. *Br J Pharmacol* 2004;142:1300–1308.

35. Song Y, Skrycok JC, Wu L, Belardinelli L. Antagonism by ranolazine of the pre-arrhythmic effects of increasing late I_{Na} in guinea-pig ventricular myocytes. *J Cardiovasc Pharmacol* 2004;44:192–199.

36. Jackson PC. Innervation of the iris by individual parasympathetic axons in the adult mouse. *J Physiol* 1986;378:485–495.

37. Gupta N, Drance SM, McAllister R, Prasad S, Rootman J, Cynader MS. Localization of M_3 muscarinic receptor subtype and mRNA in the human eye. *Ophthalmic Res* 1994;26:207–123.

38. Lin S, Kajimura M, Takeuchi K, Kodaira M, Hanai H, Kaneko E. Expression of muscarinic receptor subtypes (effect of M3 selective antagonist on gastric motility and in rat gastric smooth muscle emptying). *Dig Dis Sci* 1997;42:907–914.

39. Ross WA. Premedication for upper gastrointestinal endoscopy. *Gastrointest Endosc* 1989;32:120–126.

40. Zinner N, Susset J, Gittelman M, Arguinzoniz M, Rekeda L, Haab F. Efficacy, tolerability and safety of darifenacin, an M3 selective receptor antagonist: an investigation of warning time in patients with OAB. *Int J Clin Practice* 2006;60:119–126.

41. Carley DW. Drug repurposing: identify, develop and commercialize new uses for existing or abandoned drugs. Part I. *IDrugs* 2005;8:306–309.

42. Carley DW. Drug repurposing: identify, develop and commercialize new uses for existing or abandoned drugs. Part II. *IDrugs* 2005;8:310–313.

43. Bradley D. Why big pharma needs to learn the three "R"s. *Nat Rev Drug Discov* 2005;4:446.

44. Ashburn TT, Thor KB. Drug repositioning: identifying and developing new uses for existing drugs. *Nat Rev Drug Discov* 2004;3:673–683.

45. Winter C, Flataker L. The effect of anti-histaminic drugs on the performance of trained rats. *J Pharmacol Exp Ther* 1951;101:156–162.

46. Courvoisier S. Pharmacodynamic basis for the use of chlorpromazine in psychiatry. *J Clin Exp Psychopathol* 1956;17:25–37.

47. Domino EF. History of modern psychopharmacology: a personal view with an emphasis on anti-depressants. *Psychosom Med* 1999;61:591–598.

48. Laborit H, Huguenard P. L'hibernation artificielle par MoyEnes pharmacodynamiques et physiques En chirurgie. *J Chir* 1951;67:631–641.

49. Laborit H, Huguenard P. L'hibernation artificielle par moyenes pharmacodynamiques et physiques. *La Presse Med* 1951;59:13–29.

50. Laborit H, Huguenard P, Alluaume R. Un nouveau stabilisateur vegetatif (le 4560 RP). *La Presse Med* 1952;60:206–208.

51. Delay J, Deniker P. Le traitement des psychoses par une methode neurolytque derive de l'hibernotherapie (Le 4560 R.P. utilise seul. En cure prolongee et continue.) *CR Congress Med Alien Neruol France* 1952;50:497–502.

52. Deniker P. Introduction of neuroleptic chemotherapy into psychiatry. In Ayd FJ, Blackwell B, Eds. *Discoveries in Biological Psychiatry*. Philadelphia: Lippincott; 1970, pp 155–164.

53. Carlsson A, Lindquist M. Effect of chlorpromazine or haloperidol on the formation of 3-methoxytyramine and normetanephrine in mouse brain. *Acta Pharmacol Toxicol* 1963;20:140–144.

18

CURRENT PRACTICES IN SAFETY PHARMACOLOGY

ALAN S. BASS,[1] PETER K. S. SIEGL,[2] GARY A. GINTANT,[3] DENNIS J. MURPHY,[4] AND ROGER D. PORSOLT[5]

[1]Schering-Plough Research Institute, Kenilworth, New Jersey
[2]Merck Research Laboratories, West Point, Pennsylvania
[3]Abbott Laboratories, Abbott Park, Illinois
[4]GlaxoSmithKline Pharmaceuticals, King of Prussia, Pennsylvania
[5]Porsolt & Partners Pharmacology, Boulogne-Billancourt, France

Contents

Preclinical Development Handbook: Toxicology, edited by Shayne Cox Gad
Copyright © 2008 John Wiley & Sons, Inc.

18.1   INTRODUCTION

In the latter half of the 1960s and through the 1970s, it was recognized that contemporary approaches to toxicity testing of new pharmaceuticals were insensitive to detection of many of the severe pharmacodynamic properties, which unfortunately were ultimately realized following clinical exposure to the promising new drug. Professor Gerhard Zbinden, arguably the father of the field of safety pharmacology, said: "The adverse drug reactions which the standard toxicological test procedures do not aspire to recognize include most of the functional side-effects. Clinical experience indicates, however, that these are much more frequent than the toxic reactions due to morphological and biochemical lesions" [1]. Up to the early 1980s, pharmacodynamic testing was conducted ad hoc on selected organ systems taking into consideration the known pharmacology of the therapeutic class or concerns related to the chemical structure [2]. At that time, study protocols were not well defined and the selection of which organ systems would be evaluated did not follow a systematic approach. By the early to late 1980s, safety pharmacology programs began to appear in the pharmaceutical industry [2]. However, it was during the 1990s that the industry saw the greatest growth of these programs, with most institutions turning to the Japanese *Guidelines for General Pharmacology Studies* [3, 4] as guidance for the selection of which organ systems to evaluate and protocols to follow. By the latter part of the 1990s, regulatory bodies from around the world began to recognize the need for specific guidelines for the pharmacodynamic study of the safety of new chemical entities. This led to the preparation of draft guidelines in the

United States, Europe, and Japan [2]. Part of the drive to prepare guidelines by the regulatory bodies was the recognition of adverse events emerging during the postmarketing surveillance period with several new pharmaceuticals [5, 6]. These adverse events had not been identified during the development of these molecules based on contemporary methods of safety testing. Combining the general principles of each of these regional recommendations into a common document, a draft guideline was generated under the auspices of the International Conference on Harmonization (ICH) following the adoption of an initiative on Safety Pharmacology (Topic S7) by the ICH Steering Committee in 1998 [2]. The Expert Working Group (EWG) of Topic S7, made up of members from the regulatory community and pharmaceutical industry worldwide, deliberated for three years over the content and wording of the guidance recommendations. The document finally achieved Step 4 and was adopted by EWG members in 2000 and implemented by regulatory authorities worldwide in the summer of 2001 [7]. The suffix "A" was added to Topic ICH 7 (ICH S7A) to allow for a new initiative, which during the three years was met with a great deal of discussion and debate, Topic S7B. ICH S7B addressed the preclinical study of drug effects on cardiac ventricular repolarization as a surrogate biomarker of torsades de pointes proarrhythmic risk. This important topic is considered in detail in a later section of this chapter, but suffice it to say that this effort by the EWG members was met with a great deal of controversy, disagreement, and compromise because of the lack of definitive data informing this area of study [8–10]. In spite of these challenges, the ICH S7B guidelines were developed and revised over a period of five years, achieving Step 4 in May 2005 and being implemented in the United States and Europe in the latter part of that year. As of this publication, ICH S7B has not been implemented in Japan. [11].

As a field of study, safety pharmacology is a relatively young discipline. In many ways this is an exciting time for safety pharmacologists given the prospects for a future filled with challenges and opportunities that are clearly illustrated by the great progress that has been made during the field's brief history. Safety pharmacology is described in the ICH S7A guidelines as "those studies that investigate potential undesirable pharmacodynamic effects [of new chemical entities or biologics] on physiological functions in relation to exposure in the therapeutic range and above." More broadly, the field of safety pharmacology allows for the study of new and marketed therapeutic agents with the objectives of identifying their pharmacodynamic properties and, through detailed analysis and investigation, understanding the human risk posed by exposure to the promising new drug. These nonclinical studies can stand alone and provide critical data demonstrating the pharmacodynamic safety of a potential therapeutic agent before it progresses into clinical development. Alternatively, the results of safety pharmacology studies may serve a complementary role: providing additional data from directed studies, offering important perspectives of findings from other nonclinical or clinical investigations. In some cases, these nonclinical investigations may be immediately critical to understanding an observation of specific concern. Safety pharmacology studies may also provide data to validate a clinical strategy, which involves an intervention that may mitigate the risk to humans exposed to a new therapy (e.g., effectiveness of anticonvulsant therapy when there is a concern of seizurogenic properties). Although many examples will be cited in this chapter of the ways in which safety pharmacology serves to support the discovery and development of a new pharmaceutical agent, by no means can we be inclusive of all situations with which the reader will be faced. In fact, newly identified human health-related issues, discovery of drugs that are uniquely directed at target sites for which the safety database may be limited or completely unknown, introduction of new technologies that expand the opportunities to explore the biology and pharmacology of promising pharmaceuticals, and enhancements to technologies that improve the degree of sensitivity and specificity with which we can relate the nonclinical pharmacodynamic findings to the human response, in many ways describe the opportunities that are afforded safety pharmacology to align the growth of this emerging field with these advancements in science.

Given the broad scope of safety pharmacology to identify and further understand the potential pharmacodynamic safety or risk posed by a promising new molecule, the design of *in vitro* or *in vivo* studies may evolve from an unlimited number of decisions (e.g., species, gender, formulation, route) [7]. The ICH S7A guidelines describe three types of studies: the *core battery studies*, which include the cardiovascular, respiratory, and central nervous systems; *supplemental studies*, which include the other major organ systems (e.g., gastrointestinal, renal, immune); and *follow-up studies* of the core battery systems, which are more detailed and investigational and directed toward further defining an observation made in the core battery study or another study of a chemical agent. The focus of this chapter is on the safety pharmacology core battery systems, since these organ systems are highlighted in the ICH S7A as essential to sustaining life [7]. That is, an abrupt interruption of function of any of these organ systems may have a profound, acute, and potentially disastrous outcome, which may under extreme conditions include death. This principle articulated in the ICH S7A guidelines is not meant to diminish the importance of studying other major organ systems. The reader is referred to Refs. 12–16, which describe the study of those systems encompassed in the conduct of supplemental studies.

In the discourse of each of the presentations in this chapter, we provide guidance for many of the choices and decisions that will be made in devising an appropriate and rational study design. We focus on such issues as which models are available for studying a particular organ system, those factors that are taken into consideration in developing a study rationale, and our own personal perspective of how data from these investigations may be viewed in developing an integrated assessment of human risk. These are by no means the only approaches to the study of new pharmaceutical compounds [17–21]. In fact, several approaches to the study of each organ system presented by the different authors. That way, the reader is introduced to a diversity of approaches for considering those factors that are important in developing a rational study design. Although this chapter provides a comprehensive overview of the current technologies and approaches of investigating pharmacodynamic activity of potentially novel new drugs, as suggested earlier, the scientific fields that intersect with safety pharmacology are continuously evolving. In many ways, these advancements may complement the "established" practices of this field, but in some cases these advancements may supplant the common approaches utilized by safety pharmacologists [22]. Based on this vision of the future of safety pharmacology, the reader is encouraged to continuously view the information provided in this chapter in context with the advancements emerging from those interconnecting scientific fields.

18.2 REGULATORY GUIDELINES GOVERNING SAFETY PHARMACOLOGY

18.2.1 Introduction

Safety pharmacology studies were first referenced in the International Conference guidelines: *Safety Evaluation of Biotechnology-Derived Pharmaceuticals* and *Nonclinical Safety Studies for the Conduct of Human Clinical Trials for Pharmaceuticals* [23, 24]. In these guidelines, three categories of pharmacology studies are described for regulatory applications: primary pharmacodynamic studies, secondary pharmacodynamic studies, and safety pharmacology studies. Secondary pharmacodynamic studies (also referred to as general pharmacology studies) are described in the *Guideline for General Pharmacology* issued by the Japanese Ministry of Health and Welfare (MHW; currently referred to as the PMDA) in 1991 [3, 4]. Until 2000 there were no recognized guidelines for safety pharmacology studies.

Nonclinical toxicology studies performed to support safe conduct of clinical trials with drug candidates and registration of new drugs have traditionally used endpoints of mortality, physical signs, histopathology, and hematology/clinical chemistry. The addition of pharmacological endpoints to assess direct effects of drug candidates on major organ function (cardiovascular, respiratory, and central nervous system) complements the traditional toxicology package and provides more complete information for predicting human risk. ICH guidelines S7A and S7B were developed to provide specific information for conducting safety pharmacology studies. Compared to the earlier Japanese guidelines, the ICH safety pharmacology studies are more focused on whole organ system function and *in vivo* assays, with a prerequisite of identifying the safety or risk posed by exposure of subjects or patients to a drug candidate. Now that the ICH S7A and S7B guidelines have been adopted by all regions [7, 11], it has been assumed by some that the ICH guidelines will supersede the requirement for the PMDA general pharmacology studies for drug registration in Japan. However, data from both safety pharmacology and PMDA general pharmacology (secondary pharmacodynamic) studies to support new drug registration in Japan should be considered on a case-by-case basis and may be requested by Japanese regulatory reviewers.

Guidelines for human pharmaceuticals are created to provide both sponsors and regulators with a common reference to facilitate drug development and approval. While guidelines are not rules or absolute requirements, effective guidelines reflect current best practices and recommend approaches that regulatory agencies consider acceptable for addressing concerns about the safety of drug candidates. In developing guidelines in the ICH process, there is participation by representatives from both regulatory agencies and the pharmaceutical industry. The regulatory point of view is valuable because regulators have the opportunity to see many different types of drug applications, while the pharmaceutical industry point of view is important because sponsors provide the practical and business (resources) points of view. The Expert Working Group members from both regulatory agencies and industry provide scientific expertise. Representation from the three major regions (United States, Europe, and Japan) enables a global perspective and should result in a guideline that helps sponsors to build a new drug application package that is acceptable in all three regions. Despite efforts to harmonize the guidelines and ensure consistency in wording throughout the document, there can be regional differences in the application of the guidelines due to variations in how the regulators choose to interpret the specific text.

The two safety pharmacology ICH guidelines, S7A and S7B, share the following common objectives: (1) to provide general principles, definitions, and recommendations; (2) to minimize use of animals and resources; and (3) to provide information that is a framework which facilitates the use of scientifically valid and internationally accepted approaches for drug development. ICH S7A was created to define the safety pharmacology studies referenced in the earlier ICH guidelines and to provide specific recommendations for the series of studies that constitute a core evaluation in safety pharmacology. Adoption of ICH S7B followed that of ICH S7A with the objective to define an approach that specifically addresses the risk of a delay in cardiac ventricular repolarization (QT interval prolongation) by drug candidates. The two guidelines should be considered together since the basic principles of ICH S7A apply to ICH S7B.

18.2.2   Regulatory Strategy for Safety Pharmacology

Members of the pharmaceutical industry and regulatory community share a common goal of making safe and effective new drugs available to patients. Therefore, bringing both groups together to develop ICH guidelines is appropriate. In addition to optimizing the safety of drug candidates, industry would like to minimize failures of these promising drugs, particularly those that advance to late stage clinical development, increasing the probability that there will be an acceptable return on resource investments. Regulators look to balance clinical safety with approval of drugs that provide true benefit to patients. It is valuable for those working in the pharmaceutical industry to consider the regulator's point of view and understand that both parties share this important responsibility to patients. Providing sound rationale for the choice of assays and an integrated summary of data as it relates to human safety is very helpful for the regulators. When there are questions or concern about a strategy or data package that varies from the approach recommended in the ICH guidelines, the sponsor should engage in discussions with regulatory agencies as early as possible. The most effective strategy takes into account the concerns and needs of the regulators, engages in discussions with regulators in advance when necessary, and ensures that issues are addressed clearly and with appropriate scientific rigor.

Since safety pharmacology data contribute to the overall benefit to risk assessment of drugs, the value of these data is enhanced by inclusion of comparative data with drugs from the same class or mechanism. Results with positive controls and reference agents are very useful in supporting the data with a new drug candidate because it allows the regulators to evaluate the sensitivity of the assays and comparative pharmacodynamic profile. This is particularly important when there are no adverse effects observed with the new drug candidate since using positive controls will demonstrate the sensitivity of the assay to detect a significant pharmacodynamic change had one been detected with the new drug. As allowed within the ICH S7A guidelines, the sensitivity to a positive control can be determined at the point of establishing the *in vivo* model system or with each study of a new molecular entity when an *in vitro* model is chosen.

18.2.3 Recommended Core Safety Pharmacology Studies

In both ICH S7A and ICH S7B, there are recommended studies. In ICH S7A, assays assessing cardiovascular, respiratory, and central nervous system (CNS) effects are referred to as *core battery studies*. Although this term is not used in S7B, the *in vitro* I_{Kr} *assay* and the *in vivo QT assay* are considered equivalent to core battery assays. In most cases, these are the minimum studies that the regulators will expect to see in regulatory dossiers. There may be cases where the safety of the test substance in one or more of the organ systems is assessed with pharmacology studies used during early development (i.e., during selectivity profiling in primary or secondary pharmacodynamic studies). In most cases, these studies are not performed according to GLP. According to ICH S7A, these studies will not need to be repeated for the safety pharmacology package; however, the scientific strength of the data and conclusions from the non-GLP studies should be clearly documented (see Section 18.2.4). There may be cases where one or more of the core battery assays are not practical because unwanted effects of the test substance make interpretation of the results of the studies of very limited value. Examples mentioned in the guideline include test substances that cause tremors, changes in behavior, and cardiovascular parameters. The absence of core battery studies of a specific organ system may be acceptable if their noninclusion is clearly explained and justified.

18.2.4 Follow-Up or Supplemental Safety Pharmacology Studies

Follow-up studies are intended "to provide greater depth of understanding than, or additional knowledge to, that provided by the core battery" (ICH S7A Section 2.8.1 and ICH S7B Section 2.3.5), while supplemental studies are intended "to evaluate potential adverse pharmacodynamic effects on organ systems functions not addressed by the core battery" (ICH S7A Section 2.8.2). It is the responsibility of the sponsor to determine if follow-up or supplemental studies will provide useful information when considering results from evaluation of the test substance in core battery studies, primary or secondary pharmacodynamic studies, and clinical studies in subjects or the targeted patient population. While these studies are not required unless there is serious concern regarding the safety of the subject or patient, they provide an opportunity for the sponsor to obtain additional information that will support conclusions and strategic decisions concerning both safety and further development of the test substance. This additional information can also enable regulators to make more informed decisions regarding continuation of a clinical program.

18.2.5 Conditions Under Which Safety Pharmacology Studies Are Unnecessary

In ICH S7A, it is acknowledged that there are conditions where safety pharmacology studies "may not be needed" (ICH S7A Section 2.9). This applies to both ICH S7A and ICH S7B studies. Examples cited include locally applied agents, where there is no or very low systemic exposures, cytotoxic agents for treatment in end-stage cancer patients, and biotechnology-derived products that achieve highly specific receptor targeting. There could be other conditions not listed in the guideline where safety pharmacology studies are not needed. The key text here is "may not be needed," indicating that the absence of data from safety pharmacology studies in the regulatory dossier should be acknowledged and scientifically justified. In other words, the guideline provides flexibility to not do safety pharmacology studies if the results will be of limited value. For example, if a sponsor is developing a new cytotoxic drug for cancer, it is not appropriate to omit these data without a comment. In such a case, the sponsor should document the lack of safety pharmacology data and provide justification of how the data will not contribute to the safety profile of the test substance. In cases where discrete safety pharmacology studies are not performed, every effort should be made to include safety pharmacology parameters in the multiple dose toxicology studies.

When there are questions about the need for one or more safety pharmacology studies, discussions with the regulatory agencies will provide clarification. It is important to note that negotiating the need for, or justifying the omission of, studies with a regulatory agency in one region may not apply to all regions since there could be regional differences in the perceived need for a particular study.

18.2.6 Application of Good Laboratory Practice (GLP)

ICH S7A Section 2.11 discusses the application of GLP when performing safety pharmacology studies. The specific requirements to satisfy GLP are available from regulatory agencies in each region and have generally been harmonized [2]. Performing studies according to GLP is a requirement for nonclinical toxicity studies that support clinical trials in most regions [25]. The ICH S7A guideline recommends that the core battery safety pharmacology studies be performed in compliance with GLP and "any study or study component not conducted in compliance should be adequately justified and the potential impact on evaluation of the safety pharmacology endpoints should be explained." The purpose of GLP is to recommend procedures that will help to ensure quality and reliability of data. Components of GLP include (1) accountability (Study Director and Quality Assurance); (2) documentation with standard operating procedures (SOPs), protocols, and deviations; (3) data archiving procedures to enable accurate reconstruction of the study; and (4) independent validation of data and procedures by a Quality Assurance group. It should be pointed out that satisfying GLP requirements does not by itself guarantee scientific quality and validity. It is important for sponsors to employ scientifically robust approaches including data from positive control substances to assure assay validation and facilitate the interpretation of results. Keep in mind that the purpose of safety pharmacology studies is to generate data with conclusions that can be supported in a regulatory environment. One should follow GLP to the greatest extent possible but also be practical in the use of animals and resources. For example, there may be cases where safety pharmacology studies are performed before GMP or GLP drug substance is available. In this case, one can provide documentation according to GLP and if the study file is scientifically defendable, the assay need not be repeated merely to satisfy all GLP requirements for the drug substance. As indicated earlier, the burden of proof that the data support the conclusions is on the sponsor and one should not expect the regulatory agencies to accept the scientific interpretation of the data at face value (even if performed according to GLP). There may be some regional differences in the interpretation of need for complete compliance with GLP, and when this is the case, it might be prudent to defer replicating the studies until just prior to approval. This will minimize the use of experimental animals and resources in cases when the drug candidate is dropped from development.

In ICH S7B, there is specific reference to application of GLP for the recommended *in vitro* I_{Kr} and *in vivo* QT assays (Section 1.4), indicating that "when performed for regulatory submission, [these assays] should be conducted in compliance with GLP." This has led to confusion since one generally assumes that all safety pharmacology studies are performed for regulatory submission. The wording in ICH S7B was crafted to accommodate one region that has challenged the value of data from nonclinical studies for predicting risk of QT interval prolongation in humans. Regulators in this region prefer to rely predominantly on clinical data for this risk assessment (see ICH E14 guideline) [26] and, at present, are reluctant to consider nonclinical data to obviate the need for a thorough clinical QT/QTc study. If a sponsor chooses to rely solely on clinical data for assessment of QT safety, then the nonclinical studies do not need to conform with GLP. This approach may be complicated by regional differences in the need for data prior to initiation of clinical studies (see Section 18.2.8) and therefore availability of clinical data to justify not performing safety pharmacology studies in accordance with GLP. In practice, the sponsor should perform these assays to a sufficiently high scientific standard that they can support the clinical safety of the drug candidate. This includes documentation, computer validation [27], and archiving of data in a manner that satisfies GLP requirements. This regional difference in GLP recommendation reflects the complexity and controversy surrounding different opinions on the value of nonclinical assays to detect risk of delayed repolarization in humans. To help address this, the ICH S7B guideline recommends using an integrated risk assessment (IRA) that considers all relevant data (nonclinical and clinical) to support conclusions for predicting risk in humans. In other words, this approach allows for revision and refinement of the IRA as new data emerge to provide a different perspective of nonclinical or clinical results.

In Section 2.11 of ICH S7A, it is recommended that follow-up and supplemental studies "should be conducted in compliance with GLP to the greatest extent feasible." There is an assumption that each of these studies will be designed to address specific issues, and therefore full documentation via all aspects of GLP and 21CFRPart 11, as noted earlier, may not be practical. The guideline provides flexibility to further characterize drug candidates; however, the general principle of conducting and documenting studies in a scientifically defendable manner is expected. As mentioned earlier, the burden of proof that the data are adequately documented and strong enough to support conclusions is on the sponsor. Scientific quality and integrity are paramount.

18.2.7 Dose Levels or Concentrations of Test Substance

Recommended dose levels for *in vivo* studies and concentrations for *in vitro* studies are discussed in ICH S7A (Section 2.4) and apply to assays described in ICH S7B. The guidelines recommend defining a dose–response relationship for the adverse effects by using doses/concentrations in the therapeutic range and above. In the absence of a pharmacodynamic response on the organ system of interest, it is recommended that doses/concentrations be increased to a level that produces a moderately adverse effect or to use the maximum feasible doses. The guidelines allow exclusion of a maximum dose, where the pharmacodynamic/toxic properties may confound measurement or interpretation of safety pharmacology data (e.g., tremors interfering with interpretation of the electrocardiogram). There may be regional differences in acceptability of safety margins (ratio of exposure at a no-observed-adverse-effect level and the projected exposure at a therapeutic dose) when the maximum tolerated or maximum feasible dose is not used. In general, exploration of as large a dose level/concentration as feasible is a sound approach to a risk assessment. From a regulatory standpoint, it is preferable to identify pharmacodynamic toxicity at a defined, large margin over anticipated clinical exposure than to show no toxicity at a small multiple of exposure at a clinical dose.

18.2.8   Timing of Safety Pharmacology Studies in Relation to Clinical Development

Consistent with the stated objective of the ICH S7A guideline, "to help protect clinical trial participants and patients," the value of safety pharmacology data is greatest when it is obtained prior to first administration to humans. In ICH S7A (Section 2.10.1), it is recommended that the core assays and follow-up or supplemental studies to address specific safety issues be conducted prior to first administration to humans. When clinical studies with adequate data to address the safety of the test substance on the organ systems of interest are available, one can consider whether the nonclinical safety pharmacology studies are necessary (Section 2.10.3). There can be regional differences in the value of nonclinical data even when clinical data are available. Therefore, in cases where the sponsor chooses to propose that safety pharmacology studies are not necessary, a discussion with representatives from the regulatory agency in advance is prudent to avoid potential delays in review of the regulatory package.

Concerning the timing of ICH S7B nonclinical studies (Section 2.4), the wording is more flexible than in ICH S7A. In ICH S7A (Section 2.10.1), the recommendation is that the safety pharmacology core battery *should* be conducted prior to first administration to humans, while in ICH S7B it is stated that "conduct of S7B nonclinical studies . . . prior to first administration to humans *should be considered.*" As described in Section 18.2.6, this greater flexibility for timing of ICH S7B studies was included to accommodate the regional differences in regulatory positions on the value of nonclinical data in the risk assessment for ventricular repolarization or QT interval prolongation in humans and their value in precluding the need for a thorough clinical QT/QTc study. Regardless of these regional differences, the value of the nonclinical data is greatest when obtained prior to initiation of clinical studies because the results can be used to help in the design of clinical studies and interpretation of the results. It is also recognized that nonclinical data can provide an important perspective in situations where clinical findings suggest an issue of concern requiring resolution. Therefore, regional differences can be considered in the timing of ICH S7B nonclinical studies (in particular, the hERG assay since the *in vivo* cardiovascular study, including evaluation of QT/QTc interval, is required prior to first-in-human clinical trials in accordance with ICH S7A). However, also considered is the scientific value of having data early in development versus the commitment of animals and resources to obtaining these data.

18.2.9 Test Systems and Route of Administration

The experimental conditions and protocols should be selected to ensure that scientifically valid information is obtained. There is a preference for use of unanesthetized, unrestrained animal models and the clinical route of administration. While these conditions best replicate the clinical situation, one should consider test systems and routes of administration that can most effectively assess endpoints that reflect the safety of the test substance. For example, if the clinical route is oral but the exposure following oral dosing in the test system is poor, an intravenous infusion may yield more informative results. In some cases, conditioning and restraining animals may increase the sensitivity of the assay but may require greater resources. The guidelines provide recommendations but do allow flexibility so that sponsors can design experiments that most effectively assess the safety of test substances.

18.2.10 Duration of Studies

The recommended duration of safety pharmacology studies is generally a single-dose administration (ICH S7A Section 2.5). This approach will detect acute effects of the test substance on the organ system of interest. The rationale is that one will evaluate the direct actions of the test substance without confounding effects that are secondary to toxicities and histopathological changes that appear with repeated doses. Repeat-dose safety pharmacology studies should be considered when the data can more effectively address a specific concern that is associated with the pharmacological class, revealed in repeat-dose nonclinical studies and/or clinical studies. Good scientific judgment should guide the decision to include repeat-dose studies in the safety pharmacology package.

18.2.11 Integrated Risk Assessment

There is a well recognized, inherent uncertainty in quantitatively predicting responses to drugs in humans using nonclinical data and, as such, there is usually no single nonclinical assay or type of data that fully captures all dimensions of the clinical setting. In the ICH S7B guideline, it is recommended that the sponsor develop an integrated risk assessment for QT interval prolongation using all available data; that is, an assessment of the potential risk that a new pharmaceutical will prolong QT interval in the clinical trial subject or patient taking into account a composite analysis of all existing data (e.g., pharmacodynamic, pharmacokinetic/toxicokinetic, toxicology). This is similar to the integrated assessment of safety using toxicology data in applications for approval of new drugs. It is applicable to data from ICH S7A as well as ICH S7B studies. The integrated risk assessment is based on basic scientific principles, where results from the various nonclinical and clinical studies should complement each other and, when there are inconsistencies among the data, additional studies or information should be obtained. The integrated risk assessment is a dynamic tool and therefore should be updated as new data become available. In the ICH S7B guideline, it is suggested that the integrated risk assessment for QT interval prolongation be included in the Clinical Investigator Brochure and other regulatory documents concerning the safety of a drug candidate. The integrated risk assessment is a tool to help sponsors more effectively present all relevant data and communicate conclusions. Specifically, this will aid regulators to assess the safety of drug candidates with an integrated evaluation of available data.

18.2.12 Summary

The ICH S7A and S7B guidelines provide information and recommendations that assist both the pharmaceutical industry and regulators to bring safe and effective drugs to patients. The guidelines were designed to provide flexibility such that the assessments can best address the needs of the drug development candidate or disease as well as encourage sponsors to provide the types of data, with a level of scientific rigor, that will enable regulators to make effective decisions regarding the progression of promising new drug candidates.

18.3 *IN VIVO* CARDIOVASCULAR SAFETY PHARMACOLOGY

18.3.1 Introduction

The nonclinical study of cardiovascular function in safety pharmacology can employ both *in vitro* and *in vivo* models. *In vitro* models primarily serve to facilitate a greater understanding of potential mechanisms and sites of pharmacodynamic activity. Many institutions use *in vitro* models to prioritize predevelopment candidates during lead selection [17, 28, 29]. In contrast, *in vivo* models allow hypotheses and questions of the integrated pharmacodynamic properties, mechanisms of action, influence of indirect modulation (i.e., neuronal or hormonal), and the role of major metabolites (i.e., human metabolites) to be addressed. In addition, pharmacokinetic/ pharmacodynamic modeling and an indication of exposure multiples can be obtained from results of *in vivo* cardiovascular studies [30, 31]. The first level of a strategy for the comprehensive evaluation of the cardiovascular system includes an assessment of the major functional endpoints (i.e., heart rate, blood pressures (systolic, diastolic, and mean), and both intervals (RR, PR, QRS, and QT) and morphology of the electrocardiogram (including screening for the presence of cardiac arrhythmias)). Study in unanesthetized, unrestrained animals is a preferred methodology in the ICH guidelines and is feasible based on the availability of current radiotelemetry technologies [7, 32–35]. However, study of either restrained or anesthetized animals is also valuable under certain circumstances, as described later. Ideally, the information that is available at the time of designing the study is a complete and comprehensive package. Those factors considered may include an understanding of the physical properties of the active pharmaceutical ingredient (e.g., solubility, stability); the pharmacokinetics or toxicokinetics of the test agent in the animal species and at the doses considered for study; the metabolic profile of the test substance in various species, including human microsomes and identification of any potential major metabolites; the primary pharmacology of the test agent, including pharmacodynamic–pharmacokinetic modeling based on nonclinical data; and information regarding overt tolerance to the test agent at the doses being considered and the target organs identified in multiple-dose toxicology studies. However, as eluded to earlier in this chapter, safety pharmacology studies may be conducted at any stage of discovery (e.g., lead optimization) through the early to late clinical development phases and into the postmarketing period; as such, the amount of information available to make decisions on study design may be more limited or complete than those that have just been described.

The assays that apply to study of cardiovascular function *in vivo*, including assessment of drug effects on cardiac ventricular repolarization, are considered in this section. *In vitro* models applied to the study of drug effects on repolarization of the cardiac cycle will be deferred to next section of this chapter. As mentioned previously, the important concern of identifying drug effects on cardiac ventricular repolarization is the subject of the ICH S7B guidelines [11]. QT interval prolongation, which is a biomarker for delayed cardiac ventricular repolarization, serves as one of several risk factors for the potentially self-limiting or fatal cardiac arrhythmia, torsades de pointes [5, 8, 9]. Further consideration of this important topic will follow in this and the following section on *in vitro* cardiovascular safety pharmacology.

18.3.2 Consideration of Study Design

General Overview This section focuses on the principles and design options considered in developing a study of cardiovascular function using current methodologies and models. The reader is directed to Refs. 36–41 for a basic understanding of cardiovascular physiology and pharmacology.

At a basic first tier level, monitoring the key organ system parameters such as heart rate, arterial blood pressures (systolic, diastolic, mean) and electrocardiographic parameters (RR, PR, QRS, QT intervals) and morphology of the electrocardiogram, including surveying for the presence of arrhythmias, is essential for a general assessment of the cardiovascular properties of a promising new drug. In the absence of cardiovascular findings on these endpoints in the safety pharmacology and repeat-dose toxicity studies, there may not be a need for additional nonclinical investigation of cardiovascular risk. However, significant results from the core battery cardiovascular study or other nonclinical or clinical studies may prompt a more detailed assessment of cardiovascular function focusing on hemodynamic or electrophysiologic endpoints. At this advanced second tier level, there is a desire for greater understanding of the physiologic changes underlying these events. A more detailed evaluation may include measurements of systemic or regional blood flow (i.e., cardiac output that is the product of heart rate and stroke volume), systemic or regional vascular resistances (equivalent to systemic or regional blood pressure divided by systemic or regional flow, respectively), intracardiac dynamics (i.e., left or right atrial or ventricular pressures during systole or diastole, dynamic change in pressure (*dP/dt*, volume–pressure loops)), a temporal assessment of intracardiac and vascular changes employing echocardiography, or detailed evaluation of electrical conduction through the heart facilitated by SA- and AV-nodal recordings, His-bundle recordings, or measurement of monophasic action potentials and effective refractory period; the latter measures of electrophysiologic parameters enable a more detailed assessment concerning effects of a test substance on cardiac conduction and ventricular repolarization [38–47].

One important note to consider in incorporating many of these methodologies in the nonclinical investigation of a novel test agent is that the same technologies may also be adapted to clinical investigations. The relationship of nonclinical findings to the clinical population is an important principle that must be considered in assuring one's ability to assess potential for translation of the activity to humans. That is, critical decisions of progressing or terminating the development of a promising new drug are made based on nonclinical safety data, and so the ability to monitor the same endpoints in animals and humans and to relate these findings to an assessment of risk in humans is significantly important.

Consideration of study design is based on the available data describing the properties of the test agent being evaluated and an understanding of the target population in which this drug will be used. This information may provide some indication of whether to anticipate effects on the cardiovascular system (known pharmacologic class effects or effects related to the chemical structure) or whether modifications to the study design are in order based on the properties of the drug or the target population in which it will be used.

Selection of Gender   Consideration should be given to whether a drug will be used in a single gender or in both males and females. However, thought should also be given to whether significant exposure of the nontargeted gender is possible based on environmental exposure or the possibility of a new indication. In the case where both males and females, may be exposed to the test substance targeted for a single gender, study of that test agent in both males and females may be appropriate; although, in general, unique cardiovascular pharmacodynamic effects in males or females are not likely to occur.

On the other hand, the toxicology, pharmacokinetic/toxicokinetic, or pharmacodynamic properties of the drug may differ in males and females (i.e., higher exposure in males, greater tolerance in females) and these properties should also be taken into consideration when selecting the gender for study. If there are no preconditional factors that favor the study of one gender over the other, then the study of cardiovascular function in a single gender (males or females) should be acceptable.

Selection of Species   Species typically include mice, rats, guinea pigs, ferrets, rabbits, dogs, pigs, and nonhuman primates (i.e., cynomolgus monkeys). Selection of the species should be based on the objective of the investigation and assurance that the biology being studied in animal models can be translated to understanding the potential pharmacodynamic properties of a drug in humans. As a good example of biological differences between humans and animals, the ion channels associated with cardiac ventricular repolarization, in particular, the delayed rectifier channel, I_{Kr} [is encoded by the human-ether-a-go-go-related-gene (hERG)], are important contributors to repolarization in guinea pigs, rabbits , dogs, and monkeys, but not in mice or rats [9, 11]. Blockade of repolarizing current I_{Kr} is a prominent mechanism through which many drugs delay cardiac ventricular repolarization and cause QT interval prolongation. Therefore, evaluation of ventricular repolarization or ECGs in mice or rats will have limited value in identifying drugs with a potential to produce QT interval prolongation by this mechanism. In other words, if risk of QT interval prolongation by the test article is one of the primary objectives of the study, then the guinea pig, rabbit, dog, or nonhuman primate are more suitable species; taking into account other properties of the test agent that may allow further prioritization, such as the relationships of metabolism of the test agent to that of humans.

Given the objectives of the core battery cardiovascular study, the dog and nonhuman primate are most often employed as the test species. Some investigators advocate the use of mini-pigs in these studies; however, broad utilization of this species awaits further validation. One benefit of selecting either dogs or nonhuman primates is that they are an acceptable species and widely used in repeat-dose toxicology studies. In that case, data from the toxicology study (i.e., toxicokinetics, tolerance, generation of major metabolites) may complement the design and interpretation of results for the cardiovascular study. Furthermore, collective results of the preclinical studies may help position an integrated assessment of human risk.

Study Conditions: Unrestrained or Chemical or Physical Restraint   In most situations with few exceptions, study of a drug in unanesthetized, unrestrained animals is preferred since this allows the investigator to follow the clinical route of administration and eliminates the potential influence of the anesthetic agent or restraint procedure on the pharmacology and pharmacokinetic properties (absorption, distribution, metabolism, and excretion) of the drug. Study in unanesthetized, unrestrained animals is practical today as a result of contemporary technologies that allow collection of cardiovascular parameters through radiotelemetry [7, 32–35]. Based on this technology, continuous monitoring of cardiovascular endpoints for hours, days, and weeks is possible with the only limitation being the duration of the battery life and the stability of the model (e.g., drifting of the blood pressure signal from baseline, occlusion of the blood pressure catheter, loss of a quality electrocardiographic signal, physical condition of the animal). However, for most core battery cardiovascular studies of a relatively short duration, the limitation posed by the battery life should not be a significant impediment.

One of the drawbacks to studying unanesthetized, unrestrained animals is the confounding influences if the drug has pronounced pharmacodynamic effects (e.g., central nervous system pharmacology) and is not well tolerated at the high doses intended for study. Other factors that may potentially confound interpretation of data include those associated with the study environment (i.e., noise and activity in the animal facility). As an example, a drug that stimulates locomotor behavior may produce an increase in heart rate secondary to the increase in activity; affect the quality of the electrocardiogram (e.g., increased presence of electrocardiogram-signal artifact); and lead to sporadic alterations in blood pressure. This animal's behavior may also influence the level of activity and associated cardiovascular parameters of its study mates. These confounding changes in the cardiovascular parameters may not be easily distinguished from the pharmacodynamic activity of the drug. Thus, careful consideration of the known properties of the test agent should be made in selecting the appropriate condition for the study; including consideration of physical restraint or potential use of anesthesia.

The use of anesthetized animals may be an appropriate decision in cases where the drug is known to have profound pharmacodynamic behavioral effects that may potentially interfere with the interpretation of results. Alternatively, the behavioral properties of a drug may be the basis for defining the upper dose in the study [7], and by selecting lower doses free of these confounding effects, a study in conscious animals may be a preferred design.

However, there will be situations where chemical restraint using one of a variety of anesthetic agents is a desired approach to conducting the cardiovascular study in animals. In addition to eliminating or reducing those factors that could confound the interpretation of the results, anesthesia may be desirable where a more elaborate preparation of the animal is needed (i.e., acute placement of flow probes and intra-cardiac catheters) and recovery of the animal at the end of cardiovascular monitoring is not feasible. Chemical restraint also produces a more stable condition for cardiovascular monitoring, without the changes in cardiovascular parameters imparted by an animal's spontaneous activity. There may be conditions where this stability is desired to increase the sensitivity to detect small drug-related changes.

The reader is referred to Refs. 48 and 49 for a list of typical anesthetics and their advantages and disadvantages. Careful consideration should be given to the effects of the anesthetic agent on normal cardiovascular parameters (e.g., ECG intervals, including prolongation of QT/QTc interval; heart rate; arterial blood pressures), as well as normal physiologic hemodynamic reflexes, so that the investigator is cognizant of the limitations created by the anesthetic agent that may affect or alter the study results [48–55]. The reader is also directed to consult with the veterinary staff with regard to the preferred methodology for induction and maintenance of anesthesia, taking into consideration the specific objectives of the study. During the study it will be important that the study team carefully monitor the basal physiologic conditions of the animal (i.e., blood pressure, heart rate, electrocardiogram, blood gases, blood pH, and bicarbonate levels), adjusting those parameters (e.g., depth of anesthesia, physiologic fluids) that will assure maintenance of stable preparation through the course of the study.

There may be situations where the investigator wishes to study a test agent in conscious animals, but the parameters monitored are not accessible through radio-telemetry technology. This situation requires instrumentation of the animal and externalization of the cable and connectors through which the physiological signal will emanate to the monitoring devices [56]. Between experiments, all exteriorized cables and connectors would be protected within secure jackets. The animals will be accustomed to physical restraint procedures (i.e., restraint tubes for rodents, upright in slings, left or right lateral recumbency for dogs, and dorsal recumbency or chairs for nonhuman primates) for a period that will extend beyond the period of time intended for monitoring in the study. However, the need for training may be avoided if the technology employed in a study can be fully supported by a tethering device; in which case the animal will be free to move about the cage. The investigator should recognize that the level of complexity and number of resources and amount of time required to conduct a study using physical restraint are significantly increased over that of the other procedures that have thus far been described. This would include routine monitoring and maintenance of the hardware exiting the body surface and surgical sites.

Selection of Technologies   Introduction of radiotelemetry technologies for the study of cardiovascular function has significantly advanced the field of cardiovascular safety pharmacology and the ability to monitor core cardiovascular parameters continuously over the course of hours to days to weeks in freely moving animals. While the application of these technologies across species continues to be refined, monitoring of basic functions such as heart rate and blood pressure (systolic, diastolic, and mean) and electrocardiograms is possible in both rodent and nonrodent species and monitoring of systemic flows and cardiac dynamics in nonrodent species is also an established technology [57–59]. These technologies require surgical proficiency to implement in the laboratory; but once animals are instrumented, they can be used repeatedly over the period of years. After implantation of the radiotelemetry device, scheduled monitoring is required to assure the stability of cardiovascular parameters and electronic function of the transmitter and, importantly, the health of the animal. The latter is particularly important in advance of an upcoming study to assure that there are an adequate number of animals to assign to the study and that there were no lingering effects of a prior study agent.

With some of the technologies that require an internal implantation of vascular catheters, ECG leads, and the transmitting units, there will be a limitation of battery life and drifting of the cardiovascular signal, both indications of a deterioration of the transmitter unit. Other technologies that allow external calibration of the blood pressure and blood flow signals and the exchange of expended batteries from an external pack obviate the problems inherent in internally implanted transmitters. However, as noted earlier, there is greater commitment of resources devoted to maintaining animals that are instrumented with radiotelemetry devices that have external cables and leads.

Technologies are also available that allow monitoring of the electrocardiogram by radiotelemetry using transmitters and other hardware retained in specially designed protective jackets for dogs and nonhuman primates [60, 61]. While limited to the evaluation of the electrocardiogram, there are times when focusing on the electrocardiogram is warranted; such as a desire to expand monitoring to a larger population of animals, monitor over extended periods of time in free moving nonrodents, or alter the lead configuration.

Limitations on the number of animals studied using radiotelemetry technologies are based on the number of instrumented animals with accurately functioning transmitters in a colony, the configuration of the data acquisition system(s) (e.g., capable of simultaneously monitoring up to six to eight animals with two to four parameters per animal), the size of the technical staff required for dosing and bleeding in a relatively abbreviated period of time (i.e., completing all tasks in 15 minutes from start to finish), and practical consideration of the number of resources required for data processing and analysis. There are a number of computer-based data acquisitions technologies available on the market for monitoring cardiovascular and electrocardiographic parameters [58, 60, 62–66]. The reader is directed to the vendor websites to review the technologies and determine which system most closely aligns with the requirements of his/her program.

As described earlier, study of conscious animals in the presence of physical restraint (i.e., restraint tubes for rodents, upright in slings or left or right lateral recumbency for dogs, and dorsal recumbency or chairs for nonhuman primates) is a preferred methodology in certain situations. Once the investigator has accepted the increased complexity, the number of resources, and the amount of time devoted to a study employing physical restraint, there are several technologies that are available that allow a more detailed evaluation of the cardiovascular state. Measurement of parameters such as intracardiac dynamics, systemic blood flows, and the standard parameters (heart rate and blood pressures (systolic, diastolic, mean)) are all possible using conscious restrained procedures [67–70].

Animals that are physically restrained can be studied for hours or days, either continuously based on the length of the training or for brief periods intermittently over a longer period of time. During data collection, the requirement of close monitoring of the animal's condition limits the number of animals that can be studied at the same time.

Alternatively, the investigator may employ a tether system to acquire cardiovascular data from instrumented animals that are able to move relatively freely around their cages. However, this procedure also requires maintenance of the cables and exit wounds and training to the tether system.

The same technologies available for monitoring freely moving animals or animals under physical restraint can also be applied in an acute study under chemical restraint. In addition, the anesthetized animal allows the introduction of other technologies that may not be amendable to the chronically instrumented models, such as cardiac catheterization, echocardiography, and other more advanced procedures that allow a detailed assessment of cardiovascular function [70, 71].

Chemical restraint procedures also allow monitoring of electrophysiologic parameters such as the length of the monophasic action potential, the duration of the effective refractory period, or conduction through the SA-node, AV-node, His-bundle, and Purkinje fiber systems [43–45, 51, 72].

Chemical restraint procedures also allow for extrinsic manipulation of the cardiovascular system: for example, stimulation of pre- or postganglionic autonomic fibers innervating the heart or systemic vasculature to study the site of test article action, *in vivo* electrophysiologic techniques to maintain a constant heart rate by cardiac pacing during the evaluation of the proarrhythmic potential of a test substance that is confounded by its property of lowering heart rate, or study of the propensity for proarrhythmic activity of a test agent facilitated by programmed electrical stimulation [73–76].

Dose Selection   The ICH S7A guidelines define the basis for dose selection in the core battery cardiovascular study. The selection of doses in other cases will depend on the objective of the study and the availability of data to assist in this important decision. Both the quality and volume of data forming the basis for a rational dose selection will improve incrementally with the phase in which the study will ensue (i.e., early to late discovery; early to late development).

As described in the ICH S7A guidelines, "doses should include and exceed the primary pharmacodynamic or therapeutic range. In the absence of an adverse effect on safety pharmacology parameter(s) … , the highest tested dose should be a dose that produces moderate adverse effects in this or in other studies of similar route and duration." However, as mentioned earlier, the ICH S7A guidelines allow for doses producing biologic responses that had the potential to confound interpretation of results to be identified as a limiting dose: "In practice, some effects in the toxic range [e.g., tremors or fasciculation during ECG recording] may confound the interpretation of the results and may also limit dose levels" [7]. In this situation, the investigator will justify selection of a high dose as being absent of confounding clinical effects.

Selection of the low dose would be based on the desire to study the test substance in the therapeutic range, that is, at a onefold or greater exposure multiple of the projected or measured peak plasma exposure achieved at the clinically efficacious dose(s). The exposure multiple is most typically determined in safety pharmacology studies from comparison of peak plasma concentrations (C_{max}), but may also be based on the *area under* the plasma-drug-concentration–time *curve* [AUC]). The reader is referred to Refs. 77–79 to learn more about the pharmacokinetic/toxico-kinetic characterization of new molecules. Defining an observed-effect-level or a no-observed-effect-level based on C_{max} and/or AUC is a topic of considerable interest. Selection of a dose from C_{max} would be based on knowledge that a pharmaco-dynamic response is the result of achieving a threshold concentration (e.g., a concentration needed to activate a specific receptor subtype, thereby eliciting down-stream intracellular biochemical changes culminating in a pharmacodynamic response of the target organ). On the other hand, if it is known or suspected that the pharmacodynamic effect of the drug is the result of accumulation of a test sub-stance in the target tissue following repeated dosing to steady state or secondary to toxicity of the tissue parenchyma, then AUC may be the more appropriate basis for projecting the exposure multiple used in the selection of the low dose. However, the design of the safety pharmacology study usually follows a single dose, and, therefore, a steady-state condition is typically not achieved. A repeat-dose study would be conducted in those situations where there is a specific question or concern. If the toxicity is related to continuous intracellular exposure, but resulting from a mechanism that is dependent on a threshold-related effect, then the use of both C_{max} and AUC may be appropriate for determining the exposure multiples between a dose exposure being evaluated in the nonclinical study and the anticipated exposure achieved in the clinic. Similar considerations of dose selection should be given to assuring the evaluation of major metabolites (particularly major human metabo-lites) formed in the animal species. After having selected the low and high doses for the investigation, the choice of the mid-dose may be based on the geometric mean between the other two dose levels.

ICH S7A, which requires the core battery cardiovascular safety study to be con-ducted according to good laboratory practice (GLP), provides for a study in situa-tions where the high dose of the experimental agent is devoid of pharmacodynamic effects and, in such a case, only a vehicle and a single dose are required for testing (Section 2.4.1): "Testing of a single group at the limiting dose as described above may be sufficient in the absence of an adverse effect on safety pharmacology end-points in the test species" [7]. Application of this design may pose a risk of not being able to define a no-observed-effect-level and, therefore, a decision to follow this simplified design requires prior knowledge about the test substance suggesting a probable negative study outcome. On the other hand, this may be an acceptable level of risk for a selected test agent, given the reduced number of resources and time devoted to the conduct and reporting of an abbreviated study.

Formulation   There are several factors to consider in selection of the formulation for the cardiovascular safety pharmacology study. First, consideration is given to the properties of the formulation excipients and their ability to have an effect on car-diovascular endpoints. It will be important in the design of a cardiovascular study using a pharmacodynamically active excipient that you are able to distinguish a placebo effect from that of the active pharmaceutical ingredient.

In situations where novel excipients are employed in the formulation of the test article product, there may be a need to evaluate the cardiovascular safety of the placebo formulation by comparing its pharmacodynamic properties to an inert negative control agent (i.e., isotonic saline, isotonic dextrose). The required evaluation of a unique vehicle formulation may also occur in situations where the product formulation is being developed for oral administration in early drug safety and clinical investigations, but the design of the cardiovascular study requires a unique formulation in order to accommodate a parenteral route (i.e., for intravenous administration). Most often, for cardiovascular safety pharmacology studies, however, the formulation will be the same as that intended for early clinical administration or that devised to support the early drug safety studies.

Route of Administration   The preferred route of administration in the cardiovascular safety pharmacology study is the same route as that intended for use in the clinic. Assuming that all pharmacokinetic properties are the same between animals and humans, this approach allows the study of the test agent under similar conditions of exposure to the test substance.

However, there may be times when an alternative route of administration to that intended for clinical application of the test substance is desirable; for example, in cases where the peak plasma concentration (C_{max}) to a test substance may be enhanced by the alternate route (i.e., a test substance administered intravenously achieving a higher C_{max} than by the oral route). This may be desirable when wanting to assess cardiovascular parameters following test substance administration at peak levels greater than those achieved by the oral route.

In the study design where chemical restraint is employed, the possible routes of administration are generally limited to the parenteral or intraduodenal routes, keeping in mind in the case of intraduodenal administration that the duration of study may be important to determining the peak blood levels of the active pharmaceutical which can be achieved. As suggested in an earlier section, the duration of the study using chemical restraint will be determined by the ability to maintain stable cardiovascular parameters through the control of hydration, acid–base status, and the level of oxygenation. When administering the test article via the intravenous route, the use of an infusion, as opposed to administration as a bolus, may provide a concentration–time relationship that more closely models the plasma-concentration curve following the oral route. However, a novel development candidate with a slow rate of elimination (thereby maintaining a peak plasma concentration over a prolonged period of time) may be amenable to a study where animals are first dosed orally and then chemically restrained once peak plasma concentrations have been achieved.

Even in the case of studying cardiovascular function in conscious animals, careful consideration of the route of administration should be given. For drugs that achieve rapid peak exposures following oral administration, the early period of monitoring may be lost in the animal's cardiovascular-related stress response to the physical restraint required for dosing. In the same manner, the cardiovascular responses to bolus intravenous injection of the test substance may be lost in this early period of stress-related cardiovascular instability. For these situations, training animals to accommodate to physical restraint as described in an earlier section and maintaining this restraint position through the baseline and postdose periods will accomplish stability during which drug-related changes can be discerned from normal background variation. This same model may be used in studying drugs during a prolonged period of infusion, where having stable baseline and postdose periods is desirable.

The cardiovascular study of inhalation products is an area of limited general experience in safety pharmacology. The conditions for exposure of animals to the test substance can be the same as those used in the repeat-dose toxicology study, with the monitoring of cardiovascular and electrocardiographic parameters facilitated by radiotelemetry. Alternative routes of administration (e.g., IV dosing) may also be a means of evaluating the cardiovascular properties of the test agent. However, the unique conditions of exposure to the test substance following the inhalation route (e.g., preferential, sustained, and significantly greater exposure of the heart to the test article following administration into the lungs) may not be obtainable by the alternative route [80, 81].

Dose Regimen and Dose Groups   The objective of the core battery cardiovascular study is to identify those pharmacodynamic properties of a new test agent which may pose a risk in preparing for the early clinical trials in healthy volunteers or patients. The design of subsequent clinical studies will not only be based on the results of nonclinical safety studies but may also be tailored according to the observations (e.g., pharmacokinetics, tolerance, and biomarkers of efficacy, where possible) made during the early clinical phase. Based on this development strategy, the design of a typical core battery study uses a single-dose regimen. However, the duration of dosing may be extended to multiple daily doses or dosing over several days (1) when the objective of the nonclinical study is satisfied by achieving a higher steady-state plasma concentration of parent drug or major human metabolite(s), (2) to facilitate tissue accumulation based on a known propensity of the test substance to distribute to cardiovascular tissues or other organs or tissues affecting cardiovascular functions (i.e., central nervous system), (3) when this dosing regimen is needed to avert a dose-limiting toxicity that can be attenuated by a dose escalation design (e.g., emesis), or (4) when more than a single dose is part of the protocol design to evaluate a hypothesis or reproduce study conditions in which cardiovascular toxicity was observed following multiple doses of the experimental substance.

The number of dose groups and dosing design will be based on the objectives of the study and the pharmacokinetic, pharmacodynamic, and toxicity profile of the drug, and the statistical power of the study design (see later section on analysis of data). In the case of the core battery cardiovascular safety pharmacology study, the possible study designs may be an escalating dose or crossover design or a study in discrete groups [82–85].

When the information about tolerance to a drug is limited, the escalating dose design allows the investigator to understand the potentially adverse properties of a drug before moving to the next dose level. The dose escalation design is where one group of animals is given escalating doses of test substance and an optional parallel group is administered vehicle at each of the study intervals. This dosing design can either follow a single dose or multiple doses and decisions about the time interval between each dosing phase may be made based on the information available (e.g., pharmacokinetic/toxicokinetic, tolerance, pharmacodynamic properties). For certain drugs, where there is limited information regarding tolerance or where there is a prolonged half-life, the escalating dose design may be desirable, accepting in the latter example that there will be accumulation of drug substance with each of the subsequent doses.

The crossover design, most often a balanced Latin square crossover design [83–85], is where each of the animals is given vehicle and test substance at each of the dose levels on separate days, allowing for a washout period between each day of dosing. Animals are randomly assigned to individual dosing schedules, which in the Latin square crossover design follows an established sequence of doses (e.g., high, low, vehicle, mid-dose given on separate days to one animal; low, mid, high, vehicle dose given on separate days to another animal; and so on) such that there is a balance across the study with respect to the combinations of dosing sequences. The washout period should be at least 5 half-lives to minimize the residual drug levels remaining before administration of the next dose. The advantage of this design is that the same animal will receive each of the treatment levels on different days and the potential influences of environment are spread across groups (e.g., at least one subject receives each dose on any particular day). Using such a design, the statistical power and sensitivity to detect changes in cardiovascular parameters are enhanced when compared to the statistical power of the other designs. However, this approach cannot be used with drugs that have lingering toxicities (i.e., cytotoxic agents being developed for oncology) and may not be practical for promising drug candidates with a long half-life.

For drugs that have a long half-life, making the escalating dose and crossover designs impractical, or for those promising agents that cannot be given repeatedly to the same animal (e.g., due to residual toxicity), a study in discrete groups becomes necessary (i.e., each subject is challenged with only one dose). However, for a drug with a prolonged half-life, the long washout period between studies means that this pool of animals will be unavailable for another study for a matter of some time.

Another situation where a study in discrete groups may also be desirable, particularly in comparison to the crossover design, is where there is a need to have the entire dosing phase completed in days, rather than in weeks, which are required for the washout period in the crossover design of many test agents. The disadvantage of a study in discrete groups is the number of animals needed for this design is greater than the number needed for a study using the crossover design (e.g., vehicle and 3 treatment levels: n = 4/group, total of 16 animals for a study in discrete groups; n = 4/dose level, total of 4 animals for a study using the crossover design) and loss of the ability to look for differences in response at different dose levels within an individual subject. This also means that the size of the animal pool and the associated resources required for surgery, longitudinal monitoring, and maintenance will be greater for the animal pool required to support consecutive studies by the discrete group design.

Irrespective of the study design selected, the inclusion of a concurrent negative control (e.g., vehicle, saline, dextrose) is essential to account for time-, environment-, or individual behavior-related changes in the cardiovascular parameters. However, where the anticipated outcome of drug administration is well beyond normal variation for a significant parameter pivotal to understanding the test substance's effects in an animal species (e.g., profound increase or decrease in arterial blood pressure), the need for a concurrent negative control may not be necessary.

Pretest Monitoring   Pretest monitoring of cardiovascular parameters in chronically instrumented animals occurs at the juncture in preparing for a study where there is a need to know the animal's suitability, which is judged based on the fidelity of the electrical signal (e.g., arterial blood pressure and electrocardiogram), the relationship of the cardiovascular parameters to the baseline in that animal at the time of instrumentation and changes that have evolved over the course of the animal's residence, and the health of the animal according to a veterinary exam and evaluation of clinical pathology parameters. The duration of cardiovascular data collection during the pretest monitoring may mirror the period of data collection on the day of dosing. In addition to allowing for an assessment of the suitability of the animal for inclusion in the study, these data provide a basis for comparison should questions of preexisting conditions arise during the analysis of the study results. If animals remain unused in a study for prolonged periods of time (e.g., 2 months), periodic monitoring of cardiovascular parameters is recommended to assure that there are a minimal number of animals viewed as acceptable for a full study in the existing pool. This would include at least an additional two to four animals serving as spares.

Duration of Monitoring   Careful consideration is given to the duration of data collection during the dosing phase. Generally, data are collected prior to dosing to establish a baseline (e.g., 1–2 hours) and for a sufficient period following dosing to meet the study objectives. At a minimum, the period of data collection should be adequate to encompass the peak plasma concentration (C_{max}) of the active pharmaceutical ingredient and any of its major metabolites—particularly any major human metabolites identified in the clinical studies. In some cases, multiple days of dosing may be required to achieve higher steady-state concentrations of the test article and/or its major metabolites than that which can be achieved with a single dose. If knowledge of recovery from possible effects is an important objective, then continuous monitoring for at least 5 half-lives may provide a basis for selecting the period of postdose data collection. An understanding of the onset and duration of activity following dosing will be used to assess the safety of a test substance. In particular, knowing the duration of activity and that an observed pharmacodynamic outcome is reversible are important to devising a plan to manage a potential adverse event should this same event be observed in subjects or patients. With the ability to collect continuous cardiovascular waveforms through radiotelemetry and data acquisition technologies, an investigation can encompass continuous collection of cardiovascular parameters and post hoc on-screen review to identify discrete periods of interest for a more detailed analysis of data generated in a study.

Parameters   As described earlier in this section, *in vivo* study of conscious or anesthetized animals allows a detailed evaluation of a number of parameters that will form the basis for characterization of the cardiovascular effects of a potential new drug. Essential to this review is an understanding of the effects of the test substance on heart rate, arterial blood pressure (systolic, diastolic, mean), ECG intervals (RR, PR, QRS, QT), and ECG morphology, including knowledge related to the potential for cardiac arrhythmias. The challenge to the investigator in assessing these critical parameters is to have knowledge of the normal background incidence and variation in each of the animal populations [86–88]. This would include variations in the particular species selected for study as well as the historical control data generated within the institution. This is particularly important in distinguishing test article-related changes from artifacts associated with movement or a normal background incidence in a specific species, for example, second degree atria-ventricular blockade is a common finding in dogs [86–88]. To better understand the numerical range of normal values in the selected species, investigators are encouraged to understand the confidence limits for each cardiovascular parameter in their institutional datasets.

The study of cardiovascular parameters in addition to those already described may be facilitated by their incorporation into the safety pharmacology core battery study, when there is a known pharmacodynamic property of the test agent or its therapeutic/chemical class for which there is a concern. Additional pharmacodynamic measures may also be added to follow-up studies in order to address questions directed at better defining the conditions for safely administering a drug or understanding an underlying mechanism of action for an observed event. For example, a test substance that raises arterial blood pressure may do so by increasing systemic blood flow (cardiac output) and/or systemic vascular resistance (equivalent to arterial blood pressure divided by systemic or regional blood flow). These changes result in increased cardiac work, which may pose a significant risk to certain patient populations, such as those individuals with compromised cardiac function (e.g., congestive heart failure). In contrast, individuals with reduced blood flow to an organ (e.g., kidney) may be able to tolerate an increase in systemic flow, but not an increase in peripheral vascular resistance if this action further compromises the vulnerable organ. Understanding the hemodynamic changes elicited by a promising new drug may not only define the safety of the molecule in the particular patient population but may also form the basis for conducting a study to evaluate potential underlying mechanism(s) of action.

Drug-related changes in conduction of an electrical impulse through the heart, from the atrium to the ventricle, may also have significant life-threatening consequences. Alterations in the morphology of the electrocardiogram (or pseudo-electrocardiogram) associated with test article administration (assessed by electrodes placed on the body surface, subcutaneously, within the intrathoracic cavity around the heart, or directly on the heart) may be a harbinger of proarrhythmia and provide directions for further study. Furthermore, an understanding of cardiac depolarization and repolarization-related changes following exposure to a potential new drug, as reflected in ECG interval measurements (PR, QRS, QT, and rate corrected QT (QTc) intervals), and the test substance's ability to induce automaticity and reentrant cardiac electrical behaviors will help define the potential risks associated with its clinical exposure [8, 39, 40, 86, 87, 89].

Analysis of Data   The reader is referred to Refs. 82–85 to select a statistical application that is most appropriate to the design of the study that has been chosen. Careful attention should be paid to avoiding type 1 and 2 errors in the selection of the statistical application. Discussion with institutional biostatistics colleagues will help facilitate the selection of methodology. An analysis of the power offered by a statistical application and study design and determination of the confidence limits of the historical database will guide investigators in understanding the sensitivity of their models to detect individual changes in specific cardiovascular parameters. As suggested earlier in this chapter, this information will be of value in providing the appropriate perspective for developing an integrated assessment of risk.

Graphical views (minute-by-minute) of cardiovascular parameters over the course of the predosing and postdosing periods is easily accomplished with contemporary data acquisition technology and may identify periods that warrant a more detailed visual interrogation. Careful consideration should be given to the relationship of pharmacokinetic exposure to the drug and any coincident pharmacodynamic changes. This temporal relationship may aid in distinguishing effects related to the test agent and/or its major metabolites from those resulting from spontaneous activity. The hysteresis of this relationship may also identify findings associated with tissue accumulation, a previously unknown novel metabolite, or a mechanism that manifests long after the peak exposure to the test substance has resolved [30, 31].

Complementary to the graphical review of study findings are tabular presentations of cardiovascular parameters at specific intervals (e.g., every 5, 15, 30, or 60 minutes or a combination of intervals), depending on the route of administration and associated pharmacokinetic/toxicokinetic profile of the test agent and/or its major metabolites. Tabular data may be presented as absolute or change from baseline values. Experience has shown that baseline-corrected parameters have a lower degree of variance than data presented as absolute values and, as a result, baseline-corrected values retain a greater degree of statistical power. The reader is encouraged to work with the biostatistics group to define the best approach to the analysis of data collected under the conditions of study within his/her institution.

As described earlier in this chapter, the subject of drug-induced delay in cardiac ventricular repolarization (QT interval prolongation) has received significant attention by both the medical community and international regulators since QT interval prolongation has been identified as an important substrate contributing to the cardiac arrhythmia, torsades de pointes [5, 8, 9, 11, 90]. Measurement of cardiac ventricular repolarization (*in vivo*) on the electrocardiogram is reflected in the QT interval parameter. However, the QT interval is subject to changes in heart rate independent of other underlying mechanisms that also affect cardiac repolarization. An increase in heart rate leads to a decrease in QT interval and a decrease in heart rate leads to an increase in QT interval under normal physiologic conditions. Thus, many investigators have attempted to devise a mathematical approach to normalizing this relationship (QTc = heart rate corrected QT interval), but these attempts have met with mixed results [91–98]. At this time, it appears that correction formulas that are established specifically for the pool of animals studied or those based on the heart rate–QT interval relationships in individual animals have proved to be the best approaches to normalization, particularly for drugs that have an effect on heart rate. However, there are also laboratories that advocate collecting sufficient amounts of data such that application of rate correction formulas becomes unnecessary and that simply looking at the relationship of QT interval over a range of heart rates (binning method) becomes practical [98, 99]. Alternatively, a beat-to-beat analysis of the relationship of QT interval to TQ interval (the principle of restitution) or RR interval to QT interval have also been suggested as alternative methods of identifying new test substances that may pose a cardiac risk [100]. It should be recognized that there is no ideal method for normalizing the relationship between heart rate and QT interval and the inaccuracies of the current correction formulas appear to increase proportionally with the change in heart rate.

A discussion of rate correction formulas would not be complete without consideration of two formulas most commonly used in animal studies: that proposed by Bazett ($QTc = QT/\sqrt{RR}$) and the one proposed by Fridericia ($QTc = QT/\sqrt[3]{RR}$) in 1920 for use in clinical studies [97, 101]. Both of these formulas have an inherent problem of consistently overcorrecting QTc interval when heart rates are relatively high (tending to show a greater QTc value than that which is normal in the absence of drug-related effects) and consistently undercorrecting QTc interval when heart rates are relatively slow (tending to show a lower QTc value than that which is normal in the absence of drug-related effects) [98]. In this regard, in many preparations, the error produced by the Bazett formula is significantly greater than that derived from the Fridericia formula. As a result, several authors have suggested that the Bazett formula should not be used in animal studies [98]. On the other hand, the fact that the Fridericia formula also demonstrates a similar tendency toward overcorrection or undercorrection suggests that this method of rate correction should be used together with other formulas (i.e., pooled or individual rate correction formulas) to draw a comparison in defining the safety of a novel new drug. An additional word of caution is to establish a formula as appropriate to the conditions of a study in your laboratory and to the specific species being studied. A formula devised for one species under specific study conditions may not be applicable to another. This evaluation should be conducted at specific intervals (e.g., once per year) and the methodology revised as appropriate based on the analysis of new data.

Establishing In Vivo Cardiovascular Models by the Use of Positive Control Agents According to ICH S7A guidelines, "appropriate negative and positive control groups should be included in the experimental design." However, the guidelines go on to say that "in well-characterized *in vivo* test systems, positive controls may not be necessary. The exclusion of controls from studies should be justified" [7]. Since the pharmacodynamic effects of a test article in the multitude of possible cardiovascular parameters may change in multiple directions, the guideline requirement for "well-characterized *in vivo* test systems" is by far the only practical approach to demonstrating sensitivity and specificity of the *in vivo* model. The positive control agents chosen for such a study will accordingly be based on the parameters of interest (e.g., heart rate, arterial blood pressure, and ECG intervals) and the multitude of possible directions in which they may change, and whether this study is establishing a model that will be used in the standard "core battery cardiovascular" study or whether this study is critical to comparing the test agent to a marketed drug, for example, as an objective of a "follow-up" cardiovascular study [7]. In either situation, the positive control agent should be recognized as having been well characterized for the effect of interest by the international scientific community. The reader is directed to Ref. 37 for examples of possible positive control agents across a wide class of cardiovascular targets.

Discrete Blood Level Sampling Maintaining a controlled study environment is of paramount importance in assuring the sensitivity of the model to detect discrete cardiovascular changes. As a result of this concern, the ability to enter a study room in the midst of cardiovascular data collection in order to obtain blood samples should not be followed without careful planning as noted later. This limitation does not apply to a study conducted in the presence of chemical or physical restraint, where the investigator is continuously in close proximity to the animal. In those situations, multiple sampling of blood from the test species is possible as long as the procedures of blood collection do not interfere with the acquisition of data.

In a study in unrestrained animals, the collection of blood samples can be used to confirm exposure, as long as the time at which blood is collected does not coincide with the peak levels of either the test article or any of its major metabolites. As long as the variability of the pharmacokinetic/toxicokinetic properties of a test substance is small, as demonstrated in a formal study with a full panel of 5–12 blood samples, then the data generated from limited sampling in the cardiovascular study can be compared to the data from the full pharmacokinetic/toxicokinetic study forming the basis for an estimation of the peak plasma concentration achieved in the cardiovascular study. In order to obtain the blood sample without interfering with acquisition of cardiovascular data, the sample(s) are collected after the estimated peak concentration of the test substance and the major metabolites had been achieved; typically one or more samples are collected after cardiovascular data collection has been completed and concurrent with the elimination phase of the plasma concentration–time profile. There can be situations, however, where cardiovascular data are collected over a prolonged period following test substance administration, in which case it may become necessary to collect blood samples intermittently throughout the period of data collection, but avoiding those times in which it is critical to maintain a stable, undisturbed laboratory environment.

18.3.3 Interpretation of Results: An Integrated Assessment of Cardiovascular Risk of Human Exposure to the Test Substance

It will not be practical to comprehensively review all of those factors that can be taken into consideration in forming an integrated assessment of risk in this chapter. In the same manner, the decision to continue or discontinue development of a new molecular entity based on adverse findings in preclinical studies may differ from one institution to another based on the availability of other data (nonclinical and clinical) and the strategic interests of the organization. Because of these variables, this section does not necessarily address all situations with which an investigator may be faced or recommend a simple course of action. Rather, the purpose of this section is to list many of the critical questions that are considered in formulating a decision of the benefit–risk relationship for a drug candidate. More broadly, this careful assessment will contribute to the decision of whether a promising new drug can be safely advanced through the clinical phases and on to registration. Those pharmacodynamic properties considered in devising an integrated risk assessment may include the following.

Magnitude of Effect in the Animal Studies   Based on these data, a judgment can be made of whether a similar effect in humans might be tolerated. For example, there is currently significant discussion regarding the pro-torsadegenic risk posed by a test agent that produces an increase of QT/QTc interval having a 95% confidence interval upper bound of 10 ms in the patient population, such that changes of less than 10 ms would be considered nonproarrhythmic [26]. A similar criterion does not currently exist with regard to nonclinical studies; however, there is opportunity for questioning the relationship between findings in animals and those in humans based on a careful analysis of the outcome of clinical studies.

Dose (or Concentration)–Response Relationship   This relationship (e.g. none, shallow, or steep) is important in several respects. The absence of a dose–response relationship may suggest that the effect observed is an artifact of the experimental model, unrelated to the test substance, or that a maximum effect has been achieved. In the latter situation, administering higher doses would not be associated with a greater response and if the magnitude of the effect observed can be tolerated in the clinical studies, progression of the test article may be acceptable. On the other hand, a steep dose–response relationship is problematic as this profile suggests that an adverse event may occur without forewarning once a threshold effect has been achieved during the phase of dose escalation. This situation may warrant more extensive monitoring of the normal volunteers or patients. In extreme cases where life-threatening cardiovascular toxicity is a concern, an institution may decide to discontinue development of the promising new drug candidate.

Margin of Safety   The margin of safety (e.g., plasma concentrations eliciting an adverse cardiovascular event in the nonclinical study compared to plasma concentrations required for efficacy in clinical studies) is important in understanding the probability of achieving adequate drug level in patients to produce efficacy without placing an individual at risk of untoward cardiovascular events.

Pharmacokinetic/Toxicokinetic Properties   Several questions may emerge from understanding the pharmacokinetic/toxicokinetic properties of a new test substance. For example, was the cardiovascular event coincident with the peak levels of the test substance or its major metabolites? If the cardiovascular activity is related to concentration of the major metabolites, are these formed at concentrations in humans adequate to pose a risk? Could the effects observed in the preclinical species be attributed to either tissue (e.g., cardiac, vascular) accumulation of the test substance or the accumulation of major metabolites with repeated dosing? If these questions remain after careful review of the nonclinical and clinical data, there may be reason to consider the conduct of an additional, follow-up cardiovascular study with more extensive monitoring of pharmacokinetic/toxicokinetic parameters.

Relevance of the Nonclinical Model to Understanding Human Safety   Understanding the biology of the system and whether it is operational in humans is of paramount importance in deciding whether a test article-related observation in animals is an indication of a human risk. This topic was described earlier with regard to the differences in the contribution of repolarizing currents operative in rodents when compared to those that are operative in humans [11]. This situation may also apply to novel therapeutic targets, where there is limited data describing the relevance of a novel target to the cardiovascular system in either animals or humans. In such a situation, further nonclinical studies may be needed to understand mechanism-based effects.

Relationship of Comparable In Vitro and In Vivo Cardiovascular Findings in Terms of Concentration–Response   A cardiovascular response from one study, which is corroborated by results of another study, provides a strong indication of a potential for a cardiovascular event in humans, assuming that adequate exposures to the test substance or major metabolite(s) are achieved in the nonclinical study of the test substance. In addition, the results of the *in vitro* study may also provide a basis for a more detailed understanding of the potential underlying mechanism of the adverse event or whether a result may be produced in another species. In contrast, conflicting data between *in vitro* and *in vivo* studies may be the basis for raising questions of whether an observation will occur in humans.

Distinguishing Direct Pharmacodynamic Effects of the Test Substance from Indirect Effects Due to Toxicities   Recognizing whether a drug produces a cardiovascular adverse event as a result of its pharmacodynamic properties or as an indirect secondary event resulting from abnormal clinical or anatomic pathology is important in formulating an analysis of human risk and devising a plan for monitoring risk factor(s) in the clinical study of the test agent: for example, QT prolongation due to a direct effect of a compound on the cardiac potassium rectifying current, I_{Kr}, versus that resulting from toxicity associated with profound hypokalemia. In addition, understanding the underlying etiology of cardiovascular toxicity provides a basis for directly evaluating reversibility of the untoward effects.

Recognizing that the Targeted Patient Population May Be Highly Susceptible to a Drug-Related Toxicity   As suggested earlier in this section, ultimate decisions of the safe progression of a test article with undesirable cardiovascular pharmacodynamic properties will be based, in part, on consideration of the particular susceptibility of the patient population in which that test agent would be used (e.g., torsades de pointes in heart failure patients). In this regard, it is important to recognize that the animal models used in safety pharmacology are typically healthy animals and do not represent the underlying condition of susceptibility that may exist in that targeted patient population.

18.3.4 Summary

The objective of the cardiovascular study of a new molecular entity is to have sufficiently characterized its pharmacodynamic properties in preclinical models that emulate human physiology in order to anticipate the potential risk posed to subjects and patients following clinical exposure. A comprehensive cardiovascular study of a new test agent at the minimum would include monitoring of arterial blood pressures (systolic, diastolic, and mean), heart rate, electrocardiographic intervals, and the electrocardiogram for the presence of cardiac arrhythmias [7]. The evaluation of test article effects on QT interval *in vivo* as recommended in ICH S7B will be monitored in the core battery safety pharmacology study [11]. Additional cardiovascular endpoints may be added to the core battery study based on a cause for concern for human safety. Alternatively, the promising new test substance may be evaluated in a follow-up cardiovascular study for a more detailed understanding of test-article-induced changes in cardiovascular function. Collectively, the composite profile of preclinical and clinical data is assimilated into an integrated assessment of the potential risk posed by human exposure to the promising new drug. In addition, these data inform the clinical investigator where more detailed monitoring of cardiovascular function is needed during the course of dose escalation in early clinical trials. These data also inform the organization that is continuously judging the value and safety of continuing the development of the new molecular entity.

18.4   *IN VITRO* CARDIAC SAFETY PHARMACOLOGY (CARDIAC ELECTROPHYSIOLOGY)

18.4.1   Introduction

A number of noncardiovascular drugs from different therapeutic classes have been linked to delayed ventricular repolarization and sudden cardiac death resulting from a rare polymorphic ventricular tachyarrhythmia known as torsades de pointes [102]. The rare occurrence of TdeP for noncardiac drugs that affect ventricular repolarization (incidence likely too low to reliably detect in clinical trials) and potentially lethal consequences of this arrhythmia necessitate the use of nonclinical surrogate markers to detect drug-induced delayed repolarization (also termed acquired long QT syndrome, or aLQTS). In fact, drug-induced delay in cardiac ventricular repolarization serves not only as a surrogate marker, but also as one of several risk factors (see below) placing susceptible individuals at risk for TdeP. Numerous *in vitro* models have been described that evaluate potential proarrhythmia on subcellular, cellular, tissue, and organ levels. However, none have proved to be fully predictive of either QT prolongation or torsadogenic potential in humans. This likely reflects the extent of integration of more complex systems as one progresses from individual ionic currents to electrophysiologic interactions between different regions of the ventricular myocardium. In addition, several other risk factors (including female gender, hypokalemia, bradycardia, heart disease, excessive drug concentrations, pharmacodynamic interactions, and ion channel defects) have been identified and linked to aLQTS. These findings support the "multiple hit hypothesis" that states that the concomitant appearance of multiple risk factors may be necessary to set the stage for the initiation and perpetuation of TdeP. Thus, the successful identification (and avoidance) of aLQTS and TdeP requires a careful assessment of models of varying complexity and an appreciation of their interactions with additional risk factors. This section discusses the more widely accepted *in vitro* approaches for evaluating proarrhythmic risk of evolving compounds and their organization based on increasing levels of integration. Ionic current assays are discussed first, followed by action potential duration/repolarization studies that reflect responses of tissues, representing a higher level of integration. Finally, evaluations employing *ex vivo* whole heart preparations are described.

18.4.2   Ionic Current Assays

hERG Current   The outwardly directed delayed rectifier current I_{Kr} plays a prominent role in initiating and defining cardiac repolarization in humans and larger mammalian species. In humans, the pore forming portion of the channel that carries the I_{Kr} current is encoded by the *hERG* gene (the acronym for *human ether-a-go-go related gene*, also known as KCNH2 or Kv 11.1 9) [103, 104]. Further evidence that the hERG channel is involved in drug-induced delayed repolarization is provided by the finding that mutations of the hERG gene on chromosome 7 are associated with the congenital long QT2 syndrome [105]. Thus, block of hERG current has become an accepted surrogate marker for QT interval prolongation and a risk factor for cardiac proarrhythmia. Indeed, the evaluation of hERG current block plays a pivotal role in the nonclinical evaluation of potential proarrhythmic risk and is suggested in the ICH S7B guidance [11]. While I_{Kr} can be recorded in isolated cardiac myocytes, it is difficult to measure due to its relatively small amplitude and the presence of other time- and voltage-dependent currents that overlap the smaller I_{Kr} current. Thus, drug effects on this current are more easily assessed using human embryonic kidney (HEK) or Chinese hamster ovary (CHO) cells stably transfected with hERG [106, 107]. While transiently transfected *Xenopus* oocytes have been used, concentration–response relationships obtained with this preparation may be confounded and difficult to interpret due to drug accumulation into the yolk sac, thereby reducing drug concentrations at the vestibule of the hERG channel on the intracellular sarcolemmal surface [108].

hERG current is most easily assessed using voltage clamp techniques in which the transmembrane potential is controlled (or clamped) and changes in ionic current flowing across the cell membrane are recorded (Fig. 18.1). Voltage-dependent hERG channels are activated upon depolarization and conduct outward (repolarizing) current during each action potential. This current reflects the flow of K^+ ions through hERG channels, mimicking repolarizing I_{Kr} current flowing in native cardiac myocytes. Drug effects on hERG current are usually assessed from the reductions in the tail current amplitude (measured upon repolarization); tail currents reflect the deactivation (or decay) of hERG current activated by the preceding depolarizing (activating) voltage pulse. Voltage clamp protocols resembling square waves are usually used, although repolarizing ramp clamp pulses as well as waveforms resembling the cardiac action potential have been used when evaluating hERG current block. While no clamp protocol appears to provide significant advantages, a combined step-ramp pattern may provide a conservative estimate of hERG inhibition within a diverse panel of drugs [109].

While prior electrophysiologic experiments have employed traditional patch clamp techniques, the advent of planar patch methods (coupled with automation) holds the promise for greater throughput for functional current assays [110]. This technique allows for the simultaneous recording of currents from individual cells with gigaohm seals from multiple wells. However, issues related to the use of physiologic temperatures and validation of drug concentrations in experimental wells need to be addressed to secure this technology as a definitive safety pharmacology assay.

It is preferable to evaluate effects on hERG current at physiologic temperatures, as reducing the temperature from 35–37 °C to room temperature (22 °C) has been shown to affect potency of block for six of fifteen compounds in one experimental series (less potent for four of the six compounds, with greatest change being approximately sevenfold) [109, 112]. It is also recommended that bath concentrations be measured, as drug levels may be significantly less than anticipated due to adsorption to perfusion apparatus [11, 113].

IC_{50} values for test substance block derived from hERG current studies can be compared with anticipated clinical exposures in order to provide an assessment of relative risk. It is also important to test known hERG-blocking comparator compounds to benchmark the sensitivity of the assay. Redfern and colleagues [114] have suggested that for most compounds a 30-fold margin between hERG IC_{50} values and free C_{max} may provide an acceptable safety margin in humans for TdeP with a low risk of false positives, recognizing that drug effects on other cardiac channels as well as potential benefits of the test agent must also be considered.

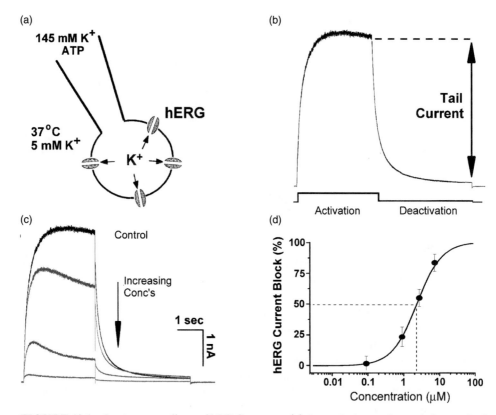

FIGURE 18.1   *In vitro* recordings of hERG current. (a) A patch clamp electrode is attached to cell stably transfected with hERG gene and expressing I_{Kr}. Typically, a glass electrode is applied to the cell membrane, forming a high resistance gigaohm seal essential for high fidelity current recordings. A pulse of suction is then applied to rupture the cell membrane under the electrode tip, providing electrical access to the cell interior through the pipette solution equilibrating with the cytoplasm. High K^+ concentrations in the cell and pipette solutions provide the driving force for outward (repolarizing) current flow. Circuitry connected with the pipette is used to control the membrane potential and record the transmembrane current in response to changes in membrane potential. (b) Records of voltage-dependent hERG current activated upon depolarization and deactivated upon repolarization. The declining outward current upon repolarization (referred to as tail current) reflects the deactivation of hERG channels opened during the prior depolarizing test pulse. A square wave voltage clamp protocol is shown in this example; typical depolarizing pulses range near 0 mV, with tail current measured near –50 mV. (c) Recordings of drug-induced block of hERG current obtained with increasing concentrations of a hERG blocking agent. While activating and tail currents are both reduced, the reduced amplitude of tail current (downward arrow) is typically measured to evaluate hERG current block. (d) IC_{50} values characterizing potency of hERG current block derived from Hill equation fit to experimental data. (From Ref. 111.)

Binding studies utilizing high-affinity radiolabeled ligands [115], atomic absorption measurement of rubidium efflux [116], and fluorescence detection of voltage-sensitive dyes [117] are used in initial screening for hERG channel block. However, these assays often demonstrate lesser sensitivity and do not directly measure functional current. Consequently, they are generally used as higher throughput screening assays to prioritize advancing candidates earlier in drug discovery rather than to provide a final evaluation of hERG channel inhibition liability.

It is also recognized that some drugs (such as fluoxetine and verapamil) are relatively potent hERG blockers, yet are not typically associated with either delayed repolarization or torsades de pointes arrhythmias. This apparent discrepancy is explained by concomitant block of the inwardly directed L-type cardiac calcium current that may mitigate the consequences of reduced hERG current [118, 119]. In such cases, changes in the action potential obtained with repolarization assays may be used to infer additional counterbalancing drug effects (see below). Drug effects on multiple cardiac ion channels (termed multichannel block) [120] emphasize the fact that hERG represents only one of multiple cardiac ionic currents that may influence cardiac repolarization.

HERG Trafficking   Recent reports have suggested that a minority of drugs may delay cardiac repolarization and predispose to TdeP not by direct block of hERG current, but rather by preventing the normal processing and cellular trafficking of the nascent hERG channel protein from the endoplasmic reticulum and reducing the surface membrane expression of functional channels. Such drug candidates may include the cancer chemotherapeutic drug arsenic trioxide [121, 122] and the antiprotozoal drug pentamidine [123, 124]. Other "conventional" hERG channel blocking drugs may also carry an additional risk of hERG trafficking inhibition [125], which may occur over the course of hours (rather than minutes as typically associated with simple block of hERG current). Further studies are necessary to define the role of assays evaluating indirect effects of drugs on ion channel protein trafficking and expression in preclinical screening.

Evaluation of Drug Effects on Other Cardiac Ion Channels   Studies of congenital long QT syndromes have also linked reduction of slowly activating repolarizing current (I_{Ks}, carried by KVLQT1/minK channels) or defective inactivation of the inwardly directed sodium current (SCN5A) to torsades de pointes proarrhythmia (long QT syndromes 1 and 3, respectively) [126, 127]. While screening of drug effects on these additional channels may be prudent, such studies are not recommended in present guidelines [11], possibly due to the likely limited number of drugs affecting these channels compared to hERG. The presumption of a testing strategy for new molecule testing is that drug-related effects on these other channels will be revealed in the *in vivo* cardiovascular studies as described in Section 18.3.

18.4.3   Repolarization (APD) Assays

I_{Kr} current (carried by hERG channels) represents only one of multiple ionic currents that are involved in cardiac repolarization. Indeed, it is the complex interplay of multiple ionic currents, pumps, and exchangers that is responsible for the generation of the action potential. Figure 18.2a illustrates a ventricular action potential—a recording of transmembrane potential versus time. From a resting membrane more negative than −80 mV, stimulation elicits a rapid upstroke (termed phase 0), with an amplitude greater than 100 mV. Repolarization ensues, consisting of three sequential phases: phase 1 represents rapid repolarization that occurs immediately following the upstroke, phase 2 defines the action potential plateau sustained by the inward

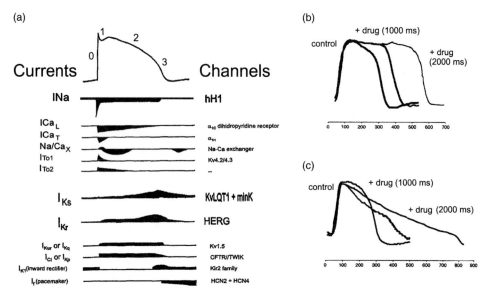

FIGURE 18.2   Repolarization assays. (a) The upper traces show a representative intracellular action potential with the phases of the action potential (0–3) labeled. Shown below are the currents that activate and inactivate during the action potential; currents are labeled on left, with corresponding channels indicated on right. Inward currents are represented by downward deflections, while outward currents are shown as upward deflections. Mutations of three channels linked to congenital long QT syndromes (I_{Na}, I_{Ks}, and I_{Kr}) are shown in bold letters. (Adapted from Ref. 243). (b, c) Monophasic action potential recordings from left ventricular epicardium of a rabbit heart Langendorff preparation. Panel (b) demonstrates drug-induced action potential prolongation without triangulation. Reverse use-dependent effects of this drug are evident, with greater prolongation at the slower (2000 ms) versus more rapid (1000 ms) pacing cycle length. Panel (c) demonstrates triangulation of the action potential with another drug; greater triangulation is evident at the slower stimulation rate. See text for further discussion. (Adapted from Ref. 130.)

calcium current, and phase 3 delineates terminal repolarization, where increasing outward currents contributed by I_{Kr}, I_{Ks}, and I_{K1} return the membrane potential to the resting potential. Reduction of these outward currents (or increased inward current through I_{Na}) reduces the "repolarization reserve" of the myocardium, predisposing to proarrhythmia [128].

Transmembrane action potentials are recorded using sharp or patch microelectrodes (the former for tissues or isolated cardiac myocytes, the latter primarily for cardiac myocytes) that provide intracellular access and allow for voltage measurements across the cell membrane (between the cell interior and a reference electrode in the recording chamber). These action potentials arise from negative potentials and have upstrokes that exceed 0 mV, with amplitudes typically greater than 100 mV.

It is also possible to record action potentials from the myocardial surface using two blunt extracellular electrodes, with one electrode depolarizing or injuring the underlying myocardium, and the second electrode recording extracellular voltages from the uninjured extracellular surface. Such recordings are termed monophasic action potentials (MAPs) [129]. MAPs are smaller in amplitude than transmembrane action potentials and do not exceed 0 mV (hence the term monophasic). Typically recorded from epicardial or endocardial surfaces, MAPs may be subject to greater motion artifacts than intracellular recordings. While MAPs represent the general time course of repolarization, they cannot be used to evaluate changes in the resting membrane potential or upstroke characteristics (the latter reflecting changes in fast inward sodium current). MAPs may be recorded from isolated Langendorff hearts, but also from intact anesthetized animals as noted in Section 18.3.

The lower portion of Fig. 18.2a displays the prominent currents involved in generating a ventricular action potential. Inward, depolarizing currents (grouped toward the top) are indicated by downward deflections, while outward, repolarizing currents (grouped toward the bottom) are indicated by upward deflections. The complexity is evident. Of particular note is the time course of activation of the outward repolarizing current I_{Kr} (hERG) during phase 2 to initiate terminal repolarizaiton of the action potential. Variations in the relative contributions of different currents are responsible for regional heterogeneity of the action potential configuration and duration across the ventricular wall. These differences also contribute to the electrical gradient responsible for the T wave of the electrocardiogram. Furthermore, differences in the configuration and duration of the action potential affect the extent of drug-induced action potential prolongation recorded from different regions of the myocardium (e.g., drug-induced delayed repolarization is typically greatest in Purkinje fibers and ventricular midmyocardium compared to epicardium or endocardium during slow stimulation) [131, 132]. Thus, the selection of tissues needs to be taken into consideration when evaluating drug effects on repolarization, and effects of known standards should be included to benchmark the sensitivity of the preparation. Selection of species is also important; for example, I_{Kr} current contributes minimally to repolarization in mouse and rat ventricular myocardium [133–136] and would be poor choices to use to detect drugs that reduced I_{Kr}. As in all scientific studies, drug effects on repolarization are most readily interpreted when parallel, vehicle-control studies demonstrate no effects on the action potential configuration over time.

Various indices of repolarization have been used to predict delayed repolarization and increased risk of torsades de pointes. Based on the link between QT interval prolongation and TdeP, prolongation of the action potential duration (APD) has been used as a measure of proarrhythmia risk. This measure is typically reported as APD_{90}, the time required for 90% repolarization. Most drugs that block I_{Kr} also demonstrate reverse use dependence, defined as greater drug-induced prolongation of the action potential at slower versus more rapid stimulation rates. An abnormal form of triggered electrical activity (termed early afterdepolarizations, or EADs) may be observed in repolarization assays during slow stimulation and the presence of QT prolonging drugs. Early afterdepolarizations are single or multiple premature depolarizations that arise during the action potential plateau. This form of triggered activity has been attributed to reactivation of inward L-type calcium current that arises during the action potential to initiate TdeP [137]. EADs are enhanced during slow stimulation and are thus considered harbingers of proarrhythmia.

More recently, drug-induced changes in the action potential configuration from a "rectangular" shape to a more triangular-shaped configuration (termed triangulation) have been implicated in proarrhythmia risk [130]. Measured as either the difference in time between 30% and 90% repolarization (or alternatively, normalized using the ratio of these values), triangulation may increase the risk of proarrhythmia in the absence of changes in the action potential duration for some drugs [130, 138, 139]; a notable exception to this rule is the hERG and calcium channel blocking drug verapamil. Other electrophysiologic indices linked to proarrhythmia risk, but not necessarily linked to altered repolarization or TdeP, may also be gleaned from intracellular recordings of the action potential; these include effects on upstroke (related to changes in conduction velocity) and changes in the resting membrane potential (related to block of the inwardly rectifying potassium current I_{K1}). Proarrhythmia associated with congenital short QT intervals has been described, linked to mutations in I_{Kr}, I_{Ks}, and I_{K1} channels [140]. Further work is necessary to evaluate the proarrhythmic risk of drugs that may mimic the short QT syndrome, and the utility of repolarization assays to evaluate clinical risk.

18.4.4   Isolated Tissue or Cell Preparations Used for Repolarization Studies

Repolarization studies have been conducted on a wide variety of isolated tissues employing intracellular recording techniques that record transmembrane potential. The mechanistic interpretation of repolarization assays may be complex, due to the multiple ionic currents contributing to the genesis of the action potential. The following sections discuss some repolarization assays in order of ascending level of complexity and integration.

Isolated Cardiac Myocytes   The cardiac myocyte represents the smallest integrated unit to evaluate ventricular repolarization. In contrast to tissues, intracellular recordings from myocytes can be attained using either sharp microelectrodes or patch pipettes. Due to intracellular dialysis associated with traditional patch pipettes, the action potential may be directly altered by the technique used, making interpretation of drug effects more difficult; this concern can be minimized through the use of the perforated patch technique [141]. Time to attain steady-state effects of drugs with isolated myocytes is typically more rapid than with superfused syncytial preparations due to diffusional barriers present in isolated tissues. However, isolated myocytes also demonstrate greater beat-to-beat variability compared to syncytial preparations, an effect attributable to a loss of cell-to-cell coupling in isolated myocytes [142]. Attention to the anatomical origin of isolated myocytes, beat-to-beat variability, as well as time and vehicle effects are necessary to properly interpret the results of repolarization assays using isolated cellular preparations. Representative repolarization studies are provided by Refs. 143–146.

Purkinje Fibers and Papillary Muscles   Purkinje fibers and papillary muscles are established, well-characterized preparations that have been widely used for electrophysiologic studies; intracellular recordings are typically obtained from these superfused preparations (see earlier discussion). Purkinje fibers are specialized conducting tissue in the ventricle. In ungulates and most mammals, fibers are free running across the ventricular surface, allowing for easy harvesting of tissues. In addition, paucity of contractile elements makes fiber impalement easy to maintain. Studies have suggested that the assay using Purkinje fibers is able to detect most drugs linked to delayed repolarization and proarrhythmia [147]. Furthermore, the Purkinje fiber assay using fibers harvested from rabbits may be more sensitive than fibers harvested from dogs [147, 148]. Some drugs (such as cisapride) elicit bell-shaped concentration–response curves, with low to intermediate concentrations eliciting prolongation, and higher concentrations eliciting lesser (or shortening) of the APD [146, 147]; these studies highlight the complexity of effects on cardiac repolarization and the need to evaluate concentration–response curves in the context of clinical exposures. For drugs highly plasma protein bound, calculated free concentrations have been used during *in vitro* studies to approximate clinical exposures. However, this approach may not be realistic, particularly if the drug is readily exchanged from plasma into the myocardium, where it may accumulate. It is possible to superfuse tissues *in vitro* with solutions containing plasma proteins to more closely approximate drug exposures *in vitro*.

Guinea pig papillary muscles have also been used to evaluate drug effects on cardiac electrical activity [149]. These preparations are typically thinner than other cardiac muscle preparations, minimizing anoxia that may occur in the center of larger syncytial preparations during bath superfusion. Studies suggest a strong correlation between hERG channel blockade and APD prolongation for a validation dataset of 21 compounds [150].

Ventricular "Wedge" Preparations   Wedge preparations are created from arterially perfused, tangentially sliced transmural sections of ventricular free wall, providing exposed transmural surfaces for electrode impalements. This preparation allows for a comparison of drug effects from different regions of the myocardium (e.g., epicardium, midmyocardium, and endocardium of the left ventricular freewall of canine or rabbit [151, 152]. Due to the vigorous activity of these contracting preparations, flexibly mounted ("floating") microelectrodes are typically used to transiently record transmembrane potentials. Wedge preparations allow for the evaluation of delayed repolarization and dispersion of repolarization between myocardial regions—factors implicated in both the genesis of TdeP as well as waveforms resembling TdeP from ECG-like traces [153]. A recent study demonstrated that despite eliciting greater APD prolongation with azimilide compared to d,l-sotalol, EADs elicited by azimilide often failed to propagate transmurally, likely due to diminished dispersion with azimilide [154]. These preparations require a relatively long equilibration period and are challenging to maintain impalements, resulting in generally low throughput as screening assays.

18.4.5 Isolated Heart Preparations Used for Repolarization Studies

While it is difficult to obtain stable intracellular recordings from the epicardium of beating hearts, it is possible to measure changes in the action potential configuration recorded from isolated, perfused (Langendorff model) hearts using monophasic action potential techniques (see Section 18.4.3). Briefly, these preparations utilize hearts rapidly excised and retrogradely perfused through the aorta with buffered salt solutions [155]; the atrioventricular node is typically ablated to allow for pacing control of ventricular rate. However, the preparation may only be stable for a few hours, especially if protein-free perfusates are used and hearts become gradually edematous [155]. Using isolated rabbit hearts, Hondeghem and colleagues [130, 156, 157] evaluated the effects of numerous compounds (many linked to proarrhythmia and TdeP) on changes in the MAP recordings from the epicardium. Based on this model, they proposed a set of repolarization parameters useful in detecting proarrhythmic risk that included *T*riangulation, *R*everse use dependence, *I*nstability, and *D*ispersion (referred to by the acronym TRIaD). Instability is defined as the extent of beat-to-beat variation in the action potential duration and was considered the most potent predictor of proarrhythmia in rabbit heart [157]. Dispersion of repolarization can be measured using multiple MAP electrodes, or (alternatively) indirectly using multiple volume-conducted ECG recordings. In blinded experiments, the SCREENIT model (system) with its multiple parameter evaluation provided a predictive qualitative assessment of potential proarrhythmia risk [156]. At present, only one laboratory routinely performs this TRIaD assay for proarrhythmic drugs; independent validation would be beneficial. In general, TRIaD is most useful for prioritizing drugs according to their probable liability for proarrhythmia, and not necessarily predicting a plasma concentration at which this liability may be manifested in the clinic.

18.4.6 *In Vitro* ECG (QT) Assays

Additional *in vitro* assays have been described that focus primarily on QT interval changes recorded from acutely isolated Langendorff perfused hearts *in vitro*. Pseudo-ECGs may be recorded with electrodes placed within the organ chamber in a configuration resembling that of the traditional ECG lead system. Alternatively, electrogram recordings may be obtained from electrodes held lightly against the epicardium of left and right ventricles to generate bipolar transcardiac electrograms [158]. These approaches afford direct measures of changes in the duration of the QT interval as well as discriminating changes in the T wave configuration to further discern proarrhythmic risk (an area of continuing research). Epicardial and endocardial MAPs may also be recorded, providing further information on repolarization dispersion. It is also possible to control heart rate by external pacing, thus providing the ability to evaluate QT interval changes at selected heart rates (thus avoiding the use of correction formulas, see Section 18.3). A number of published studies have demonstrating the sensitivity and specificity of isolated perfused hearts from rabbit [159, 160] and guinea pig hearts [158] to drugs that prolong the QT interval clinically.

18.4.7 *In Vitro* Proarrhythmia Models

While the proarrhythmia model of methoxamine-treated female rabbit hearts are generally recognized as the more sensitive model, other recognized risk factors may also be applied to exaggerate drug effects (e.g., hypokalemia). Using these torsadogenic models, the relationship between the specificity and magnitude of drug effects with human proarrhythmia is uncertain. Hearts from smaller mammals (rats, mice) may be inappropriate for these studies due to the minimal role of I_{Kr}/hERG current in facilitating ventricular repolarization in these species as well as the rapid heart rates compared to humans.

18.4.8   Conclusions

Numerous *in vitro* models representing various levels of complexity and integration have been described that detect a drug's ability to affect and delay ventricular repolarization, a surrogate marker of proarrhythmia and TdeP. Block of hERG current remains a cornerstone in this collection of *in vitro* cardiac safety testing. It should be recognized that the sensitivity of this assay to detect a positive signal of QT risk is high, while specificity may not be sufficiently high to avoid false positives (e.g., drugs such as verapamil that produce multichannel blockade). Repolarization assays provide evidence of more integrated responses, providing further insights into multichannel block and torsadogenic effects such as EADs, instability, triangulation, and reverse use dependence, as well as the increased dispersion of repolarization resulting from a heterogeneous electrophysiologic substrate. Finally, ECG recordings from isolated hearts provide for evaluation of direct effects on the duration (and configuration) of the QT interval. The challenge of the present is to improve the ability of preclinical studies to predict torsadogenic risk through the use and balanced interpretation of multiple models. The challenge of the future is to develop preclinical models that provide further mechanistic insights into the initiation and perpetuation of TdeP, as a direct measure of torsadogenic risk.

18.5   RESPIRATORY SAFETY PHARMACOLOGY

18.5.1   Introduction

A study designed to evaluate the potential for new drugs to produce adverse effects on respiratory function must first determine whether the drug can produce a change in respiratory function and then establish whether this change is a liability. Such changes can result either from the primary or secondary pharmacological properties of a drug or from organ dysfunction resulting from its toxicological properties. Drugs from a variety of pharmacological classes are known to adversely affect the respiratory system (see Tables 18.1 and 18.2). Most drug-induced effects on the lung involve the parenchyma, or alveolar region, and produce changes involving alveolar proteinosis, interstitial and intra-alveolar edema, as well as interstitial pneumonitis and fibrosis [161, 162]. Drugs can also influence the pleura and airways, producing effects that include pleural effusion, pneumothorax, bronchospasm, and bronchiolitis obliterans [161, 162]. Drugs from at least 23 different pharmacological classes are also known to influence the neuromuscular control of pulmonary ventilation. Such drugs can be classified as respiratory stimulants or depressants and produce their effects primarily through mechanisms involving the central nervous system [163, 164], peripheral arterial chemoreceptors [165, 166], or pulmonary chemo- and mechanoreceptors [167].

Agencies that regulate drug testing and marketing have recognized the importance of conducting respiratory function safety studies. The International Conference on Harmonization (ICH), which represents regulatory agencies from the United States, Europe, and Japan, has established guidelines for the safety testing of pharmaceuticals on organ functions. This document (ICH S7A), entitled *Safety Pharmacology Studies for Human Pharmaceuticals*, states that the respiratory system is a vital organ system whose function is critical for life and, as such, must

TABLE 18.1 Drugs Known to Cause Bronchoconstriction and/or Pulmonary Injury

Chemotherapeutics	Analgesics
Carmustine (BCNU)	Heroin
Azathioprine	Morphine
Bleomycin	Methadone
Busulfan	Naloxone
Cyclophosphamide	Ethchlorvynol
Mitomycin	Propoxyphene
Nitrosoureas	Salicylates
Procarbazine	Cardiovascular drugs
Lomustine	Amiodarone
Methotrexate	ACE inhibitors
Cytosine arabinoside	Endothelin antagonists
Mercaptopurine	Anticoagulants
Procarbazine	Beta-blockers
Vinblastine	Fibrinolytics
Immunosuppressives	Dipyridamole
Cyclosporine	Protamine
Interleukin-2	Tocainide
Antivirals	Adenosine agonists
Interferons	Miscellaneous drugs
Antibiotics	Muscarinic (M_3) agonists
Ampicillin	Serotonin agonists
Amphotericin B	Histamine (H_1) agonists
Cephalosporines	Ergotamine
Cyclines	Bromocriptine
Furazolidone	Paracetamol
Nitrofurantoin	Polymyxins
Sulfasalazine	Myorelaxants
Sulfonamides	Dantrolene
Pentamidine	Hydrochlorothiazide
Anti-inflammatories	Methylsergide
Gold salts	Oral contraceptives
NSAIDs	Tocolytic agents
Penicillamine	Tricyclics
Beclomethasone	Tazanolast
Acetylsalicyclic acid	

be evaluated in safety pharmacology studies. As part of the core battery of safety pharmacology studies, the ICH guideline requires that the effect of drugs on respiratory function be evaluated prior to first human administration.

The objective of this section is to provide a brief overview of the functional disorders of the respiratory system and to present the strategy and techniques considered to be most appropriate for detecting and characterizing drug-induced respiratory disorders in nonclinical safety studies.

TABLE 18.2   Drugs Known to Influence Ventilatory Control

Depressants	Tranquilizers/analgesics
Inhaled anesthetics	Chlorpromazine
Aspartic acid analogues	Rompum (xylazine)
Barbiturates	Nalorphine
Benzodiazepines	Antibiotics
Diazepam	Macrolides
Temazapan	Aminoglycosides
Flunitrazepam	Endothelins
Chlordiazepoxide	Nitric oxide synthase inhibitors
Serotonin analogues	Stimulants
Methoxy(dimethyl)tryptamine	Alkaloids
Dopamine analogues	Nicotine
Apomorphine	Lobeline
Adenosine analogues	Piperidine
2-Chloroadenosine	Xanthine analogues
R-Phenylisopropyl-adenosine (R-PIA)	Theophylline
N-ethylcarboxamide (NECA)	Caffeine
β-Adrenergic antagonists	Theobromine
Timolol maleate	Analeptics
GABA analogues	Doxapram
Muscimol	Salicylates
Baclofen	Progesterone analogs
Calcium channel blockers	Almitrine
Daurisoline	Glycine analogues
Antimalarials	Strychnine
Chloroquine	GABA antagonists
Opiates	Picrotoxin
Morphine	Bicuculline
Codeine	Serotonin synthesis inhibitors
Methadone	ρ 18-Chlorophenylalanine
Meperidine	Reserpine
Phenazocine	
Anticholinergics	
M_1 selective	
M_2 selective	

18.5.2   Functional Disorders of the Respiratory System

The respiratory system can be divided functionally into a pumping apparatus and a gas exchange unit. The pumping apparatus includes those components of the nervous and muscular systems that are responsible for generating and regulating breathing patterns, whereas the gas exchange unit consists of the lung with its associated airways, alveoli, and interstitial area that contains blood and lymph vessels and an elastic fibrous network.

Pumping Apparatus   The pumping apparatus of the respiratory system is responsible for generating and regulating the pleural pressures needed to inflate and deflate the lung. Normal gas exchange between the lung and blood requires breathing patterns that ensure appropriate alveolar ventilation. Ventilatory disorders that alter alveolar ventilation are defined as hypoventilation or hyperventilation syndromes. Hypoventilation is defined as an increase in the partial pressure of arterial CO_2 ($Paco_2$) above normal limits and can result in acidosis, pulmonary hypertension, congestive heart failure, headache, and/or disturbed sleep [168]. Hyperventilation is defined as a decrease in $Paco_2$ below normal limits and can result in alkalosis, syncope, epileptic attacks, reduced cardiac output, and/or muscle weakness [169, 170].

Mechanisms responsible for ventilatory disorders may involve muscle and/or neural dysfunction. Those dysfunctions involving the nervous system are categorized as either central or peripheral. Central mechanisms involve the neurological components of the pumping apparatus that are located within the central nervous system and include the medullary central pattern generator (CPG) and the integration centers that regulate the output of the CPG. Integration centers are located in the medulla, pons, hypothalamus, and cortex of the brain [171]. The major neurological inputs from the peripheral nervous system that influence the CPG are arterial chemoreceptors [171] and respiratory tract chemo- and mechanoreceptors [161]. Drugs can stimulate or depress ventilation by selective interaction with the central nervous system [163, 164, 172], arterial chemoreceptors [165, 166], and/or espiratory tract chemo- and mechanoreceptors [161].

Gas Exchange Unit   The primary function of the respiratory system is the exchange of gases (O_2 and CO_2) between the environment and blood. Functional disorders of the respiratory system are defined, therefore, as changes in the respiratory system that reduce the efficiency of gas exchange. Airway narrowing or blockade can reduce the efficiency of gas exchange by decreasing or preventing airflow between the upper or central airways and the alveoli. Functional changes of this type are called obstructive disorders [173]. Airway narrowing can result from airway smooth muscle contraction or hypertrophy, accumulation of mucus or edema fluid in the airway, luminal cell hyperplasia, or breakdown in elastic support tissue [174]. An obstructive disorder also creates a resistive load during ventilation and, by increasing the work of breathing, can lead to respiratory fatigue and failure [175].

A reduction in the normal elasticity, or a "stiffening," of the lung increases the work (or pressure) required to expand the lung. This decrease in lung compliance generally produces a rapid shallow breathing pattern [175], which can reduce ventilatory efficiency by lowering alveolar ventilation and, ultimately, can lead to respiratory fatigue and failure [174]. Functional changes of this type are called restrictive disorders and can result from changes involving interstitial thickening due to edema, hemorrhage, cellular infiltration, or fibrosis, or from intra-alveolar changes caused by edema, cellular infiltration, or abnormal surfactant production [176]. These interstitial and intra-alveolar changes also affect lung function by increasing the diffusion barrier for CO_2 and O_2 between the pulmonary blood vessels and the alveolar surface [176].

18.5.3   Techniques for Measuring Changes in Respiratory Function

Ventilatory Disorders   A plethysmograph chamber or facemask with a pneumotachometer is generally used to measure ventilatory patterns in humans and conscious animal models. Plethysmograph chambers that most accurately measure ventilatory patterns are designed to directly monitor lung volume changes or airflows generated by thoracic movements. Such chambers isolate openings to the upper airways (mouth and nose) from the thorax and are referred to as "head-out" or "head-enclosed" chambers (Fig. 18.3). The pressure changes in these chambers are a direct measure of lung airflow and, consequently, can accurately measure both the duration and volume of each breath (Fig. 18.4). These measurements are required for determining the various parameters needed to characterize breathing patterns (see below). Whole body (barometric) plethysmograph chambers are often used to monitor ventilatory patterns and offer the advantage that the subject does not have to be restrained [177] (Fig. 18.5b). This method, however, is limited in that the volume of each breath is determined indirectly from the relatively minor increase in chamber pressure resulting from the expansion of inhaled gases due to a decrease in intrapulmonary pressure and to increases in intrapulmonary temperature and humidity. Furthermore, the reliability of this estimated tidal volume is rather low since it is highly dependent on a number of variables including breathing rate and pattern, chamber temperature and humidity, and nasal air temperature [178]. Altering these variables can produce significant effects. For example, increasing the breathing rate of a rat from 40 to 70 breaths per minute caused an underestimation of actual tidal volume by up to 30% [178]. Other indirect methods for estimating lung volume changes in animal models include the use of induction, bioimpedence, or sonomicrometry. These methods utilize induction coils, biopotential electrodes, or piezoelectric crystals either placed in a strap on the skin surface or implanted subcutaneously to measure the linear expansion of the thorax and abdomen during breathing. These methods can accurately measure respiratory rate; however, they are limited in that lung volume is generally estimated from a single dimensional measurement. As such, these estimated volume measurements are highly dependent of body position (e.g., standing, sitting, or recumbent), which can alter the three-

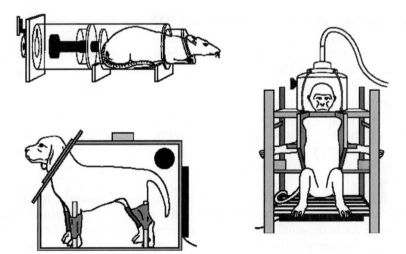

FIGURE 18.3 Plethysmograph chambers for the direct measurement of ventilatory parameters. The rat and dog are in "head-out" chambers, while the monkey is in a "head-enclosed" chamber. For all chambers, an airtight seal is made around the neck using a rubber collar.

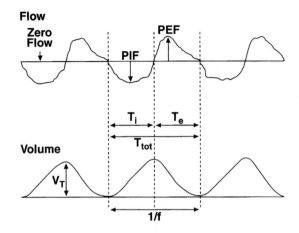

Functional Endpoints

V_E -   Minute Volume (V_T x f)

f   -   Breathing Rate

V_T -   Tidal Volume

PIF   -   Peak Inspiratory Flow

PEF   -   Peak Expiratory Flow

FIT   -   Fractional Inspiratory Time $\dfrac{(T_i)}{(T_{tot})}$

FIGURE 18.4   Tracings of lung airflow and lung volume changes during spontaneous breathing in a conscious rat. Airflow was measured directly using a "head-out" plethysmograph chamber. The functional endpoints are automatically calculated for each breath using an analog/digital converter and a data acquisition and analysis software system.

dimensional shape of the thorax or abdomen [179]. The accuracy and reliability of these methods have not yet been demonstrated in animal models.

Because most anesthetics, analgesics, and sedatives alter ventilatory reflexes and drive, studies evaluating the effects of drugs on ventilation should use conscious animals. It is also essential that animals be appropriately acclimated to the experimental apparatus to ensure normal (resting) ventilatory patterns. Proper characterization of a breathing pattern must include measurements of respiratory rate, tidal volume, and minute volume. Other parameters such as inspiratory flow (peak or mean), expiratory flow (peak or mean), inspiratory time, expiratory time, and total breath time can be used to help define mechanisms of ventilatory change (Fig. 18.4).

Respiratory rate, tidal volume, and minute volume are essential measurements since normal ventilation requires that the pumping apparatus provide both adequate total pulmonary ventilation (minute volume) and the appropriate depth (tidal volume) and frequency of breathing. The depth and frequency of breathing required for alveolar ventilation are determined primarily by the anatomic dead space of the lung. In general, a rapid shallow breathing pattern (tachypnea) is less efficient than a slower deeper breathing pattern that achieves the same minute volume. Thus, any

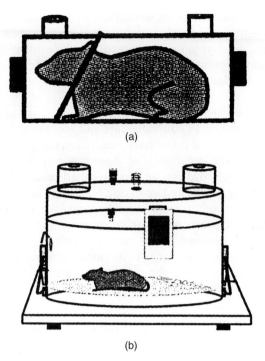

(a)

(b)

FIGURE 18.5 Plethysmograph chambers for obtaining indirect measures of airway resistance: (a) a dual-chamber (Pennock box) that separates the head and thorax into two separate compartments; (b) a whole-body (barometric) chamber.

change in minute volume, tidal volume, or the rate of breathing can influence the efficiency of ventilation [175].

An additional reason for measuring both respiratory rate and tidal volume is that these parameters are independently controlled [171] and can be selectively altered by drugs. Thus, monitoring changes in tidal volume or respiratory rate alone cannot be used to evaluate drug-induced effects on pulmonary ventilation. For example, the phosphodiesterase inhibitor and adenosine antagonist theophylline increases minute volume by increasing tidal volume without affecting respiratory rate [180], whereas the opioid morphine depresses minute volume by reducing respiratory rate without affecting tidal volume [181, 182]. Other drugs such as adenosine agonists depress respiratory rate but have no effect on minute volume since there is a compensatory increase in tidal volume [181].

The inspiratory and expiratory phases of individual breaths are also independently controlled [171] and, by characterizing changes in these parameters, mechanisms responsible for ventilatory changes can be determined. Thus, by measuring changes in the airflow rate and duration of each of these phases, mechanisms responsible for changes in tidal volume or respiratory rate can be identified [175]. For example, a selective decrease in airflow during inspiration (the active phase) is generally indicative of a decrease in respiratory drive, whereas a selective decrease in airflow during expiration (the passive phase) is generally indicative of an obstructive disorder. Furthermore, a change in the ratio of inspiratory to expiratory time can be used to differentiate effects on stretch and irritant pulmonary receptors [171]. The examples presented above clearly demonstrate that measurements of both respiratory rate and tidal volume are critical for the evaluation of drug-induced effects on pulmonary ventilation and that airflow and time measurements of individual breaths are needed to help define mechanisms of change in ventilatory control.

Moderate to marked changes in pulmonary ventilation can result in hypo- or hyperventilation syndromes. In conscious rats and monkeys, decreases of approximately 30% or greater in total pulmonary ventilation can produce hypoventilation [181, 183]. To establish the occurrence of these syndromes, $Paco_2$ is measured. In humans and large animals, this can be accomplished readily by collecting arterial blood with a catheter or needle and analyzing for $Paco_2$ using a blood gas analyzer. In conscious rodents (or other small animals), however, obtaining arterial blood samples by needle puncture or catheterization is generally disruptive of normal breathing patterns and often invalidates the measurement. An alternative and noninvasive method for monitoring $Paco_2$ is the measurement of peak expired (end-tidal) CO_2 concentrations. This technique has been used successfully in humans [184], pigs [185], and conscious rats [181].

Obstructive Disorders

Forced Maneuvers   An obstructive disorder is defined functionally by the American Thoracic Society (ATS) as "a disproportionate reduction of maximum airflow from the lung with respect to the maximum volume that can be displaced from the lung" [186]. In human clinical studies, obstructive disorders are detected by measuring maximum (forced) expiratory airflows following maximal inspiration. Spirometry is used to measure volume and flow changes, and the functional endpoints include forced expiratory volume after 1 second (FEV1), peak expiratory flow (PEF), forced expiratory flows at 25 and 75% of expired volume ($FEF_{25\%}$ and $FEF_{75\%}$), mean mid-expiratory flow (MMEF) and total expired gas volume or forced vital capacity (FVC). Decreases in FEV_1, PEF, and $FEF_{25\%}$ indicate central (or large) airway narrowing, while $FEF_{75\%}$ and MMEF are used to detect peripheral (or small) airway narrowing [186]. Since airflow is dependent on the starting volume, the flow parameters are normalized to FVC. A disproportionate reduction in flow relative to lung volume distinguishes an obstructive from a restrictive disorder [186].

Experimental systems that can simulate the flow–volume maneuver performed by humans have been developed for use in animals. A pressure panel has been developed that controls lung inflation and deflation rates of anesthetized animals (Buxco Electronics, Inc., Sharon, CT). The animal's lung is inflated to a maximum volume or inspiratory capacity (IC), as determined by the inflation pressure (generally 30 cm H_2O), and then is rapidly deflated by switching to a vacuum reservoir (generally at −50 cm H_2O) using a solenoid valve. A plethysmograph chamber is required to measure lung volume and airflow changes, and a pressure-sensitive catheter is required to measure airway or transpulmonary (i.e., airway pressure – pleural pressure) pressure changes. Details of the equipment used for conducting this maneuver in rats and dogs have been described [187, 188]. Analyzers are also available (Buxco Electronics, Inc.) that will calculate IC, FVC, FEV, PEF, MMEF, and FEF values for each flow–volume maneuver. Evaluating obstructive disorders in animals using the flow–volume maneuver offers a high degree of sensitivity since changes are measured at maximum attainable flow rates and lung volumes. In addition, this procedure provides functional endpoints similar to human measurements. The disadvantages of this procedure are that it generally requires an anesthetized/paralyzed animal and is limited to a single time point measurement. The latter limitation excludes this as a procedure for measuring acute dynamic changes in lung airflow as might occur following administration of a drug given intravenously or by inhalation.

Dynamic Measurements—Direct   Drug-induced lung airflow disorders can also be evaluated in animal models by measuring total pulmonary resistance or conductance during tidal breathing or mechanical ventilation (i.e., dynamically) (Fig. 18.6). Total pulmonary resistance defines the change in pleural, airway, or transpulmonary pressure (ΔP) required to produce a defined change in lung airflow (ΔF) and is calculated as $\Delta P/\Delta F$, while conductance is calculated as $\Delta F/\Delta P$. To determine dynamic resistance or conductance, the ΔP and ΔF are measured for each breath at the same lung volume during inspiration and expiration (usually between 50% and 70% of tidal volume). By selecting isovolumetric points, the dependence of ΔP on the elastic component of the lung is removed, leaving ΔP dependent on resistance to the flow of gas in the airways. This procedure requires the use of a plethysmograph chamber

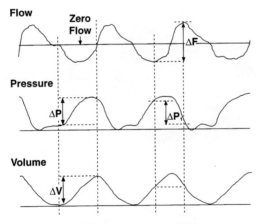

Functional Endpoints

Dynamic Compliance $= \dfrac{\Delta V}{\Delta P}$ (At zero flow points)

Dynamic Resistance $= \dfrac{\Delta P_1}{\Delta F}$ (At isovolume points)

Dynamic Conductance $= \dfrac{\Delta F}{\Delta P_1}$ (At isovolume points)

FIGURE 18.6 Tracings of lung airflow, transpulmonary pressure, and lung volume changes during spontaneous breathing in a rat. Airflow was measured directly using a "head-out" plethysmograph chamber, while pleural pressure was measured using a pressure-sensitive catheter placed into the esophagus within the thoracic cavity. The functional endpoints are automatically calculated for each breath using an analog/digital converter and a data acquisition and analysis software system.

or facemask with pneumotachometer for volume and flow measurements, and a pressure-sensitive catheter for the measurement of pleural, airway, or transpulmonary pressure (Fig. 18.6). The methods for conducting these measurements have been established in guinea pigs [189], rats [190], and dogs [191].

Because dynamic measurements of airflow resistance in a spontaneously breathing animal require a pressure-sensitive catheter to be inserted into the esophagus or pleural cavity, animals are generally anesthetized and the measurements are collected over a period of minutes to hours. Attempts to develop a method for measuring pleural pressure chronically in conscious animals have involved surgical implantation of pressure-sensitive catheters directly into the pleural cavity. The success of these techniques has been limited by lung damage [189] and/or tissue growth and encapsulation of the pressure-sensitive catheter with a damping or loss of the signal [189, 192, 193]. To overcome these limitations, Murphy et al. [194, 195] developed a novel surgical procedure for placement of a pressure-sensitive catheter beneath the pleural surface. The catheter (attached to a radiotelemetry transmitter) is surgically implanted beneath the serosal layer of the esophagus within the thoracic cavity (Fig. 18.7). Using this technique, the pleural pressure changes have remained constant for at least 1 year in rats and 2 years in monkeys following surgery (personal observation). By combining this procedure with the use of a plethysmograph chamber, dynamic measurements of lung airflow resistance can

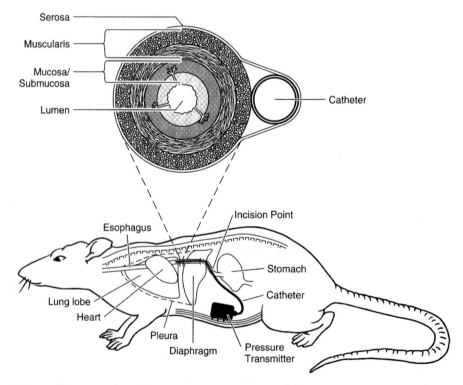

FIGURE 18.7   Drawing of a rat showing placement of the pressure-sensitive subpleural catheter and radiotelemetry transmitter for chronic measurement of pleural pressure in conscious animals. The enlargement is a cross section through the esophagus showing the position of the catheter between the serosal and muscularis layers.

be obtained repeatedly and chronically in conscious animals (Fig. 18.3). This procedure has been used successfully in rats [194], monkeys [195], and dogs (personal experience, data not published).

Dynamic Measurements—Indirect   Noninvasive procedures have been developed that can detect changes in resistance to lung airflow indirectly in conscious animals by measuring changes in airflow patterns. A plethysmograph chamber that separates the head and trunk into separate compartments has been used to measure the time delay between thoracic and nasal airflows in a spontaneously breathing animal [196] (Fig. 18.5a). A prolongation of this delay is related to the product of airway resistance and thoracic gas volume (specific airway resistance). The primary limitation of this procedure is that it is an indirect measure of airway resistance with the estimated value (specific airway resistance) dependent on a number of variables including respiratory rate, lung volume, and the temperature and humidity differences in the head and trunk chambers. Furthermore, the reliability of specific airway resistance measurements appears to decrease as resistance to lung airflow increases [196].

A procedure using barometric whole-body plethysmography has been developed for noninvasively detecting changes in the resistance to lung airflow of conscious, nonrestrained animals [197] (Fig. 18.5b). Estimated airway resistance (airway responsiveness) is determined for each breath by calculating an expiratory pause, which is dependent on differences in peak inspiratory and expiratory flows, and the duration of the early and late phases of expiration. This measurement is not influenced significantly by changes in respiratory rate and lung volume and appears to be a reliable method for measuring acute, severe bronchoconstriction. However, the scientific validity of this method has been challenged [198]. Furthermore, the method appears to be less sensitive than direct measurements of lung airflow resistance [197], false-positive results can occur for drugs that alter flow patterns by influencing respiratory drive, and the value of this procedure for chronic (repeated) measurements of mild to moderate lung airflow changes has yet to be established.

Restrictive Disorders   A restrictive disorder is defined functionally either as a reduction in total lung capacity (TLC) or as a decrease in lung compliance [176, 186, 199]. In human clinical studies, TLC is determined either by using a gas dilution technique or by combining the volumes obtained for inspiratory capacity (IC) and functional residual capacity (FRC) [200]. IC is the increase in volume of gas in the lung following inflation from resting expiration to maximum inspiration and is measured using spirometry. FRC is the volume of gas remaining in the lung at resting expiration and is obtained by a maneuver that involves breathing against an occluded airway at resting expiration and recording the pressure and volume changes generated. Boyle's law ($PV = P_1V_1$) is used to calculate the volume of gas at end-expiration [201]. Lung compliance is a measure of the change in airway or transpulmonary pressure (ΔP) resulting from a given change in lung volume (ΔV) and is calculated as $\Delta V/\Delta P$. A pressure-sensitive catheter is required to measure airway or transpulmonary pressure, and a plethysmograph chamber or facemask with pneumotachometer is used to measure lung volume.

Forced Maneuvers   Forced maneuver procedures are available for determining TLC [41], FRC [202], IC [188], and quasistatic lung compliance [188] in animal models. A pressure panel has been developed (Buxco Electronics, Inc., Sharon, CT) that can perform a pressure–volume maneuver in anesthetized animals. The animal's lung is inflated to IC, as determined by the inflation pressure (generally 30 cm H_2O), and then slowly deflated at a constant rate using a solenoid valve and a vacuum reservoir. During deflation, lung volumes and airway or transpulmonary pressures are measured. This technique also requires a plethysmograph chamber for measuring lung volumes and a pressure-sensitive catheter for measuring airway or transpulmonary pressures. Details of the equipment used for conducting this maneuver in rats and dogs have been described [187, 188]. Analyzers are also available (Buxco Electronics, Inc., Sharon, CT) that will calculate IC, FRC, TLC, and quasistatic lung compliance values during each pressure–volume maneuver.

Evaluating restrictive disorders in animals using the pressure–volume maneuver offers a high degree of sensitivity since changes are measured at maximum attainable lung volumes and transpulmonary pressures. In addition, this method provides functional endpoints similar to human measurements (e.g., IC, FRC, TLC, and compliance). As described under the section on resistance measurements, the limitations of this technique are that it generally requires the use of anesthetized/paralyzed animals and is a single time point measurement. The latter limitation excludes this as a procedure for measuring acute dynamic changes in lung compliance as might occur following administration of a drug given intravenously or by inhalation.

Dynamic Measurements   Restrictive disorders can also be evaluated in animal models by measuring dynamic lung compliance during tidal breathing or mechanical ventilation. Dynamic compliance is obtained by measuring the differences in airway or transpulmonary pressure (ΔP) and volume (ΔV) that occur at the beginning and end of each inspiration (i.e., at zero flow points) (Fig. 18.6). By selecting zero flow points, the dependence of ΔP on tissue and airflow movement is removed, leaving ΔP dependent on the elastic component of the lung. This procedure requires the use of a plethysmograph chamber or facemask with pneumotachometer for volume measurements and a pressure-sensitive catheter for airway or transpulmonary pressure measurements. Methods for measuring dynamic lung compliance acutely have been established in guinea pigs [29], rats [190], and dogs [191]. Murphy et al. [194, 195] recently developed a procedure that allows for chronic measurement of dynamic compliance in conscious animals.

Dynamic lung compliance measurements are required for evaluating rapid, transient changes in compliance. This procedure can be used in conscious animals, which also allows for repeated measurements over prolonged periods of time. Changes in dynamic lung compliance, however, need to be interpreted with caution since changes in small airway patency can alter dynamic compliance measurements by changing the time constant for alveolar filling [187].

18.5.4   Design of Respiratory Function Safety Studies

General Approach

Tier 1 Evaluation (Core Battery Safety Pharmacology Studies)   Because the respiratory system consists of two functional units—the pumping apparatus and the gas exchange unit—a study designed to evaluate the potential for new drugs to produce adverse effects on respiratory function must evaluate both of these components. Evaluating dose–response relationships, determining the degree of change in specific respiratory parameters, and characterizing changes in arterial blood gases and pH are used to establish the liability associated with the functional changes. Because the safety profile defined by this type of study can have a significant impact on the successful development of new therapeutic agents, it is important that the techniques and assays used in this type of study minimize the occurrence of false-negative and false-positive results. For this reason, techniques that provide direct measures of respiratory parameters should be used. A direct measure is one that provides the endpoint of interest, in contrast to an indirect measure that provides a surrogate endpoint, which requires certain assumptions and/or calculations to estimate the true endpoint. Furthermore, because most drugs are intended for use in conscious patients, and because most anesthetics, analgesics, and sedatives can alter ventilatory reflexes, respiratory drive, and airway reactivity, nonclinical studies evaluating the effects of drugs on respiratory function should utilize conscious animal models. Nonclinical safety studies evaluating the potential adverse effects of new therapeutic agents on respiratory function should be conducted prior to human exposure since acute changes in respiratory function can be life threatening [7].

The core (Tier 1) test for evaluating drug-induced effects on the neuromuscular components of the pumping apparatus is the measurement of ventilatory patterns in conscious animals (Fig. 18.8). Parameters to be initially measured should include respiratory rate, tidal volume, and minute volume. If a change in these parameters occurs, inspiratory flow (mean or peak), expiratory flow (mean or peak), fractional inspiratory time (inspiratory time/total breath time), and time between breaths (expiratory pause or apnea) should be evaluated to help define the mechanism. Measurement of arterial gases (Pao_2, $Paco_2$) and arterial pH should also be conducted to help define the extent or severity of the ventilatory change.

The Tier 1 test for evaluating drug-induced effects on the gas exchange unit is the measurement of the mechanical properties of the lung (Fig. 18.8). This is most effectively accomplished by obtaining the dynamic measurements of total pulmonary resistance and lung compliance. The advantages of this method are that measurements can be obtained repeatedly and continuously in conscious animals and that both ventilatory and lung function parameters can be evaluated simultaneously. Evaluating a drug-induced effect on both ventilation and lung mechanics will establish whether a drug can alter respiratory function and will determine whether a ventilatory change results from pulmonary or extrapulmonary factors.

Tier 2 Evaluation (Follow-up Studies)   Follow-up (Tier 2) respiratory function tests should be initiated to further investigate mechanisms or liabilities (Fig. 18.8) [7]. Studies to investigate mechanisms of ventilatory change should initially determine whether the effect was due to respiratory muscle or neural function change. This can be accomplished by assessing the effect of drug treatment on efferent phrenic nerve activity [203, 204]. Changes in phrenic nerve activity (action potential burst frequency or intensity) are indicative of an effect on the nervous system. Direct stimulation of the phrenic nerve and assessment of its effect on respiratory muscle function (e.g., transdiaphragmatic function) can also be used to detect muscle defects [205]. A neurological effect is further classified as either central or peripheral. Peripheral nervous system effects are generally mediated by peripheral arterial

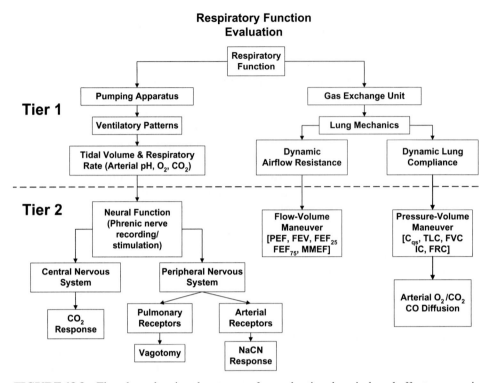

FIGURE 18.8   Flowchart showing the strategy for evaluating drug-induced effects on respiratory function. Tier 1 tests are conducted to detect and quantify functional changes of the respiratory system, while Tier 2 tests are conducted to investigate mechanisms or further characterize effects associated with a functional change. Abbreviations are described in the text.

chemoreceptors or respiratory tract chemo- and mechanoreceptors. Exposure to CO_2 gas stimulates ventilation primarily through a central mechanism [206], while injection of NaCN produces a transient stimulation of ventilation through a mechanism that involves selective stimulation of peripheral chemoreceptors [166]. Based on these responses, a noninvasive method for distinguishing central from peripheral nervous system effects in conscious animals has been developed [181]. Cervical vagotomy can be used to determine whether pulmonary chemo- or mechanorecep-tors are involved in chemical-induced effects on ventilatory control (e.g., see Ref. 48).

Tier 2 studies to further investigate lung mechanical changes include forced maneuver procedures that can distinguish central from peripheral airway obstruc-tion [161], identify the presence of gas trapping (FRC) [164], establish changes in lung compliance [163], and provide measures of lung capacities [164]. Acute drug-induced changes in lung compliance often result from pulmonary edema and/or interalveolar septal thickening [161, 162]. Procedures for identifying these effects include measurement of CO diffusion from alveoli to blood or changes in the ratio of arterial P_{O_2} to P_{CO_2} [188, 190, 207]. Decreases in CO diffusion or the ratio of arterial P_{O_2}/P_{CO_2} are generally indicative of pulmonary edema, thickening of interalveolar septa, or the loss of normal alveolar architecture [161, 162].

Dosing and Dose Level Selection   Nonclinical safety studies of respiratory function are designed to support initial administration of a new chemical entity to
humans. The primary safety concerns in the initial single rising dose human studies
are acute life-threatening changes in major organ systems. As such, single-dose
studies are generally appropriate for addressing these concerns. However, respiratory disorders that are associated with multiple-dose treatment can occur and should
be addressed in a multiple-dose safety study. Since pharmacological and toxicological effects can be route specific, the test drugs should be given by the intended
clinical route. Furthermore, to evaluate dose–response relationships, three or more
dose levels and a vehicle control should be used. If possible, selection of the high
dose should be based on acute toxicological findings and should be a dose that
produces evidence of toxicity. This dose level, however, must not be associated with
toxicological changes in secondary organ systems, which may compromise the respiratory function measurements. For example, effects such as emesis, hyperactivity,
tremors, or muscle hypertonia would be unacceptable, whereas a slight increase in
serum ALT or a slight decrease in body weight is generally acceptable. Selecting the
maximum possible dose level is important for safety evaluation since secondary
pharmacological effects are often associated with nonspecific receptor interactions
where affinity for the drug may be 100–1000-fold lower than the intended target
(e.g., receptor, ion channel, or enzyme). The middle and low doses should generally
be log or half-log decrements of the high dose, with the low dose no less than that
required to produce systemic exposure similar to that at the primary pharmacological or anticipated human dose. In the absence of toxicology data, multiples of the
pharmacological dose (e.g., ED_{50}) should be used. If toxicity is not limiting, the
highest multiple should be at least 100 times the pharmacologically active dose.

Species Selection   The rat is considered an appropriate species for general use in
studies designed to evaluate the potential adverse effects of drugs on respiratory
function. The physiology of the respiratory system has been well characterized in
this species [208, 209] and much of the information on drug-induced effects on
ventilatory control and mechanisms of airway disease has been obtained in the rat
[164, 210]. The rat is also readily available from animal vendors, is easy to handle
and train, has a relatively stable breathing pattern, and has the appropriate tempera-
ment for conscious respiratory measurements. Furthermore, the techniques for measuring respiratory functions in rats are well established, and the rat is commonly
used in toxicology studies. For safety pharmacology studies that are conducted after
a compound has been selected for development, selecting a species that is used in
toxicology studies provides additional supportive information including pharmacokinetic data [161] that can be used to define the test measurement intervals,
acute toxicity data [162] that can be used to select the appropriate high dose, and
toxicology/pathology findings [163] that can be used to help define the mechanism
of the functional changes measured in safety pharmacology studies.

Alternate species may be required to address specific study requirements. For
example, the development of humanized monoclonal antibodies or other biotechnology-derived proteins requires species that have homologous target proteins and
do not produce an antigenic response to the drug. In such cases, transgenic mice or
nonhuman primates are generally required. Similarly, if the test compound has
known histamine or leukotriene activity, the guinea pig should be considered.

18.6   CENTRAL NERVOUS SYSTEM (CNS) SAFETY PHARMACOLOGY

18.6.1   Introduction

For many years the principal official recommendations for safety pharmacology studies were contained in the Japanese guidelines, the most recent version of which was published in 1995 [4]. The latest guidelines are those proposed by the *European Agency for the Evaluation of Medicinal Products*, ICH S7A [211], which have been in operation in Europe since June 2001 and have also been adopted by the United States and Japan. These guidelines describe a core battery of CNS studies that can be considered mandatory and include "motor activity, behavioral changes, coordination, sensory/motor reflex responses and body temperature" with the remark that "the central nervous system should be assessed appropriately." Core battery studies should be carried out before proceeding to first studies in humans (Phase I) and it is recommended that they be conducted in compliance with internationally recognized standards of Good Laboratory Practice (GLP). A further series of studies, follow-up or supplementary studies, should be carried out where indicated and include "behavioral pharmacology, learning and memory, ligand-specific binding, neurochemistry, visual, auditory and/or electrophysiology examinations." In general, follow-up studies are conducted prior to product approval and, because of their unique characteristics, require only assurance of "data quality and integrity" rather than full compliance with GLP.

The following sections describe CNS studies of both kinds. For further discussion the reader is referred to other publications [212, 213] on this subject.

18.6.2   Core Battery CNS Safety Pharmacology Procedures

Core battery CNS procedures are typically simple tests, using traditional techniques, which can be carried out rapidly in a routine fashion. They are the first techniques to be employed in CNS safety assessment. Indeed, they are frequently applied at the very beginning of the discovery process as a screen to eliminate substances with a potential for CNS risk. There is, however, a difference in emphasis between early CNS safety screening and core battery CNS safety tests as defined by ICH S7A. Initial screening studies are more exploratory in nature, investigate a wider range of doses using a limited number of procedures, and are seldom conducted according to GLP. In contrast, pre-Phase I core battery studies investigate a more restricted dose range selected in relation to the doses active in the primary indication. Whereas early screening is frequently conducted in the mouse because smaller quantities of test substance are required, pre-Phase I core battery studies are usually conducted in the rat to provide data more comparable with that obtained in other domains (toxicology, pharmacokinetics, biochemistry). At this stage of drug development, the required quantity of test substance is not a primary consideration.

ICH S7A requirements   ICH S7A recommends that a core battery should cover a range of simple tests measuring the effects of test substances on motor activity, behavior, coordination, sensory/motor reflex responses and body temperature. These effects can be covered by the battery of tests described below. In addition, we believe that it is useful, for little extra cost, to evaluate the effects of test substances on the convulsive threshold and their interaction with a standard CNS depressant such as a barbiturate. The former is primarily useful for detecting proconvulsive activity whereas the later is very sensitive for unmasking latent sedative or psychostimulant effects. Both kinds of test were included in the Japanese guidelines but were dropped in ICH S7A.

General Behavioral Observation   A first approach is to assess the global behavioral profile of a test substance using either a systematic observation procedure following that originally described in the mouse by Irwin [214] or the more recently described functional observation battery (FOB) [215]. Both are specifically mentioned in ICH S7A, but the FOB is more frequently used for assessing neurotoxicity and is less suitable for serial observations over several hours. As psychopharmacologists rather than toxicologists, we have preferred to use the Irwin test for initial screening of novel substances because of its rapidity and simplicity. In screening applications, the test substance is usually investigated over a wide dose range (6–8 doses) with few animals per dose ($N = 3$) investigated sequentially, starting at a high and potentially lethal dose and working upwards or downwards according to a bracketing prodecure to determine the first lethal dose, the active dose range, and the principal behavioral and physiological effects. In core battery applications, the test substance is usually evaluated over a smaller predetermined dose range (3–4 doses) with more animals per dose ($N = 4$–10), ranging from the dose known to be active in tests for the primary indication and ascending to a given multiple (30–100 times the low dose depending on feasibility). In a core battery evaluation, the test substance is rarely administered at potentially lethal doses because these are already known from available toxicological data.

In the Irwin procedure, rats or mice are given the test substance and are repeatedly observed over a 3–4 hour period followed by daily observations up to 72 hours using a standardized observation grid containing most or all of the following items: mortality, sedation, excitation, stereotypies, aggressiveness, reaction to touch, pain sensitivity, muscle relaxation, loss of righting reflex, changes in gait and respiration, catalepsy, ptosis, corneal reflex, pupil diameter, and rectal temperature.

The effects of a standard benzodiazepine (diazepam) in the Irwin test in the rat are shown in Table 18.3.

Locomotor Activity Tests   Locomotor activity can be quantified in rodents in a variety of ways (interruptions of photoelectric beams, activity wheels, changes in electromagnetic fields, Doppler effects, video-image analysis, telemetry) [216]. Animals are administered the test substance and are placed in standardized enclosures for a limited observation period (10–40 minutes). Unlike the Irwin test, where animals are observed continuously from the moment of administration, locomotor activity tests are usually conducted at a fixed time after administration, the time being selected as a function of the test substance kinetics to approximate maximum exposure during the test. This avoids interpretational difficulties related to interactions between the onset of drug action and behavioral habituation to the test environment. In contrast to the Irwin test, which is labor intensive, most locomotor activity tests are automated and permit several animals to be tested simultaneously. Although different authors quantify different aspects of locomotion (small displacements, large displacements, rearing), the basic information yielded by activity meter tests is whether a test substance increases or decreases locomotion. Data obtained should be correlated with that obtained from direct observation (Irwin

TABLE 18.3   Effects of Diazepam (Oral Dose) in the Primary Observation (Irwin) Test in the Rat[a]

1 (mg/kg)	2 (mg/kg)	4 (mg/kg)	8 (mg/kg)	16 (mg/kg)	64 (mg/kg)
No change	Hypothermia + at 30 min	Sedation + ↓ Traction Hypothermia (++ → 30 min) (+ at 60 and 120 min)	Sedation + ↓ Traction Hypothermia (++ → 60 min) (+ at 120 min)	Sedation ++ ↓ Traction ↓ Reactivity to touch ↓ Muscle tone Abnormal gait Hypothermia ++ (+++ at 30 min) (+ at 120 min)	Sedation ++ ↓ Traction ↓ Reactivity to touch ↓ Muscle tone Abnormal gait Hypothermia (+++ → 120 min) (++ at 180 min) (+ at 24 h)

[a]Note the dose-dependent increase in sedation and decreases in reactivity to touch, traction, and muscle tone accompanied by abnormal gait. $N = 4$ for each treatment group. + = slight; ++ = moderate; +++ = marked. Observations were performed at 15, 30, 60, 120, and 180 minutes after administration. Symptoms that did not necessitate handling were also observed up to 15 min immediately following administration.

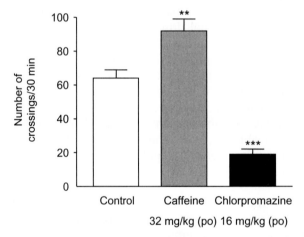

FIGURE 18.9   Effects of caffeine and chlorpromazine (oral administration) on locomotion in the rat.

test) to ensure that apparent decreases are not due to motor incapacity or even to overexcitation.

The effects of a standard psychostimulant (caffeine) and a standard CNS depressant (chlorpromazine) in the activity meter test in the rat are shown in Fig. 18.9.

Motor Coordination Tests   Locomotor coordination is most commonly assessed using a rotarod [217]. Rats or mice are placed onto a rod rotating either at a fixed speed or at a constantly increasing speed. The time taken for the animal to fall off the rod, or the number of animals remaining on the rod over a set duration, is mea-

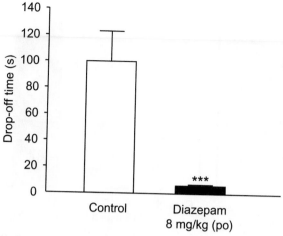

FIGURE 18.10   Effects of diazepam (oral administration) on rotarod performance in the rat.

sured. To decrease test variability, the animals are usually given prior habituation to the rotarod before receiving the test substance. With most setups, several animals are tested simultaneously on the same rod, separated physically and visually by partitions with automated scoring of performance. When used in conjunction with locomotor activity tests, the rotarod test provides a useful quantification of the margin of safety between doses that alter spontaneous activity and those that disturb motor function. Unlike locomotor activity tests, which show bi-directional drug effects, rotarod tests are seldom capable of showing facilitation of motor performance.

The effects of a standard benzodiazepine (diazepam) in the rotarod test in the rat are shown in Fig. 18.10.

Effects on the Convulsive Threshold   Test substances can induce frank convulsions when given at sufficiently high doses, but can also lower the convulsive threshold without inducing frank convulsions. Surprisingly, the ICH S7A core battery does not include tests for the convulsive threshold, although such tests were included in the earlier Japanese guidelines. We have criticized this absence [218] because we consider the existence of proconvulsant activity an important CNS risk. Furthermore, although anticonvulsant activity is not in itself a risk, it is known that several anticonvulsants (benzodiazepines, NMDA antagonists) cause memory disturbance. Thus, the presence of anticonvulsant activity could constitute a first marker for cognition impairment, with obvious implications for CNS safety. Both kinds of activity can be seen with chemically induced convulsions such as with pentylenetetrazole (PTZ), where a shortened or lengthened latency or a higher or lower frequency of convulsions/deaths can be observed with pro- and anticonvulsants, respectively [219]. A variant of the electroconvulsive shock (ECS) method, whereby successive animals are subjected to increasing or decreasing intensities of ECS depending on the occurrence of convulsions with the preceding shock level, permits a sensitive measure of the electroconvulsive threshold. It is important for safety pharmacology purposes that convulsive threshold tests can vary in both directions.

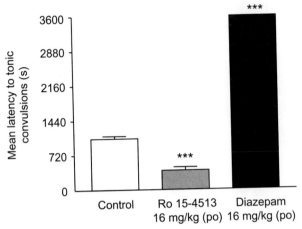

FIGURE 18.11   Effects of Ro 15-4513 and diazepam (oral administration) on the latency to tonic convulsions induced by PTZ (120 mg/kg subcutaneous) in the rat.

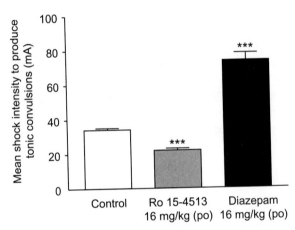

FIGURE 18.12   Effects of Ro 15-4513 and diazepam (oral administration) on the mean shock intensity required to induce tonic convulsions in the rat.

The effects of a standard proconvulsant benzodiazepine (Ro13–4513) and an anticonvulsant benzodiazepine (diazepam) in the PTZ test in the rat are shown in Fig. 18.11 and in the ECS threshold test in the rat in Fig. 18.12.

Interaction with Hypnotics   Another risk factor that is not life threatening in itself but can have life threatening consequences is the induction of drowsiness or sleep. Sleep induction in rodents can be evaluated by loss of the righting reflex. Intrinsic sleep-inducing activity can be observed during the Irwin test or FOB (see earlier discussion). A more sensitive index of sleep enhancement can, however, be obtained by observing the interaction of the test substance with sleep induced by standard hypnotics such as barbiturates [220]. Such procedures can also unmask psychostimu-lant activity not always evident from direct observation (decrease in barbiturate-induced sleep). Barbiturate interaction studies therefore provide a useful complement to studies of general behavior and spontaneous locomotion.

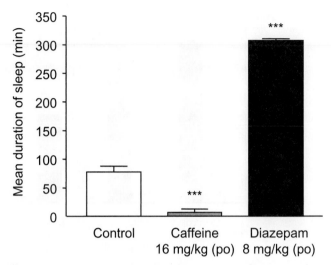

FIGURE 18.13   Effects of caffeine and diazepam (oral administration) on the duration of sleep induced by barbital (150 mg/kg intraperitoneal) in the rat.

The effects of a standard psychostimulant (caffeine) and a standard CNS depressant (diazepam) in the barbital interaction test in the rat are shown in Fig. 18.13.

18.6.3   Follow-up CNS Safety Pharmacology Procedures

Follow-up CNS safety pharmacology involves more complex and time-consuming experimental procedures and includes methods for evaluating drug effects on cognitive function, the electroencephalogram (EEG), and the potential for the new substance to cause drug abuse or dependence.

Cognitive Function   Included under the term cognitive function are learning, memory, attention, and general intellectual activity. New drugs should be devoid of impairing effects on these functions, whatever their indication. Indeed, package inserts for many kinds of drugs contain warnings about the use of the drug while driving, working, or engaging in various daily occupations, referring mainly to an attentional deficit. Drug-induced impairment of learning and memory can also be troublesome side effects of certain agents, even if not life threatening. It is therefore important that CNS safety pharmacology provide procedures for evaluating these effects in animals. The following section provides an indication of the kinds of experiment that could be undertaken. The list is by no means exhaustive.

Passive Avoidance   One of the simplest procedures for looking for adverse effects on learning/memory is the one-trial passive avoidance task [221]. There are several variants of this procedure, but the basic principle is that a rat or a mouse receives an aversive stimulation in a recognizable environment and on a later occasion shows it has remembered by not going there (passive avoidance). For example, a rat placed into the light compartment of a two-compartment box will explore the apparatus and eventually enter the dark compartment, where it receives a brief electric shock [222]. When placed again into the light compartment 24 or 48 hours later, the animal will avoid going into the dark compartment despite a natural preference for the dark. Amnesia-inducing drugs (benzodiazepines, anticholinergics, NMDA

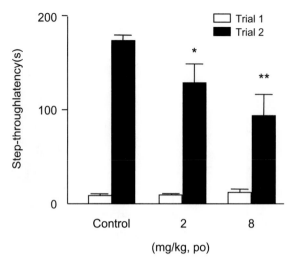

FIGURE 18.14   Effects of diazepam (oral administration) on passive avoidance behavior in the rat. Note the absence of effects of diazepam on the step-through latency at Trial 1 and the presence of a dose-dependent decrease in step-through latency at Trial 2 in the absence of diazepam.

antagonists), administered before the first exposure, will attenuate the animal's memory for the shock as shown by a decreased latency to enter the dark compartment on the test day.

The effects of a standard benzodiazepine (diazepam) in the passive avoidance test in the rat are shown in Fig. 18.14.

Passive avoidance is a fairly simple and rapid procedure because it involves learning obtained in a single trial. It is therefore suitable as a first screen for potential cognition impairing activity. On the other hand, it is not clearly interpretable in terms of the cognitive function involved as it is not possible to distinguish a drug's effects on learning or memory, or whether the drug influenced performance by impairing attention or even pain sensitivity during the learning trial.

Morris Maze   Another procedure, which allows a greater degree of interpretation, is the Morris water maze [223]. In this test a rat or a mouse is placed into a circular tank containing opacified water and has to find an escape platform just beneath the surface and therefore invisible to the animal. After swimming around for a certain time (usually limited to 2 minutes), the animal will eventually come across the hidden platform and climb onto it to escape from the water. When placed again in the water on subsequent occasions, the animal will find the platform with increasing rapidity, indicating that it has learned the position of the platform.

Morris maze learning involves spatial navigation and the capacity of the animal to attend to extra-maze cues. Furthermore, the procedure can be modulated to examine the effects of drugs on both short-term memory (within-day learning) and longer term memory (day-to-day learning).

The effects of different neuroleptics (tiapride, haloperidol, and risperidone) on short-term memory and on longer term memory in the Morris maze test in the rat are shown in Figs. 18.15 and 18.16.

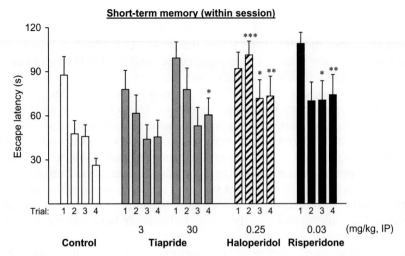

FIGURE 18.15 Effects of three neuroleptics (intraperitoneal administration), tiapride, haloperidol, and risperidone, on escape latencies during the first session of the Morris maze task in the rat. Note the clear decrease in escape latencies in the vehicle control group (short-term memory) and the absence of effect of the three substances on performance at the first trial (absence of intrinsic effects on swimming performance). Tiapride slightly but dose-dependently attenuates the decrease in escape latency from trial to trial, whereas haloperidol and risperidone clearly attenuate this decrease (perturbing effect on short-term memory).

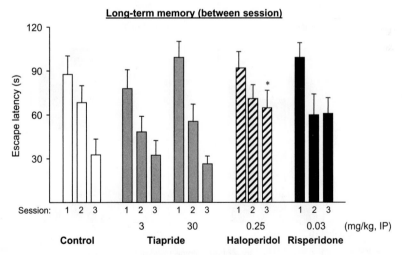

FIGURE 18.16 Effects of three neuroleptics (intraperitoneal administration), tiapride, haloperidol, and risperidone, on escape latencies during the same Morris maze task on three consecutive days (first trial of each day). Note the clear decrease in escape latencies in the vehicle control group from day to day (long-term memory). Tiapride has no effect on the decrease in the first trial escape latency from day to day (absence of effect on long-term memory), whereas haloperidol clearly attenuates this decrease with a similar tendency for risperidone (perturbing effect on long-term memory).

Radial Maze   Another task in which short-term memory can be differentiated from long-term memory is the radial maze [224]. This apparatus consists of a central platform with arms radiating from it like the spokes of a wheel. A hungry rat or a mouse is placed in the center of the maze and can find food at the end of each arm. Before drug testing, animals are usually given initial maze training to learn that food is available at the end of each arm. Once trained in the maze, an ideal performance during a trial would be for the animal to visit each arm once to collect food. This task therefore requires that, during a trial, the animal remembers the arms already visited (short-term or "working" memory). Longer term memory can also be investigated by arranging that only some of the arms are baited, but always the same ones, during repeated sessions. In this case the animal, in addition to always choosing a new arm ("working" memory), must visit only the arms previously associated with food (long-term or "reference" memory). Amnesia-inducing drugs, such as anticholinergics or benzodiazepines, clearly impair radial maze performance, in particular, "working" memory.

With the radial maze, other aspects of performance can also be measured. These include running times and response choice strategy. The strategy parameter assesses the degree to which the animal uses behavioral routines for selecting arms. For example, when animals are highly trained in the maze, they will tend to select subsequent arms always in a particular direction (left or right) and thereby minimize errors without using working memory at all. Assessing the effects of test substances on the different parameters can therefore permit a more accurate interpretation of the behavioral changes observed.

The effects of MK-801 (dizocilpine) in the radial maze test in the rat are shown in Fig. 18.17.

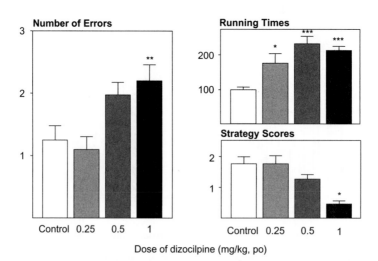

FIGURE 18.17   The effects of MK-801 (dizocilpine) (oral administration) on the three parameters measured (errors, running times, response strategy) during the radial maze task in the rat (mean of three sessions). Note the dose-dependent increase in the number of errors with no effect on running times. A decrease in response strategy occurs only at the highest dose. Taken together, these data suggest a specific impairment of "working" memory by MK-801.

The radial maze requires considerable training and is therefore more time consuming than either passive avoidance or the Morris maze. On the other hand, by means of the different parameters measured, it offers data that are more clearly interpretable. Furthermore, the radial maze is based on a different motivational system (food reward). Radial maze data can thus usefully complement those obtained in the other procedures.

Operant Behavior Techniques: Delayed Responding   In delayed responding procedures, the animal is required to retain information over a short period (usually seconds) and then to show, by pressing an appropriate lever, whether it has correctly remembered it [225]. In a typical example, a rat in a Skinner box is presented with a lever, either on the left or the right side of the food dispenser. The rat presses the lever and the lever is withdrawn. Five seconds later, two levers are presented and the rat has to press the lever opposite to that which was presented previously to obtain a food reward (delayed alternation, delayed nonmatching to sample). If the rat presses the same lever as that previously presented, the lever will be withdrawn but no food will be given. In this fashion, the animal can be trained to retain a piece of spatial information (position of a lever), and thereby demonstrate its short-term memory capacity over time. Using the same apparatus, it is possible to measure the animal's reaction times, both to the single lever presentations (simple reaction time) and to the two-lever presentations (choice reaction time), and thereby provide additional information about other aspects of cognitive performance more related to attention and information processing speed.

The effects of a standard benzodiazepine (diazepam) and a standard anticholinergic (scopolamine) in the delayed alternation test in the rat are shown in Fig. 18.18.

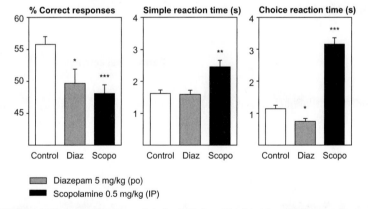

FIGURE 18.18   Effects of diazepam (oral administration) and scopolamine (intraperitoneal administration) on the 3 parameters measured during the acquisition of a delayed alternation task in the rat (mean performance over 10 sessions). Note that both diazepam and scopolamine significantly decrease the number of correct responses (impairment of learning/memory). Diazepam has no effect on simple reaction times, whereas scopolamine significantly increases it (impairment of attention). Diazepam significantly decreases choice reaction times, whereas choice reaction times are clearly increased by scopolamine. The increased choice reaction times with scopolamine probably reflect an impairment of information processing speed, whereas the decrease observed with diazepam probably reflects the disinhibitory effects of diazepam.

Although most of the published work with delayed responding concerns studies performed in the rat [226], similar tasks can be performed in monkeys [227] and in humans [228].

EEG Studies   Electroencephalogram (EEG) investigations are recommended as possible follow-up studies in both ICH S7A and the previous Japanese guidelines. An EEG provides a useful means of evaluating the effects of a test substance on brain activity in freely moving conscious animals. As far as CNS follow-up safety pharmacology is concerned, three major EEG applications (EEG trace monitoring, quantified EEG (QEEG), and the sleep/wake cycle) appear to be of particular relevance.

EEG Trace Monitoring   If initial experiments on the convulsive threshold suggest potential proconvulsant activity, follow-up studies using visual monitoring of the EEG traces can be employed to determine whether paroxysmal activity (spikes) can be detected [229]. Certain substances induce clear paroxysmal activity on the EEG at doses that have no observable effects or before these effects become clearly apparent in behavior. It is thus possible to confirm the existence of proconvulsant activity from the EEG traces and even to identify the locus of such activity from differential placement of the EEG electrodes within the brain, for example, cortex or hippocampus.

Trace monitoring studies, for economic reasons, are performed mainly in the rat but can also be conducted in the dog using telemetric devices. Dog studies are particularly useful if the primary therapeutic activity of the test substance, for example, effects on the cardiovascular system, have been established in the same species.

The effects of a standard convulsant (PTZ) on the cortical EEG trace in the dog are shown in Fig. 18.19.

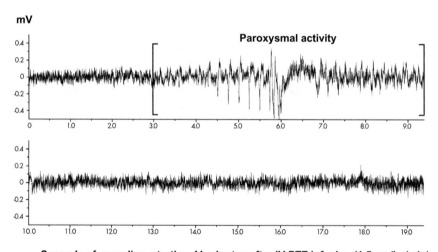

Seconds of recording, starting 41 minutes after IV PTZ infusion (1.5 mg/kg/min)

FIGURE 18.19   Effects of an intravenous infusion of PTZ (1.25 mg/kg/min) on the EEG trace in the conscious freely moving beagle dog measured via telemetry. Note the sequence of paroxysmal activity (marked by the square brackets). This occurred in the absence of overt convulsive phenomena.

QEEG   QEEG makes use of the Fourier theorem to analyze the amount of electrical power in the different frequency bands of the EEG [230]. Animals, with electrodes fixed to the skull (cortical leads) and sometimes also implanted stereotaxically in selected structures (e.g., hippocampus, striatum), are exposed to brief measurement periods (1–2 hours) during which they are either left free to move spontaneously or activated by means of a treadmill to ensure a stable heightened level of vigilance. The EEG is recorded and is subjected, via appropriate software, to a fast Fourier transformation.

While there is debate as to whether QEEG, by virtue of the different profiles observed, is capable of identifying specific classes of psychotropic agents, there is general consensus that the QEEG can detect basic stimulant, sedative, or even convulsant activity [231]. This could have clear relevance for drug safety by corroborating, in terms of brain activity, data obtained from behavioral observation. A more clearly safety pharmacology application is to determine the highest dose that can be administered without affecting the QEEG.

The effects of a standard psychostimulant (amphetamine) on the QEEG power spectrum in the rat are shown in Fig. 18.20.

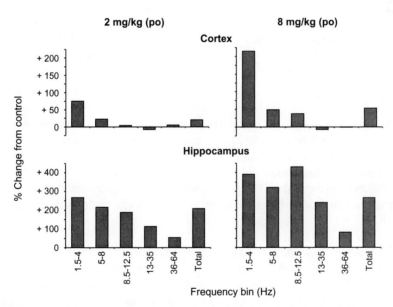

FIGURE 18.20   Effects of d-amphetamine (oral administration) on the power spectrum of the QEEG. Note that amphetamine dose-dependently increases power over the whole frequency range, more markedly so at low frequencies and particularly in the hippocampus. Similar profiles are observed with other psychostimulants such as methylphenidate or nomifensine (data not shown).

Sleep/Wake Cycle   Studies of the sleep/wake cycle are to be distinguished from QEEG by the fact that spontaneous as opposed to induced changes are studied over longer periods of time [232]. Such studies determine whether the test substance induces alterations in the architecture of natural sleep [233]. Although sleep patterns differ between rodents and humans, rodents being mostly awake during the

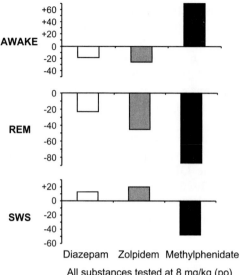

FIGURE 18.21   Effects of diazepam, zolpidem, and methylphenidate (oral administration) on the sleep/wake cycle in the rat during the first 4 hours after drug administration. Note that both diazepam and zolpidem decrease the amount of wakefulness and increase the amount of slow wave sleep, whereas opposite effects are observed with methylphenidate. All substances decrease the amount of REM sleep, with the most marked effects being observed on this parameter with methylphenidate.

dark phase of the light/dark cycle, drug effects appear to be highly comparable between the species. From a safety pharmacology standpoint, as for QEEG, the aim of this type of study is to determine up to which dose the test substance is devoid of effects on sleep function.

The effects of two standard sleep-enhancing agents (diazepam and zolpidem) and a psychostimulant (methylphenidate) on the sleep/wake cycle in the rat are shown in Fig. 18.21.

Drug dependence and abuse   Another subject, clearly within the notion of safety, is the assessment of a novel substance's potential to induce problems of dependence or abuse. These are mentioned briefly in ICH S7A ("other organ systems"), but more complete guidelines have been proposed recently in Europe [234] and North America [235].

Although dependence and abuse frequently occur together, they are not synonymous [236]. Drug dependence refers to the inability of the dependent individual to function normally without the drug. Drug abuse, as its name implies, refers to misuse or overuse of a drug and is generally covered under the notion of drug seeking behavior. Dependence can be both physical and psychological and is usually manifested on drug discontinuation. Psychological dependence is indicated by craving for the drug, whereas physical dependence is demonstrated more objectively by signs ranging from changes in body temperature to life-threatening conditions such as status epilepticus or delirium tremens. Withdrawal symptoms are readily demonstrated in animal models, whereas drug craving is more problematic. The difference between dependence and abuse can be illustrated pharmacologically. For example, marihuana and LSD are frequently abused, but it is difficult to show any clear signs of withdrawal on drug discontinuation. In contrast, selective serotonin reuptake inhibitors (SSRIs) do induce discontinuation signs, but have not been subject to abuse. On the other hand, drugs such as heroin and cocaine cause both abuse and marked signs of physical and psychological dependence.

Drug Dependence   Tests for drug dependence consist mainly of repeated treatment studies, followed by drug discontinuation, where withdrawal symptoms occur either spontaneously (nonprecipitated withdrawal) or after administration of specific antagonists, for example, naloxone (opiates) or flumazenil (benzodiazepines).

In the absence of a known mechanism, the most convincing evidence of drug dependence liability comes from studies where the test substance is repeatedly administered at high doses and is then simply discontinued. Under these conditions, clear withdrawal signs (weight loss, decreased food consumption, hyperthermia) can be observed after a variety of substances, for example, benzodiazepines, morphine, and cocaine [237]. If it can be shown that a test substance can be repeatedly administered at maximally tolerated doses and then be discontinued without observable symptoms under conditions where similar treatment with an appropriately chosen reference substance induces clear withdrawal signs, then it seems reasonable to conclude that the test substance is unlikely to cause physical dependence.

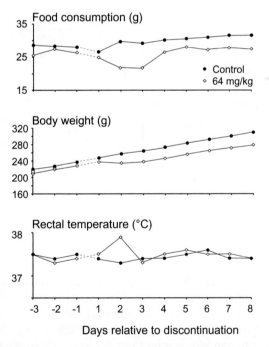

FIGURE 18.22   Effects of drug discontinuation after 10 days of twice daily treatment with chlordiazepoxide (oral administration) on food consumption, body weight gain, and rectal temperature in the rat. Note a decrease in food consumption and an increase in rectal temperature during the first 2 days after drug discontinuation with recovery toward vehicle control values thereafter. Similar but less marked effects are observed on body weight.

Withdrawal effects in the rat after discontinuing repeated treatment with a standard benzodiazepine (chlordiazepoxide) are shown in Fig. 18.22.

Drug Abuse   Drug abuse represents a more serious social problem than drug dependence because it involves a greater variety of substances. Tests for abuse are generally of two kinds. The first kind assesses whether a new substance resembles a known drug of abuse. The second kind assesses whether the test substance possesses positive reinforcing properties and can thereby sustain drug seeking behavior.

SIMILARITY TO KNOWN DRUGS OF ABUSE

Direct Observation Tests   A first approach to assessing similarity is simply to compare the behavioral effects of the test substance with those of a known drug of abuse using an Irwin-style observation procedure.

The effects of two NMDA antagonists (PCP and MK-801) in the mouse Irwin test are shown in Fig. 18.23.

Irwin Test in the Mouse

MK 801 (p.o.)

0.125 (mg/kg)	1 (mg/kg)	4 (mg/kg)	32 (mg/kg)
No change	Excitation +++	Excitation +++	Sedation ++
	Straub	Straub	Straub
	Stereotypies	Stereotypies	Stereotypies
	Convulsions	Convulsions	Convulsions
	Hyperthermia +	Hyperthermia +	Tremor
			↓ Reactivity to touch
			Motor incoordination
			↓ Muscle tone

Phencyclidine (p.o.)

1 (mg/kg)	4 (mg/kg)	16 (mg/kg)	64 (mg/kg)
↓ Reactivity	Excitation ++	Excitation +++	Convulsions
	↓ Traction	Stereotypies	Death (3/3)
	↓ Reactivity to touch	Convulsions	
		Tremor	
		↓ Fear	
		↓ Traction	
		Motor incoordination	
		↓ Muscle tone	
		↑ Respiration	

FIGURE 18.23   Effects of PCP and MK-801 (dizocilpine) in the Irwin test in the mouse. Note the large overlap in behavioral signs (excitation, stereotypies, motor incoordination, convulsions) between the two substances.

Drug Discrimination Tests   A more sensitive approach to assessing drug similarity is the use of drug discrimination procedures where animals, by pressing on one of two levers in a Skinner box, can show that they can discriminate the presence of a particular drug of abuse (training drug) from vehicle [238]. They are then given the new substance and can indicate by their choice of lever, whether the new substance resembles the training drug. A test substance that is perceived as being subjectively similar to a drug of abuse is also likely to be abused. An advantage of drug discrimination paradigms is that similar methodology can be used in monkeys [239] and even humans [240].

An interesting variant of the drug discrimination procedure is to use the test substance as the training drug. If the test substance can be shown to serve as a discriminative stimulus, it can be supposed that the test substance induces identifiable subjective effects. If the substance cannot be discriminated, it is less likely to be abused because of its subjective effects. On the other hand, the existence of a drug-induced discriminative stimulus with a test substance is no proof that substance will be abused. For example, naloxone can clearly be discriminated but is never abused. If clear discrimination can be established with the test substance, using the test substance as the training drug becomes particularly useful because the same trained animals can subsequently be tested for generalization to a range of drugs of abuse. This represents a more economical approach than using independent groups of animals, each trained to recognize a particular class of drug. It must be remembered, however, that drug discrimination procedures represent only an indirect approach toward predicting whether a test substance will be abused. They cannot predict the abuse potential of a drug inducing totally novel sensations.

The effects of three standard psychostimulants (amphetamine, cocaine, and methylphenidate) in rats trained to discriminate amphetamine are shown in Fig. 18.24.

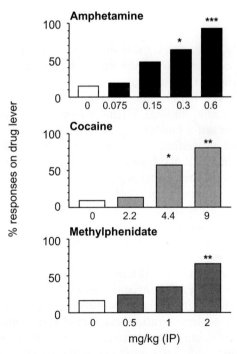

FIGURE 18.24 Effects of d-amphetamine, cocaine, and methylphenidate (intraperitoneal administration) on drug discrimination in rats trained to discriminate 0.6 mg/kg (IP) d-amphetamine from saline. Note the dose-dependent generalization of lower doses of amphetamine toward responding on the lever associated with the training dose of amphetamine, with similar generalization curves for cocaine and methylphenidate.

TESTS FOR POSITIVE REINFORCING PROPERTIES

Place Preference Tests   A relatively simple paradigm is conditioned place preference, where it can be shown that an animal, which has been repeatedly exposed to
an identifiable environment in the presence of a drug of abuse, will show preference
for that environment when later given a choice [241].

The effects of two standard drugs of abuse (cocaine and morphine) in the conditioned place preference test in the rat are shown in Fig. 18.25.

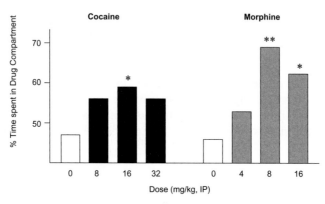

FIGURE 18.25   Effects of cocaine and morphine (intraperitoneal administration) in the
conditioned place preference test in the rat.

Self-Administration Procedures   The most direct tests of abuse potential are
self-administration procedures, where the animal, by pressing on a lever, causes itself
to receive an IV infusion of the test substance via a pump system connected to an
indwelling catheter [242]. Parallel methods exist in both rats and monkeys and
provide substantially similar findings. Virtually all drugs that are abused in humans
will induce or maintain self-administration behavior in animals.

Generally, two basic procedures are used. The most common is the substitution
procedure, where an animal is first trained to self-administer a known drug of abuse
such as cocaine or heroin. The animal is then tested to see whether a test substance
will substitute for the training drug, that is, whether the animal will continue to
self-administer the test substance. Another procedure is to assess whether a test
substance can initiate self-administration behavior in drug-naive animals. The substitution procedure is probably the more sensitive for detecting self-administration
potential, because the test animal can already be considered a "drug abuser." A test
substance that does not maintain self-administration in this procedure is therefore
unlikely to do so in any other variant and thus can be considered devoid of abuse
potential. Another advantage of the substitution procedure is that it permits a
quantification of the self-administration level in individual animals before assessing
the test substance. This is important because there exist marked individual differences between animals, particularly monkeys, in their inclination to self-administer
drugs, as there are in humans. A final advantage of the substitution procedure is that
it permits the animal, particularly the monkey, to be used repeatedly for drug evaluation programs, which represents an important economic consideration for these
time-consuming and costly procedures.

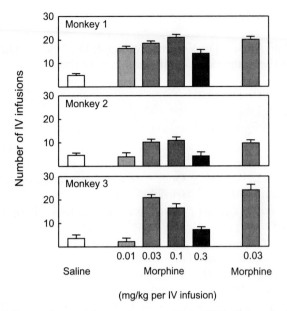

FIGURE 18.26 Effects of morphine and a standard SSRI (fluoxetine) in three rhesus monkeys habituated to self-administer 0.1 mg/kg/infusion morphine (substitution procedure). Fluoxetine does not maintain self-administration in contrast to heroin.

The effects of a standard drug of abuse (morphine) and a standard SSRI (fluoxetine) in a self-administration procedure in the rhesus monkey are shown in Fig. 18.26.

18.6.4 General Conclusions

This section has provided an overview of the kinds of studies that can be carried out to evaluate the risk of adverse effects of a novel substance on CNS function. The basic routines useful for core battery CNS safety assessment, mainly in the rodent, were covered. Additional and more complex procedures were also included to provide a more comprehensive review relevant to CNS safety prior to drug registration. For this reason, an important part of the present section was devoted to methods for evaluating higher CNS function (cognitive behavior and electrical brain activity), because adverse effects at this level could radically affect the safety of many substances in everyday use. Methods for evaluating drug abuse and dependence were also included, despite the fact that these problems generally concern only CNS-active drugs.

A final point is that no guidelines can provide a complete recipe for the studies that should be undertaken to establish a drug's CNS safety. The considerable latitude of ICH S7A is a reflection of changing official attitudes toward defining the precise methods to be employed. It is now up to the individual drug developers to decide and justify which specific procedures are included. The present section has attempted to illustrate some of the possibilities beyond routine core battery studies, to ensure that a novel substance is devoid of risk on higher CNS function.

ACKNOWLEDGMENTS

We thank Dr. Paul Moser, Dr. Vincent Castagné, Dr. Niklaus Dürmüller, and Ms. Julie Presher for their comments on the contents of this chapter.

REFERENCES

1. Zbinden G. *Pharmacological Methods in Toxicology.* Elmsford, NY: Pergamon Press; 1979.
2. Bass AS, Kinter L, Williams P. Origins, practices and future of safety pharmacology. *J Pharmacol Toxicol Methods* 2004;49:145–151.
3. Anon. *Guidelines for General Pharmacology Studies.* Tokyo, Japan: Ministry of Health and Welfare; 1991.
4. Anon. *General Pharmacology Japanese Guidelines for Nonclinical Studies of Drugs Manual,* Tokyo, Japan: Yakuji Nippo Limited; 1995.
5. Shah RR. Drug-induced QT interval prolongation: regulatory perspectives and drug development. *Ann Med* 2004;36 (Suppl 1):47–52.
6. Gardin JM, Schumacher D, Constantine G, Davis KD, Leung C, Reid CL. Valvular abnormalities and cardiovascular status following exposure to dexfenfluramine or phentermine/fenfluramine. *Multicenter Study JAMA* 2000;283:1703–1709.
7. Anon. *ICH Guidance for Industry—S7A Safety Pharmacology Studies for Human Pharmaceuticals.* Washington, DC: US Department of Health and Human Services, Food and Drug Administration; 2001.
8. Bass AS, Tomaselli G, Bullingham R III, Kinter LB. Drug effects on ventricular repolarization: a critical evaluation of the strengths and weaknesses of current methodologies and regulatory practices. *J Pharmacol Toxicol Methods* 2005;52:12–21.
9. Kinter LB, Siegl PK, Bass AS. New preclinical guidelines on drug effects on ventricular repolarization: safety pharmacology comes of age. *J Pharmacol Toxicol Methods* 2004;49:153–158.
10. Baillie M, Bass AB, Darpo B, Engwall M, Garnes D, Gintant G, Hammond T, Hanson LA, Mittelstadt S, Rampe D, Sarazan RD, Siegl P, Thomas K. International Life Sciences Institute/Health & Environmental Sciences Institute Cardiovascular Risk Assessment, Cardiovascular Risk Assessment Workshop Proceedings; 2007.
11. Anon. *ICH Guidance for Industry—S7B Nonclinical Evaluation of the Potential for Delayed Ventricular Repolarization (QT Interval Prolongation) by Human Pharmaceuticals.* Washington, DC: US Department of Health and Human Services, Food and Drug Administration; 2005.
12. Harrison AP, Erlwanger KH, Elbrond VS, Andersen NK, Unmack MA. Gastrointestinal-tract models and techniques for use in safety pharmacology. *J Pharmacol Toxicol Methods* 2004;49:187–99.
13. Kinter LB. Safety pharmacology of the renal and gastro-intestinal systems. In: Williams PD, Bass AS, Eds. *Safety Pharmacology: A Practical Guide.* Gaithersburg, MD: TherImmune Research Corporation; 2003.
14. Gray LE. Jr, Kelce WR, Wiese T, Tyl R, Gaido K, Cook J, Klinefelter G, Desaulniers D, Wilson E, Zacharewski T, Waller C, Foster P, Laskey J, Reel J, Giesy J, Laws S, McLachlan J, Breslin W, Cooper R, Di Giulio R, Johnson R, Purdy R, Mihaich E, Safe S, Sonnenschein C, Welshons W, Miller R, McMaster S, Colborn T. Endocrine Screening Methods Workshop report: detection of estrogenic and androgenic hormonal and

antihormonal activity for chemicals that act via receptor or steroidogenic enzyme mechanisms. *Reprod Toxicol* 1997;11:719–750.

15. Emeigh Hart SG. Assessment of renal injury *in vivo. J Pharmacol Toxicol Methods* 2005;52:30–45.

16. Descotes J. Developments in biological standardization. *Immunotoxicol Immunomodulators* 1992;77:99–102.

17. Whitebread S, Hamon J, Bojanic D, Urban L. *In vitro* safety pharmacology profiling: an essential tool for successful drug development. *Drug Discov Today* 2005;10:1421–1433.

18. Friedrichs GS, Patmore L, Bass AS. Non-clinical evaluation of ventricular repolarization (ICH S7B): results of an interim survey of international pharmaceutical companies. *J Pharmacol Toxicol Methods* 2005;52:6–11.

19. Kinter LB, Valentin JP. Safety pharmacology and risk assessment. *Fundam Clin Pharmacol* 2002;16:175–182.

20. Matsuzawa T, Hashimoto M, Nara H, Yoshida M, Tamura S, Igarashi T. Current status of conducting function tests in repeated dose toxicity studies in Japan. *J Toxicol Sci* 1997;22:375–382.

21. Gad SC. *Safety Pharmacology in Pharmaceutical Development and Approval.* Boca Raton, FL: CRC Press; 2004.

22. Bass AS, Darpo B, Breidenbach A, Bruse K, Feldman HS, Garnes D, Hammond T, Haverkamp W, January C, Koerner J, Lawrence C, Leishman D, Roden D, Valentin JP, Vos MA, Zhou YY, Thomas K, Sager P. Recommendations for areas of investigation from the Workshop Breakout Sessions. Workshop: Moving Towards Better Predictors of Drug-Induced Torsades de Pointes (TdP); 2005.

23. Anon. *ICH Guidance for Industry—S6 Safety Evaluation of Biotechnology-Derived Pharmaceuticals.* Washington, DC: US Department of Health and Human Services, Food and Drug Administration; 1997.

24. Anon. *ICH Guidance for Industry—M3 NonClin Safety Studies for the Conduct of Human Clinical Trials for Pharmaceuticals.* Washington, DC: US Department of Health and Human Services, Food and Drug Administration; 1997.

25. Anon. Title 21 Code of Federal Regulations (21 CFR Part 58). *Good Laboratory Practice for NonClinical Laboratory Studies.* Washington, DC: US Department of Health and Human Service, Food and Drug Administration; revised 1 April 2006.

26. Anon. *ICH Guidance for Industry—E14 Clinical Evaluation of QT/QTc Interval Prolongation and Proarrhythmic Potential for Non-Antiarrhythmic Drugs.* Washington, DC: US Department of Health and Human Services, Food and Drug Administration; 2005.

27. Anon. Title 21 Code of Federal Regulations (21 CFR Part 11). *Electronic Records; Electronic Signatures.* Washington, DC: US Department of Health and Human Service, Food and Drug Administration, 2000.

28. Wakefield ID, Pollard C, Redfern WS, Hammond TG, Valentin JP. The application of *in vitro* methods to safety pharmacology. *Rev Fundam Clin Pharmacol* 2002;16:209–218.

29. Suter W. Predictive value of *in vitro* safety studies. *Curr Opin in Chem Biol* 2006;10:362–366.

30. Ollerstam A, Visser SA, Persson AH, Eklund G, Nilsson LB, Forsberg T, Wiklund SJ, Gabrielsson J, Duker G, Al-Saffar A. Pharmacokinetic-pharmacodynamic modeling of drug-induced effect on the QT interval in conscious telemetered dogs. *J Pharmacol Toxicol Methods* 2006; 53:174–183.

31. Sheiner LB, Steimer JL. PharmacokInetic/pharmacodynamic ModelIng In drug development. *Annu Rev Pharmacol Toxicol* 2000;40:67–95.

32. Hanson LA, Bass AS, Gintant G, Mittelstadt S, Rampe D, Thomas K. ILSI-HESI cardiovascular safety subcommittee initiative: evaluation of three non-clin models of QT prolongation. *J Pharmacol Toxicol Methods*. 2006;54:116–129.

33. Klumpp A, Trautmann T, Markert M, Guth B. Optimizing the experimental environment for dog telemetry studies. *J Pharmacol Toxicol Methods* 2006;54:141–149.

34. Chaves AA, Keller WJ, O'Sullivan S, Williams MA, Fitzgerald LE, McPherson HE, Goykhman D, Ward PD, Hoe CM, Mixson L, Briscoe RJ. Cardiovascular monkey telemetry: sensitivity to detect QT interval prolongation. *J Pharmacol Toxicol Methods* 2006;54:150–158.

35. Swissa M, Zhou S, Paz O, Fishbein MC, Chen LS, Chen PS. Canine model of paroxysmal atrial fibrillation and paroxysmal atrial tachycardia. *Am J Physiol Heart Circ Physiol* 2005;289:H1851–H1857.

36. Acosta D Jr, Ed. *Cardiovascular Toxicology*. London: Taylor & Francis; 2001.

37. *Goodman and Gilman's The Pharmacological Basis of Therapeutics*. New York: McGraw-Hill; 2006.

38. Berne RM, Levy MN. *Cardiovascular Physiology*, 8th ed. St Louis, MO: Mosby; 2001.

39. De Mello WC, Janse MJ. Heart cell coupling and impulse propogation [sic] in health and disease. Boston: Kluwer Academic Pubulishers; 2002.

40. Levy MN, Pappano AJ. *Cardiovascular Physiology*, 9th ed. Philadelphia, PA: Mosby Elsevier; 2007.

41. Opie LH. *Heart Physiology: From Cell to Circulation*, 4th ed. Philadelphia: Lippincott Williams & Wilkins; 2004.

42. Pypendop BH, Verstegen JP. Hemodynamic effects of medetomidine in the dog: a dose titration study. *Vet Surg* 1998;27:612–622.

43. Gomez De Segura IA, Vazquez Moreno-Planas I, Benito J, Galiano A, De Miguel E. Electrophysiologic cardiac effects of the new local anesthetic IQB-9302 and of bupivacaine in the anesthetised dog. *Acta Anaesthesiol Scand* 2002;46:666–673.

44. Beckman KJ, Parker RB, Hariman RJ, Gallastegui JL, Javaid JI, Bauman JL. Hemodynamic and electrophysiological actions of cocaine. Effects of sodium bicarbonate as an antidote in dogs. *Circulation* 1991;83:1799–1807.

45. Bicer S, Nakayama T, Hamlin RL. Effects of chronic oral amiodarone on left ventricular function, ECGs, serum chemistries, and exercise tolerance in healthy dogs. *J Vet Intern Med* 2002;16:247–540.

46. Lee JD, Tajimi T, Patritti J, Ross J Jr. Preload reserve and mechanisms of afterload mismatch in normal conscious dog. *Am J Physiol* 1986;250(3 Pt 2):H464–H473.

47. Boon JA. *Manual of Veterinary Echocardiology*. Philadelphia: Lippincott Williams & Wilkins; 1998.

48. Kohn DF, Wixson SK, White WJ, Benson GJ. *Anesthesia and Analgesia in Laboratory Animals*. San Diego, CA: Academic Press; 1997.

49. Muir WW. III, Hubbell JAE, Skarda RT, Bednarski RM. *Handbook of Veterinary Anesthesia*, 3rd ed. St Louis, MO: Mosby; 2000.

50. Riley DC, Schmeling WT, al-Wathiqui MH, Kampine JP, Warltier DC. Prolongation of the QT interval by volatile anesthetics in chronically instrumented dogs. *Anesth Analg* 1988;67:741–749.

51. Gallagher JD. Effects of halothane and quinidine on intracardiac conduction and QTc interval in pentobarbital-anesthetized dogs. *Anesth Analg* 1992;75:688–695.

52. Shimizu W, McMahon B, Antzelevitch C. Sodium pentobarbital reduces transmural dispersion of repolarization and prevents torsades de pointes in models of acquired and congenital long QT syndrome. *J Cardiovasc Electrophysiol* 1999;10:154–164.

53. Takahara A, Sugiyama A, Satoh Y, Wang K, Honsho S, Hashimoto K. Halothane sensitizes the canine heart to pharmacological I_{Kr} blockade. *Eur J Pharmacol* 2005;507:169–177.

54. Shimosato S, Etsten BE. Effect of anesthetic drugs on the heart: a critical review of myocardial contractility and its relationship to hemodynamics. *Clin Anesth* 1969;3:17–72.

55. Picker O, Scheeren TWL, Arndt JO. Inhalation anaesthetics increase heart rate by decreasing cardiac vagal activity in dogs. *Br J Anaesth* 2001;87:748–754.

56. Picker O, Schindler A, Scheeren TW. Accuracy and reproducibility of long-term implanted transit-time ultrasound flow probes in dogs. *Intensive Care Med* 2000;26:601–607.

57. www.dissdata.com.

58. Data Sciences International (www.datasci.com).

59. www.transonic.com.

60. Emka Technologies (www.emkatech.com).

61. www.vivometrics.com.

62. Buxco Electronics, Inc. (www.buxco.com).

63. Data Integrated Scientific Systems (www.itstelemetry.com).

64. LDS Test and Measurement (PoNeMah; http://www.lds-group.com).

65. Modular Instruments Inc. (www.mi2.com).

66. Notocord Systems (www.notocord.com).

67. Miura T, Miyazaki S, Guth BD, Indolfi C, Ross J Jr. Heart rate and force-frequency effects on diastolic function of the left ventricle in exercising dogs. *Circulation* 1994;89:2361–2368.

68. Kingma JG Jr, Armour JA, Rouleau JR. Left ventricular intramyocardial pressure determination using two different solid-state micromanometric pressure sensors. *Can J Physiol Pharmacol* 1996;74(6):701–705.

69. Hamlin B, Guth B, Sarazan D, Picker O, Schindler A, Scheeren TW. Accuracy and reproducibility of long-term implanted transit-time ultrasound flow probes in dogs. *Intensive Care Med* 2000;26:601–607.

70. Hamlin RL, Nakayama T, Nakayama H, Carnes CA. Effects of changing heart rate on electrophysiological and hemodynamic function in the dog. *Life Sci* 2003;72:1919–1930.

71. Oyama MA, Sisson DD, Bulmer BJ, Constable PD. Echocardiographic estimation of mean left atrial pressure in a canine model of acute mitral valve insufficiency. *J Vet Intern Med* 2004;18:667–672.

72. Goldberger JJ, Kadish AH, Johnson D, Qi X. New technique for vagal nerve stimulation. *J Neurosci Methods* 1999;91:109–114.

73. Bass AS, Robie NW. Stereoselectivity of S- and R-sulpiride for pre- and postsynaptic dopamine receptors in the canine kidney. *J Pharmacol Exp Ther* 1984;229:67–71.

74. Bass AS, Murphy MB, Kohli JD, Goldberg LI. Potentiation by dopexamine of the cardiac responses to circulating and neuronally released norepinephrine: a possible mechanism for the therapeutic effects of the drug. *J Cardiovasc Pharmacol* 1989;13:667–671.

75. Nolan ER, Feng MR, Koup JR, Liu J, Turluck D, Zhang Y, Paulissen JB, Olivier NB, Miller T, Bailie M/B. A novel predictive pharmacokinetic/pharmacodynamic model of repolarization prolongation derived from the effects of terfenadine, cisapride and E-4031 in the conscious chronic AV node—ablated, His bundle-paced dog. *J Pharmacol Toxicol Methods* 2006;53:1–10.

76. Toshida N, Hirao K, Yamamoto N, Tanaka M, Suzuki F, Isobe M. Ventricular echo beats and retrograde atrioventricular nodal exits in the dog heart: multiplicity in their electrophysiologic and anatomic characteristics. *J Cardiovasc Electrophysiol* 2001; 12:1256–1264.

77. Smith DA, van de Waterbeemd, Walker DK. *Pharmacokinetics and Metabolism in Drug Design*, 2nd ed. Weinheim: Wiley-VCH; 2006.

78. Schoenwald RD, ed. *Pharmacokinetics in Drug Discovery and Development*. Boca Raton, FL: CRC Press; 2002.

79. Boroujerdi M. *Pharmacokinetics: Principles and Applications*. New York: McGraw-Hill Medical Publications Division; 2001.

80. Markert M, Klumpp A, Trautmann T, Guth B. A novel propellant-free inhalation drug delivery system for cardiovascular drug safety evaluation in conscious dogs. *J Pharmacol Toxicol Methods* 2004;50:109–119.

81. Petruska JM, Beattie JG, Stuart BO, Pai S, Walters KM, Banks CM, Lulham GW, Mirro EJ. Cardiovascular effects after inhalation of large doses of albuterol dry powder in rats, monkeys, and dogs: a species comparison. *Fundam Appl Toxicol* 1997;40:52–62.

82. Gad SC. *Statistics and Experimental Design for Toxicologists and Pharmacologists*, 4th ed. Boca Raton, FL: CRC Press; 2005.

83. Jones B, Kenward MG. *Design and Analysis of Cross-over Trials*. London: Chapman & Hall; 1989.

84. Winer BJ, Brown DR, Michels KM. *Statistical Principles in Experimental Design*, 3rd ed. New York: McGraw Hill; 1991.

85. Snedecor GW, Cochran WG. *Statistical Methods*, 6th ed. Ames: Iowa State University Press; 1967.

86. Detweiler DK. Electrocardiographic monitoring in toxicological studies: principles and interpretations. *Adv Exp Med Biol* 1983;161:579–607.

87. Tilley LP, Burtnick NL. *ECG for the Small Animal Practitioner*. Jackson WY: Teton NewMedia; 1999.

88. Hanton G, Rabemampianina Y. The electrocardiogram of the beagle dog: reference values and effect of sex, genetic strain, body position and heart rate. *Lab Anim* 2006;40:123–136.

89. Roden DM, Anderson ME. Proarrhythmia. In Starke FK, Ed., *Handbook of Experimental Pharmacology*, Vol. 171. New York; Springer 2006, pp 73–97.7.

90. Fenichel RR, Malik M, Antzelevitch C, Sanguinetti M, Roden DM, Priori SG, Ruskin JN, Lipicky RJ, Cantilena LR. Independent Academic Task Force. Drug-induced torsades de pointes and implications for drug development. *J Cardiovasc Electrophysiol* 2004;15:475–495.

91. Soloviev MV, Hamlin RL, Shellhammer LJ, Barrett RM, Wally RA, Birchmeier PA, Schaefer GJ. Variations in hemodynamic parameters and ECG in healthy, conscious, freely moving telemetrized beagle dogs. *Cardiovasc Toxicol* 2006;6:51–62.

92. Watanabe H, Miyazaki H. A new approach to correct the QT interval for changes in heart rate using a nonparametric regression model in beagle dogs. *J Pharmacol Toxicol Methods* 2006;53:234–241.

93. Tattersall ML, Dymond M, Hammond T, Valentin JP. Correction of QT values to allow for increases in heart rate in conscious beagle dogs in toxicology assessment. *J Pharmacol Toxicol Methods* 2006;53:11–19.

94. Batey AJ, Doe CP. A method for QT correction based on beat-to-beat analysis of the QT/RR interval relationship in conscious telemetred beagle dogs. *J Pharmacol Toxicol Methods* 2002;48:11–19.

95. Raunig D, Depasquale MJ, Huang CH, Winslow R, Fossa AA. Statistical analysis of QT interval as a function of changes in RR interval in the conscious dog. *J Pharmacol Toxicol Methods* 2001;46:1–11.

96. Malik M, Camm AJ. Evaluation of drug-induced QT interval prolongation: implications for drug approval and labelling. *Drug Safety* 2001;24:323–351.

97. Fridericia LS. Die systolendauer im elektrokardogramm bei normalen menchen und bei Herzkranken. *Acta Med Scand* 1920;53:469–486.

98. Spence S, Soper K, Hoe CM, Coleman J. The heart rate-corrected QT interval of conscious beagle dogs: a formula based on analysis of covariance. *Toxicol Sci* 1998;45:247–258.

99. Osborne BE, Leach GDH. The beagle electrocardiogram. *Fundam Cosmet Toxicol* 1971;9:2857–2864.

100. Fossa AA, Wisialowski T, Crimin K. QT prolongation modifies dynamic restitution and hysteresis of the beat-to-beat QT-TQ interval relationship during normal sinus rhythm under varying states of repolarization. *J Pharmacol Exp Ther* 2006;316:498–506.

101. Bazett HC. An analysis of the time-relations of electrocardiograms. *Heart* 1920;7:353–370.

102. Dessertenne F. La tachycardia ventriculaire a deux foyers opposes variables. *Arch Mal Coeur* 1996;59:263–272.

103. Sanguinetti MC, Jiang C, Curran ME, Keating MT. A mechanistic link between and inherited and acquired cardiac arrhythmia: HERG encodes the iKr potassium channel. *Cell* 1995;81:299–307.

104. Trudeau MC, Warmke JW, Ganetzky B, Robertson GA. HERG, a human inward rectifier in the voltage-gated potassium channel family. *Science* 1995;269:92–95.

105. Curran ME, Splawski I, Timothy KW, Vincent GM, Green ED, Keating MT. A molecular basic for cardiac arrhythmia: HERG mutations cause long QT syndrome. *Cell* 1995;80:795–803.

106. Zhou Z, Gong Q, Ye B, Fan Z, Makielski JC, Robertson GA, January CT. Properties of HERG channels stably expressed in HEK293 cells studied at physiological temperature. *Biophys J* 1998;74:230–241.

107. Walker BD, Valenzuela SM, Singleton CB, Tie H, Bursill JA, Wyse KR, Qiu MR, Breit SN, Campbell TJ. Inhibition of HERG channels stably expressed in a mammalian cell line by the antianginal agent perhexiline maleate. *Br J Pharmacol* 1999;127:243–251.

108. Witchel HJ, Milnes JT, Mitcheson JS, Hancox JC. Troubleshooting problems with *in vitro* screening of drugs for QT interval prolongation using HERG K+ channels expressed in mammalian cell lines and Xenopus oocytes. *J Pharmacol Toxicol Methods* 2002;48:65–80.

109. Kirsch GE, Trepakova ES, Brimecombe JC, Sidach SS, Erickson HD, Kochan MC, Shyjka LM, Lacerda AE, Brown AM. Variability in the measurement of hERG potassium channel inhibition: effects of temperature and stimulus pattern. *J Pharmacol Toxicol Methods* 2004;50:93–101.

110. Guo L, Guthrie H. Automated electrophysiology in the preclinical evaluation of drugs for potential QT prolongation. *J Pharmacol Toxicol Methods* 2005;52(1):123–135.

111. Gintant GA, Su Z, Martin RL, Cox BF. Utility of hERG assays as surrogate markers of delayed cardiac repolarization and QT safety. *J Toxicol Pathol* 2006;34:81–90.

112. Yao J-A, Du X, Lu D, Baker RL, Daharsh E, Atterson P. Estimation of potency of HERG channel blockers: impact of voltage protocol and temperature. *J Pharmacol Toxicol Methods* 2005;52:146–153.

113. Herron W, Towers C, Templeton A. Experiences in method development for the analysis of *in vitro* study solutions for content. *J Pharmacol Toxicol Methods* 2004;49:211–216.

114. Redfern WS, Carlsson L, Davis AS, Lynch WG, MacKenzie I, Pelethorpe Sl, Siegl PKS, Strang I, Sullivan AT, Wallis R, Camm AJ, Hammond TG. Relationships between preclinical cardiac electrophysiology, clinical QT interval prolongation and torsades de pointes for a broad range of drugs: evidence for a provisional safety margin in drug development. *Cardiovasc Res* 2003;58:32–45.

115. Diaz GJ, Daniell K, Leitza ST, Martin RL, Su Z, McDermott JS, Cox BF, Gintant GA. The [^{3}H] dofetilide binding assay is a predictive screening tool for hERG blockade and proarrhythmia: comparison of intact cell and membrane preparations and effects of altering [K^+]$_o$. *J Pharmacol Toxicol Methods* 2004;50:187–199.

116. Chaudhary KW, O'Neal JM, Mo Z-L, Fermini B, Gallavan RH, Bahinski A. Evaluation of the rubidium efflux assay for preclinical identification of hERG blockade. *Assay Drug Dev Technol* 2006;4(1):73–82.

117. Baxter DF, Kirk M, Garcia AF, Raimondi A, Holmqvist MH, Flint KK, Bojanic D, Distefano PS, Curtis Rl, Xie Y. A novel membrane potential-sensitive fluorescent dye improves cell-based assays for ion channels. *J Biomol Screen* 2002;7(1):79–85.

118. Bril A, Gout B, Bonhomme M, Landais L, Faivre J, Linee P, Poyser RH, Ruffolo RR Jr. Combined potassium and calcium channel blocking activities as a basis for antiarrhythmic efficacy with low proarrhythmic risk: experimental profile of BRL-32872. *J Pharmacol Exp Ther* 1996;509:129–137.

119. Zhang S, Zhou Z, Gong Q, Makielski JC, January CT. Mechanism of block and identification of the verapamil binding domain to HERG potassium channels. *Circ Res* 1999;84:989–998.

120. Martin RL, McDermott JS, Salmen HJ, Palmatier J, Cox BF, Gintant GA. The utility of hERG and repolarization assays in evaluating delayed cardiac repolarization: Influence of multi-channel block. *J Cardiovasc Pharmacol* 2004;43:369–379.

121. Ficker El, Kuryshev YA, Dennis AT, Oberjero-Paz C, Wang L, Hawryluk P, Wible BA, Brown AM. Mechanisms of arsenic-induced prolongation of cardiac repolarization. *Mol Pharmacol* 2004;66:33–44.

122. Drolet B, Simard C, Roden DM. Unusual effects of a QT-prolonging drug, arsenic trioxide, on cardiac potassium currents. *Circulation* 2004;109:26–29.

123. Kuryshev YA, Ficker E, Wang L, Hawryluk P, Dennis AT, Wible BA, Brown AM, Kang J, Chen XL, Sawamura K, Reynolds Wl, Rampe D. Pentamidine-induced long QT syndrome and block of HERG trafficking. *J Pharmacol Exp Ther* 2005;312(1):316–323.

124. Cordes JS, Sun Z, Lloyd DB, Bradley JA, Opsahl AC, Tengowski MW, Chen X, Zhou J. Pentamidine reduces hERG expression to prolong the QT interval. *Br J Pharmacol* 2005;145(1):15–23.

125. Wible BA, Hawryluk P, Ficker E, Kuryshev YA, Kirsch G, Brown AM. HERG-lite: a novel comprehensive high throughput screen for drug-induced hERG risk. *J Pharmacol Toxicol Methods* 2005;52(1):136–145.

126. Glaaser IW, Kass RS, Clancy CE. Mechanisms of genetic arrhythmias: from DNA to ECG. *Prog Cardiovasc Dis* 2003;46(3):259–270.

127. Roden DM, Viswanathan PC. Genetics of acquired long QT syndrome. *J Clin Invest* 2005;115(8):2025–2032.

128. Roden DM. Long QT syndrome: reduced repolarization reserve and the genetic link. *J Intern Med* 2006;259:59–69.

129. Franz MR. Current status of monophasic action potential recording: theories measurements and interpretations. *Cardiovasc Res* 1999;41:25–40.

130. Hondeghem LM, Carlsson L, Duker G. Instability and triangulation of the action potential predict serious proarrhythmia but APD prolongation is antiarrhythmic. *Circulation* 2001;103:2004–2013.

131. Strauss HC, Bigger JT Jr, Hoffman BF. Electrophysiological and beta-receptor blocking effects of MJ 1999 on dog and rabbit cardiac tissue. *Circ Res* 1970;26(6):661–678.

132. Sosunov EA, Anyukhovsky EP, Rosen MR. Effects of quinidine on repolarization in canine epicardium midmyocardium, and endocardium. I. *In vitro* study. *Circulation* 1997;96:4011–4018.

133. Wang L, Feng Z-P, Kondo CS, Sheldon RS, Duff HJ. Developmental changes in the delayes rectifier K+ channels in mouse heart. *Circ Res* 1996;79:79–85.

134. Liu GX, Zhou J, Nattel S, Koren G. Single-channel recordings of a rapid delayed rectifier current in adult mouse ventricular myocytes; basic properties and effects of divalent cations. *J Physiol (London.)* 2004;556(2):401–413.

135. Wymore RS, Gintant GA, Wymore RT, Dixon JE, McKinnon D, Cohen IS. Tissue and species distribution of mRNA for the iKr-like K^+ channel, erg. *Circ Res* 1997;80:261–268.

136. McDermott JS, Salmen HJ, Cox BF, Gintant GA. Importance of species selection in arrhythmogenic models of QT interval prolongation. *Antimicrob Agents Chemother* 2002;46(3):938–939.

137. January CT, Riddle JM. Early afterdepolarizations: mechansim of induction and block. A role for L-type Ca2+ current. *Circ Res* 1999;64(5):977–990.

138. Lu HR, Vlaminckx E, Van Ammel K, De Clerck F. Drug-induced long QT in isolated rabbit Purkinje fibers; importance of action potential duration, triangulation and early afterdepolarizations. *Eur J Pharmacol* 2002;452(2):183–192.

139. Hondeghem LM. TRIad; foundation for proarrhythmia (triangulation, reverse use dependence and instability). *Novartis Found Symp* 2005;266:235–244.

140. Brugada R, Hong K, Cordeiro JM, Dumaine R. Short QT syndrome. *CMAJ* 2005;173(11):1349–1354

141. Horn R, Marty A. Muscarinic activation of ionic currents measured by a new whole-cell recording method. *J Gen Physiol* 1988;92:145–159.

142. Zaniboni M, Pollard AE, Yang L, Spitzer KW. Beat-to-beat repolarization variability in ventricular myocytes and its suppression by electrical coupling. *Am J Physiol Heart Circ Physiol* 2000;278(3):H677–H687.

143. Sawanobori T, Adaniya H, Namiki T, Hiraoka M. Rate-dependent effects of sematilide on action potential duration in isolated guinea pig ventricular myocytes. *J Pharmacol Exp Ther* 1994;271(1):302–310.

144. Salata JJ, Jurkiewicz NK, Wallace AA, Stupienski RF 3rd, Guinosso PJ Jr, Cardiac electrophysiological actions of the histamine H1-receptor antagonists astemizole and terfenadine compared with chlorpheniramine and pyrilamine. *Circ Res* 1995;76:110–119.

145. Gintant GA. Azimilide causes reverse rate-dependent block while reducing both components of delayed rectifier current in canine ventricular myocytes. *J Cardiovasc Pharmacol* 1998;31:945–953.

146. Davie C, Pierre-Valentin J, Pollard C, Standen N, Mitcheson J, Alexander P, Thong B. Comparative pharmacology of guinea pig cardiac myocyte and cloned hERG (IKr) channel. *J Cardiovasc Electrophysiol* 2004;15:1302–1309.

147. Gintant GA, Limberis JT, McDermott JS, Wegner CD, Cox BF. The canine Purkinje fiber: an *in vitro* model system for acquired long QT syndrome and drug-induced arrhythmogenesis. *J Cardiovasc Pharmacol* 2001;37:607–618.

148. Lu HR, Vlaminckx E, Teisman A, Gallacher DJ. Choice of cardiac tissue plays an important role in the evaluation of drug-induced prolongation of the QT interval *in vitro* in rabbit. *J Pharmacol Toxicol Methods* 2005;52(1):90–105.

149. Varro A, Nakaya Y, Elharrar V, Surawicz B. The effects of amiodarone on repolarization and refractoriness of cardiac fibers. *Eur J Pharmacol* 1988;154(1):11–18.

150. Kii Y, Hayashi S, Tabo M, et al. QT PRODACT. Evaluation of the potential of compounds to cause QT interval prolongation by action potential assays using guinea-pig papillary muscles. *J Pharmacol Sci* 2006;99(5):449–457.

151. Yan G-X, Shimizu W, Antzelevitch C. Characteristics and distribution of M cells in arterially perfused canine left ventricular wedge preparations. *Circulation* 1998;98:1921–1927.

152. Yan G-X, Rials SJ, Wu Y, Liu T, Xu X, Marinchak RA, Kowey PR. Ventricular hypertrophy amplifies transmural repolarization dispersion and induces early afterdepolarization. *Am J Physiol Heart Circ Physiol* 2001;281:H1968–H1975.

153. Di Diego JM, Belardinelli L, Antzelevitch C. Cisapride-induced transmural dispersion of repolarization and torsades de pointes in the canine left ventricular wedge preparation during epicardial stimulation. *Circulation* 2003;108:1027–1033.

154. Yan G-X, Wu Y, Liu T, Wang J, Marinchak RA, Kowey PR. Phase 2 early afterdepolarizations as a trigger of polymorphic ventricular tachycardia in acquired long-QT syndrome. Direct evidence from intracellular recordings in the intact left ventricular wall. *Circulation* 2001;103:2851–2856.

155. Sutherland FJ, Hearse DJ. The isolated blood and perfusion fluid perfused heart. *Pharmacol Res* 2000;41(6):613–627.

156. Hondeghem LM, Hoffmann P. Blinded test in isolated female rabbit heart reliably identifies action potential duration prolongation and proarrhythmic drugs: importance of triangulation, reverse use-dependence, and instability. *J Cardiovasc Pharmacol* 2003;41:14–24.

157. Shah RR, Hondeghem LM. Refining detection of drug-induced proarrhythmia: QT interval and TRIaD. *Heart Rhythm* 2005;2:758–772.

158. Hamlin RL, Cruze CA, Mittelstadt SW, Kijtawornrat A, Keene BW, Roche BM, Takayama T, Nakayama H, Hamlin DM, Arnold T. Sensitivity and specificity of isolated perfused guinea pig heart to test for drug-induced lengthening of QTc. *J Pharmacol Toxicol Methods* 2004;49:15–23.

159. Eckardt L, Haverkamp W, Mertens H, Johna R, Clague JR, Borggrefe M, Beirthardt G. Drug-related torsades de pointes in the isolated rabbit heart: comparison of clofilium D,L-sotalol, and erythromycin. *J Cardiovasc Pharmacol* 1998;32:425–434.

160. Johna R, Mertens H, Haverkamp W, Eckardt L, Niederboker T, Borggrefe M, Breithardt G, Clofilium in the isolated perfused rabbit heart: a new model to study proarrhythmia induced by class III antiarrhythmic drugs. *Basic Res Cardiol* 1998;93:127–135.

161. Akoun GM, Milleron BJ, Mayaund CM, Francois TJ. Natural history of drug-induced pneumonitis. In Akoun GM, White PJ, Eds. Drug Induced Disorders, Vol. 3. Elsevier Scientific Publishers; 1989, pp 3–9.

162. Rosenow EC, Myers JL, Swensen SJ, Pisani RJ. Drug induced pulmonary disease: an update. *Chest* 1992;102:239–250.

163. Eldridge FL, Millhorn DE. Central regulation of respiration by endogenous neurotransmitters and neuromodulators. *Annu Rev Physiol* 1981;43:121–135.

164. Mueller RA, Lundberg DBA, Breese GR, Hedner J, Hedner T, Jonason J. The neuropharmacology of respiratory control. *Pharmacol Rev* 1982;34:255–285.

165. Heymans C. Action of drugs on carotid body and sinus. *Pharmacol Rev* 1955;7:119–142.

166. Heymans C, Neil E. The effects of drugs on chemoreceptors. In Heymans C, Neil E, eds. *Reflexogenic Areas of the Cardiovascular System*. London: Churchill Ltd; 1958; pp 192–199.

167. Sant'Ambrogio G. Nervous receptors of the tracheobronchial tree. *Annu Rev Physiol* 1987;49:611–627.

168. Phillipson EA. Disorders in the control of breathing: hypoventilation syndromes. In Murray JF, Nadal JA, eds. *Textbook of Respiratory Medicine*. Philadelphia: Saunders; 1988, pp 1831–1840.

169. Cherniack NS. Disorders in the control of breathing: hyperventilation syndromes. In Murray JF, Nadal JA, eds. *Textbook of Respiratory Medicine*. Philadelphia: Saunders; 1988, pp 1861–1866.

170. Laffey JG. Kavavagh BP. Hypocapnia. *N Engl J Med* 2002;347(1):43–53.

171. Boggs DF. Comparative control of respiration. In Parent RA, ed. *Comparative Biology of the Normal Lung*, Vol I. Boca Raton FL: CRC Press; 1992, pp 309–350.

172. Keats AS. The effects of drugs on respiration in man. *Annu Rev Pharmacol Toxicol* 1985;25:41–65.

173. McCarthy DS. Airflow obstruction. In Kryger MH, eds. *Pathophysiology of Respiration*. Hoboken, NJ: Wiley; 1981, pp 7–42.

174. Rochester DF, Arora NS. Respiratory muscle failure. *Med Clin Studies North Am* 1983;67:573–597.

175. Milic-Emili J. Recent advances in clinical assessment of control of breathing. *Lung* 1982;160:1–17.

176. Warren CPW. Lung restriction. In Kryger MH, ed. *Pathophysiology of Respiration*. Hoboken, NJ: Wiley; 1981, pp 43–69.

177. Drorbaugh JE, Fenn WO. A barometric method for measuring ventilation in newborn infants. *Pediatrics* 1955;16:81–86.

178. Jacky JP. Barometric measurement of tidal volume: effects of pattern and nasal temperature. *J Appl Physiol Respir Environ Exere Physiol* 1980;49(2):319–325.

179. Zimmerman PV, Connellan SJ, Middleton HC, Tabona MV, Goldman MD, Pride N. Postural changes in rib cage and abdominal volume-motion coefficients and their effect on the calibration of a respiratory inductance plethysmograph. *Am Rev Respir Dis* 1983;127:209–214.

180. Murphy DJ, Joran ME, Renninger JE. Effects of adenosine agonists and antagonists on pulmonary ventilation in conscious rats. *Gen Pharmacol* 1993;24(4):943–954.

181. Murphy DJ, Joran ME, Grando JC. Microcapnometry: a non-invasive method for monitoring arterial CO_2 tension in conscious rats. *Toxicol Methods* 1994;4(3):177–187.

182. Murphy DJ, Joran ME, Grando JC. A non-invasive method for distinguishing central from peripheral nervous system effects of respiratory depressant drugs in conscious rats. *Gen Pharmacol* 1995;26(3):569–575.

183. Watchko JF, Standaert TA, Mayock DE, Twiggs G, Woodrum DE. Ventilatory failure during loaded breathing: the role of central neural drive. *J Appl Physiol* 1988;65(1):249–255.

184. Nuzzo PF, Anton WR. Practical applications of capnography. *Respir Therapy* 1986;16:12–17.

185. Lucke JN, Hall GM, Lister D. Porcine malignant hyperthermia I: metabolic and physiologic changes. *Br J Anesthesiol* 1976;48:297–304.

186. Becklake M, Crapo RO. American Thoracic Society Statement: Lung function testing: selection of reference values and interpretative strategies. *Am Rev Respir Dis* 1991;144:1202–1218.

187. Diamond L, O'Donnell M. Pulmonary mechanics in normal rats. *J Appl Physiol Respir Environ Exerc Physiol* 1977;43:942–948.

188. Mauderly JL. Effect of inhaled toxicants on pulmonary function. In McClellan RO, Henderson RF, eds. *Concepts in Inhalation Toxicology*. New York: Hemisphere Publishing; 1989, pp 347–401.

189. Amdur MO, Mead J. Mechanics of respiration in unanesthetized guinea pigs. *Am J Physiol* 1958;192:364–368.

190. O'Neil JJ, Raub JA. Pulmonary function testing in small laboratory animals. *Environ Health Perspect* 1984;56:11–22.

191. Mauderly JL. The influence of sex and age on the pulmonary function of the beagle dog. *J Gerontol* 1974;29:282–289.

192. Douglas JS, Dennis MW, Ridgeway P, Bouhuys A. Airway dilation and constriction in spontaneously breathing guinea pigs. *J Pharmacol Exp Ther* 1971;180:98–109.

193. Kruger JJ, Bain T, Patterson JL Jr. Elevation gradient of intrathoracic pressure. *J Appl Physiol* 1961;16:465–468.

194. Murphy DJ, Renninger JP, Gossett KA. A novel method for chronic measurement of pleural pressure in conscious rats. *J Pharmacol Toxicol Methods* 1998;39:137–141.

195. Murphy DJ, Renninger JP, Coatney RW. A novel method for chronic measurement of respiratory function in the conscious monkey. *J Pharmacol Toxicol Methods* 2001;46:13–20.

196. Pennock BE, Cox CP, Rogers RM, Cain WA, Wells JH. A noninvasive technique for measurement of changes in specific airway resistance. *J Appl Physiol* 1979;46:39–406.

197. Hamelmann E, Schwarze J, Takeda K, Oshiba A, Larsen GL, Irvin CG, Gelfand EW. Noninvasive measurement of airway responsiveness in allergic mice using barometric plethysmography. *Am J Respir Crit Care Med* 1997;156:766–775.

198. Lundblad LKA, Irvin CG, Adler A, Bates JHT. A re-evaluation of the validity of unrestrained plethysmography in mice. *J Appl Physiol* 2002;93:1198–1207.

199. Celli BR. American Thoracic Society Statement: Standards for the diagnosis and care of patients with chronic obstructive pulmonary disease. *Am J Respir Crit Care Med* 1995;152 (5) Suppl:S78–S121.

200. Brown LK, Miller A. Full lung volumes: functional residual capacity, residual volume and total lung capacity. In Miller A, ed. *Pulmonary Function Tests: A Guide for the Student and House Officer*. New York: Grune & Stratton; 1987, pp 53–58.

201. King TKC. Measurement of functional residual capacity in the rat. *J Appl Physiol* 1966;21:233–236.

202. Palecek F. Measurement of ventilatory mechanics in the rat. *J Appl Physiol* 1969;27:149–156.

203. Smolders FDJ, Folgering HTh, Bernards JA. Ventilation estimated from efferent phrenic nerve activity in the paralyzed cat. *Pflugers Arch* 1975;359:157–169.

204. Chitravanshi VC, Sapru HN. Phrenic nerve responses to chemical stimulation of the sub regions of ventral medullary respiratory neuronal group in the rat. *Brain Res* 1999;821:443–460.

205. Syabbalo N. Assessment of respiratory muscle function and strength. *Postgrad Med J* 1998;74:208–215.

206. Borison HL. Central nervous system depressants: control-systems approach to respiratory depression. *Pharmacol Ther B* 1997;3:211–226.

207. Trenchard D, Gardner D, Guz A. Role of pulmonary vagal afferent nerve fibers in the development of rapid shallow breathing in lung inflammation. *Clin Sci* 1972;42:251–263.

208. Drazen JM. Physiological basis and interpretation of indices of pulmonary mechanics. *Environ Health Perspect* 1984;56:3–9.

209. Costa DL, Raub JA, Tepper JS. Comparative respiratory physiology of the lung. In Parent RA, ed. *Comparative Biology of the Normal Lung*, Vol I. Boca Raton, FL: CRC Press; 1992, pp 175–402.

210. Hakkinen PJ, Witschi HP. Animal models. In Witschi HP, Brain JD, eds. *Handbook of Experimental Pharmacology*, Vol 75. New York: Springer-Verlag; 1985, pp 95–114.

211. Anon. *ICH S7A: Safety Pharmacology Studies for Human Pharmaceuticals*. European Agency for the Evaluation of Medicinal Products. Evaluation of Medicines for Human Use. CPMP/ICH/539/00, London, 16 November 2000.

212. Porsolt RD, Lemaire M, Dürmüller N, Roux S. New perspectives in CNS safety pharmacology. *Fundam Clin Pharmacol* 2002;16:197–207.

213. Porsolt RD. Central nervous system (CNS) safety pharmacology studies. In Vogel GH, Hock FJ, Maas J, Mayer D. eds. *Drug Discovery and Evaluation: Safety and Pharmacokinetic Assays*. Heidelberg: Springer Verlag; 2006, pp 15–60.

214. Irwin S. Comprehensive behavioral assessment: a systematic quantitative procedure for assessing the behavioral and physiologic state of the mouse. *Psychopharmacologia* 1968;13:222–257.

215. Mattson JL, Spencer PJ, Albee RR. A performance standard for clinical and functional observational battery examination of rats. *J Am Coll Toxicol* 1996;15:239–250.

216. Reiter LR, McPhail RC. Motor activity: a survey of methods with potential use in toxicity testing. *Neurobehav Toxicol* 1979;1 (Suppl):53–66.

217. Dunham NW, Miya TS. A note on a simple apparatus for detecting neurological deficit in mice and rats. *J Am Pharm Assoc* 1957;46:208–209.

218. Porsolt RD, Picard S, Lacroix P. International safety pharmacology guidelines (ICH S7A and S7B): where do we go from here? *Drug Dev Res* 2005;64:83–89.

219. Krall E. Antiepileptic drug development: anticonvulsant drug screening. *Epilepsia* 1978;19:409–428.

220. Simon P, Chermat R, Doaré L, Bourin M, Farinotti R. Interactions imprévues de divers psychotropes avec les effets du barbital et du pentobarbital chez la souris. *J Pharmacol (Paris)* 1982;13:241–252.

221. Bammer C. Pharmacological investigations of neurotransmitter involvement in passive avoidance responding: a review and some new results. *Neurosci Biobehav Rev* 1982;6:247–296.

222. Glick SD, Zimmerberg D. Amnesic effects of scopolamine. *Behav Biol* 1972;7:2445–2454.

223. Morris RGM. Spatial localization does not require the presence of local cues. *Learn Motiv* 1981;12:239–260.

224. Olton DS. The radial maze as a tool in behavioral pharmacology. *Physiol Behav* 1986;40:793–797.

225. Dunnett SB, Evenden JL, Iversen SD. Delay-dependent short-term memory deficits in aged rats. *Psychopharmacology* 1988;96:174–180.

226. Porsolt RD, Roux S, Wettstein JG. Animal models of dementia. *Drug Dev Res* 1995;35:214–229.

227. Prendergast MA, Jackson WJ, Terry AV, Decker MW, Arneric SA, Buccafusco JJ. Central nicotinic receptor agonists ABT-418, ABT-089, and (–)-nicotine reduce distractibility in young-adult monkeys. *Psychopharmacology* 1998;136:50–58.

228. Bartus RT, Flicker C, Dean RL. Logical principles for the development of animal models of age-related memory impairments. In Crook T, Bartus RT, Ferris S, Gershon S, eds. *Assessment in Psychopharmacology*. Madison, WI: Mark Powley Associates; 1983, pp 263–299.

229. Dürmüller N, Guillaume P, Lacroix P, Porsolt RD, Moser P. Use of dog EEG in safety pharmacology. *J Pharmacol Toxicol Methods* 2007.

230. Itil TM. The discovery of psychotropic drugs by computer-analyzed cerebral bioelectrical potentials (CEEG). *Drug Dev Res* 1981;1:373–407.

231. Van Riezen H, Glatt AF. Introduction and history of the use of electroencephalography in animal drug studies. *Neuropsychobiology* 1993;28:118–125.

232. Jouvet M. Biogenic amines and the states of sleep. *Science* 1969;163:32–41.

233. Ruigt GSF, van Proosdij JN, van Delft AML. A large scale, high resolution automated system for rat sleep staging. *EEG Clin Neurophysiol* 1989;73:52–71.

234. Anon. *Guideline on the Non-clinical Investigation of the Dependence Potential of Medicinal Products*. EMEA/CHMP/SWP/94227/2004, London, 23 March 2006.

235. Balster RL, Bigelow GE. Guidelines and methodological reviews concerning drug abuse liability assessment. *Drug Alcohol Assess* 2003;70 (Suppl 3):S13–S40.

236. Balster RL. Drug abuse potential evaluation in animals. *Br J Addiction* 1991;86:1549–1558.

237. Goudie AJ, Harrison AA, Leathley MJ. Evidence for a dissociation between benzodiazepine withdrawal signs. *NeuroReport* 1993;4:295–299.

238. Lal H, ed. *Discriminative Stimulus Properties of Drugs*. New York: Plenum Press; 1977.

239. Gerak LR, France CP. Discriminative stimulus effects of nalbuphine in rhesus monkeys. *J Pharmacol Exp Ther* 1996;276:523–531.

240. Foltin RW, Fischman MW. The cardiovascular and subjective effects of intravenous cocaine and morphine combinations in humans. *J Pharmacol Exp Ther* 1992;261:623–632.

241. Schechter MD, Calcagnetti DJ. Trends in place preference conditioning, with a cross-indexed bibliography 1957–1991. *Neurosci Biobehav Rev* 1993;17:21–41.

242. Brady JV, Fischman MW. Assessment of drugs for dependence potential and abuse liability: an overview. In Seiden LS, Balster RL, eds. *Behavioral Pharmacology: The Current Status*. New York: Alan R Liss; 1985, pp 361–382.

243. Fozzard HA, Task Force of the Working Group on Arrhythmias of the European Society of Cardiology. The Sicilian gambit: A new approach to the classification of antiarrhthmic drugs based on their actions on arrhythmogenic mechanisms. *Circulation* 1991;84:1831–1851.

19

SAFETY ASSESSMENT OF BIOTECHNOLOGY-DERIVED THERAPEUTICS

Mary Ellen Cosenza

Amgen Inc., Thousand Oaks, California

Contents

19.1   INTRODUCTION

Over the course of the last 20 years, the biotechnology field has grown and is now a large part of pharmaceutical therapeutics development. According to a 2006 report from the Pharmaceutical Research and Manufacturers of America (PhRMA)

Preclinical Development Handbook: Toxicology, edited by Shayne Cox Gad
Copyright © 2008 John Wiley & Sons, Inc.

TABLE 19.1 Categories of Biotechnology-Derived Pharmaceuticals

Proteins
   Hormones
   Blood products
   Cytokines
   Growth factors
   Ligands and receptors
Modified human proteins
Antibodies
   Murine
   Chimeric
   Humanized
   Fully human
   Fragments
Gene therapies
Cellular therapies
Engineered tissue products
Vaccines

[1], approximately 125 biotechnology-derived pharmaceuticals have been approved and are on the market. In addition, over 418 biotechnology-derived pharmaceuticals are in development for over 100 different diseases, and many of these potential therapeutics are being developed for grievous illnesses such as cancer, autoimmune diseases, and AIDS/HIV. Therapeutics derived from biotechnology (often referred to simply as "biologics") fall into several categories, including growth factors, hormones, enzymes, receptors, monoclonal antibodies, cytokines, vaccines, and gene and cell therapies (Table 19.1).

Many of the early biotechnology-derived therapeutics were replacement molecules, that is, recombinant-derived proteins largely unaltered from the endogenous counterparts. These included recombinant forms of human insulin, human growth hormone, interferon, erythropoietin, clotting factors, and colony stimulating factors (G-CSF and GM–CSF). Enzymes such as Activase (TPA) and Pulmozyme (DNAase) were developed in the late 1980s to early 1990s. Over time, modified versions of these proteins have been developed (e.g., pegylated proteins) as well as humanized and fully human monoclonal antibodies. More complicated molecules have been developed as well, such as fusion molecules (e.g., Enbrel, a peptide fused to a human IgG Fc) and conjugated antibodies (e.g., Mylotarg, a recombinant humanized antibody conjugated to a cytotoxic antibiotic) (Table 19.2). Early monoclonal antibodies were murine derived and chimerized; with the advent of more advanced technologies, monoclonal antibodies recently approved or currently in development are more humanized or fully human. These molecules bind to a specific antigen or epitope on a cell receptor. In addition, biotechnology-derived molecules are being designed to address more complicated diseases. New molecules are being developed to subtly alter immune function and to target specific ligand and receptor interactions. The background disease states are also more complicated and many molecules will be used in combinations with traditional pharmaceuticals or other biologics.

The regulation of these products differs by region and by type of product (e.g., replacement proteins versus DNA vaccines). Several years ago, a guidance from the

TABLE 19.2   Examples of Marketed Biotechnology Products[a]

Year of Approval	Approved Biologics	Trade Name
1982	Insulin	Humulin®
1985	Growth hormone	Protropin®
1986	Interferon alfa	Roferon®, Intron A®
1986	Muromonab-CD3	Orthoclone OKT® 3
1987	Alteplase (TPA)	Activase®
1989	Epoetin alfa	Epogen®
1990	Interferon gamma	Actimmune®
1991	Filgrastim (G-CSF)	Neupogen®
	Sargramostim (GM-CSF)	Leukine®
1992	Aldesleukin (IL-2)	Proleukin®
1993	Interferon beta	Betaseron®
	Dornase alfa (DNase)	Pulmozyme®
1994	Imiglucerase (β-glucocerebrosidase)	Cerezyme®
	Abciximab	ReoPro®
1997	Rituximab	Rituxan®
	Daclizumab	Zenapax®
	Oprelvekin (IL-11)	Neumega®
1998	Trastuzumab	Herceptin®
	Infliximab	Remicade®
	Basiliximab	Simulect®
	Palivizumab	Synagis®
2001	Pegfilgrastim (pegylated G-CSF)	Neulasta®
	Darbepoetin alfa	Aranesp®
	Alemtuzumab	Campath®
2003	Alefacept	Amevive®
	Tositumomab	Bexxar®
	Efalizumab	Raptiva®
2004	Bevacizumab	Avastin®
	Natalizumab	Tysabri®
	Palifermin (KGF)	Kepivance®

[a]DNase, deoxyribonuclease I; G-CSF, granulocyte colony-stimulating factor; GM-CSF, granulocyte-macrophage colony-stimulating factor; IL-2, interleukin 2; IL-11, interleukin 11; KGF, keratinocyte growth factor; TPA, tissue plasminogen activator.
Source: www.fda.gov.

International Congress on Harmonisation was developed to address the preclinical development and safety issues of most of these types of products (ICH S6 *Preclinical Safety Evaluation of Biotechnology-Derived Pharmaceuticals*). ICH S6 defined biotechnology-derived pharmaceuticals as "products derived from characterized cells through the use of a variety of expression systems including bacteria, yeast, insect, plant, and mammalian cells." The scope of this guidance included proteins, peptides, derivatives of these, or products of which they are components. It also states that these principles may apply to "recombinant DNA protein vaccines, chemically synthesized peptides, plasma derived products, endogenous proteins extracted from human tissues, and oligonucleotide drugs," but does not cover "antibiotics, allergenic extracts, heparin, vitamins, cellular blood components, conventional bacterial or viral vaccines, DNA vaccines, or cellular and gene therapies."

Regulatory agencies throughout the world define some of these products differently, which may affect how they are regulated. The main theme of the ICH S6 guidance is to create a case-by-case, science-driven approach to biotechnology preclinical product development. Each molecule should be fully examined for both its physical and pharmacologic properties. Its pharmacologic attributes need to be understood before embarking on a preclinical safety assessment development plan. The goal of any preclinical development plan is the same: to provide information for designing and conducting clinical trials. The biggest challenge is to use all of the information available and to conduct the best preclinical, *in vitro* and *in vivo*, experiments to best predict what will happen in humans. A rational, science-based approach is the best way to develop biotechnology-derived products [2].

Many traditional small-molecule studies are not very appropriate for biologics [3]: some for "technical" reasons (the protein may be too large to enter an ion channel) and other studies for scientific reasons (monoclonal antibodies would not be expected to have direct genotoxic effects on DNA or chromosomes). Carcinogenicity studies are also not generally conducted for biotechnology-derived therapeutics unless there is a "cause for concern." In the early days of biotechnology development, there was greater concern for the technical issues of conducting these types of studies. These concerns included immunogenicity of human proteins in rodents and the technical challenge of parenteral administration in rats and mice over a 2 year time period. Over time some of these concerns have been diminished as immunogenicity can sometimes be addressed via dosing changes.

Early concerns for biotechnology products focused on "quality" issues [4] or process-related impurities. The concerns at that time were for carry-over of DNA or other cellular proteins, endotoxins, chemical contaminants, and viruses. Of course, these concerns still exist, but methods for purification and assays for evaluation of clearance have alleviated the need for the safety assessment scientist to focus on contaminants; current safety assessments focus on the pharmacologic activity of the molecules. This chapter therefore does not address the standard assays and methods (e.g., viral clearance) used to address purity issues. There are several guidances that address these issues, especially the FDA's Guidance for Industry on content and format of investigational new drug (IND) applications for Phase I studies of drugs, including well-characterized therapeutic, biotechnology-derived products [5] and the ICH's Q6B Specifications: *Test Procedures and Acceptance Criteria for Biotechnological/Biological Products* [6]. Other product-related impurities that do need to be considered by the safety assessment scientist include genetic variants, aggregate forms, chemical linkers, and differences in glycosylation patterns.

The assessment of safety in the preclinical development of biotechnology-derived therapeutics differs from that of traditional small molecules primarily in the species specificity and the potential for immunogenicity of the former. In addition, clinical indications, length of exposure, route of administration, and dosing intervals can be very different between biologics and traditional small-molecule pharmaceuticals. Determining safety margins can be challenging in a situation where "toxicity" is mainly due to exaggerated pharmacology. It is also not unusual to have trouble establishing "no effect" (NOEL) doses with these highly selective and potent molecules. The development plans for traditional pharmaceuticals are more routine and driven by well-established guidelines, while the development plans for biologics are

TABLE 19.3   Differences Between Small-Molecule and Biotechnology-Derived Pharmaceuticals

Parameter	Small-Molecule Pharmaceuticals	Biotechnology-Derived Pharmaceuticals
Size	<500 daltons	>1 kD (macromolecules)
Immunogenicity	Nonimmunogenic	Potential for immunogenicity
Metabolism	Metabolized	Degraded
Frequency of dosing	Daily	Variable
Toxicity	Often structurally based	Exaggerated pharmacology
Half-life	Short	Long
Route of administration	Oral, some IV	Parenteral
Species specificity	Active in several species	Species specific
Synthesis	Organic chemistry (synthesized)	Genetic engineering (derived from living material)
Structure	Well defined	Often not fully characterized

TABLE 19.4   Typical Toxicology Studies for Small-Molecule and Protein Therapeutics

Small-Molecule Therapeutics	Protein Therapeutics
Screening studies	Range-finding studies
Range-finding studies	One month studies
Acute GLP studies	Three/six month studies
One month studies	Safety pharmacology
Safety pharmacology	Reproductive studies
Mutagenicity studies	Tissue cross-reactivity studies
Three month studies	Irritation/tolerance
Reproductive studies	Others as needed
Six month—rat	
One year—dog/monkey	
Industrial toxicology	
Diet RF studies	
Carcinogenicity studies	
Total cost: 5.0–6.5 million	*Total cost*: 2.5–3.0 million
Linear time: 4.5–5 years	*Linear time*: 2–2.5 years

more driven by the pharmacology of the molecule under investigation (Tables 19.3 and 19.4).

This chapter focuses on the standard approaches to safety assessment and toxicity evaluation of biotechnology-derived therapeutics and current issues in the field.

19.2   SPECIES SPECIFICITY AND SELECTION

Perhaps the greatest challenge in the preclinical development of biotechnology-derived therapeutics is species specificity. As therapeutics have become more specific over the years, this has become an even greater challenge. Unlike the pharmaceutical development of traditional small molecules, one cannot assume that a biotechnology-derived therapeutic will be active in a standard species used for toxicity testing. Rats and dogs are often selected for the assessment of safety of small molecules without regard to pharmacologic activity, the focus being on off-target toxicity due to structural effects. Species selection for small-molecule toxicity studies is often based on ADME considerations, particularly metabolite formation (i.e., which species has a metabolite profile most like humans). Only in recent years, with companies developing both traditional pharmaceuticals and biologics, has more emphasis been placed on testing for pharmacologic activity in species for standard toxicity assessments. This has always been an issue for biologics, for which lack of pharmacologic activity in a species leads to no effects in that species. In addition, the use of standard studies in standard species for biologics had little purpose and was of questionable use (except for potential effects of containments). The early work performed on interferons is a classic example; studies performed in nonrelevant species gave misleading information [7–9]. Several studies were conducted in rodents with recombinant human interferons. No evidence of toxicity was noted in many of these studies; these results later proved to be not predictive of what was to occur in humans. Activity in monkeys was more predictive, but there was a relative difference in the level of activity between primates and humans, indicating again how complex these assessments can be. Further work was performed on many of the interferons using homologous (surrogate) molecules.

19.2.1   Species Selection

There are several ways to determine whether a preclinical species is appropriate for safety assessment. If the therapeutic target is a replacement protein, the sequencing of the protein across species is a good place to start. Sequencing of related targets (e.g., ligands and receptors) can also be compared. If the therapeutic target is a receptor, receptor or ligand distribution between species can be investigated even before developing or testing the molecule. Often, *in vitro* studies are done first to look at cross-reactivity. Receptor binding can be a start, but binding itself is not sufficient. There are human or humanized molecules that demonstrate binding in primate cells but have no bioactivity. Receptor affinity and then occupancy or binding should be compared across species. Often there are log-fold differences between humans and nonhuman primates or lower species, especially in the immune system [10].

Assays for biologic activity should be available to test potency and specificity. Assays used for characterization in Good Laboratory Practice (GLP) test species should be validated. Assays can be cell culture-based or biochemical in nature. They may measure physiologic responses or enzymatic reaction rates. *In vitro* assays can be used to compare the potency and specificity across species and to predict what will happen in humans by correlating the responses *in vitro* with *in vivo* pharmacodynamic studies. There are instances when *in vitro* assay data does not correlate with *in vivo* data; this is sometimes the case when a protein is pegylated (i.e., is conjugated to polyethylene glycol (PEG) and activity is related to pharmacokinetics [11]. In these cases, the *in vitro* activity of the molecule is actually reduced due to steric hindrance from the large (PEG) moiety added to the protein. The *in vitro* results would lead one to believe that the potency of the linked molecule is less than the unlinked molecule. In actuality, because of the extended *in vivo* pharmacokinetic half-life of the linked molecule, the *in vivo* potency is greater than the original molecule.

Tissue cross-reactivity studies have traditionally been performed on monoclonal antibodies as described in the FDA guidance *Points to Consider in the Manufacture and Testing of Monoclonal Antibody Products for Human Use* [12]. These studies are usually conducted with tissues from three unrelated human donors. Comparison of the binding in tissues from different species can be helpful in determining the most relevant animal species for *in vivo* toxicology studies. These studies can help determine if an antibody binds to tissues in different species, and whether the distribution (which tissues show significant binding) is similar between human tissues and preclinical species. Unintended binding can also be evaluated and may give clues of what to look for in future *in vivo* studies (e.g., which target organs). These types of studies have several limitations, and better information can often be derived from studies examining mRNA across tissues and species. As stated in the FDA document [12], newer technologies should be employed as they become available and validated.

At one time, lack of binding in these studies led to the consideration of not performing any *in vivo* studies with the clinical molecule. If the target is not found in any appropriate animal species, then surrogates or other approaches may need to be considered. Lack of binding may also reflect a technical issue, and other methods to determine if the test species are relevant should be employed as well. Many targets in recent years are soluble receptors and traditional immunohistochemistry studies do not detect these receptors well (low receptor density, or the receptor is not easily accessible) [13]. Differences in target expression and binding in different species may be compensated for by altering doses, but these differences need to be identified before starting the safety assessment studies.

In vivo studies also have applicability in the selection of test species. If there are disease models in the potential safety assessment species and activity can be determined with the molecule intended for humans, safety assessment plans become more straightforward. The doses with activity can help determine margins of safety from the toxicology studies. Comparisons of *in vitro* data from human cells/tissues with data from the pharmacologically active species can greatly aid in the dose selection for early human studies. Animal models of disease often have provided useful information for safety assessment. When there are no disease models, pharmacologic activity can be measured using biomarkers or surrogate markers in normal animals. If this is not feasible, then receptor occupancy *in vitro* may be compared to *in vitro* activity. Other strategies may be needed if the molecule does not cross-react with an appropriate species. This is where exaggerated pharmacology and target liability (i.e., toxicity inherent to the receptor, ligand, enzyme, etc. being targeted) may need to be evaluated with a surrogate molecule, knock-out animals, or knock-in models (in which the human receptor/target is spliced into the genome of the test species) [13].

19.2.2 Nonhuman Primates

Many biologics are only active in primates; this is especially common with monoclonal antibodies. There are many challenges for programs that are limited to testing in nonhuman primates. These include the availability of nonhuman primates and the availability of laboratories and historical databases. This is particularly true for reproduction toxicology (see Section 19.4.2). Although more safety pharmacology (see Section 19.4.4) parameters are now validated in non-human primates, there are some that are not testable in this model. This is particularly true for developmental CNS/behavioral measurements that are well validated in rodents. Other challenges are in the immunotoxicology arena, where intended or unintended effects on the immune system are measured using flow cytometry, cytokine measurements, and functional assays. These have been validated in rodents over the years, and only a few laboratories have been able to validate these assays in primates. The historical databases for T-cell-dependent antibody response (TDAR) and keyhole limpet hemocyanin (KLH) assays in nonhuman primates are still small.

Marmosets were gaining popularity a few years ago due to their small size, hence reducing the amount of compound needed for chronic studies. This size advantage can be outweighed by other factors, such as the small amount of blood available in these animals. In addition, marmosets are sensitive to stress [14]. Few laboratories have much experience with these animals and there is only a small historical database available.

Some molecules are even more specific and are only active in humans and chimpanzees (*Pan troglodytes*), severely limiting the types of testing that can be conducted preclinically. This situation will lead the safety assessment scientist to consider the use of surrogate molecules and/or the use of transgenic or knock-out animals. The use of chimpanzees for safety assessment is often impractical [15] because of the limitations of the testing laboratories. There are very few such laboratories available, and they are not resourced sufficiently to run multiple complicated studies concurrently. These laboratories also are not equipped to run toxicity studies at the same standards for GLPs as traditional toxicology laboratories. Chimpanzees are a protected and endangered species and cannot be bred. Few tests and bleedings can be conducted as each of these requires sedation of the animals. They are also very expensive studies to conduct, they are nonterminal (i.e., animals are not euthanized at the end of the study), and only a small number of animals can be separately housed at any time, making long-term monitoring difficult. Because chimpanzees often weigh more than 45 kg, they require large amounts of test material [16]. Many of the chimps available in the United States have been infected with HIV, which can complicate test results especially for compounds that have effects on the immune system. Special studies such as reproductive toxicology and carcinogenicity cannot be conducted in chimpanzees for numerous ethical, technical, and logistical reasons.

19.2.3   Surrogates and Other Alternatives

Surrogates or homologous proteins have their own issues. They can be difficult to develop in the desired species and by definition will be different from the molecules being developed for humans. They may have different affinity for receptors, different epitopes, different half-lives, and so on, all of which may change the dynamics and alter the pharmacologic and toxicologic effects of the molecules. They can delay the development of other programs because they will use the same manufacturing facilities. Surrogates provide little or no information on the final human product contaminants and degradation products. Overall, the decision whether to investigate a surrogate or homologous protein is the balance between the time, cost, and delay to other programs versus getting target liability information. In general, any of these molecules need to undergo the same rigorous evaluation as the clinical agent [17].

Other methods of getting target liability information include literature reviews and knock-out animals. Surrogate antibodies can help elucidate the mechanism of action [18]. Other tactics include the use of homologous ligands or the use of transgenics expressing human receptors. This allows the use of human-specific molecules but may not address off-mechanism toxicities. Knock-out models also have been used to mimic the suppression of endogenous cytokines or proteins. Disease models have also been used for safety assessment [19], especially when compound availability is a concern.

All of these strategies have their challenges, advantages, and disadvantages. In evaluating all of these data, it is important to bear in mind the goals of preclinical safety of biologics: to determine the pharmacologic and toxicologic attributes and activities of the molecule to be tested in humans, to determine the target organs, and to assess the potential similarities and differences. This information will be used to predict appropriate doses (safe starting doses as well as maximal doses) for clinical testing and to determine what parameters may need to be measured in early clinical trials. In some cases, one species may be sufficient if there is only one species that has activity or if the biologic activity or the molecule and its target are well understood.

19.3   IMMUNOGENICITY

It is generally well accepted that immunogenicity is not well predicted across species. It has also been well documented that many biologic compounds intended for human use are immunogenic in animals [20]. ICH S6 states that "most biotechnology-derived pharmaceuticals intended for humans are immunogenic in animals." Traditional antigenicity studies or guinea pig anaphylaxis studies are not useful for predicting immunogenicity in humans and are now generally recognized (ICH S6) as not being appropriate studies for biologics. When these studies were conducted years ago, at the request of regulators, they were generally positive and led to adverse effects in animals. Since these studies have no predictive value, they are no longer considered appropriate and may be an unnecessary use of animals.

19.3.1   Types of Antibodies to Biotechnology-Derived Pharmaceuticals

All preclinical (and clinical) studies with biologics should include measurements of total incidence of antibodies and whether these antibodies are neutralizing. Assays to determine antibodies have become more sophisticated over the years, and the newest technologies allow detection at lower levels than were achievable with traditional enzyme-linked immunoassays (ELISAs) [21]. The technology exists today to measure and characterize the production of antibodies and to evaluate their effects on pharmacokinetics and pharmacodynamics. Clinically relevant antibodies are those that clear, sustain, neutralize, or cross-react with an endogenous protein. It is important to screen for the presence and development of antibodies to the test molecule throughout development. Since the consequence of these antibodies may range from no clinically significant effects to serious safety effects, assays need to be developed to determine if the antibodies that appear are able to block the biologic activity of the test compound. This may occur either by direct binding to an epitope with activity or by blocking the active site through steric hindrance after binding to a site in close proximity [21].

A "clearing antibody" is one that results in more rapid clearance of test molecule: that is, the binding of the antibody to the test molecule causes the test molecule to be removed more quickly from the circulation. This type of antibody can be detected by comparing the pharmacokinetic profiles of the test molecule in animals with and without antibodies, or by comparing the pharmacokinetic profile of the first dose (at which time no antibodies are expected) with a subsequent dose (see Fig. 19.1). A clearing antibody may or may not have a direct neutralizing effect, but the consequence of the rapid clearance may eradicate any pharmacologic activity of the test compound. This type of antibody can make the toxicology studies invalid; if there is not adequate exposure to the test molecule, then the lack of toxicity does not give assurance of lack of effect from the pharmacologic activity of the molecule itself.

A "sustaining antibody" is one that delays the clearance of the test molecule: that is, the binding of the antibody to the test molecule keeps the test molecule in the circulation longer. This type of antibody also can be determined by measuring the serum or blood concentrations in animals with and without antibodies (see Fig. 19.2). The binding of a sustaining antibody to the test compound may or may not be neutralizing. When there are sustaining antibodies, the recovery period of the toxicology studies may need to be extended to see true reversibility of effects. These types of antibodies can lead to even greater exaggeration of pharmacology, and dose levels may need to be altered to account for unanticipated accumulation.

Both clearing and sustaining antibodies may also be "neutralizing antibodies": that is, the binding of the antibody to the test molecule changes the ability of the test molecule to produce its pharmacologic activity. The most worrisome type of antibodies are those that cross-react with an endogenous protein (see Fig. 19.3). In this case, the individual's own endogenous proteins can no longer function pharmacologically because the antibody response is binding and neutralizing its

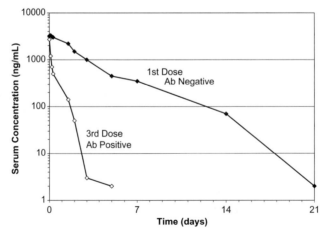

FIGURE 19.1   Clearing antibody.

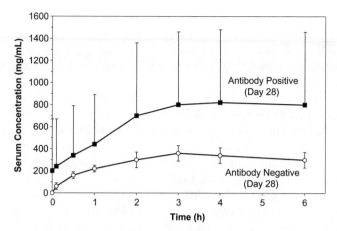

FIGURE 19.2   Sustaining antibody.

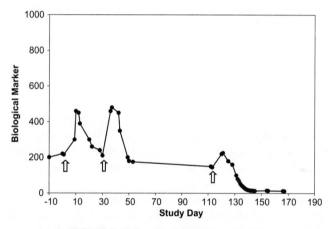

FIGURE 19.3   Neutralizing antibody.

activity as well. These types of antibodies can have devastating effects in the clinic [22–24].

There are ways to alter the incidence and robustness of antibodies in preclinical studies. Altering the dosing regimen and route is the most obvious manner. The subcutaneous and intramuscular routes are the most immunogenic with the intravenous route being the least immunogenic [25]. This may be due to aggregation at the injection sites. The frequency and duration of dosing also can affect immunogenicity. The longer the dosing period, the greater the probability of an immunogenic response and the greater the response may be. The dosing frequency may also have an effect, but there is a balance between more immunogenicity due to greater exposure versus a frequency that mimics a pulse effect [23].

One of the most controversial topics in this area is the ability or lack of ability of animal immunogenicity results to predict immunogenicity in humans. Generally, it has been accepted that an antibody response in animals cannot directly predict such a response in humans. But recent studies have shown that animal studies may be able to predict relative immunogenicity of different compounds (e.g., modified versions of a protein) and the potential subsequent effects of antibody production [20, 26]. There is also evidence that glycosylated proteins are less immunogenic than nonglycosylated proteins [22, 27]. Other effects that need to be assessed include those due to antibody–drug complexes. These complexes can deposit in tissues and organs [28] and cause glomerulonephritis [29]. Infusion reactions and anaphylactic responses also need to be monitored [24].

In summary, immunogenicity is a substantial complication for preclinical safety assessment studies. It can invalidate the model species, but antibody production alone should not stop the conduct of these studies. The antibodies need to be measured with reproducible assays [30]. Longer recovery periods are often needed for these studies to wash out the drug from the test animals. This can greatly increase the ability of the assays to detect antibodies to the drug. If there are active drug levels in the blood samples, they can interfere with the ability to measure true antibody levels [21]. The effects on pharmacokinetics and pharmacodynamics need to be measured and evaluated. The potential consequences of the antibodies on endogenous molecules need to be evaluated as well. The secondary effects, such as antibody deposition, should be measured. The lack of ability to predict human immunogenicity and the relative potential to predict this should be considered on a case-by-case basis.

19.3.2   Study Design Issues

Unlike most traditional small molecules, biologics are not given once or twice a day, orally, in a pill or capsule. They are almost all dosed via a parenteral route, are not given (or "taken") daily, and some are given in hospital settings or in clinician offices (e.g., monoclonal antibodies for the treatment of solid tumors such as Avastin® and Erbitux®). Several are now self-administered on a weekly or even less frequent basis (e.g., TNF inhibitors such as Enbrel® and Remicade®). The dose regimen for the safety assessment studies should reflect the dosing regimen plan for the human studies. The dosing interval in animals may be different from that planned for humans, depending on the half-life of the molecule in animals versus humans. Also, the development of antibodies in animals may alter the pharmacokinetics, and modifying the dosing interval may reduce the incidence of antibodies.

Other design issues include dose level selection. Often when the dose-limiting toxicity is related to the pharmacology (often referred to as "exaggerated pharmacology") it is difficult to establish a large margin of safety. The difference between the intended level of effect and an effect that leads to toxicity, even if it is the same effect, may be very small.

Other factors that need to be considered in dose selection are those that fall under the category of pharmacokinetics and drug metabolism. These factors will not be considered in any great depth in this chapter, but a few points to consider are listed here:

- Route of dosing (IV, SQ, infusion)
- Half-life of the molecule (e.g., IgG isotypes)
- PK/PD modeling (very useful for growth factors such as Epogen® and Neupogen®)

- Dosing regimen in the clinic (weekly, monthly, once per cycle)
- Length of intended clinical use (acute vs. chronic)

One study type generally not deemed relevant for biologics is metabolism studies. Mass balance studies have not proved useful when performed with proteins. Radio-labeled studies have limited usefulness as these labeled molecules undergo rapid metabolism and the label is often unstable. Protein biologics undergo proteolytic degradation into smaller peptides and then into individual amino acids. Distribution is viewed more from the perspective of target distribution, except for gene and cell therapies or vectors.

Toxicokinetics must be assessed in these studies, as with traditional pharmaceuticals. These data are necessary to prove exposure (which may differ with route) and to monitor the potential effects of antibodies on the exposure levels over time. One of the greatest differences between small molecules and biologics is the potential for immunogenicity, which can greatly affect pharmacokinetics, as previously discussed.

Recovery periods are very important in studies with biologics for several reasons. As already discussed, it is important to have a wash-out period of the drug to properly test for antibody levels. This works best with samples that are clear of the test compound itself (assay interference).

19.4 SPECIAL STUDIES

19.4.1 Genotoxicity

It is generally accepted now that these studies are not applicable for biotechnology-derived products, unless there is a "chemical" linker or toxic conjugate to the molecule. This is clearly stated in ICH S6 as well as the FDA document for monoclonal antibodies [12].

19.4.2 Reproductive Toxicology

When a biologic cross-reacts with traditional reproductive toxicology species, then these studies should be conducted as appropriate for the intended clinical population. The main consideration for these studies, if conducted in rodents and rabbits, is the dosing regimen and immunogenicity. The regimen should be carefully chosen to ensure pharmacokinetic coverage during the pivotal parts of gestation. The frequency of dosing in these studies might need to be closer to ensure that there is adequate exposure. Also, this may address the potential immunogenicity as discussed earlier. The exposure period for the Segment II studies in rodents and rabbits is usually short enough to avoid a strong immunogenic response, but samples should be taken to measure drug levels and antibodies in the dose range-finding studies.

The more complicated situation is with those molecules that only work in nonhuman primates. Here a decision must be made as to whether to conduct these studies in primates or to create a rodent surrogate. The decision should be based on good science as well as the practical and technical issues. There is no right or wrong answer to this question, but there are several factors that need to be considered. There are differences between non-human primate subspecies to consider as well. For example, rhesus monkeys are seasonal breeders and cynomolgus monkeys are not. Cynomolgus monkeys also have a similar duration of menstrual cycle and placental morphology and physiology similar to humans. Human IgGs are known to cross the placental barrier, and their response to teratogens has been shown to be similar to humans [31]. On the other hand, compared with rodents, nonhuman primates have a small number of offspring (usually just one offspring per mother), they are very expensive, and their gestation period is 150 days long. They have a low conception rate and a high spontaneous abortion rate. In addition, there are only a small number of laboratories that have the capabilities of conducting primate reproductive studies. The historical database is not that large.

As for specific studies, male fertility is easier to test in cynomolgus monkeys [32], and these assays (e.g., hormones, sperm count) can often be incorporated into standard toxicology studies [33]. Mating studies are much more difficult, but fertility parameters can be measured in females as well (e.g., menstrual cycle, FSH, LH). Segment II studies are usually dosed during organogenesis (days 20 to 50), and the mothers are C-sectioned on day 100 [34]. Placental transfer can also be measured with continuous dosing.

19.4.3   Carcinogenicity

Unless there is a specific "cause for concern," these studies are generally considered inappropriate for biologics (ICH S6). This issue is also addressed in ICH S1A [35], which states that these studies are not generally needed for molecules that are developed as replacement therapy (e.g., insulin and certain hormones). This guidance also recognizes that neutralizing antibodies may "invalidate" the results. As with the S6 document, ICH S1A suggests that these studies be considered depending on the clinical indication, patient population, and treatment duration. Further reasons to consider these studies might include modifications made to the molecule or indications of potential effects based on subchronic studies (e.g., unexpected hyperplasia).

For molecules that are only pharmacologically active in non-human primates, there are additional technical issues. Carcinogenicity studies would not be feasible in non-human primates due to the long life span, nor are they practical due to the large number of animals that would be needed for statistics. The alternative would be to develop a surrogate that would be active in rodents. This would carry the same issues as already discussed. In addition, the longer time span needed for testing would only increase the chance for neutralizing antibody production. Alternative approaches, such as *in vitro* proliferation studies or receptor binding studies, may be informative but still not definitive. Another complication is with molecules that are immunosuppressive, as these might increase the incidence of any background tumors.

19.4.4   Safety Pharmacology

Often, parameters assessed in safety pharmacology studies can be incorporated into standard toxicology studies, including single-dose studies. For molecules that cross-react in traditional species (rodents and dogs), study designs can be more flexible, while study designs for molecules that are active only in nonhuman primates have more challenges. Non-human primates can be telemeterized for cardiovascular assessments if there are concerns and even many CNS evaluations can be performed in non-human primates as well now.

19.4.5   Local Tolerance

Local tolerance assessments can usually be conducted as part of subchronic or chronic toxicity studies, by taking sections from injection sites. They are often used to test formulation changes as well.

19.5   FUTURE TRENDS

In the future, biotechnology products are going to become more complex. We will see more conjugated monoclonal antibodies, oligonucleotides, fusion molecules, and gene or plural: cell therapies. The need to address the basic questions with these products will remain the same, but the challenges will be greater. There are new tools becoming available to the toxicologist to address these concerns. Global development strategies for development of biotechnology products will be more science driven, more problem focused, and with additional regulatory challenges. The overall goal should still be to evaluate preclinically the potential effects of these molecules in humans in the diseases of interest. The safety assessment scientist should develop a plan with a strong scientific rationale, using all of the necessary tools and good justification for the animal model chosen.

REFERENCES

1. Pharma Org. www.pharma.org.
2. Cavagnaro JA. Preclinical safety evaluation of biotechnology-derived pharmaceuticals. *Nat Rev* 2002;1:469.
3. Griffiths SA, Lumley CE. Non-clinical safety studies for biotechnologically-derived pharmaceuticals: conclusions from an International Workshop. *Hum Exp Toxicol* 1998;17:63.
4. Dayan AD. Safety evaluation of biological and biotechnology-derived medicines. *Toxicology* 1995;105:59.
5. FDA IND Guidelines. www.fda.gov.
6. ICH Q6B Specifications: *Test Procedures and Acceptance Criteria for Biotechnological/ Biological Products* 1999.
7. Green JD, Terrell TG. Utilization of homologous proteins to evaluate the safety of recombinant human proteins—case study: recombinant human interferon gamma (rhIFN-γ). *Toxicol Lett* 1992;64/65:321.
8. Serabian MA, Pilaro AM. Safety assessment of biotechnology-derived pharmaceuticals: ICH and beyond. *Toxicol Pathol* 1999;27:2.
9. Ryan AM, Terrell TG. Biotechnology and its products. In Haschek W, Ed. *Handbook of Toxicologic Pathology*, 2nd ed. London: Academic Press; 2002, p 479.
10. Hart TK, et al. Preclinical efficacy and safety of pascolizumab (SB 240683): a humanized anti-interleukin-4 antibody with therapeutic potential in asthma. *Clin Exp Immunol* 2002;130:93.

11. Elliott S, Lorenzini T, Asher S, et al. Enhancement of therapeutic protein in vivo activities through glycoengineering. *Nat Biotechnol* March 2003;21:414–421.

12. *Points to Consider in the Manufacture and Testing of Monoclonal Antibody Products for Human Use.* Washington, DC: FDA, CBER; 1997.

13. Bolon B, et al. Genetic engineering and molecular technology. In Krinke G, Ed. *The Laboratory Rat.* London: Academic Press; 2000, p 603.

14. Zuhlke U, et al. The common marmoset (*Callithrix jacchus*) as a model in biotechnology. In Korte R, Vogel F, Weinbauer GF, Eds. *Primate Models in Pharmaceutical Drug Development.* Munster, Germany: Waxmann; 2002, p 119.

15. Klingbeil C, Hsu D. Pharmacology and safety assessment of humanized monoclonal antibodies for therapeutic use. *Toxicol Pathol* 1999;27:1.

16. Tony Ndifor Presentation at CRL Biotechnology Symposium 2003.

17. Clarke J, et al. Evaluation of a surrogate antibody for preclinical safety testing of an anti-CD11a monoclonal antibody. *Regul Toxicol Pharmacol* 2004;40:219.

18. Treacy G. Using an analogous monoclonal antibody to evaluate the reproductive and chronic toxicity potential for a humanized anti-TNFa monoclonal antibody. *Hum Exp Toxicol* 2000;19:226.

19. Sato K, et al. Efficacy of intracoronary versus intravenous FGF-2 in a pig model of chronic myocardial ischemia. *Ann Thorac Surg* 2000;70:2113–2118.

20. Bugelski PJ, Treacy G. Predictive power of preclinical studies in animals for the immunogenicity of recombinant therapeutic proteins in humans. *Curr Opin Mol Ther* 2004;6:10.

21. Gupta S, et al. Recommendations for the design, optimization, and qualification of cell-based assays used for the detection of neutralizing antibody responses elicited to biological therapeutics. *J Immunol Methods* 2006;321:1–18.

22. Koren E, Zuckerman LA, Mire-Sluis AR. Immune responses to therapeutic proteins in humans—clinical significance, assessment and prediction. *Curr Pharm Biotechnol* 2002;3:349.

23. Schellekens H. Immunogenicity of therapeutic proteins: clinical implications and future prospects. *Clin Ther* 2002;24:1720.

24. Rosenburg AS. Immunogenicity of biological therapeutics: a hierarchy of concerns. In Brown F, Mire-Sluis A, Eds. *Immunogenicity of Therapeutic Biological Products.* Basel: Karger AG; 2003, p 15.

25. Working PK. Potential effects of antibody induction by protein drugs. In Ferraiolo BL, Mohler MA, Gloff CA, Eds. *Protein Pharmacokinetics and Metabolism.* New York: Plenum Press; 1992, p 73.

26. Wierda D, Smith HW, Zwickl CM. Immunogenicity of biopharmaceuticals in laboratory animals. *Toxicology* 2001;158:71.

27. Gribben JG, et al. Development of antibodies to unprotected glycosylation sites on recombinant human GM-CSF. *Lancet* 1990;335:434.

28. Henck JW, et al. Reproductive toxicity testing of therapeutic biotechnology agents. *Teratology* 1996;53:185.

29. Terrell TG, Green JD. Comparative pathology of recombinant murine interferon-γ in mice and recombinant human interferon-γ in cynomolgus monkeys. In Richter GW, Solez K, Ryffel B, Eds. *International Review of Experimental Pathology: Cytokine-Induced Pathology Part A: Interleukins and Hematopoietic Growth Factors.* San Diego: Academic Press; 1993, p 73.

30. Mire-Sluis AR. Progress in the use of biological assays during the development of biotechnology products. *Pharm Res* 2001;18:1239.

31. Weinbauer GF. The nonhuman primate as a model in developmental and reproductive toxicology. In Korte R, Weinbauer GF, Eds. *Primate Models in Pharmaceutical Drug Development*. Munster, Germany: Waxmann; 2002, p 49.

32. Vogel F. How to design male fertility investigations in the cynomolgus monkey. In Korte R, Weinbauer GF, Eds. *Towards New Horizons in Primate Toxicology*. Munster, Germany: Waxmann; 2000, p 43.

33. Weinbauer GF, Cooper TG. Assessment of male fertility impairment in the macaque model. In Korte R, Weinbauer GF, Eds. *Towards New Horizons in Primate Toxicology*. Munster, Germany: Waxmann; 2000, p 13.

34. Weinbauer GF. The nonhuman primate as a model in developmental and reproductive toxicology. In Korte R, Weinbauer GF, Eds. *Primate Models in Pharmaceutical Drug Development*. Munster, Germany: Waxmann; 2002, p 49.

35. ICH S1A: *The Need for Long-Term Rodent Carcinogenicity Studies of Pharmaceuticals* 1995.

20

PRECLINICAL DEVELOPMENT OF PROTEIN PHARMACEUTICALS: AN OVERVIEW

DIPANKAR DAS AND MAVANUR R. SURESH

University of Alberta, Edmonton, Alberta, Canada

Contents

Preclinical Development Handbook: Toxicology, edited by Shayne Cox Gad
Copyright © 2008 John Wiley & Sons, Inc.

20.1   INTRODUCTION

Protein pharmaceuticals can broadly be classified into three main categories—namely, recombinant proteins and enzymes, monoclonal antibodies (MAbs) and their derivatives, and synthetic peptides. The development of hybridoma technology for the generation of monospecific antibodies by Kohler and Milstein [1] in 1975 was a landmark technological achievement to harness unique specific antibodies. This technology and the development and refinement of recombinant DNA technology also in the early 1970s form the two pillars for the emergence of protein pharmaceuticals. Another important related technique is the solid phase peptide synthetic approach for production of pure shorter peptides. This synthetic strategy is often limited by the size, secondary modifications, and lack of glycosylation. However, it has the unique advantage of being able to incorporate synthetic analogues and derivatives that cannot be developed biologically. This chapter deals primarily with antibodies and recombinant protein pharmaceuticals. Readers are directed to several comprehensive reviews and books on solid phase synthetic strategies, a technique invented by Merrifield [2, 3]. The majority of currently approved pharmaceuticals and generics are small molecular weight (MW) compounds. The major differences between small MW pharmaceuticals and the larger proteins are summarized in Table 20.1. Biogeneric protein pharmaceuticals are a new category of therapeutics that are likely to be a new class in the next few years.

20.2   MACROMOLECULAR DRUGS

Two major technological advances ushered in the era of large molecular weight protein drugs. In the early 1970s advances in the development of recombinant DNA

TABLE 20.1   Differences Between Traditional Drugs and Protein Pharmaceuticals

Small Molecular Weight Pharmaceuticals	Protein Pharmaceuticals
1. Mostly synthetic	1. Biology-based production
2. Uniquely pure entities (with exception of enantiomers)	2. Microheterogeneity in glycosylation and other posttranslation modifications
3. Rarely form aggregates	3. Protein aggregates are common
4. Nonimmunogenic	4. Immunogenic to different degrees
5. Rarely an issue with adventitious agents	5. Adventitious agents can be an issue
6. Generally stable	6. Susceptible to denaturation and physical and chemical instabilities
7. Unique metabolic pathways for each class of drugs	7. Universal protease-based cleavage, metabolism, and reabsorption
8. Generally lack targeting properties	8. Often with targeting capabilities

technology allowed the expression and purification of mammalian proteins in pro-karyotic systems. *Escherichia coli* has been used extensively to generate recombi-nant proteins for a variety of biopharmaceutical productions. Expression in this simple platform, however, has two major drawbacks. First, this prokaryote can only express nonglycosylated proteins; and second, the bulk of the recombinant protein is obtained as denatured aggregate of inclusion bodies. Structural and functional information is either lost or distorted as a result and relatively laborious extraction and refolding strategies are required to renature the protein from the inclusion bodies [4]. Recent advances have resulted in the development of secreted recombi-nant proteins from *E. coli* with substantial native activity [5]. The limitations of the prokaryotic expression platforms have led to the development of yeast, insect cell, and mammalian expression platforms [6–11]. A number of biopharmaceuticals are produced in yeast including human insulin and hepatitis A vaccine, providing thera-peutic proteins to millions of people around the world. The advantages of the yeast platform include the high level production of the recombinant protein and the wealth of large scale fermentation expertise in the brewery industry, which was the natural starting point for bulk production of biopharmaceuticals. However, yeast and insect cells impart a different glycosylation footprint on the expressed protein. For example, the recombinant proteins expressed in yeast are of the high mannose glycoprotein product. In a pharmaceutical context, the pharmacokinetics of aglyco-syl and glycosylated proteins are significantly different, with the latter being cleared rapidly by the liver asialoglycoprotein receptor [12].

The most ideal platform for expression of biopharmaceuticals is the mammalian cell. The CHO (Chinese hamster ovary) cells have been one of the platforms exploited for protein expression. This platform provides a biopharmaceutical product that closely mimics the natural protein with minimal differences compared to the other prokaryotic, yeast, and insect platforms. Production of biopharmaceuticals in mammalian platforms is expensive and generally provides comparatively lower yield of product. However, unique amplification strategies using the dihydrofolate reductase (DHFR) or the glutamine synthetase (GS) systems have provided yields that are significantly higher for commercial viability.

Almost all of the current approved biopharmaceuticals are therapeutic proteins and vaccines. Several other proteins are used in nonpharmaceutical applications, such as in industrial uses, including detergents, leather tanning, meat and cheese processing, beverage production, and the baking industry. Currently, there are several hundred protein pharmaceuticals in various stages of clinical trials. The excellent safety and therapeutic properties have resulted in choices made by patients and health care professionals to prefer biopharmaceuticals over small molecular weight drugs. A case in point in therapeutic options in our province (Alberta, Canada) is the use of Herceptin, a monoclonal antibody targeting the Her-2neu receptor positive aggressive breast cancer. A few years ago the provincial body approved reimbursement or use of the MAb only as a third line therapy after anthracycline treatment of recurrent metastatic breast cancer. This year all women in the Province of Alberta can access MAb treatment for Her-2neu receptor positive breast cancer as the primary first line therapy. While proteins dominate biopharma-ceuticals as the largest category, several other promising large MW drugs are in clinical trials or in early preclinical development, including DNA vaccines, antisense oligonucleotides, RNAi, polysaccharides, cells, and organs as well as novel delivery

TABLE 20.2   Classification of Biopharmaceuticals

Category	Example
1. Monoclonal antibody	1. Rituxan, Synagis, Simulect (18 approved by FDA)
2. Polyclonal antibody	2. Respigam, Thymoglobulin
3. Antisense oligonucleotide	3. Vitravene
4. Hormones	4. Insulin
5. Enzymes	5. Asparaginase, Raspuricase
6. Interferons	6. Interferons α, β, γ
7. Interleukin	7. Interleukin 2
8. Tumor necrosis factor	8. TNF-α
9. Vaccines	9. Hepatitis B surface antigen
10. Hematopoietic growth factor	10. Erythropoeitin, colony stimulating factor
11. Blood factors	11. Factors VIII, IX
12. Nonrecombinant proteins	12. Sucraid, Wellferon
13. Thrombolytic agents	13. Tissue plasminogen activator

systems such as nasal therapeutics and even skin patch vaccines. Table 20.2 has a summary of the categories of approved biopharmaceutical drugs.

20.3   GENES, DIRECTED EVOLUTION, AND GENE SHUFFLING

The advent of genomics and proteomics along with the complete sequence information of over several hundred organisms including *Homo sapiens* has provided new insights and opportunities for the future of biopharmaceuticals. The 2000 version of the human genome sequence had estimated that we harbored ~40,000–50,000 genes. A more recent version [13] of the human genome has narrowed this to about 25,000–30,000 genes. Classical recombinant strategies of cloning and expression of proteins have been refined with the emergence of new gene modifications for overexpression of pharmaceuticals as well as redesigning the natural proteins for new and improved properties. At least four innovative strategies can be recognized in the context of optimization of biopharmaceutical production. They are codon optimization, directed evolution, gene shuffling, and enhanced expression platforms.

Codon optimization is a strategy that has been introduced to exploit two technological developments. The first relates to the refinement of automated synthesis and sequencing of genes, including large DNA molecules in a relatively short time. We recently obtained the large synthetic spike gene of SARS-coronavirus consisting of ~4000 nucleotides in a few weeks from a commercial outfit (www.Geneart.com). This is a significant technological resource that has evolved from the very first aminoacyl t-RNA synthetase gene constructed manually by a group of several scientists over a period of one year [14]. Similarly, on the sequencing end we are now routinely able to sequence genes with the help of automated gene sequencers within days, a far cry from the first gene sequence of a phage gene in the 1970s [15, 16]. In the recent SARS virus outbreak in several countries, the combined efforts of two laboratories in Canada resulted in the complete genome sequence of the whole virus within a week [17].

The second innovation toward codon optimizing genes is the detailed understanding of the patterns of t-RNA composition in the most common host expression systems. Many a gene expression fails to generate the desired product or barely produces the recombinant protein. The causes of such diminished production are several and key among them is the paucity of certain species of t-RNA in the cell used for expression. As a result, the cellular translation machinery is less efficient in production of the recombinant biopharmaceutical. Hence, modifying the specific codons in the synthetic gene to match the abundant species of t-RNA permits efficient protein synthesis. In a recent study, we have successfully utilized the codon optimized nucleoprotein gene of SARS-CoV for 10–20-fold overexpression at ~30–55 mg/L of *E. coli* culture (Fig. 20.1) [18].

Another major gene improvement strategy is rational design of neobiopharmaceuticals, but it requires in-depth understanding of structure, function, and mechanisms. The technique of site-directed mutagenesis is an elegant method of specific sequence modification of biopharmaceuticals for improved characteristics, including function, biodistribution, and immunogenicity. Random site-directed mutagenesis of proteins has evolved into directed evolution and gene shuffling to make improved biopharmaceuticals. Unlike rational design, which requires a thorough understanding of the protein, the directed evolution approach requires only minimal knowledge of its structure and function [19]. The strategy in directed evolution is based on either random mutagenesis of the gene or recombination of homologous gene segments followed by specific screening based on desired functional characteristics.

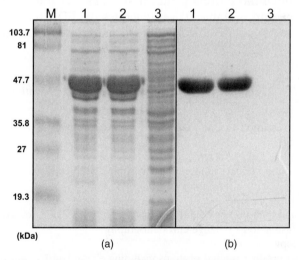

FIGURE 20.1 Analysis of codon optimized SARS-CoV NP gene expression in *E. coli*. Total cell protein analysis by SDS-PAGE and Western blot. The 10% polyacrylamide gel was stained with Coomassie Brilliant Blue (a). Proteins transferred to nitrocellulose membrane were subsequently probed with anti-His₆ MAb followed by goat anti-mouse-HRPO (b). Lane M: standard prestained molecular weight markers; lanes 1 and 2: induced culture; lane 3: uninduced culture. Note the overproduction of the protein and its detection by Western blot.

This is akin to Darwinian evolution, which requires generation of diversity by mutagenesis and selection of exploiting assays for improved protein characteristics. A particularly useful technique in the above approach is DNA shuffling. A whole range of gene fragments are generated following initial incorporation of point mutations into a gene. The new variant is generated by reassembly of the fragments and functional selection for desired property. Exploiting the above methods, many proteins and biopharmaceuticals with improved catalytic activity, enzyme stability, thermostability, enzyme substrate specificity, new substrate activity, and stereoselectivity have been developed. Altering the *in vivo* biological properties of a therapeutic protein is also an important objective, which includes pharmacokinetics and immunogenicity. Retavase is a modified form of tPA (tissue plasminogen activator), which is used during myocardial infarction to initiate the activation of plasminogen to promote fibrinolytic reactions. This modified protein has only two of the five structural domains of native tPA along with increased half-life in blood.

20.4   MOLECULAR AND BIOCHEMICAL CHARACTERIZATION OF PROTEIN DRUGS

The initial identification and development of a protein pharmaceutical starts from early seminal discoveries on a potential protein candidate exploiting classical methods or using genomics and proteomics. Biomarker identification from the latter methods is an exciting protein mining prospect today. Classical approaches rely on the identification of candidate proteins with specific properties such as hormones, interleukins, monoclonals, toxins, and other effectors. Early laboratory data from investigators is often the starting point for systematic characterization of a single candidate pharmaceutical. Table 20.3 enumerates the FDA requirements for characterizing a protein pharmaceutical. Genomic and proteomic chip or microarray-

---

TABLE 20.3   FDA Requirements for Physicochemical Characterization of Biologicals

1. Amino acid analysis
2. Amino acid sequencing, entire sequence, or C- and N-terminal sequences
3. Peptide mapping
4. Determine disulfide linkage if any
5. SDS-PAGE (sodium dodecyl sulfate–polyacrylamide gel electrophoresis) reduced and nonreduced
6. Isoelectric focusing
7. Conventional and high pressure liquid chromatography (HPLC), for example, reverse phase, size exclusion, ion-exchange chromatography
8. Mass spectroscopy
9. Assays to detect product-related proteins including deamidated, oxidized, cleaved, and aggregated forms and other variants, for example, amino acid substitutions and adducts/derivatives
10. Assays to detect residual host proteins, DNA, and reagents
11. Immunochemical analyses
12. Assays to quantitate bioburden and endotoxin

Source: http://www.fda.gov/.

based identification often differentiates several potential candidates. However, even among the few candidate markers, one would have to be selected based on the efficacy and the feasibility of pharmaceutical development. Classical approaches of marker identification will often provide some degree of characterization of the protein. *In vitro* bioassays for the protein or *in vivo* animal-based therapeutic endpoints are often developed to test the potency and efficiency. One of the first objectives in preclinical development and characterization requires the purification of the protein from bulk raw materials. In the last few decades the refinement of techniques in recombinant DNA cloning and expression of pure proteins has revolutionized protein pharmaceuticals including monoclonal antibodies. Enumerated below is a series of preclinical steps to be undertaken although the order of some of the steps may be altered. Table 20.4 lists the properties of proteins and methods to obtain the parameters.

1. *Gene Sequence.* Knowledge of the entire human genome provides the sequence of the gene for any human protein for expression in a heterologous system. Monoclonal antibodies useful for human therapeutics can also be analyzed to obtain the primary gene sequence of the variable H and L chains from hybridomas. Hence, one of the first steps is to decide the gene or gene segment to be cloned and the choice of the expression system. The gene of interest could be synthesized using codon optimization to maximize the yield.

2. *Expression Platform and Vectors.* An early choice must be made for the type of plasmid vector appropriate to the expression platform. The most common expression systems are based on *E. coli*, yeast, and mammalian CHO cells. The choices of plasmid vectors are numerous and require careful consideration for the type of drug resistant selection, promoters, and enhancers along with the genes of interest. An important practical issue in biopharmaceutical development is the practical yields of the protein in a given expression system. Two well developed approaches for

---

TABLE 20.4   Some Key Analytical Methods for Preclinical Studies

Characterization of Proteins

Structure, amino acid composition, prosthetic group, disulfide and free SH group, metals, confirmation, p*I*, aggregation, mass, two-dimensional fragmentation pattern, fluorescence, light scattering, sedimentation pattern, charge and electrophoretic properties, UV extinction coefficient, enzymatic activity, biological assays and potency, immunological properties and stability (denaturation, aggregation, oxidation), carbohydrate composition and sequence.

Methods for Protein Analysis

Spectroscopy (UV-Visible), fluorescence spectroscopy, affinity, avidity, size exclusion chromatography, circular dichroism (CD), high performance liquid chromatography, SDS-PAGE, IEF, Fourier transform—infrared, nuclear magnetic resonance (NMR), light scattering, ELISA, MS or LC/MS (Q-TOF), bioassays, stress tests–shake test, surfactant test, freeze–thaw test, heat stability.

Source: Adapted from Ref. 20.

enhanced expression in mammalian systems are the DHFR- and GS-based amplification strategies. The preclinical development of cells expressing the desired protein could be optimized early by the above strategies. This can be further enhanced in process development for further enhancement of yield.

3. *Purification Strategies.* The small scale purification methodology is often the starting point for future scale-up of the protein. The myriad of protein purification strategies can broadly be classified into two categories—namely, general protein chromatography techniques that are applicable to all types of proteins and affinity chromatography methods that apply to specific proteins or to certain groups of proteins. General chromatography techniques include methods based on charge hydrophobicity or size of the protein. The addition of sophisticated instrumentation and protein monitoring methods along with purification supports provide the means to purify almost any protein in several steps. Affinity chromatography can be divided broadly into the group-specific and ligand-specific methods. Both have distinct advantages over the multistep traditional chromatography approaches in being able to substantially purify specific proteins in one step. Group-specific affinity chromatography utilizes affinity ligands that can bind and purify specific classes of proteins [21]. The protein G affinity support can purify all types of monoclonal IgG irrespective of the specificity of the antibody. This is due to the ability of the immobilized protein G to bind to the Fc part of all subclasses of IgG. The popular immobilized metal affinity chromatography (IMAC) columns can bind to metalloproteins and recombinant hexa histidine (His) tag incorporated peptides. Ligand-specific affinity columns are more specific and can purify a specific receptor protein, providing almost pure protein in one step.

4. *Preclinical Protein Characterization.* An in-depth description of the biochemical, biophysical, and molecular preclinical characterization of proteins is an essential part of the development of new biopharmaceuticals. This is an extensive systematic study of the future product prior to formulation and early Phase I and II clinical trials. The key data obtained from this preclinical study will also be the basis of future specifications of the key raw materials and the protein product derived from the early production process. The FDA website provides the detailed analytical testing to be done for a candidate prepharmaceutical (http://www.fda.gov/cber/gdlns/cmcdna.pdf). Table 20.3 lists the data required for the drug substance defined as the unformulated active ingredient. Based on this data, the finished drug product is developed with the addition of excipients.

A protein drug can be a simple polypeptide consisting of only amino acids without any higher order structure or with homo or hetero multimeric quarternary structure. More complex proteins may have prosthetic or coenzyme moieties as well as posttranslational modifications including glycosylation, sulfation, phosphorylation, and/or formylation. Conjugation of some of the categories of biopharmaceuticals with radioisotope, drugs, or toxins is also common. Thus, unique biologicals will require the design of special analyses as well as assays to confirm integrity of the pharmaceutical in later stages of development. In addition, data on the optimal storage conditions and data on aggregation, stability, and degradation are also required. This could include both accelerated and real-time stability that would impact on product development, shipping, and marketing strategies. Technological advancements in protein identification and characterization have expanded the scope of preclinical analysis listed in Table 20.2. A detailed enumeration of each is beyond the scope of this chapter and is discussed extensively in a recent book chapter [20].

It is also important to recognize that the boundaries are not rigid between preclinical characterization of biopharmaceuticals and formulation studies. Thus, detailed understanding of the properties of the biopharmaceutical at an early stage is an advantage in the eventual formulation of the final product. Addition of excipients is common and can include human albumin, amino acids, carbohydrates, detergents, chelates, and other chemicals and preservatives.

20.5 INFLUENCE OF CARBOHYDRATE IN PROTEIN DRUGS

Many protein pharmaceuticals are glycoproteins and hence have special properties and pharmacokinetic profiles compared to nonglycosylated proteins. Glycosylated proteins are expressed in yeast, insect cells, or mammalian platforms. The carbohydrate chains are linked to specific amino acids and include N-linked asparagine and the O-linked carbohydrate chains linked to either serine or threonine. The presence of carbohydrates can have an impact on its biodistribution in the body depending on the route of administration and the lack of sialic acid in the side chain. The asialoglycoprotein receptor is a major sink for glycoproteins that lack sialic acid or have lost their sialic acid as a result of degradation or senescence. In some of our early studies using radioactively labeled proteins in mice and rabbits, we demonstrated that intra-venous (IV) injection of asialoglycoproteins results in them being taken up by the liver almost on the first pass, presumably by the hepatocytes [12]. It is estimated that ~40,000 copies of such receptors are on the surface of each hepatocyte and hence the liver has an enormous capacity to clear glycoproteins. Modulation of protein drugs for enhanced delivery to target cells and organs can also be achieved by altering the carbohydrate modeling composition of the glycan chains. This is elegantly shown in the case of enhanced targeting of β-glucocerebrosidase to the macrophages of the reticuloendothelial system to treat Gaucher disease, which is characterized by the accumulation of glucosylceramide. The therapeutic recombinant enzyme (Cerezyme) incorporates the carbohydrate modeling process to generate mannose terminated oligosaccharides to enhance the uptake of the enzyme by the macrophages of the reticuloendothelial system in which Gaucher disease is manifested.

20.6 ANTIBODIES

Antibodies are a group of glycoproteins produced by B-lymphocytes in response to foreign antigens. Natural or deliberate immunization of foreign antigens results in specific antibody production recognizing several epitopes of the antigens. Immunogenicity of the foreign antigen dictates the magnitude of the immune responses in an animal. Antibodies produced in this way are referred to as polyclonal antibodies. Antitoxin or venom antidotes are in this category, which is available commercially. They exhibit heterogeneity in binding avidity, specificity, immunoglobulin class, and isotype. Repeated immunizations or natural exposure to the antigens results in an improved high affinity immunoglobulin response as a result of maturation of the B-cell immune responses. A single B-cell isolated from the polyclonal humoral response and immortalized results in a monoclonal colony secreting identical pure monoclonal antibodies. Each B-cell has the capacity to produce an antibody that recognizes a single epitope. Conferring immortality to a B-cell is accomplished by fusion to a myeloma cell (immortal B-cell cancer), which results in a hybridoma line combining the key properties of the two parental cells of unlimited cell division and secreting a single antibody species.

In the last 30 years since this method was introduced, monoclonal antibodies have become invaluable tools in diagnostic immunoassays and therapeutics of various human diseases [22–26]. Most immunodiagnostic kits now use monoclonal antibodies instead of the polyclonal antibodies. Recombinant DNA technology has also contributed to the development of a new generation of antibody pharmaceuticals for treatment of human diseases and various therapeutic proteins. Most protein pharmaceuticals today are produced recombinantly using *E. coli*, yeast, insect, or mammalian cells. They are safe, convenient, and less expensive to produce, and an abundant supply can be produced within a short period of time. Antibodies and their derivative fragments have also been used as tools in a variety of applications, such as fundamental research work, as well as in diagnosis and human therapeutics. Antibody pharmaceuticals constitute at least 25% of the proteins in different phases of clinical trials [27, 28]. Utilization of antibodies as drug delivery vehicles or as triggers for human immune responses in cancer therapy is clearly promising in future applications [29].

Steps in Hybridoma Production

1. Immunization of mice with antigens.
2. Check of antibody titer in mouse blood.
3. Spleen removal and preparation of a single cell suspension.
4. Myeloma cell (SP2/0) preparation.
5. Fusion of spleen cells and myeloma cells with polyethylene glycol (PEG).
6. Hybridoma selection in selective (HAT) medium.
7. Observation and maintenance of different hybridoma clones (7–15 days postfusion).
8. Screen for specific antibody secretion by ELISA.
9. Expansion of positive clones.
10. Recloning of all positive hybridoma clones by limiting dilution technique.
11. To ensure monoclonality, recloning to >90% positive clones and storage of ~10 vials in liquid N_2.
12. Isotype determination.
13. Small scale cell culture and purification on protein G.
14. Characterization.

20.7 HYBRIDOMA-DERIVED MONOCLONALS

20.7.1 Immunization

Immunization of the animals with the desired antigen is the first step in monoclonal antibody development. Conventionally, this is done by the immunization of BALB/c mice with the antigen followed by repeated booster injections until a suitable serum titer has been obtained. Typically, 6–8 week old female mice are initially immunized and the fusion is performed within 6 months. The planned immunization schedule is very important for the development of the antibody. Collecting a small amount of the serum prior to immunization and storage at $-20\,°C$ is standard practice. This should be used as a negative control for screening assays. At least three to four injections with a maximum of 100–200 µL of volume per mouse are administered, with 1–2 week intervals between the injections. Approximately 20–50 µg of antigen, emulsified with complete Freund's adjuvant (CFA) for primary immunization, should be used for subcutaneous (SC) or intraperitoneal (IP) administration. Subsequent IP injections of 10–25 µg antigen should be emulsified with incomplete Freund's adjuvant (IFA). A final boost 2–3 days prior to fusion should be administered with the antigen in phosphate buffer saline (PBS). An intravenous or intrasplenic injection may be given to maximize the amount of immunogen reaching the spleen and activating B-cells [30–34]. Adequate immunization time is required for affinity maturation and isotype class switching to occur. The first exposure of a naive immune system to a specific immunogen will primarily result in production of IgM antibodies. Subsequent repeated immunizations induce the B-cells to undergo a class switch of the immunoglobulin isotype. The interval between the immunizations can also greatly affect the affinity of antibody produced. As the interval is increased, the antigen level decreases and only higher affinity B-cells remain ready to respond to a subsequent boost. Therefore, the immune response is mostly directed against the more immunogenic antigen or domain. The use of insufficient or excessive amounts of antigen can lead to immune tolerance. Excessive immunization can also block lymphocyte antigen receptors and produce immune paralysis. Overimmunization has also been implicated in the production of relatively low avidity antisera by selecting for low affinity B-lymphocyte clones.

It is apparent that mice consistently do not respond well to certain antigens or small peptides, or antigens that are not immunogenic. In order to generate an immune response to small molecules, also known as haptens, conjugation to larger carrier proteins is essential. Keyhole limpet hemocyanin (KLH) is mostly used as a carrier protein to conjugate synthetic peptides or small molecules and subsequently used as the immunogen to inject mice [35–38].

20.7.2 Isolation of B-Cells from the Spleen

The immunized mouse exhibiting high antibody titers against the antigen is euthanized in a CO_2 chamber. The blood is quickly collected from the heart and the serum is separated and stored at $-20\,°C$ as a positive control. The mouse is completely submerged in a beaker containing 70% alcohol to maintain aseptic conditions and the beaker is placed in a biosafety hood. The mouse is placed on a petri dish so that its left side is facing upward. The area is washed with 70% alcohol or betadine and cut open to isolate the spleen. Using sterile scissors and forceps, the connective tissue and fat are trimed off from around the spleen. The spleen is placed in the petri dish containing 10 mL of RPMI-1640. The spleen is injected with culture medium to release the cells. Using a syringe and a cell strainer, a single cell suspension is obtained. The cell pellets are resuspended in 5 mL of ice cold lysing buffer (0.15 M NaCl, 10 mM $KHCO_3$, 0.1 mM EDTA pH 7.3) to remove the red blood cells. The cell pellet should be erythrocyte-free and the spleen cells are now ready for fusion with myeloma cells.

20.7.3 Fusion and Postfusion

The development of the drug selection procedure employing HAT (hypoxanthine, aminopterin, and thymidine) in the early 1960s by Littlefield's group [39] and the construction of appropriate myeloma cells devoid of HGPRT (hypoxanthine guanine phosphoribosyl transferase) were critical to development of hybridoma technologies to usher in the monoclonal revolution as a new class of protein therapeutics. Currently, the SP2/0 myeloma cell deficient in the HGPRT enzyme is one of the common choices for fusion with spleenocytes. Several other myeloma cells have been made including rat and human myelomas. While mouse and rat myelomas have been used successfully to generate hybridoma secreting mouse and rat antibodies, respectively, the human myelomas have been problematic, including hybridoma yield and stability. An inherent and key limitation of cell fusion hybridoma technology is that the fusion is random and the frequency is low (<1% to 5%) [40]. As a result, many a good, specific, high affinity antibody secreting B-cell may not fuse with the myeloma cell. This problem is mitigated in phage display and other technologies described in subsequent sections. The myeloma cells should be in the log phase of growth when used for the fusion. It is also essential to check the HGPRT deficiency of the SP2/0 cells by growing them in media with 8-azaguanine. Since the SP2/0 cells are HGPRT deficient, SP2/0 cells should not die in 8-azaguanine.

Spontaneous fusions of cultured cells rarely occur; however, the addition of certain viruses or chemical fusogens can markedly increase the rate at which they fuse. Electrofusion methods have also been developed as alternative strategies. PEG (polyethylene glycol) is the chemical fusogen most commonly used for cell fusion. Cell membranes adhere because of hydrophobic interactions between membrane phospholipids and a small proportion of them break down and reform so that fused cells are formed. Early techniques employed addition of peritoneal macrophages as feeder cells for promoting the growth of hybridoma cells. Alternatively, the HAT medium is supplemented with 50 μg/mL of LPS and 20 μg/mL of dextran sulfate. These agents stimulate the spleen cells to respond well to these mitogens. In about 7–10 days hybridoma clones start to appear.

Following the hybridoma fusion, the first 10 days appear to be the most critical to cell survival in HAT selection medium. The cell population consists of fused and unfused B and myeloma cells. Although the unfused lymphocytes die rapidly, it is necessary to introduce a selective mechanism to separate unfused myeloma cells from fused heterohybrid cells. HGPRT is the key enzyme of the salvage pathway for DNA synthesis. Fusion of myeloma cells with the B-cells compensates for their deficiency of HGPRT. Aminopterin blocks the *de novo* DNA synthesis pathway and since unfused myeloma cells cannot use the *de novo* pathway for DNA synthesis, they subsequently die due to the lack of the salvage pathway HGPRT enzyme. Heterohybrid (myeloma fused with lymphocytes) fused cells are able to bypass the *de novo* pathway blockage due to the functional HGPRT in the lymphocyte and survive only through the salvaged pathways. In this selection mechanism, only fused cells are able to grow in the HAT medium.

Due to great variation in growth at this critical time, it is extremely important to care for the hybrids within individual wells. Each plate should be microscopically checked often following fusion for colony formation as well as potential contamination problems. Many wells may not show any growth and others may contain more than one hybrid cell. Nonproducing hybrids usually outgrow the producing hybrids in the same well and eventually completely overtake them; therefore, care must be taken to avoid this with early recloning at limited dilutions of <1 cell per well. Nonproducers are hybrid cells that may have received enough genetic information from both cells to survive selection and remain viable, but lack antibody production. Since immunoglobulin synthesis represents ~30% of the total B-cell protein synthesis, nonsecretory hybrid cells have lesser metabolic burden and hence can have a selective advantage to outgrow in the wells.

Some hybrids grow slower than others and may not initially produce antibodies within the detection limits of the screening method. A well that initially appears to be slightly positive and then becomes negative is most likely due to the production of immunoglobulin from unfused B-cells before they die. When a third of the well is covered with clones or the color of medium changes to orange or yellow, clones are ready for screening using ELISA. Solid phase ELISA is the most common method for selecting desired clones. This method of screening involves coating the ELISA plate with the desired antigen (1 μg/well). Following a blocking step, an aliquot of the clone supernatant (100 μL) is incubated with the antigen coated plate and the antigen–antibody complex is detected using an enzyme-labeled antibody capable of binding to the Fc region of the mouse antibody. Clones showing ELISA values five times higher than the negative control are considered positive. The serum of unimmunized mice and irrelevant antibody are used as negative controls. A positive serum from immunized mice is generally used as positive control. The strong positive clones are cultured and expanded in 24 well tissue culture plates. All the positive clones should be cultured for at least 10 days in HT medium (hypoxanthine and thymidine) to utilize the salvage pathway for synthesizing nucleic acids and to ensure that all traces of aminopterin have been removed from the wells.

20.7.4 Cloning

When a microtiter well tests positive for the antibody of interest, it is important to reclone as soon as possible to avoid the potential loss of the positive clone due to overgrowth by nonsecreting cells. Cloning is the isolation and propagation of a hybridoma cell at limiting dilution of less than one hybridoma per well to reach monoclonality of the culture. The application of the MAb technique can only be realized if the cell culture producing the antibody is truly monoclonal, consisting solely of cells derived from a single precursor hybrid cell. Successive recloning two to four times can ensure monoclonality and the isolation of the stable clone. In the soft agar method, the heterogeneous population is dispersed in warm, molten agar and poured into petri dishes. As the cells begin to divide, individual colonies can be selected and transferred to tissue culture plates for expansion and screening. Cloning by limiting dilution is less labor intensive and more widely used, since the primary hybridoma is merely diluted in media and aliquoted at less than one cell per well. Limiting dilution recloning requires an accurate cell count of the viable hybridoma cells suspended in the medium of the microtiter well in which the cells are growing. If less than 80% of the clones tested are positive in the second recloning step, the hybridoma should be recloned until 90–100% cloning efficiency is reached. The two best clones with the highest ELISA values are chosen and a cell bank is prepared for long-term storage in liquid N_2. Valuable therapeutic hybridoma clones should also be protected by storage at the ATCC, USA which is an excellent repository for a variety of biologicals. Alternatively, advances in DNA sequencing by automated machines allow rapid determination of the variable heavy and light chains of the monoclonal antibody for long-term protection of valuable clones. Such sequence information can utilize total synthesis of the gene and cloning for possible resurrection of the valuable antibodies by recombinant DNA techniques.

20.7.5 Cell Line Characterization and Cryopreservation

Once a hybridoma has been cloned and recloned, it is necessary to characterize the line to determine the conditions for optimal growth and good antibody secretion. Mycoplasma contamination of any line needs to be tested. A number of commercial tests are available to detect mycoplasma. These include general mycoplasma tests to specific PCR detection of individual species. The master hybridoma cell lines are cryopreserved to allow for long-term storage. Generally, a freezing medium (90% FBS and 10% DMSO) is used for long-term storage in liquid N_2. A simple commercial device is available (Freezing container, Nalgene Inc.) to gradually cool the hybridoma cells to $-80\,°C$ for 24–48 h, and then transfer to liquid N_2 is essential. Thawing of stored hybridoma cells in primary or secondary banks is a rapid procedure. Unlike slow cryopreservation of cell lines, thawing must occur very quickly to minimize damage to the cells. The stored cell line is thawed in a $37\,°C$ water bath for 1 min and subsequently cultured for expanding the clone.

20.7.6 Small Scale Bioreactor Culture

The thawed hybridoma cell line is cultured and expanded for generating small amounts of the MAb. Early methods routinely injected hybridomas into pristane primed mice to generate ascites fluid to purify the MAb. Such methods are currently discouraged due to animal care concerns. In addition, the ascites could also harbor small amounts of endogenous mouse polyclonal antibodies that copurify with the monoclonal antibody. This defeats the very purpose of the development of monoclonal antibodies. Hence, *in vitro* culture of hybridomas in any one of the commerical small scale bioreactors is recommended to prepare pure MAb for preclinical characterization of the biopharmaceutical.

The I-MAb™ bioreactor bag is a monoclonal antibody production system we routinely use to make laboratory amounts of MAbs (~25–50 mg). This is based on the feature of high surface area/gas exchange of CO_2/O_2 in a closed environment for increased cell growth, metabolism, and decreased risk of contamination. The bag is incubated until the cell viability falls to 10–20%. This is usually reached at the mid 3–4 week incubation period. Antibody production continues during the declining phase of growth and is often maximal during this phase. This is supported by two theories: viable cells secrete antibodies and dead cells release the antibodies. After an incubation period of 25–30 days, the I-MAb bag is harvested and clarified by centrifugation. We have successfully reutilized the bioreactors for several cycles to minimize the cost of antibody production.

20.7.7 Purification

Generally, the desired species of MAbs are of the IgG class. Often the subclass of the IgG is determined by the subtype of specific commercial reagents. Purifying MAbs from a small scale bioreactor can be performed by a number of methods. Classical biochemical methods exploited ethanol precipitation, salt precipitation, PEG precipitation, caprylic acid precipitation, ion exchange chromatography, thiophilic gel chromatography, or affinity chromatography. Among these methods, only affinity chromatography gives high purity of IgG in one simple step. Affinity chromatography is of two broad types—namely, group-specific and ligand-specific strategies. In the former, the purification is based on the binding of the Fc domain to affinity supports such as protein G [41] and protein A [42]. The second strategy exploits the specific antigen or mimetic as ligand to bind the antibody via the antigen combining site. Protein G is the most common affinity matrix and is derived from a cell wall protein of type G streptococci that has an affinity for the Fc region of immunoglobulin G (IgG). Protein G also has a binding site for albumin; however, it has been deleted in recombinant forms of protein G so that it only has affinity for IgG. Protein A does not have a comparable binding affinity or diversity in subclass binding that is found in protein G; many mouse IgG subclass antibodies will not bind to protein A. Protein L is a newer isolated affinity matrix from *Peptostreptococcus magnus*. It binds to the kappa light chain of all antibody classes including IgG. Hence, it is the most versatile of the three proteins [43]. protein L is especially useful for purification of Fab and scFv fragments. Another advantage of protein L is that it does not bind to bovine antibody, which is found in trace amounts in extensively used fetal bovine serum (FBS). The technique of affinity chromatography relies on the ability of proteins to recognize and bind to specific ligands in a reversible manner. Affinity chromatography uses an adsorbent comprised of a matrix to which the ligand is attached. The attachment or bonding is performed so that the immobilized ligand is still able to interact with the protein. An affinity separation is then performed by passing the impure protein over the adsorbent. The target protein is adsorbed, and contaminants pass through. Following adsorption, the adsorbent is washed to remove residual contaminants and the bound protein is eluted in a pure form. Elution is normally achieved by changing the buffer or salt composition so the protein can no longer interact with the immobilized ligand. MAbs differ in their biochemical and ligand characteristics, making it necessary to develop individual protocols for their purification; however, due to the existence of common constant domains (Fc and light chains), group-specific affinity chromatography can be utilized for MAb purification. The immobilized ligands commonly used are protein G, protein A, and protein L. A variation of affinity chromatography is the technique of affinity cochromatography. In this technique, antibody is purified indirectly [21, 44, 45]. The antigen is captured on an affinity support and this complex is used to isolate antibody specific to the antigen.

20.7.8 Applications

Monoclonal antibodies (MAbs) are used extensively in most immunoassays, such as radioimmunoassays, enzyme linked immunosorbant assay (ELISA), immunohistology, and flow cytometry for *in vitro* diagnosis. Several MAbs are also used for *in vivo* diagnostic imaging and immunotherapy of different human diseases. Currently, applications of MAbs fall within four main areas: diagnosis, imaging, therapy, and affinity purification.

Disease Diagnosis   Polyclonal antibodies have been used in the diagnosis of diseases for several decades; however, they have inherent limitations due to their polyvalent nature of cross-reacting with irrelevant antigens to some extent. MAbs are particularly useful in diagnostics, where monospecificity is the most important criterion [26]. The use of MAbs in the analysis of cell surface antigens is also important in tissue typing for transfusion and qualitative and quantitative analysis of specific cell populations in blood in normal and disease states.

Molecular Imaging   Imaging is the *in vivo* use of specific or antibody probes to identify and localize disease. Imaging can be considered intermediate to diagnosis and therapy. Its purpose is to search for and localize antigens such as tumor location within the body, for treatment decisions to be made. Imaging antibodies need to meet a stringent set of criteria: they must be stable during labeling and after administration and be of sufficiently high affinity to localize in small tumors. Several radiolabled antibodies are approved by the FDA for *in vivo* imaging. A more recent innovation is fluorescence-based imaging.

Therapy   A variety of protein and carbohydrate molecules on the surface of cancer cells are potential targets for antibody-directed therapies [22, 24, 25, 46–49]. Clinically useful targets may be uniquely expressed by cancer cells or expressed at higher levels by cancer cells than by normal cells. Consequently, antibodies will selectively bind to or accumulate in cancer cells. The antibody can act in several ways including the induction of apoptosis, the blocking of growth factor receptors, induction of cell- or complement-mediated cytotoxicity, or the blocking of angiogenesis. Targeting strategies can be an antibody linked to a radioactive particle, drug loaded liposome immunotoxin, or a chemotherapeutic agent. Targeting a receptor that internalizes upon antibody binding will lead to intracellular delivery of the toxic agents. By attaching liposomes containing cytotoxic drugs to MAbs or smaller fragments, anticancer drugs can be delivered to the cell interior [29]. The treatment of solid tumors with such relatively large molecules as immunoglobulin presents certain challenges, especially since direct action requires the antibody to penetrate the tumor mass. Penetration may be facilitated by the use of antibody fragments, which can be made by recombinant technology.

The potential use of MAbs in therapeutics was quickly recognized and the first MAb was approved for therapeutic use in 1986. This was a mouse monoclonal to CD3 antigen for the prevention of transplantation rejection. The U.S. FDA has since approved 18 different MAbs for treating different human diseases [50]. Current sales of the antibody-based protein pharmaceuticals exceed $10 B and is expected to grow to $16.7 B in 2008 [51] and to $26B by 2010 (http://www.drugresearcher.com/news/ng.asp?id=60408-worldwide-antibody-market).

20.7.9   Immunogenicity Issues and Humanization

Following the discovery of hybridoma technology, murine monoclonal antibodies have proved useful in *in vitro* diagnostics of various diseases; however, when used *in vivo* for the treatment of patients with various ailments, their effect is not always sustained [22, 25, 26]. When mouse antibodies are administered to patients, human immune systems elicit human antibodies against the foreign mouse domains. The specific response of human antibodies directed against mouse antibodies is referred to as HAMA (human anti-mouse antibody) [52, 53]. The HAMA response can complex and neutralize the mouse antibodies by rapid clearance from the blood, thus preventing the mouse antibody from binding to its target. In addition, mouse antibodies only weakly recruit the human immune system components that may be necessary to clear the targeted antigens or tumors. Rodent antibodies tend to provoke strong HAMA responses, which restrict their usefulness for repeated application in the same patient. Hence, current MAb pharmaceuticals would have to be at least a chimeric antibody with a substantial human constant domain.

The first chimeric antibodies were developed in 1984 to solve the problem of the HAMA response [54]. Chimeric antibodies are antibodies in which the constant regions (H and L chains) of a mouse or rat antibody are replaced with human constant regions by recombinant DNA technology. This provides the antibody with human effector functions and also reduces immunogenicity (HAMA) caused by the rodent Fc region. While chimeric antibodies solved the problem of efficient interaction with the human immune system, these antibodies, which have about 30% mouse and 70% human protein sequence, could still elicit a HACA (human anti-chimeric antibody) response against the chimeric mouse part, therefore limiting the use of MAbs as human therapeutics [53, 55].

The next step in MAb evolution was the further humanization beyond the chimeric antibodies. The technology of antibody humanization was developed in 1986 in which only those parts of a mouse antibody that are directly involved in binding to its specific target are transplanted from the mouse antibody to a human antibody framework or CDR grafting [56]. It was thought that humanization would remove much of the immunogenicity remaining with chimeric antibodies; however, human anti-human antibody (HAHA) responses were also observed, although with a reduced incidence compared with HAMA and HACA [53]. An optimal humanized antibody would contain the minimum number of mouse domains required to reproduce the binding strength and specificity of the original mouse antibody and can still be capable of recruiting components of the human immune system. Humanization or fully human antibodies can be developed in several ways: (1) humanized/CDR grafted/reshaped antibodies, (2) human antibodies from immune donors, (3) fully human antibodies from phage libraries, (4) humouse technology, and (5) deimmunization [57].

The ongoing immunogenicity problems of using MAbs as human therapeutics have continued to be an issue [58]. The evolution of MAb technology that began with the generation of rodent chimeric and then humanized MAbs has culminated with the development of fully human MAbs [59]. Human B-cells are immunized *ex vivo* in the presence of human antigens and then immortalized by means of cell fusion. The group has generated MAbs specific to a number of human antigens and some of them show neutralizing activity against human proteins [60].

20.8 BISPECIFIC MONOCLONAL ANTIBODIES

Bispecific monoclonal antibodies (BsMAbs) have distinct binding specificities to two different antigens incorporated in the same molecule. The early bispecific antibodies were designed by chemically coupling two distinct polyclonal antibodies [61]. Cell fusion of two hybridomas to generate hybrid hybridomas or quadroma secreting bispecific antibodies was an alternate convenient strategy [62]. Triomas are BsMAb secreting cells derived by fusing a hybridoma with spleen cells derived from a mouse immunized with a second antigen. The coexpression of two different IgGs in triomas and quadromas result in the assembly of bispecific MAbs as well as unwanted MAb species resulting from random pairing of heavy and light chains. These unwanted contaminants compete with the activity of the bispecific antibody and must be removed from the mixture, posing a significant challenge for purification. Exploiting elegant protein engineering techniques, it is now possible to engineer the inter-CH3 domain disulfide bonds of heavy chains so that they preferentially form heterodimers over homodimers [63]. The light chain mispairing problem is resolved by using an identical light chain for each arm of the bispecific antibodies. By these methods, nine unwanted H and L chain pairings were eliminated from the population and only one pure product was obtained for further use. Recombinant DNA strategies have also been used to generate bispecific antibodies. The heavy and light chains of the two immunoglobulin binding regions are independently linked by a (Gly-Gly-Gly-Gly-Ser)$_3$ linker and two single chain antibodies are linked by a different peptide to generate a bispecific single chain MAb.

BsMAbs are unique heterobifunctional nano cross-linkers that remove chemical conjugation steps to cross-link any two desired antigens or cells in a predetermined fashion. Such probes have a variety of applications in immunohistology, immunoassays, immunoimaging, immunotherapy, and even retargeting of cytotoxic or dendritic cells to cancer sites [64–67]. Full length bispecific antibodies forming heterodimers based on the knobs-in-holes concept has also been described for therapeutic applications [68].

The use of bispecific molecules in therapy is based on the selective recruitment of an effector mechanism against a defined disease-related biomarker. Hence, bispecific molecules serve as bridges or mediators between an effector and a target. Bispecific molecules are capable of recruiting effector molecules (toxins, drugs, prodrugs, cytokines, and radionuclides), effector cells (NK cells, macrophages, cytotoxic T lymphocytes, or dendritic cells), and the retargeted carrier systems (viral vectors for gene therapy). Therapeutically useful bispecific antibodies should also have the following criteria for *in vivo* uses: (1) be nonimmunogenic to avoid neutralizing immune responses, (2) have a defined structure and bind to the effector cells to induce activation only after binding to the target cells, (3) have a minimum size to allow penetration into the tumor tissues and exhibit sufficiently long half-lives to induce prolonged therapeutics effects, and (4) be flexible if possible to accommo-date a variety of biologicals.

20.9 RECOMBINANT ANTIBODY

20.9.1 Phage Display

In classical hybridoma technology, hetero fusion efficiency between a B-cell and myeloma is low. Consequently, many of the valuable B-cells secreting high affinity and high specificity antibodies fail to form viable hybridomas. Attempts have been made to improve fusion efficiency with polyethylene glycol, electrofusion, and affin-ity strategies, but these approaches do not encompass the entire antibody repertoire generated by the mammalian immune system upon immunization with a specific antigen. To overcome this limitation and to minimize the immunogenicity issues of full length murine antibodies, recombinant DNA technology introduced phage display technology for the surface expression of the Fab or scFv libraries derived from total splenic mRNA.

Phage display technology is a very powerful technique for generating recombi-nant libraries containing millions of different peptides, proteins, or small molecules. Phage display has been used to define epitopes for monoclonal antibodies, select enzyme substrates, and screen cloned antibody repertoires for affinity screening of combinatorial peptide libraries to identify ligands for peptide receptors [69]. Phage display technology provides a very effective means to identify proteins that bind to a target molecule of interest [69–73]. A large variety of phage display systems have been developed. The most common is the phagemid vector-based system, where the gene that codes for the protein of interest is genetically cloned in frame into the viral gene 3 protein (g3p). The proteins encoded by the library are expressed on the surface of the phage and designed to select those that bind to the target molecule of interest by a simple panning step. Phages that bind the specific target molecule contain the gene for the protein and have the ability to replicate and propagate in the proper host cell.

Bacteriophage display of combinatorial antibody libraries can select monoclonal antibody reductants of a desired specificity without the use of conventional hybrid-oma technology. Two general methods have been used to generate phage display libraries. One technique utilizes immunized animals, while the other uses naive Ab genes. With the first technique, an animal is immunized with a target molecule of interest and a phage display library is constructed using the total complement of sequences from the antibody mRNA in the lymphocytes of the immunized animal. The isolation of specific antibodies from a cloned immunological repertoire requires a large, diverse library, as well as an efficient selection procedure. To achieve this goal, a natural strong immune response must be generated in mice and the quality of the total splenic mRNA and cDNA from which the library is constructed must be high. A high serum antibody titer against the immunizing antigen usually indi-cates that there is enrichment for antigen-specific clones. The second method to generate a phage display library uses germline antibody genes to construct a naive phage display library [74, 75]. This library is not initially enriched with antibody sequences that bind to a particular molecule; therefore, it is more challenging to isolate the antibodies of interest. The advantage of a naive library is that it only needs to be synthesized once and can be used to isolate a clone and improve the binding affinity by random and selective modifications. The applications of phage technology include the creation and screening of libraries to discover novel therapeutic targets and methods for selection of biologically active ligands.

20.9.2 Yeast Display

Saccharomyces cerevisae is useful as a host for the recombinant eukaryotic protein expression, since it allows the proper folding and glycosylation of expressed heterologous proteins [76–78]. The rigid structure of the cell makes yeast suitable for several genetic applications especially cell surface display of foreign proteins. Yeast display exploits the agglutinin adhesion receptor protein to display recombinant protein on the surface of the yeast [79, 80]. The receptor consists of two proteins: Aga1 and Aga2. Aga1 is secreted from the cell and becomes covalently attached to β-glucan in the extracellular matrix of the yeast cell wall. Aga2 is also secreted by the cell and binds Aga1 through two disulfide bonds and remains attached to the cell wall via Aga1. The yeast display system takes advantage of the association between Aga1 and Aga2 by fusing heterologous proteins to the C terminus of the Aga2 protein within a yeast display vector. The resulting construct is then transformed into the yeast strain, which only contains the Aga1 gene. Expression of both proteins results in the association of Aga2 fusion protein to Aga1. Consequently, the tagged heterologous molecule is displayed on the cell surface at 10,000–100,000 copies per cell and can be monitored by fluorescent labeled antibodies recognizing the tags encoded by the display vector.

20.9.3 Ribosome and mRNA Display

Unlike the phage display and yeast display technology, *in vitro* display technology can be used to generate and select the ligands by evolutionary strategies. In the phage display system, the whole library is transformed into *E. coli*, generating the recombinant phage particles displaying the target heterologous molecules. In contrast, DNA library molecules are first transcribed into mRNA *in vitro* and then translated by the ribosome machinery [81]. In this system, the library size is small, which represents the number of different full length protein molecules coupled to the encoded mRNA molecules in the complex. In both the ribosome and mRNA display systems, the functional library size is limited by the amount of *in vitro* translation mixture. The difference between the two methods is how the protein is connected to the mRNA molecules.

In ribosome display, the DNA library is transcribed first to mRNA and then translated *in vitro* with a stoichiometric quantity of ribosomes [82]. Since the DNA has no stop codon, the translation process continues to the end of the mRNA molecule, which results in the nascent polypeptide being bound to the ribosome. The phenotype of the complex is represented by the protein, while the genotype is represented by the mRNA. In order to bind the nascent protein to the target, it has to be properly folded while still attached to the ribosome. Exploiting recombinant DNA technology, the C-terminal region of the DNA library is connected to the ribosome, subsequently providing flexibility for the protein to be folded and be available as a free unit for binding to the target. The ribosomal complex is captured by the target and the mRNA is isolated by destabilizing the complex. RT-PCR and PCR provide the DNA template for further characterization.

In mRNA display [83–85], the DNA library, which is free of stop codons, is transcribed *in vitro* to mRNA. Each mRNA molecule is then ligated to a short DNA linker containing the adaptor molecule. The modified mRNA is then translated into protein and the translation process will stall at the mRNA–DNA junction. During this step, a peptide bond will form between the adaptor molecule and the nascent peptide by the complex translational machinery. The resulting mRNA and protein complex is purified from the ribosome and subjected to reverse transcription (RT-PCR). The cDNA/mRNA–protein complex is then subjected to selective binding to the target. The isolated enriched complex is hydrolyzed by NaOH and the single stranded DNA is recovered. The recovered DNA is then PCR amplified for the next round of selection and further characterization.

20.10   HIGH LEVEL MAMMALIAN EXPRESSION OF RECOMBINANT ANTIBODIES AND PROTEINS BY GENE AMPLIFICATION SYSTEM

The selection of a candidate preclinical antibody or protein product also requires bulk production for eventual characterization and clinical trials. At least two novel mammalian expression systems have been developed that can amplify the production/secretion of the recombinant antibodies. The range of secretion varies from 100 to 1000 mg/L of mammalian culture. The dihydrofolate reductase (DHFR) gene is used as the amplification vector. It catalyzes the chemical reaction of dihydrofolate to tetrahydrofolate and, at a much slower rate, the conversion of folate to tetrahydrofolate. It has been found that chemical compounds such as methotrexate, pyrimethamine, and trimethoprim inhibit the catalysis. The dihydrofolate reductase system is exploited for high level expression of recombinant antibodies [86]. The most widely used mammalian expression system is the gene amplification procedure utilizing DHFR deficient Chinese hamster ovary (CHO) cells [87–89]. Methotrexate binds to the DHFR enzyme, but DHFR deficient CHO cells, which have taken up mammalian expression vector containing the DHFR gene, can develop resistance to methotrexate by amplifying the DHFR gene. Since the antibody gene of interest is also colinked with the DHFR gene in the mammalian expression vector, it is subsequently coamplified. When the cells are subjected to successive rounds of selection in medium containing stepwise increments in methotrexate levels, recombinant CHO cells with specific antibody productivity also increase. The magnitude of specific productivity of the recombinant CHO cells progressively increases with gene copy number [88]. It has been reported [90] that using the DHFR amplification system with CHO cells resulted in specific antibody productivity as high as $100 \mu g/10^6$ cells/day.

Another gene amplification system for high levels of protein biopharmaceutical is the glutamine synthetase based amplification system [91–93]. The CHO cells growing in culture require glutamine for their growth and survival. Glutamine can either be obtained from the medium or be synthesized by the cells from glutamate and ammonia through catalysis by the enzyme glutamine synthetase. The CHO cells grown in a selection medium that is glutamine free and contains methionine sulfoximine (MSX is an inhibitor of GS) do not survive. Specific antibody gene expression can be achieved by plating the CHO cells in MSX solution medium and then transfecting the cells with a mammalian expression vector that coded for the GS gene along with the foreign gene of interest. Only those cells that incorporate the vector and express GS at levels sufficiently high to overcome the MSX block will survive. Expression of the foreign gene can be amplified by growing the cells in successively higher concentrations of MSX. The specific gene of interest that is colinked to the GS gene in the same vector or adjacently in the host chromosome is coamplified. As a result of these two amplification strategies based on DHFR or GS vectors, significantly higher levels of antibodies have been obtained for preclinical and eventual clinical use.

20.11   SPECIAL CONSIDERATIONS

Many protein pharmaceuticals are formulated naturally occurring human proteins such as hormones, cytokines, and enzymes. However, several therapeutic proteins are also derived from nonhuman sources such as microbes and animals. Examples include several monoclonals and enzymes such as urate oxidase from *Saccharomyces cerevisiae*, L-asparaginase from *E. coli*, and streptokinase from *Streptococcus hemolyticus*. These foreign therapeutic proteins can elicit significant immunogenic responses upon administration to humans. These include strong humoral and cell-mediated immune responses. As a result, two types of biomedical responses can occur. First, such proteins can elicit allergic reactions, compromising the safety of the patient. Second, the antibodies generated against the nonhuman protein therapeutic can complex and inactivate the pharmaceutical. Two strategies have been adopted to mitigate the immunogenicity of such proteins. The first approach with therapeutic enzymes incorporates the attachment of polyethylene glycol chains on the surface of the therapeutic proteins. This imparts several beneficial characteristics such as reduced immunogenicity, toxicity, clearance, and proteolysis as well as enhanced bioavailability with slower clearance.

Early therapeutic monoclonal antibodies were mouse proteins and hence generated human anti-mouse antibodies (HAMA) against the constant mouse regions as well as against the variable regions. This led to the development of chimeric antibodies incorporating human constant regions in place of the mouse domains. These chimeric antibodies reduced the immunogenicity of such therapeutics. The introduction of fully human therapeutic antibodies has further minimized the immunogenicity but has not eliminated it altogether. A new technique of deimmunization has been introduced to selectively replace the T-cell and B-cell epitopes of preclinical pharmaceutical candidates to mitigate immune responses by rational design [57]. This new approach to designing therapeutic proteins is emerging due to an improved understanding of T-cell modulation of the immune response and new methods for modeling T-cell epitopes using different bioinformatics tools. Potential T-cell epitopes present in the antibody or in any protein are identified using bioinformatics software (EpiMatrix) to analyze the protein sequence for known human HLA class I and/or II epitopes. Once these epitopes are identified, substitution of key amino acids in the T-cell epitopes may alter or attenuate the immunogenicity of the protein. Modification of the key amino acids can abolish binding to human class II MHC molecules and presentation of the peptides, in the context of MHC, to T-helper cells. Following substitution of the key amino acids, immunogenicity of the modified protein can also be evaluated *in vitro*.

20.12 SUPRAMOLECULAR THERAPEUTICS: CELLS, TISSUES, AND ORGANS

A unique new category of biopharmaceuticals is the use of whole cells as therapeutics, which has already became a reality. The U.S. FDA has approved the use of a magnetic device for the isolation and purification of CD34 antigen positive bone marrow cells for bone marrow therapy. This device is an affinity column that has the anti-CD34 antibody coated with paramagnetic particles as the affinity reagent to isolate highly purified bone marrow cells using a magnet free of contaminating cancer and other immune cells for transplantation.

Pioneering work in our university has isolated and purified human islets from both cadaver and live donor pancreas can be transplanted to diabetics [94–97]. Several patients injected with the islet cells into the liver via the portal vein have been free of daily injections of insulin. Advances in tissue therapeutics have also made artificial skin for grafting in burn injury as well as regeneration and reconstruction of the artificial bladder using the three-dimensional growth of bladder cells. In the future, the horizons of therapeutic possibilities will merge with several novel nonbiological materials including nanotechnologies. A case in point is the cardiovascular stents coated with biologicals to prevent clotting, encapsulation of islet cells in microbeads, implantable devices, targeted nanodevices, and biologicals.

ACKNOWLEDGMENTS

This work was supported by NIH grant # 5U01AI061233-02 and an NSERC strategic grant.

REFERENCES

1. Kohler G, Milstein C. Continuous cultures of fused cells secreting antibody of predefined specificity. *Nature* 1975;256(5517):495–497.
2. Merrifield RB. Solid-phase peptide synthesis. 3. An improved synthesis of bradykinin. *Biochemistry* 1964;3:1385–1390.
3. Merrifield RB. Automated synthesis of peptides. *Science* 1965;150(693):178–185.
4. Das D, Kriangkum J, Nagata LP, Fulton RE, Suresh MR. Development of a biotin mimic tagged ScFv antibody against western equine encephalitis virus: bacterial expression and refolding. *J Virol Methods* 2004;117(2):169–177.
5. Zhang G, Brokx S, Weiner JH. Extracellular accumulation of recombinant proteins fused to the carrier protein YebF in *Escherichia coli. Nat Biotechnol* 2006;24(1):100–104.
6. Bendig MM. The production of foreign proteins in mammalian cells. *Genet Eng* 1988;7:91–127.

7. Colosimo A, Goncz KK, Holmes AR, Kunzelmann K, Novelli G, Malone RW, Bennett MJ, Gruenert DC. Transfer and expression of foreign genes in mammalian cells. *Biotechniques* 2000;29(2):314–318, 320–322, 324 passim.

8. Hinnen A, Buxton F, Chaudhuri B, Heim J, Hottiger T, Meyhack B, Pohlig G. Gene expression in recombinant yeast. *Bioprocess Technol* 1995;22:121–193.

9. Hinnen A, Meyhack B, Heim J. Heterologous gene expression in yeast. *Biotechnology* 1989;13:193–213.

10. Jarvis DL. Foreign gene expression in insect cells. *Bioprocess Technol* 1993;17:195–219.

11. Kost TA, Condreay JP, Jarvis DL. Baculovirus as versatile vectors for protein expression in insect and mammalian cells. *Nat Biotechnol* 2005;23(5):567–575.

12. Boniface GR, Selvaraj S, Suresh MR, Longenecker BM, Noujaim AA. Synthetic glycosylated-HSA analogues for hepatocyte receptor imaging. In Billinghurst MW, Ed. *Current Applications in Radiopharmacology*. Oxford: Pergamon; 1986, pp 157–164.

13. Finishing the euchromatic sequence of the human genome. *Nature* 2004;431(7011): 931–945.

14. Agarwal KL, Buchi H, Caruthers MH, Gupta N, Khorana HG, Kleppe K, Kumar A, Ohtsuka E, Rajbhandary UL, Van de Sande JH, Sgaramella V, Weber H, Yamada T. Total synthesis of the gene for an alanine transfer ribonucleic acid from yeast. *Nature* 1970;227(5253):27–34.

15. Sanger F, Air GM, Barrell BG, Brown NL, Coulson AR, Fiddes CA, Hutchison CA, Slocombe PM, Smith M. Nucleotide sequence of bacteriophage phi X174 DNA. *Nature* 1977;265(5596):687–695.

16. Sanger F, Nicklen S, Coulson AR. DNA sequencing with chain-terminating inhibitors. *Proc Natl Acad Sci USA* 1977;74(12):5463–5467.

17. Marra MA, Jones SJ, Astell CR, Holt RA, Brooks-Wilson A, Butterfield YS, Khattra J, Asano JK, Barber SA, Chan SY, Cloutier A, Coughlin SM, Freeman D, Girn N, Griffith OL, Leach SR, Mayo M, McDonald H, Montgomery SB, Pandoh PK, Petrescu AS, Robertson AG, Schein JE, Siddiqui A, Smailus DE, Stott JM, Yang GS, Plummer F, Andonov A, Artsob H, Bastien N, Bernard K, Booth TF, Bowness D, Czub M, Drebot M, Fernando L, Flick R, Garbutt M, Gray M, Grolla A, Jones S, Feldmann H, Meyers A, Kabani A, Li Y, Normand S, Stroher U, Tipples GA, Tyler S, Vogrig R, Ward D, Watson B, Brunham RC, Krajden M, Petric M, Skowronski DM, Upton C, Roper RL. The genome sequence of the SARS-associated coronavirus. *Science* 2003;300(5624):1399–1404.

18. Das D, Suresh MR. Copious production of SARS-CoV nucleocapsid protein employing codon optimized synthetic gene. *J Virol Methods* 2006;137(2):343–346.

19. McGrath BM, Walsh G, Eds. *Directory of Therapeutic Enzymes*. London: CRC/Taylor & Francis; 2005.

20. Niazi SK. *Handbook of Preformulation: Chemical, Biological, and Botanical Drugs*. London: Taylor & Francis/CRC Press; 2006.

21. Gupta S, Suresh M. Affinity chromatography and co-chromatography of bispecific monoclonal antibody immunoconjugates. *J Biochem Biophys Methods* 2002;51(3):203–216.

22. Adams GP, Weiner LM. Monoclonal antibody therapy of cancer. *Nat Biotechnol* 2005;23(9):1147–1157.

23. Carter P. Improving the efficacy of antibody-based cancer therapies. *Nat Rev Cancer* 2001;1(2):118–129.

24. Gatto B. Monoclonal antibodies in cancer therapy. *Curr Med Chem Anticancer Agents* 2004;4(5):411–414.

25. von Mehren M, Adams GP, Weiner LM. Monoclonal antibody therapy for cancer. *Annu Rev Med* 2003;54:343–369.

26. Waldmann TA. Monoclonal antibodies in diagnosis and therapy. *Science* 1991;252(5013):1657–1662.

27. Glennie MJ, Johnson PW. Clinical trials of antibody therapy. *Immunol Today* 2000;21(8):403–410.

28. Hudson PJ. Recombinant antibody fragments. *Curr Opin Biotechnol* 1998;9(4):395–402.

29. Allen TM. Ligand-targeted therapeutics in anticancer therapy. *Nat Rev Cancer* 2002;2:750–763.

30. Nilsson BO, Larsson A. Intrasplenic immunization with minute amounts of antigen. *Immunol Today* 1990;11(1):10–12.

31. Spitz M. "Single-shot" intrasplenic immunization for the production of monoclonal antibodies. *Methods Enzymol* 1986;121:33–41.

32. Spitz M, Spitz L, Thorpe R, Eugui E. Intrasplenic primary immunization for the production of monoclonal antibodies. *J Immunol Methods* 1984;70(1):39–43.

33. Svalander PC, Andersson J, Nilsson BO. Intrasplenic immunization for production of monoclonal antibodies against mouse blastocysts. *J Immunol Methods* 1987;105(2):221–227.

34. Thorpe R, Perry MJ, Callus M, Gaffney PJ, Spitz M. Single shot intrasplenic immunization: an advantageous procedure for production of monoclonal antibodies specific for human fibrin fragments. *Hybridoma* 1984;3(4):381–385.

35. Erlanger BF. The preparation of antigenic hapten-carrier conjugates: a survey. *Methods Enzymol* 1980;70(A):85–104.

36. Harris JR, Markl J. Keyhole limpet hemocyanin (KLH): a biomedical review. *Micron* 1999;30(6):597–623.

37. Harris JR, Markl J. Keyhole limpet hemocyanin: molecular structure of a potent marine immunoactivator. A review. *Eur Urol* 2000;37(Suppl 3):24–33.

38. Kerr DE, Garrigues US, Wallace PM, Hellstrom KE, Hellstrom I, Senter PD. Application of monoclonal antibodies against cytosine deaminase for the *in vivo* clearance of a cytosine deaminase immunoconjugate. *Bioconjug Chem* 1993;4(5):353–357.

39. Littlefield JW, Gould EA. The toxic effect of 5-bromodeoxyuridine on cultured epithelial cells. *J Biol Chem* 1960;235:1129–1133.

40. Coligan JE, Kruisbeek AM, Margulies DH, Shevach EM, Strober W. *Current Protocols in Immunology*. New York: Greene Publishing/Wiley-Interscience; 1992.

41. Bjorck L, Kronvall G. Purification and some properties of streptococcal protein G, a novel IgG-binding reagent. *J Immunol* 1984;133(2):969–974.

42. Forsgren A, Sjoquist J. "Protein A" from *S. aureus*. I. Pseudo-immune reaction with human gamma-globulin. *J Immunol* 1966;97(6):822–827.

43. Kastern W, Sjobring U, Bjorck L. Structure of peptostreptococcal protein L and identification of a repeated immunoglobulin light chain-binding domain. *J Biol Chem* 1992;267(18):12820–12825.

44. Husereau DR, Suresh MR. A general affinity method to purify peroxidase-tagged antibodies. *J Immunol Methods* 2001;249(1–2):33–41.

45. Xu D, Leveugle B, Kreutz FT, Suresh MR. Mimetic ligand-based affinity purification of immune complexes and immunoconjugates. *J Chromatogr B Biomed Sci Appl* 1998;706(2):217–229.

46. Alpaugh K, Von Mehren M. Monoclonal antibodies in cancer treatment: a review of recent progress. *Biodrugs* 1999;12(3):209–236.

47. Batra JK, FitzGerald D, Gately M, Chaudhary VK, Pastan I. Anti-Tac(Fv)-PE40, a single chain antibody *Pseudomonas* fusion protein directed at interleukin 2 receptor bearing cells. *J Biol Chem* 1990;265(25):15198–15202.

48. Cheng JD, Rieger PT, von Mehren M, Adams GP, Weiner LM. Recent advances in immunotherapy and monoclonal antibody treatment of cancer. *Semin Oncol Nurs* 2000;16(4 Suppl 1):2–12.

49. Suresh MR. *Handbook of Immunoassay: Cancer Markers*, 2nd ed. Nature Publishing Group, UK; 2005, pp 635–663.

50. Carter PJ. Potent antibody therapeutics by design. *Nat Rev Immunol* 2006;6(5):343–357.

51. Pavlou AK, Belsey MJ. The therapeutic antibodies market to 2008. *Eur J Pharm Biopharm* 2005;59(3):389–396.

52. Brekke OH, Sandlie I. Therapeutic antibodies for human diseases at the dawn of the twenty-first century. *Nat Rev Drug Discov* 2003;2(1):52–62.

53. Mirick GR, Bradt BM, Denardo SJ, Denardo GL. A review of human anti-globulin antibody (HAGA, HAMA, HACA, HAHA) responses to monoclonal antibodies. Not four letter words. *Q J Nucl Med Mol Imaging* 2004;48(4):251–257.

54. Morrison SL, Johnson MJ, Herzenberg LA, Oi VT. Chimeric human antibody molecules: mouse antigen-binding domains with human constant region domains. *Proc Natl Acad Sci USA* 1984;81(21):6851–6855.

55. Hanauer SB. Review article: safety of infliximab in clinical trials. *Aliment Pharmacol Ther* 1999;13 (Suppl 4):16–22; discussion 38.

56. Jones PT, Dear PH, Foote J, Neuberger MS, Winter G. Replacing the complementarity-determining regions in a human antibody with those from a mouse. *Nature* 1986; 321(6069):522–525.

57. Presta LG. Engineering of therapeutic antibodies to minimize immunogenicity and optimize function. *Adv Drug Deliv Rev* 2006;58(5–6):640–656.

58. Amin T, Carter G. Immunogenicity issues with therapeutic proteins. *Curr Drug Discov* 2004;20–24.

59. Trikha M, Yan L, Nakada MT. Monoclonal antibodies as therapeutics in oncology. *Curr Opin Biotechnol* 2002;13(6):609–614.

60. Li J, Sai T, Berger M, Chao Q, Davidson D, Deshmukh G, Drozdowski B, Ebel W, Harley S, Henry M, Jacob S, Kline B, Lazo E, Rotella F, Routhier E, Rudolph K, Sage J, Simon P, Yao J, Zhou Y, Kavuru M, Bonfield T, Thomassen MJ, Sass PM, Nicolaides NC, Grasso L. Human antibodies for immunotherapy development generated via a human B cell hybridoma technology. *Proc Natl Acad Sci USA* 2006;103(10):3557–3562.

61. Nisonoff A, Rivers MM. Recombination of a mixture of univalent antibody fragments of different specificity. *Arch Biochem Biophys* 1961;93:460–462.

62. Cao Y, Suresh MR. Bispecific antibodies as novel bioconjugates. *Bioconjug Chem* 1998;9(6):635–644.

63. Merchant AM, Zhu Z, Yuan JQ, Goddard A, Adams CW, Presta LG, Carter P. An efficient route to human bispecific IgG. *Nat Biotechnol* 1998;16(7):677–681.

64. Cao Y, Lam L. Applications of bispecific antibodies in therapeutics. *Drugs Future* 2002;27(1):33–41.

65. Cao Y, Lam L. Bispecific antibody conjugates in therapeutics. *Adv Drug Deliv Rev* 2003;55(2):171–197.

66. Kontermann RE. Recombinant bispecific antibodies for cancer therapy. *Acta Pharmacol Sin* 2005;26(1):1–9.

67. Segal DM, Weiner GJ, Weiner LM. Bispecific antibodies in cancer therapy. *Curr Opin Immunol* 1999;11(5):558–562.

68. Carter P. Bispecific human IgG by design. *J Immunol Methods* 2001;248(1–2):7–15.

69. Griffiths AD, Duncan AR. Strategies for selection of antibodies by phage display. *Curr Opin Biotechnol* 1998;9(1):102–108.

70. Hill HR, Stockley PG. Phage presentation. *Mol Microbiol* 1996;20(4):685–692.

71. McGregor D. Selection of proteins and peptides from libraries displayed on filamentous bacteriophage. *Mol Biotechnol* 1996;6(2):155–162.

72. Rader C, Barbas CF 3rd. Phage display of combinatorial antibody libraries. *Curr Opin Biotechnol* 1997;8(4):503–508.

73. Winter G, Griffiths AD, Hawkins RE, Hoogenboom HR. Making antibodies by phage display technology. *Annu Rev Immunol* 1994;12:433–455.

74. Gram H, Marconi LA, Barbas CF 3rd, Collet TA, Lerner RA, Kang AS. *In vitro* selection and affinity maturation of antibodies from a naive combinatorial immunoglobulin library. *Proc Natl Acad Sci USA* 1992;89(8):3576–3580.

75. Nissim A, Hoogenboom HR, Tomlinson IM, Flynn G, Midgley C, Lane D, Winter G. Antibody fragments from a "single pot" phage display library as immunochemical reagents. *EMBO J* 1994;13(3):692–698.

76. Boder ET, Wittrup KD. Yeast surface display for screening combinatorial polypeptide libraries. *Nat Biotechnol* 1997;15(6):553–557.

77. Boder ET, Wittrup KD. Optimal screening of surface-displayed polypeptide libraries. *Biotechnol Prog* 1998;14(1):55–62.

78. Boder ET, Wittrup KD. Yeast surface display for directed evolution of protein expression, affinity, and stability. *Methods Enzymol* 2000;328:430–444.

79. Feldhaus MJ, Siegel RW. Yeast display of antibody fragments: a discovery and characterization platform. *J Immunol Methods* 2004;290(1–2):69–80.

80. Kondo A, Ueda M. Yeast cell-surface display—applications of molecular display. *Appl Microbiol Biotechnol* 2004;64(1):28–40.

81. Lipovsek D, Pluckthun A. *In-vitro* protein evolution by ribosome display and mRNA display. *J Immunol Methods* 2004;290(1–2):51–67.

82. Zahnd C, Amstutz P, Pluckthun A. Ribosome display: selecting and evolving proteins *in vitro* that specifically bind to a target. *Nat Methods* 2007;4(3):269–279.

83. Nemoto N, Miyamoto-Sato E, Husimi Y, Yanagawa H. *In vitro* virus: bonding of mRNA bearing puromycin at the 3′-terminal end to the C-terminal end of its encoded protein on the ribosome *in vitro*. *FEBS Lett* 1997;414(2):405–408.

84. Roberts RW. Totally *in vitro* protein selection using mRNA–protein fusions and ribosome display. *Curr Opin Chem Biol* 1999;3(3):268–273.

85. Roberts RW, Szostak JW. RNA–peptide fusions for the *in vitro* selection of peptides and proteins. *Proc Natl Acad Sci USA* 1997;94(23):12297–12302.

86. Kim SJ, Kim NS, Ryu CJ, Hong HJ, Lee GM. Characterization of chimeric antibody producing CHO cells in the course of dihydrofolate reductase-mediated gene amplification and their stability in the absence of selective pressure. *Biotechnol Bioeng* 1998; 58(1):73–84.

87. Gu X, Wang DI. Improvement of interferon-gamma sialylation in Chinese hamster ovary cell culture by feeding of *N*-acetylmannosamine. *Biotechnol Bioeng* 1998;58(6):642–648.

88. Pendse GJ, Karkare S, Bailey JE. Effect of cloned gene dosage on cell growth and hepatitis B surface antigen synthesis and secretion in recombinant CHO cells. *Biotechnol Bioeng* 1992;40(1):119–129.

89. Van Hove JL, Yang HW, Wu JY, Brady RO, Chen YT. High-level production of recombinant human lysosomal acid alpha-glucosidase in Chinese hamster ovary cells which

targets to heart muscle and corrects glycogen accumulation in fibroblasts from patients with Pompe disease. *Proc Natl Acad Sci USA* 1996;93(1):65–70.

90. Page MJ, Sydenham MA. High level expression of the humanized monoclonal antibody Campath-1H in Chinese hamster ovary cells. *Biotechnology* (*NY*) 1991;9(1):64–68.

91. Blochberger TC, Cooper C, Peretz D, Tatzelt J, Griffith OH, Baldwin MA, Prusiner SB. Prion protein expression in Chinese hamster ovary cells using a glutamine synthetase selection and amplification system. *Protein Eng* 1997;10(12):1465–1473.

92. Brown ME, Renner G, Field RP, Hassell T. Process development for the production of recombinant antibodies using the glutamine synthetase (GS) system. *Cytotechnology* 1992;9(1–3):231–236.

93. Cockett MI, Bebbington CR, Yarranton GT. High level expression of tissue inhibitor of metalloproteinases in Chinese hamster ovary cells using glutamine synthetase gene amplification. *Biotechnology* (*NY*) 1990;8(7):662–667.

94. Shapiro AM, Lakey JR, Ryan EA, Korbutt GS, Toth E, Warnock GL, Kneteman NM, Rajotte RV. Islet transplantation in seven patients with type 1 diabetes mellitus using a glucocorticoid-free immunosuppressive regimen. *N Engl J Med* 2000;343(4):230–238.

95. Shapiro AM, Ricordi C, Hering BJ, Auchincloss H, Lindblad R, Robertson RP, Secchi A, Brendel MD, Berney T, Brennan DC, Cagliero E, Alejandro R, Ryan EA, DiMercurio B, Morel P, Polonsky KS, Reems JA, Bretzel RG, Bertuzzi F, Froud T, Kandaswamy R, Sutherland DE, Eisenbarth G, Segal M, Preiksaitis J, Korbutt GS, Barton FB, Viviano L, Seyfert-Margolis V, Bluestone J, Lakey JR. International trial of the Edmonton protocol for islet transplantation. *N Engl J Med* 2006;355(13):1318–1330.

96. Shapiro AM, Ryan EA, Lakey JR. Clinical islet transplant—state of the art. *Transplant Proc* 2001;33(7–8):3502–3503.

97. Shapiro AM, Ryan EA, Lakey JR. Pancreatic islet transplantation in the treatment of diabetes mellitus. *Best Pract Res Clin Endocrinol Metab* 2001;15(2):241–264.

21

THE PHARMACOGENOMICS OF PERSONALIZED MEDICINE

Ronald E. Reid

University of British Columbia, Vancouver, British Columbia, Canada

Contents

21.1 INTRODUCTION

According to the European Agency for Evaluation of Medicinal Products (EMEA, http://www.emea.eu.int/), *pharmacogenetics* is defined as "the study of inter-individual variations in DNA sequence related to drug response." This definition emphasizes the studies on allelic variation of metabolic enzymes involved in drug metabolism and points to the early successes in correlating the alterations in drug metabolism with variations in the genes responsible for production of the metabolic enzymes.

A first indication of the individuality of disease biochemistry appeared in an article by A. E. Garrod in 1902 in which he described the high concentrations of homogentisic acid in the urine of those patients suffering from alkaptonuria. Garrod believed this could arise from a congenital defect in a particular enzyme at some stage in the metabolism of the amino acids tyrosine and phenylalanine [1]. Garrod also suggested that drug idiosyncracies might also be attributed to inherited differences, thus setting the stage for the scientific investigation of gene–drug interactions.

Some 50 years later A. Forbat, the Anaesthetic Registrar at St. James Hospital in London, reported an incident where a patient undergoing surgery was treated with the muscle relaxant succinyldicholine and showed "no sign of returning respiration at the conclusion of the operation." He concluded that the patient's sensitivity to succinyldicholine was due to a lowered pseudocholinesterase level and he suggested that "further cases of sensitivity to succinyldicholine should be published, and if a low pseudocholinesterase level is found which cannot be explained by disease, malnutrition, or poisoning, their families should be investigated for a hereditary or racial basis of abnormally low pseudocholinesterase level" [2]. Subsequent studies confirmed this conclusion [3–5] and publications on similar "familial" related abnormal responses to primaquine therapy of malaria [6] and isoniazid therapy of tuberculosis [5] established the gene–drug interaction in disease therapy. R. J. Williams's book on biochemical individuality [7] and the introduction of the term "pharmacogenetics" in papers by A. Motulsky [8] and F. Vogel [9], describing genetically determined variability in the effects of drugs on animal species, initiated a philosophy of genetic biomarkers that would be valuable in decisions on specific drug therapies based on the genetic makeup of the individual patient.

Watson and Crick's seminal paper on the structure of deoxyribonucleic acid (DNA) [10] led to a plethora of research into the structure of DNA and the mechanisms by which information was stored and transmitted. Eventually, the analysis of genes and gene products led to the principles that one gene produces one protein. It also led to the principle that the genetic code links the sequence of bases in DNA to the sequence of amino acids in proteins and hence to the structure of proteins which is instrumental in determining protein function. The "Central Dogma" propounded the directional nature of the flow of information in the genome from DNA to messenger RNA to proteins and it became obvious that informational errors in DNA in the form of mutations would show up in the structure of proteins and ultimately the function of these proteins in the cell. Therefore, it appears logical that the normal or abnormal structure of proteins is related to the normal or abnormal function of a cell, which in turn is related to the normal or diseased function of an organism.

The Human Genome Project has demonstrated that the genome sequence is 99.9% identical in all humans. The remaining 0.1% genetic variation provides the basis upon which individuals differ in physical characteristics, susceptibility to disease, and response to drug therapy. Genetic variations or mutations can occur in coding or noncoding regions of the genome. The coding region variations (Fig. 21.1) include (1) *silent mutations* that produce no change in the amino acid sequence of the expressed protein; (2) *conservative missense mutations* that result in a codon specifying an amino acid with a side chain that has similar physicochemical properties to the amino acid that appears in the normal (*wild-type*) sequence; (3) *noncon-*

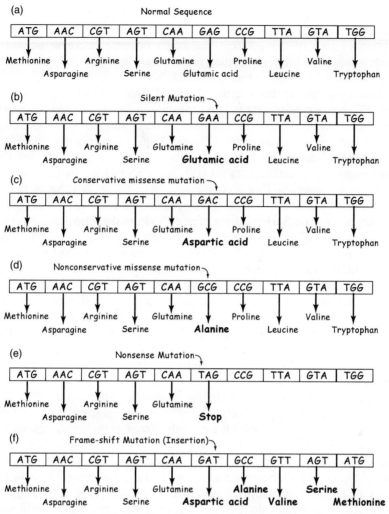

FIGURE 21.1 The effects of different types of single nucleotide polymorphisms: (a) the normal genomic DNA sequence and the protein sequence encoded; (b) a silent mutation; (c) a conservative missense mutation where glutamic acid is replaced by aspartic acid through an A/G mutation but both amino acids are acidic residues; (d) a nonconservative missense mutation where glutamic acid (an acidic residue) is replaced by alanine (a hydrophobic residue) through an A/C mutation; (e) a missense mutation where a G/T mutation results in a stop codon, thus truncating the protein; (f) an insertion of a T between the A and G of the GAG glutamic acid codon, thus shifting the reading frame so that all amino acids downstream (including the glutamic acid) are changed. (Adapted from Ref. 11.)

servative missense mutations that result in a codon specifying an amino acid with a side chain that has distinctly different physicochemical properties to the wild-type amino acid; (4) *nonsense mutations* that result in a stop codon leading to truncation of the protein; and (5) *frame-shift mutations*, where the addition or deletion of a number of bases that are not a multiple of three (in this example, one base) causes a shift in the reading frame of the gene, thus changing the amino acid sequence of the protein from the point of insertion onwards, and usually creates a stop codon somewhere in the sequence. Noncoding variations usually occur in the 5'- or 3'-untranslated regions of the genome, causing a possible decrease or increase in expression levels, or in other noncoding regions such as the introns where alternate splice junctions could alter the final protein.

The common forms of "informational errors" found in the human genome are (1) indels, (2) microsatellites or tandem repeats, and (3) single nucleotide polymorphisms. *Single nucleotide polymorphisms* (SNPs), defined as single base pair positions in genomic DNA at which different sequence alternatives (alleles) exist wherein the least frequent allele has an abundance of 1% or greater, are the most commonly occurring genetic variations [12]. These SNPs have two important applications in genome research. First, a polymorphism by nature is a change in the DNA that might alter amino acid coding, gene splicing, or gene expression and hence directly alter phenotype. Second, the nature of SNPs makes them powerful markers for the variants that affect phenotype (see Section 21.2, HapMap discussion).

The Human Genome Project (HGP) was built on the potential for the application of genetic information to the human condition that would go a long way to opening up the black boxes of disease diagnosis and therapy. Completion of the HGP [13] has changed the focus of genomic research from that of gene identification to that of examining gene structure and function. The relation of gene function and functional variation to disease and drug action and the application of this relationship to disease diagnosis (*D*X) and therapy (*R*X) at the molecular level is the major medical related outcome expected from the billions of dollars spent on sequencing the human genome.

Current pharmacogenetic research has established the importance of genetic information in drug therapy involving the genes expressing drug metabolizing enzymes in the liver. It is now well established that genetic differences between individuals can explain some of the variability seen in the pharmacokinetics of drug therapy, which in turn alters the efficacy and toxicity of certain drugs [14]. Many of these variations are highly penetrant, single gene traits involving the phase I (oxidation) and phase II (conjugation) metabolic enzymes [15] (*penetrance* is the frequency with which individuals who carry a given gene variant will show the manifestations associated with that variant; if penetrance of an allele is 100% then all individuals carrying that allele will express the associated disorder).

In principle, one is able to manipulate the therapeutic outcome of a patient population by separating the patients who will not respond normally to a particular drug therapy from those who will, based on an analysis of established genetic biomarkers related to the drug's metabolic profile (Fig. 21.2). The patients homozygous for the genetic biomarkers associated with poor metabolism of the recommended therapeutic agent may, depending on the therapeutic window of the drug, exhibit a response resembling an overdose to the "normal" drug dose. These individuals will require a reduced dose to achieve therapeutic levels (see Patient A in Fig. 21.3). Meanwhile those patients carrying biomarkers associated with extensive metabolism may exhibit a lack of efficacy at "normal" doses and therefore would require an increased dose of the drug to achieve therapeutic activity (see Patient D in Fig. 21.3). The patients who are homozygous or heterozygous for the normal (wild-type) genetic biomarker (see Patients B and C, respectively, in Fig. 21.3) may require no alteration of the "normal" dose of the drug for adequate therapeutic outcome.

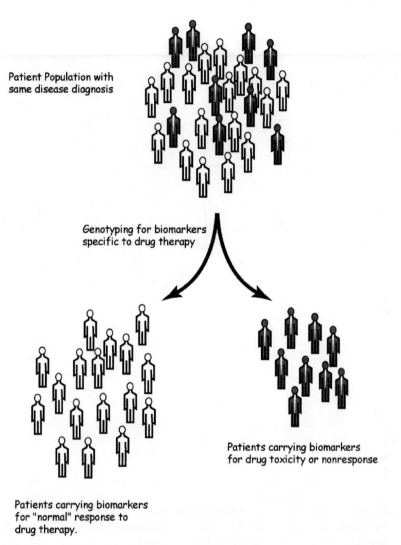

Patient Population with
same disease diagnosis

Genotyping for biomarkers
specific to drug therapy

Patients carrying biomarkers
for drug toxicity or nonresponse

Patients carrying biomarkers
for "normal" response to
drug therapy.

FIGURE 21.2 Manipulating therapeutic outcomes through pharmacogenetic analysis of a population with the same disease diagnosis to eliminate those patients with genetic biomarkers indicating an adverse response to a particular drug therapy.

Documented success in correlating the therapeutic activity of a number of drugs with allelic differences in the genes for such common metabolic enzymes as cytochrome P450 2D6 (CYP2D6), CYP2C19, CYP2C9, thiopurine methyltransferase (TPMT), and *N*-acetyltransferase type 2 (NAT2) (Fig. 21.4) has led to the appearance of pharmacogenetic information on drug labels for aripiprazole, atomoxetin, and celecoxib. The U.S. Food and Drug Administration (USFDA) has set up guidelines for the drug industry to submit voluntary pharmacogenetic data on drugs for which they are seeking approval (http://www.fda.gov/cber/gdlns/pharmdtasub.pdf). In response, a number of companies have developed instrumentation and assays for pharmacogenetic tests, including the analytical instrument division of Roche, which

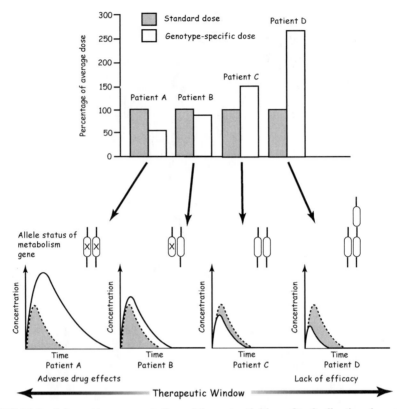

FIGURE 21.3   Schematic representation of the potential benefit of adjusting dose to geno-type. The dashed line in the concentration–time curves for Patients A–D is the theoretical "normal" drug concentration–time curve, while the solid line is the theoretical "genetic" drug concentration–time curve for each patient. The allele status for each patient is shown above the theoretical plots. The oval containing the X indicates the presence of the detrimental allelic variation. The extra oval in Patient D indicates a duplication of one of the normal alleles. The top bar graph indicates the normal doses (shaded) compared to the dose adjustments that should be made based on the patient's allele status. (Adapted from Ref. 16 with permission of the author and Nature Publishing Group.)

is marketing a gene chip for the analysis of CYP2D6 genetic polymorphisms; Applied Biosystems, which has developed a TaqMan™ assay targeting 220 genes in phase I and II metabolic enzymes and drug transport proteins; and Third Wave, which has recently received FDA clearance for *in vitro* diagnostic testing of UGT1A1 polymorphisms using their Invader™ assay. Finally, it has been proposed that drug dosing adjustments based on genotype could be beneficial if the pharmacokinetic differences in the genetic variants fall outside the acceptable range for stating bioequivalence (*bioequivalence* of two formulations of a given drug occurs if the area under the curve, maximum blood concentrations, and times of maximum blood concentrations differ by no more than 80–125%), unless sufficiently powerful studies can show that the pharmacokinetic differences do not affect the clinical outcome [17].

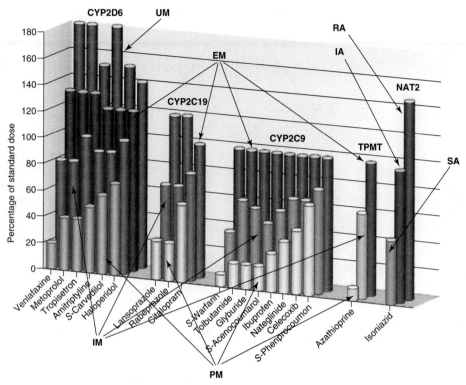

FIGURE 21.4 Examples of dose adjustments based on pharmacogenetic information. The influence of genetic polymorphisms in CYP2D6, CYP2C19, CYP2C9, TPMT, and NAT2 is expressed as subpopulation-specific dosages, according to the difference in pharmacokinetic parameters from clinical studies. Substantial adjustments need to be made to the drug dose to achieve the same level of drug exposure in individuals with different genotypes. EM, extensive metabolizer; IA, intermediate acetylator; IM, intermediate metabolizer; PM, poor metabolizer; RA, rapid acetylator; SA, slow acetylator; UM, ultrarapid metabolizer. (From Ref. 17 with permission of the author and Nature Publishing Group.)

21.2 PHARMACOGENOMICS

The failure of pharmacogenetics to make major inroads in clinical applications has led many to question whether or not pharmacogenetics is more a product of hype than science. In spite of the success of the single gene approach (Fig. 21.5) in correlating the genotype of some drug metabolic enzymes with the dose of drug necessary for effective therapeutic activity, it is a rare occasion that a discrete biological activity such as drug response can be attributed to an individual molecule such as a metabolic enzyme.

Drug action is a reflection of the multifactorial polygenic pharmacokinetic and pharmacodynamic parameters of the drug (Fig. 21.6). The pharmacokinetic parameters determine the eventual distribution of the drug in the body including the concentration of the drug at the site of pharmacodynamic action. The enzyme action of drug metabolism has already been discussed and is the cornerstone of pharmacogenetics. Other pharmacokinetic parameters include drug absorption,

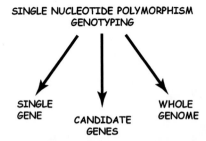

FIGURE 21.5   Approaches to genotyping for drug therapy. The single gene approach has been used successfully in pharmacogenetic studies of a number of phase I and II metabolic enzymes. The candidate gene approach involves the selection of the genes for proteins that are demonstrated to be involved in a particular drug action including metabolic enzymes, transport proteins, drug targets, and proteins involved in modular drug response pathways. The whole genome approach utilizes single nucleotide polymorphisms throughout the genome.

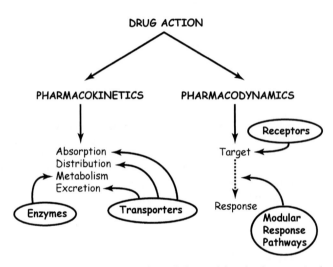

FIGURE 21.6   Schematic representation of the multigenic *therapeutic drug pathway*.

distribution, and excretion, all of which may be affected by transport proteins to some extent.

The pharmacodynamics of drug action is a description of the effect of the drug on the body and is a result of complex interactions involving drug targets and the subsequent biochemical reactions, which eventually produce a biological response. The modular nature of biochemical systems lends itself to application in the drug response mechanism in that it is possible to describe the response of many drug–target interactions through linked modules of biochemical systems. The genes involved in drug metabolism, drug transport, and drug responses are considered the *candidate genes* for the therapeutic drug pathway.

The suggestion of genome-wide searches for gene effects using large scale testing of single nucleotide polymorphisms (SNPs) has led to considerable discussion of the efficiency of different approaches [18]. The candidate gene approach [19] suggested a study of coding and/or promoter variants with potential functional significance in disease diagnosis and drug therapy. The whole genome approach [20] suggested that a high density of coding and noncoding SNPs evenly spaced throughout the genome could be used to determine optimal drug therapy. The use of *linkage disequilibrium* (LD; the observation that two or more alleles, usually at loci that are physically close together on a chromosome, are not inherited independently but are observed to occur together more frequently than predicted under Mendel's Law of Independent Assortment) to map SNP loci that may be relevant to disease therapy found that the extent of LD in different parts of the genome is highly variable and those fragments of the genome that appear to be inherited in blocks, indicating a high degree of LD, are known as *haplotype blocks* [21, 22]. Investigations into this haplotype diversity have culminated in the HapMap Project (www.hapmap.org), which will map all haplotype blocks in the human genome and validate the map in four populations: the Yoruba in Nigeria; the Han Chinese in Beijing, China; the Japanese in Tokyo, Japan; and residents in Utah, USA with ancestry from northern and central Europe [23]. It has been demonstrated that, while a haplotype block may contain several hundred SNPs, only a few of the SNPs in a given haplotype block are needed to identify that particular block. These SNPs are known as *haplotype tag SNPs (htSNPs)* and tend to capture most of the variation of a particular region of the genome [24, 25]. This concept of htSNPs has been further extended in the pharmacogenetics of candidate genes such that the number of SNPs needed to characterize a therapeutic drug pathway is reduced by limiting the htSNP variations to those SNPs in genes involved in the therapeutic drug pathway [26–30].

Although recent studies indicate that LD is structured into discrete blocks in the human genome [21, 31, 32], the range and distribution of LD in different populations is largely unknown. Furthermore, the effect of genotype on disease phenotype varies between disorders and populations owing to genetic and environmental heterogeneity [33]. For these reasons, it is difficult to estimate the number of SNPs or the number of samples that would be required for a successful genome-wide LD study. The estimates that have been made vary widely, from 1 million [34] or 0.5 million [35] to as little as 30,000 SNPs [36]. If 0.5 million SNPs were to be analyzed in, for example, 1000 individuals, and if the project was to be carried out in a year, then approximately 1.5 million SNP genotypes per day would need to be produced. At genotyping costs as low as 10 cents per SNP, this example project would cost $50 million (U.S.).

The individual's genotype is only part of the equation for predicting individual drug response and other factors play a contributory role in the individual's response to drug therapy. If one takes the complexity of disease diagnosis, the environment, and drug therapy into consideration, a new definition of the pharmacogenetics concept is required (Fig. 21.7).

Since *genomics* is defined as a study of the full complement of genetic information both coding and noncoding in an organism (genome), this holistic view of pharmacogenetics is termed *pharmacogenomics*, which is defined as the application of information from the human genome, transcriptome, proteome, metabolome, and envirome to drug design, discovery, and clinical development, reflecting the state of

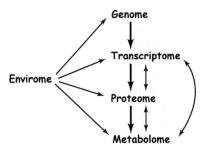

FIGURE 21.7   A schematic representation of the biological organization of the "-omes" describing an individual phenotype. The classical view of biological organization is to consider the flow of information from the genome to the transcriptome, to the proteome and then the metabolome (heavy arrows). However, each tier of the organization depends on the other, so a perturbation in one network can affect another (bidirectional light arrows). Furthermore, the environment has a crucial impact on not only expression and concentrations of transcripts, proteins, and metabolites, but also on the genome by selecting from adaptive changes in subpopulations of cells (light unidirectional arrows). Metabolomics can potentially probe much more than classical metabolism and metabolic disorders: it can also be used to monitor changes in the genome or to measure the effects of downregulation or upregulation of a specific gene transcript. (Adapted from Ref. 37 with permission of Nature Publishing Group.)

drug responses at cellular, tissue, individual, or population levels. Pharmacogenomics is a specialized branch of functional genomics reflecting the application of structural genomics to drug therapy. In this context, *structural genomics* is defined as the construction of high resolution genetic, physical, and transcript maps of an organism [38] and *functional genomics* refers to the development and application of global (genome-wide or system-wide) experimental approaches to assess gene function by making use of the information and reagents provided by structural genomics. Functional genomics is characterized by high throughput or large scale experimental methodologies combined with statistical and computational analysis of the results. The fundamental strategy in a functional genomics approach is to expand the scope of biological investigation from studying single genes, proteins, or metabolites to studying all genes, proteins, or metabolites at once in a systematic fashion [38]. Pharmacogenomics, then, aims to study all genes, proteins, and metabolites relevant to drug therapy and its successful outcome.

21.3   PERSONALIZED MEDICINE

Evidence-based medicine is predicated on a standardized application of the scientific principles of unbiased observation and experiment to disease diagnosis and drug therapy. The techniques involved are derived from randomized and double-blind clinical trials and are inconsistent with the treatment of an individual patient [39]. The application of statistical information derived from clinical trials on large populations results in a standard dose range for the population, which either overdoses or underdoses a small but significant portion of that population. The failure to recognize patients as individuals is likely a factor in adverse drug and toxic drug–drug interactions that account for 100,000 patient deaths, 2 million hospitalizations, and $100 billion in health care costs in the United States yearly [40–43].

With the completion of the Human Genome Project, there has been as shift in research from gene identification to the study of gene structure and function [44]. The early successes in the application of genetic information to disease diagnosis and the estimation of drug efficacy and toxicity have evolved into the concept of *personalized medicine*. This is defined as the utilization of molecular biomarkers from an individual's genome, transcriptome, proteome, and metabolome under the influence of the envirome in the assessment of that individual's health and treatment choices. This includes the predisposition to disease, screening and early diagnosis of disease, assessment of prognosis, pharmacogenomic prediction of therapeutic drug efficacy and risk of toxicity, and monitoring the illness until the final therapeutic outcome is determined (Fig. 21.8) [39, 43, 45–49].

A *biomarker* is defined as a characteristic that is objectively measured and evaluated as an indicator of normal biologic processes, pathogenic processes, or pharmacologic responses to a therapeutic intervention [50]. A *molecular biomarker* is defined as a specific subset of small molecule (metabolite) or large molecule (protein or DNA) biomarkers that may be discovered using genomic or proteomic technologies as opposed to *clinical biomarkers* arising from imaging technologies [51]. The U.S. Food and Drug Administration elaborates on a *valid biomarker* as a biomarker that is measured in an analytical test system with well-established performance characteristics and for which there is an established scientific framework or body of evidence that elucidates the physiologic, toxicologic, pharmacologic, or clinical significance of the test results [52].

Molecular profiling (the application of genomic, transcriptomic, proteomic, and metabolomic technologies to the development of *in vitro* molecular biomarkers) of

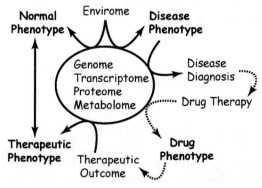

FIGURE 21.8 Schematic representation of the concept of molecular profiling for personalized medicine. The dashed arrows indicate the critical components of pharmacogenomics: disease diagnosis, drug therapy, drug phenotype, and therapeutic outcome.

a patient's phenotype (Fig. 21.8) utilizes molecular biomarkers of the genome, transcriptome, proteome, and metabolome to provide a molecular basis for the normal or healthy patient phenotype in a particular envirome and thereby provides many opportunities for improving the choice of therapy and the prediction of drug response as well as disease pathology [53]. Alteration of molecular biomarkers in the diseased state compared to the normal state (characterized by the normal molecular phenotype) provides a molecular characterization of the disease phenotype, which is utilized in the diagnosis. The disease phenotype is then utilized to choose the best drug therapy, which will alter the molecular biomarkers to a drug therapy phenotype (Fig. 21.8). The difference between the biomarkers used in the diagnosis and drug phenotype descriptions will be the result of drug therapy. The molecular biomarkers present at assessment of the therapeutic outcome will provide a therapeutic phenotype for that particular drug profile.

In principle, if a drug therapy has been successful in restoring the patient's phenotype to normal, the diagnostic biomarkers for the disease that appear in the drug phenotype, therapeutic phenotype, and normal phenotype should be similar. Attainment of this ideal outcome is heavily dependent on the disease diagnosis, patient biomarker variance, and therapeutic outcome assessment. It is suggested here that the failure of many pharmacogenomic-based therapies is likely the result of inconsistencies in the disease diagnosis and/or assessment of therapeutic outcomes through a lack of sufficient molecular biomarkers or lack of proper interpretation of the biomarkers.

Finally, the interplay between complex genetic factors and the equally complex environmental factors (envirome) is an important yet poorly understood area of research in pharmacogenomics. The genetic regulation of metabolic pathways is also complicated by the fact that they are polygenic or oligogenic, with many different genes interacting in the regulatory process. These genes may also exhibit allelic heterogeneity with many different predisposing risk alleles. Different individuals may also exhibit locus heterogeneity with different or overlapping sets of genes being important in a particular pathway, which is additionally complicated if the gene interactions are additive, synergistic, or epistatic. A further complication arises with individuals when resulting pathologies are qualitative rather than all or nothing traits, with thresholds determining clinical manifestations. It is quite obvious that the application of personalized medicine in the health care environment will require extensive education and training of health care professionals as well as politicians and the public in general.

Walter Fierz has developed the concept of personalized medicine through six dimensions, which I have listed and taken liberty with in my presentation (Fig. 21.8) [39].

1. *Genome, Transcriptome, Proteome, and Metabolome.* An individual is characterized by a *phenotype*, which is defined as the observable characteristics of an organism, either in total or with respect to one or more particular named characteristics and the phenotype is a manifestation of gene expression in that organism under the influence of the environmental conditions [54]. The observable characteristics of an organism are a product of the molecular state of the individual's genome, transcriptome, proteome, and metabolome in the envirome. The application of molecular biomarkers and molecular profiling of an individual's genome through

SNP analysis and htSNP determination; an individual's transcriptome through mRNA microarray analysis, an individual's proteome through microcharacterization, differential display, and protein–protein interactions; and an individual's metabolome through metabolite profiling provides an accurate molecular description of the individual's phenotype (either normal or diseased), the preferred drug therapy, or therapeutic outcome.

2. *Envirome.* The transcriptome, proteome, and metabolome are a direct result of genome expression; however, modifications to these components and to the genome occur as a result of effects from the individual's environment. It is assumed here that a complete description of the effects of the envirome on the genome, transcriptome, proteome, and metabolome through molecular biomarker assessment, as far as technology will allow, is then a description of the individual's molecular phenotype from which all other higher order characteristics such as disease diagnosis and therapeutic outcomes are derived. The envirome includes the individual's geographical location, lifestyle, and the total ensemble of environments, both current and in earlier life, that may affect the occurrence of disease and drug therapy. This includes predisposing risk factors like type of neighborhood, family income, intrauterine exposure to teratogens such as maternal cocaine misuse, and exposure to radiation, and provoking environmental factors that can act as triggers of various disorders, such as crises in personal relationships and social stressors [55]. The consistently accurate assessment of such diverse factors is a true challenge to the success of pharmacogenomics and personalized medicine.

3. *Disease Diagnosis.* Individuals are differentially predisposed and susceptible to disease and disease will progress differently depending on personal factors. The application of molecular markers to the pathology and etiology of disease complicates the already difficult process of accurate disease diagnosis and treatment. The application of laboratory tests to disease diagnosis is not a new concept; however, the application of molecular biomarkers provides a plethora of new tests that must be considered in a description of the pathology and etiology of the disease. Personalized medicine will not be successful without a consistent, accurate application of the information in the genome, transcriptome, proteome, and metabolome to the disease diagnosis.

4. *Medication.* The *therapeutic drug index* (TI) is equal to the effective dose (drug efficacy)/toxic dose (drug toxicity) and is an indicator of the drug's *therapeutic window* (the smaller the TI, the wider the window). Obviously, the ability to robustly predict efficacy and toxicity will go a long way to improving the drug development process in terms of success versus dollars spent. The development of specific, reliable biomarkers that can predict efficacy and toxicity should reduce the time, size, and cost of clinical trials. The identification of biomarkers that predict a response to drug therapy will provide tests for predicting an individual patient's response to a particular drug therapy. The major problem with biomarkers is that their usefulness falls off rapidly with their lack of accessibility. Clinically useful biomarkers should be obtained in the least invasive manner possible [51].

The importance of molecular biomarkers for the selection and dose of therapeutic agent is where we began this chapter. The application of genome biomarkers in the form of SNPs in the genes for metabolic enzymes provides the success that has been attained in pharmacogenetics to date, by predicting the efficacy and toxicity of therapeutic agents (Table 21.1). Pharmacogenomics expands this early approach to include therapeutic drug pathways that are made up of the proteins involved in the pharmacokinetics and pharmacodynamics of drug therapy (Fig. 21.6). Considerable expertise will be required to obtain and apply the information from molecular biomarkers to the choice and delivery of the correct therapeutic agent to the patient at the proper dose at the right time. Assessing the outcome of therapy will also be critical to determining the correct application of molecular biomarkers. Pharmacists, with specialized knowledge and expertise, will be critical participants in the health care arena and the resulting partnership between physicians and pharmacists will create an environment for optimal application of personalized medicine.

5. *Health Care.* The United States Pharmacopoeial Convention held a meeting in 1992 to discuss the future of health care technologies, focusing on the design of an optimal system of health care delivery and what that system might mean to drug standards-setting and drug information development [56]. The participants very perceptively compiled a list of five forces that would be driving health care technology development between 1992 and 2020: (1) globalization, (2) cost containment and outcomes, (3) advanced personalized therapies, (4) advances in information infrastructure, and (5) the predict-and-manage paradigm in health care, all of which are beginning to surface in the development of personalized medicine.

The international effort to complete the Human Genome Project has now led to international efforts to study gene function and will only contribute more to the international harmonization of drug/technology regulation and standards. The cost of tests for molecular biomarkers is at odds with the potential that these tests have to reduce the cost of health care. Yet as technology progresses, these tests will be well within the realm of routine use. The application of genomic data to drug therapy has already emphasized the advance of personalized medicine in this genomic age and this will only become a greater part of health care as the developing technologies force novel approaches to genetic counseling, patient education, evaluating risk profiles, medical decision making, monitoring treatment, privacy and regulatory issues, and patient empowerment [39]. The individual's access to information through home computers and the Internet has already changed the way we shop and entertain ourselves and will also bring tremendous advances in the individual's access to medical information, thus empowering people to take responsibility for their own health care. The advances in biomedical knowledge and information systems will shift the emphasis of health care from the reactive response to illness to the proactive minimization of unnecessary morbidity over an individual's lifetime [56].

6. *Information Management.* The development of information infrastructure capable of managing the genomic, transcriptomic, proteomic, and metabolomic data that will arise through personalized medical therapy as well as managing the environmental influences on each of these groups of data is critical to the success of personalized medicine. Personalized medicine is all about connecting patient-specific information with knowledge-based information [39] and requires a management system that can be readily accessed and interpreted by health care professionals. The success of personalized medicine depends on information management systems (both bioinformatic and healthinformatic) that are rapid and user friendly. This also

TABLE 21.1 Specific Examples of the Application of Allelic Variation in Drug Therapy

Gene	Action	Drug	Therapy	Efficacy/Toxicity
Cytochrome P450 2D6	Drug metabolism	Codeine	Pain	Efficacy
Cytochrome P450 2C9	Drug metabolism	Warfarin	Coagulation	Toxicity (hemorrhage)
Thiopurine S-methyltransferase	Drug metabolism	Mercaptopurine	Acute lymphoblastic leukemia	Toxicity (myelotoxic)
HER2/neu	Drug target	Herceptin	Breast cancer	Efficacy
bcr/abl	Drug target	Gleevec	Chronic myelogenous leukemia	Efficacy
EFGR	Drug target	Erbitux	Colon cancer	Efficacy
Apolipoprotein E-4	Marker	Tacrine	Alzheimer disease	Efficacy
Cholesteryl ester transferase	Marker	Statins	Atherosclerosis	Efficacy
ATP binding cassette B1	Drug transport	Saqinavir, indinavir, ritonavir; daunorubicin, etoposide	HIV; leukemia	Efficacy
UDP-glucuronosyltransferase 1A1	Drug metabolism	Irinotecan	Cancer	Toxicity (myelotoxic)
N-acetyltransferase 2	Drug metabolism	Isoniazid	Tuberculosis	Toxicity (hepatotoxic)
Pseudocholinesterase	Drug metabolism	Suxamethonium	Muscle relaxation during surgery	Toxicity (prolonged apnea)

means the storage and transmission of personal data, which brings ethical, social, and legal issues to bear on health care development.

21.4   MOLECULAR PROFILING TECHNOLOGIES

21.4.1   Genotyping Technologies—Genomics

Genomics [53, 57–60] is defined as the study of the full complement of genetic information, both coding and noncoding, in an organism (genome).

Most genotyping assays currently used to screen for polymorphic variations involve amplification by the polymerase chain reaction (PCR) and specific methods for discriminating and detecting the amplified product. SNP detection can involve either scanning DNA sequences for previously unknown polymorphisms or screening individuals for known polymorphisms. The latter is commonly known as genotyping (Fig. 21.9).

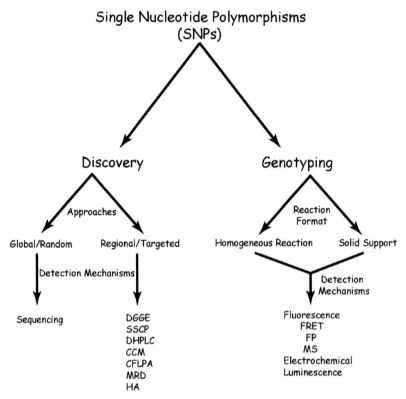

FIGURE 21.9   SNP analysis technologies. DGGE, denaturing gradient gel electrophoresis; SSCP, single strand conformation polymorphism; DHPLC, denaturing high performance chromatography; CCM, chemical cleavage of mismatch; CFLPA, cleavage fragment length polymorphism analysis; MRD, mismatch repair detection; HA, heteroduplex analysis; FRET, fluorescence resonance energy transfer; FP, fluorescence polarization; MS, mass spectrometry.

DNA Scanning for New Polymorphisms   DNA scanning for new polymorphisms is further subcategorized into a global, or random, approach and the regional, or targeted, approach [58]. The random global approach is typified by the variation in restriction enzyme site sequences resulting in restriction fragment length polymorphisms that are detected by Southern blotting. However, whole genome shotgun sequencing was the best technique for global polymorphism detection and discovery [60, 61].

While the global, random approach to SNP discovery seeks high density markers throughout the genome, the targeted, regional approach focuses on identification of all SNPs in particular candidate genes [62, 63]. The technologies developed for the targeted approach exploit the difference between mismatched heteroduplex DNA and the perfectly matched homoduplex DNA and include such techniques as denaturing gradient gel electrophoresis (DGGE), single strand conformation polymorphism (SSCP), and denaturing high performance liquid chromatography (DHPLC). These techniques will detect the presence of sequence variation but will not determine the base change; sequencing of the product is required. These and many other techniques for targeted approach SNP analysis are described in a more specialized article [58].

Genotyping Known SNPs   The application of molecular biomarkers such as single nucleotide polymorphisms toward *in vitro* diagnostic assays is developing into a critical technology in disease therapy [57, 58, 64–66]. These molecular biomarkers will inform physicians about subtypes of disease at the molecular level that require differential treatment. They will provide the pharmacist with information for choice of the best therapeutic methodology for effectively managing the disease and can indicate which individual patients are at the highest risk of experiencing either an adverse reaction or a lack of response to a given drug, thereby identifying those patients likely to respond optimally to a given therapy [53].

Selection of a genotype assay is critical if one is to advance from a preclinical to a clinical setting. The assay must be cheap, high throughput (highly multiplexed), easily and reliably developed from sequence information, robust (specific genotyping of all SNPs under similar reaction conditions), automated, accurate, reproducible, homogeneous (self-contained assay requiring minimal handling for sample analysis), small footprint for the hardware (must easily fit on a lab bench), reliable and easy to use software, and simple (or not complex) in terms of performing the assay (designing primers and probes) as well as interpreting the results.

The general genotyping procedure consists of PCR amplification of the region of interest, allele discrimination, and detection of the discrimination product. Allele discrimination generally falls into one of five techniques illustrated in Fig. 21.10 [57, 58, 64–67]: differential hybridization, allele-specific PCR, oligonucleotide ligation assay (OLA), nuclease cleavage (flap cleavage, 5'-nuclease cleavage, restriction enzyme cleavage), and minisequencing or primer extension. Each detection reaction may be carried out in homogeneous reaction medium, on a solid support, or one may use technology that will carry out the detection reaction in a homogeneous medium and then utilize a solid support to capture the product.

Amplification   Most methods used for genotyping SNPs in large diploid genomes depend on PCR amplification of the genomic regions that span the SNPs before the

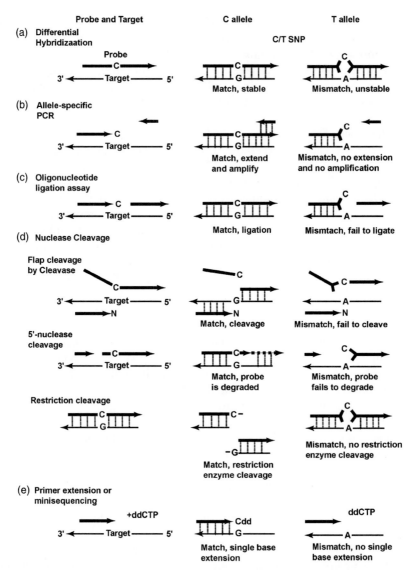

FIGURE 21.10   Allele discrimination strategies for the detection of the C allele of a C/T transition: a summary of the five main biochemical reaction principles that underlie the SNP genotyping technologies. The bold arrows indicate the probes while the thinner arrows indicate the target. (Adapted from Refs. 64 and 66.)

actual genotyping or detection reaction is implemented [68]. The PCR provides the required sensitivity and specificity for distinguishing between heterozygous and homozygous SNP genotypes in large, complex genomes and the difficulties in designing and carrying out multiplex PCR reactions is a critical factor limiting the throughput of the current SNP-genotyping assays [66].

Allele Discrimination   The allele discrimination (Fig. 21.10 and Table 21.2) component of the genotyping technology can be divided into five general categories based on the biochemical reaction principles that underlie the technology: differential hybridization, allele-specific PCR (AS-PCR), the oligonucleotide ligation assay (OLA), the cleavage assays, and the primer extension or minisequencing assay.

1. Differential hybridization using allele-specific oligonucleotides (ASOs) (Fig. 21.10a) was first demonstrated in 1979 [127] and used in 1983 [128] to detect the sickle-cell mutation in the β-globin gene using Southern blot hybridization to genomic DNA. Differential hybridization relies on the differential interaction between the amplified target (amplicon) and a specific labeled oligonucleotide (probe).

The use of ASOs in solution as hybridization probes is considered homogeneous because no purification steps are required and monitoring is done in real time during the amplification process. The most common homogeneous ASO hybridization techniques employ SNP detection in real time during the PCR amplification process in homogeneous solution using fluorescence detection. Applied Biosystems' TaqMan (http://www.appliedbiosystems.com/) and Public Health Research Institute's (PHRI) Molecular Beacons (http://www.molecular-beacons.org/) provide technology for the real-time PCR detection of SNPs. The Molecular Beacon probes have a tendency to adopt a stem–loop structure that destabilizes mismatched hybrids, thereby increasing their power of allele discrimination compared with linear ASO probes [74, 129, 130]. Other techniques for improving the discrimination power of homogeneous reactions include the TaqMan probes modified with minor groove-binder molecules that increase their affinity for the target [131] and the use of two probes, each labeled with a different reporter fluorophore, which allows both SNP alleles to be detected in a single tube [66].

The homogeneous reactions are robust, flexible, and not labor intensive. The thermal stability of a hybrid between an ASO probe and its SNP-containing target sequence is determined by the stringency of the reaction conditions as well as by the nucleotide sequence that flanks the SNP and the secondary structure of the target sequence. Prediction of the reaction conditions or the sequence of the ASO probe that will allow the optimal distinction between two alleles that differ at a single nucleotide position using ASO hybridization is extremely difficult. These parameters must be established separately for each SNP. As a result, there is no single set of reaction conditions that would be optimal for genotyping all SNPs, which makes the design of multiplex assays based on hybridization with ASO probes in solution an almost impossible task [66].

A common technique to circumvent some of the design problems of the homogeneous reaction is to use microarrays where either the probe or target oligonucleotide is immobilized on a solid support. There is some inconsistency in nomenclature of the probe and target in the microarray technology. Some authors name the target as the immobilized oligonucleotide and the probe as the labeled oligonucleotide, while others give the impression that the probe is immobilized on the solid support while the target is hybridized to the probe array [114, 132, 133]. I will use the latter definition (Fig. 21.11).

The reactions on solid support are carried out on glass slides, silicon chips, latex beads, or on the walls of a microtiter plate. The dot blot [134] is a form of differential hybridization where the probe oligonucleotide is labeled and the target or amplicon

TABLE 21.2   Genotyping Technologies

Technique[a]	Mechanism of Allele Discrimination	Reaction Format	Detection Mechanism	References
Reverse dot blot	Hybridization	Solid support	Colorimetric	69
Microarray	Hybridization	Solid support	Fluorescence	12, 70, 71
DASH	Hybridization	Solid support	Fluorescence	72, 73
Molecular Beacons	Hybridization	Homogeneous reaction	FRET	74, 75
5′-Nuclease cleavage (TaqMan)	Hybridization	Homogeneous	FRET or FP	76, 77
Cleavase (Invader assay)	Hybridization	Homogeneous reaction	FRET, FP, MS	78–82
Biosensor Microchip	Hybridization	Solid support	Electrochemical and fluorescence	83–89
AS-PCR	Primer extension	Homogeneous reaction	Fluorescence or FRET	90–95
AS-PE	Primer extension	Solid support	Fluorescence	96
APEX	Primer extension	Solid support	Fluorescence	97–100
FP-TDI	Primer extension	Homogeneous reaction	FRET or FP	101–104
MALDI-TOF MS	Primer extension	Homogeneous reaction	MS	105–108
Pyrosequencing	Primer extension	Homogeneous reaction or solid support	Luminescence	109–113
BioBeads and TagArrays	Primer extension	Homogeneous reaction and solid support capture	Fluorescence	114–117
OLA	Ligation	Homogeneous reaction and solid support	Colorimetric and fluorescence	118–120
RCA	Ligation	Solid support	Fluorescence	121–124
Closed tube	Ligation	Homogeneous reaction	FRET	125
Microsphere/ microarray ligation	Ligation	Homogeneous reaction	Fluorescence	115, 126

[a]Abbreviations: DASH, dynamic allele-specific hybridization; AS-PCR, allele-specific polymerase chain reaction; AS-PE, allele-specific primer extension; APEX, arrayed primer extension; FP-TDI, fluorescence polarization template directed dye terminator incorporation; MALDI-TOF-MS, matrix assisted laser desorption/ionization time-of-flight mass spectrometry; OLA, oligonucleotide ligation assay; RCA, rolling circle amplification.

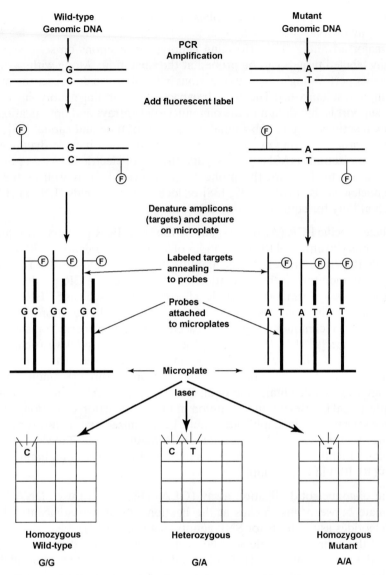

FIGURE 21.11 Schematic representation of the reverse blot microarray technology. The amplicons or "targets" are represented by thin lines while the synthetic "probes" covalently linked to the microplate are represented by thick lines. Note in this figure that the probes select for one strand of the fluorescently labeled amplified targets.

is immobilized on a solid support. Gene chips are a form of reverse dot blot where the amplicon is fluorescently tagged and hybridized to an immobilized array of oligonucleotide probes (Fig. 21.11) [69]. Because the oligonucleotide sequences are SNP specific, each chip has a unique design, and the cost and effort involved in the manufacture of unique chips can be prohibitive. The identity of an oligonucleotide at a particular location on the microarray is known and the genotypes are inferred by determining which immobilized oligonucleotide is associated with a positive signal (Fig. 21.11). The GeneChip from Affymetrix (http://www.affymetrix.com/

index.affx) uses this principle. The probes are synthesized on the glass chip by photolithography or solid-phase DNA synthesis [135].

The major advantage of performing genotyping reactions on solid supports is that many labeled targets can be probed at the same time. Along with saving time and reagents, performing numerous reactions in parallel also decreases the probability of sample/result mix-ups. The main drawback of performing genotyping reactions on solid support is that design of the oligonucleotide arrays and optimization of the multiplex reactions require substantial investment of time and capital [58].

Other approaches using microarray ASO hybridization include dynamic allele-specific hybridization (DASH) [72, 136] and the use of electric field strength instead of temperature to denature the probe–target hybrids [83] as well as the use of peptide nucleic acids (PNAs) [137, 138] or locked nucleic acids (LNAs) [139, 140] with high affinity for complementary DNA.

2. Allele-specific PCR (AS-PCR) (Fig. 21.10b) uses PCR primers with the 3′-end complementary to either of the nucleotides of a SNP in combination with a common reverse PCR primer to selectively amplify the SNP alleles [141]. The simplest approach for monitoring the formation of allele-specific PCR products using a homogeneous assay format is to include a fluorescent dye such as SYBR Green that intercalates with the double-stranded PCR products in the reaction mixture [92]. Other detection techniques include fluorescence resonance energy transfer (FRET) and fluorescence [91, 94, 95]. Roche's LightCycler™ (http://www.roche-applied-science.com/sis/rtpcr/lightcycler/), Perkin Elmer's AlphaScreen (http://las.perkinel-mer.com/), and adaptations of the Molecular Beacon are three techniques using this technology. In general, a limitation of all the variations of AS-PCR is similar to the ASO differential hybridization in solution in that the reaction conditions or primer design for selective allele amplification must be optimized empirically for each SNP. Therefore, homogeneous allele-specific PCR methods like TaqMan, Molecular Beacon, and LightCycler assay are best suited for the analysis of a limited number of SNPs (10–100) in large sample collections [66].

3. The oligonucleotide ligation assay (OLA) (Fig. 21.10c) uses DNA ligase to discriminate between mismatches at the ligation site of two adjacent hybridized oligonucleotides as the basis for SNP genotyping (Fig. 21.12).

One of the hybridized allele-specific nucleotides carries a donor dye while the other carries an acceptor dye [125, 142, 143]. In order to detect both alleles, one donor dye (e.g., FAM or 5-carboxy-fluorescine) and two acceptor dyes (e.g., ROX or 6-carboxy-X-rhodamine and TAMRA or N,N,N', N'-tetramethyl-6-carboxyrho-damine) are required (Fig. 21.12). A 5′-donor dye-labeled common probe is designed to terminate one base immediately upstream of the polymorphic site. The 5′-phosphorylated probes carrying the 3′-acceptor dyes are designed to anneal with the allelic bases at the 5′-end. The PCR primers are designed to anneal with high melting temperatures while the 5′- and 3′-labeled probes are designed to have a matching but low melting temperature. The reaction is carried out with a thermostable DNA polymerase with no 5′-nuclease activity and a thermostable DNA ligase. These reactions can be carried out in a single sealed tube since the PCR amplification is carried out at high temperature where the ligation probes will not anneal and be removed from the ligation reaction. When the amplification is complete, the temperature is lowered and the ligation reaction is carried out. Fluorescence reso-

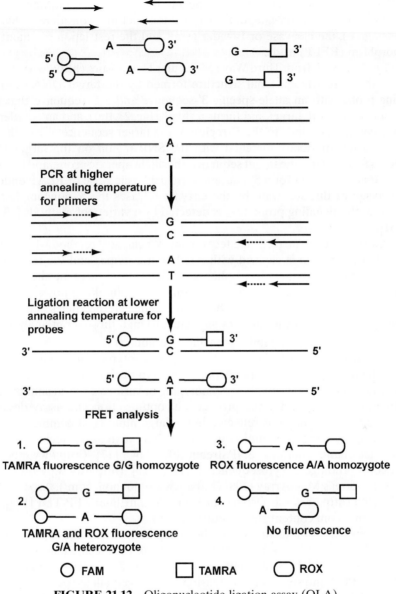

FIGURE 21.12   Oligonucleotide ligation assay (OLA).

nance energy transfer (FRET) is measured in real time and the genotypes are determined by measuring the rate of emergence of fluorescence for the two dyes found on the ligation probes.

Variations on this theme include colorimetric detection in microtiter plate wells [118, 120], multiplex detection using fluorescently labeled ligation probes with different electrophoretic mobilities that can be analyzed in a sequencing instrument [119], one immobilized ligation probe [122], immobilized single stem–loop probes [144], padlock probes and the rolling circle amplification [121, 123, 145–147], and homogeneous reaction with tag-capture [126, 148].

4. The cleavage assays (Fig. 21.10d) include the 5′-nucelase TaqMan assay (discussed in the hybridization category because it is sometimes considered a hybridization technique), the cleavase or Invader assay, and the restriction fragment length polymorphism (RFLP) assay.

The Invader assay from Third Wave Molecular Diagnostics (http://www.twt.com/) is based on a three-dimensional structure formed by the target DNA sequence, a signaling probe with an allele-specific 3′-sequence and a 5′-sequence that is noncomplementary to the target and forms a "flap" (Fig. 21.10d), and an invader probe oligonucleotide that binds to the 3′-region of the target sequence. When the allele-specific probe is perfectly matched with the SNP region on the target DNA, a complex is formed with the target sequence, the allele-specific probe, and the invader probe that is a substrate for a 5′-endonuclease called cleavase or FLAP endonuclease. Cleavage of this substrate by the enzyme releases the 5′-noncomplementary sequence of the signaling probe that is detected by a variety of methods [78, 80–82, 149–151].

The restriction enzyme cleavage technology is a classical method where the PCR amplified target region is cleaved with restriction enzymes and the resulting fragments are separated by gel electrophoresis. Allelic variations that either create or remove restriction sites can be detected using this technology; however, the need for gel separation of fragments and the requirement that the alleles being analyzed be located at restriction sites are not amenable to high throughput analysis.

5. The primer extension/minisequencing technique (Fig. 21.10e) has become the reaction principle of choice for high throughput genotyping due to the advantages of using the high specificity of DNA-polymerase to distinguish between SNPs and the fact that primer extension allows genotyping of various SNPs at similar reaction conditions, thereby reducing the problems of optimization and assay design. The versatility of this technique is reflected in the large number of commercially available systems utilizing the minisequencing primer extension technology. These include Beckmann-Coulter's SNPStream [96, 114, 117] (http://www.beckman-coulter.com), Biotage's Pyrosequencing [112, 113] (http://www.pyrosequencing.com/), Sequenom's MassArray [108] (http://www.sequenom.com/), Asper Biotech's Apex [98, 99] (http://www.asperbio.com/), and PerkinElmer's FP-TDI [104] (http://las.perkinelmer.com/content/snps/fp-tdi.asp#).

The primer extension technique has been augmented with the 5′-tag technology to permit the purification of the extended products via specific tags, which in turn allows for versatile high throughput genotyping (Fig. 21.13). The genomic DNA is amplified by PCR and single base extension with tagged allele-specific primers and fluorescent-labeled ddNTPs is carried out in solution to detect the SNP. The resulting labeled and tagged fragments are captured by complementary tags on microtiter plates or color-coded beads. Fluorescence resulting from laser excitation of the plates or beads is read by a detector and fed to the computer database for analysis and storage. Most companies providing the single base extension (SBE) tag-capture technology also provide a primer design service so that users can take advantage of multiplexing limited only by the capacity to design effective primers for the amplification and detection steps.

The choice of genotyping technology just described will be governed by the nature of the analysis being carried out. If one is interested in a small number of

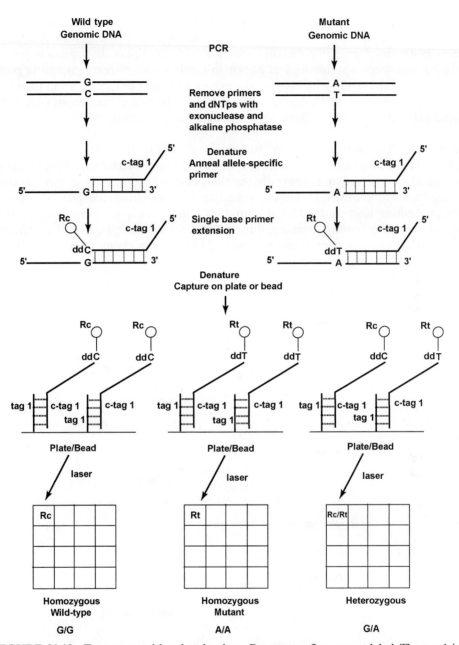

FIGURE 21.13 Tag-array and bead technology. R, reporter fluorescent label. The tag 1 is specific for the G/A mutation at a particular position in the gene under investigation. Other tags can be designed for other SNPs to permit multiplexing in the same well of the microtiter plate to produce an "array of arrays" [96].

biomarkers, then PCR analytical techniques like ABI's TaqMan assay or Roche's LightCycler assay are useful. When more complex assays that can analyze large populations for dozens of polymorphisms in a single multiplex analysis are required, the 12- and 48-plex technology of Beckman-Coulter's SNPStream microtiter plate tag-array technology, the bead-based tag-array technology of Luminex and Illumina, the Affymetrix oligonucleotide arrays, or ABI's PinPoint and Sequenom's MassExtend mass spectrometry technology are more accommodating.

Detection   The different formats for detection [64] of the allele discrimination product include gel electrophoresis, microtiter plate or closed tube, and the microarray bead or chip format. Historically, the allele discrimination product was detected using radioisotopic methods but the technique has been almost completely replaced by monitoring light emitted by the product (fluorescence, luminescence, fluorescence resonance energy transfer, fluorescence polarization; Fig. 21.14 and Table 21.2) or a change in mass (mass spectrometry) or electrochemical conductivity of the product (Table 21.2).

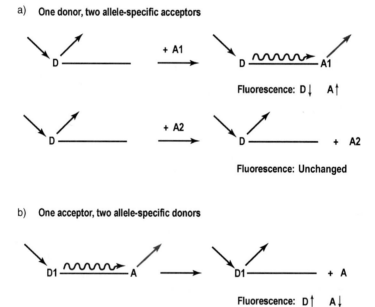

FIGURE 21.14 Fluorescence-based techniques for genotype scoring. The alleles can be detected using allele-specific acceptors or allele-specific donors: (a) two allele-specific acceptors with one donor, examples of which occur in minisequencing and the oligonucleotide ligation assay; and (b) two allele-specific donors with one acceptor, examples of which occur in the TaqMan assay, the Invader assay, and Molecular Beacons. (Adapted from Ref. 64.)

21.4.2   Gene Expression Profiling—Transcriptomics

Transcriptomics is defined as the study of the full complement of RNA in the cell, including mRNA transcripts (transcriptome).

Technologies that examine gene expression profiles are at the core of functional genomics and differential gene expression (DGE) is at the center of the functional genomics technology. Genes that are expressed or transcribed from genomic DNA are collectively known as the "transcriptome" and are considered to be a major determinant of cellular phenotype and function. Methods of expression profiling are classified into two types: open and closed. Open systems do not require any advance knowledge of the sequence of the genome being examined. Closed systems require some advance knowledge of the genes being examined and usually involve the use of gene chip technology.

Closed Gene Expression Profiling—Microarray Technologies   The most common methods of closed system analyses [152] are oligonucleotide or cDNA array hybridization technologies and quantitative polymerase chain reaction. The arrays detect mRNA levels that can be confirmed by RTQ-PCR (real-time quantitative polymerase chain reaction) or *in situ* hybridization [51]. Closed system profiling technologies are used for analysis of a known subset of genes, where there is a solid understanding of such global genetic complexities as splice variants, polymorphisms, and RNA editing [153].

cDNA arrays (Fig. 21.15) are prepared by spotting gene-specific PCR products including full-length cDNAs, collections of partially sequenced cDNAs (or expressed sequence tags—ESTs), or randomly chosen cDNAs from any library of interest onto a matrix consisting of glass, silicon, nylon or nitrocellulose membranes, gels, or beads. Glass is particularly suitable because of its durable and nonporous properties and low background fluorescence. The glass-based matrix is coated with polylysine, amino silanes, or amino-reactive silanes to aid in the attachment of the cDNA sample. PCR products are spotted onto the matrix by robots through contact printing or noncontact piezo or ink-jet devices. The probe DNA is cross-linked to the matrix by UV irradiation and rendered single stranded by heat or alkali treatment. The array is used to analyze mRNA expression. Total mRNA from both a test and reference sample is reverse transcribed to produce cDNA, during which the product is individually labeled with either fluorescent Cye3- or Cye5-dUTP. The fluorescent targets are pooled and allowed to hybridize under stringent conditions to the clones on the array. Laser excitation of the incorporated targets yields an emission with a characteristic spectra, which is measured using a scanning confocal laser microscope. The fluorescence analysis of the test and reference sample allows comparison of the gene expression of one to the other, thus identifying up- and downregulated genes. The rather large amount of RNA required per hybridization (50–200 µg of target per array) is a limiting factor in the use of this technology [132]. Whole genome high density tiling arrays (WGAs) are a variation of the microarray technology that provides a universal data capture platform for a variety of genomic information [154].

Data collection is obviously very complex and computer algorithms for analyzing the data fall into four methods: hierarchic clustering, self-organizing maps, multidimensional scaling, and pathway associations. Cluster analysis of microarrays consists

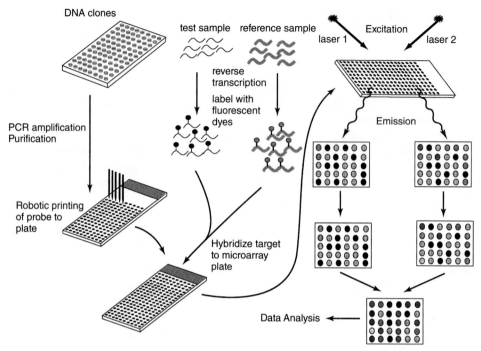

FIGURE 21.15   Schematic representation of a cDNA microarray. Templates for genes of interest are obtained from DNA clones and amplified by PCR. Following the purification and quality control, aliquots are printed on coated glass microscope slides using a computer-controlled, high speed robot. The array is used to analyze mRNA expression. Total mRNA from both a test and reference sample is fluorescently labeled with either Cye3- or Cye5-dUTP using a single round of reverse transcription. The fluorescent targets are pooled and allowed to hybridize under stringent conditions to the clones on the array. Laser excitation of the incorporated targets yields an emission with a characteristic spectra, which is measured using a scanning confocal laser microscope. (From Ref. 132 with permission of the author and Nature Publishing Group.)

of arranging the hybridization data into a cluster order based on color-coded intensities, which in turn provides clues as to which genes are being regulated in groups [155].

Comparisons of test and control expression profiles provide useful insights into the molecular pathologies of a variety of diseases and drug therapies [49]. It will not, however, deliver the kind of intimate understanding of the highly interrelated control circuitry that is necessary to achieve true understanding of genome function [132]. Duggan et al. [132] have suggested that we should reconsider our perception of transcriptional control as a simple on–off switch to a model, whereby control is analogous to a highly gated logic circuit, where numerous, often contradictory, inputs are summed to produce a final response.

There has been considerable enthusiasm in the scientific community in promoting the application of DNA microarray technology for the analysis of genetic variation aimed at identifying molecular biomarkers for application to personalized medicine and drug development. The U.S. Food and Drug Administration has issued a draft regarding guidance on the submission of pharmacogenomic data for drug development by the pharmaceutical industry (http://www.fda.gov/cber/gdlns/pharmdtasub.pdf). However, variations in the technical, instrumental, computational, and interpretative aspects of microarray technologies are causing serious concerns and the lack of reproducibility and accuracy of microarray studies within and between facilities are just some of the challenges and pitfalls facing the microarray community and regulatory agencies before microarray data can be reliably applied to support regulatory decision making. Problems in intralaboratory data quality have been observed, and the microarray community and regulatory agencies must work together to identify critical factors affecting data quality, and to optimize and standardize microarray procedures to make certain that biologic interpretation and decision making are based on reliable data [156]. These fundamental issues must be adequately addressed before microarray technology can be transformed from a research tool to clinical practice.

Open Gene Expression Profiling   The open systems for detecting differential gene expression [153] are distinct from the closed systems in that no preexisting biological or sequence information is necessary. These technologies will not be discussed in detail here since they are not extensively used in the molecular biomarker field of pharmacogenomics. A brief description of some of the major open system technologies is given in Table 21.3 with appropriate references.

21.4.3   Protein Analysis—Proteomics

Proteomics [166–168] is defined as the study of the total protein complement of a genome, or the complete set of proteins expressed by a cell, tissue, or organism (proteome).

The detection of an open reading frame (ORF) is an indication of the presence of a gene but does not indicate transcription, RNA editing, or translation. Verification of a gene product by proteomic technology is important to confirm the above as well as determine posttranslational modifications and the presence of protein isoforms. Transcriptome analysis does not indicate alteration in protein levels by proteolysis, recycling, and sequestration of proteins; therefore, proteomics is important in determining the levels of proteins in a cell as well as protein localization, protein expression, and protein–protein interaction. Hence, an understanding of the complex relationship between proteins and genes on a genomic scale is vital to understanding protein function in disease and disease therapy.

Proteomics can be divided into three main areas [166]: (1) protein microcharacterization for large scale identification of proteins and their posttranslational modifications; (2) "differential display" proteomics for comparison of protein levels with potential application in a wide range of diseases; and (3) studies of protein–protein interactions using techniques such as protein chips, the mass spectrometry ICAT technology, or the yeast two-hybrid system.

Routine microcharacterization of proteins using gel electrophoresis will only detect the most abundant proteins and a purification strategy is required to reduce the complexity of the proteome and allow visualization of the less abundant proteins. This is especially important when analyzing the signaling and regulatory proteins that are of critical importance to understanding drug action.

TABLE 21.3   Comparison of Different Open System Technologies

Expression Analysis Technology	Amount of Template Required (μg)	Sensitivity	N-fold Difference Detection Limit	Genes Covered (%)[a]	References
Differential display	0.5 (mRNA)	NA	NA	96	157
Arbitrarily Primed Polymerase Chain Reaction (AP-PCR)	0.012 (total RNA)	NA	NA	NA	158
Serial Analysis of Gene Expression (SAGE)	5 (total RNA)	<1:10,000	NA	92 (of transcripts at ≥3/cell)	159, 160
Representational Difference Analysis (RDA)	0.02 (mRNA estimated from 10,000 cells)	<1:300,000	NA	N/A	161
Gene Calling®	0.02 (mRNA)	1:125,000	1.5	~95	162
Restriction Enzyme Analysis of Differentially Expressed Sequences (READS™)	10 (total RNA; 100 pg/reaction)	1:100,000	NA	90	163
Total Gene Expression Analysis (TOGA)	NA	<1:100,000	60–98	60% coverage using one enzyme, 98% using four (4 × 256 reactions)	164
Tandem Arrayed Ligation of Expressed Sequence Tags (TALEST)	2 (mRNA)	1:200,000	NA	85	165

[a]For many of the techniques the reported coverage percent is not correlated to mRNA abundance. Coverage of rare transcripts may be considerably lower. NA, information not available.

Differential Gel Electrophoresis   Proteins isolated from cells or tissues that have been subjected to different conditions (experimental and control) are separated by their "isoelectric point" in the first dimension and by size in the "second dimension" (Fig. 21.16) [51, 166, 167, 169, 170]. The technology relies on excising the spots from the gels, proteolytically digesting the protein, and extracting the

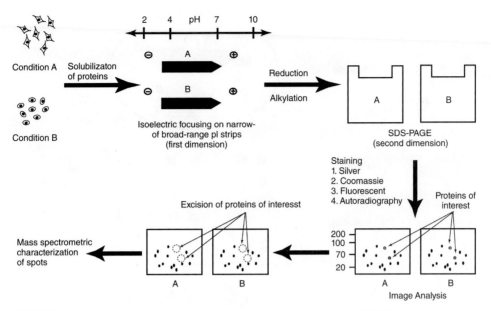

FIGURE 21.16   A schematic representation of the two-dimensional (2D) gel approach to protein separation. Cells (or tissues) derived from two different conditions, A and B, are harvested and the proteins solubilized. The crude protein mixture is then applied to a "first dimension" gel strip that separates the proteins based on their isoelectric points. After this step, the strip is subjected to reduction and alkylation and applied to a "second dimension" SDS-PAGE gel where proteins are denatured and separated on the basis of size. The gels are then fixed and the proteins visualized by silver or Coumassie staining or by fluorescence (if the proteins had been fluorescently labeled) or autoradiography (also depending on the nature of the label). After visualization, the resulting protein spots are recorded and quantified. Image analysis requires sophisticated software. Finally, the spots of interest are excised from the gel and subjected to mass spectrometric analysis. (Adapted from Ref. 166 with permission of the author and Nature Publishing Group.)

peptide fragments produced. The peptide fragments produced are analyzed by mass spectrometry or tandem mass spectrometry and the data derived is correlated with database information of protein sequence, genomic sequence, or expressed sequence tags.

Protein Chips   The protein chip approach to simplification of the protein mixture utilizes a variety of "bait" molecules that are ligands, such as proteins, peptides, antibodies, antigens, allergens, and small molecules immobilized in high density on modified surfaces to form functional and analytical protein microarrays (Fig. 21.17) [171–174]. The cell lysate is passed over the surface of the solid support immobilizing the bait molecules to allow it to capture its counterpart in the cell lysate. The most common bait protein used in the protein chip technology is the antibody [175–182]. The protein chip technique has been coupled with a direct matrix assisted laser desorption/ionization (MALDI) mass spectrometric detection of the material bound to the bait protein [183–186].

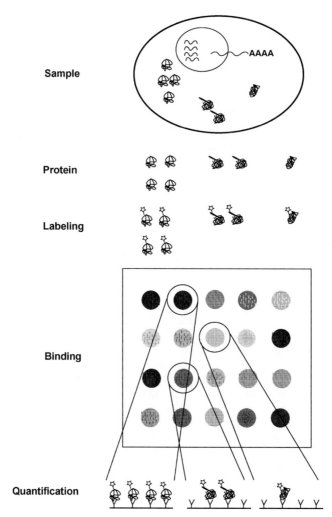

FIGURE 21.17 Parallel quantification of proteins by antibody microarray. Different proteins labeled with fluorochromes can be detected in parallel with a microarray-based assay. Specific capture antibodies immobilized in an array interact with their respective target proteins present in the solution. The resulting signal intensity correlates with the amount of captured target. Within each microarray, different kinds of control spots can be included, such as positive and negative control spots and/or internal calibration spots. This will allow accurate signal quantification. (From Ref. 171. Copyright © 2002, with permission from Elsevier.)

Isotope Coded Affinity Tag (ICAT) ICAT is a chromatography–mass spectrometry-based technology where two samples are labeled with tags that differ in their incorporation of a heavy label (deuterium for hydrogen or ^{13}C for ^{12}C) (Fig. 21.18). The labeling reagent is typically a thiol-specific reagent with an alkyl linker containing either nine ^{12}C or nine ^{13}C atoms and a biotin moiety for avidin chromatography [187–190].

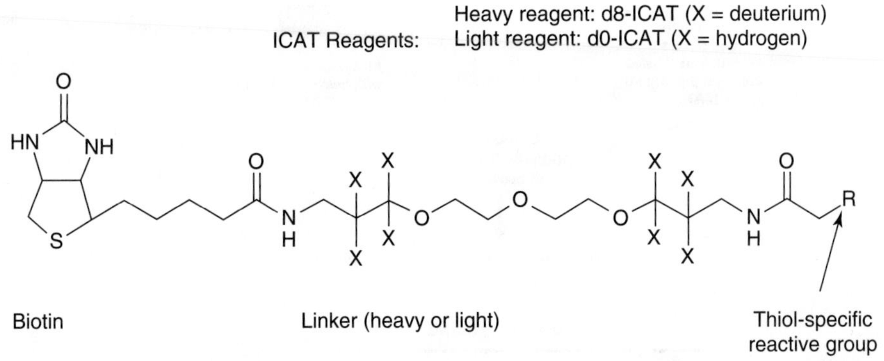

ICAT Reagents: Heavy reagent: d8-ICAT (X = deuterium)
Light reagent: d0-ICAT (X = hydrogen)

Biotin   Linker (heavy or light)   Thiol-specific
reactive group

FIGURE 21.18   Isotope coded affinity tag labeling reagent. (From Ref. 171 with permission of the author and Nature Publishing Group.)

Two protein mixtures representing two different cell states are treated with the isotopically labeled light and heavy ICAT reagents (Fig. 21.18), respectively; an ICAT reagent is covalently attached to each cysteinyl residue in every protein. The protein mixtures are combined and proteolyzed to peptides, and ICAT-labeled peptides are isolated utilizing the biotin tag. These peptides are separated by microcapillary high performance liquid chromatography. A pair of ICAT-labeled peptides is chemically identical and is easily visualized because they essentially coelute and there is an 8 Da mass difference (depending on the tag) measured in a scanning mass spectrometer (four m/z unit difference for a doubly charged ion) (Fig. 21.19). The ratios of the original amounts of proteins from the two cell states are strictly maintained in the peptide fragments. The relative quantification is determined by the ratio of the peptide pairs. Every other scan is devoted to fragmenting and then recording sequence information about an eluting peptide (tandem mass spectrum). The protein is identified through a computer search of the recorded sequence information against large protein databases [166].

Yeast Two-Hybrid System   The yeast two-hybrid system (Fig. 21.20) [191] is one of the best *in vitro* approaches to mapping protein–protein interactions. Using this technique, the protein of interest or "bait" protein is fused to a protein containing a DNA-binding domain. Proteins being screened for interaction with the bait protein are fused to proteins containing a transcriptional activating domain. If the bait protein binds to the protein being screened, the DNA-binding domain is brought into proximity of the transcriptional activating domain and the activation of transcription of a reporter construct occurs resulting in reporter gene product (Fig. 21.20).

This technology can be used to identify compounds and peptides that disrupt protein–protein interactions [192] and is amenable to automation and high throughput. One of the main consequences of the forward and reverse techniques shown in Fig. 21.20 is that once a positive interaction is detected (in either the forward or reverse systems), simple sequencing of the relevant clone identifies the open reading frame and thereby identifies the proteins interacting (forward) or those whose interaction has been disrupted (reverse).

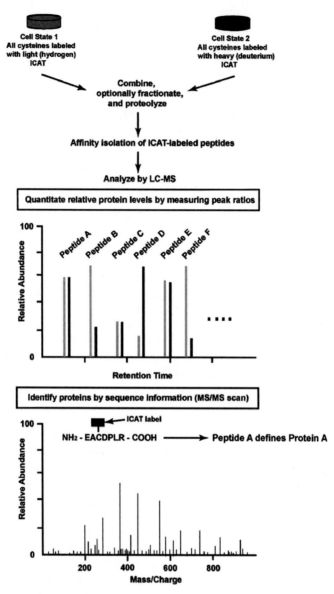

FIGURE 21.19   The ICAT strategy for quantifying differential protein expression. (Adapted from Ref. 166 with permission of the author and Nature Publishing Group.)

21.4.4   Metabolomics

Metabolomics is defined as the measurement of metabolite concentrations, fluxes, and secretions in cells and tissues in which there is a direct connection between genetic activity (transcriptome), protein activity (proteome), and the metabolic activity itself [193, 194]. There is some multiplicity in the nomenclature in this area and one will also encounter "metabonomics" [195] as well as "metabolic profiling" [196].

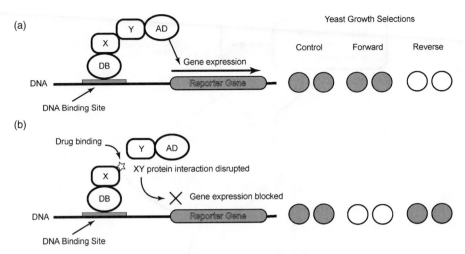

FIGURE 21.20   Schematic representations of the way two-hybrid systems work. DB, DNA binding domain; AD, activating domain; X and Y are the proteins under investigation for interaction. The grey and white patches on the right-hand side represent growing and non-growing yeast cells, respectively; under normal conditions (control), the yeast cells grow whether or not a two-hybrid interaction takes place. In the forward two-hybrid selections, potential interactions (a) are identified by the transcriptional activation of a reporter gene required for growth, which confers a selective advantage. In the reverse two-hybrid selections, the interaction activates the expression of a "toxic gene" and so prevention of the interaction (b) provides a selective advantage. (From Ref. 192. Copyright © 1999, with permission from Elsevier.)

In our effort to precisely link the organism's gene function to phenotype, we arrive at the complex analysis of the metabolome. Metabolites have been characterized as "the ultimate gene product" [197] and are at the cross-roads of genotype–phenotype interactions. Under our definition of phenotype [54], metabolomics is considered here to be a form of molecular phenotyping. If we consider the organism's phenotype to be composed of cellular phenotypes and the cellular phenotype to be composed of metabolic networks, then the interrelationship of metabolic pathways is considered the fundamental component of an organism's phenotype [198].

It is the description of the metabolic profile of the organism that is critical to a phenotypic description of that organism's physiology and pathophysiology. Phenotype cannot rely solely on a description dictated by predicted proteins encoded by the genome of the organism but must include metabolic transformations that are stoichiometrically, thermodynamically, and kinetically possible (Fig. 21.21) [198]. This is the level at which we see the implications of allelic variations occurring in the genome. The identification of an allelic variation in a gene producing an enzyme that has an altered activity is the basis of functional genomics but the question remains: Does the allelic variation alter phenotype and, if so, how? The complex flow of metabolites in an organism has a robustness that arises from the extensive redundancy in metabolic pathways. There are often a number of isozymes that catalyze the same reaction and the alteration of one isozyme at the genetic level may

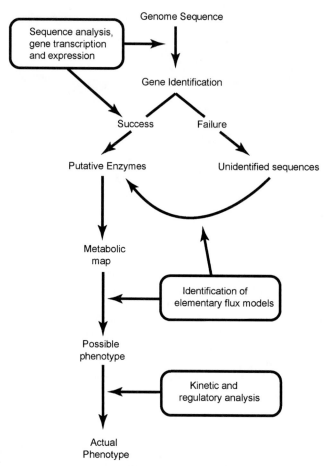

FIGURE 21.21 The necessary steps to convert a genome sequence into a phenotypic description include not only the early stages of identifying the genes and investigating their transcription and expression, but also later events that include assembling the enzyme-catalyzed reactions into a metabolic map, determining what kinds of metabolic activity are stoichiometrically possible, and, finally, determining which of these are kinetically possible. Identification of elementary flux modes is especially useful for defining the stoichiometric structure of the map, but it can also aid in identifying the roles of orphan genes remaining after bioinformatics studies have permitted the identification of other genes by comparison with the sequences of known enzymes. (Adapted from Ref. 198 with permission of Nature Publishing Group.)

not alter the metabolic system to any great extent. Alternatively, the allelic variation may result in a metabolic flux in another closely linked pathway that is totally unexpected and not seen until an identification and comparison of the metabolic profiles of the wild type and mutant is made (Fig. 21.22).

Distinguishing features of the metabolome include the fact that metabolites are not directly linked to the genetic code but are actually products of a concerted action of several networks of enzymes and other regulatory proteins [199]. Metabolites are also structurally far more complex than the four-letter code describing

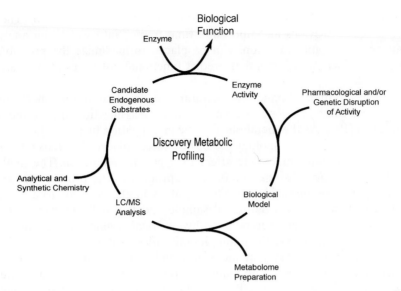

FIGURE 21.22   Connecting the proteome and metabolome through discovery metabolite profiling (DMP). Assigning the enzyme function using DMP begins by disruption of the enzyme activity of interest through either pharmacological or genetic means. Differences in the metabolome between wild-type and enzyme-disrupted systems are then identified using untargeted LC/MS methods and converted into chemical structures using more detailed analytical methods (tandem MS, NMR) and chemical synthesis. These compounds are then directly examined as substrates for the enzyme of interest. (From Ref. 199. Copyright © 2005, with permission from Elsevier.)

genes or the 20-letter code describing proteins [194]. As a result, metabolites cannot be sequenced like genes or proteins and their characterization requires that the structure of each metabolite be determined individually through a description of elemental composition and stereochemical orientation of functional groups.

The metabolome is complicated by the interactive nature of the biochemical systems that produce the metabolites, and the environmental conditions under which a metabolomic experiment is carried out need to be accurately specified. Also, it is obvious that metabolites are not just steps in a metabolic cycle but are also sensors and regulators in a complex series of molecular interactions in the whole organism [200]. Therefore, metabolic studies are severely limited by the knowledge of the biochemical systems of the organism under investigation as well as the "state" of the specific individual under investigation. This individuality further complicates the metabolomic study since individuals are not only genetically unique but are also environmentally unique. It is also important to note that the complexity of the metabolome may mean that variation in specific genes reflected in the metabolome will not be reflected by a concomitant change in the morphological or physiological phenotype (a phenotypically silent variation) until it is accompanied by additional variations in the genome, transcriptome, proteome, metabolome, or envirome [201]. Some unique biochemical pathways will be affected by allelic variation in the genes responsible for the regulators of the pathway, but those metabolic reaction pathways that can be accommodated by other pathways will not necessarily be altered by an allelic variation until a combination of variations in both pathways occurs. The study of metabolomics provides an important "time frame" into which the analysis of genomic and proteomic variations can be placed to maximize the probability of observing biological transitions that predict functional outcomes of the variations [195].

Approaches to metabolomic investigations are classified in a manner similar to the single gene, candidate gene, and whole genome classification of genomic studies (see Fig. 21.5) [194]. As the metabolic/genetic investigation increases in complexity so does the protocol and technology used. The strategy of *target analysis* is to directly investigate the primary metabolic effect of a genetic alteration. The analysis is usually limited to the substrate and/or direct product of the protein expressed by the altered gene. The *metabolite profiling* strategy limits the study to a number of predefined metabolites in a biological sample and is usually narrowed down to metabolites in a particular metabolic pathway. *Metabolomics* defines the strategy for a comprehensive analysis, including identification and quantification, of all the metabolites in a biological system and is designed to investigate the possible multiple effects of genetic variation on many different biochemical pathways. The technology behind metabolomics will often be called upon to identify unknown metabolites as well as handle the complex datasets of multiple interacting biochemical systems. Finally, the strategy of *metabolic fingerprinting* is to screen a large number of metabolites for biological relevance in diagnostics or other analytical procedures where it is important to rapidly distinguish between individuals in a population.

The main analytical technologies used in metabolomic investigations are nuclear magnetic resonance (NMR) and mass spectrometry (MS) alone or in combination with liquid (LC-MS) or gas chromatographic (GC-MS) separation of metabolites [37, 193–197, 199, 201–207]. Other techniques include thin layer chromatography [208], Fourier transform infrared (FT-IR) spectrometry [209], metabolite arrays [210], and Raman spectroscopy [211].

21.4.5   Enviromics

The analysis of gene–environment interactions is relatively new and mainly in the area of disease diagnosis. The term enviromics was first used in the field of psychiatric epidemiology and defined the study of "the total ensemble of environments, both current and in earlier life, that affect the occurrence of mental and behavioural disturbances" [55]. A more generalized definition of enviromics that would be applicable to pharmacogenomics would be the total ensemble of environments both current and in earlier life that can be identified to affect disease development and therapeutic outcomes. This would include such variables as physical environment for work and relaxation, lifestyle, social stressors, patient demographics, diet, and exposure to other drugs and toxic agents including pathogens. The critical problem to development of enviromics in the description of pharmacogenomics is to accurately describe and adequately quantify the environmental factors under consideration in the drug study. *Genetic epidemiology* is the discipline that seeks to explain the extent to which genetic and environmental factors that people are exposed to influence their risk of disease, by means of population-based investigations.

Some relatively simple examples of gene–environment interactions and their correlation with particular diseases are listed in Table 21.4. The concept of pharmacogenetics could be considered a special example of the binary nature of gene–environment interaction, where the environmental exposure is a drug. The allelic variation of genes involved in the metabolism of the particular drug are used to identify individuals who are at risk for adverse drug reactions or treatment failure. The population can then be divided into those who should avoid taking the drug or those who should have their dose modified [15]. However, it would be naive to assume that the drug is the only environmental factor to play a role during disease therapy. Indeed, under the holistic view of pharmacogenomics, there are a number of complicating factors leading to a successful drug therapy.

Enviromics is a relatively new and undocumented area in pharmacogenomics and considerable research must be done, selecting critical environmental factors affecting personalized medicine and examining their interaction with the genome, transcriptome, proteome, and metabolome in the production of molecular biomarkers. Without a thorough understanding of the effects of the envirome, one will have only limited success with the application of the concept of personalized medicine.

21.5 ASSOCIATIVE ANALYSIS

Ultimately there are four phenotypes that must be described to adequately assess the affect of the envirome, genome, transcriptome, proteome, and metabolome on disease development, initiation of therapy, and therapeutic outcome: the disease and normal phenotypes, the drug phenotype, and the therapeutic phenotype (see Fig. 21.8). The molecular profile of the disease will play a major role in the selection of therapies that are available to the physician. The relationship between the molecular profiles of the normal phenotype and the disease phenotype will provide a valuable source of detailed molecular information for the predict-and-manage paradigm of health care, outlined by the United States Pharmacopoeial Convention [56]. It should also be mentioned here that the genetic basis of complex phenotypes are often "modifier" variations in that changes in expression levels of multiple genes contribute to the phenotypic outcome.

The complexity of gene–environment interactions and their effect on the disease phenotype is summed up in a quote from D. J. Weatherall [224]: "A central problem for the medical sciences in general, and for clinical genetics in particular, is the extent to which it will be possible to relate findings at the molecular level to clinical phenotype."

The association of genetic variation with environmental influences is a rather new field for drug therapy but it has been extensively studied with respect to the disease phenotype, although the effect of environment has usually been limited to a single variable. An example of the complexity that exists in genetic influences on the disease phenotype alone has been impressively demonstrated for the β-thalassemias (Fig. 21.23) [224]. Weatherall [224] has pointed out that the mechanisms underlying the phenotypic diversity of the β-thalassemias can be classified as follows: *primary causes* that are the many genetic variations that occur in the β-globin genes that underlie the β-thalassemias; *secondary causes* that result from variations at other genetic loci involved in globin synthesis; and *tertiary causes* resulting from variations

TABLE 21.4 Selected Examples of Gene–Environment Interactions Observed in at Least Two Studies

Gene Symbol[a]	Variant(s)	Environmental Exposure	Outcome and Nature of Interaction	References
Genes for skin pigmentation (e.g., MC1R)	Variants for fair skin color	Sunlight or ultraviolet light B	Risk of skin cancer is higher in people with fair skin color who are exposed to higher amounts of sunlight	212
CCR5	Δ-32 deletion	HIV[a]	Carriers of the receptor deletion have lower rates of HIV infection and disease progression	213
MTHFR	Ala222Val polymorphism	Folic acid intake	Homozygotes for the low activity Ala222Val variant are at different risk of colorectal cancer and adenomas if nutritional folate status is low	214
NAT2	Rapid versus slow acetylator SNPs	Heterocyclic amines in cooled meat	Red meat intake is more strongly associated with colorectal cancer among rapid acetylators	215
F5	Leiden prothrombotic variant	Hormone replacement	Venous thromboembolism risk is increased in Factor V Leiden carriers who take exogenous steroid hormones	216
UGT1A6	Slow metabolism SNPs	Aspirin	Increased benefit of prophylactic aspirin use in carriers of the slow metabolism variants	217
APOE	E4 allele	Cholesterol intake	Exaggerated changes in serum cholesterol in response to dietary cholesterol changes in APOE4 carriers	218
ADH1C	γ-2 alleles	Alcohol intake	Inverse association between ethanol intake and myocardial infarction; risk is stronger in carriers of slow-oxidizing γ-2 alleles	219
PPARG2	Pro12Ala	Dietary fat intake	Stronger relation between dietary fat intake and obesity in carriers of the Pro12Ala allele	220
HLA-DPB1	Glu69	Occupational beryllium	Exposed workers who are carriers of the Glu69 allele are more likely to develop chronic beryllium lung disease	221
TPMT	Ala154Thr and Tyr240Cys	Thiopurine drugs	Homozygotes for the low-activity alleles of TPMT are likely to experience severe toxicity when exposed to thiopurine drugs	222
ADRB2	Arg16Gly	Asthma drugs	Arg16Gly homozygotes have a greater response in the airway to albuterol	223

[a]Abbreviations: ADH1C, alcohol dehydrogenase 1C (class 1), γ-polypeptide; ADRB2, adrenergic β-2 receptor; CCR5, chemokine (C–C motif) receptor 5; APOE, apolipoprotein E; F5, coagulation factor V; HIV, human immunodeficiency virus; HLA-DPB1, major histocompatibility complex, class II, DP β-1; MC1R, melanocortin receptor 1; MTHFR, 5,10-methylenetetrahydrofolate reductase (NADPH); NAT2, N-acetyltransferase 2; PPARG2, peroxisome proliferative activated receptor-γ; TPMT, thiopurine-S-methyltransferase; UGT1A6, UDP-glycosyltransferase-1 family, polypeptide A6.
Source: From Ref. 15.

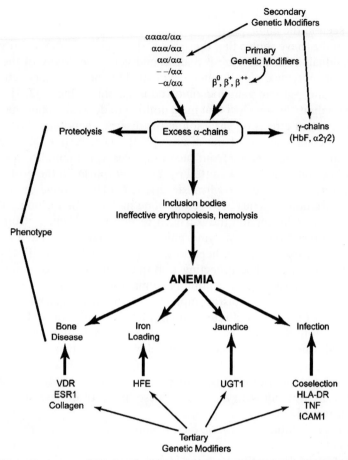

FIGURE 21.23 Summary of the genetic contributions to phenotypic diversity of the β-thalassemias. The secondary modifiers, the α- and γ-globin genes, are shown at the top of the figure. The tertiary modifiers are shown at the bottom of the figure. VDR, vitamin D receptor; ESR1, estrogen receptor; collagen, several genes determined in collagen synthesis; HFE, the locus for hereditary hemochromatosis; UGT1, UGT glucuronyltransferase involved in bilirubin glucuronidation; HLA-DR, major histocompatibility complex locus; TNF, tumor necrosis factor-α; ICAM1, intercellular adhesion molecule 1. (Adapted from Ref. 224 with permission of the author and Nature Publishing Group.)

at genetic loci that are not involved in globin production but that might modify the complications of the disease in many different ways (Fig. 21.23).

Well over 200 different mutations have been identified in the β-globin genes of β-thalassemia patients with the majority being point mutations or the deletion of one or two bases [225, 226]. The primary genetic cause of the resulting phenotypes is described by the complete loss of β-globin gene product (β°) and the moderate or marked reduction in the normal output of β-globin gene product (β+ and β++, respectively) (Fig. 21.23). The location of the mutation in the genomic DNA as well as the degree of recessive or dominant mode of inheritance of these mutations and the stability of the gene products play major roles in the primary cause of the final phenotype seen in the clinic [224].

Clinical studies have shown that there is a wide diversity in the severity of disease among individuals with the same β-thalassemia genotype. Many of these unusual examples of phenotypic diversity can be explained by the secondary action of products of the α- and γ-globin gene loci involved in globin synthesis [224].

Finally, variability at gene loci that have nothing to do with globin chain synthesis may have important effects on variation in the disease phenotype, particularly with respect to the complications of the disease [224]. These tertiary genetic causes of phenotypic diversity may come from such examples as (1) jaundice resulting from the alteration of bilirubin levels caused by a polymorphism in the promoter region of the gene for UDP-glucuronosyltransferase (UGT1); (2) bone disease resulting from allelic variation in genes involved in bone metabolism, including the vitamin D receptor gene, collagen, and the estrogen receptor; (3) damage from variations in iron loading resulting from polymorphisms in the HFE locus and causing such complications as cardiac disease, hepatic disease, and diabetes; and (4) phenotypic variation due to coselection reflecting a β-thalassemia heterozygote advantage against malaria. The varying susceptibility to malaria is also reflected by polymorphic variation in the major histocompatibility complex loci (HLA-DR), tumor necrosis factor-α (TNF-α), and intercellular adhesion molecule 1 (ICAM1).

Molecular profiles of the primary, secondary, and tertiary genetic variables for the β-thalassemias are obviously complex and mechanistically incomplete. Therefore, the major task of including enviromic data in these molecular profiles is still a daunting undertaking and will be a major obstacle to overcome in the associative analyses leading to a complete description of disease, drug, and therapeutic phenotypes [224].

A similar classification of genetic factors could be devised for the general drug phenotype category in pharmacogenomics. The candidate gene approach and the modular biology of drug action both lend themselves to a division of genetic factors into primary, secondary, and tertiary causes. Polymorphisms altering drug metabolism, transport, or target function could be considered the primary factors.

The association of primary genetic factors with phenotype in pharmacogenomics is currently restricted to polymorphic variation in drug metabolizing enzymes in accessible tissues like erythrocytes and leukocytes [59]. Phenotyping involves direct measurement of enzyme activity or the determination of the metabolic ratio of a probe drug (Table 21.5). Since determination of enzyme activity can be problematic, the administration of probe drugs to the patient and determination of drug and metabolite levels resulting from metabolism of the probe drug in the liver is the common technique for determination of drug phenotype [59]. The majority of phenotyping studies have analyzed the levels and polymorphic variations of metabolizing enzymes, and there have been few such studies on the effects of variation in drug transport proteins or receptor proteins. Application of the candidate gene approach and the modular biology concept in the therapeutic drug pathway to pharmacogenomics will begin to correct this shortfall.

The interaction between genes and the environment in which they exist is not only a cornerstone to evolutionary theory but plays a critical role in disease pathology and drug therapy. A study of the effect of genes and environment on disease development and drug therapy requires a serious effort to assess environmental risk

TABLE 21.5   Phenotyping Methods for Analysis of Pharmacogenetic Polymorphisms

Gene[a]	Method or Probe Drug	Type of Sample	References
Cholinesterase	Enzyme inhibition	Plasma	227
COMT	Enzyme levels	Erythrocytes	228
CYP1A1	Induced enzyme activity	Lymphocytes	229
CYP1A2	Caffeine	Blood, urine, and saliva	230, 231
CYP2A6	Coumarin	Urine	232
CYP2C9	Tolbutamide	Urine	233
CYP2C19	Mephenytoin	Urine	234
CYP2C19	Omeprazole	Urine	235
CYP2D6	Debrisoquine	Urine	236
CYP2D6	Sparetine	Urine	237
CYP2D6	Dextromethorphan	Urine	238
CYP2D6	Metoprolol	Urine	239
CYP2E1	Chlorzoxazone	Blood	240
CYP2E1	Direct measurement	Lymphocytes	241
CYP 3A4	Midazolam	Blood	242
CYP 3A4	6-Hydroxycortisol	Urine	243
CYP 3A4	Erythromycin breath test	Breath test	244
FMO3	Trimethylamine	Urine	245
GSTM1	Enzyme levels	Leukocytes	246
GSTT1	Enzyme levels	Erythrocytes	247
NAT1	4-Aminobenzoate	Urine	248
NAT2	Caffeine	Urine	249
Paraoxonase	Enzyme levels	Plasma	250
Sulfotransferase	Enzyme levels	Platelet	251, 252
TPMT	Enzyme levels	Erythrocytes	253
P-glycoprotein	Digoxin	Blood	254

[a]Abbreviations: COMT, catechol-*O*-methyltransferase; CYP, cytochrome P450; FMO, flavin-linked monooxygenase; GST, glutathione *S*-transferase; NAT, *N*-acetyltransferase; TPMT, thiopurine methyltransferase.
Source: Adapted from Ref. 59 with kind permission of the author and Springer Science and Business Media.

factors and not to simply treat them as a "binary indicator variable for 'exposed or not' or as a black box of correlated residual variation. It entails serious consideration of exogenous exposures as complex, multivariate, time-dependent variables, along with an understanding of the metabolic pathways that influence the internal environment and the genes that regulate these pathways" [255]. Obtaining high quality information on environment and lifestyle in conjunction with biological samples to assess genetic variants in genes responsible for producing the proteins of a therapeutic drug pathway, as well as a consistent and accurate evaluation of therapeutic outcomes, will be a difficult and complex, but crucial, task in the assessment of gene–environment interactions for drug therapy [15].

Well designed studies of gene–environment interactions are assessed using either a qualitative (Table 21.6) [15, 256–258] or statistical model [15, 259]. However, the complexity of screening a large number of potential gene–environment interactions in populations with a large number of genotypes and many variables of environmental exposure greatly increases the chance of finding false-positive results at

TABLE 21.6 Some Patterns of Relative Risk in Gene–Environment Interactions for Three Classical Genetic Diseases that Have an Environmental Component, Assuming Dichotomous Genetic Susceptibility and Environmental Exposure.

Gene Variant	Environmental Exposure	Relative Risk (XP)[a]	Relative Risk (PKU)[b]	Relative Risk (Emphysema)[c]
Absent	Absent	1.0	1.0	1.0
Present	Absent	~1.0	1.0	Modest
Absent	Present	Modest	1.0	Modest
Present	Present	Very high	Very high	High

[a] In the XP (xeroderma pigmentosum) example, exposure to ultraviolet light increases the risk of developing skin cancer in noncarriers of XP mutations. The combination of these mutations and exposure to ultraviolet light vastly increases the risk of skin cancer. In theory, if individuals with XP mutations completely avoid ultraviolet light, their risk of skin cancer becomes close to the background risk.
[b] In the PKU (phenylketonuria) example, only individuals with recessive mutations in the causative gene (phenylalanine hydroxylase) who are exposed to phenylalanine in the diet are susceptible to PKU.
[c] In the emphysema example, with a deficiency in the α-1 antitrypsin gene, both nonsmokers who are at genetic risk and smokers who are not at genetic risk have an increased risk of developing emphysema, and the combination (smokers who are at genetic risk) is associated with the highest risk.
Source: From Ref. 15. Data from Refs. 256 and 257.

conventional levels of statistical significance [15]. Most studies are not powerful enough to detect modest interactions and demanding small p values to counteract this problem will result in a lower probability of declaring true-positive interactions as "significant." A plausible option is to restrict the search for gene–environment interactions to those that involve gene products and environmental exposures that interact in the same biological pathways. Further restricting analysis to gene variants that alter gene function within the biological pathways may also reduce the complexity of the analysis, although for variants that affect gene regulation this science is in its infancy [260]. Therefore, the application of the candidate gene approach to pharmacogenomic analysis may prove useful in the analysis of gene–environment interactions as well, especially when one utilizes the "modular biology" concept to simplify the biochemical pathways of drug response [261, 262].

21.6 CONCLUSION

The preclinical development of genetic data for application in the pharmacogenomics of disease therapy and management has become far more complex than the earlier studies had suggested. The Mendelian single gene pharmacogenetic approach to personalized medicine will be limited to a small number of phase I (CYP2D6, CYP2C9, CYP2C19) and phase II (TPMT, UGT) metabolic enzymes that can be directly linked to toxicity or efficacy problems through a demonstration of a genetic link to "poor metabolism" or "ultra metabolism" of a particular drug. The next stages beyond the single gene approach are the candidate genes and the whole genome approaches to pharmacogenomics. While the application of linkage disequilibrium to SNP analysis and the development of the HapMap in the whole genome approach to pharmacogenomics is conceptually the most comprehensive application of allelic variation to disease diagnosis and drug therapy in personalized medicine, the number of SNPs that must be determined for each patient may be a prohibitive factor. The current application of htSNPs in candidate genes, determined through the development of a drug therapeutic pathway using the modular biology approach to assess the pharmacokinetic and pharmacodynamic parameters, may be the technique that reduces the number of SNPs that must be determined to a level that is financially feasible and sufficiently reproducibly accurate to apply to the clinical environment of personalized medicine.

The correlation of genetic variation in the genes involved in a drug's pharmacokinetics of distribution in the body and pharmacodynamics of action on the body is not likely to provide sufficient information for successful personalized medicine. One must also accept the fact that gene transcription, translation, and protein function involve genetically independent mechanisms that will modify the correlation of genotype with phenotype. As a result, it will be important to augment the genetic biomarkers with transcriptomic, proteomic, and metabolomic biomarkers in order to assure a successful application of personalized medicine in a clinical environment.

While the technology for the high throughput genotyping required of candidate gene analysis is highly developed, there is room for cheaper high throughput methods with more effective elimination of false positives while maintaining sensitivity. Also, extensive technology development will be required to get the application of high throughput in transcriptomics, proteomics, and metabolomics to acceptable standards for the clinic. The main hurdle looming on the pharmacogenomic horizon is the envirome. The genotype–phenotype correlation in disease diagnosis and therapy cannot escape interaction with the environment. And nowhere will the effects of environment be felt greater than in disease diagnosis and assessment of therapeutic outcome. Health care professionals will become more adept at selecting and accurately assessing critical environmental factors and their interactions with the many genomic, transcriptomic, proteomic, and metabolomic molecular biomarkers in the diagnosis of disease, choice of therapeutic agent (or not), and assessment of therapeutic outcome or proactive predict-and-manage approach.

This endeavor will require the education of health care professionals in the application of these technologies and education of the public on what it means to have a genetic test. It will also require the education of politicians and policy makers on the efficient utilization of the technology to both reduce health care costs, over the long term, and at the same time protect the individual's personal information and right to privacy. There will also be a large requirement for health informatics to handle the huge amount of data that will arise from the various clinical studies in developing the pharmacogenomics database, as well as a demand for user friendly access to the information by health care professionals who do not have the time nor the inclination to spend hours learning a computer program. Some of the biggest challenges for pharmacogenomics lie in handling the information. Innovation and technology tend to outstrip the development of good algorithms and software to complement them. There is a need for better software to collect, organize, and interpret data. Since pharmacogenomics is a combination of several different areas of research, we need to work on sharing and combining different types of biological information, rather than trying to generate it faster. The development of pharmacogenomics for effective and efficient disease diagnosis and therapy in the clinic will depend heavily on the cooperation and collaboration of a number of different scientific communities involved in the many aspects of genome research.

ACKNOWLEDGMENTS

I am deeply in debt to a number of individuals who have taken time out of their busy schedules to read and comment on this chapter. The quality of the content and presentation of the information in this chapter was greatly improved by the criticisms and corrections provided by Dan Koboldt, David Wishart, Zhming Jiang, and Tom Pfeifer, for which I thank them profusely. In the final judgment, however, the responsibility for any remaining errors and omissions is mine.

REFERENCES

1. Garrod AE. The incidence of alkaptonuria: a study in chemical individulity. *Lancet* 1902;2:1616–1620.
2. Forbat A, Lehmann H, Silk E. Prolonged apoena following injection of succinyldicholine. *Lancet* 1953;Nov 21:1067–1068.
3. Kalow W. Familial incidence of low pseudocholinesetrase level. *Lancet* 1956;Sept 15:576–577.
4. Lehmann H, Ryan E. The familial incidence of low pseudocholinesterase level. *Lancet* 1956;July 21:124.
5. Price Evans DA, Manley KA, McKusick VA. Genetic control of isoniazid metabolism in man. *Br Med J* 1960;Aug 13:485–491.
6. Carson PE, Flanagan CL, Ickes CE, Alving AS. Enzymatic deficiency in primaquine-sensitive erythrocytes. *Science* 1956;124:484–485.
7. Williams RJ. *Biochemical Individuality. The Basis of the Genetotrophic Concept.* Austin: University of Texas Press;1956.
8. Motulsky AG. Drug reactions, enzymes and biochemical genetics. *JAMA* 1957;165:835–837.
9. Vogel F. Moderne probleme der humangenetik. *Ergebnisse der Innere Medizinische und Kinderheilkunde* 1959;12:52–62.
10. Watson JD, Crick FHC. Molecular structure of nucleic acids. *Nature* 1953;171:737–738.
11. Guttmacher AE, Collins FS. Genomic medicine—a primer. *N Engl J Med* 2002;347:1512–1520.
12. Wang J, Fan JB, Siao CJ, Berno A, Young P, Saplosky R, Ghandour G, Perkins N, Winchester E, Spenser J, Kruglyak L, Stein L, Hsie L, Topaloglou T, Hubbell E, Robinsion E, Mittmann M, Morris MS, Shen N, Kilburn D, Rioux J, Nusbaum C, Rozen S, Hudson TJ, Lander ES. Large-scale identification, mapping, and genotyping of single-nucleotide polymorphisms in the human genome. *Science* 1998;280:1077–1082.
13. HGP. The human genome. Science genome map. *Science* 2001;291:1218.
14. Brockmoller J, Kirchheiner J, Meisel C, Roots I. Pharmacogenetic diagnostics of cytochrome P450 polymorphisms in clinical drug development and in drug treatment. *Pharmacogenomics* 2000;1:125–151.
15. Hunter DJ. Gene–environment interactions In human diseases. *Nat Rev Genet* 2005;6:287–298.
16. Kirchheiner J, Fuhr U, Brockmoller J. Opinion: Pharmacogenetics-based therapeutic recommendations—ready for clinical practice? *Nat Rev Drug Discov* 2005;4:639–647.
17. Kirchheiner J, Brockmoller J. Clinical consequences of cytochrome P450 2C9 polymorphisms. *Clin Pharmacol Ther* 2005;77:1–16.

18. Roses AD. Pharmacogenetics and the practice of medicine. *Nature* 2000;405:857–865.

19. Risch N, Merikangas K. The future of genetic studies of complex human diseases. *Science* 1996;273:1516–1517.

20. Collins FS, Guyer MS, Charkravarti A. Variations on a theme: cataloging human DNA sequence variation. *Science* 1997;278:1580–1581.

21. Daly MJ, Rioux JD, Schaffner SF, Hudson TJ, Lander ES. High-resolution haplotype structure in the human genome. *Nat Genet* 2001;29:229–232.

22. Gabriel SB, Schaffner SF, Nguyen H, Moore JM, Roy J, Blumenstiel B, Higgins J, DeFelice M, Lochner A, Faggart M, Liu-Cordero SN, Rotimi C, Adeyemo A, Cooper R, Ward R, Lander ES, Daly MJ, Altshuler D. The structure of haplotype blocks in the human genome. *Science* 2002;296:2225–2229.

23. Consortium TIH. The International HapMap Project. *Nature* 2003;426:789–796.

24. Taillon-Miller P, Saccone SF, Saccone NL, Duan S, Kloss EF, Lovins EG, Donaldson R, Phong A, Ha C, Flagstad L, Miller S, Drendel A, Lind D, Miller RD, Rice JP, Kwok PY. Linkage disequilibrium maps constructed with common SNPs are useful for first-pass disease association screens. *Genomics* 2004;84:899–912.

25. Johnson GC, Esposito L, Barratt BJ, Smith AN, Heward J, Di Genova G, Ueda H, Cordell HJ, Eaves IA, Dudbridge F, Twells RC, Payne F, Hughes W, Nutland S, Stevens H, Carr P, Tuomilehto-Wolf E, Tuomilehto J, Gough SC, Clayton DG, Todd JA. Haplotype tagging for the identification of common disease genes. *Nat Genet* 2001;29:233–237.

26. Ahmadi KR, Weale ME, Xue ZY, Soranzo N, Yarnall DP, Briley JD, Maruyama Y, Kobayashi M, Wood NW, Spurr NK, Burns DK, Roses AD, Saunders AM, Goldstein DB. A single-nucleotide polymorphism tagging set for human drug metabolism and transport. *Nat Genet* 2005;37:84–89.

27. Goldstein DB, Ahmadi KR, Weale ME, Wood NW. Genome scans and candidate gene approaches in the study of common diseases and variable drug responses. *Trends Genet* 2003;19:615–622.

28. Deloukas P, Bentley D. The HapMap project and its application to genetic studies of drug response. *Pharmacogenomics J* 2004;4:88–90.

29. Lin M, Aquilante C, Johnson JA, Wu R. Sequencing drug response with HapMap. *Pharmacogenomics J* 2005;5:149–156.

30. Kamatani N, Sekine A, Kitamoto T, Iida A, Saito S, Kogame A, Inoue E, Kawamoto M, Harigai M, Nakamura Y. Large-scale single-nucleotide polymorphism. (SNP) and haplotype analyses, using dense SNP Maps, of 199 drug-related genes in 752 subjects: the analysis of the association between uncommon SNPs within haplotype blocks and the haplotypes constructed with haplotype-tagging SNPs. *Am J Hum Genet* 2004;75:190–203.

31. Reich DE, Cargill M, Bolk S, Ireland J, Sabeti PC, Richter DJ, Lavery T, Kouyoumjian R, Farhadian SF, Ward R, Lander ES. Linkage disequilibrium in the human genome. *Nature* 2001;411:199–204.

32. Sachidanandam R, Weissman D, Schmidt SC, Kakol JM, Stein LD, Marth G, Sherry S, Mullikin JC, Mortimore BJ, Willey DL, Hunt SE, Cole CG, Coggill PC, Rice CM, Ning Z, Rogers J, Bentley DR, Kwok PY, Mardis ER, Yeh RT, Schultz B, Cook L, Davenport R, Dante M, Fulton L, Hillier L, Waterston RH, McPherson JD, Gilman B, Schaffner S, Van Etten WJ, Reich D, Higgins J, Daly MJ, Blumenstiel B, Baldwin J, Stange-Thomann N, Zody MC, Linton L, Lander ES, Altshuler D. A map of human genome sequence variation containing 1.42 million single nucleotide polymorphisms. *Nature* 2001;409:928–933.

33. Weiss KM, Terwilliger JD. How many diseases does it take to map a gene with SNPs? *Nat Genet* 2000;26:151–157.

34. Roberts L. Human genome research. SNP mappers confront reality and find it daunting. *Science* 2000;287:1898–1899.

35. Kruglyak L. Prospects for whole-genome linkage disequilibrium mapping of common disease genes. *Nat Genet* 1999;22:139–144.

36. Collins A, Lonjou C, Morton NE. Genetic epidemiology of single-nucleotide polymorphisms. *Proc Natl Acad Sci USA* 1999;96:15173–15177.

37. Griffin JL, Shockcor JP. Metabolic profiles of cancer cells. *Nat Rev Cancer* 2004;4:551–561.

38. Hieter P, Boguski M. Functional genomics: it's all how you read it. *Science* 1997;278:601–602.

39. Fierz W. Challenge of personalized health care: to what extent is medicine already individualized and what are the future trends? *Med Sci Monit* 2004;10:RA111–RA123.

40. Bordet R, Gautier S, Le Louet H, Dupuis B, Caron J. Analysis of the direct cost of adverse drug reactions in hospitalised patients. *Eur J Clin Pharmacol* 2001;56:935–941.

41. Suh DC, Woodall BS, Shin SK, Hermes-De Santis ER. Clinical and economic impact of adverse drug reactions in hospitalized patients. *Ann Pharmacother* 2000;34:1373–1379.

42. du Souich P. In human therapy, is the drug–drug interaction or the adverse drug reaction the issue? *Can J Clin Pharmacol* 2001;8:153–161.

43. Ginsburg GS, McCarthy JJ. Personalized medicine: revolutionizing drug discovery and patient care. *Trends Biotechnol* 2001;19:491–496.

44. Collins FS, Green ED, Guttmacher AE, Guyer MS. A vision for the future of genomics research. *Nature* 2003;422:835–847.

45. Ross JS, Ginsburg GS. The integration of molecular diagnostics with therapeutics. Implications for drug development and pathology practice. *Am J Clin Pathol* 2003;119:26–36.

46. Meyer JM, Ginsburg GS. The path to personalized medicine. *Curr Opin Chem Biol* 2002;6:434–438.

47. Senn S. Individual response to treatment: is it a valid assumption? *BMJ* 2004;329:966–968.

48. Jain KK. From molecular diagnostics to personalized medicine. The IBC Workshop, London, UK, 1st May 2002. *Expert Rev Mol Diagn* 2002;2:299–301.

49. Evans WE, Relling MV. Moving towards individualized medicine with pharmacogenomics. *Nature* 2004;429:464–468.

50. Group BDW. Biomarkers and surrogate endpoints: preferred definitions and conceptual framework. *Clin Pharmacol Ther* 2001;69:89–95.

51. Lewin DA, Weiner MP. Molecular biomarkers in drug development. *Drug Discov Today* 2004;9:976–983.

52. Lesko LJ. *Guidance for Industry: Pharmacogenomic Data Submissions*. Washington, DC: US Department of Health and Human Services, Food and Drug Administration, CDER, CBER, CDRH; 2003. http://www.fda.gov/cder/guidance/5900dfp.pdf.

53. Koch WH. Technology platforms for pharmacogenomic diagnostic assays. *Nat Rev Drug Discov* 2004;3:749–761.

54. Singleton P, Sainsbury D. *Dictionary of Microbiology and Molecular Biology*. Hoboken, NJ: Wiley-Interscience;1994.

55. Anthony JC. The promise of psychiatric enviromics. *Br J Psychiatry Suppl* 2001;40:s8–s11.

56. Bezold C, Halpern JA, Eng JL. *2020 Visions: Health Care Information Standards and Technologies*. Rockville, MD: The United States Pharmacopoeial Convention, Inc; 1993.

57. Romkes M, Buch SC. Genotyping technologies: application to biotransformation enzyme genetic polymorphism screening. *Methods Mol Biol* 2005;291:399–414.

58. Kwok P-Y, Chen X. Detection of single nucleotide polymorphisms. *Curr Issues Mol Biol* 2003;5:43–60.

59. Daly AK. Development of analytical technology in pharmacogenetic research. *Naunyn Schmiedebergs Arch Pharmacol* 2004;369:133–140.

60. Twyman RM. SNP discovery and typing technologies for pharmacogenomics. *Curr Top Med Chem* 2004;4:1423–1431.

61. Shi MM. Enabling large-scale pharmacogenetic studies by high-throughput mutation detection and genotyping technologies. *Clin Chem* 2001;47:164–172.

62. Cargill M, Altshuler D, Ireland J, Sklar P, Ardlie K, Patil N, Lane CR, Lim EP, Kalayanaraman N, Nemesh J, Ziaugra J, Friedland L, Rolfe A, Warrington J, Lipshutz RJ, Daley GQ, Lander ES. Characterization of single-nucleotide polymorphisms in coding regions of human genes. *Nat Genet* 1999;22:231–238.

63. Halushka MK, Fan JB, Bentley K, Hsie L, Shen N, Weder A, Cooper R, Lipshutz RJ, Chakravarti A. Patterns of single-nucleotide polymorphisms in candidate genes for blood-pressure homeostasis. *Nat Genet* 1999;22:239–247.

64. Carlson CS, Newman TL, Nickerson DA. SNPing in the human genome. *Curr Opin Chem Biol* 2001;5:78–85.

65. Kirk BW, Feinsod M, Favis R, Kliman RM, Barany F. Single nucleotide polymorphism seeking long term association with complex disease. *Nucleic Acids Res* 2002;30:3295–3311.

66. Syvanen AC. Accessing genetic variation: genotyping single nucleotide polymorphisms. *Nat Rev Genet* 2001;2:930–942.

67. Kwok P-Y. High-throughput genotyping assay approaches. *Pharmacogenomics* 2000;1:95–100.

68. Mullis KB, Faloona FA. Specific synthesis of DNA *in vitro* via a polymerase-catalyzed chain reaction. *Methods Enzymol* 1987;155:335–350.

69. Saiki RK, Walsh PS, Levenson CH, Erlich HA. Genetic analysis of amplified DNA with immobilized sequence-specific oligonucleotide probes. *Proc Natl Acad Sci USA* 1989;86:6230–6234.

70. Mei R, Galipeau PC, Prass C, Berno A, Ghandour G, Patil N, Wolff RK, Chee MS, Reid BJ, Lockhart DJ. Genome-wide detection of allelic imbalance using human SNPs and high-density DNA arrays. *Genome Res* 2000;10:11126–11137.

71. Hacia JG, Sun B, Hunt N, Edgemon K, Mosbrook D, Robbins C, Fodor SP, Tagle DA, Collins FS. Strategies for mutational analysis of the large multiexon ATM gene using high-density oligonucleotide arrays. *Genome Res* 1998;8:1245–1258.

72. Emahazion T, Feuk L, Jobs M, Sawyer SL, Fredman D, St Clair D, Prince JA, Brookes AJ. SNP association studies in Alzheimer's disease highlight problems for complex disease analysis. *Trends Genet* 2001;17:407–413.

73. Howell WM, Jobs M, Gyllensten U, Brookes AJ. Dynamic allele-specific hybridization. A new method for scoring single nucleotide polymorphisms. *Nat Biotechnol* 1999;17:87–88.

74. Tyagi S, Bratu DP, Kramer FR. Multicolor molecular beacons for allele discrimination. *Nat Biotechnol* 1998;16:49–53.

75. Kostrikis S, Tyagi S, Mhlanga MM, Ho DD, Kramer FR. Spectral genotyping of human alleles. *Science* 1998;279:1228–1229.

76. Livak KJ. Allelic discrimination using fluorogenic probes and the 5′-nuclease assay. *Genet Anal* 1999;14:143–149.

77. Latif S, Bauer-Sardina I, Ranade K, Livak K, Kwok P-Y. Fluorescence polarization in homogeneous nucleic acid analysis II: 5′-nuclease assay. *Genome Res* 2001;11:436–440.

78. Hsu TM, Law SM, Duan S, Neri B, Kwok P-Y. Genotyping single nucleotide polymorphisms by the Invader assay with dual-color fluorescence polarization detection. *Clin Chem* 2001;47:1373–1377.

79. Kaiser MW, Lyamicheva N, Ma W, Miller C, Neri B, Fors L, Lyamichev VI. A comparison of eubacterial and archaeal structure-specific 5′-exonucleases. *J Biol Chem* 1999;274:21387–21394.

80. Kwiatkowksi RW, Lyamichev VI, de Arruda M, Neri B. Clinical, genetic, and pharmacogenetic applications of the Invader assay. *Mol Diagn* 1999;4:353–364.

81. Lyamichev VI, Kaiser MW, Lyamicheva NE, Vologodskii AV, Hall JG, Ma WP, Allawi HT, Neri B. Experimental and theoretical analysis of the invasive signal amplification reaction. *Biochemistry* 2000;39:9523–9532.

82. Hall JG, Eis PS, Law SM, Reynaldo LP, Prudent JR, Marshall DJ, Allawi HT, Mast AL, Dahlberg JE, Kwiatkowski RW, de Arruda M, Neri BP, Lyamichev VI. Sensitive detection of DNA polymorphisms by the serial invasive signal amplification reaction. *Proc Natl Acad Sci USA* 2000;97:8272–8277.

83. Sosnowski RG, Tu E, Butler WF, O'Connell JP, Heller MJ. Rapid determination of single base mismaatch mutations in DNA hybrids by electric field control. *Proc Nat Acad Sci USA* 1997;94:1119–1123.

84. Edman CF, Raymond DE, Wu DJ, Tu E, Sosnowski RG, Butler WF, Nerenberg M, Heller MJ. Electric field directed nucleic acid hybridization by electric fleld control. *Nucleic Acids Res* 1997;25:4907–4914.

85. Cornell BA, Braach-Maksvytis VL, King LG, Osman PD, Raguse B, Wieczorek L, Pace RJ. A biosensor that uses ion channel switches. *Nature* 1997;387:580–583.

86. Wang J, Cai X, Rivas G, Shiraishi H, Dontha N. Nucleic-acid immobilization, recognition and detection at chronopotentiometric DNAchips. *Biosens Bioelectron* 1997;12:587–599.

87. Heller MJ, Forster AH, Tu E. Active microeletronic chip devices which utilize controlled electrophoretic fields for multiplex DNA hybridization and other genomic applications. *Electrophoresis* 2000;21:157–164.

88. Radtkey R, Feng L, Muralhidar M, Duhon M, Canter D, DiPierro D, Fallon S, Tu E, McElfresh K, Nerenberg M, Sosnowski R. Rapid, high fidelity analysis of simple sequence repeats on an electronically active DNA microchip. *Nucleic Acids Res* 2000;28:E17.

89. Westin L, Xu X, Miller C, Wang L, Edman CF, Nerenberg M. Anchored multiplex amplification on a microelectronic chip array. *Nat Biotechnol* 2000;18:199–204.

90. Todd AV, Fuery CJ, Impey HL, Applegate TL, Haughton MA. DzyNA-PCR; use of DNAzymes to detect and quantify nucleic acid sequences in a real-time fluorescent format. *Clin Chem* 2000;46:625–630.

91. Myakishev MV, Khripin Y, Hu S, Hamer DH. High-throughput SNP genotyping by allele-specific PCR with universal energy-transfer-labeled primers. *Genome Res* 2001;11:163–169.

92. Germer S, Higuchi R. Single-tube genotyping without oligonucleotide probes. *Genome Res* 1999;9:72–78.

93. Beaudet L, Bedard J, Breton B, Mercuri RJ, Budarf ML. Homogeneous assays for single-nucleotide polymorphism typing using AlphaScreen. *Genome Res* 2001;11:600–608.

94. Nazarenko IA, Bhatnagar SK, Hohman RJ. A closed tube format for amplification and detection of DNA based on energy transfer. *Nucleic Acids Res* 1997;25:2516–2521.

95. Whitcombe D, Theaker J, Guy SP, Brown T, Little S. Detection of PCR products using self-probing amplicons and fluorescence. *Nat Biotechnol* 1999;17:804–807.

96. Pastinen T, Raitio M, Lindroos K, Tainola P, Peltonen L, Syvanen AC. A system for specific, high-throughput genotyping by allele-specific primer extension on microarrays. *Genome Res* 2000;10:1031–1042.

97. Tonisson N, Kurg A, Kaasik K, Lohmussaar E, Metspalu A. Unravelling genetic data by arrayed primer extension. *Clin Chem Lab Med* 2000;38:165–170.

98. Shumaker JM, Metspalu A, Caskey CT. Mutation detection by solid phase primer extension. *Hum Mutat* 1996;7:346–354.

99. Pastinen T, Kurg A, Metspalu A, Peltonen L, Syvanen AC. Minisequencing: a specific tool for DNA analysis and diagnostics on oligonucleotide arrays. *Genome Res* 1997;7:606–614.

100. Dubiley S, Kirillov E, Mirzabekov A. Polymorphism analysis and gene detection by minisequencing on an array of gel-immobilized primers. *Nucleic Acids Res* 1999;27:E19.

101. Hsu TM, Chen X, Duan S, Miller R, Kwok P-Y. A universal SNP genotyping assay with fluorescence polarization detection. *BioTechniques* 2001;31:560–570.

102. Chen X, Kwok P-Y. Template-directed dye-terminator incorporation (TDI) assay: a homogeneous DNA diagnostic method based on fluorescence energy transfer. *Nucleic Acids Res* 1997;25:347–353.

103. Chen X, Zehnbauer B, Gnirke A, Kwok P-Y. Fluorescence energy transfer detection as a homogeneous DNA diagnostic method. *Proc Nat Acad Sci USA* 1997;94: 10756–10761.

104. Chen X, Levine L, Kwok P-Y. Fluorescence polarization in homogeneous nucleic acid analysis. *Genome Res* 1999;9:492–498.

105. Buetow KH, Edmonson M, MacDonald R, Clifford R, Yip P, Kelley J, Little DP, Strausberg R, Koester H, Cantor CR, Braun A. High-throughput development and characterization of a genome wide collection of gene-based single nucleotide polymorphism markers by chip-based matrix-assisted laser desorption/ionization time-of-flight mass spectrometry. *Proc Nat Acad Sci USA* 1996;98:581–584.

106. Ross P, Hall L, Smirnov I, Haff L. High level multiplex genotyping by MALDI-TOF mass spectrometry. *Nature Biotechnol* 1998;16:1347–1351.

107. Sauer S, Lechner D, Berlin K, Lehrach H, Escary JL, Fox N, Gut IG. A novel procedure for efficient genotyping of single nucleotide polymorphisms. *Nucleic Acids Res* 2000;28:E13.

108. Braun A, Little DP, Koster H. Detecting CFTR gene mutations by using primer oligo base extension and mass spectrometry. *Clin Chem* 1997;43:1151–1158.

109. Nordstrom T, Nourizad K, Ronaghi M, Nyren P. Method enabling pyrosequencing on double-stranded DNA. *Anal Biochem* 2000;282:186–193.

110. Ahmadian A, Gharizadeh B, Gustafsson AC. Single-nucleotide polymorphism analysis by pyrosequencing. *Anal Biochem* 2000;280:103–110.

111. Ronaghi M. Pyrosequencing sheds light on DNA sequencing. *Genome Res* 2001;11:3–11.

112. Alderborn A, Kristofferson A, Hammerling U. Determination of single-nucleotide polymorphisms by real-time pyrophosphate DNA sequencing. *Genome Res* 2000;10: 1249–1258.

113. Nyren P, Pettersson B, Uhlen M. Solid phase DNA minisequencing by an enzymatic luminometric inorganic pyrophosphate detection assay. *Anal Biochem* 1993;208: 171–175.

114. Fan JB, Chen X, Halushka MK, Berno A, Huang X, Ryder T, Lipshutz RJ, Lockhart DJ, Chakravarti A. Parallel genotyping of human SNPs using generic high-density oligonucleotide tag arrays. *Genome Res* 2000;10:853–860.

115. Chen J, Iannone MA, Li MS, Taylor JD, Rivers P, Nelsen AJ, Slentz-Kesler KA, Roses A, Weiner MP. A microsphere-based assay for multiplexed single nucleotide polymorphism analysis using single base chain extension. *Genome Res* 2000;10:549–557.

116. Cai H, White PS, Torney D, Deshpande A, Wang Z, Keller RA, Marrone B, Nolan JP. Flow cytometry-based minisequencing: a new platform for high-throughput single-nucleotide polymorphism scoring. *Genomics* 2000;66:135–143.

117. Hirschhorn JN, Sklar P, Lindblad-Toh K, Lim YM, Ruiz-Gutierrez M, Bolk S, Langhorst B, Schaffner S, Winchester E, Lander ES. SBE-TAGS: an array-based method for efficient single-nucleotide polymorphism genotyping. *Proc Natl Acad Sci USA* 2000; 97:12164–12169.

118. Nickerson DA, Kaiser R, Lappin S, Stewart J, Hood L, Landegren U. Automated DNA diagnostics using an ELISA-based oligonucleotide ligation assay. *Proc Natl Acad Sci USA* 1990;87:8923–8927.

119. Grossman PD, Bloch W, Brinson E, Chang CC, Eggerding FA, Fung S, Iovannisci DM, Woo S, Winn-Deen ES. High-density multiplex detection of nucleic acid sequences: oligonucleotide ligation assay and sequence-coded separation. *Nucleic Acids Res* 1994;22:4527–4534.

120. Samiotaki M, Kwiatkowski M, Parik J, Landegren U. Dual-color detection of DNA sequence variants by ligase-mediated analysis. *Genomics* 1994;20:238–242.

121. Baner J, Nilsson M, Mendel-Hartvig M, Landegren U. Signal amplification of padlock probes by rolling circle replication. *Nucleic Acids Res* 1998;26:5073–5078.

122. Lizardi PM, Huang X, Zhu Z, Bray-Ward P, Thomas DC, Ward DC. Mutation detection and single-molecule counting using isothermal rolling-cycle amplification. *Nat Genet* 1998;19:225–232.

123. Nilsson M, Malmgren H, Samiotaki M, Kwiatkowski M, Chowdhary BP, Landegren U. Padlock probes: circularizing oligonucleotides for localized DNA detection. *Science* 1994;265:2085–2088.

124. Zhang DY, Brandwein M, Hsuih TC, Li H. Amplification of target-specific, ligation-dependent circular probe. *Gene* 1998;211:277–285.

125. Chen X, Livak KJ, Kwok PY. A homogeneous, ligase-mediated DNA diagnostic test. *Genome Res* 1998;8:549–556.

126. Gerry NP, Witowski NE, Day J, Hammer RP, Barany G, Barany F. Universal DNA microarray method for multiplex detection of low abundance point mutations. *J Mol Biol* 1999;292:251–262.

127. Wallace RB, Shaffer J, Murphy RF, Bonner J, Hirose T, Itakura K. Hybridization of synthetic oligodeoxyribonucleotides to phi chi 174 DNA: the effect of single base pair mismatch. *Nucleic Acids Res* 1979;6:3543–3557.

128. Conner BJ, Reyes AA, Morin C, Itakura K, Teplitz RL, Wallace RB. Detection of sickle cell beta S-globin allele by hybridization with synthetic oligonucleotides. *Proc Natl Acad Sci USA* 1983;80:278–282.

129. Bonnet G, Tyagi S, Libchaber A, Kramer FR. Thermodynamic basis of the enhanced specificity of structured DNA probes. *Proc Natl Acad Sci USA* 1999;96:6171–6176.

130. Tyagi S, Kramer FR. Molecular beacons: probes that fluoresce upon hybridization. *Nat Biotechnol* 1996;14:303–308.

131. Kuimelis RG, Livak KJ, Mullah B, Andrus A. Structural analogues of TaqMan probes for real-time quantitative PCR. *Nucleic Acids Symp Ser* 1997;255–256.

132. Duggan DJ, Bittner M, Chen Y, Meltzer P, Trent JM. Expression profiling using cDNA microarrays. *Nat Genet* 1999;21:10–14.

133. Maughan NJ, Lewis FA, Smith V. An introduction to arrays. *J Pathol* 2001;195:3–6.

134. Saiki RK, Chang CA, Levenson CH, Warren TC, Boehm CD, Kazazian HH Jr, Erlich HA. Diagnosis of sickle cell anemia and beta-thalassemia with enzymatically amplified DNA and nonradioactive allele-specific oligonucleotide probes. *N Engl J Med* 1988; 319:537–541.

135. Blohm DH, Guiseppi-Elie A. New developments in microarray technology. *Curr Opin Biotechnol* 2001;12:41–47.

136. Prince JA, Feuk L, Howell WM, Jobs M, Emahazion T, Blennow K, Brookes AJ. Robust and accurate single nucleotide polymorphism genotyping by dynamic allele-specific hybridization (DASH): design criteria and assay validation. *Genome Res* 2001; 11:152–162.

137. Ross PL, Lee K, Belgrader P. Discrimination of single-nucleotide polymorphisms in human DNA using peptide nucleic acid probes detected by MALDI-TOF mass spectrometry. *Anal Chem* 1997;69:4197–4202.

138. Griffin TJ, Tang W, Smith LM. Genetic analysis by peptide nucleic acid affinity MALDI-TOF mass spectrometry. *Nat Biotechnol* 1997;15:1368–1372.

139. Orum H. Purification of nucleic acids by hybridization to affinity tagged PNA probes. *Curr Issues Mol Biol* 1999;1:105–110.

140. Orum H, Jakobsen MH, Koch T, Vuust J, Borre MB. Detection of the factor V Leiden mutation by direct allele-specific hybridization of PCR amplicons to photoimmobilized locked nucleic acids. *Clin Chem* 1999;45:1898–1905.

141. Newton CR, Graham A, Heptinstall LE, Powell SJ, Summers C, Kalsheker N, Smith JC, Markham AF. Analysis of any point mutation in DNA. The amplification refractory mutation system (ARMS). *Nucleic Acids Res* 1989;17:2503–2516.

142. Day DJ, Speiser PW, White PC, Barany F. Detection of steroid 21-hydroxylase alleles using gene-specific PCR and a multiplexed ligation detection reaction. *Genomics* 1995;29:152–162.

143. Khanna M, Park P, Zirvi M, Cao W, Picon A, Day J, Paty P, Barany F. Multiplex PCR/ LDR for detection of K-ras mutations in primary colon tumors. *Oncogene* 1999;18:27–38.

144. Broude NE, Woodward K, Cavallo R, Cantor CR, Englert D. DNA microarrays with stem-loop DNA probes: preparation and applications. *Nucleic Acids Res* 2001;29:E92.

145. Faruqi AF, Hosono S, Driscoll MD, Dean FB, Alsmadi O, Bandaru R, Kumar G, Grimwade B, Zong Q, Sun Z, Du Y, Kingsmore S, Knott T, Lasken RS. High-throughput genotyping of single nucleotide polymorphisms with rolling circle amplification. *BMC Genomics* 2001;2:4.

146. Nilsson M, Krejci K, Koch J, Kwiatkowski M, Gustavsson P, Landegren U. Padlock probes reveal single-nucleotide differences, parent of origin and *in situ* distribution of centromeric sequences in human chromosomes 13 and 21. *Nat Genet* 1997;16:252–255.

147. Fire A, Xu SQ. Rolling replication of short DNA circles. *Proc Natl Acad Sci USA* 1995;92:4641–4645.

148. Iannone MA, Taylor JD, Chen J, Li MS, Rivers P, Slentz-Kesler KA, Weiner MP. Multi-plexed single nucleotide polymorphism genotyping by oligonucleotide ligation and flow cytometry. *Cytometry* 2000;39:131–140.

149. Lyamichev V, Mast AL, Hall JG, Prudent JR, Kaiser MW, Takova T, Kwiatkowski RW, Sander TJ, de Arruda M, Arco DA, Neri BP, Brow MA. Polymorphism identification and quantitative detection of genomic DNA by invasive cleavage of oligonucleotide probes. *Nat Biotechnol* 1999;17:292–296.

150. Mein CA, Barratt BJ, Dunn MG, Siegmund T, Smith AN, Esposito L, Nutland S, Stevens HE, Wilson AJ, Phillips MS, Jarvis N, Law S, de Arruda M, Todd JA. Evaluation of single nucleotide polymorphism typing with invader on PCR amplicons and its automation. *Genome Res* 2000;10:330–343.

151. Wilkins Stevens P, Hall JG, Lyamichev V, Neri BP, Lu M, Wang L, Smith LM, Kelso DM. Analysis of single nucleotide polymorphisms with solid phase invasive cleavage reactions. *Nucleic Acids Res* 2001;29:E77.

152. Lockhart DJ, Winzeler EA. Genomics, gene expression and DNA arrays. *Nature* 2000;405:827–836.

153. Green CD, Simons JF, Taillon BE, Lewin DA. Open systems: panoramic views of gene expression. *J Immunol Methods* 2001;250:67–79.

154. Mockler TC, Ecker JR. Applications of DNA tiling arrays for whole-genome analysis. *Genomics* 2005;85:1–15.

155. Ross JS, Schenkein DP, Kashala O, Linette GP, Stec J, Symmans WF, Pusztai L, Hortoba-gyi GN. Pharmacogenomics. *Adv Anat Pathol* 2004;11:211–220.

156. Shi L, Tong W, Goodsaid F, Frueh FW, Fang H, Han T, Fuscoe JC, Casciano DA. QA/QC: challenges and pitfalls facing the microarray community and regulatory agencies. *Expert Rev Mol Diagn* 2004;4:761–777.

157. Liang P, Pardee AB. Differential display of eukaryotic messenger RNA by means of the polymerase chain reaction. *Science* 1992;257:967–971.

158. Welsh J, Chada K, Dalal SS, Cheng R, Ralph D, McClelland M. Arbitrarily primed PCR fingerprinting of RNA. *Nucleic Acids Res* 1992;20:4965–4970.

159. Bertelsen AH, Velculescu VE. High-throughput gene expression analysis using SAGE. *Drug Discov Today* 1998;3:152–159.

160. Velculescu VE. Serial analysis of gene expression. *Science* 1995;270:484–487.

161. Hubank M, Schatz DG. Identifying differences in mRNA expression by representational difference analysis of cDNA. *Nucleic Acids Res* 1994;22:5640–5648.

162. Shimkets RA, Lowe DG, Tai JT, Sehl P, Jin H, Yang R, Predki PF, Rothberg BE, Murtha MT, Roth ME, Shenoy SG, Windemuth A, Simpson JW, Simons JF, Daley MP, Gold SA, McKenna MP, Hillan K, Went GT, Rothberg JM. Gene expression analysis by transcript profiling coupled to a gene database query. *Nat Biotechnol* 1999;17:798–803.

163. Prashar Y, Weissman SM. READS: a method for display of 3′-end fragments of restriction enzyme-digested cDNAs for analysis of differential gene expression. *Methods Enzymol* 1999;303:258–272.

164. Sutcliffe JG, Foye PE, Erlander MG, Hilbush BS, Bodzin LJ, Durham JT, Hasel KW. TOGA: an automated parsing technology for analyzing expression of nearly all genes. *Proc Natl Acad Sci USA* 2000;97:1976–1981.

165. Spinella DG, Bernardino AK, Redding AC, Koutz P, Wei Y, Pratt EK, Myers KK, Chap-pell G, Gerken S, McConnell SJ. Tandem arrayed ligation of expressed sequence tags (TALEST): a new method for generating global gene expression profiles. *Nucleic Acids Res* 1999;27:E22.

166. Pandey A, Mann M. Proteomics to study genes and genomes. *Nature* 2000;405: 837–846.

167. Hunter TC, Andon NL, Koller A, Yates JR, Haynes PA. The functional proteomics toolbox: methods and applications. *J Chromatogr B Analyt Technol Biomed Life Sci* 2002;782:165–181.

168. Zhu H, Bilgin M, Snyder M. Proteomics. *Annu Rev Biochem* 2003;72:783–812.

169. Tonge R, Shaw J, Middleton B, Rowlinson R, Rayner S, Young J, Pognan F, Hawkins E, Currie I, Davison M. Validation and development of fluorescence two-dimensional differential gel electrophoresis proteomics technology. *Proteomics* 2001;1:377–396.

170. Unlu M, Morgan ME, Minden JS. Difference gel electrophoresis: a single gel method for detecting changes in protein extracts. *Electrophoresis* 1997;18:2071–2077.

171. Templin MF, Stoll D, Schrenk M, Traub PC, Vohringer CF, Joos TO. Protein microarray technology. *Trends Biotechnol* 2002;20:160–166.

172. Zhu H, Snyder M. Protein arrays and microarrays. *Curr Opin Chem Biol* 2001;5:40–45.

173. Zhu H, Snyder M. "Omic" approaches for unraveling signaling networks. *Curr Opin Cell Biol* 2002;14:173–179.

174. Seetharaman S, Zivarts M, Sudarsan N, Breaker RR. Immobilized RNA switches for the analysis of complex chemical and biological mixtures. *Nat Biotechnol* 2001;19:336–341.

175. Lueking A, Horn M, Eickhoff H, Bussow K, Lehrach H, Walter G. Protein microarrays for gene expression and antibody screening. *Anal Biochem* 1999;270:103–111.

176. Wiese R, Belosludtsev Y, Powdrill T, Thompson P, Hogan M. Simultaneous multianalyte ELISA performed on a microarray platform. *Clin Chem* 2001;47:1451–1457.

177. Moody MD, Van Arsdell SW, Murphy KP, Orencole SF, Burns C. Array-based ELISAs for high-throughput analysis of human cytokines. *Biotechniques* 2001;31: 186–190,192–194.

178. Huang RP, Huang R, Fan Y, Lin Y. Simultaneous detection of multiple cytokines from conditioned media and patient's sera by an antibody-based protein array system. *Anal Biochem* 2001;294:55–62.

179. Sreekumar A, Nyati MK, Varambally S, Barrette TR, Ghosh D, Lawrence TS, Chinnaiyan AM. Profiling of cancer cells using protein microarrays: discovery of novel radiation-regulated proteins. *Cancer Res* 2001;61:7585–7593.

180. Robinson WH, DiGennaro C, Hueber W, Haab BB, Kamachi M, Dean EJ, Fournel S, Fong D, Genovese MC, de Vegvar HE, Skriner K, Hirschberg DL, Morris RI, Muller S, Pruijn GJ, van Venrooij WJ, Smolen JS, Brown PO, Steinman L, Utz PJ. Autoantigen microarrays for multiplex characterization of autoantibody responses. *Nat Med* 2002;8:295–301.

181. Hiller R, Laffer S, Harwanegg C, Huber M, Schmidt WM, Twardosz A, Barletta B, Becker WM, Blaser K, Breiteneder H, Chapman M, Crameri R, Duchene M, Ferreira F, Fiebig H, Hoffmann-Sommergruber K, King TP, Kleber-Janke T, Kurup VP, Lehrer SB, Lidholm J, Muller U, Pini C, Reese G, Scheiner O, Scheynius A, Shen HD, Spitzauer S, Suck R, Swoboda I, Thomas W, Tinghino R, Van Hage-Hamsten M, Virtanen T, Kraft D, Muller MW, Valenta R. Microarrayed allergen molecules: diagnostic gatekeepers for allergy treatment. *FASEB J* 2002;16:414–416.

182. Joos TO, Schrenk M, Hopfl P, Kroger K, Chowdhury U, Stoll D, Schorner D, Durr M, Herick K, Rupp S, Sohn K, Hammerle H. A microarray enzyme-linked immunosorbent assay for autoimmune diagnostics. *Electrophoresis* 2000;21:2641–2650.

183. Davies H, Lomas L, Austen B. Profiling of amyloid beta peptide variants using SELDI Protein Chip arrays. *Biotechniques* 1999;27:1258–1261.

184. Nelson RW. The use of bioreactive probes in protein characterization. *Mass Spectrom Rev* 1997;16:353–376.

185. Xiao Z, Prieto D, Conrads TP, Veenstra TD, Issaq HJ. Proteomic patterns: their potential for disease diagnosis. *Mol Cell Endocrinol* 2005;230:95–106.

186. Semmes OJ, Feng Z, Adam BL, Banez LL, Bigbee WL, Campos D, Cazares LH, Chan DW, Grizzle WE, Izbicka E, Kagan J, Malik G, McLerran D, Moul JW, Partin A, Prasanna P, Rosenzweig J, Sokoll LJ, Srivastava S, Thompson I, Welsh MJ, White N, Winget M, Yasui Y, Zhang Z, Zhu L. Evaluation of serum protein profiling by surface-enhanced laser desorption/ionization time-of-flight mass spectrometry for the detection of prostate cancer: I. Assessment of platform reproducibility. *Clin Chem* 2005;51:102–112.

187. Gygi SP, Rist B, Gerber SA, Turecek F, Gelb MH, Aebersold R. Quantitative analysis of complex protein mixtures using isotope-coded affinity tags. *Nat Biotechnol* 1999;17:994–999.

188. Han DK, Eng J, Zhou H, Aebersold R. Quantitative profiling of differentiation-induced microsomal proteins using isotope-coded affinity tags and mass spectrometry. *Nat Biotechnol* 2001;19:946–951.

189. Michaud GA, Snyder M. Proteomic approaches for the global analysis of proteins. *Biotechniques* 2002;33:1308–1316.

190. Smolka MB, Zhou H, Purkayastha S, Aebersold R. Optimization of the isotope-coded affinity tag-labeling procedure for quantitative proteome analysis. *Anal Biochem* 2001;297:25–31.

191. Uetz P, Giot L, Cagney G, Mansfield TA, Judson RS, Knight JR, Lockshon D, Narayan V, Srinivasan M, Pochart P, Qureshi-Emili A, Li Y, Godwin B, Conover D, Kalbfleisch T, Vijayadamodar G, Yang M, Johnston M, Fields S, Rothberg JM. A comprehensive analysis of protein–protein interactions in *Saccharomyces cerevisiae*. *Nature* 2000;403: 623–627.

192. Vidal M, Endoh H. Prospects for drug screening using the reverse two-hybrid system. *Trends Biotechnol* 1999;17:374–381.

193. Nicholson JK, Wilson ID. Opinion: understanding "global" systems biology: metabonomics and the continuum of metabolism. *Nat Rev Drug Discov* 2003;2:668–676.

194. Fiehn O. Metabolomics—the link between genotypes and phenotypes. *Plant Mol Biol* 2002;48:155–171.

195. Nicholson JK, Connelly J, Lindon JC, Holmes E. Metabonomics: a platform for studying drug toxicity and gene function. *Nat Rev Drug Discov* 2002;1:153–161.

196. Kell DB. Metabolomics and systems biology: making sense of the soup. *Curr Opin Microbiol* 2004;7:296–307.

197. Fiehn O, Kloska S, Altmann T. Integrated studies on plant biology using multiparallel techniques. *Curr Opin Biotechnol* 2001;12:82–86.

198. Cornish-Bowden A, Cardenas ML. From genome to cellular phenotype—a role for metabolic flux analysis? *Nat Biotechnol* 2000;18:267–268.

199. Saghatelian A, Cravatt BF. Discovery metabolite profiling—forging functional connections between the proteome and metabolome. *Life Sci* 2005;77:1759–1766.

200. Trethewey RN. Metabolite profiling as an aid to metabolic engineering in plants. *Curr Opin Plant Biol* 2004;7:196–201.

201. Saghatelian A, Cravatt BF. Global strategies to integrate the proteome and metabolome. *Curr Opin Chem Biol* 2005;9:62–68.

202. Fernie AR, Trethewey RN, Krotzky AJ, Willmitzer L. Metabolite profiling: from diagnostics to systems biology. *Nat Rev Mol Cell Biol* 2004;5:763–769.

203. Bino RJ, Hall RD, Fiehn O, Kopka J, Saito K, Draper J, Nikolau BJ, Mendes P, Roessner-Tunali U, Beale MH, Trethewey RN, Lange BM, Wurtele ES, Sumner LW. Potential of metabolomics as a functional genomics tool. *Trends Plant Sci* 2004;9:418–425.

204. Jenkins H, Hardy N, Beckmann M, Draper J, Smith AR, Taylor J, Fiehn O, Goodacre R, Bino RJ, Hall R, Kopka J, Lane GA, Lange BM, Liu JR, Mendes P, Nikolau BJ, Oliver SG, Paton NW, Rhee S, Roessner-Tunali U, Saito K, Smedsgaard J, Sumner LW, Wang T, Walsh S, Wurtele ES, Kell DB. A proposed framework for the description of plant metabolomics experiments and their results. *Nat Biotechnol* 2004;22:1601–1606.

205. Raamsdonk LM, Teusink B, Broadhurst D, Zhang N, Hayes A, Walsh MC, Berden JA, Brindle KM, Kell DB, Rowland JJ, Westerhoff HV, van Dam K, Oliver SG. A functional genomics strategy that uses metabolome data to reveal the phenotype of silent mutations. *Nat Biotechnol* 2001;19:45–50.

206. Watkins SM, German JB. Toward the implementation of metabolomic assessments of human health and nutrition. *Curr Opin Biotechnol* 2002;13:512–516.

207. Shockcor JP, Holmes E. Metabonomic applications in toxicity screening and disease diagnosis. *Curr Top Med Chem* 2002;2:35–51.

208. Tweeddale H, Notley-McRobb L, Ferenci T. Effect of slow growth on metabolism of *Escherichia coli*, as revealed by global metabolite pool ("metabolome") analysis. *J Bacteriol* 1998;180:5109–5116.

209. Oliver SG, Winson MK, Kell DB, Baganz F. Systematic functional analysis of the yeast genome. *Trends Biotechnol* 1998;16:373–378.

210. Bochner BR, Gadzinski P, Panomitros E. Phenotype microarrays for high-throughput phenotypic testing and assay of gene function. *Genome Res* 2001;11:1246–1255.

211. Hanlon EB, Manoharan R, Koo TW, Shafer KE, Motz JT, Fitzmaurice M, Kramer JR, Itzkan I, Dasari RR, Feld MS. Prospects for *in vivo* Raman spectroscopy. *Phys Med Biol* 2000;45:R1–59.

212. Rees JL. The genetics of sun sensitivity in humans. *Am J Hum Genet* 2004;75:739–751.

213. Smith MW, Dean M, Carrington M, Winkler C, Huttley GA, Lomb DA, Goedert JJ, O'Brien TR, Jacobson LP, Kaslow R, Buchbinder S, Vittinghoff E, Vlahov D, Hoots K, Hilgartner MW, O'Brien SJ. Contrasting genetic influence of CCR2 and CCR5 variants on HIV-1 infection and disease progression. Hemophilia Growth and Development Study (HGDS), Multicenter AIDS Cohort Study (MACS), Multicenter Hemophilia Cohort Study (MHCS), San Francisco City Cohort (SFCC), ALIVE Study. *Science* 1997;277:959–965.

214. Chen J, Giovannucci EL, Hunter DJ. MTHFR polymorphism, methyl-replete diets and the risk of colorectal carcinoma and adenoma among U.S. men And women: an example of gene–environment interactions in colorectal tumorigenesis. *J Nutr* 1999;129: 560S–564S.

215. Chen J, Stampfer MJ, Hough HL, Garcia-Closas M, Willett WC, Hennekens CH, Kelsey KT, Hunter DJ. A prospective study of *N*-acetyltransferase genotype, red meat intake, and risk of colorectal cancer. *Cancer Res* 1998;58:3307–3311.

216. Bloemenkamp KW, Rosendaal FR, Helmerhorst FM, Buller HR, Vandenbroucke JP. Enhancement by factor V Leiden mutation of risk of deep-vein thrombosis associated with oral contraceptives containing a third-generation progestagen. *Lancet* 1995;346: 1593–1596.

217. Chan AT, Tranah GJ, Giovannucci EL, Hunter DJ, Fuchs CS. Genetic variants in the UGT1A6 enzyme, aspirin use, and the risk of colorectal adenoma. *J Natl Cancer Inst* 2005;97:457–460.

218. Lehtimaki T, Moilanen T, Porkka K, Akerblom HK, Ronnemaa T, Rasanen L, Viikari J, Ehnholm C, Nikkari T. Association between serum lipids and apolipoprotein E phenotype

is influenced by diet in a population-based sample of free-living children and young adults: the Cardiovascular Risk in Young Finns Study. *J Lipid Res* 1995;36:653–661.

219. Hines LM, Stampfer MJ, Ma J, Gaziano JM, Ridker PM, Hankinson SE, Sacks F, Rimm EB, Hunter DJ. Genetic variation in alcohol dehydrogenase and the beneficial effect of moderate alcohol consumption on myocardial infarction. *N Engl J Med* 2001;344: 549–555.

220. Memisoglu A, Hu FB, Hankinson SE, Manson JE, De Vivo I, Willett WC, Hunter DJ. Interaction between a peroxisome proliferator-activated receptor gamma gene polymorphism and dietary fat intake in relation to body mass. *Hum Mol Genet* 2003;12:2923–2929.

221. Maier LA. Genetic and exposure risks for chronic beryllium disease. *Clin Chest Med* 2002;23:827–839.

222. Weinshilboum R. Thiopurine pharmacogenetics: clinical and molecular studies of thiopurine methyltransferase. *Drug Metab Dispos* 2001;29:601–605.

223. Israel E, Drazen JM, Liggett SB, Boushey HA, Cherniack RM, Chinchilli VM, Cooper DM, Fahy JV, Fish JE, Ford JG, Kraft M, Kunselman S, Lazarus SC, Lemanske RF, Martin RJ, McLean DE, Peters SP, Silverman EK, Sorkness CA, Szefler SJ, Weiss ST, Yandava CN. The effect of polymorphisms of the beta(2)-adrenergic receptor on the response to regular use of albuterol in asthma. *Am J Respir Crit Care Med* 2000;162:75–80.

224. Weatherall DJ. Phenotype–genotype relationships in monogenic disease: lessons from the thalassaemias. *Nat Rev Genet* 2001;2:245–255.

225. Huisman TH, Carver MFH., Baysai E. *A Syllabus of Thalassemia Mutations*. Augusta, GA: The Sickle Cell Anemia Foundation; 1997.

226. Weatherall DJ, Clegg JB. *The Thalassemia Syndromes*. Oxford, UK: Blackwell Science; 2001.

227. Whittaker M, Britten JJ, Dawson PJG. Comparison of a commercially available assay system with two reference methods for the determination of cholinesterase variants. *Clin Chem* 1983;29:1746–1751.

228. Weinshilbom RM, Raymond FA. Inheritance of low erythrocyte catechol-O-methyltransferase activity in man. *Am J Hum Genet* 1977;29:125–135.

229. Kouri RE, McKinney CE, Slomiany DJ, Snodgrass DR, Wray NP, McLemore TL. Positive correlation between high aryl hydrocarbon hydroxylase activity and primary lung cancer as analysed in cryopreserved lymphocytes. *Cancer Res* 1982;42:5030–5037.

230. Fuhr U, Rost K. Simple and reliable CYP1A2 phenotyping by the paraxanthine/caffeine ration in plasma and saliva. *Pharmacogenetics* 1994;4:109–116.

231. Campbell ME, Spielberg SP, Kalow W. A urinary metabolite ratio that reflects systemic caffeine clearance. *Clin Pharmacol Ther* 1987;42:157–165.

232. Cholerton S, Idle ME. Comparison of a novel thin-layer chromatographic-flourescence detection method with a spectrofluorometric method for the determination of 7-hydroxycoumarin in human urine. *J Chromatogr* 1992;575:325–330.

233. Veronese ME, Miners JO, Randles D, Gregov D, Birkett DJ. Validation of the tolbutamide metabolic ratio for population screening with the use of sulfaphenazole to produce model phenotypic poor metabolizers. *Clin Pharmacol Ther* 1990;47:403–411.

234. Wedlund PJ, Aslanian WS, McAllister CB, Wilkinson GR, Branch RA. Mephenytoin hydroxylation deficiency in Caucasians: frequency of a new oxidative drug metabolism polymorphism. *Clin Pharmacol Ther* 1984;36:773–780.

235. Chang M, Dahl ML, Tybring G, Gotharson E, Bertilsson L. Use of omeprazole as a probe drug for CYP2C19 phenotype in Swedish Caucasians: comparison with *S-*

methylphenytoin hydroxylation phenotype and CYP2C19 genotype. *Pharmacogenetics* 1995;5:358–363.

236. Idle JR, Mahgoub A, Angelo MM, Dring LG, Lancaster R, Smith RL. The metabolsim of [^{14}C] debrisoquine in man. *Br J Clin Pharmacol* 1979;7:257–266.

237. Eichelbaum M, Spannbrucker N, Steincke B, Dengler HJ. Defective N-oxidation of sparteine in man: a new pharmacogenetic defect. *Eur J Clin Pharmacol* 1979;17:153–155.

238. Jacqz-Aigrain E, Menard Y, Popon M, Mathieu H. Dextromethorphan phenotypes determined by high-performance liquid chromatography and fluorescence detection. *J Chromatogr* 1989;495:361–363.

239. Lennard MS. Quantitative-analysis of metoprolol and 3 of its metabolites in urine and liver-microsomes by high-performance liquid-chromatography. *J Chromatogr* 1985;342:199–205.

240. Kim RB, O'Shea D, Wilkinson GR. Interindividual variability of chlorzoxazone 6-hydroxylation in men and women and its relationship to CYP2E1 genetic polymorphisms. *Clin Pharmacol Ther* 1995;57:645–655.

241. Raucy JL, Schultz ED, Wester MR, Arora S, Johnson DE, Omdahl JL, Carpenter SP. Human lymphocyte cytochrome P450 2E1, a putative marker for alcohol-mediated changes in hepatic chlorozoxazone activity. *Drug Metab Dispos* 1997;25:1429–1435.

242. Thummel KE, Shen DD, Podoll TD, Kunze KL, Trager WF, Hartwell PS, Raisys VA, Marsh CL, McVicar JP, Barr DM, Perkins JD, Carithers RL. Use of midazolam as a human cytochrome-P450 3A pobe. I. *In-vitro, in-vivo* correlations in liver-transplant patients. *J Pharmacol Exp Ther* 1994;271:549–556.

243. Zhiri A, Mayer HA, Michaux V. 6-Beta-hydroxycortisol in serum and urine as determined by enzyme-immunoassay on microtitre plates. *Clin Chem* 1986;32:2094–2097.

244. Watkins PB, Hamilton TA, Annesley TM, Ellis CN, Kolars JC, Voorhees JJ. The erythromycin breath test as a predictor of cyclosporine blood-levels. *Clin Pharmacol Ther* 1990;48:120–129.

245. Alwaiz M, Ayesh R, Mitchell SC, Idle ME, Smith RL. Trimethylaminuria—the detection of carriers using a trimethylamine load test. *J Inherit Metab Dis* 1989;12:80–85.

246. Sieidegard J, Pero RW. The hereditary transmission of high glutathione transferase-activity towards *trans*-stilbene oxide in human mononuclear leukocytes. *Hum Genet* 1985;69:66–68.

247. Hallier E, Langhof T, Dannaappel D, Leutbecher M, Schroder K, Goergens HW, Muller A, Bolt HM. Polymorphism of glutathione conjugation of methyl-bromide, ethylene-oxide and dichloromethane in human blood—influence on the induction of sister chromatid exchanges (SCE) in lymphocytes. *Arch Toxicol* 1993;67:173–178.

248. Cribb AE, Isbrucker R, Levatte T, Tsui B, Gillespie CT. Acetylator phenotyping: the urinary caffeine metabolite ratio in slow acetylators correlates with a marker of systemic NAT1 activity. *Pharmacogenetics* 1994;4:166–170.

249. Grant DM, Tang BK, Kalow W. Polymorphic N-acetylation of a caffeine metabolite. *Clin Pharmacol Ther* 1983;33:355–359.

250. Playfer JR, Eze LC, Bullen MF, Evans DAP. Genetic polymorphism and inter-ethnic variability of plasma paraozonase activity. *J Med Genet* 1976;13:337–342.

251. Price RA, Cox NJ, Spielman RS, Van Loon JA, Maidak BL, Weinshilbom RM. Inheritance of human platelet thermolabile phenol sulphotransferase (TLPST) activity. *Genet Epidemiol* 1988;5:1–15.

252. Price RA, Spielman RS, Lucena AL, Van Loon JA, Maidak BL, Weinshilbom RM. Genetic polymorphism for human platelet thermostable phenol sulphotransferase (TSPST) activity. *Genetics* 1989;122:905–914.

253. Weinshilbom RM, Sladek SL. Mercaptopurine pharmacogenetics: monogenic inheritance of erythrocyte thiopurine methyltransferase activity. *Am J Hum Genet* 1980;32:651–662.

254. Greiner B, Eichelbaum M, Fritz P, Kreichgauer HP, VonRichter O, Zundler J, Kroemer HK. The role of intestinal P-glycoprotein in the interaction of digoxin and rifampin. *J Clin Invest* 1999;104:147–153.

255. Thomas DC. Genetic epidemiology with a capital "E." *Genet Epidemiol* 2000;19:289–300.

256. Botto LD, Khoury MJ. Commentary: facing the challenge of gene–environment interaction: the two-by-four table and beyond. *Am J Epidemiol* 2001;153:1016–1020.

257. Khoury MJ, Adams MJ Jr, Flanders WD. An epidemiologic approach to ecogenetics. *Am J Hum Genet* 1988;42:89–95.

258. Ottman R. An epidemiologic approach to gene–environment interaction. *Genet Epidemiol* 1990;7:177–185.

259. Rothman KJ, Greenland S. *Modern Epidemiology*. Philadelphia: Lippincott-Raven; 1998.

260. Rebbeck TR, Spitz M, Wu X. Assessing the function of genetic variants in candidate gene association studies. *Nat Rev Genet* 2004;5:589–597.

261. Ge H, Walhout AJ, Vidal M. Integrating "omic" information: a bridge between genomics and systems biology. *Trends Genet* 2003;19:551–560.

262. Hartwell LH, Hopfield JJ, Leibler S, Murray AW. From molecular to modular cell biology. *Nature* 1999;402:C47–C52.

22

GENOMICS

DIMITRI SEMIZAROV AND ERIC A. G. BLOMME

Global Pharmaceutical Research and Development, Abbott Laboratories, Abbott Park, Illinois

Contents

22.1 INTRODUCTION

In the past five to ten years a growing number of new drugs have been discovered using a target-based approach [1], implying a significant paradigm shift in the pharmaceutical industry. This shift has been facilitated by the decoding of the complete sequence of the human genome [2–4]. Today, a significant portion of the research and development (R&D) effort in the pharmaceutical industry is focused on drug target identification and validation. This paradigm change also requires that new

Preclinical Development Handbook: Toxicology, edited by Shayne Cox Gad
Copyright © 2008 John Wiley & Sons, Inc.

methodologies be used in preclinical development. The preclinical development process for targeted agents involves genomic analysis of preclinical model systems to elucidate the mechanism of target inhibition, delineate off-target effects, and identify biomarkers.

Genomic technologies may potentially play an important role at all stages of drug discovery. For example, target identification in cancer often involves large scale genomic screens for genes or their products that alter cell proliferation and survival. Identification of genes frequently amplified at the chromosomal level may reveal a target for therapeutic intervention, whose inhibition by small molecules or antibodies may deprive the cancer cell of its proliferation/survival advantage. Because gene amplification often leads to overexpression [5–7], the search for genes overexpressed in cancer cells is a logical and common strategy for target identification.

Genomic technologies are now frequently utilized in lead selection and compound optimization. They are routinely used to profile candidate compounds in order to identify the pathways activated and thus delineate the on-target and off-target effects. Large databases are being created to correlate the chemical structures of compounds and their toxicogenomic profiles. An important component of preclinical development is biomarker discovery. The increasing importance of biomarkers is closely connected with the exponential growth in R&D costs currently experienced by the pharmaceutical industry [8]. An early discovery of an efficacy biomarker could substantially decrease development costs and cut the development time, thus allowing an earlier market entry and hence an improved patent life cycle [9]. Therefore, biomarker discovery programs are now incorporated early into the discovery process, typically at the lead optimization or preclinical testing stages. So-called patient stratification biomarkers, that is, markers correlated with the disease type or response to a drug candidate, are particularly valuable in oncology development, as cancer represents a heterogeneous genetic disease. In one of the recent successful examples of patient stratification strategies, the response to a drug called Herceptin was found to correlate with the amplification of the *HER2* gene [10–12]. These biomarkers offer the possibility of rationally selecting patients for clinical trials and are now being pursued early in the discovery process. For example, cell culture screens for target inhibition are often accompanied by detailed genomic analysis of the cell lines to identify genetic markers correlating with the response in the assay.

Several genomic technologies are used in biomarker discovery. Gene expression and CGH microarrays are used to determine the molecular profiles that predict the outcome in various cancers and correlate with the response to the drug (for examples see Refs. 13–21). Microarrays can also be utilized to determine the molecular signatures of the response to the agent, leading to discovery of efficacy biomarkers [22].

In the following sections, we describe the current state of the aforementioned microarray technologies, as well as several methods for manipulating gene activity, and review the applications of these tools in preclinical drug development. The objective of this chapter is to introduce to the reader the most common genomic technologies, to describe the relevant protocols, and to briefly summarize their applications in preclinical drug development. Chapter 24 comprehensively reviews the applications of DNA microarrays in the field of toxicology.

22.2   GENE EXPRESSION MICROARRAYS

22.2.1   Technology

We define some of the microarray terms used in this chapter.

Probe. A DNA fragment attached to the microchip and used to detect transcripts in the test sample.

Reverse Transcriptase. An enzyme capable of synthesizing DNA using RNA as a template.

DNA Polymerase. An enzyme capable of synthesizing DNA on a DNA template.

cDNA. DNA synthesized off an mRNA template.

cDNA. RNA synthesized in an *in vitro* transcription reaction using cDNA as a template.

Standard Microarray Protocol   Generally, gene expression microarrays represent microchips containing thousands of DNA probes, which are used to analyze the abundance of multiple transcripts in a sample. Based on the type of probe, microarrays can be classified into oligonucleotide and cDNA arrays. While cDNA microarrays may potentially offer higher sensitivity of mRNA detection, difficulties in manufacturing and deposition of cloned and purified long DNA sequences have limited the use of cDNA arrays largely to academic laboratories. In this chapter, we focus on the more commonly used oligonucleotide microarrays.

Figure 22.1 presents an outline of a typical microarray experiment. Total RNA is isolated from the test sample using one of the known techniques [23, 24] and is used as a template to synthesize cDNA. An oligo(dT) primer with an attached T7 sequence is used as a primer for reverse transcription. An enzyme called reverse transcriptase catalyzes the synthesis of cDNA using the input RNA as a template. The resulting cDNA is then subjected to one round of DNA replication to generate double-stranded DNA. This reaction is catalyzed by a DNA polymerase. The resulting double-stranded DNA then serves as a template for T7 RNA polymerase, which recognizes the T7 sequences in the cDNA [25]. The *in vitro* transcription is performed in the presence of biotinylated rNTPs to label the cRNA. The cRNA is fragmented and hybridized to the array.

After array hybridization, the array is washed to remove unbound molecules, stained using streptavidin-phycoerythrin and a bioinylated anti-streptavidin antibody, and scanned in a fluorescent scanner in order to quantify the signal for all the probes. After the acquisition of the image by the scanner, a specialized program overlays a grid on the array to identify the spots and generates a table of signal intensities. A different program then processes the signal intensities for individual probes to generate the intensities for each individual gene, determine the background, and perform normalization. The signal intensity for each gene serves as a measure of the abundance of the corresponding transcript in the initial sample.

The quantity of the test RNA sample is an important factor in microarray analysis. The RNA polymerase synthesizes multiple copies of cRNA from each cDNA molecule, and the target preparation protocol results in an amplification of the original sample. For RNA quantities $> 1\,\mu g$, the above-described protocol typically

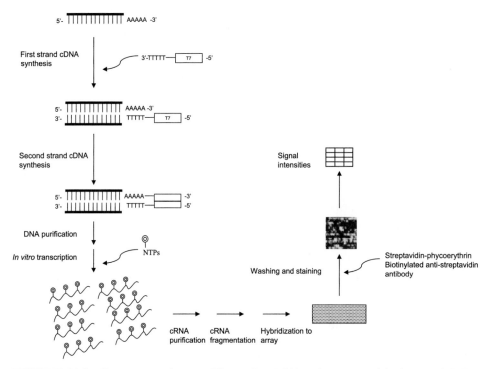

FIGURE 22.1   Gene expression profiling using DNA microarrays (single-round RNA amplification protocol). The total RNA sample is amplified to generate biotin-labeled cRNA, which is fragmented and hybridized to a microarray.

produces enough cRNA for at least one or two array hybridizations. Another important consideration is the integrity of the sample. If the total RNA is degraded, the reverse transcriptase will not be able to synthesize sufficiently long cDNAs and the cRNA products will not hybridize to all the probes for the transcript. Although 3′-bias is an important consideration in microarray probe design, many probes on a microarray are removed by hundreds of nucleotides from the 3′-terminus of the transcript. Probes that are distant from the 3′-terminus will not hybridize if the cRNA products are of insufficient length. Similarly, suboptimal functioning of the reverse transcriptase may lead to shortened cDNAs and cRNAs and hence will result in an underestimation of the abundance of the transcripts. As microarray applications expand, more different sample types will need to be analyzed. Next, we consider two special situations with regard to the sample type.

Microarray Analysis of Archived and Small Samples   The standard expression microarray protocol requires high quality intact RNA. However, as microarrays became an important tool in biomarker research, the researchers started looking for ways to apply the microarray technology to retrospectively analyze archived human tissue samples. Freezing of a sample immediately after surgical resection typically preserves RNA. Therefore, such samples can be analyzed with a standard microarray protocol. It is critical that the sample be frozen immediately, because even quick manipulation of tissue results in changes in gene expression [26, 27] that may be mistaken for true characteristics of the sample. However, the most difficult challenge is presented by formalin-fixed paraffin-embedded (FFPE) samples, as formalin fixation results in irreversible modification and degradation of RNA [28, 29]. It is noteworthy that formalin fixation results in a wide spectrum of RNA modifications, including cross-linking, addition of monomethylol residues to the nucleic bases, and adenine dimerization [28]. Until recently, such samples were deemed unsuitable for microarray analysis. In 2003, a specialized microarray for analysis of FFPE samples was developed [30]. It contains mostly probe sets that are directed against the three hundred 3'-terminal nucleotides of the transcripts (instead of the 600 nucleotide limit set for regular microarrays). The increased 3'-bias is intended to facilitate binding of shortened cRNAs synthesized off truncated cDNAs. However, a solution remains to be found for analysis of highly modified RNA, as RNA with modified nucleic bases has a limited capacity to produce cDNA in the reverse transcription reaction. The chip is designed for use with a reagent system [31], which enables RNA isolation from FFPE tissues as well as its amplification and labeling.

Significant progress has also been made in analysis of small samples. The progress in this area was fueled by the introduction of a tissue dissection technology called laser capture microdissection [26, 32]. The technique involves placing a transparent film over a tissue section and selectively adhering the cells of interest to the film with a fixed-position, short-duration, focused pulse from an infrared laser (Fig. 22.2). During the procedure, the tissue is visualized microscopically. The film with the

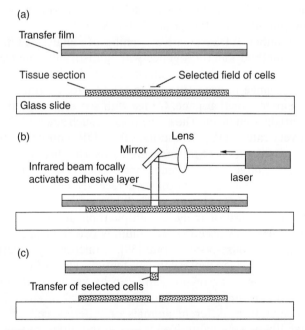

FIGURE 22.2 [32] Laser capture microdissection protocol. (a) A tissue section is mounted on a microscope slide and covered with transparent film. Cells of interest are selected visually under a microscope. (b) A laser beam focused on the cells of interest is activated, causing the film to adhere to the selected cells. (c) The film is removed together with the attached cells. At this point, the cells of interest can be lysed and further processed.

procured tissue is then removed from the section and used to isolate DNA or RNA [32]. As laser capture microdissection of tissue samples became common, an urgent need arose for a microarray protocol suitable for analysis of samples ranging from 100 to 1000 cells. The problem was solved by introducing an additional round of RNA amplification. In a two-round amplification protocol (Fig. 22.3), the first round is performed with regular rNTPs, while the second round uses labeled rNTPs as in the single-round amplification protocol described in the previous subsection. Today, protocols involving laser capture microdissection and RNA isolation from single cells followed by gene expression analysis have become routine. They made possible the analysis of pure tumor cells and comparison with adjacent normal tissue [33–35].

Microarray Data Analysis   Most microarray experiments involve either a comparison between a treatment and the baseline or a comparison between the test sample and a reference. Therefore, the first level of data analysis almost inevitably involves building gene expression ratios, that is, calculating the ratios between the intensity values for the same gene from two different chips. A *t*-test is typically used to determine the significance of the difference between the control and the test values for each gene. The data can then be filtered to remove insignificant changes. Methods based on conventional *t*-tests provide the probability (p) that a difference in gene expression occurred by chance. It is common to set up a significance threshold at p-value ≤ 0.01. Although $p = 0.01$ is a reasonably stringent cut-off for experiments designed to evaluate small numbers of genes, a microarray experiment measuring the expression of 20,000 genes (such as an experiment using Affymetrix U133A arrays) would identify 200 genes by chance.

To reduce the number of false positives, significance analysis of microarrays [36] can be used. This method identifies genes with statistically significant changes in expression by assimilating a set of gene-specific *t*-tests. Each gene is assigned a score on the basis of its change in gene expression relative to the standard deviation of repeated measurements for that gene. Genes with scores greater than a threshold are deemed potentially significant. The percentage of such genes identified by chance is the false discovery rate (FDR). To estimate the FDR, nonsense genes are identified by analyzing permutations of the measurements. The threshold can be adjusted to identify smaller or larger sets of genes, and FDRs are calculated for each set. Other false discovery analysis methods have recently been introduced, some of which include analysis of false negatives [37, 38].

To improve the robustness of analysis, multiple replicates of the same sample are typically run. The commonly accepted minimum is two replicates; however, use of triplicates minimizes the false-positive rate [39]. A microarray experiment consists of multiple steps, and each step represents a potential source of variation. The variation of the measured gene expression data can be categorized into two generic sources: biological and technical variations. The biological variation in gene expression measured comes from different animals or different cell lines or tissues. It reflects the variability in gene expression between the different biological samples used in the experiment. Biological variation can be assessed only by using independent biological replicates. If all biological samples are pooled, the biological variation is minimized, but the potentially useful information on the variability in gene expression between different animals or cells is lost. The technical variation accounts

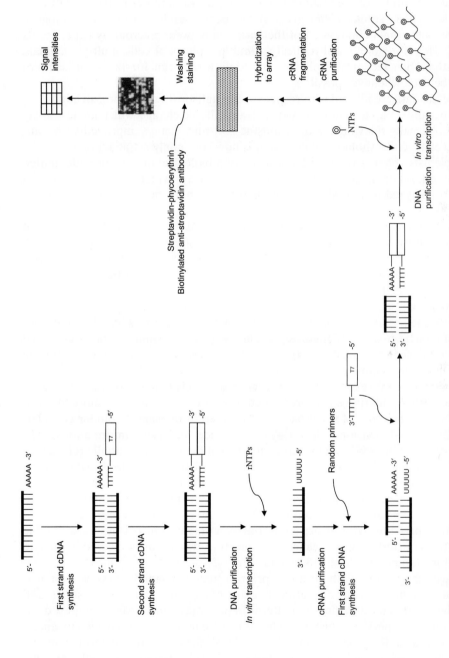

FIGURE 22.3 Gene expression profiling of small samples using DNA microarrays. Unlike the standard protocol outlined in Fig. 22.1, this procedure involves two rounds of RNA amplification. The first round is performed in the presence of regular rNTPs, while the second round involves biotin-modified rNTPs to label the cRNA product.

for the variation associated with the use of microarray techniques unrelated to the biological samples. The biological, technical, and residual variations are mutually independent. The variation in a measured intensity is the sum of these two variations.

The contributions of the technical and biological variabilities to the overall variability have been studied extensively. It has been established that the biological variation is the main component of the variation between microarray experiments [40, 41]. Therefore, biological replicates (multiple plates of cells, multiple animals, etc.) rather than technical replicates (multiple arrays run for the same sample) should be used whenever possible.

Once the data are filtered with respect to the statistical significance, an additional filter is usually set up to remove genes with a small fold change, which are less likely to be biologically relevant. As the robustness of microarrays improved with time, the fold change threshold was lowered; it is now commonly set at 1.5 or 2.

Simple lists of genes regulated as a result of a biological process provide limited information. As applications of expression microarrays widened and the numbers of genes analyzed increased, the analysis methods have become more and more complex.

One of the most common tasks in microarray data analysis is identification of common patterns of gene regulation in a population of samples. An example of such a task would be identification of genes coinduced in a series of treatments or discovery of genes associated with a particular biological characteristic of the samples (disease category, tissue type, etc.). Problems of this type are commonly solved by two-dimensional clustering, a statistical procedure whereby samples (each represented by one or more microarrays) are aggregated into clusters based on the similarity of their expression "signatures," while the genes are simultaneously clustered based on the similarity of their expression levels across the samples. The rationale behind clustering samples according to their expression profiles is simple: samples with similar gene expression "signatures" are more likely to have common biological characteristics. Similarly, genes coregulated in a series of samples are more likely to be part of a common biological pathway activated in the samples under consideration. Thus, two-dimensional clustering may provide very useful information on the degree of relatedness between samples and reveal the genes potentially relevant to the classification. Clustering results can be conveniently visualized using a gene expression matrix, or a heatmap, in which each column represents an experiment and each row represents a gene (Fig. 22.4). Each element of the heatmap is colored based on the expression level, thus providing a convenient visual representation of the gene expression patterns across all the experiments. One of the most notable applications of clustering is in cancer classification, which was pioneered in the late 1990s (for examples see Refs. 18 and 42–44).

If clustering is done without any a priori introduced sample classification, it is referred to as unsupervised clustering. Because of its unbiased nature, unsupervised clustering is often used to identify patterns in previously unclassified complex datasets. Several unsupervised clustering algorithms are used for microarray data analysis (reviewed in Refs. 45 and 46). Hierarchical clustering is the most common algorithm. It uses an agglomerative approach, whereby expression profiles are successively joined to form groups based on similarity between them, thus forming a hierarchical tree, or dendrogram [47]. The latter presents a convenient visualization

Genes

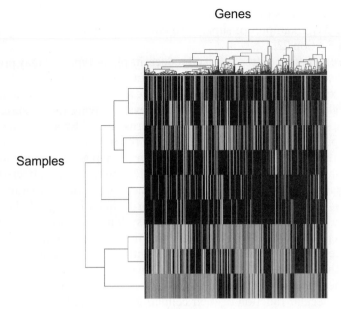

Samples

FIGURE 22.4   An example of a heatmap obtained by hierarchical two-dimensional cluster-ing of nine samples. Each row represents a sample and each column represents a gene. (Although not visible here, a red color is used for upregulation and a blue color is used for downregulation of genes, with black reserved for unaffected genes.) The dendrogram on the left illustrates the degree of relatedness between the expression profiles of the samples and the dendrogram on the top reflects the similarity of the expression levels for each gene across the samples.

option and is often presented together with a heatmap (Fig. 22.4). An alternative algorithm is k-means clustering, a divisive approach based on partitioning the dataset into a predefined number (k) of clusters [48]. Obviously, it requires some a priori knowledge of the biology of the dataset so that the number of clusters could be preset. When the researcher can specify in advance not only the number of clus-ters but also the relationships between them, self-organizing maps (SOMs) can be used, which organize the clusters into a "map" where similar clusters are close to each other [49].

Unsupervised algorithms can find novel patterns in datasets but are not designed to classify data according to known classes. On the contrary, supervised clustering approaches, such as support vector machines (SVMs) [50], take known classes and create rules for assigning genes or experiments into these classes. The user initially runs microarrays for a training set with known class labels and enters the gene expression profiles together with the classification information into the algorithm. This "trains" the algorithm or teaches it to associate certain gene expression patterns with the predefined sample class labels. The next step is to profile samples from a new set of samples, the test set, and input the gene expression data into the algo-rithm. The latter will then classify the samples using the knowledge on class–expres-sion pattern associations learned from the training set. SVMs have been used to identify genes with similar expression patterns, but their most powerful application is in classification of samples. They have been used extensively in cancer classification and in some cases proved to be more reliable than the traditional diagnostic methods [42, 51]. Examples of supervised clustering relevant to drug discovery are discussed in Section 22.2.2.

The gene expression pattern of a cell reflects its phenotype and may provide information on the intracellular signaling pathways functioning in the cell. A comparison of the gene expression profiles for diseased tissue and the adjacent normal tissue may provide insight into the mechanisms and pathways driving the disease. In *in vitro* experiments, studying the gene induction patterns caused by a treatment may help identify the pathways activated or repressed by the treatment. A prerequisite for all these applications is the ability of the researcher to map gene expression profiles to signaling pathways, that is, identify the associations between the affected genes and the known pathways for the entire signature. There are several programs that allow association of gene expression patterns with predefined biological classes [52–60]. They use one of the existing gene classification systems, such as Gene Ontology [61, 62], Biocarta [63], or KEGG [64], to determine the enrichment of an expression signature in a certain motif, such as "cell cycle control" or "DNA biosynthesis." Gene Ontology is the most commonly used annotation system, which classifies a significant fraction of the genome (~15,000 genes) according to their involvement in a biological process or molecular function or their cellular localization. It is built hierarchically and involves a parent–child relationship between its terms. Programs such as MappFinder allow the researcher to identify the GO terms that show correlated gene expression changes in a microarray experiment. The affected GO terms can then be rank-ordered based on the Z-score, a statistic that reflects the number of genes in the term meeting the criteria for fold change in the microarray experiment [52]. MappFinder was one of the first GO-based programs designed for analysis of gene expression data. It has since been used to study the effects of various factors on intracellular pathways *in vitro* [65, 66] and *in vivo* [67]. Combined use siRNA-mediated gene silencing and MappFinder analysis of expression signatures has been suggested as an approach to pathway profiling [65]. Other pathway analysis programs have been developed in the past several years, which allow convenient visualization of the pathway analysis results [55–60]. Many of them use manually curated pathways instead of Gene Ontology, which permits greater focus and lower redundancy, especially when studying specific disease-related pathways.

Given the large amounts of gene expression data accumulated in the literature, integrative analysis of multiple datasets related to the same disease represents a very attractive idea. The precedent for such analysis was established when Rhodes et al. [68] performed so-called meta-analysis of four different gene expression datasets for prostate cancer. The authors identified a molecular signature common to the datasets, thus generating a robust signature of the disease. The signature was then mapped to KEGG pathways [64] to reveal a common biological motif, activation of polyamine biosynthesis [68]. Other studies identified common gene signatures in different breast and lung cancer datasets [69–71]. The existence of common motifs in datasets from different laboratories despite the well-publicized problem of interplatform variability presents strong evidence in favor of microarrays as tools for identification of drug targets and biomarkers.

As the amount of information derived from microarrays continues to increase, new and more complex data analysis procedures will emerge that will facilitate the current and future applications of the technology.

22.2.2   Applications of Microarrays in Preclinical Development

The applications of gene expression microarrays in drug discovery are summarized in Fig. 22.5. Chronologically, the first application of gene expression microarrays in drug discovery was in the area of identification of therapeutic targets.

Target Identification and Validation   One of the most obvious and logical strategies for target identification is a genome-wide scan for genes or their protein products overexpressed in the diseased tissue relative to its normal counterpart. Gene expression microarrays are ideally suited for this purpose because they provide wide genome coverage and permit efficient screening of hundreds of samples using a standardized reproducible protocol. To date, they have been most widely used to identify drug targets in cancer.

The development of sophisticated data analysis methods, such as two-dimensional clustering, has permitted cancer classification on the genomic basis and identification of groups of genes overexpressed in subsets of target cancers. Hematological cancers were historically the first group of cancers to be subjected to microarray classification, because of the better availability of homogeneous tumor cell populations. In a pioneering study of 72 acute leukemia samples, Golub et al. [42] identified a gene expression signature that reliably determined the disease type. The signature correctly assigned the samples into the acute myeloid leukemia (AML) or acute lymphoid leukemia (ALL) categories and further determined the subtype in the ALL category (B cell and T cell). In another study, Yeoh et al. [72] profiled 360 ALL blasts and identified gene expression patterns associated with the 6 known clinical subgroups of disease. While these and other works produced robust gene expression-based disease classifiers, no members of these classifiers appeared suitable as therapeutic targets. A recent exemplary microarray study of the mixed-lineage leukemia (MLL) [73, 74] went one step further. Armstrong et al. [73] not only identified a distinct gene expression profile that distinguishes leukemias with MLL translocations, but also identified a single gene that is consistently overexpressed in this leukemia type and validated it as a therapeutic target [74]. Mixed-lineage leukemia has traditionally been defined as a subtype harboring specific chromosomal translocations, so-called MLL translocations. The first study established a globally distinct nature of this disease by identifying its characteristic gene expression profile [73]. The authors then analyzed the MLL signature and identified

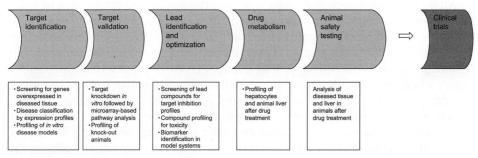

FIGURE 22.5   Applications of expression microarrays at different stages of drug discovery and development.

one gene consistently overexpressed in most MLLs compared to other acute leukemias [74]. This gene codes for a receptor tyrosine kinase, FLT3, which plays an important role in hematopoietic development. The authors then determined that many MLLs also carry mutations in the FLT3 gene, which result in constitutive activation of the kinase. An inhibitor of FLT3 was shown to differentially kill cells carrying MLL translocations *in vitro* and inhibit MLL development in a mouse model, thus validating FLT3 as a therapeutic target for MLL. This study truly demonstrates the power of gene expression microarrays in drug target discovery.

Microarrays have also been used for target identification is solid tumors. Expression profiling of medulloblastoma, a highly invasive tumor of the cerebellum, revealed expression signatures of the metastatic and nonmetastatic subtypes of the disease [75]. Several genes, including PDGFRA and members of the downstream RAS/mitogen-activated protein kinase pathway, were found to be upregulated in the metastatic tumors. The study thus yielded several potential therapeutic targets. Dhanasekaran et al. [76] have profiled over 50 normal and neoplastic prostate samples and three common prostate cell lines. Characteristic expression signatures were identified for localized prostate cancer, metastatic hormone-refractory prostate cancer, and benign prostatic hyperplasia. Two genes were consistently overexpressed in prostate cancer samples, hepsin (a transmembrane serine protease) and PIM1 (a serine/threonine kinase). The expression of the protein products of these genes was examined on a tissue microarray containing 738 tissues and found to be elevated in prostate cancer. An independent microarray screen of 11 malignant and 4 normal prostate samples also revealed hepsin overexpression in prostate cancer and implicated hepsin as a promising drug target [77]. Other studies later confirmed the conclusions on hepsin as a promising therapeutic target [78].

It is important to note here that target identification by microarrays should not be limited to direct identification of genes overexpressed in diseased tissue. Most genes in the disease signature encode proteins that are not druggable. Moreover, overexpression of certain genes in a disease signature only represents the bottom part of the signaling pathway modulating the disease process. Recent bioinformatics developments described in the preceding subsection permitted mapping of gene expression signatures to signaling pathways. Thus, an alternative approach to target identification may involve identification of pathways activated in diseased tissue and a search for druggable targets within the pathways. Subsequent target validation steps may involve modulation of the target activity *in vitro* followed by microarray profiling to determine whether the target-related signature is affected.

All the aforementioned studies have been performed in patient samples. In many cases patient samples are not available and therefore target discovery has to be performed in preclinical model systems, such as cultured cells or animal models of disease. However, these systems may produce a lot of noise, because cultured cells accumulate a lot of secondary genetic changes (such as gene amplifications/deletions), which are not relevant to the initial disease-originating events. Therefore, microarray-based target discovery in cultured cells requires inventive experimental design and careful validation. In an example from the oncology area, Sarang et al. [79] performed a rescue screen in neuroblastoma cells for approximately 900 known therapeutic agents. They found that 26 of these agents are capable of rescuing the cells from oxidant stress. The compounds were profiled by microarrays to identify the common gene expression signature. One of the genes in the signature codes for a secreted peptide called galanin. In a series of validation experiments, galanin was found to reverse cell death cased by oxidant stress. It was thus concluded that galanin receptor may represent a therapeutic target. Indirect identification of therapeutic targets has been performed by analyzing pathways activated by expression of known oncogenes [80, 81].

Although microarrays can reliably associate gene overexpression with disease, they cannot tell whether the overexpression is the cause or an effect of the disease. In most cases, microarray screens generate long lists of overexpressed genes and thus necessitate complex hypothesis-driven follow-up experiments aimed at selecting the genes that have a causative role in the disease process. Target validation is often performed in model systems using a loss-of-function or gain-of-function approach. Microarrays can also be used at this stage to assess the global effects of target knock-down or target overexpression. An example of such application is a study by Cho et al. [82], who knocked down the protein kinase RIα gene with an antisense oligonucleotide in cultured cells and subjected the cells to microarray analysis. It was found that suppression of the protein kinase RIα gene causes coordinated changes in gene expression that can be mapped to cell growth, differentiation, and activation pathways. The genes that compose the proliferation–transformation signature were downregulated, whereas those that defined the differentiation signature were upregulated in antisense-treated cancer cells and tumors, but not in host livers, thus validating the mechanism of protein kinase RIα. Short interfering RNA (siRNA) has recently emerged as a promising tool in target validation [83, 84]. Gene silencing with siRNA followed by microarray experiments and systematic pathway analysis may prove to be a powerful strategy in functional genomics. Early studies established the feasibility of this approach [65, 85]. One should expect that this approach will be actively used in target validation in the near future.

Compound Characterization   More recently, DNA microarrays have become an important tool in compound selection and optimization. Since microarrays are capable of generating a genome-wide view of the physiological state of the cell, they are well suited for characterization of compounds and elucidating their mechanism. A global approach to the problem would be to create a database of expression signatures associated with compound treatments in a relevant model system (Fig. 22.6). If such database is sufficiently populated with compounds with known mechanisms, one could envision its use as a look-up table: a series of novel compounds can be profiled by microarrays and their expression signatures can be plugged into the table. One of the available clustering algorithms would then be used to determine which of the known compounds have the most similar signatures to the test compounds.

Although more effort is needed to compile a comprehensive activity/expression signature database, numerous studies have used microarray profiling to determine the mechanism of known and novel agents. In an early example of microarray-based compound profiling, Glaser et al. [86] profiled three known histone deacetylase (HDAC) inhibitors in two cell lines to generate an HDAC inhibition signature. The gene expression signatures of the three active HDAC inhibitors were generally similar to each other and differed significantly from the signatures for inactive analogues, suggesting that the expression signatures are mechanism based. A core signature of 13 genes was identified that was common to all the HDAC inhibitors and

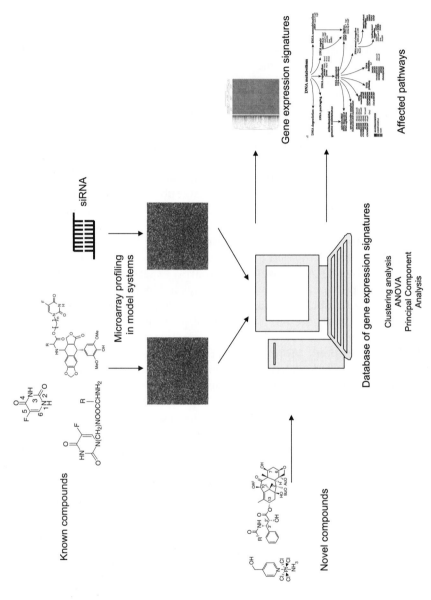

FIGURE 22.6 Creation of a genomics database for compound selection and optimization. Gene expression signatures of target inhibition and elimination are obtained using known inhibitors and siRNA, respectively, for multiple targets. Novel compounds synthesized to inhibit the target are profiled using the same microarray and their gene expression signatures are utilized to identify the affected pathways and targets.

all the cell lines used. The inhibitors were structurally different, implying that the signatures reflect the HDAC inhibition mechanism rather than off-target effects of the compounds.

An inhibitor of cyclooxygenase 1 (COX1) and cyclooxygenase 2 (COX2), sulindac sulfide, has been profiled in colorectal carcinoma cells, which express the COX1 enzyme but little COX2 [87]. A group of 11 genes was identified; their expression was further analyzed in another colon cancer cell line, HCT116, which expresses very low levels of both enzymes. The drug did not affect the expression of these 11 genes in HCT116, suggesting that their induction is COX dependent. This study is important because COX inhibitors have been shown to induce growth arrest and apoptosis of colon cancer cells. Elucidation of the mechanism of this potential anticancer effect could result in either selection of one of the known COX inhibitors for preclinical studies or optimization of the structure and creation of new COX inhibitors with potential anticancer activity. More compound profiling studies are analyzed in a very comprehensive review by Clarke et al. [88].

In an example from a different therapeutic area, Gunther et al. [22] have profiled multiple classes of antidepressants, antipsychotics, and opioid receptor agonists in primary human neurons. The gene expression patterns obtained for these groups of drugs were then used to construct statistical models capable of predicting drug efficacy. Several supervised classification algorithms were shown to reliably predict the functional group of each of the drugs based on their expression signatures.

A similar approach can be taken with respect to toxicity if the appropriate model system is used (hepatocytes, liver of model animals, etc.). This application of DNA microarrays will be comprehensively covered in Chapter 24. The toxic mechanism of a new compound can be determined from the database by association with the toxicity signatures of known compounds. In an early proof-of-concept study, Waring et al. [89] treated rats with 15 different known hepatotoxins, which are known to cause a variety of hepatocellular injuries including necrosis, DNA damage, cirrhosis, hypertrophy, and hepatic carcinoma. Gene expression signatures of the livers of treated rats were clustered and compared to the histopathology findings and clinical chemistry values. The results show strong correlation between the histopathology, clinical chemistry, and gene expression profiles induced by the agents. Other studies also demonstrated the feasibility of predicting the toxicity of compounds using microarray gene expression signatures [90–94]. A recent publication describes the creation of a comprehensive chemogenomics database [95]. The authors have profiled approximately 600 known compounds, including over 400 FDA-approved drugs in up to seven different tissues of rats. It was demonstrated that gene expression signatures, when used in conjunction with the database, can be used to predict the toxicity of a compound.

Biomarker Discovery   Biomarker identification is a major application for DNA microarrays in preclinical development, which often parallels and aids compound optimization. A biomarker is "a characteristic that is objectively measured and evaluated as an indicator of normal biologic processes, pathogenic processes, or pharmacologic responses to a therapeutic intervention" [96]. An early identification of a useful biomarker could result in substantial savings in the development process. Therefore, a substantial amount of effort has been devoted to biomarker discovery at the preclinical development stage, using model systems, such as cultured cells and animal models. Studies similar to the ones described in the previous subsection may yield useful pharmacodynamic biomarkers related to the mechanism. However, if the goal is to identify patient stratification biomarkers—that is, biomarkers that can predict a patient's response to the drug—one needs to screen basal levels of expression and then relate them to the sensitivity or resistance of the system to the drug. Early attempts to correlate gene expression signatures with drug sensitivity have been done in cultured cell lines [97–99]. Gene expression microarrays have been used to generate basal expression profiles of the 60 cell lines used by the NCI for cancer drug discovery screens (NCI-60 panel) [97]. The gene expression profiles were then correlated with the sensitivity of the cells to several common drugs, such as 5-fluorouracil and L-asparaginase [98]. The authors then correlated the expression of certain genes to the mechanisms of drug resistance. Gene expression signatures were used to predict the chemosensitivity of the cell lines. Staunton et al. [99] developed an algorithm to predict the sensitivity of the NCI-60 cell lines to 232 known agents. All 232 compounds were profiled in the 60 cell lines and the data were divided into a training set and a test set. The training set was used to develop classifiers and the test set was used to test the accuracy of the classifiers. The study yielded accurate classifiers ($p \leq 0.05$) and thus proved the feasibility of chemosensitivity prediction by microarrays.

Correlations between drug sensitivity and expression signatures have also been determined in more complex model systems, such as animal cancer models [100, 101]. Zembutsu et al. [100] profiled 85 cancer xenografts derived from nine human organs. The xenografts, implanted into nude mice, were examined for sensitivity to nine anticancer drugs (5-fluorouracil, 3-[(4-amino-2-methyl-5-pyrimidinyl)methyl]-1-(2-chloroethyl)-1-nitrosourea hydrochloride, adriamycin, cyclophosphamide, cisplatin, mitomycin C, methotrexate, vincristine, and vinblastine). The authors identified gene expression signatures, which correlated with drug sensitivity of the xenografts, and established an algorithm to calculate the drug sensitivity score based on the gene expression pattern.

Studies of this type have established the feasibility of predicting response to the drug based on the expression profile. However, it remains to be proved that correlations established in model systems will reproduce in patient samples. To date, only a limited number of studies correlated drug response with the basal expression profile in human samples [20, 21, 102–104]. Cell culture and xenograft-based models have a number of limitations. Most importantly, cultured cells undergo multiple rounds of selection, acquire additional genetic abnormalities, and therefore may poorly represent the original tumor, both in terms of their genomic patterns and their drug sensitivity profile. Future research will show whether gene expression profiles obtained in preclinical model systems can be used to predict patient response in clinical trials.

22.3 COMPARATIVE GENOMIC HYBRIDIZATION

22.3.1 Technology

Chromosomal aberrations are detrimental events associated with a number of developmental diseases, such as Down syndrome. Amplifications and deletions of chromosomal regions occurring in somatic cells are believed to be one of the main factors leading to cancer. Although fluorescent *in situ* hybridization (FISH; for a recent review, see Ref. 105) has been effectively applied to analyze known genetic aberrations for decades, until recently there was no method for detecting gene copy number alterations on a whole-genome scale. Comparative genomic hybridization (CGH), a technique that enables genome-wide analysis of chromosomal aberrations, was first described by Kallioniemi and colleagues in 1992 [106]. The method involves hybridization of the test DNA (sometimes mixed with reference DNA) to a complete representation of the genome attached to a solid support. Originally, CGH was performed on metaphase chromosome spreads, but in the past five to seven years, microarray-based CGH has become dominant (reviewed in Refs. 107 and 108). An overview of the array CGH procedure is shown in Fig. 22.7.

The original array CGH protocols have employed a two-color hybridization scheme, whereby the test DNA is labeled with a red fluorescent dye, while the reference normal DNA is labeled green. Although genomic DNA can be labeled and hybridized directly, many CGH protocols involve a PCR-based amplification step. Once the DNA is labeled, the test and the reference samples are mixed and hybridized to the array. Cot-1 DNA is typically added to suppress the hybridization of

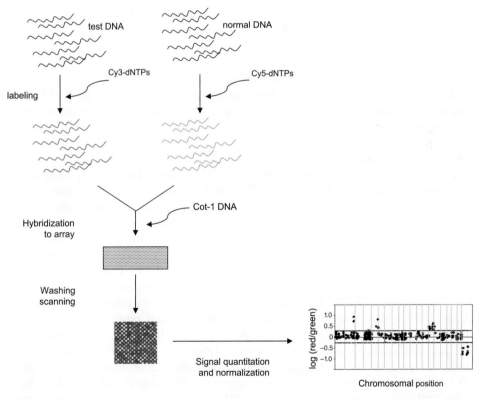

FIGURE 22.7 Two-color procedure for comparative genomic hybridization. The test gDNA is labeled red and the reference normal gDNA is labeled green. The gDNA samples are mixed and hybridized to a CGH array. Cot-1 DNA is added to eliminate the signal from repetitive sequences. After hybridization, the array is washed and scanned to generate signal intensities for all regions of interest.

repetitive sequences. After hybridization, the array is washed and scanned to generate the fluorescent intensity values for each probe on the array. The data are then normalized and presented as ratios of test/normal (usually on a log scale). An example of the CGH output for one chromosome in one sample is shown in Fig. 22.7. Ratios between the test and reference samples for multiple positions on a chromosome provide information on the copy number for each region measured. The copy number profile of a sample typically consists of a series of plateaus corresponding to regions with a constant copy number, flanked by abrupt transitions. An important limitation on the use of CGH is that it can measure changes in copy number, but it cannot detect balanced chromosomal translocations or changes in ploidy.

The value of CGH arrays increases with an improvement in genome coverage, resolution, and reproducibility. Several types of array platforms are currently used for CGH. Historically, the genome was represented on CGH arrays as a collection of bacterial artificial chromosomes (BACs) (e.g., see Refs. 109 and 110). Thousands of BACs were propagated and used as templates to generate PCR products. The PCR products were purified and deposited on a microarray. BAC arrays provide sufficiently high sensitivity to detect single copy amplifications and deletions [109]. The main drawback of the earlier BAC arrays was low resolution. Spotting 2460 BAC clones in triplicate provided an average resolution of 1.4 MB across the genome [109]. However, a high density BAC array was recently developed that contains approximately 30,000 clones arranged in a tiling fashion and covering the entire genome [109]. The array provided a significantly higher resolution and made possible detecting amplifications as small as 300 kb [109].

Arrays containing cDNAs have been used extensively for CGH [4, 6, 111, 112]. The advantages of cDNA arrays include higher reproducibility, easier manufacturing, and better representation of the genome [108]. However, multiple probes are required to detect small copy number changes, and more sample needs to be used (several micrograms), due to the lower sensitivity of the array [108].

A significant breakthrough was achieved in 2004 when two oligonucleotide-based platforms were developed for CGH [113, 114]. One of them was a microarray containing over 21,000 60-mer probes synthesized *in situ* by an ink jet technology [113]. The array provided a significant improvement in resolution and was shown to reliably detect single-copy losses, homozygous deletions, and various types of amplifications. It used the two-color protocol outlined in Fig. 22.7, with the addition of a PCR step to amplify the test and control DNAs. The other platform represented a high density microarray originally designed for detection of single nucleotide polymorphisms (SNPs) [114]. The array covered over 10,000 SNPs distributed across the genome. Each SNP was interrogated by multiple 25 mers synthesized *in situ* by a photolithographic method. Unlike the two-color CGH protocol described in Fig. 22.7, the SNP array protocol involves labeling DNA by incorporation of biotinylated dNTPs (Fig. 22.8). After array hybridization, the array is stained using streptavidin-phycoerythrin and a biotinylated anti-streptavidin antibody. Signal intensities from individual SNP measurements are smoothed across a user-defined smoothing window using a specialized algorithm. The resulting values are then compared to a preloaded reference dataset for normal DNA to produce an estimate of the copy number in the experimental sample. The array was used to evaluate chromosomal aberrations on a genome-wide scale in a number of cancer cells. It reliably detected

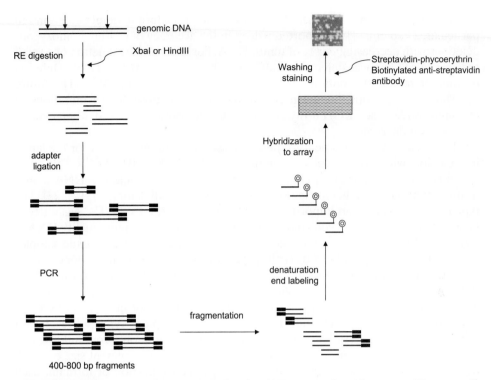

FIGURE 22.8 Gene copy number analysis using SNP genotyping microarrays. The genomic DNA sample is digested with a restriction endonuclease for complexity reduction. Adapters are ligated to the restriction fragments and the fragments are amplified by PCR. The PCR products are denatured, labeled, and hybridized to a microarray. The array is washed and stained to produce signal intensities for each probe. The data for multiple SNPs are smoothed and compared to an internal control to generate an estimate of the copy number for the chromosomal region.

chromosomal amplifications as well as homozygous and hemizygous deletions simultaneously with LOH detection [114]. The arrays produced results generally comparable with those obtained on BAC and cDNA arrays, but the authors reported a substantially lower noise level and a much higher resolution, averaging approximately 300 kb [114].

The next generation of SNP microarray has an increased SNP coverage (approximately 114,000 SNPs), which corresponds to a resolution of <100 kb. The software used for data analysis smoothes the signals for all the SNPs and compares the data with the internal reference dataset for over 100 individuals. The output of the software is the absolute copy number for each SNP position on the chip [115]. The new microarray has been validated in a large study of 101 lung carcinoma samples (tumors and cell lines) [116]. The increased resolution of the array enabled identification of several small amplifications and homozygous deletions that had not previously been detected by other CGH protocols.

One possible limitation on the use of high density oligonucleotide arrays for CGH is the requirement for high purity of the target tissue in the sample. The SNP array protocol uses a PCR amplification step, which may produce nonlinear amplification effects and thus diminish the ability of the procedure to detect deletions. In particular, Zhao et al. [114] reported a drop in the accuracy of scoring homozygous deletions with decreasing purity of tumor DNA. For example, the deletion of a small region in a cell line was detectable only with ≥90% purity of tumor DNA. Deletion of another region was only detected at 100% purity of tumor DNA. The future will show whether this limitation can be overcome in subsequent generations of oligonucleotide-based CGH arrays, but it should be considered today when making the platform decision.

Most existing CGH protocols require at least 500 ng of input DNA for the labeling reaction, which is equivalent to approximately 50,000–100,000 cells. This often presents a constraint as many clinical specimens are small. Numerous DNA amplification methods have been suggested for CGH on small samples [117–123]. The type of sample is also an important consideration in array CGH. The easiest type of sample to work with is cell culture, because the isolation of high quality DNA is routine and the cell population is homogeneous. Analysis of frozen tissue samples presents more difficulties because of the potential sample heterogeneity. For example, tumor samples often contain significant amounts of normal tissue, and this dilutes the signal obtained for aberrations in the tumor. Profiling of archived FFPE samples by CGH presents the greatest challenges, because of the poor quality of DNA isolated from such samples. Fixation protocols used in hospitals typically result in a number of known alterations in DNA, including degradation, cross-linking, and modification or loss of nucleic bases [124–126]. The average fragment size of DNA decreases with increasing fixation time [127]. The concentration of formalin used for tissue fixation and the age of the sample also affect the quality of the genomic DNA preparation [128].

Archived tissue samples represent an invaluable resource for genetic analysis because the existence of large banks of FFPE tissues with clinical annotation makes possible retrospective analysis of correlation between the genomic profile of the disease and the outcome or response to treatment. This goal undoubtedly justifies the amount of effort devoted to the optimization of FFPE CGH protocols. Additionally, the task of genomic analysis would be significantly facilitated if the fixation protocols used by hospitals were standardized, thus eliminating the variation in the DNA quality. Obviously, a protocol minimizing DNA degradation would be preferred.

22.3.2   Applications of CGH in Preclinical Development

Unlike gene expression microarrays, CGH has not yet become a mainstream tool in drug discovery, mostly because it was not commercially available until recently. However, we believe that CGH has a great potential to become a dominant tool in the next decade, particularly in cancer. Indeed, CGH detects alterations at the DNA level, which are believed to be fundamental to the disease. Chromosomal alterations are the main genetic feature of cancer; they often play a causative role in tumorigenesis by altering intracellular signaling and gene expression.

In preclinical development of oncology compounds, one frequently has to face decisions on selecting the appropriate *in vitro* and *in vivo* model systems. The genetic heterogeneity of cancer necessitates stratification of patients on the basis of the predominant genetic aberrations. The susceptibility to novel targeted agents correlates with the presence and the amount of the target, which may in turn be determined by the presence of a genetic aberration. Therefore, the genomic profile of the preclinical model system needs to reflect that of the target patient population. For example, Herceptin, an approved agent for the treatment of breast cancer, was developed using cell lines with a HER2 amplification as a model system [129, 130].

Herceptin acts by binding to the HER2 receptor and causing its internalization and the blockage of signal transduction [10–12, 131]. The *HER2* gene is frequently amplified in breast cancer; its amplification status is determined by FISH [132]. When a monoclonal antibody was developed against the extracellular domain of HER2, it was first tested on cultured breast cancer cells [129]. Of six mammary carcinoma cell lines tested, only the lines with HER2 amplification (SK-BR3, MBA-MB-175, and MDA-MD-361) were sensitive to the antibody. The established correlation between HER2 amplification and sensitivity to Herceptin was later used in the clinical development of the drug [10, 11].

In most cases, however, *in vitro* and *in vivo* model systems for compound screening are used without consideration for their genomic profile. Most commonly, oncology drug candidates are screened using cultured cancer cells and rodent xenografts that comprise the same cell lines grown subcutaneously in immunocompromised mice. One issue with using tumor cell lines is that the cells have been cultured on plastic for many generations, have acquired additional chromosomal aberrations, and therefore are not representative of the original tumor. In most cases, the main (and the only) selection criterion for cells to be used as model systems is their tissue origin. Such indiscriminate selection of model systems is one of the factors behind the current low success rate in the clinic [133, 134].

Most transformed cell lines used in preclinical development possess multiple secondary chromosomal aberrations that have been acquired during their propagation on plastic. These aberrations are not reflective of the genomic profile of the tumor of origin, but they may affect the sensitivity of cells to drugs. We have recently screened 23 small cell lung carcinoma cell lines previously used for compound screening *in vitro* and detected numerous large chromosomal amplifications and deletions that have not been detected in the target tumor [135]. In other studies, concurrent CGH screening of primary tumors and cultured cell lines of the same origin revealed gene copy number changes in the cell lines that were not present in the tumor samples [116].

In the near future, the adoption of whole-genome CGH screens should enable rational selection of model systems based on their genomic profiles. The first step in the selection process should be a comprehensive analysis of the genetic heterogeneity of the target population (Fig. 22.9). Model systems would then be selected whose genomic profiles reflect those found in the patient population (e.g., primary cell lines established from tumors). If the selected model systems vary in their sensitivity to the lead compounds, their genomic profiles need to be correlated with the sensitivity/resistance status. One of the established statistical procedures (e.g., analysis of variance, or ANOVA) can be used for this correlation. Once genomic features are identified that correlate with the sensitivity to the lead compounds, they can be used to stratify patients. If the correlation is confirmed in the early phases of clinical development, then enrollment of patients into Phase III should be based on the presence of this key genomic feature. Patient stratification based on genomic bio-

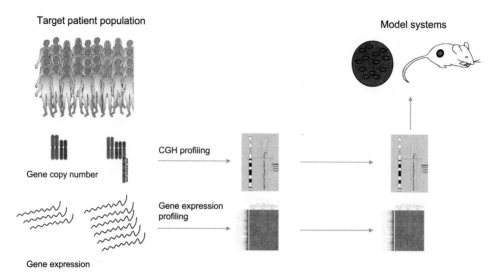

Target patient population

Model systems

CGH profiling

Gene copy number

Gene expression
profiling

Gene expression

FIGURE 22.9 Genomics-based selection of model systems for preclinical drug development in oncology. The genetic heterogeneity of the patient population is examined by comprehensive genomic profiling with CGH and expression microarrays. A preclinical model is selected based on the similarity of its genomic profile to that of the target patient population, in particular, with respect to the key genomic aberrations that affect the sensitivity to the drugs under development. Testing of the compounds in the preclinical models is accompanied by detailed genomic analysis of the models to identify the key genomic features that correlate with the sensitivity to the compounds. The presence of these genomic features will then serve as a criterion for selecting patients for clinical trials.

markers would improve the response rate in clinical trials and decrease the duration of the trial and its cost.

A number of recent studies have proved the feasibility of comprehensive profiling of cancers for gene copy number. For several types of cancer, correlation has been established between the genetic profile and the outcome or susceptibility to existing treatments. For example, neuroblastoma, a childhood tumor derived from neural crest cells, displays remarkable genetic heterogeneity, with several well-known recurrent aberrations, such as MYCN amplification, 17q gains, and 1p losses [136, 137]. The presence of these aberrations correlates with the outcome [136, 137], raising a possibility of patient stratification and creation of targeted therapies. This suggests that any neuroblastoma drug development program would benefit from a stratification scheme, whereby the model system would be screened for genetic abnormalities and the response to the agent would be correlated with the genomic profile.

A number of studies have been performed to identify genes amplified in specific tumors. Cheng et al. [138] have profiled ovarian and breast cancers using array CGH and identified a recurrent amplification on chromosome 1q22. The amplification was centered on the gene coding for a small GTPase called RAB25. The aberration was associated with decreased survival in both types of cancer. RAB25 was then shown to increase anchorage-independent cell proliferation and suppress apoptosis and anoikis. The authors concluded that RAB25 represents an attractive therapeutic target. Chibon et al. [139] used BAC-based CGH arrays to characterize the genomic profiles of malignant fibrous histiocytoma, an aggressive tumor, which shows no distinct line of differentiation. The 6q23 band was found to be frequently amplified in this type of cancer. The authors characterized the genes residing in the amplified region and identified ASK1 (MAP3K5) as a candidate target for therapeutic intervention. Tonon et al. [140] profiled 44 lung adenocarcinomas and small cell carcinomas and determined the most frequent aberrations in these tumors. Two genomic regions, 8p12 and 20q11, were found to be frequently amplified in both types of cancer. Several genes residing in these regions were identified, and their overexpression was confirmed by quantitative RT-PCR. Ehlers et al. [141] used both CGH and gene expression microarrays to study uveal melanoma and determined that the gain of chromosome 8 correlates most strongly with the expression of DDEF1, a gene located at 8q24. It was shown that overexpression of DDEF1 results in increased cell motility. The authors concluded that DDEF1 represents an attractive therapeutic target.

In the past few years, CGH has been used to discover patient stratification biomarkers for several types of cancer. Paris et al. [142] profiled archived tumors from 64 prostate cancer patients, 32 of whom had recurred postoperatively. The authors identified a loss at 8p23.2 that was associated with advanced disease, but most importantly, they discovered a chromosomal gain at 11q13.1 that was predictive of postoperative recurrence, independent of the stage of the disease. One gene (MEN1) coding for a nuclear protein menin was mapped to the amplified region, and its expression was correlated with disease recurrence, thus establishing the gene as a biomarker of the aggressive recurrent disease. In another study, 35 gastric carcinomas were profiled on ~2400-element BAC CGH arrays, and the patterns of chromosomal aberrations were correlated with the clinical history of the patients [16]. Hierarchical clustering of the CGH profiles revealed three predominant groups. Membership in these groups correlated with lymph node status and survival. Patients from cluster 3 had a significantly better prognosis than patients from clusters 1 and 2. Although no commonly amplified genes were identified, this study clearly demonstrates the power of genome-wide CGH in patient stratification and biomarker discovery.

A study by Wreesmann et al. [143] dealt with papillary thyroid cancer (PTC). Two distinct variants of this disease exist, the more aggressive tall-cell thyroid cancer (TCV) and conventional thyroid cancer (cPTC). A panel of 25 TCV and 45 cPTCs was profiled by CGH and gene expression microarrays to identify genomic features that would distinguish between the two subtypes of the disease. Significant differences were identified in the patterns of chromosomal gains and losses. One gene, MUC1, was of particular interest because it was both amplified and overexpressed in TCV. Its overexpression was confirmed by immunohistochemistry on independent TCV samples. Multivariate analysis showed a significant correlation between MUC1 expression level and the outcome of treatment, establishing the gene as a prognostic marker in PTC.

Diffuse large B-cell lymphoma is a highly heterogeneous disease that displays significant diversity with respect to clinical presentation and outcome. Different subtypes of the disease require different therapeutic approaches. A recent report [144] described CGH profiling of 224 diffuse large B-cell lymphomas previously examined by expression microarrays. The authors reported a high degree of correlation between the gene copy number and the expression data and identified a chromosomal region (3p11-p12) that provided prognostic information that is statistically independent of the previously built gene expression-based model.

The first steps have been taken toward developing a diagnostic tool based on a CGH array. Schwaenen et al. [145] reported a novel CGH chip that can detect recurrent chromosomal abnormalities in B-cell chronic lymphocytic leukemia (B-CLL). The chip contained a total of 644 DNA elements and covered all the known regions frequently altered in B-CLL, as well as some other B-cell neoplasms. The array was tested and validated in 106 primary B-CLL tumor samples.

Although the bulk of the CGH work has been of an exploratory nature, one can expect that comprehensive CGH profiling of preclinical development models will become routine in the near future. Once the recurrent aberrations are identified for the tumor type of interest, a focused array similar to that described earlier can be developed to routinely interrogate preclinical model systems and stratify patients in clinical trials according to their genomic profile. Thus, the use of CGH in preclinical development will facilitate development of agents targeted to specific patient populations.

22.4   GENE SILENCING

We define some of the gene silencing terms used in this chapter.

Antisense Oligonucletide. A short DNA fragment complementary to the target mRNA sequence.

RnaseH. An enzyme that specifically binds to and degrades RNA–DNA duplexes.

Dicer. An RNase III-type endonuclease that processes long double-stranded RNA into siRNA.

RISC. An RNA–protein complex containing an siRNA molecule and effector proteins that unwind the siRNA and catalyze the cleavage of the target mRNA.

Transfection. Transfer of nucleic acids into the cell.

Electroporation. Transfection of cells with nucleic acids by using electric current to increase the permeability of the cells.

High throughput alteration of gene activity has recently emerged as a powerful tool in drug discovery. Gene knock-down screens are often performed in cell culture to identify therapeutic targets, and gene overexpression is a common tool in target validation. In the area of preclinical development, manipulation of the target gene's activity is used in compound optimization and selection. In this section we describe gene silencing, a set of techniques frequently used in drug development to identify therapeutic targets and optimize candidate compounds.

22.4.1   Antisense Oligonucleotides and Ribozymes

Antisense oligonucleotides were historically the first tool for targeted gene silencing. Their initial applications were focused on inhibiting the replication of viruses in cell culture [146]. Typically, antisense oligonucleotides ~20 nucleotides in length are used. To increase stability and prevent enzymatic degradation, antisense oligonucleotides are usually modified, for example, by introducing phosphorothioate groups [147]. Other common types of modification include morpholino [148] and methoxyethyl [149] groups and peptide nucleic acids (PNAs) [150].

The mechanism of gene silencing by antisense oligonucleotides is illustrated in Fig. 22.10. They act by hybridizing to mRNA and causing RNaseH-mediated degradation of the transcript or creating a steric hindrance for the enzymes that catalyze translation and splicing [151].

In more than 20 years since the first use, antisense oligonucleotides have produced notable successes, including an approved therapeutic agent (Vitravene™ by Isis Pharmaceuticals), but their applications were limited by several drawbacks of the technology. Most importantly, antisense oligonucleotides have revealed significant nonspecific effects [82, 147, 152, 153]. In particular, phosphothioate oligonucleotides have been shown to bind various proteins and thus cause off-target effects [153]. Some oligonucleotides also induce expression of interferons through binding to Toll-like receptors [154, 155]. The potency of antisense oligonucleotides is determined by many factors, including the type of modification and accessibility of the target. Overall, they are less potent as the more recently discovered gene silencing tools [156–159].

Ribozymes also hybridize to mRNA through Watson–Crick base pairing and catalyze its degradation through hydrolysis of the phosphodiester bonds (reviewed in Ref. 160). The most commonly used type is the hammerhead ribozyme. The catalytic sequence of a ribozyme is flanked by sequences complementary to the target transcript, a feature that provides target specificity. The accessibility of the target sequence is an important factor, which determines the potency of silencing [161].

22.4.2 Short Interfering RNA

Mechanism of Gene Silencing   A breakthrough in the field of functional genomics was achieved with the discovery of RNA interference in the late 1990s. In 1998, Fire et al. [162] showed that double-stranded RNA causes specific gene silencing when injected into *Caenorhabditis elegans*. Several years later it was found that in *Drosophila melanogaster* embryo extracts, long double-stranded RNA is cleaved into

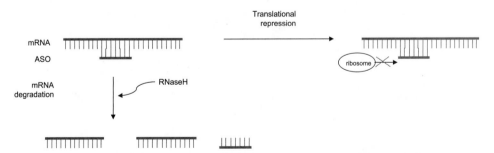

FIGURE 22.10   Mechanism of gene silencing by antisense oligonucleotides. Binding of an antisense oligonucleotide to the target mRNA results in target degradation by RNaseH and translational repression due to steric hindrances.

fragments containing approximately 22 base pairs by an enzyme complex called Dicer [163]. This observation prompted the first use of synthetic RNA fragments to induce RNA interference. Elbashir et al. [83, 84] demonstrated that chemically synthesized 21 and 22 nucleotide RNA duplexes cause degradation of homologous mRNA when introduced into cultured cells. These duplexes were named short interfering RNAs (siRNAs). The mechanism of gene silencing by siRNA is illustrated in Fig. 22.11 (for a recent review, see Ref. 164). Long dsRNA is processed in the cell by the Dicer. The enzyme cleaves long dsRNA strands into fragments 21–28 nucleotides long, which contain two-nucleotide overhangs. The siRNA duplexes are then incorporated into an enzymatic complex called RNA-induced silencing complex (RISC). Within the silencing complex, the siRNA duplex is unwound in an ATP-dependent manner. Once the duplex is unwound, the antisense strand guides the

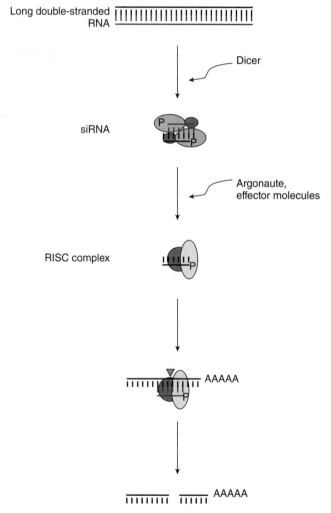

FIGURE 22.11   Mechanism of gene silencing by siRNA. Long double-stranded RNA is cleaved by the Dicer complex. The resulting siRNA binds to the RISC complex and is guided to the target site to degrade the target mRNA.

RISC complex to the target site on the mRNA. The latter then causes endonucleolytic cleavage of the target mRNA sequence [164, 165].

In a typical *in vitro* siRNA experiment, the researcher transfects cells with chemically synthesized siRNA duplexes (typically 22 nucleotides long with two-nucleotide overhangs on both ends) and 24–48 hours later measures the effects of the siRNA on the target levels by either QPCR or Western blot. Alternatively, a vector coding for a so-called short hairpin RNA (shRNA) can be transiently or stably transfected into cells to produce a more lasting silencing effect [166]. Several reports have addressed the issue of differential siRNA potency [167, 168]. Duplexes that target different regions of the same gene vary significantly in their potency. The potency of siRNA is likely to be determined by the primary and secondary structures of the target site [164]. More research is necessary to clearly define the rules for designing potent siRNAs.

Another important consideration in gene silencing is the specificity of the silencing tool. In the case of siRNA, the low concentrations used and the enzymatic nature of its mechanism are factors that diminish the potential for nonspecific effects. There are several types of nonspecific effects that could be displayed by siRNAs, including (1) degradation of mRNAs other than the target due to cross-hybridization, (2) binding to cellular proteins in a sequence-specific manner (aptamer effect), (3) translational silencing through the miRNA effect, and (4) induction of the "dsRNA response" that is nonspecific with respect to the siRNA sequence. Several recent studies have demonstrated that transfection of siRNA into the cell does not cause global nonspecific effects on gene expression [169, 170]. However, other studies have described nonspecific effects caused by siRNA, which depended on the concentration, cell type, and the type of siRNA [171, 172]. Overall, the combination of high potency, relatively higher specificity, and ease of finding accessible target sites have quickly made siRNA the preferred gene silencing tool.

Use of siRNA for Target Identification   One of the major applications of siRNA is in drug discovery. The initial application was in target identification and validation. A typical siRNA-based target identification screen involves high throughput transfection of a large siRNA library into cultured cells and observation of the resulting phenotypes, most often by an established assay. Such screens are most common in cancer drug discovery. Prerequisites for a successful screen include a representative cell culture model, a robust transfection protocol, and a reliable quantitative assay for the desired phenotype. In cancer drug discovery, the desired phenotype is typically cell death, apoptosis, or inhibition of cell proliferation. Other assays are currently being adapted to high throughput siRNA screens, including cell migration, invasion, and colony formation assays. Cells that are hard to transfect, for example, primary cells, may be subjected to electroporation. Electroporation has been shown to be amenable to high throughput screening [173]. While the results of a comprehensive cancer drug discovery screen are yet to be published, several focused studies have been reported. Berns et al. [174] used a set of retroviral vectors targeting approximately 8000 different human genes for suppression. This RNAi library was used in human cells to identify five new modulators of the p53-dependent proliferation arrest. Suppression of these genes confers resistance to both p53-dependent and p19ARF-dependent proliferation arrest and abolishes a DNA-damage-induced G1 cell-cycle arrest.

To facilitate high throughput screening with siRNA libraries, an siRNA microarray has recently been developed [175]. The siRNAs are deposited onto a microchip, which is then used for reverse transfection of mammalian cells, thus facilitating high throughput screening of hundreds of genes in multiple cell types. The technique has shown significant promise for drug discovery, but it has several limitations. In particular, only adherent cells can be used in the screen and the transfection conditions need to be optimized for each cell type.

Use of siRNA for Target Validation   Short interfering RNA has recently been shown to be an extremely useful tool for target validation. It has been applied to validate targets identified in DNA microarray experiments [176, 177]. Indeed, DNA microarrays identify genes overexpressed in the diseased tissue, but they do not prove the functional involvement of the genes into the disease process. Meanwhile, if silencing these genes with siRNA reverses the disease phenotype, the target candidate is typically taken to the next stage of validation. In a recent study from the oncology area, Williams et al. [176] used DNA microarrays to profile colon tumors from 20 patients alongside with normal colon tissue samples. Over 500 genes were found to be consistently overexpressed in one-third of the cancer samples, and 13 of them were confirmed by quantitative real-time PCR. To identify genes that play an important role in colorectal carcinogenesis, siRNA was used to disrupt expression of several of the overexpressed genes in a colorectal carcinoma cell line, HCT116. Silencing of one of these genes (survivin) severely reduced tumor growth both *in vitro* and in an *in vivo* xenograft model, thus validating the target in colorectal cancer.

In a recent study, Li and colleagues [178] used siRNA to validate a target *in vivo*. They used inducible RNA interference in mice to silence hypoxia-inducible factor-1α (HIF-1α) in established xenograft tumors. It was shown that HIF-1α inhibition results in transient tumor stasis or tumor regression. A differential requirement of HIF-1α for tumor growth was also observed among different tumor types. Examination of tumors resistant to HIF-1α inhibition suggested that the resistance might result from a less hypoxic tumor environment and that the level of HIF-1α expression in tumors may be a useful marker for predicting tumor response to HIF-1α inhibition. This study demonstrated the versatility of inducible RNAi as a tool for evaluating cancer targets *in vivo*.

Overall, siRNA and DNA microarrays are highly complementary technologies, when used successively in the target discovery process. First, DNA microarrays can be used to identify genes overexpressed in a diseased tissue. Then siRNA can be used to silence these genes in a disease model system, while the phenotype is observed. If silencing of a gene affects the disease phenotype, then the gene may indeed have functional involvement in the disease process. This would warrant further investigation, primarily in an *in vivo* system.

Use of siRNA for Compound Characterization   The application of siRNA in compound selection and optimization is rapidly gaining momentum. Several possible schemes have been developed for compound selection that involve combined use of siRNA-based gene silencing and DNA microarrays. siRNA against the chosen target can be used to generate gene expression signatures associated with target knock-down. Candidate compounds can then be screened in the same system and their microarray signatures can be compared with that of the siRNA (Fig. 22.6). Theoretically, if the compounds inhibit the target, the overlap of the compound and the siRNA signatures should represent the target inhibition signature, while the signatures unique to the compounds represent their off-target effects. In our experience, however, an siRNA against a gene and an inhibitor of the gene product do not always produce similar signatures. This could be explained by the fact that silencing of a gene and inhibiting its product are fundamentally different events. Indeed, inhibitors are often directed against one specific site of a protein, leaving the possibility that the other sites may still maintain their function or interact with other proteins. Meanwhile, silencing the gene results in the elimination of the entire protein. The time course of the two events is almost certainly different as well: 24 hours after the addition of the inhibitor one should not expect to see the same effects as 24 hours after the siRNA transfection. Additionally, either silencing or inhibition may be incomplete, with the residual activity responsible for the differences in the gene expression effects between the silencing agent and the inhibitor. Nonspecific effects of both the inhibitor and the siRNA may also contribute to the divergence. While nonspecific effects are expected from the compound, the siRNA is meant to serve as the gold standard of specificity in this type of experiment. One approach to selecting only the specific effects of siRNA is to profile several siRNAs against the target and then select the overlap of their signatures as the target silencing profile.

Overall, manipulation of gene activity has become a routine tool in drug discovery. Today, it is hard to imagine a target identification or validation strategy without a step that would involve manipulation of the target activity. The approach is becoming more common with each new technique developed, as the techniques provide higher potency and specificity.

22.5 CONCLUSION

In the years following the publication of the human genome sequence, genomic technologies have begun to revolutionize drug discovery and development. Drug development has undergone a major paradigm change, whose essence is in shifting from the trial-and-error approach to an innovative, hypothesis-driven, and systematic strategy based on target selection and validation, followed by selection and optimization of a compound that would modulate the activity of the target with minimal side effects.

Today, the initial stages of the drug development process, target identification and validation, almost always involve analysis of gene content or expression or manipulation of gene activity. Genomic technologies are also beginning to be used in preclinical and clinical development, following innovative proof-of-concept studies published in the past few years. As we have demonstrated in this chapter, the use of genomics in preclinical development may help bridge the gap between the preclinical and clinical stages of drug development by helping select preclinical models more relevant to the target disease. Thus, genomics may solve one of the most significant problems in today's drug development, the high failure rate in clinical trials of drugs that have been selected based on their activity in preclinical systems. One of the implications of this upcoming change for pharmaceutical research and development organizations is the necessity of organizational changes to facilitate close collaboration between discovery and development. Just as the promise of the biomarker research compelled the managers of many pharmaceutical companies to create cross-functional translational biology teams, the new strategies for genomics-based preclinical development may necessitate formation of groups dedicated to the genomic analysis of target patient population and the appropriate selection of preclinical model systems. It is not always easy to quantify the benefits of genomics in the drug development process. The list of purely genomics-based drugs remains short. However, the success of the new drug development paradigm is dependent on the genomic data and therefore there is no alternative to continuing and expanding the use of genomic technologies in drug discovery and development.

REFERENCES

1. Orth AP, et al. The promise of genomics to identify novel therapeutic targets. *Expert Opin Ther Targets* 2004;8(6):587–596.
2. Lander ES, et al. Initial sequencing and analysis of the human genome. *Nature* 2001;409(6822):860–921.
3. Venter JC, et al. The sequence of the human genome. *Science* 2001;291(5507): 1304–1351.
4. Pollack JR, et al. Genome-wide analysis of DNA copy-number changes using cDNA microarrays. *Nat Genet* 1999;23(1):41–46.
5. Linn SC, et al. Gene expression patterns and gene copy number changes in dermatofibrosarcoma protuberans. *Am J Pathol* 2003;163(6):2383–2395.
6. Pollack JR, et al. Microarray analysis reveals a major direct role of DNA copy number alteration in the transcriptional program of human breast tumors. *Proc Natl Acad Sci USA* 2002;99(20):12963–12968.
7. Heidenblad M, et al. Microarray analyses reveal strong influence of DNA copy number alterations on the transcriptional patterns in pancreatic cancer: implications for the interpretation of genomic amplifications. *Oncogene* 2005;24(10):1794–1801.
8. Lewin DA, Weiner MP. Molecular biomarkers in drug development. *Drug Discov Today* 2004;9(22):976–983.
9. Frank R, Hargreaves R. Clinical biomarkers in drug discovery and development. *Nat Rev Drug Discov* 2003;2(7):566–580.
10. Cobleigh, MA, et al. Multinational study of the efficacy and safety of humanized anti-HER2 monoclonal antibody in women who have HER2-overexpressing metastatic breast cancer that has progressed after chemotherapy for metastatic disease. *J Clin Oncol* 1999;17(9):2639–2648.
11. Vogel CL, et al. Efficacy and safety of trastuzumab as a single agent in first-line treatment of HER2-overexpressing metastatic breast cancer. *J Clin Oncol* 2002;20(3):719–726.
12. Carter P, et al. Humanization of an anti-p185HER2 antibody for human cancer therapy. *Proc Natl Acad Sci USA* 1992;89(10):4285–4289.
13. Singh D, et al. Gene expression correlates of clinical prostate cancer behavior. *Cancer Cell* 2002;1(2):203–209.

14. Shipp MA, et al. Diffuse large B-cell lymphoma outcome prediction by gene-expression profiling and supervised machine learning. *Nat Med* 2002;8(1):68–74.

15. Weiss MM, et al. Genomic alterations in primary gastric adenocarcinomas correlate with clinicopathological characteristics and survival. *Cell Oncol* 2004;26(5–6):307–317.

16. Weiss MM, et al. Genomic profiling of gastric cancer predicts lymph node status and survival. *Oncogene* 2003;22(12):1872–1879.

17. Pomeroy SL, et al. Prediction of central nervous system embryonal tumour outcome based on gene expression. *Nature* 2002;415(6870):436–442.

18. vant Veer LJ, et al. Gene expression profiling predicts clinical outcome of breast cancer. *Nature* 2002;415(6871):530–536.

19. Khan J, et al. Classification and diagnostic prediction of cancers using gene expression profiling and artificial neural networks. *Nat Med* 2001;7(6):673–679.

20. Bohen SP, et al. Variation in gene expression patterns in follicular lymphoma and the response to rituximab. *Proc Natl Acad Sci USA* 2003;100(4):1926–1930.

21. Takata R, et al. Predicting response to methotrexate, vinblastine, doxorubicin, and cisplatin neoadjuvant chemotherapy for bladder cancers through genome-wide gene expression profiling. *Clin Cancer Res* 2005;11(7):2625–2636.

22. Gunther EC, et al. Prediction of clinical drug efficacy by classification of drug-induced genomic expression profiles *in vitro*. *Proc Natl Acad Sci USA* 2003;100(16):9608–9613.

23. Chomczynski P, Sacchi N. Single-step method of RNA isolation by acid guanidinium thiocyanate-phenol-chloroform extraction. *Anal Biochem* 1987;162(1):156–159.

24. Chomczynski P. A reagent for the single-step simultaneous isolation of RNA, DNA and proteins from cell and tissue samples. *Biotechniques* 1993;15(3):532–534, 536–537.

25. Van Gelder RN, et al. Amplified RNA synthesized from limited quantities of heterogeneous cDNA. *Proc Natl Acad Sci USA* 1990;87(5):1663–1667.

26. Perou CM, et al. Molecular portraits of human breast tumours. *Nature* 2000;406(6797):747–752.

27. Huang J, et al. Effects of ischemia on gene expression. *J Surg Res* 2001;99(2):222–227.

28. Masuda N, et al. Analysis of chemical modification of RNA from formalin-fixed samples and optimization of molecular biology applications for such samples. *Nucleic Acids Res* 1999;27(22):4436–4443.

29. Cronin M, et al. Measurement of gene expression in archival paraffin-embedded tissues: development and performance of a 92-gene reverse transcriptase–polymerase chain reaction assay. *Am J Pathol* 2004;164(1):35–42.

30. Erlander MG, et al. Global gene expression profiling from formalin-fixed paraffin-embedded (FFPE) tissues: implications for retrospective and prospective clinical studies. *Proc Am Soc Clin Oncol* 2003;22:125.

31. http://www.arctur.com/research_portal/products/paradise_main.htm.

32. Emmert-Buck MR, et al. Laser capture microdissection. *Science* 1996;274(5289):998–1001.

33. Ma XJ, et al. A two-gene expression ratio predicts clinical outcome in breast cancer patients treated with tamoxifen. *Cancer Cell* 2004;5(6):607–616.

34. Fuller AP, et al. Laser capture microdissection and advanced molecular analysis of human breast cancer. *J Mammary Gland Biol Neoplasia* 2003;8(3):335–345.

35. Ma XJ, et al. Gene expression profiles of human breast cancer progression. *Proc Natl Acad Sci USA* 2003;100(10):5974–5979.

36. Tusher VG, Tibshirani R, Chu G. Significance analysis of microarrays applied to the ionizing radiation response. *Proc Natl Acad Sci USA* 2001;98(9):5116–5121.

37. Tsai CA, Hsueh HM, Chen JJ. Estimation of false discovery rates in multiple testing: application to gene microarray data. *Biometrics* 2003;59(4):1071–1081.

38. Delongchamp RR, et al. Multiple-testing strategy for analyzing cDNA array data on gene expression. *Biometrics* 2004;60(3):774–782.

39. Lee ML, et al. Importance of replication in microarray gene expression studies: statistical methods and evidence from repetitive cDNA hybridizations. *Proc Natl Acad Sci USA* 2000;97(18):9834–9839.

40. Novak JP, Sladek R, Hudson TJ. Characterization of variability in large-scale gene expression data: implications for study design. *Genomics* 2002;79(1):104–113.

41. Chen JJ, et al. Analysis of variance components in gene expression data. *Bioinformatics* 2004;20(9):1436–1446.

42. Golub TR, et al. Molecular classification of cancer: class discovery and class prediction by gene expression monitoring. *Science* 1999;286(5439):531–537.

43. Ramaswamy S, et al. Multiclass cancer diagnosis using tumor gene expression signatures. *Proc Natl Acad Sci USA* 2001;98(26):15149–15154.

44. Bittner M, et al. Molecular classification of cutaneous malignant melanoma by gene expression profiling. *Nature* 2000;406(6795):536–540.

45. Quackenbush J. Computational analysis of microarray data. *Nat Rev Genet* 2001;2(6):418–427.

46. Raychaudhuri S, et al. Basic microarray analysis: grouping and feature reduction. *Trends Biotechnol* 2001;19(5):189–193.

47. Eisen MB, Brown PO. DNA arrays for analysis of gene expression. *Methods Enzymol* 1999;303:179–205.

48. Tavazoie S, et al. Systematic determination of genetic network architecture. *Nat Genet* 1999;22(3):281–285.

49. Toronen P, et al. Analysis of gene expression data using self-organizing maps. *FEBS Lett* 1999;451(2):142–146.

50. Brown MP, et al. Knowledge-based analysis of microarray gene expression data by using support vector machines. *Proc Natl Acad Sci USA* 2000;97(1):262–267.

51. Nutt CL, et al. Gene expression-based classification of malignant gliomas correlates better with survival than histological classification. *Cancer Res* 2003;63(7):1602–1607.

52. Doniger SW, et al. MAPPFinder: using Gene Ontology and GenMAPP to create a global gene-expression profile from microarray data. *Genome Biol* 2003;4(1):R7.

53. Volinia S, et al. GOAL: automated Gene Ontology analysis of expression profiles. *Nucleic Acids Res* 2004;32(Web Server issue):W492–W49.

54. http://david.niaid.nih.gov/david/.

55. Vaquerizas JM, et al. GEPAS, an experiment-oriented pipeline for the analysis of microarray gene expression data. *Nucleic Acids Res* 2005;33(Web Server issue):W616–W620.

56. Al-Shahrour F, et al. BABELOMICS: a suite of web tools for functional annotation and analysis of groups of genes in high-throughput experiments. *Nucleic Acids Res* 2005;33(Web Server issue):W460–W464.

57. Al-Shahrour F, Diaz-Uriarte R, Dopazo J. FatiGO: a web tool for finding significant associations of Gene Ontology terms with groups of genes. *Bioinformatics* 2004;20(4):578–580.

58. Mlecnik B, et al. PathwayExplorer: web service for visualizing high-throughput expression data on biological pathways. *Nucleic Acids Res* 2005;33(Web Server issue):W633–W637.

59. www.ingenuity.com.

60. www.genego.com.

61. Harris MA, et al. The Gene Ontology (GO) database and informatics resource. *Nucleic Acids Res* 2004;32(Database issue):D258–D261.

62. Ashburner M, et al. Gene ontology: tool for the unification of biology. The Gene Ontology Consortium. *Nat Genet* 2000;25(1):25–29.

63. www.biocarta.com.

64. Kanehisa M, et al. The KEGG resource for deciphering the genome. *Nucleic Acids Res* 2004;32(Database issue):D277–D280.

65. Semizarov D, Kroeger P, Fesik S. siRNA-mediated gene silencing: a global genome view. *Nucleic Acids Res* 2004;32(13):3836–3845.

66. Zucchini C, et al. Identification of candidate genes involved in the reversal of malignant phenotype of osteosarcoma cells transfected with the liver/bone/kidney alkaline phosphatase gene. *Bone* 2004;34(4):672–679.

67. Meyer MH, Dulde E, Meyer RA Jr. The genomic response of the mouse kidney to low-phosphate diet is altered in X-linked hypophosphatemia. *Physiol Genomics* 2004;18(1):4–11.

68. Rhodes DR, et al. Meta-analysis of microarrays: interstudy validation of gene expression profiles reveals pathway dysregulation in prostate cancer. *Cancer Res* 2002;62(15):4427–4433.

69. Jiang H, et al. Joint analysis of two microarray gene-expression data sets to select lung adenocarcinoma marker genes. *BMC Bioinformatics* 2004;5(1):81.

70. Sorlie T, et al. Repeated observation of breast tumor subtypes in independent gene expression data sets. *Proc Natl Acad Sci USA* 2003;100(14):8418–8423.

71. Shen R, Ghosh D, Chinnaiyan AM. Prognostic meta-signature of breast cancer developed by two-stage mixture modeling of microarray data. *BMC Genomics* 2004;5(1):94.

72. Yeoh EJ, et al. Classification, subtype discovery, and prediction of outcome in pediatric acute lymphoblastic leukemia by gene expression profiling. *Cancer Cell* 2002;1(2):133–143.

73. Armstrong SA, et al. MLL translocations specify a distinct gene expression profile that distinguishes a unique leukemia. *Nat Genet* 2002;30(1):41–47.

74. Armstrong SA, et al. Inhibition of FLT3 in MLL. Validation of a therapeutic target identified by gene expression based classification. *Cancer Cell* 2003;3(2):173–183.

75. MacDonald TJ, et al. Expression profiling of medulloblastoma: PDGFRA and the RAS/MAPK pathway as therapeutic targets for metastatic disease. *Nat Genet* 2001;29(2):143–152.

76. Dhanasekaran SM, et al. Delineation of prognostic biomarkers in prostate cancer. *Nature* 2001;412(6849):822–826.

77. Magee JA, et al. Expression profiling reveals hepsin overexpression in prostate cancer. *Cancer Res* 2001;61(15):5692–5696.

78. Fromont G, et al. Differential expression of 37 selected genes in hormone-refractory prostate cancer using quantitative taqman real-time RT-PCR. *Int J Cancer* 2005;114(2):174–181.

79. Sarang SS, et al. Discovery of molecular mechanisms of neuroprotection using cell-based bioassays and oligonucleotide arrays. *Physiol Genomics* 2002;11(2):45–52.

80. Huang E, et al. Gene expression phenotypic models that predict the activity of oncogenic pathways. *Nat Genet* 2003;34(2):226–230.

81. Svaren J, et al. EGR1 target genes in prostate carcinoma cells identified by microarray analysis. *J Biol Chem* 2000;275(49):38524–38531.

82. Cho YS, et al. Antisense DNAs as multisite genomic modulators identified by DNA microarray. *Proc Natl Acad Sci USA* 2001;98(17):9819–9823.

83. Elbashir SM, et al. Duplexes of 21-nucleotide RNAs mediate RNA interference in cultured mammalian cells. *Nature* 2001;411(6836):494–498.

84. Elbashir SM, Lendeckel W, Tuschl T. RNA interference is mediated by 21- and 22-nucleotide RNAs. *Genes Dev* 2001;15(2):188–200.

85. Ziegelbauer J, Wei J, Tjian R. Myc-interacting protein 1 target gene profile: a link to microtubules, extracellular signal-regulated kinase, and cell growth. *Proc Natl Acad Sci USA* 2004;101(2):458–463.

86. Glaser KB, et al. Gene expression profiling of multiple histone deacetylase (HDAC) inhibitors: defining a common gene set produced by HDAC inhibition in T24 and MDA carcinoma cell lines. *Mol Cancer Ther* 2003;2(2):151–163.

87. Bottone FG Jr et al. Gene modulation by the cyclooxygenase inhibitor, sulindac sulfide, in human colorectal carcinoma cells: possible link to apoptosis. *J Biol Chem* 2003;278(28):25790–25801.

88. Clarke PA, Te Poele R, Workman P. Gene expression microarray technologies in the development of new therapeutic agents. *Eur J Cancer* 2004;40(17):2560–2591.

89. Waring JF, et al. Clustering of hepatotoxins based on mechanism of toxicity using gene expression profiles. *Toxicol Appl Pharmacol* 2001;175(1):28–42.

90. Burczynski ME, et al. Toxicogenomics-based discrimination of toxic mechanism in HepG2 human hepatoma cells. *Toxicol Sci* 2000;58(2):399–415.

91. Thomas RS, et al. Identification of toxicologically predictive gene sets using cDNA microarrays. *Mol Pharmacol* 2001;60(6):1189–1194.

92. Thomas RS, et al. Developing toxicologically predictive gene sets using cDNA microarrays and Bayesian classification. *Methods Enzymol* 2002;357:198–205.

93. Hamadeh HK, et al. Prediction of compound signature using high density gene expression profiling. *Toxicol Sci* 2002;67(2):232–240.

94. Waring JF, et al. Microarray analysis of hepatotoxins *in vitro* reveals a correlation between gene expression profiles and mechanisms of toxicity. *Toxicol Lett* 2001;120(1–3):359–368.

95. Ganter B, et al. Development of a large-scale chemogenomics database to improve drug candidate selection and to understand mechanisms of chemical toxicity and action. *J Biotechnol* 2005;119(3):219–244.

96. Biomarkers and surrogate endpoints: preferred definitions and conceptual framework. *Clin Pharmacol Ther* 2001;69(3):89–95.

97. Ross DT, et al. Systematic variation in gene expression patterns in human cancer cell lines. *Nat Genet* 2000;24(3):227–235.

98. Scherf U, et al. A gene expression database for the molecular pharmacology of cancer. *Nat Genet* 2000;24(3):236–244.

99. Staunton JE, et al. Chemosensitivity prediction by transcriptional profiling. *Proc Natl Acad Sci USA* 2001;98(19):10787–10792.

100. Zembutsu H, et al. Genome-wide cDNA microarray screening to correlate gene expression profiles with sensitivity of 85 human cancer xenografts to anticancer drugs. *Cancer Res* 2002;62(2):518–527.

101. Zembutsu H, et al. Gene-expression profiles of human tumor xenografts in nude mice treated orally with the EGFR tyrosine kinase inhibitor ZD1839. *Int J Oncol* 2003;23(1):29–39.

102. Oshita F, et al. Genomic-wide cDNA microarray screening to correlate gene expression profile with chemoresistance in patients with advanced lung cancer. *J Exp Ther Oncol* 2004;4(2):155–160.

103. Chen X, et al. Variation in gene expression patterns in human gastric cancers. *Mol Biol Cell* 2003;14(8):3208–3215.

104. Leung SY, et al. Phospholipase A2 group IIA expression in gastric adenocarcinoma is associated with prolonged survival and less frequent metastasis. *Proc Natl Acad Sci USA* 2002;99(25):16203–16208.

105. Levsky JM, Singer RH. Fluorescence *in situ* hybridization: past, present and future. *J Cell Sci* 2003;116(Pt 14):2833–2838.

106. Kallioniemi A, et al. Comparative genomic hybridization for molecular cytogenetic analysis of solid tumors. *Science* 1992;258(5083):818–821.

107. Pinkel D, Albertson DG. Array comparative genomic hybridization and its applications in cancer. *Nat Genet* 2005;37(Suppl):S11–S17.

108. Albertson DG, Pinkel D. Genomic microarrays in human genetic disease and cancer. *Hum Mol Genet* 2003;12(Spec No 2):R145–R152.

109. Snijders AM, et al. Assembly of microarrays for genome-wide measurement of DNA copy number. *Nat Genet* 2001;29(3):263–264.

110. Pinkel D, et al. High resolution analysis of DNA copy number variation using comparative genomic hybridization to microarrays. *Nat Genet* 1998;20(2):207–211.

111. Clark J, et al. Genome-wide screening for complete genetic loss in prostate cancer by comparative hybridization onto cDNA microarrays. *Oncogene* 2003;22(8):1247–1252.

112. Hyman E, et al. Impact of DNA amplification on gene expression patterns in breast cancer. *Cancer Res* 2002;62(21):6240–6245.

113. Barrett MT, et al. Comparative genomic hybridization using oligonucleotide microarrays and total genomic DNA. *Proc Natl Acad Sci USA* 2004;101(51):17765–17770.

114. Zhao X, et al. An integrated view of copy number and allelic alterations in the cancer genome using single nucleotide polymorphism arrays. *Cancer Res* 2004;64(9):3060–3071.

115. www.affymetrix.com.

116. Zhao X, et al. Homozygous deletions and chromosome amplifications in human lung carcinomas revealed by single nucleotide polymorphism array analysis. *Cancer Res* 2005;65(13):5561–5570.

117. Hosono S, et al. Unbiased whole-genome amplification directly from clinical samples. *Genome Res* 2003;13(5):954–964.

118. Devries S, et al. Array-based comparative genomic hybridization from formalin-fixed, paraffin-embedded breast tumors. *J Mol Diagn* 2005;7(1):65–71.

119. Lage JM, et al. Whole genome analysis of genetic alterations in small DNA samples using hyperbranched strand displacement amplification and array-CGH. *Genome Res* 2003;13(2):294–307.

120. Daigo Y, et al. Degenerate oligonucleotide primed-polymerase chain reaction-based array comparative genomic hybridization for extensive amplicon profiling of breast cancers: a new approach for the molecular analysis of paraffin-embedded cancer tissue. *Am J Pathol* 2001;158(5):1623–1631.

121. Wang G, et al. Balanced-PCR amplification allows unbiased identification of genomic copy changes in minute cell and tissue samples. *Nucleic Acids Res* 2004;32(9):E76.

122. Tanabe C, et al. Evaluation of a whole-genome amplification method based on adaptor-ligation PCR of randomly sheared genomic DNA. *Genes Chromosomes Cancer* 2003;38(2):168–176.

123. Guillaud-Bataille M, et al. Detecting single DNA copy number variations in complex genomes using one nanogram of starting DNA and BAC-array CGH. *Nucleic Acids Res* 2004;32(13):E112.

124. Giannella C, et al. Comparison of formalin, ethanol, and Histochoice fixation on the PCR amplification from paraffin-embedded breast cancer tissue. *Eur J Clin Chem Clin Biochem* 1997;35(8):633–635.

125. Koshiba M, et al. The effect of formalin fixation on DNA and the extraction of high-molecular-weight DNA from fixed and embedded tissues. *Pathol Res Pract* 1993;189(1):66–72.

126. Tbakhi A, et al. The effect of fixation on detection of B-cell clonality by polymerase chain reaction. *Mod Pathol* 1999;12(3):272–278.

127. Ghazvini S, et al. Comparative genomic hybridization analysis of archival formalin-fixed paraffin-embedded uveal melanomas. *Cancer Genet Cytogenet* 1996;90(2):95–101.

128. Semizarov D, unpublished observations.

129. Hudziak RM, et al. p185HER2 monoclonal antibody has antiproliferative effects *in vitro* and sensitizes human breast tumor cells to tumor necrosis factor. *Mol Cell Biol* 1989;9(3):1165–1172.

130. Lupu R, et al. Direct interaction of a ligand for the erbB2 oncogene product with the EGF receptor and p185erbB2. *Science* 1990;249(4976):1552–1555.

131. Harris M. Monoclonal antibodies as therapeutic agents for cancer. *Lancet Oncol* 2004;5(5):292–302.

132. Hicks DG, Tubbs RR. Assessment of the *HER2* status in breast cancer by fluorescence *in situ* hybridization: a technical review with interpretive guidelines. *Hum Pathol* 2005;36(3):250–261.

133. Kola I, Landis J. Can the pharmaceutical industry reduce attrition rates? *Nat Rev Drug Discov* 2004;3(8):711–715.

134. Kamb A. What's wrong with our cancer models? *Nat Rev Drug Discov* 2005;4(2):161–165.

135. Semizarov D, unpublished observations.

136. Maris JM. The biologic basis for neuroblastoma heterogeneity and risk stratification. *Curr Opin Pediatr* 2005;17(1):7–13.

137. Mosse YP, et al. High-resolution detection and mapping of genomic DNA alterations in neuroblastoma. *Genes Chromosomes Cancer* 2005;43(4):390–403.

138. Cheng KW, et al. The RAB25 small GTPase determines aggressiveness of ovarian and breast cancers. *Nat Med* 2004;10(11):1251–1256.

139. Chibon F, et al. ASK1 (MAP3K5) as a potential therapeutic target in malignant fibrous histiocytomas with 12q14-q15 and 6q23 amplifications. *Genes Chromosomes Cancer* 2004;40(1):32–37.

140. Tonon G, et al. High-resolution genomic profiles of human lung cancer. *Proc Natl Acad Sci USA* 2005;102(27):9625–9630.

141. Ehlers JP, et al. DDEF1 is located in an amplified region of chromosome 8q and is overexpressed in uveal melanoma. *Clin Cancer Res* 2005;11(10):3609–3613.

142. Paris PL, et al. Whole genome scanning identifies genotypes associated with recurrence and metastasis in prostate tumors. *Hum Mol Genet* 2004;13(13):1303–1313.

143. Wreesmann VB, et al. Genome-wide profiling of papillary thyroid cancer identifies MUC1 as an independent prognostic marker. *Cancer Res* 2004;64(11):3780–3789.

144. Bea S, et al. Diffuse large B-cell lymphoma subgroups have distinct genetic profiles that influence tumor biology and improve gene expression-based survival prediction. *Blood* 2005;106(9):3183–3190.

145. Schwaenen C, et al. Automated array-based genomic profiling in chronic lymphocytic leukemia: development of a clinical tool and discovery of recurrent genomic alterations. *Proc Natl Acad Sci USA* 2004;101(4):1039–1044.

146. Zamecnik PC, Stephenson ML. Inhibition of Rous sarcoma virus replication and cell transformation by a specific oligodeoxynucleotide. *Proc Natl Acad Sci USA* 1978;75(1):280–284.

147. Stein CA. Does antisense exist? *Nat Med* 1995;1(11):1119–1121.

148. Summerton J, Weller D. Morpholino antisense oligomers: design, preparation, and properties. *Antisense Nucleic Acid Drug Dev* 1997;7(3):187–195.

149. Dorn G, et al. Specific inhibition of the rat ligand-gated ion channel P2X3 function via methoxyethoxy-modified phosphorothioated antisense oligonucleotides. *Antisense Nucleic Acid Drug Dev* 2001;11(3):165–174.

150. Egholm M, et al. PNA hybridizes to complementary oligonucleotides obeying the Watson–Crick hydrogen–bonding rules. *Nature* 1993;365(6446):566–568.

151. Dias N, Stein CA. Antisense oligonucleotides: basic concepts and mechanisms. *Mol Cancer Ther* 2002;1(5):347–355.

152. Fisher AA, et al. Evaluating the specificity of antisense oligonucleotide conjugates. A DNA array analysis. *J Biol Chem* 2002;277(25):22980–22984.

153. Lebedeva I, Stein CA. Antisense oligonucleotides: promise and reality. *Annu Rev Pharmacol Toxicol* 2001;41:403–419.

154. Roman M, et al. Immunostimulatory DNA sequences function as T helper-1-promoting adjuvants. *Nat Med* 1997;3(8):849–854.

155. Hafner M, et al. Antimetastatic effect of CpG DNA mediated by type I IFN. *Cancer Res* 2001;61(14):5523–5528.

156. Kretschmer-Kazemi Far R, Sczakiel G. The activity of siRNA in mammalian cells is related to structural target accessibility: a comparison with antisense oligonucleotides. *Nucleic Acids Res* 2003;31(15):4417–4424.

157. Grunweller A, et al. Comparison of different antisense strategies in mammalian cells using locked nucleic acids, 2′-O-methyl RNA, phosphorothioates and small interfering RNA. *Nucleic Acids Res* 2003;31(12):3185–3193.

158. Miyagishi M, Hayashi M, Taira K. Comparison of the suppressive effects of antisense oligonucleotides and siRNAs directed against the same targets in mammalian cells. *Antisense Nucleic Acid Drug Dev* 2003;13(1):1–7.

159. Xu Y, et al. Effective small interfering RNAs and phosphorothioate antisense DNAs have different preferences for target sites in the luciferase mRNAs. *Biochem Biophys Res Commun* 2003;306(3):712–717.

160. Doudna JA, Cech TR. The chemical repertoire of natural ribozymes. *Nature* 2002;418(6894):222–228.

161. Kuwabara T, Warashina M, Taira K. Cleavage of an inaccessible site by the maxizyme with two independent binding arms: an alternative approach to the recruitment of RNA helicases. *J Biochem (Tokyo)* 2002;132(1):149–155.

162. Fire A, et al. Potent and specific genetic interference by double-stranded RNA in Caenorhabditis elegans. *Nature* 1998;391(6669):806–811.

163. Zamore PD, et al. RNAi: double-stranded RNA directs the ATP-dependent cleavage of mRNA at 21 to 23 nucleotide intervals. *Cell* 2000;101(1):25–33.

164. Dorsett Y, Tuschl T. siRNAs: applications in functional genomics and potential as therapeutics. *Nat Rev Drug Discov* 2004;3(4):318–329.

165. Dykxhoorn DM, Novina CD, Sharp PA. Killing the messenger: short RNAs that silence gene expression. *Nat Rev Mol Cell Biol* 2003;4(6):457–467.

166. Lee NS, et al. Expression of small interfering RNAs targeted against HIV-1 rev transcripts in human cells. *Nat Biotechnol* 2002;20(5):500–505.

167. Vickers TA, et al. Efficient reduction of target RNAs by small interfering RNA and RNase H-dependent antisense agents. A comparative analysis. *J Biol Chem* 2003;278(9):7108–7118.

168. Holen T, et al. Positional effects of short interfering RNAs targeting the human coagulation trigger tissue factor. *Nucleic Acids Res* 2002;30(8):1757–1766.

169. Semizarov D, et al. Specificity of short interfering RNA determined through gene expression signatures. *Proc Natl Acad Sci USA* 2003;100(11):6347–6352.

170. Chi JT, et al. Genomewide view of gene silencing by small interfering RNAs. *Proc Natl Acad Sci USA* 2003;100(11):6343–6346.

171. Jackson AL, et al. Expression profiling reveals off-target gene regulation by RNAi. *Nat Biotechnol* 2003;21(6):635–637.

172. Persengiev SP, Zhu X, Green MR. Nonspecific, concentration-dependent stimulation and repression of mammalian gene expression by small interfering RNAs (siRNAs). *Rna* 2004;10(1):12–18.

173. Walters DK, Jelinek DF. The effectiveness of double-stranded short inhibitory RNAs (siRNAs) may depend on the method of transfection. *Antisense Nucleic Acid Drug Dev* 2002;12(6):411–418.

174. Berns K, et al. A large-scale RNAi screen in human cells identifies new components of the p53 pathway. *Nature* 2004;428(6981):431–437.

175. Wheeler DB, Carpenter AE, Sabatini DM. Cell microarrays and RNA interference chip away at gene function. *Nat Genet* 2005;37(Suppl):S25–S30.

176. Williams NS, et al. Identification and validation of genes involved in the pathogenesis of colorectal cancer using cDNA microarrays and RNA interference. *Clin Cancer Res* 2003;9(3):931–946.

177. Zhou A, et al. Identification of NF-kappa B-regulated genes induced by TNFalpha utilizing expression profiling and RNA interference. *Oncogene* 2003;22(13):2054–2064.

178. Li L, et al. Evaluating hypoxia-inducible factor-1alpha as a cancer therapeutic target via inducible RNA interference in vivo. *Cancer Res* 2005;65(16):7249–7258.

23

PROTEOMICS

JUAN CASADO AND J. IGNACIO CASAL

Spanish National Cancer Center (CNIO), Madrid, Spain

Contents

Preclinical Development Handbook: Toxicology, edited by Shayne Cox Gad
Copyright © 2008 John Wiley & Sons, Inc.

23.1   INTRODUCTION

The term *proteomics* was first coined in the mid-1990s [1] and has become a key research area during the last decade. It is dedicated to study the biological implication of proteins in disease, pathologies, or alterations of living organisms. The *proteome* was first defined as the protein complement of the genome [1]. The proteome is dynamic and its composition changes as a consequence of alterations in an effort to adapt to environmental changes and keep the homeostasis of living systems. There are at least four main questions that proteomic studies aim to find a response for: (1) How many proteins change as a consequence of an alteration? (2) How much do these proteins change? (3) Did the changes observed involve the regulation of any biochemical pathways? (4) What is the biological relevance or can we take advantage of that information to solve the alteration? To answer these questions, a number of techniques are routinely used to comprehensively and systematically separate, visualize, identify, and quantify the plethora of proteins coexisting in tissues and cells.

Two-dimensional polyacrylamide gel electrophoresis (2D-PAGE), high performance liquid chromatography (HPLC), and mass spectrometry (MS) are the most important tools in proteomics. The combination of all these techniques allows the identification and quantification of up to thousands of proteins, the identification of proteins differentially expressed in normal versus altered organisms/tissues, and the characterization of posttranslational modification of proteins.

23.2 PROTEIN EXTRACTION AND PURIFICATION

One of the most important steps in a proteomic study is the selection of the biological material to work with. Whole proteome analysis of any organism, cell, organelle, biological fluid, or a single protein can be considered. Therefore, due to the great diversity of protein samples used, the optimal procedure must be determined empirically for each sample. Here, we provide some general guidelines.

23.2.1 Disruption of Tissues and Solubilization of Proteins

The proteins of interest must be completely soluble. A number of chemicals are frequently found in literature for protein solubilization, the most frequently used being 8 M urea or 6 M guanidine hydrochloride.

Proteomic experiments can also focus on the identification and characterization of a subset of proteins of interest, such as membrane proteins [2, 3] or glycoproteins. A wide number of chemicals have been described to be useful for the extraction of membrane proteins including treatment with alkaline pH, N-acetyl trimethylammonium, and different concentrations of detergents, such as Triton X-100, Triton X-114 [4], N-lauroylsarcosine, N-octylglucoside, and sodium dodecyl sulfate (SDS) among others. The enrichment of glycoproteins is achieved by two different methods, using hydrazide chemistry or lectin binding.

23.2.2 Depletion of Abundant Proteins

Some of the proteins with meaningful biological information can be present at low concentrations in the experimental samples. One example is the identification of proteins present in human plasma, containing six abundant proteins (albumin, IgG, IgA, haptoglobin, transferrin, and alpha-1 anti-trypsin) that can be depleted from the sample by selective immunodepletion of the proteins using chromatographic columns containing antibodies against everyone of the six proteins [5]. The selective removal of the most abundant "housekeeping" proteins favors the enrichment of proteins present at a lower abundance in the sample that can be visualized by 2D-PAGE and identified with mass spectrometry.

23.3 TWO-DIMENSIONAL POLYACRYLAMIDE GEL ELECTROPHORESIS

Two-dimensional polyacrylamide gel electrophoresis (2D-PAGE) allows the separation of hundreds (up to thousands) of proteins in a single experiment. The result is a gel matrix where proteins appear as single spots that can be visualized after a protein staining procéss. After digitalization of the gel to obtain an image with the help of transmission light scanners, the subsequent images can be processed for spot analysis. It can be used to find differential expression profiles between normal versus altered protein patterns and to quantify these changes by densitometric measurement of the intensity of the protein spots observed in the gel. The quality and biological significance of the results are compromised by the protein sample preparation and the reproducibility of the experiments. The main steps involved in 2D-PAGE analysis and some of the potential problems are described next.

23.3.1 Protein Sample Preparation

Proteins can be found soluble in the cytosol, embedded in cell membranes, and bound to nucleic acids or to other proteins. For 2D-PAGE, it is necessary that the pool of proteins submitted be completely soluble. Different treatments can be used to solubilize different types of proteins. The choice of cell/tissue disruption method, composition of lysis buffer, and the use of detergents directly affect the solubilization of proteins.

Since proteases are normally present in biological samples and proteolysis may cause undesired results in the 2D gels, cocktails of protease inhibitors should be added during the protein extraction steps. Some of the protease inhibitors frequently used include 4-(2-aminoethyl) benzenesulfonyl fluoride (AEBSF), ethylenediaminetetraacetic acid (EDTA), bestatin, E-64, leupeptin, aprotinin, and phenylmethylsulfonyl fluoride (PMSF), among others.

If only a subset of proteins from the biological sample is of interest (i.e., subcellular proteins), prefractionation methods need to be employed [6]. This is normally achieved by differential solubilization or ultracentrifugation in sucrose gradients. Once the proteins of interest have been extracted, it is common to include some steps to remove contaminants. Dialysis for salt removal, lyophilization, precipitation of proteins with trichloroacetic acid–cold acetone [7], or DNA removal with the use of endonucleases are among the current procedures.

Protocol A: Protein Cleaning and Preparation for Isoelectrofocusing Sample volumes corresponding to 100 μg of protein, previously quantified [8], are pelleted by centrifugation at 13,000 rpm after addition of 6% trichloroacetic acid in chilled acetone and incubation at 4 °C for 30 min [7]. The addition of 0.2% deoxycholate usually facilitates the precipitation of proteins. The precipitation can be repeated several times if there is an excess of salts in the sample of interest. After removal of the supernatant, the protein pellet is dried under a nitrogen stream at room temperature. The appearance of several spots corresponding to the same protein is frequently observed in 2D gels. This can be attributed most times to the oxidation state of thiol groups in the protein of interest. This problem is solved by oxidizing the thiol groups, for instance, adding chemicals, such as DeStreak (Amersham Biosciences), prior to or during the rehydration of immobilized pH gradient (IPG) strips.

23.3.2 First Dimension: Isoelectrofocusing

Prior to the isoelectrofocusing (IEF), dry and clean precipitates need to be solubilized in a rehydration solution (typically 100–300 μL) containing 8 M urea, 2% 3-[(3-cholamidopropyl)dimethylamonio]-1-propanesulfonate (CHAPS), 2 mg/mL dithiothreitol (DTT), 0.0125 g/mL iodoacetamide (IAM), a trace of bromophenol blue, and carrier ampholytes IPG buffer (commercially available depending on the pH range of the IPG strip). Proteins are embedded in the IPG strip at low voltages (50 V per IPG strip) and are ready for IEF. It consists of different steps: a first step of 500V for 1h, a second step of 1000V for 1h. The final step requires 8,000V for 4h, until a total voltage of about 40,000 (volt × hour)V·h. After completion of the IEF, each strip is deposited in a vial with 5mL of equilibrating solution and left with agitation for 15min.

23.3.3 Second Dimension: Polyacrylamide Gel Electrophoresis—Choice of Gel Size, Concentration, and Protein Molecular Weight Range

After the IEF, the IPG strip must be equilibrated by covering it with a solution containing 50mM tris(hydroxymethyl)aminomethane (Tris-base) pH 8.8, 6M urea, 30% glycerol, 2% SDS, 0.01g bromophenol blue, and 10mg/mL DTT. Proteins are separated according to their molecular weight under denaturing conditions in the presence of SDS [9].

Protocol B: Standard SDS-PAGE Gel Solution for 100 mL

Solution for 12.5% Acrylmide-Bisacrylamide Gels	Volume
Stock solution 40% acrylamide/bisacrylamide (37.5:1, 2.6% C)	41.7mL
1.5M Tris-HCl pH 8.8	25mL
10% Sodium dodecyl sulfate (SDS)	1mL
Water	31.8mL
10% Ammonium persulfate	0.5mL
N,N,N′,N′-tetramethylethylenediamine (TEMED)	33μL

Once the gel is polymerized, the IPG strips, containing the proteins focused at their isoelectric point (p*I*) and equilibrated, are placed on top of the gel and the proteins are separated according to their molecular weight in a chamber containing running buffer (25mM Tris-HCl, 192mM glycine, and 0.1% SDS).

23.4   GEL STAINING AND IMAGE PROCESSING

The staining of 2D gels is a crucial step in proteomic analysis. It allows the visualization of protein spots resolved on the 2D gel and enables further analysis, including the identification of differential proteins among samples, densitometric quantification, and recovery of proteins of interest.

23.4.1   Coomassie Brilliant Blue and Silver Staining

An improved method for Coomassie Brilliant Blue (CBB) stained gel is the colloidal Coomassie Brilliant Blue [10]. Silver staining is used to visualize proteins that are present at a low concentration in the gel (2ng/spot) (Fig. 23.1a).

Protocol C: Colloidal Coomassie Brilliant Blue G-250 Staining   Fix the gels with 40% methanol and 10% acetic acid for 30min. Prepare a stock solution of colloidal Coomassie Brilliant Blue G-250 staining as follows: mix 4g of Brilliant Blue G-205 with 230mL of 85% phosphoric acid and stir. Add 640mL of saturated ammonium sulfate solution and stir. Add distilled water to 4L. Prepare 100mL of staining

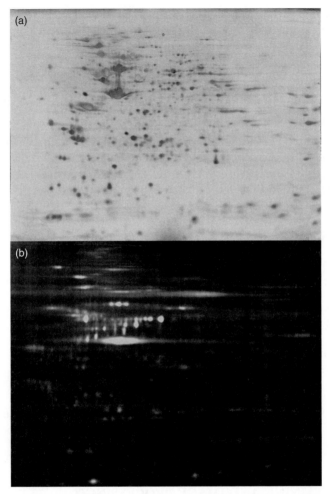

FIGURE 23.1 Representative images corresponding to (a) silver stained 2D gels (14 × 16 cm) and (b) DIGE stained corresponding to the overlapping Cy3 + Cy5 images. Protein spots appear all over the gel matrix separated according to their isoelectric point and molecular weight. After staining, the spots of interest (differential spots) can be recovered and further processed for protein identification and characterization using mass spectrometry and database searches.

solution by adding 20 mL methanol to 80 mL of the stock solution. The staining solution should be prepared immediately before use, as the colloid only lasts for a few hours. Stain gels overnight (if maximum sensitivity is required) using a rocking platform to avoid colloidal stain sticking to the surface of the gel. Finally, destain the gels with 3–5 changes of 25% methanol until the spots appear clearly defined in the gel. The use of rocking platforms during the staining is crucial, because the staining of gels without agitation can cause the appearance of noise and background during software-based image densitometry of the gels. The duration and temperature of staining and destaining steps are also crucial in order to obtain reproducible results.

Protocol D: Silver Staining/Destaining of Proteins in Polyacrylamide Gels   Cover the gel with fixing solution (50% methanol, 10% acetic acid), remove the fixing solution, cover gel with 5% methanol for 15 min, and wash 3 times with distilled water. Cover the gel with sensitizing solution 0.2 g/L of $Na_2S_2O_3$ freshly prepared for 2 min and wash with distilled water. Cover gel with 0.2 g/L of silver nitrate ($AgNO_3$) for 25 min and wash 3 times with distilled water. Cover gel with developing solution containing 3 g/100 mL Na_2CO_3, 50 µL/100 mL of 37% HCOH, and 2 mL of sensitizing solution. Allow staining until the protein spots are visible over the background of the gel (10 min maximum). Remove the developing solution and stop with 14 g/L Na_2-ethylenediaminetetraacetic acid (EDTA) for 10 min. Finally, wash with distilled water.

Once stained, the gels can be destained by covering the gels with 0.2 g potassium ferricyanide ($K_3Fe(CN)_6$) in 100 mL of sensitizing solution, leaving a yellow background in the gel. Restaining is also possible starting the protocol again by adding the silver nitrate solution (adapted from Ref. 11).

23.4.2   Fluorescent Dyes

Silver staining, while sensitive, exhibits a low dynamic range. Handling may significantly change the results and the background of the gels frequently interferes with further characterization of silver-stained proteins using mass spectrometry. Fluorescent staining is superior in sensitivity and linear response as compared to Coomassie Brilliant Blue and silver staining, respectively [12]. A range of fluorescent dyes are commercially available for different purposes, including Sypro[r] Ruby, Deep purple, 5-hexadecanoylamino-fluorescein [13]. Sypro Ruby is a sensitive fluorescent stain for detecting proteins separated by polyacrylamide gel electrophoresis. This fluorescent stain does not interfere with subsequent analysis of proteins by mass spectrometry and is quantitative over three orders of magnitude. Apart from its high sensitivity, Sypro Ruby will not stain nucleic acids [14].

Other specific applications of fluorescent dyes for the detection of subsets of proteins have also been developed; such as the case of ProQ diamond for phosphoproteins.

Protocol E: Sypro Ruby Staining of Proteins in Polyacrylamide Gels   It is highly recommended to bind the gel to one of the glass plates prior to running the electrophoresis as follows: prepare a Bind-Silane working solution by mixing 8 mL of ethanol, 200 µL of acetic acid, 10 µL of Bind-Silane, and 1.8 mL of distilled water. Cover the inner surface of one of the glass plates used to polymerize the acrylamide gel and dry to room temperature for 1–2 h. Perform the assembly and polymerization of the gels as usual. The gels will stay attached to the glass during electrophoresis, staining procedures, scanning, and storage.

Incubate the gel in fixing solution (30% methanol, 7.5% acetic acid) for at least 2 h. Remove fixing solution and cover the gel with Sypro Ruby stain. Incubate 3 h or overnight with gentle shaking protected from direct light. Wash extensively with distilled water (at least 4 changes of 20 min). Finally, scan the gels and select the spots of interest. Sypro Ruby protein gel stain can be imaged using laser-based imaging systems equipped with 450, 473, 488, or 532 nm laser lines. For further details on Sypro Ruby staining you may access http://probes.invitrogen.com/lit/bioprobes31/section1.html.

23.4.3 Differential In-Gel Electrophoresis Staining

An outstanding application of fluorescent dyes to proteomics using 2D gels is the differential in-gel electrophoresis (DIGE) technology, which is based on the use of three CyDye™ fluorochroms, Cy2, Cy3, and Cy5, for protein labeling (Fig. 23.1b). It allows one to label up to three samples that can be separated in a 2D gel in order to search for differential protein profiles, thus avoiding experimental variations from gel to gel and increasing the accuracy of the results. A pooled internal standard, containing equal amounts of protein from each sample, should also be created as a reference for normalization in these experiments.

Fluorescent two-dimensional DIGE constitutes the proteomic equivalent to gene expression analysis by DNA microarrays. Even minor differences of protein expression can be detected across multiple samples simultaneously with statistical confidence by using the DeCyder software [15, 16]. The comparison of spot intensities using the DIGE approach and the DeCyder software is more objective than the conventional approach based on the comparison of the brightness of gel images obtained by conventional staining. The quantification of abundance changes are obtained over a linear dynamic range of almost four orders of magnitude for the Cy dyes [15]. This novel technology is being applied to the analysis of differential protein expression in different neoplasia for the search of cancer markers [17–19] or to study drug resistance [20].

Protocol F: DIGE Protein Labeling   Reconstitute each vial of commercial CyDye in high quality N,N-dimethylformamide (DMF) to a final concentration of 400 pmol/µL. After complete resuspension, each dye gives a visible color, Cy2—yellow, Cy3—red, and Cy5—blue. Add the proper amount of dye to the different protein (up to three) extracts. Normally, 400 pmol of dye is used to label 50 µg of protein, although higher concentration of protein can be efficiently labeled by adding proportional amounts of each dye. Let dyes react with the sample during 30 min at room temperature in the dark and quench the labeling reaction by adding 10 mM lysine. Combine the labeled samples into a single microfuge tube and mix. Centrifuge for 10 min at 13,000 rpm to pellet any particles not dissolved. Add to each labeled sample and pooled samples 100–300 µL (depending on drystrip length) of rehydration solution, containing 8 M urea, 2% CHAPS, 2 mg/mL DTT, 0.0125 g/mL iodoacetamide, a trace of bromphenol blue, and carrier ampholytes IPG buffer (commercially available depending on the pH range of the IPG strip). The following steps of the 2D electrophoresis are performed as described in Section 23.3.2.

23.4.4 Software-Based Image Analysis for Quantification and Comparison of Protein Patterns

Software-based analysis of conventional (non-DIGE) 2D gels includes the detection of spots (individual proteins) present inside the gel matrix. Although the reproducibility from gel to gel is relatively high, some degree of experimental variability can be observed from gel to gel (even if the same protein mixture is analyzed). For this reason, triplicates (at least) of 2D gels should be run for every individual sample in order to compare the pattern of spots that appear in each of the gels. In this way, the software is able to measure the average "volume" of each spot, measured as the area (in dots per square area of the gel surface) by the intensity of the same spot (the value of intensity assigned to each spot) assigned as a percentage of the total intensity of the surface of the 2D gel. The scanner-densitometer used has been calibrated by assigning an algorithm able to transform the transmission light that reaches the detectors through the gel [21]. Therefore, the software can reveal the differences in protein profiles and measure changes in the intensity of spots from each sample.

23.4.5 Drawbacks and Limitations of 2D-PAGE

2D-PAGE gels can resolve a limited range of proteins, in terms of molecular weight and isoelectric point. In general, high range (above 150 kDa) or low range (below 12 kDa) molecular weight proteins are difficult to detect with this technique. The same limitations apply to hydrophobic proteins (e.g., membrane proteins), which normally migrate very poorly in these gels. Finally, it should be taken into account that only relatively abundant proteins can be visualized.

Commercial p*I* strips including immobilized ampholites range from 3 (most acidic) to 11 (most basic). Although these p*I* values cover a wide range of the proteins present in living organism, it is not possible to include proteins with higher or lower p*I* points in a 2D gel.

The size of the gel needs to be considered. Larger 2D gels allow a better resolution of proteins that could appear as overlapped spots in small 2D gels, but they require longer p*I* strips and considerable consumption of acrylamide and other reagents (especially when replicates of the experiments are necessary), and the handling for staining and scanning is a hurdle.

On the other hand, conventional staining approaches have a limited dynamic range. The use of sensible staining using fluorescent dyes requires the use of equipment such as laser scanners and robotized spot-pickers to pick up the spots of interest for further analysis. This instrumentation is expensive and not available in every lab.

23.5 IN-GEL AND IN-SOLUTION ENDOPROTEASE DIGESTION OF PROTEINS

In most proteomic studies, the start-up material used for high throughput protein identification is a proteolytic mixture of the proteins. Here we describe some of the current methods for protein digestion.

23.5.1 Reduction and Alkylation of Proteins

Reduction with 10 mM DTT is necessary to break disulfide bonds and to unfold the protein. Alkylation with 50 mM iodoacetamide is an efficient reaction that yields carboxyamidomethylated residues and keeps the protein unfolded. This allows the endoprotease to access all the cleavage sites efficiently.

23.5.2   Trypsin Digestion

Trypsin is the most frequently used endoprotease for proteomic analyses for several reasons. It possesses high cleavage specificity after Lys or Arg residues (provided Pro is not the following amino acid in the protein sequence). The frequency of appearance of Lys and Arg residues inside proteins is relatively high compared to other amino acids. Modified trypsins that reduce the autoproteolysis and increase the efficiency of the reaction are readily available in the market. Moreover, trypsin cleaves after basic residues, which favors the protonation of the peptides under low acidic conditions (which is crucial for mass spectrometry in positive ionization mode). The amount of trypsin added to samples must be proportional to the amount of protein, normally 1:20 or even 1:50 (w/w) trypsin:protein ratio is a suitable ratio.

23.5.3   Alternative Proteases

In some cases, tryptic digestion is not sufficient to characterize the protein of interest because the resulting peptides are too small or too large for their separation with C18 reverse phase columns and subsequent analysis with mass spectrometry. In these cases, the combination of two (or more) endopeptidase digestions with mass spectrometric analysis of the resulting peptides enables the comprehensive identification or proteins present in complex mixtures. It is advisable to use combinations of proteases with different specificities, such as trypsin combined with chymotrypsin, Asp-N, or Glu-C.

23.5.4   In-Gel Digestion of Proteins

This method is based on the behavior of gel plugs to act as a "sponge," shrinking when acetonitrile is added or swelling when aqueous buffer or other reagents are added to the piece of gel [22].

Protocol G: In-Gel Digestion of Proteins   Cover the gel plug containing the protein of interest with acetonitrile for 10 min; remove the acetonitrile. Cover the gel with 10 mM DTT in 50 mM ammonium bicarbonate and store at 56 °C for 30 min; remove the DTT. Cool to room temperature. Alkylate the sample by covering the gel with 50 mM iodoacetamide in 50 mM ammonium bicarbonate and keep at room temperature in the dark for 15 min; remove the iodoacetamide. Add trypsin at a 1:20 ratio and store at 37 °C for 8 hours. Stop the endoprotease reaction by adding 1 µL of concentrated acetic acid. Remove the supernatant and place it in a new clean tube. Cover the plug with acetonitrile for 10 min and recover the supernatant. Mix both supernatants and lyophilize the peptide mixture. The peptide mixture will be ready for mass spectrometry after resuspension in appropriate buffer.

23.5.5   In-Solution Digestion of Proteins

Proteins in solution in different buffers can be lyophilized to dryness and redissolved in 50 mM ammonium bicarbonate containing relatively high concentrations of urea (4–8 M) to help the solubilization of the proteins at basic pH, necessary for tryptic or chymotryptic endoprotease digestion. When 8 M urea is used to solubilize proteins, the concentration of urea should be diluted to 2 M prior to endoprotease digestion in order to maintain the protease activity.

Protocol H: In-Solution Digestion of Proteins   Lyophilize the sample to dryness and redissolve in a small volume (10 μL of 50 mM ammonium bicarbonate). Vortex and/or bath sonicate to ensure the solubilization of your protein(s) of interest. Add 10 μL of DTT in 50 mM ammonium bicarbonate and store at 56 °C for 30 min. Cool to room temperature. Alkylate by adding 10 μL of iodoacetamide in ammonium bicarbonate and keep at room temperature in the dark for 15 min. Dilute in one volume of 50 mM ammonium bicarbonate to reduce the urea concentration to 2 M. Add trypsin at a 1:20 ratio and store at 37 °C for 8 h. Your peptide mixture will be ready for mass spectrometry analysis after resuspension in the appropriate buffer.

23.6   PRINCIPLES OF MASS SPECTROMETRY: IONIZATION SOURCES AND DIFFERENT MASS ANALYZERS

Mass spectrometry has become a key area in proteomic studies [23]. Several sources of soft ionization for peptides and proteins have been developed during the last decades to allow high throughput analysis of peptides and routine identification and characterization of proteins (or their proteolytically derived peptides) present at very low concentrations in biological samples (even attomoles / nanograms of protein). Moreover, tandem mass spectrometry (MS/MS) approaches enable the confident identification of mixtures of proteins based on amino acid sequence information. Mass spectrometers are composed of three parts: the ionization source, the mass analyzer, and the detector. Several mass analyzers can be found in mass spectrometers, including triple quadrupoles (Q), time-of-flight (TOF) analyzers, ion traps (IT), Fourier cyclotron resonance (FCR), and combinations such as quadrupole time-of-flight (Q-TOF). All these analyzers are able to accurately measure the mass of compounds (proteins or peptides) that enter the analyzer in gas phase as a function of their charge state (mass-to-charge (m/z) ratio).

23.6.1   Matrix Assisted Laser Desorption Ionization–Time of Flight (MALDI-TOF): Spotting on MALDI Plates and Use of Different Matrices

The MALDI technique [24] has primarily been used in conjunction with TOF analyzers for molecular mass determination. For MALDI, peptides are mixed with a matrix that transfers the energy of a laser beam to the peptides embedded in the crystallized matrix. The resulting spectra, characterized by singly charged precursor ions, present high energy collision fragments, which are readily interpretable.

Protocol I: Dried Droplet Method for Spotting of Samples on MALDI Plates   After tryptic digestion and lyophilization, the resulting peptides are resuspended in 5 μL water with 0.1% trifluoroacetic acid. It is advisable to introduce desalting steps by using Zip-tips® containing C18 beads (commercially available). The solution containing the peptides is mixed with 5 μL of MALDI-TOF matrix. Normally, 1% α-cyano-4-hydroxy-cinnamic acid dissolved in 90% acetonitrile and 10% trifluoroacetic acid is used as matrix for peptide mass fingerprinting of proteins. Normally, 1 μL of the mixture (peptides and matrix) is spotted on the MALDI plate and allowed to dry for 5 min before MALDI analysis.

23.6.2 Acquisition of Peptide Mass Fingerprints (PMFs) for Protein Identification

Peptide mass fingerprinting is the most common strategy for identifying proteins proceeding from SDS-PAGE separations, either 1D or 2D. The proteins are usually in-gel digested with trypsin or other endoproteases (e.g., Lys C or Glu C). The resulting proteolytic peptides are extracted from the gel piece and analyzed by MALDI-TOF MS [25]. The peptide masses contained in the resulting spectra are the peptide mass fingerprints. This mass profile is matched against the theoretical masses obtained from the *in silico* digestion of all proteins contained in the database. This interrogation is made with algorithms such as MASCOT (http://www.matrixscience. co.uk), or Profound (http://prowl.rockefeller.edu/profound_bin) among others. The choice of the algorithm may influence the final identification. A combination of several search algorithms is advisable [26]. The results of the matching are ranked according to the number of peptide masses matching their sequence within a given mass error tolerance. Successful protein identification requires several factors: (1) mass accuracy of the instrument, (2) ratio of assigned versus nonassigned peaks in the spectrum, and (3) quality and size of the database used [27]. Common databases used for the analysis are SwissProt or NCBI. The whole process is now automated and hundreds of samples can be analyzed per day. As a general rule, when MASCOT is used for identification, protein identification is considered as significant when the MASCOT score is higher than 66 and the sequence coverage is higher than 15%.

23.6.3 Time of Flight–Time of Flight (TOF-TOF) Analysis of Precursor Ions

TOF-TOF instruments combine the high throughput of the PMF analysis with the increased confidence given by peptide fragmentation that extends protein identification coverage. This approach is particularly useful when complex mixtures of peptides are analyzed. These instruments have the ability to acquire MALDI-TOF mass spectra followed by high energy collision-induced dissociation (CID) and to perform subsequent MS/MS analysis of fragment ions for more definitive protein identification. The peptide sequence information gained in MS/MS experiments leads to higher confidence in the database search results and identification of more proteins. The acquisition queue is automated in such a way that the five or ten most prominent ions of every spectrum are subjected to further MS/MS fragmentation. The accuracy of these instruments has improved considerably in the last few years; 2.5 parts per million (ppm) are now easily achieved. This accuracy is very useful for the study of proteomes from unknown genomes and the *de novo* sequencing approaches.

Although MALDI instruments are very useful for classical gel-based proteomics and protein identification, they are not the best option for the analysis of complex proteomes, since they lack multidimensionality. On the other hand, they are not particularly appropriate for the study of posttranslational modifications and more specifically phosphoproteome analysis. For these cases, other mass spectrometry techniques based on electrospray ionization coupled to liquid chromatography are more efficient.

23.7 ELECTROSPRAY IONIZATION OF PROTEINS AND TANDEM MASS SPECTROMETRY

In electrospray ionization, proteins present in aqueous buffers are desolvated into a gas phase when flowing through a narrow capillary and are subjected to high voltage [28]. Contrary to other ionization techniques, such as fast atom bombardment (FAB), electrospray ionization (ESI) is more efficient and robust for the ionization of large organic molecules, including peptides. Therefore, it has become widely used in proteomics. Basically, the mechanism underlying ESI is that the application of voltage to a capillary (made of metal or silica), at atmospheric pressure and containing proteins or peptides in solution, produces charged tiny droplets that form a spray. As droplets evaporate, charged peptides pass from the aqueous phase to the gas phase.

23.7.1 Basic Concepts of Electrospray-Based Mass Analyzers

The basic principle of electrospray-based mass spectrometers is that ions, produced in an ESI source, can be isolated as a function of voltage applied to opposite electrodes and radiofrequency. By controlling these variables, ions can be stored, fragmented, or forced to hit a detector in order to measure their mass-to-charge ratio (m/z). Once peptides are charged and in the gas phase, they enter the mass spectrometer with the aid of rotary vacuum pumps. Basic amino acid residues become protonated when solved in low acidic buffers. Therefore, proteins and peptides in low acidic buffers become multiply charged and can be analyzed as positive ions.

ESI sources are usually coupled to ion traps, triple quadrupoles, and Q-TOF instruments. Ion traps and quadrupoles are able to isolate ions of interest and perform tandem mass spectrometry (MS/MS or MS^n) at high speed and resolution rates. In order to choose what kind of mass analyzer is more appropriate for a certain experimental approach, three issues need to be considered: mass resolution, scan speed, and accuracy of mass measurement. Ion traps are composed of a three-dimensional (3D) chamber (3D traps) or linear ion traps (i.e., LTQ, Thermo Finnegan), where ions can be stored, isolated, and fragmented in order to achieve structural information on those. Ion traps are capable of performing multiple stages of precursor ion fragmentation (MS^n, where n = number of sequential fragmentation) in a single experiment. Linear ion traps are characterized by higher ion capacity and scan rates, compared to 3D ion traps. Triple quadrupoles can be used to detect, isolate, and fragment specific precursor ions that produce a selected product ion of interest, such as a neutral loss.

During the last few years, ultrahigh resolution equipment has been developed, including Orbitrap or Fourier transform (FT) ion cyclotron resonance technologies, which are able to reach up to sub-ppm mass accuracy.

23.7.2   Mass Determination of Intact Proteins

A direct measurement of the molecular weight of proteins can be performed with ESI-equipped mass spectrometers. In this approach, proteins of interest are resuspended in low acidic buffers (0.1% acetic or formic acid) and placed inside small capillaries with metallic tips to facilitate the appearance of a spray with the aid of voltage. Protein ions spraying from the ESI source are normally detected as a mixture of different charge states, which is called a charge envelope. The mass determination is performed by deconvoluting the set of mass-to-charge ratios, corresponding to consecutive charged species, detected for a specific protein, with specific algorithms such as MagTran (free software available at http://www.geocities.com/SiliconValley/Hills/2679/magtran.html) or Maxent software (http://www.cs.princeton.edu/~schapire/maxent/). Mass determination of intact proteins can routinely be performed on purified proteins in solution. Protein purifications using chromatographic procedures usually contain certain amounts of salt or other impurities that can dramatically affect the mass measurement of the protein of interest. Desalting steps prior to mass determination are carried out by dialysis or by reverse phase chromatography with hydrophobic columns (C2, C4, or C8 depending on the size of the protein).

Using Fourier transform ion cyclotron resonance (FTICR), the mass determination of whole intact proteins ranging from 10,000 to 100,000 Da may be provided with an accuracy near 1 ppm. Protein masses of up to 229 kDa have also been reported [29]. In some cases, this data can lead to unambiguous protein identification. However, the mass of the intact protein is compromised by posttranslational modifications or partial proteolysis of the purified protein [30]. In that case, ions corresponding to the intact protein are subsequently fragmented in the mass spectrometer, yielding the molecular masses of both the protein and the fragment ions. If a sufficient number of informative fragment ions are observed, this analysis can provide a complete description of the primary structure of the protein and reveal all of its primary structure and its modifications.

Many proteomic studies, including the ability to fragment and analyze large intact proteins for protein characterization, protein–protein interaction, and chemical cross-link location inside proteins, are called *top–down* approaches. A second widely used alternative is the *bottom–up* approach, in which complex mixtures of peptides are analyzed by mass spectrometry in two stages. In the first stage, the masses of peptides are determined; in a second stage, peptides are fragmented to produce information on the sequence of the peptides to reconstruct the primary structure of the original protein.

23.7.3   Peptide Bond Fragmentation Using Collision Energy

Peptide structure determination using mass spectrometry is based on ionization of peptides and subsequent fragmentation of the peptide amide bonds after collision-induced dissociation (CID) by controlled collision with an inert gas (such as He or Ar). The collision of ionized peptide molecules against the inert gas inside a collision chamber is sufficient to overcome the energetic threshold of the amide bonds. After fragmentation, the series of fragment ions generated from the N and C termini, respectively, are scanned, which leads to the elucidation of the primary structure backbone of the peptide. The series of fragment ions derived from the N terminus are designated as *a*, *b*, or *c* ions, whereas the ions derived from the C terminus are *x*, *y*, or *z* ions. This is a nomenclature widely accepted for the fragmentation of peptides, first proposed in 1984 and modified four years later [31].

23.7.4   Electron Transfer Dissociation

Two highly effective methods for fragmenting large peptides and proteins, electron capture dissociation (ECD) and electron transfer dissociation (ETD) [32, 33], have emerged as promising alternatives for protein and peptide characterization, in both, top–down and bottom–up approaches. Electron transfer dissociation is an alternative to CID fragmentation that fragments the backbone of peptides with the aid of anthracene anions. Anthracene is introduced in the collision chamber of ion traps and transfers electrons to multiply protonated peptides, leading to their eventual fragmentation. ETD fragmentation technologies are still in development and require the improvement of new software bioinformatic tools to aid in the interpretation of ETD-derived MS/MS spectra. Although quite recent, ETD seems particularly well suited for characterization of posttranslational modifications, particularly phosphorylation. Therefore, it is foreseeable that ETD may become an indispensable tool for posttranslational modification and protein sequence analysis in the near future.

23.8   MULTIDIMENSIONAL LIQUID CHROMATOGRAPHY COUPLED TO MASS SPECTROMETERS

23.8.1   Multidimensional LC-ESI-Q-TRAP

Here we focus on the analysis of complex mixtures of peptides by coupling an ESI source at the end of a separation step using high performance liquid chromatography (HPLC). Although ESI was originally designed to be performed at a few microliters per minute flow rate (micro HPLC), separation techniques have rapidly evolved to run at nano-flow rates below 100 nL per minute using nanocolumns with diameters ranging from 1.5 to 3 μm. The major advantage of using nano-LC flow rates is the significant increase in the sensitivity of the identification.

Peptide mixtures can routinely be separated using reverse phase (RP) chromatographic columns packed with, normally, C18. Peptides elute as independent chromatographic peaks as long as an increasing concentration of acetonitrile is pumped through the reverse phase column. As soon as the peptides elute from the RP column and reach the ESI source, ions are produced and can readily be scanned and fragmented. If the mixture of peptides of interest is more complex, a prefractionation can be achieved by coupling a strong cation exchange (SCX) column before the RP. This is called two-dimensional liquid chromatography (2D-LC) or multidimensional protein identification (MudPit) [34]. In this approach, after injecting the peptide mixture, increasing concentrations of salt (normally from 0.05 mM up to 2 M NaCl or ammonium formate) are pumped first through the SCX column. The eluting peptides from each salt concentration go through a second separation through the RP column. Chromatographic runs from 30 min up to 6 hours can be performed, depending on the complexity of the peptide mixture. Modern HPLC instruments allow one to configure this experimental approach online, which permits a comprehensive identification of proteins derived from tryptic digestions with a high degree of automation. Nevertheless, if high concentrations of peptides need to be analyzed, the first fractionation using SCX may be performed offline using capillary or even preparative columns and salt gradients, instead of salt plugs.

The recent development of C18 beads smaller than 2 μm, together with ultrahigh pressure liquid chromatrography (UPLC) (Waters Corp.) has led to better separation and resolution during chromatographic runs and has been shown to be very advantageous for both peptide and metabolite screening.

23.8.2   LC- MALDI-TOF(-TOF)

The same principle of "divide and conquer" can be applied for MALDI-TOF analysis. Complex mixtures of peptides can be separated through RP columns and directly spotted as independent spots onto the surface of a MALDI plate, where an appropriate matrix is added for subsequent analysis. This process can be automated using specific robots such as Probot (LC-Packings). Contrary to what happens during peptide mass fingerprint analysis, where all the peptides derived from a unique protein are spotted in a single position, in this new approach the peptides belonging to the same protein are usually spotted in consecutive positions of the MALDI plate. Hence, a correction in the acquisition and search algorithm needs to be introduced in order to take into account this possibility. TOF instruments are characterized by a high sensitivity and accuracy to measure the m/z ratios of peptides quickly and reliably, but when coupled to peptide fractionation using HPLC, these capabilities significantly improve.

23.9   DATABASE SEARCH AND USE OF BIOINFORMATIC TOOLS FOR PROTEIN IDENTIFICATION

23.9.1   Search Engines Against Nucleotide and Amino Acid Databases

The analysis of even a single protein tryptic digest yields a vast amount of fragmentation data after analysis with a mass spectrometer. Manual sequencing of peptides and subsequent identification of the original protein would be a major constraint. Several search engines have been developed to help in this task, including MS-Fit, MASCOT, OMSSA, PHENYX, SEQUEST, and X! Tandem, among others. Basically, search engines compare the experimental mass-to-charge ratios measured by mass spectrometers with *in silico* mass-to-charge ratios derived from the fragmentation of amino acid sequence databases. Nucleotide databases can also be used for protein identification as long as protein sequence can be derived from nucleotides.

Most proteomic studies are therefore biased toward the identification of peptides and proteins contained in databases (either as nucleic acid or as amino acid sequences). Hence, most "shotgun" protein identification experiments, aimed at the successful identification of as many proteins present in the sample as possible, are constrained to organisms whose genomes have been sequenced, or at least partially sequenced.

Annotated databases, including functional information of proteins as well as their modifications, are rapidly improving and new nucleotide databases from several organisms are also emerging. The Human Genome Project and other genome sequencing projects are turning out in rapid succession the complete genome sequences of specific species and thus, in principle, the amino acid sequence of every protein potentially encoded [35].

23.9.2 Use of Customized Databases for Tagged Recombinant Proteins and *De Novo* Sequencing

Mass spectrometry is also useful to characterize the quality and sequence content of recombinant proteins that contain peptide tags (His-tag, GST-tag, etc.) for their purification after expression in *E. coli* or other systems. In these cases, where the exact amino acid sequence of the recombinant protein is known, customized databases can be prepared in order to identify all the proteolytic peptides of the protein of interest. The goal is to detect the possible occurrence of deletions or partial degradation from the N or C terminus or the loss of the tags.

An alternative to protein identification using search algorithms is the identification of unknown proteins, from unknown genomes, by *de novo* sequencing. There are two things that need to be considered in *de novo* sequencing experiments. First, better accuracy of the measured mass leads to better sequence information from the fragmented peptide. Second, appropriate software (i.e., PEAKS, http://www.bioinfor.com) needs to be used to gather all the information detected after fragmentation of the peptides of interest.

23.10 IDENTIFICATION OF POSTTRANSLATIONAL MODIFICATION OF PROTEINS

Many critical events involved in cellular responses (control of enzymatic activity, protein–protein interaction, cellular localization, signal transduction) are mediated by changes in posttranslational protein modifications rather than transcriptional changes [36]. More than 300 modifications have been reported on proteins and peptides both in prokaryotic and eukaryotic cells (http://www.abrf.org/index.cfm/dm.home). Currently, mass spectrometry is considered as the most appropriate approach for the identification and characterization of posttranslational modification of proteins [37]. It can unambiguously identify the occurrence of posttranslational modifications at the residue level.

Almost 2% of the human genome encodes protein kinases [38], and it is estimated that protein phosphorylation can affect up to one-third of all proteins [39], due to the relative abundance of phosphorylated residues near 1% pTyr, 12% pThr, and 87% pSer [40]. Phosphorylation analysis of proteins is made by cleavage into their constituent peptides using endopeptidase digestion, generally trypsin, separation, and analysis of the resulting peptides by LC-MS/MS. The high sensitivity and the ability to isolate and fragment peptides of ion traps and triple quadrupoles serves as a quick and reliable method for the detection of phosphorylations [41–43].

The use of nano-HPLC coupled to mass spectrometers with high ion capacity and fast scan rates enhances the detection of phosphorylated peptides and enables the determination of the phosphorylation at the residue level [44, 45].

In order to detect phosphorylation sites on protein digests, data-dependent mass analysis is frequently used to trigger MS^3 scans, where specific neutral losses (98.0, 49.0, 32.7 Da) are observed. This is called data-dependent neutral loss (DDNL) analysis. Nevertheless, phosphopeptide analysis with mass spectrometry has to face the inherent problem of low concentrations inside the peptide mixture [46]. Therefore, several enrichment strategies have been developed to favor their analysis using mass spectrometry. These methods include the use of immobilized metal ion (Fe^{3+} or Ga^{3+}) affinity chromatography (IMAC), zirconium dioxide [47], or titanium dioxide [45, 48]. Phosphopeptides can also be collected in a few fractions by strong cation exchange (SCX) chromatography using a salt gradient (e.g., 1 mM to 1 M NaCl or ammonium formate). Another strategy for tyrosine kinases is the use of immunological methods based on anti-phosphotyrosine antibodies, which are sufficiently specific for the enrichment of phosphotyrosine-containing peptides by affinity or immunoprecipitation.

As an example of the identification of phosphorylation using mass spectrometry, Fig. 23.2 shows the identification of a chymotryptic peptide from Cdc25 protein, involved in cell cycle regulation in *Xenopus laevis*, after HPLC separation using a reverse phase column online with linear ion trap mass spectrometry. The fragmentation spectrum shows an MS^2 event of the triply charged precursor ion $[M+3H]^{3+}$ m/z = 843.4 that corresponds to the singly phosphorylated peptide, SVSNKENEGEL-FKpSPNCKPVAL. The peptide sequence and the occurrence of the phosphorylated residue can be derived from the singly and doubly charged y and b ion series. A diagnostic prominent neutral loss as phosphoric acid (-98 Da) is also observed. The expected ion masses are listed above the sequence.

On the other hand, acetylation and methylation patterns of chromatin proteins (most times on the N terminus and/or lysine residues of histones) has become an increasingly important aspect of epigenetics and cancer biology [49, 50].

23.11   PROTEIN QUANTITATION

Until recently, the quantitative study of the pool of proteins expressed in biological samples using differential display was restricted to 2D gel analyses. Protein quantitation using the 2D gel-based approach consists of the measurement of the volume (area in pixels by intensity of the spots) of spots identified as a single protein in different gels. A significant statistical variation of the amount of protein measured in gels corresponding to drug treatments or specific biological alterations of interest with respect to a control can therefore be expressed in terms of quantitative variation. An alternative non-gel-based approach has been the use of isotope coded affinity tags (ICAT) for the quantitative study of protein expression at the proteome level [51]. Recently, an improved approach, analogous to ICAT, has been developed. It is called iTRAQ™ (Applied Biosystems) and consists of a range of up to eight different amine-specific, stable isotope tags that label all peptides in up to eight different biological samples, enabling simultaneous identification and quantitation of the whole set of proteins.

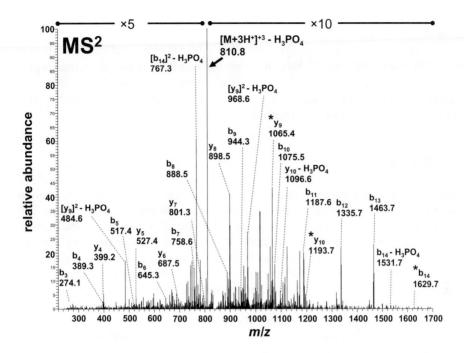

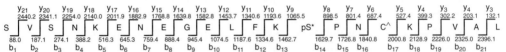

FIGURE 23.2 Identification of a chymotryptic peptide by RP-HPLC online with linear ion trap mass spectrometry. The fragmentation spectrum shows an MS^2 event of the triply charged precursor ion $[M + 3H]^{3+}$ $m/z = 843.4$ that corresponds to the singly phosphorylated peptide SVSNKENEGELFKpS*PNC^KPVAL, where p shows the presence of a phosphorylated Ser and ^ indicates carboxyamidomethylated Cys. The peptide sequence and the occurrence of the phosphorylated residue can be derived from the singly and doubly charged y and b ion series. The loss of the a phosphoric acid molecule in the MS^2 event yielded a prominent neutral loss (black arrow) with m/z ratio 810.8. The phosphorylated serine (pS) residue is indicated and the diagnostic ions bearing phosphorylations are indicated with an asterisk (*). The peptide sequence and the assignment of the fragmentation series are also indicated. The expected ion masses have been listed above the sequence. Loss of phosphate from the ions is indicated by H_3PO_4.

A more recent and powerful alternative is the stable isotope labeling with amino acids in cell culture (SILAC) [52–54], which can be used mainly in cell cultures because it is based on the metabolic incorporation of labeled amino acids containing heavy isotopes (i.e., ^2H instead of ^1H, ^{13}C instead of ^{12}C, or ^{15}N instead of ^{14}N) in living cells. After at least five cell population turnovers, complete labeling of all the proteins is achieved. The cell cultures to be compared are mixed and the changes in the expression of proteins versus the control can be quantified because the peptides containing the different isotopes coelute simultaneously from the C18 column, leading to a mass shift that is observed in the mass spectrometer. A major limitation of the iTRAQ and SILAC approaches is the cost of the reagents necessary to perform these experiments.

A more economical approach for isotopic peptide labeling and quantification is based on the enzymatic $^{16}O/^{18}O$ labeling. This methodology is based on the trypsin catalyzed oxygen exchange at the free terminus from a peptide [55, 56]. Proteins are digested initially with normal water and they are further incubated either with $H_2 {}^{16}O$ or with $H_2 {}^{18}O$ for the differential labeling.

23.12 PROTEIN ARRAYS

Protein microarrays represent an innovative and versatile approach to study protein abundance, function, and protein–protein interaction at an unprecedented scale. The molecular characteristics of proteins make construction of protein arrays much more challenging than building DNA microarrays. The major obstacle to the development of this field is the content of the microarrays. In contrast to the PCR technique for nucleic acids that can generate large quantities of virtually any DNA, there is no counterpart for protein amplification. Protein expression or production systems are difficult to automate and always unpredictable. Many proteins are unstable, which complicates microarray shelf life. Finally, in contrast to the simple hybridization procedures for nucleic acids, proteins have shown a wide range of chemistries and specificities that complicate substantially any interaction study at the multiplex level.

Two major approaches have been followed for the production of protein microarrays: abundance-based microarrays and function-based microarrays.

23.12.1 Abundance-Based Microarrays

There are two types of abundance-based microarrays: (1) antibody or antibody-like microarrays and (2) reverse phase protein microarrays. Antibody microarrays are the most popular option given the stability, selectivity, and high affinity of the antibodies as well as the high number of antibodies commercially available. Therefore, this option has been the fastest growing in the field. In any case, some precautions should be taken into account: not all the antibodies are actually functional in the microarray format, and even monospecific antibodies can show cross-reaction on the microarray when confronted with complex protein mixtures. The most practical approach for the use of capture microarrays is the direct labeling of the analytes with one or two fluorochroms. This approach can be used for the analysis of differential expression of proteins in different conditions (e.g., for the analysis of tumor tissues versus normal tissues in cancer). This approach has recently been reported by a number of authors in prostate cancer [57] and breast cancer [58].

Reverse phase protein microarrays rely entirely on the existence of analyte-specific reagents [59]. This is particularly important as the concentration of analytes in the spots is locally high and may facilitate spurious interactions. Other authors [60] used reverse phase microarrays to classify different types of cancer using the NCI-60 cell lines. The cell lines were spotted as lysates and then probed with antibodies. More than 200 antibodies were tested to finally select 52 that gave a reliable signal. Also, some interference problems may appear from the locally high concentration of analytes. This might be alleviated by prefractionation of the samples before spotting.

23.12.2   Function-Based Protein Microarrays

Function-based microarrays consist of panels of proteins spotted at defined positions. They are used to study the biochemical properties and activities of the target proteins spotted on the microarray. Thus, protein microarrays are mainly used to examine protein interactions with other proteins or other molecules [61]. There are also other arrays used for studying the enzyme activity and substrate specificity. Proteins have to be printed in the right conditions to maintain conformation, integrity, and activity. In some cases, the integrity of the protein requires it to be printed as a complex of several proteins to remain active and functional. The major challenge about this type of microarray continues to be the production of the proteins. It is time consuming and costly to produce proteins of good purity and yield.

Generally, these arrays are made by using three different approaches: (1) chemical linkage [62], (2) peptide fusion tag [61], and (3) self-assembling protein arrays [63]. All three methods have advantages and disadvantages [64]. Alternatively, it may be simpler to study protein domains rather than the full length proteins, because small domains are usually simple to express and purify [65]. Self-assembling microarrays, also called nucleic acid programmable protein arrays (NAPPAs), are a new and interesting alternative based on the printing of cDNAs on the microarray surface and expressed *in situ* using a mammalian cell-free expression system. The nascent molecule, labeled with a tag, is captured by an adjacent antibody against the tag printed on the chip surface. This approach is very promising because it excludes the necessity of expressing, purifying, and storing the proteins. Also, it opens new avenues to prepare custom-made protein microarrays.

There is great enthusiasm about this new area of protein microarrays. Still, major efforts need to be made in different areas of production before these tools become commonly used in laboratories, as happens with DNA chips. Few articles have reported original findings of proteomic interest and most of the communications to date have been based more on technology optimization than in solving real problems. Therefore, the utility of protein microarrays remains to be fully determined.

23.13   LINKS OF INTERESTS

Metabolic Pathways

http://expasy.org/tools/pathways/
http://www.genome.ad.jp/kegg/kegg2.html

Protocols Online

http://www.protocol-online.org/
www.thermo.com/eThermo/CMA/PDFs/Articles/articlesFile_21631.pdf
www.bio-rad.com/cmc_upload/Literature/13023/4006173B-wMS.pdf
http://probes.invitrogen.com/lit/bioprobes31/section1.html
www.fluorotechnics.com/content/documents/ap_dp_comp_sypro.pdf
http://www5.amershambiosciences.com/APTRIX/upp00919.nsf/Content/
    Proteomics+DIGE

Reference Books for Proteomics

http://www.proteinsandproteomics.org/

Handbook of 2D-PAGE

http://www6.amershambiosciences.com/aptrix/upp01077.nsf/Content/Products?
OpenDocument&parentid=575392&moduleid=164456&zone=Proteomics

2D Gels and Gel Repository

http://expasy.org/ch2d/
www.apczech.cz/pdf/DF_DeStreak.pdf

HPLC and Mass Spectrometry Resources

http://www.ionsource.com/
http://www.lcgcmag.com/LC%2FHPLC

Nucleic Acid and Protein Databases

http://www.ebi.ac.uk/FTP/
http://www.uniprot.o
http://www.tigr.org/

Bioinformatic Tools

http://expasy.org/tools/
http://ncrr.pnl.gov/software/
http://www.ionsource.com/links/programs.htm
http://www.geocities.com/SiliconValley/Hills/2679/magtran.html
http://www.cs.princeton.edu/~schapire/maxent/

Search Engines Used in Mass Spectrometry

MS-Fit: (http:/prospector.ucsf.edu) University of California (San Francisco,
EEUU)
MASCOT: (www.matrixscience.com) Imperial Cancer Research Fund (London,
UK)
OMSSA: http://pubchem.ncbi.nlm.nih.gov/omssa/
PHENYX: http://www.phenyx-ms.com/
SEQUEST: http://fields.scripps.edu/sequest/
X! Tandem: http://www.thegpm.org/TANDEM/index.html

Posttranslational Modifications

http://expasy.org/tools/findmod/findmod_masses.html
http://www.abrf.org/index.cfm/dm.home

Proteomic Forums and Survey Studies

http://www.abrf.org/index.cfm/group.show/Proteomics.34.htm

http://www.swissproteomicsociety.org/digest/

23.14 CONCLUSION

The measurement of changes in gene expression as a response to the appearance of an alteration/disease is not sufficient in many cases. It is estimated that only 50% of the measured increments of mRNA are directly correlated to an increase in the amount of the corresponding expressed protein, as observed in human [66], yeast [67, 68], bacteria [69], and other cell lines [70]. Therefore, changes detected at the protein level using proteomic techniques could be more indicative of the existence of alterations and modifications.

The classical approach to study proteins and biological processes, which was based on purification to homogeneity followed by biochemical assays of the specific activity of the purified proteins, has been replaced today by a tremendous increase in the application of proteomic technologies to the study and characterization en masse of proteins and complete proteomes. Although the analysis of full proteomes remains a formidable task, the new generation of multidimensional chromatographic steps coupled to the unprecedented resolution of the new mass spectrometers allows optimism for the future. Technological advances have translated into major improvements in the three major branches of the current proteomics: two-dimensional electrophoresis, mass spectrometry, and protein/antibody microarrays. Increased reproducibility, better statistical analysis, and improvements in mass accuracy, resolving power, and accuracy of quantifications is giving proteomics a major impulse within the life sciences.

REFERENCES

1. Wilkins MR, Sanchez JC, Gooley AA, Appel RD, Humphery SI, Hochstrasser DF, Williams KL. Progress with proteome projects: why all proteins expressed by a genome should be identified and how to do it. *Biotechnol Genet Eng Rev* 1996;13:19–50.

2. Wu CC, MacCoss MJ, Howell KE, Yates JR. A method for the comprehensive proteomic analysis of membrane proteins. *Nat Biotechnol* 2003;21:532–538.

3. Alfonso P, Dolado I, Swat A, Núñez A, Cuadrado A, Nebreda A, Casal JI. Membrane protein alterations induced by oncogenic H-ras transformation of p38 MAPK-deficient fibroblasts. *Proteomics* 2006;6(Supp 1):S262–S271.

4. Bordier C. Phase separation of integral membrane proteins in Triton X-114 solution. *J Biol Chem* 1981;256:1604–1607.

5. States DJ, Omenn GS, Blackwell TW, Fermin D, Eng J, Speicher DW, Hanash SM. Challenges in deriving high-confidence protein identifications from data gathered by a HUPO plasma proteome collaborative study. *Nat Biotechnol* 2006;24:333–338.

6. Foster LJ, de Hoog CL, Zhang YL, Zhang Y, Xie XH, Mootha VK, Mann M. A mammalian organelle map by protein correlation profiling. *Cell* 2006;125:187–199.

7. Bensadoun A, Weinstein D. Assay of proteins in the presence of interfering materials. *Anal Biochem* 1975;70:241–250.

8. Bradford M. A rapid and sensitive method for the quantitation of microgram quantities of protein utilizing the principle of protein-dye binding. *Anal Biochem* 1976;72: 248–254.

9. Laemmli UK. Cleavage of structural proteins during assembly of head of bacteriophage-T4. *Nature* 1970;227:680–685.

10. Neuhoff V, Arold N, Taube D, Ehrhardt W. Improved staining of proteins in polyacrylamide gels including isoelectric focusing gels with clear background at nanogram sensitivity using Coomassie Brilliant Blue G-250 and R-250. *Electrophoresis* 1988;9:255–262.

11. Blum H, Beier H, Gross HJ. Improved silver staining of plant proteins, RNA and DNA in polyacrylamide gels. *Electrophoresis* 1987;8:93–99.

12. Lanne B, Panfilov O. Protein staining influences the quality of mass spectra obtained by peptide mass fingerprinting after separation on 2-D gels. A comparison of staining with Coomassie brilliant blue and SYPRO Ruby. *J Proteome Res* 2005;4:175–179.

13. Chevalier F, Rofidal V, Vanova P, Bergoin A, Rossignol M. Proteomic capacity of recent fluorescent dyes for protein staining. *Phytochemistry* 2004;65:1499–1506.

14. White IR, Pickford R, Wood J, Skehel JM, Gangadharan B, Cutler P. A statistical comparison of silver and SYPRO Ruby staining for proteomic analysis. *Electrophoresis* 2007;25:3048–3054.

15. Tonge R, Shaw J, Middleton B, Rowlinson R, Rayner S, Young J, Pognan F, Hawkins E, Currie I, Davison M. Validation and development of fluorescence two-dimensional differential gel electrophoresis proteomics technology. *Proteomics* 2001;1:377–396.

16. Alban A, David SO, Bjorkesten L, Andersson C, Sloge E, Lewis S, Currie I. A novel experimental design for comparative two-dimensional gel analysis: two-dimensional difference gel electrophoresis incorporating a pooled internal standard. *Proteomics* 2003;3:527–533.

17. Gharbi S, Gaffney P, Yang A, Zvelebil MJ, Cramer R, Waterfield MD, Timms JF. Evaluation of two-dimensional differential gel electrophoresis for proteomic expression analysis of a model breast cancer cell system. *Mol Cell Proteomics* 2002;1:91–98.

18. Friedman DB, Hill S, Keller JW, Merchant NB, Levy SE, Coffey RJ, Caprioli RM. Proteome analysis of human colon cancer by two-dimensional difference gel electrophoresis and mass spectrometry. *Proteomics* 2004;4:793–811.

19. Alfonso P, Núñez A, Madoz-Gurpide J, Lombardia L, Sánchez L, Casal JI. Proteomic expression analysis of colorectal cancer by two dimensional gel electrophoresis. *Proteomics* 2005;5:2602–2611.

20. González-Santiago L, Alfonso P, Suárez Y, Núñez A, García-Fernández LF, Alvarez E, Muñoz A, Casal JI. Proteomic analysis of the resistance to Aplidin in human cancer cells. *J Proteome Res* 2007;6:1286–1294.

21. Rauman B, Cheung A, Marten M. Quantitative comparison and evaluation of two commercially available, two-dimensional electrophoresis image analysis software packges, Z3 and Melanie. *Electrophoresis* 2002;23:2194–2202.

22. Shevchenko A, Wilm M, Vorm O, Mann M. Mass spectrometric sequencing of proteins from silver stained polyacrylamide gels. *Anal Chem* 1996;68:850–858.

23. Domon B, Aebersold R. Mass spectrometry and protein analysis. *Science* 2006;212–217.

24. Karas M, Hillenkamp F. Laser desorption ionization of proteins with molecular masses exceeding 10,000 daltons. *Anal Chem* 1988;60:2299–2301.

25. Mann M, Hojrup P, Roepstorff P. Use of mass spectrometric molecular weight information to identify proteins in sequence databases. *Biol Mass Spectrom* 1993;22:338–345.

26. Chamrad DC, Korting G, Stuhler K, Meyer HE, Klose J, Bluggel M. Evaluation of algorithms for protein identification from sequence databases using mass spectrometry data. *Proteomics* 2004;4:619–668.

27. Baldwin MA. Protein identification by mass spectrometry: issues to be considered. *Mol Cell Proteomics* 2004;3:1–9.

28. Fenn JB, Mann M, Meng CK, et al. Electrospray ionisation for mass spectrometry of large biomolecules. *Science* 1989;246:64–71.

29. Han XM, Jin M, Breuker K, McLafferty FW. Extending top–down mass spectrometry to proteins with masses greater than 200 kilodaltons. *Science* 2006;314:109–112.

30. Hayter JR, Robertson DHL, Gaskell SJ, Beynon RJ. Proteome analysis of intact proteins in complex mixtures. *Mol Cell Proteomics* 2003;2:85–95.

31. Biemann K. Contributions of mass spectrometry to peptide and protein structure. *Biomed Environ Mass Spectrom* 1988;16:99–111.

32. Syka JEP, Coon JJ, Schroeder MJ, Shabanowitz J, Hunt DF. Peptide and protein sequence analysis by electron transfer dissociation mass spectrometry. *Proc Natl Acad Sci USA* 2004;101:9528–9533.

33. Coon JJ, Ueberheide B, Syka JEP, Dryhurst DD, Ausio J, Shabanowitz J, Hunt DF. Protein identification using sequential ion/ion reactions and tandem mass spectrometry. *Proc Natl Acad Sci USA* 2005;102:9463–9468.

34. Washburn MP, Wolters D, Yates JR. Large-scale analysis of the yeast proteome by multi-dimensional protein identification technology. *Nat Biotechnol* 2001;19:242–247.

35. Peri S, Navarro JD, Amanchy R, Kristiansen TZ, Jonnalagadda CK, Surendranath V, Niranjan V, Muthusamy B, Gandhi TKB, Gronborg M, Ibarrola N, Deshpande N, Shanker K, Shivashankar HN, Rashmi BP, Ramya MA, Zhao ZX, Chandrika KN, Padma N, Harsha HC, Yatish AJ, Kavitha MP, Menezes M, Choudhury DR, Suresh S, Ghosh N, Saravana R, Chandran S, Krishna S, Joy M, Anand SK, Madavan V, Joseph A, Wong GW, Schiemann WP, Constantinescu SN, Huang LL, Khosravi-Far R, Steen H, Tewari M, Ghaffari S, Blobe GC, Dang CV, Garcia JGN, Pevsner J, Jensen ON, Roepstorff P, Deshpande KS, Chinnaiyan AM, Hamosh A, Chakravarti A, Pandey A. Development of human protein reference database as an initial platform for approaching systems biology in humans. *Genome Res* 2003;13:2363–2371.

36. Olsen JV, Blagoev B, Gnad F, Macek B, Kumar C, Mortensen P, Mann M. Global, *in vivo*, and site-specific phosphorylation dynamics in signaling networks. *Cell* 2006;127: 635–648.

37. Mann M, Jensen ON. Proteomic analysis of post-translational modifications. *Nat Biotechnol* 2003;21:255–261.

38. Manning G, Whyte DB, Martinez R, Hunter T, Sudarsanam S. The protein kinase complement of the human genome. *Science* 2002;298:1912–1934.

39. Cohen P. The role of protein phosphorylation in human health and disease. *Eur J Biochem* 2001;268:5001–5010.

40. Hunter T, Sefton BM. Transforming gene product of Rous sarcoma virus phosphorylates tyrosine. *Proc Natl Acad Sci USA Biol Sci* 1980;77:1311–1315.

41. Mann M, Hendrickson RC, Pandey A. Analysis of proteins and proteomes by mass spectrometry. *Annu Rev Biochem* 2001;70:437–473.

42. Meng FY, Forbes AJ, Miller LM, Kelleher NL. Detection and localization of protein modifications by high resolution tandem mass spectrometry. *Mass Spectrom Rev* 2005;24:126–134.

43. Villar M, Ortega-Perez I, Were F, Cano E, Redondo JM, Vazquez J. Systematic characterization of phosphorylation sites in NFATc2 by linear ion trap mass spectrometry. *Proteomics* 2006;6(Suppl 1):S16–S27.

44. Beausoleil SA, Jedrychowski M, Schwartz D, Elias JE, Villen J, Li JX, Cohn MA, Cantley LC, Gygi SP. Large-scale characterization of HeLa cell nuclear phosphoproteins. *Proc Natl Acad Sci USA* 2004;101:12130–12135.

45. Larsen MR, Thingholm TE, Jensen ON, Roepstorff P, Jorgensen TJD. Highly selective enrichment of phosphorylated peptides from peptide mixtures using titanium dioxide microcolumns. *Mol Cell Proteomics* 2005;4:873–886.

46. Steen H, Jebanathirajah JA, Rush J, Morrice N, Kirschner MW. Phosphorylation analysis by mass spectrometry—myths, facts, and the consequences for qualitative and quantitative measurements. *Mol Cell Proteomics* 2006;5:172–181.

47. Kweon HK, Hakansson K. Selective zirconium dioxide-based enrichment of phosphorylated peptides for mass spectrometric analysis. *Anal Chem* 2006;78:1743–1749.

48. Pinkse MWH, Uitto PM, Hilhorst MJ, Ooms B, Heck AJR. Selective isolation at the femtomole level of phosphopeptides from proteolytic digests using 2D-nanoLC-ESI-MS/MS and titanium oxide precolumns. *Anal Chem* 2004;76:3935–3943.

49. Fraga MF, Ballestar E, Villar-Garea A, Boix-Chornet M, Espada J, Schotta G, Bonaldi T, Haydon C, Ropero S, Petrie K, Iyer NG, Perez-Rosado A, Calvo E, Lopez JA, Cano A, Calasanz MJ, Colomer D, Piris MA, Ahn N, Imhof A, Caldas C, Jenuwein T, Esteller M. Loss of acetylation at Lys16 and trimethylation at Lys20 of histone H4 is a common hallmark of human cancer. *Nat Genet* 2005;37:391–400.

50. Boix-Chornet M, Fraga MF, Villar-Garea A, Caballero R, Espada J, Nunez A, Casado J, Largo C, Casal JI, Cigudosa JC, Franco L, Esteller M, Ballestar E. Release of hypoacetylated and trimethylated histone H4 is an epigenetic marker of early apoptosis. *J Biol Chem* 2006;281:13540–13547.

51. Shiio Y, Aebersold R. Quantitative proteome analysis using isotope-coded affinity tags and mass spectrometry. *Nat Protocols* 2006;1:139–145.

52. Ong SE, Blagoev B, Kratchmarova I, Kristensen DB, Steen H, Pandey A, Mann M. Stable isotope labeling by amino acids in cell culture, SILAC, as a simple and accurate approach to expression proteomics. *Mol Cell Proteomics* 2002;1:376–386.

53. Gruhler A, Olsen JV, Mohammed S, Mortensen P, Faergeman NJ, Mann M, Jensen ON. Quantitative phosphoproteomics applied to the yeast pheromone signaling pathway. *Mol Cell Proteomics* 2005;4:310–327.

54. Mann M. Functional and quantitative proteomics using SILAC. *Nat Rev Mol Cell Biol* 2006;7:952–958.

55. Yao X, Freas A, Ramirez J, Demirev PA, Fenselau C. Proteolytic ^{18}O labeling for comparative proteomics: model studies with two serotypes of adenovirus. *Anal Chem* 2001;73:2836–2842.

56. Yao X, Afonso C, Fenselau C. Dissection of proteolytic ^{18}O labeling: endoprotease-catalyzed ^{16}O-to-^{18}O exchange of truncated peptide substrates. *J Proteome Res* 2003;2:147–152.

57. Miller JC, Zhou H, Kwekel J, Cavallo R, Burke J, Butler EB, Teh BS, Haab BB. Antibody microarray profiling of human prostate cancer sera: antibody screening and identification of potential biomarkers. *Proteomics* 2003;3:56–63.

58. Celis JE, Moreira JM, Cabezon T, Gromov P, Friis E, Rank F, Gromova I. Identification of extracellular and intracellular signaling components of the mammary adipose tissue and its interstitial fluid in high risk breast cancer patients: toward dissecting the molecular circuitry of epithelial–adipocyte stromal cell interactions. *Mol Cell Proteomics* 2005;4:492–522.

59. Speer R, Wulfkuhle JD, Liotta LA, Petricoin EF3. Reverse-phase protein microarrays for tissue-based analysis. *Curr Opin Mol Ther* 2005;7:240–245.

60. Nishizuka S, Charboneau L, Young L, Major S, Reinhold WC, Waltham M, Kouros-Mehr H, Bussey KJ, Lee JK, Espina V, Munson PJ, Petricoin E3, Liotta LA, Weinstein JN. Proteomic profiling of the NCI-60 cancer cell lines using new high-density reverse-phase lysate microarrays. *Proc Natl Acad Sci USA* 2003;100:14229–14234.

61. Zhu H, Bilgin M, Bangham R, Hall D, Casamayor A, Bertone P, Lan N, Jansen R, Bidlingmaier S, Houfek T, Mitchell T, Miller P, Dean RA, Gerstein M, Snyder M. Global analysis of protein activities using proteome chips. *Science* 2001;293:2101–2105.

62. MacBeath G, Schreiber SL. Printing proteins as microarrays for high-throughput function determination. *Science* 2000;289:1760–1763.

63. Ramachandran N, Hainsworth E, Bhullar B, Eisenstein S, Rosen B, Lau AY, Walter JC, LaBaer J. Self-assembling protein microarrays. *Science* 2004;305:86–90.

64. LaBaer J, Ramachandran N. Protein microarrays as tools for functional proteomics. *Curr Opin Chem Biol* 2005;9:14–19.

65. Espejo A, Cote J, Bednarek A, Richard S, Bedford MT. A protein-domain microarray identifies novel protein–protein interactions. *Biochem J* 2002;367:697–702.

66. Varambally S, Yu JJ, Laxman B, Rhodes DR, Mehra R, Tomlins SA, Shah RB, Chandran U, Monzon FA, Becich MJ, Wei JT, Pienta KJ, Ghosh D, Rubin MA, Chinnaiyan AM. Integrative genomic and proteomic analysis of prostate cancer reveals signatures of metastatic progression. *Cancer Cell* 2005;8:393–406.

67. Griffin TJ, Gygi SP, Ideker T, Rist B, Eng J, Hood L, Aebersold R. Complementary profiling of gene expression at the transcriptome and proteome levels in *Saccharomyces cerevisiae*. *Mol Cell Proteomics* 2002;1:323–333.

68. Washburn MP, Koller A, Oshiro G, Ulaszek RR, Plouffe D, Deciu C, Winzeler E, Yates JR. Protein pathway and complex clustering of correlated mRNA and protein expression analyses in *Saccharomyces cerevisiae*. *Proc Natl Acad Sci USA* 2003;100:3107–3112.

69. Baliga NS, Pan M, Goo YA, Yi EC, Goodlett DR, Dimitrov K, Shannon P, Aebersold R, Ng WV, Hood L. Coordinate regulation of energy transduction modules in *Halobacterium* sp analyzed by a global systems approach. *Proc Natl Acad Sci USA* 2002;99: 14913–14918.

70. Tian Q, Stepaniants SB, Mao M, Weng L, Feetham MC, Doyle MJ, Yi EC, Dai HY, Thorsson V, Eng J, Goodlett D, Berger JP, Gunter B, Linseley PS, Stoughton RB, Aebersold R, Collins SJ, Hanlon WA, Hood LE. Integrated genomic and proteomic analyses of gene expression in mammalian cells. *Mol Cell Proteomics* 2004;3:960–969.

24

TOXICOGENOMICS IN PRECLINICAL DEVELOPMENT

ERIC A. G. BLOMME, DIMITRI SEMIZAROV, AND JEFFREY F. WARING

Global Pharmaceutical Research and Development, Abbott Laboratories, Abbott Park, Illinois

Contents

Preclinical Development Handbook: Toxicology, edited by Shayne Cox Gad
Copyright © 2008 John Wiley & Sons, Inc.

24.1   INTRODUCTION

24.1.1   Toxicogenomics and Other Emerging Technologies in Perspective

The cost of drug discovery and development has risen exponentially in the last decades. According to the Pharmaceutical Research and Manufacturers of America (PhRMA), the industry's trade group, pharmaceutical companies spent $33 billion on R&D in 2003, a threefold rise since 1990 and nearly 30-fold since 1977 [1]. This increase in investment has so far failed to deliver a surge of new medicines, and this is reflected by a concerning low productivity of pharmaceutical R&D [1, 2]. The cost of developing a new chemical entity (NCE) ranges from $800 million (U.S.) to $1.1 billion [1, 3]. These rising R&D costs are not sustainable and the lack of productivity of pharmaceutical R&D units has to be addressed. There are several factors underlying this change in the drug development economics. First, pharmaceutical companies are now tackling diseases of greater complexity than in the past and the industry's interest in the development of blockbusters requires running longer and more expensive clinical trials [1]. Second, the requirements for approval are notably higher than in the past because of the enhanced standard of care for most diseases and more stringent regulations intended to improve drug quality and safety [4].

One striking aspect of the drug discovery and development process is the high failure rate of compounds with an estimated 99.9% of compounds eliminated from the discovery and development pipeline [1]. Obviously, the vast majority of these compounds are eliminated very early in the process because of suboptimal pharmacological, physicochemical, pharmacokinetic, or toxicologic properties. Nevertheless, failure rates in the subsequent, more costly stages of development are substantially high with the vast majority of clinical attrition occurring in Phases IIb and III [4]. Eliminating unsuccessful drugs earlier than in full development is definitely a prerequisite for a decrease in the overall R&D costs. Indeed, the recently implemented laboratory technologies (such as combinatorial chemistry, genomics tools, or high throughput screening) driving discovery efforts are resulting in a constantly increasing number of novel compounds being synthesized and a similarly rising number of therapeutically interesting targets. Therefore, approaches that allow for an earlier, multidirectional characterization of compounds are needed to face these major challenges.

The major causes of attrition in the clinic in 2000 were lack of efficacy and safety, both accounting for approximately 30% of failures, respectively [4]. This is in contrast to what was occurring in the late 1980s when poor pharmacokinetic properties were the main reason for termination (around 40%), while lack of clinical safety already accounted for 30% of failures [5]. This remarkable improvement in the pharmacokinetic properties of advanced compounds was mostly the result of a significant effort by the pharmaceutical industry to develop preclinical tools to better predict the pharmacokinetic properties of experimental compounds. While the industry has successfully addressed the failures related to pharmacokinetics, it has not significantly improved its ability to better characterize early the toxicologic properties of compounds. In fact, one may argue that with an increased number of compounds to be evaluated, less toxicologic characterization has been possible, and often compounds are selected for animal testing without sufficient data regarding their toxicologic potential. Furthermore, traditional toxicologic evaluation through *in vivo* studies typically creates a bottleneck in the R&D process because of its length and cost, and due to the requirement for significant amounts of compound. Approaches designed to characterize the toxicologic profile of compounds earlier would allow discovery scientists to select the molecules with an optimal, or at least adequate, toxicological profile for these costly studies. To be cost effective and applicable in the drug discovery setting, these approaches must use small amounts of compounds (typically an amount that would not require scale-up chemistry), have acceptable accuracy (the level of acceptability being dependent on the stage of testing) and reproducibility, and have an appropriate throughput [6]. Various technologies, including the "omics" technologies, potentially meet these criteria and are addressed in this textbook in various chapters.

24.1.2   Definition and Basics of Toxicogenomics

In this chapter, we use the term *toxicogenomics* to refer to the use of gene expression analysis in the field of toxicology. The sequencing of several whole genomes has led to the development of methodologies that make it feasible to monitor in several animal species (humans, mice, rats) the expression levels of large numbers of genes expressed in a specific tissue at a certain time, an activity referred to as *gene expression profiling* or simply expression profiling. Among these laboratory tools reviewed in Chapter 22, molecular toxicologists have mostly used *DNA microarrays* to generate transcription profiles from tissues collected from *in vivo* studies or cells derived from *in vitro* experiments. Consequently, this chapter heavily emphasizes the use of microarrays in toxicology studies. It is noteworthy, however, that other technologies are available or may become available in the future for gene expression profiling. In particular, for specific applications, it is generally agreed that more cost-effective platforms with a higher throughput will be needed for toxicogenomics to realize its full potential in drug discovery and development [7].

Toxicogenomics is based on the relatively simple assumption that toxicants acting through a similar mechanism of action will generate similar gene expression profiles or at least affect similar pathways, leading to common gene expression changes (Fig. 24.1). In other words, these expression changes (either upregulation or downregulation) induced in common by toxicants with similar toxicologic properties could represent an easy and sensitive endpoint to identify and classify toxicants.

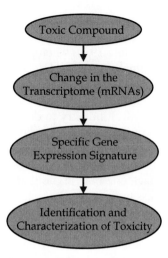

FIGURE 24.1   Principle of toxicogenomics. Toxic compounds induce changes in the cellular transcriptome, including changes in the expression of particular gene sets that correlate with the mechanism of toxicity. These gene sets are typically referred to as signatures. These signatures can be used for the identification and characterization at the molecular level of toxic changes.

These common gene expression changes are typically referred to as *fingerprints* or *signatures* of toxicity. Proof-of-principle for the signature concept has already been nicely demonstrated in various types of cancer, as mentioned in Chapter 22. Using gene expression analysis, investigators have identified new classes of hematological malignancies or predicted prognosis in lung cancer and breast cancer [8]. Furthermore, because microarrays allow for the global evaluation of the cell transcriptome, the assumption is also that the identified gene expression changes will allow toxicologists to understand better the molecular mechanisms whereby toxicants injure cells. Again, this is clearly supported by the numerous mechanistic observations made in various diseases using microarrays [8]. These observations are typically a stepping stone for the articulation of new hypotheses on the mechanism of action, which can then be evaluated and confirmed by subsequent, appropriately designed experiments.

The use of most of the early microarray platforms was associated with reproducibility and accuracy issues. Since then, the technology has rapidly improved and several recent studies have demonstrated the reproducibility and accuracy of gene expression data [9–11]. This rapid improvement has led to a change of practices. For instance, it was initially recommended to confirm specific gene expression changes observed with microarrays with techniques that were considered more accurate, such as real-time reverse transcription-PCR (RT-PCR) [12]. In our laboratory, we do use RT-PCR to validate microarray data, but this confirmation step is now only occasional. An example demonstrating the good correlation between a microarray platform and RT-PCR is illustrated in Fig. 24.2. For gene expression profiling to reliably identify and characterize toxicity, gene expression data must be sufficiently reproducible following exposure to chemicals. The consistency and reproducibility were evaluated by different industrial, governmental, and academic laboratories

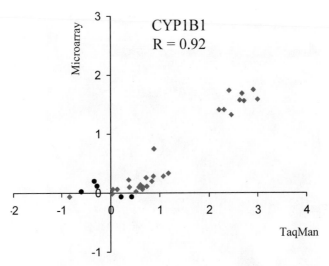

FIGURE 24.2 Correlation between expression levels of cytochrome P450, 1b1 (CYP1B1) measured with Affymetrix microarrays and RT-PCR (TaqMan). The log10 values of the fold changes determined by Affymetrix microarrays (*Y* axis) are plotted against those determined by RT-PCR (*X* axis). Included are the gene expression levels from 32 hepatocyte treatments measured by both platforms. The values represented by squares indicate genes that exhibit the same directionality in terms of gene expression changes using both technologies. Circles indicate genes that exhibit different directionality between the two platforms.

using various commercial and customized microarray platforms and shown to be sufficient for assessing toxic reactions in tissues such as liver, kidney, and heart [9, 13, 14].

Any experimental *in vivo* study is associated with some degree of interindividual variability. This is the reason behind the use of treatment groups of appropriate size in toxicology studies. Developing an understanding of the interindividual variability in gene expression data was critical to fully understanding the optimal number of animals per group to be used in toxicogenomic studies. Clearly, gene expression data are also subject to interindividual variability inherent to any *in vivo* model. In our experience, gene expression data generated following short *in vivo* exposures (typically less than 24 hours) are typically quite variable. However, gene expression profiles from tissues exposed for longer periods of time (1–5 days) are usually less variable than other endpoints typically used in toxicological assessment, such as serum chemistry, hematology, or histopathology. Figure 24.3 illustrates this concept using liver as an example. This low variability has clear implications and advantages, as it allows the toxicologist to use as few as 2–3 rats/group to generate interpretable and reliable data.

The question of species extrapolation has been evaluated and studied by toxicologists for decades. In most instances, especially in the case of pharmaceuticals, the objective of the toxicologist is to identify hazards and assess their risks for humans. A particular interest with toxicogenomics is to understand if this technology can lead to an improved prediction of toxicologic reactions in humans, and in particular whether gene expression profiling allows toxicologists to reliably deter-

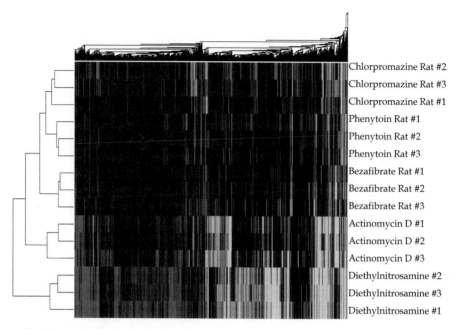

FIGURE 24.3 Heatmap with hierarchical clustering illustrating gene expression changes in the liver of rats treated for 3 days with various hepatotoxicants at toxic doses. Genes shown include genes that were up- or downregulated by at least two fold with a $p < 0.01$. Despite significant variability in response observed with clinical pathology and histopathology, there is limited interindividual variability in gene expression profiles.

mine which of the changes occurring in traditional toxicologic preclinical species would not be relevant to humans. Several studies have shown that, in general, toxicogenomics improves the robustness of cross-species extrapolation [15]. Indeed, despite the differences in genomes, many responses to toxicants are evolutionary conserved. Therefore, since analysis of gene expression changes following the exposure to a toxicant improves the understanding of the mechanism of toxicity and of the major cellular subsystems affected, it becomes easier to assess the relevance of a specific toxic change or to predict how a specific species would react to a compound. However, it is important to point out that most of these studies have focused on a specific class of toxicants or a particular mechanism of toxicity. Furthermore, *in vitro* studies have mostly been used to evaluate how humans may react to a specific compound and these studies make it difficult to fully comprehend a cause-and-effect relationship. Consequently, it is prudent to state that while a toxicogenomic analysis in the context of a particular toxicologic study can and will ultimately improve the overall risk assessment to humans, it is likely that exceptions will remain.

24.1.3 History of Toxicogenomics

Soon after the microarray technology was first invented in 1995, toxicologists and molecular biologists rapidly realized its potential to generate large amounts of valuable molecular data, which could help in understanding the pathogenesis of various toxic changes [16, 17]. This technology has rapidly been embraced by the pharmaceutical industry as a potentially useful tool to identify safer drugs in a faster, more cost-effective manner [18]. Almost all major pharmaceutical companies now have dedicated groups applying gene expression analysis in toxicology. Academic and governmental institutions have also aggressively adopted this technology, and the regulatory community has clearly identified toxicogenomics as an important part for the success of its critical path initiative [19]. Growing interest in this field is best exemplified by the vast numbers of workshops, committees, and consortia created to address various technical issues, to improve the science base of the community, to allow contributors to keep pace with these new emerging technologies, and to establish guidelines for determining how genomic data should be submitted to regulatory agencies. An exponentially growing number of studies are being published on this topic. Some studies have used microarrays to identify the mechanism of toxicity of pharmaceutical agents or standard toxicants [20–22]. Other studies have evaluated the predictive power of toxicogenomics by identifying potential toxic liabilities before the development of other manifestations of toxicity, such as clinical chemistry or histopathology [23–25]. Finally, several investigators have used this technology in an attempt to identify new markers of toxicity [26]. The majority of published studies have evaluated reference and tool compounds that induce well-characterized, general, or specific toxicities. These compounds either have been on the market for many years or have never been developed as pharmaceutical agents. However, in the last few years, several pharmaceutical companies have clearly moved beyond this proof-of-concept stage and have applied this technology to drug development programs to address critical, development-limiting toxicologic issues, as indicated by recent submissions of gene expression profiling datasets to regulatory agencies as well as by various published studies.

24.1.4 Applications of Toxicogenomics

It would clearly be beyond the scope of this chapter to provide an in-depth review of all published studies using toxicogenomics. Rather, in this chapter, we focus on potential applications of toxicogenomics using selected examples as illustrations. Regrettably, numerous very valuable published studies have not been referenced here because of space limitations, and therefore, we encourage the reader interested in a specific application to proceed to a more elaborate literature search.

In the drug discovery and development process, toxicogenomics has been or can be applied at different stages to address different issues (Fig. 24.4). Its applications include the following:

- Prediction and characterization of the toxic properties of experimental compounds from short-term *in vivo* studies or *in vitro* systems. This activity typically takes place in the discovery setting at the lead identification, lead optimization, and candidate selection stages.
- Elucidation of the mechanism of toxic changes. These types of studies are more often conducted on candidate compounds that do induce unexpected changes of unknown mechanism in repeat-dose toxicology studies. The objectives are to develop an understanding of the relevance of these changes for humans or

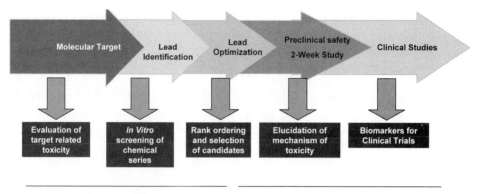

Predictive Toxicology   Mechanistic Toxicology

FIGURE 24.4   Use of toxicogenomics in drug discovery and development. In drug discovery and development, toxicogenomics can be applied at different stages. An understanding of potential target-related toxicity with gene expression profiling can help to prioritize for the most drugable targets. Toxicogenomic studies using short-term *in vivo* studies or *in vitro* assays (predictive toxicology) are useful for the early characterization of the toxic properties of compounds at the lead identification/lead optimization stages. Toxicogenomics can also be used to elucidate the mechanism of toxicity associated with compounds. These mechanistic studies typically take place after candidate selection but are also useful to establish appropriate counterscreens for backup compound selection. Finally, gene expression profiling studies can help identify novel biomarkers for the identification and monitoring of toxicologic changes, in both preclinical and clinical studies.

to generate mechanistic data for the establishment of appropriately designed counterscreens for selecting backup compounds.

- Characterization of new therapeutic targets and the proactive identification of potential toxicity issues associated with their modulation (also referred to as toxicity related to primary pharmacology or on-target toxicity). The purpose is to investigate further the biology of the target as early as the target selection stage. Given the rising number of targets that pharmaceutical companies are working with, learning what makes a good or bad target at the gene expression level with respect to toxicology can lead to better target prioritization in the discovery pipeline.

- Identification of selective gene expression signatures that could be used as sensitive biomarkers. There is a definite need for additional biomarkers that could help in the identification and monitoring of specific toxicologic changes, in both preclinical and clinical studies. In the last few years, very few additional sensitive and specific correlates of particular toxic changes have been made available to the toxicology community. Whole-genome analysis represents an ideal approach for the identification of genes or signaling pathways whose deregulation leads to specific toxic effects.

- Molecular characterization of compounds associated with idiosyncratic reactions in the clinic. Idiosyncratic toxic events are low-incidence toxic events of unknown mechanism that occur in humans, usually in a non-dose-dependent manner and that were not observed in preclinical species. This type of toxicity leads to costly failures of drugs in clinical trials or market withdrawal. Approaches that would allow for understanding the mechanism of idiosyncratic adverse events could have an enormous impact on the productivity of the pharmaceutical industry. They could rescue useful drugs through identification of populations sensitive to the toxic effects or through early prediction of idiosyncratic adverse events.

24.2 PRACTICAL AND LOGISTIC ASPECTS OF TOXICOGENOMICS

24.2.1 Technical Considerations

At the time when this chapter is written, gene expression profiling is still a rapidly evolving discipline for which efforts have so far essentially focused on addressing key technical issues and on validating approaches through proof-of-concept studies. Because of the immaturity of the microarray technology, there are many different technical issues, including external or internal control selection, probe design, platform variation and comparison, scanner performance characteristics, data normalization, or analysis software packages. These technical issues are being aggressively addressed by various academic, governmental, and industry groups, often in the form of consortia or collaborations [9, 10, 14, 27, 28]. While technical issues are critical to the reliability and correct interpretation of microarray data, most of them are closely related to the instrumentation being used and are consequently rapidly evolving and becoming obsolete. For this reason, in this chapter, we only address technical issues that will have some relevance for a significant period of time and that need to be understood by molecular toxicologists. For other issues, the reader is referred to Chapter 22 or other existing publications [10,12, 27–30].

24.2.2 Species Considerations

The vast majority of toxicogenomic studies are conducted using rat tissues or cell lines of rat or human origin. The major reason is that the rat is the most commonly used small laboratory animal species for toxicology testing in the pharmaceutical industry. Another reason is the incomplete genome annotation for other species (dog or monkey) and the lack of historical gene expression data for these species. Nevertheless, gene expression studies have been conducted in large animal species (dog and monkey) and several investigators have experimental microarray platforms available for these large species [31, 32].

24.2.3 Toxicogenomics in *In Vitro* and *In Vivo* Studies

Tissue Considerations Toxicogenomic studies have been performed using cell cultures and tissues from *in vivo* studies. Cell cultures are very homogeneous, and gene expression changes induced by toxicants can be reproduced reliably in a laboratory under similar experimental conditions. The use of tissues can be more challenging. Several tissues, such as liver or heart, are relatively homogeneous in their phenotypes and transcriptomes, and robust, consistent changes in gene expression can reliably be detected, as long as a consistent tissue collection protocol is followed.

Other tissues, such as brain or testis, are more heterogeneous and complex, and their gene expression profiles are therefore less consistent. For instance, the brain is composed of various cell types (neurons, glia) with immense phenotypic and transcriptional diversity [33, 34]. In addition, depending on the region of the brain, marked differences in functions and transcriptomes are present between cells of the same origin. This complexity explains the limited number of attempts to apply toxicogenomics to these tissues. Technologies, such as laser capture microdissection (LCM) and RNA amplification protocols, have greatly enhanced the ability to perform expression analysis on single cell populations [35]. However, these technologies also require a more extensive investment of time and labor with an overall reduced capacity. In addition, the analysis of gene expression changes in single cell populations may limit one's ability to fully understand major interactions between cells that may play a significant role in the pathogenesis of a toxicologic change. These limitations will be illustrated in our section covering testicular toxicity (Section 24.6.2). Finally, it should be reemphasized that an accurate interpretation of gene expression changes can only succeed if tissue collection protocols are sufficiently consistent. Even in the case of rather homogeneous tissues like heart or kidney, it is critical to collect samples for gene expression analysis in a consistent manner [36]. Likewise, relatively homogeneous tissues like kidney contain several compartments that are clearly different in structure, function, and transcriptome. Toxicants may induce changes in only specific compartments or cellular subpopulation. Failure to cover all compartments of a tissue would limit one's ability to detect toxicant-induced gene expression changes. In our laboratory, we have established collection protocols for all tissues that we routinely evaluate. For example, we collect kidneys in a manner such that appropriate and consistent proportions of cortex and medulla are included for RNA extraction. Inappropriate collection procedures would lead to the identification of gene expression changes related to the collection procedure rather than to the toxicity being evaluated.

Samples for gene expression analysis should be collected immediately after sacrifice and flash frozen in liquid nitrogen or preserved in an appropriate RNA stabilization solution. They can then be stored for a prolonged period of time at −80 °C without significant RNA degradation. Inappropriate collection procedures or storage conditions will result in RNA degradation, as typically revealed by an overall poor RNA quality after RNA extraction procedures (Fig. 24.5). It is therefore recommended to always evaluate RNA quality after extraction to ensure that the quality is sufficient to justify the costly step of hybridization to microarrays, but also to ensure that interpretation of the microarray data is feasible.

Hybridization Design in Toxicogenomic Studies   Three common hybridization designs are used in experiments using two-color or two-channel microarrays. These designs do not pertain to experiments using one-color microarrays. These designs are referred to as *direct, reference*, and *loop* [37, 38]. In the *direct design*, the test article-treated samples are hybridized against their appropriate control samples. This allows for the identification of differentially expressed genes at a specific time. In the *reference design*, which is the most commonly used design within the biological community, all study samples are hybridized against a common reference sample, and this can be useful in the case of a study containing one control group for several treatment groups. This design is also well suited for the characterization of the

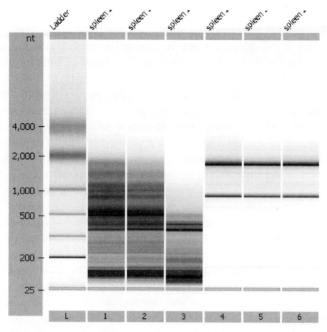

FIGURE 24.5 Evaluation of RNA quality after extraction using an Agilent Bioanalyzer. Rat spleens were collected after sacrifice and flash frozen. For samples 1–3, the collection procedure was inappropriate, resulting in RNA degradation as evidenced by the multiple bands and smear observed on the Bioanalyzer-generated electrophoretic image. These samples should not be used for hybridization to microarrays. Note the sharp contrast with samples 4 and 5, where RNA quality is optimal for microarray experiments.

magnitude of gene expression changes and temporal relationships. The *loop design* is seldom used, although it has been shown to attain a higher precision [30, 38]. It entails sequential hybridization of all study samples against one another; it may offer advantages for time course experiments where one needs to understand expression changes over time.

Experimental Design in Toxicogenomic Studies The design of *in vivo* and *in vitro* toxicogenomic studies is determined by the questions to be answered or the issues to be addressed. Specific design will be discussed as different applications are reviewed. However, several considerations are relevant to the current discussion.

Duration of Dosing In the case of a study to address the mode of action of a specific toxicologic change, a time-course experiment may be very appropriate to identify gene expression changes linked to the development of the toxicity. Time points are selected based on the particular toxicologic change to be investigated. An important aspect to remember is that gene expression changes are transient and therefore timing is of critical importance. Changes that are more relevant to generate a mechanistic understanding of toxicologic effects are typically those occurring before the effects are fully developed. Therefore, it is usually more insightful to evaluate gene expression during the development of a tissue change, rather than when the change has already occurred and is fully established. In the case of a study used to rank-order several potential lead molecules for candidate selection, the study needs to be designed with a consideration for compound availability, reference database, performance characteristics of the predictive signatures of interest, and so on. For instance, in our laboratory, an *in vivo* toxicogenomic hepatic reference database has been generated based on 3-day repeat-dose studies in rats. Consequently, we typically assess our compounds for hepatotoxicity in 3-day repeat-dose studies. In several companies, toxicogenomic analysis is now integrated in most 2–4 week rat repeat-dose toxicology studies. The objective is usually to be proactive in case unexpected toxicologic changes occur in the studies or to enhance knowledge and expertise in gene expression analysis. In addition, these types of practice are useful to promote a better acceptance of these new technologies in a company.

Dose   In a mechanistic *in vivo* study, the dose will be selected based on the best chance to consistently reproduce the toxicologic change of interest. In contrast, the method used to develop the predictive signatures will dictate the dose to be used in a predictive study. Validation of predictive signatures should address to some extent their predictive power and accuracy for various dose levels. For instance, in our laboratory, our *in vivo* databases and signatures have been developed based on a low and a high dose. The low dose corresponds to an estimated pharmacological dose (a dose resulting in an exposure similar to that achieved in the ED_{50} in the most appropriate animal model), while the high dose corresponds to a maximal tolerated dose (MTD) for a 3-day study (defined by the highest dose before rats exhibit clinical signs of toxicity, lack of body weight gain, or a significant decrease in food consumption). It is clear that in the vast majority of cases, because these studies are typically conducted early in a project, only limited information is available for selecting the doses. Consequently, dose setting can be a challenging task and requires extensive communication among all project stakeholders. An adequate dose selection is, however, crucial for proper decision making and, in our experience, is central to a successful prediction of toxicologic changes.

Samples   When conducting an *in vivo* study, we strongly recommend that all major tissues, including blood, be collected for concurrent histopathologic and clinical pathologic examinations. The latter are relatively inexpensive compared to the current cost of microarrays, can be performed quickly in a discovery setting, and provide critical information that helps interpret gene expression data in the context of changes in the homeostasis of the tissue being analyzed and in the context of the overall status of the animal. For instance, if clinical observations and analysis of the clinical pathology and histopathology changes suggest that an animal is moribund, gene expression changes may be more reflective of the overall poor condition of the animal than of a specific mechanism of toxicity. In our laboratory, for predictive studies, we typically select or prioritize the tissues to be evaluated with microarrays based on a prior histopathologic and clinical pathologic evaluation. For instance, if a test article demonstrates dose-limiting hepatotoxicity as evidenced by hepatocellular necrosis and elevations of serum transaminases, it would be moot and redundant to evaluate the liver by gene expression analysis. However, if the project team considers it important to understand the pathogenesis of this hepatoxicity, microarray analysis of the liver may be warranted.

24.3   TOXICOGENOMIC REFERENCE DATABASES

24.3.1   The Need for Toxicogenomic Reference Databases

Gene expression changes, when viewed in isolation, can often lead to more questions than answers [39]. Furthermore, although changes in expression of individual genes may be of importance, it is usually more appropriate to examine gene expression changes by looking at pathways being regulated. The analysis of pathways increases the confidence that a change in expression of specific genes has biological implications, but increases the accuracy of the overall interpretation. Abundant historical data are not yet available and general experience is still insufficient for the meaningful interpretation of thousands of simultaneous gene expression changes, which may often appear disconnected. Only after a specific toxicologic change has been observed consistently can its real toxicologic significance be understood. The same holds true for gene expression changes. A recent study nicely illustrated this aspect. In this study, over 300 liver microarray experiments covering three different classes of compounds (genotoxic carcinogens, nongenotoxic carcinogens, and noncarcinogens) were clustered across 72 putative oncogenes [40]. The three classes of compounds were strikingly interdispersed within the cluster, indicating that upregulation of oncogene expression was not a surrogate marker for carcinogenesis, as both noncarcinogens and carcinogens were upregulating the expression of these selected genes. This study also reiterates the danger of focusing on the change in expression of single or a limited set of genes in a microarray experiment.

Gene expression changes induced by toxicants typically reflect a large number of complex pharmacological, physiological, and biochemical processes [18, 41]. To generate a plausible mechanistic hypothesis for the pathogenesis of a toxicologic change, the gene expression changes related to the toxicity need to be identified and separated from those that are adaptive, beneficial, or unrelated to the development of the toxicologic change. This requires an appropriate study design, including the evaluation of multiple time points, but mostly the access to reference data. The use of reference compounds may clarify or confirm which gene expression changes are related to a specific lesion or how the lesion develops. However, contextual information from large, established reference databases is optimal to properly interpret gene expression data by correlating unique gene changes to those associated with treatment with a large repository of compounds or with specific toxicologic mechanisms [39]. The large number of compounds, tissues, corroborative toxicologic and pathologic changes, and gene expression data in these reference databases allow one to strengthen statistical inferences [42]. The concept of databases in toxicology is not novel, and as an illustration, one can think of databases for serum chemistry, hematology, pathology, or carcinogenesis.

24.3.2   Design and Development of Toxicogenomic Reference Databases

The ideal toxicogenomic database contains gene expression profiles induced in various tissues following the treatment of the reference species (most often rats) with a variety of reference toxicants (known pharmaceutical agents, prototypical toxicants) and control compounds, at multiple doses and time points [23, 43–47].

The reference compounds profiled in the database should reflect a variety of toxic mechanisms and represent different structure–activity relationships [42]. The use of multiple doses of the reference compounds (e.g., an efficacious dose and a maximum tolerated dose) is extremely useful to distinguish a pharmacological effect from a toxicological effect. In some situations, time-course data can be very useful to identify gene expression changes linked to a time-dependent toxic response and can increase the chances of observing a true toxic response. The number of animals required for each time point or dose is also an important consideration. Biological replicates are useful to establish both the biological and technical variability. As mentioned earlier, when rats are exposed for a sufficient period of time to toxicants, the interindividual variability of gene expression changes is relatively small, so that 3 animals per group and per time point are usually considered sufficient for the generation of meaningful gene expression profiles.

In addition to gene expression profiles, a useful database also contains sufficient technical and biological information. The realization by the scientific community that gene expression data can only be correctly understood and put in a perspective if the critical amount of associated information is available had led to the publication in 2001 by the Microarray Gene Expression Data Society of the minimum information about a microarray experiment (MIAME) guidelines for the reporting and publication of microarray experiments [48]. These guidelines have become a reference for the submission of gene expression data to scientific journals and are used as standards by some public and commercial databases.

Experimental inconsistencies can lead to some confusion, as not all datasets relate to one another. In particular, the platform used to generate the reference profiles can limit the value of some experimental datasets. While some marked improvements have been achieved in the ability to extrapolate data from one platform to another and in establishing more consistent gene nomenclature, different platforms still generate slightly different datasets or may be evaluating different genes [49]. Furthermore, even when the same platform is used, gene expression data have been shown to vary across laboratories because of differences in protocols or instrumentations [37]. These issues are the focus of several major initiatives involving academic, industry, and government laboratories with the objectives of identifying, validating, and implementing standards that could be used for gene expression analysis [9, 10, 14]. Overall, however, several confounding factors still exist that currently limit the comparison of gene expression data from one laboratory to another. These experimental aspects should be carefully evaluated when selecting the database to work with.

The nature of the species or strain used can also be a limitation. Ideally, one should compare gene expression profiles generated in a particular species with those generated in the same species or even strain. Practically, this may not always be feasible because of a lack of reference data in some species or strains. Therefore, certain circumstances require extrapolating across species. There have been significant improvements in the annotations of the genome of the major preclinical species currently used in toxicology [15]. However, the mapping of orthologous genes should still be viewed as approximate and needs considerable additional effort to be optimized. Furthermore, not all species react similarly to a specific toxicant and this difference in response also limits the ability to extrapolate from one species to another. Different rat strains may also have different responses to some toxicity and the difference in response at the transcriptome level has also been addressed. Overall, the transcriptome response following exposure to toxicants has been shown to be usually very similar across different rat strains [50].

24.3.3   Existing Toxicogenomic Databases

Several publicly available, commercial or proprietary databases exist for the analysis of gene expression datasets [28]. Although not all of these repositories are specific to toxicology, they can still represent a useful source of data for the analysis of gene expression. Several recently developed databases are mostly focused on toxicology. For instance, the National Institute of Environmental Health Sciences has recently established the National Center for Toxicogenomics to create a reference knowledge database (Chemical Effects in Biological Systems or CEBS) that would ultimately allow scientists to understand mechanisms of toxicity through the use of gene expression analysis as well as proteomics and metabolite profiling [51, 52]. Companies such as GeneLogic (Gaithersburg, MD) or Iconix (Mountain View, CA) have created large toxicogenomic reference databases containing gene expression profiles induced by prototypical reference compounds with corroborating toxicologic and pathologic endpoints [42, 53]. A list of selected public databases with a brief description of their general attributes is presented in Table 24.1.

24.4   TOXICOGENOMICS IN DRUG DISCOVERY

24.4.1   Predictive Toxicology

In this chapter, the term *predictive toxicology* is used to refer to the use of short-term assays that allow the toxicologist to predict with sufficient accuracy toxic changes that would occur after longer exposure and to extrapolate toxic reactions from preclinical species to humans [54, 55]. Predictive toxicology assays can be in the form of *in vitro* assays or short-term *in vivo* studies. Because most attempts to use toxicogenomics in predictive toxicology have so far focused on the use of short-term *in vivo* studies, we limit our discussion to this approach. The use of cell cultures is covered later in this chapter.

Large-scale expression analysis is an extremely sensitive approach to detect deregulated genes and signaling pathways that contribute to toxic changes. The main assumption of toxicogenomics is that following exposure to toxicants at relevant doses, transcriptional changes occur before the development of a toxic phenotype as assessed by traditional endpoints, such as clinical observations, hispathologic examination, or clinical pathology measurements. In our experience, this assumption is accurate for the vast majority of toxicities with few exceptions. For this reason, toxicogenomics offers the unique opportunity to reliably identify compounds with toxic liabilities early in the drug discovery process, and to thus significantly improve the productivity of drug discovery [18, 54, 55]. As mentioned earlier, the development of more sensitive and predictive technologies that would allow for the characterization of toxicology early is critical for the selection of molecules with an optimal toxicologic profile. Pharmaceutical R&D units and private toxicogenomics companies have consequently invested significant resources in the development of

TABLE 24.1   Some Public Databases

Database	Attributes	URL
Gene Expression Omnibus (GEO)	World's largest public repository Adherence to MIAME guidelines Toxicology data available Exploration, analysis, and visualization tools	http://www.ncbi.nlm.nih.gov/projects/geo/
ArrayExpress	Large public repository Adherence to MIAME guidelines Toxicology data available in Tox-MIAMExpress Expression data from normal human and mouse tissues	http://www.ebi.ac.uk/arrayexpress/
Chemical Effects in Biological Systems (CEBS)	Evolving public toxicogenomics repository from the National Institute of Environmental Sciences (NIEHS) National Center for Toxicogenomics (NCT) Designed to house data from complex studies having multiple data steams (genetic, proteomic, metabonomic data) Exploration and analysis tools	http://cebs.niehs.nih.gov/
Environment, Drugs, and Gene Expression (EDGE)	Public toxicogenomics repository Standardized experimental conditions including standardized microarray platform Mostly focused on mouse liver microarray data Useful bioinformatics tools (clustering, BLAST searching, rank analysis, classification tools)	http://edge.oncology.wisc.edu/
Symatlas	Product of the Genomics Institute of the Novartis Research Foundation Expression data from a large panel of normal human and mouse tissues or cell culture models	http://symatlas.gnf.org/SymAtlas/
DbZach System	Toxicogenomic database allowing data mining and full knowledge-based understanding of toxicologic mechanisms Contains correlating clinical chemistry parameters and histopatholigc data	http://dbzach.fst.msu.edu/

predictive gene expression-based assays. However, relatively few of these efforts have been formerly published, such that the majority of the information used here is based on personal experience.

Predictive toxicology should ideally be applied at the lead selection and lead optimization stages, concurrently with the other assays used to assess drug-like properties of molecules (pharmacologic and physicochemical properties, ADME pharmacokinetic characterization). Predictive toxicogenomics is not yet amenable to such an early stage because of its relative immaturity, low throughput, and significant cost. In addition, while most available data suggest that expression analysis will allow for the use of gene expression-based assays early in the discovery process, not enough data related to the accuracy of this approach are available to fully assess the value added by this technology. Nevertheless, several companies are using gene expression analysis to rank-order or prioritize compounds using short-term rat studies based on their toxic potential in specific tissues, in particular, liver.

24.4.2 Development of Predictive Gene Expression Signatures

As pointed out earlier, changes in expression of single genes are typically not sufficient to predict or identify existing toxic changes. Rather, changes in the expression of a gene set are more likely to correlate with toxicity. Consequently, the first step in predicting toxic changes entails the development of gene expression signatures that strongly correlate with toxic changes. Albeit simple in concept, this task has proved to be substantially more difficult and more resource intensive than initially anticipated. Not all recently developed genomics approaches have demonstrated superiority compared to traditional methods or have been able to adequately validate signatures based on external samples (forward validation process). Indeed, sophisticated statistical tools and biostatistical expertise are needed to address the complexity of the various changes in the transcriptome and to develop predictive toxicogenomic signatures [18, 53, 56]. Some of the most commonly used statistical methods are briefly reviewed next.

Toxicants typically induce hundreds to thousands of gene expression changes, a large number difficult to manage for most statistical methods. Therefore, the first step in developing predictive signatures is to reduce the number of parameters, focusing on the ones relevant to the classification model. Two major approaches are traditionally used for dimensionality reduction. The most commonly used approach is to rank genes with respect to differences in expression between experimental groups using parametric or nonparametric statistical tests, such as standard or permutation t- or F-test, Wilcoxon statistics, or significance analysis of microarrays (SAMs) [43, 44, 57, 58]. The genes that are differentially expressed at a specified significance level or a fixed number of top ranking genes are then selected for inclusion in the prediction model. The second approach for dimension reduction is to use noise reduction methods, such as principal component analysis (PCA) [59]. The PCA method reduces a large set of genes into several components, where each new component is a weighted linear combination of all genes. These components are rank-ordered according to the amount of variance, and the first component represents the greatest variability among the samples. By selecting the first n components as most informative, the dimension of gene expression data is vastly reduced.

Once data have been reduced and informative genes have been selected, predictive models can be developed with the objective of classifying compounds as toxic or nontoxic in the relevant tissue. This step requires a training set consisting of a repository of gene expression profiles encompassing both toxic and nontoxic compounds, and the use of computational algorithms that will allow for the accurate classification of unknown samples. These computational methods require significant numbers of gene expression profiles to generate useful predictive models. Several computational algorithms have been used for the analysis of microarray-generated gene expression data. They include logistic regression, linear discriminant analysis (LDA), naive Bayesian classifiers, artificial neural networks (ANNs), and support vector machines (SVMs). Both logistic regression and LDA use statistical inference to weigh the contributions of each signature gene expression value in sample prediction and typically require tens to hundreds of datasets, depending on the variability of the gene expression data. In situations where there is a clear difference between groups, these methods can be quite robust [43, 53]. Naive Bayesian classification is a popular approach for classification. In one study, gene expression profiles were generated from the liver of mice treated with 12 compounds, representing 5 well-characterized classes of hepatotoxicants (peroxisome proliferators, aryl hydrocarbon receptor agonists, noncoplanar polychlorinated biphenyls, inflammatory agents, and hypoxia-inducing agents) [45]. Using a naive Bayesian classification, a predictive signature consisting of 12 genes accurately classified all samples into their chemical groups. Artificial neural networks (ANNs) are analogous in concept to a biological nervous system. They are composed of a number of highly interconnected processing elements called neurons or nodes tied together with weighted connections. An iterative learning process begins by feeding input data into the network, which calculates the predicted output based on predetermined weights. Comparison of the predicted output and the targeted output leads to adjustment of the weights of the connections, and a new output is calculated. This process is reiterated until the network output closely matches the targeted output. ANNs have the advantage of learning complex patterns and of learning from new information; they have gained increasing popularity for the classification of gene expression profiles in many disciplines. In our laboratory, as illustrated later, the ANN approach has proved to be extremely powerful for the generation of predictive signatures of hepatotoxicity in rats. Support vector machines (SVMs) are a relatively new type of learning algorithm with robust performance with respect to sparse and noisy data [60]. SVMs operate by finding an optimal demarcation that most distantly separates positive and negative samples. Unlike other classification algorithms, SVMs perform very well with a large number of data and this feature makes SVMs especially attractive for the classification of gene expression data, which usually have a large number of gene expression endpoints and a limited number of samples [61, 62]. One can easily be confused with the choice and complexity of these various classification algorithms. The ultimate criterion to select an optimal prediction model is the prediction accuracy, which is estimated using a testing set that is different from the training set during a validation step. Although most studies evaluate the robustness of predictive models using various validation approaches, no exhaustive survey of the various prediction methods is available in the literature. For predictive toxicogenomics, the choice of methods is likely dependent on the experimental design. For instance, an LDA approach is an easy alternative and performs very well if there is a clear difference between the classes of toxicants and/or the sample size is relatively large. However, in the case of a more complex system, such as general hepatotoxicity, with a limited number of gene expression profiles, a machine learning approach, like SVMs or ANNs, could be more appropriate [18, 62].

24.4.3 Case Examples

Prediction of Hepatotoxicity Hepatotoxicity has been the toxicity of choice for most toxicogenomic studies. Indeed, the liver is a common target organ for many toxicants and has been extensively studied. This has promoted the generation of comprehensive gene expression databases that facilitate interpretation of liver-derived gene expression profiles. Additionally, the liver is a rather homogeneous tissue, as opposed to tissues such as intestines or brain, for instance. The liver is composed mostly of hepatocytes sharing similar biochemical functions that translate into relatively uniform gene expression profiles. This homogeneity makes identification and interpretation of gene expression changes easier. For these reasons, a wealth of published and proprietary gene expression information is available for the liver, and hepatotoxicity can now be relatively well predicted and understood with gene expression profiling.

As a proof-of-concept, our laboratory has developed, a few years ago, a quantitative approach to predict hepatotoxicity based on gene expression profiles [18]. We first constructed an internal database containing microarray-generated liver gene expression profiles from 3-day rat toxicology studies using over 50 hepatototoxicants and nonhepatotoxicants. All compounds were administered to 3 male rats/group at a high dose (a dose expected to induce hepatotoxicity after 1 week of treatment) and at a lower, nonhepatotoxic dose. A set of marker genes was identified that distinguished the hepatotoxicants from the nonhepatotoxicants using ANOVA analysis. Using an artificial neural network algorithm coupled with principal component analysis for dimensionality reduction, a quantitative model was established to classify compounds according to a composite toxicity score (Fig. 24.6). A forward validation step was conducted using additional compounds that were not part of the original database. The neural network algorithm could successfully classify these compounds based on their potential to cause hepatotoxicity with a high degree of sensitivity and specificity. This predictive hepatotoxicity assay is now routinely used to prioritize compounds using exploratory 3-day repeat-dose rat studies for various projects.

Prediction of Nephrotoxicity A recent publication illustrates how microarray-generated gene expression profiles from the kidneys of rats treated for short periods of time with various nephrotoxicants and nonnephrotoxicants can be used to predict toxic changes in longer term studies [25]. In this study, using a large commercial reference database, a predictive gene expression signature of renal tubular toxicity was developed and shown to predict with good accuracy renal tubular changes that would typically occur after longer exposure to the toxicants. These gene expression profiles were derived from the kidneys of rats treated for 5 days, a time point where no obvious toxic changes were evident, as evidenced by the lack of histopathologic observations and the lack of changes in serum chemistry parameters (most notably serum creatinine and blood urea nitrogen). In a step to confirm that tubular injury would ultimately occur in longer term studies, the authors dosed rats up to 28 days with the 15 nephrotoxicants used in their positive class, as a phenotypic anchor to the predictive signature. In addition, the signature was validated using compounds naive and not structurally related to the training set. These test compounds included

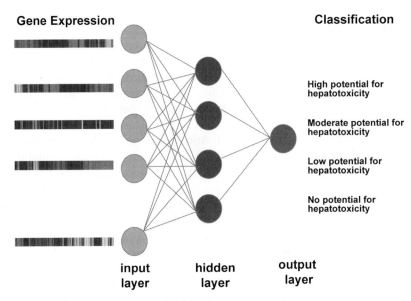

FIGURE 24.6 Schematic representation of the ANN-based approach used for the development of a predictive hepatotoxicity toxicogenomic assay. An internal rat liver gene expression database was first constructed. Reference gene expression profiles were then reduced in dimensionality using PCA. The filtered gene expression profiles were fed into an ANN, which processes the information from one layer to the next using multiple weighting factors and transfer functions. The output of the ANN is compared with the ideal toxicity classification and the model is readjusted. This learning process is repeated until the model is able to make an accurate prediction. Using microarray-generated gene expression profiles from male Sprague–Dawley rats treated for 3 days with experimental compounds, the neural network algorithm classifies the compounds based on their potential to cause hepatotoxicity in rats on a four-category scale ranging from no potential to high potential. (From Ref. 18, with permission from Elsevier.)

9 nephrotoxicants and 12 nonnephrotoxicants. The signature correctly predicted the future presence or absence of renal tubular injury in 76% of the compound treatments.

Another study used a similar, yet slightly different, approach to study time- and dose-dependent gene expression changes associated with proximal tubular injury in the rat [63]. In this study, Sprague–Dawley rats were treated with a wide variety of classical nephrotoxicants and renal gene expression profiles were evaluated 1, 3, and 7 days after initiation of dosing. The gene expression profiles nicely clustered based on the severity and nature of the pathologic changes and were consistent with tubular degeneration, regeneration, and necrosis. In addition, using an SVM-based approach and a training set of 120 gene expression profiles, a predictive classifier was developed that was able to predict the type of pathology of a testing set composed of 28 gene expression profiles with 100% selectivity and 82% sensitivity.

These two studies are good illustrations of the validity of the toxicogenomic approach for predictive toxicology but are also a good indication of the scale involved in the generation of predictive signatures of sufficient accuracy to be useful.

Both studies required the use of significant numbers of prototypical toxicants for both the training and testing sets, multiple time points, 3 or 4 rats/treatment group/ time point, and sophisticated computational algorithms. In other words, such studies are associated with a significant investment of resources, and it is likely that continued validation of these early signatures by a combined effort of the broad scientific community will be required to improve accuracy, but also to better estimate their predictivity and suitability in early toxicology testing.

Prediction of Carcinogenicity   Assessment of the carcinogenic potential of compounds in the rodent bioassay is expensive and lengthy and cannot be performed until late in a program. In addition, the endpoint of the rodent bioassay consists essentially of macroscopically and microscopically detectable tumors, which may spontaneously occur in naive, aging animals and whose incidence varies tremendously among animals, thereby requiring a significant number of animals to obtain sufficient statistical power [64]. Toxicogenomics applied in a predictive mode would allow for a profound reduction in the duration of dosing, thereby reducing the amount of compound required and permitting an earlier assessment of the compound. Furthermore, a response at the transcriptome level more homogeneous than the development of tumors could be expected, thereby allowing for a significant reduction in the number of animals to be dosed. It is obvious that any predictive signature of a carcinogenic effect would not dispense with the requirement to conduct the regulatory carcinogenicity studies. However, such predictive signatures would clearly be valuable when applied early to make more informed decisions on compounds.

Using a 5-day repeat-dose toxicity study in rats, Kramer et al. [65] evaluated whether gene expression profiling could help identify candidate molecular markers that may predict hepatic carcinogenicity induced by either nongenotoxic or genotoxic compounds. They hypothesized that there might exist a small number of critical genes whose expression may be predictive of the early events of carcinogenesis initiated by multiple mechanisms. Their study included three dose levels of a number of well-characterized compounds, including five nongenotoxic carcinogens, one genotoxic carcinogen, one carcinogen that may act via genotoxicity, a mitogen, and a noncarcinogenic hepatotoxicant. Analysis of the hepatic gene expression profiles resulted in the identification of several genes (including CYP-R and TSC-22, which were upregulated and downregulated, respectively) whose expression correlated well with the estimated carcinogenic potential. CYP-R catalyzes the transfer of electrons from NADPH to heme oxygenase, cytochrome-b_5, and a variety of cytochromes P450. As correctly stated by the authors, the upregulation of this gene may simply represent a surrogate marker for cytochrome P450 induction, since many nongenotoxic carcinogens are also cytochrome inducers. Alternatively, CYP-R induction may reflect a role for oxidative stress in rodent hepatocarcinogenesis. TSC-22 belongs to a subfamily of leucine zipper transcription factors and had been previously shown to be regulated by various treatments, such as TGF-β, phorbol ester, progesterone, or vesnarionone. Although the exact role of TSC-22 is uncertain, its repression may reflect regulation mediated directly by the test articles or an adaptive response to these compounds. In either case, its regulation supports an altered balance between proliferation and apoptosis, consistent with what would be expected with carcinogens.

A second study used gene expression profiling to evaluate whether known genotoxic carcinogens would induce a common set of genes belonging to defined biological pathways and whether these genes could be used as a predictive signature for hepatic genotoxic carcinogens [44]. This study used potent carcinogens (such as dimethylnitrosamine or 2-nitrofluorene) dosed daily for up to 14 days in rats. Gene expression analysis of livers indicated that the following biological pathways were mostly deregulated: DNA damage response, specific detoxification response, proliferation and survival, and structural changes. This common pattern of deregulation is consistent with what would be expected in the early events of tumorigenesis and could be predictive of later tumor development. The same investigators followed up on these encouraging preliminary results with a study incorporating nongenotoxic carcinogens [66]. In contrast to what was seen with the genotoxic compounds, nongenotoxic carcinogens impacted distinct cellular pathways/response (including oxidative DNA or protein damage, cell cycle progression, tissue regeneration) that were consistent with compound-specific mechanisms and the two-stage model of carcinogenesis.

Several important lessons can be learned from these pioneering studies. First, neither a single gene nor a single pathway will be sufficient to predict and discriminate the two classes of carcinogens. Second, a predictive gene expression signature of relatively good accuracy can likely be generated once a sufficient repository of gene expression profiles from a larger variety of carcinogens at different doses and different time points become available. Indeed, for a project of that scale, it is likely that a collaborative effort from the scientific community will be necessary for the refinement and validation of any predictive signature of carcinogenicity.

24.4.4   Predicting Species-Specific Toxicity

Toxicologic changes occurring in preclinical species are not necessarily relevant to humans because of species differences in cell biology, physiology, or responses to changes induced by compounds [67]. A classic example of a toxicity with no relevance to humans involves the peroxisome proliferators, such as the fibrate class of cholesterol-lowering drugs, that activate the peroxisome proliferator-activated receptor-α (PPAR-α). Upon chronic administration, these compounds cause hepatomegaly and eventually hepatic neoplasms in rats [68, 69]. There are marked species differences in the response to peroxisome proliferators, with mice and rats being highly responsive in contrast to humans. This differential species response correlates directly with the number of hepatic PPAR-α; PPAR-α is expressed in human liver at only 5–10% of rodent liver levels. Consequently, humans are at minimal or no risk to develop hepatic tumors following chronic exposure to peroxisome proliferators. Toxicogenomics has furthered the understanding of the molecular mechanisms associated with the various effects of several peroxisome proliferators [23, 70, 71]. This allows one to more specifically demonstrate the mechanisms of action by which certain compounds lead to rodent hepatomegaly and hepatic carcinogenesis, thereby improving overall risk assessment. The value of toxicogenomics to understand species-specific responses is also illustrated with the case of cyclosporine-induced nephrotoxicity [72, 73]. In the kidneys of cyclosporin A-treated rats, a marked downregulation of calbindin-D28kDa, a calcium binding protein, correlates with and causes the accumulation of calcium in tubules and ultimately renal tubular calcification in this species. In contrast, cyclosporine does not regulate calbindin-D28kDa expression in the kidneys of dogs and monkeys, two species resistant to cyclosporine-mediated renal toxicity.

24.5 *IN VITRO* TOXICOGENOMICS

24.5.1 Objectives of *In Vitro* Toxicogenomics

Compounds are ultimately assessed in animal toxicology studies. Not surprisingly, the vast majority of published toxicogenomic studies to date have been using tissue from animals dosed *in vivo*. *In vivo* studies require large amounts of compound and consequently do not allow for an early characterization of the toxicologic profiles of compounds. Moreover, the number of compounds that can be analyzed in animal studies is limited, in part because of the cost and practicalities of these studies. Thus, *in vitro* systems may significantly improve the throughput and increase the value of toxicogenomics in drug discovery by allowing for an early toxicological character-ization of compounds. In addition, gene expression profiling using *in vitro* systems may identify biomarkers of toxicity in the form of gene sets that could be transferred and investigated in preclinical or clinical studies to monitor possible toxic reactions. Finally, gene expression studies in human cells, such as primary human hepatocytes, may, in some cases, be more relevant to the clinical situation or allow for a better understanding of the relevance of toxic changes and for a better assessment of safety risks for humans.

The selection of an appropriate cell system should be guided by the questions to be addressed. If one desires to identify the mechanism of toxicity of a compound, using a cell system that most closely mimics the target organ, such as a primary cell system, would be preferable. However, if one wishes to identify markers of general toxicity, then the cell type may not be as important. In fact, it is likely that identifying general markers of toxicity (such as DNA damage, apoptosis, or oxida-tive stress) would be feasible using cell lines of various origins, such as HeLa or Jurkat cells.

The major limitation of *in vitro* systems is their inability to recapitulate the overall complexity of the living organism, which limits their potential in detecting lesions associated with multicellular interactions. Most *in vitro* systems are also short term and therefore inadequate to detect chronic effects [74]. Understanding the predictive value of *in vitro* systems has remained a major challenge for toxicologists for decades and *in vitro* toxicogenomics falls into the same predicament. Several studies have addressed the relationship between *in vitro* and *in vivo* toxicogenomic results. These studies have demonstrated that different mechanisms of toxicity can be identified using gene expression profiles generated from *in vitro* systems and that consequently the concept of predictive signatures was also relevant to *in vitro* systems [75, 76].

Although gene expression profiling using *in vitro* systems can distinguish com-pounds with different mechanisms of toxicity, signatures of satisfactory accuracy and cost-effective gene expression platforms with adequate throughput are necessary for its implementation in a discovery setting. For an *in vitro* toxicogenomic assay to have practical applications in drug discovery, gene expression signatures need to be generated and validated for several relevant toxicologic endpoints. In addition, in order to increase the throughput of gene expression profiling (e.g., adapting it to a 96- or 384-well format), it would be advantageous to reduce the number of genes being monitored. Ideally, one would want to rapidly evaluate compounds for several toxicologic endpoints in a simultaneous fashion in a limited number of wells.

The selection of an appropriate dose represents a critical issue. At this point, there is no clear consensus of what represents an ideal dose for *in vitro* toxicogenomic assessment, and it is likely that the dose selection will depend on the cell type. In our experience, development of robust predictive signatures and characterization of the toxicologic profiles of compounds require the use of relatively high doses, sufficient to cause cytotoxicity. For instance, in our primary rat hepatocyte model, we typically characterize compounds at concentrations sufficient to cause death of 20% of cells. Failure to reach these cytotoxic concentrations will result in an insensitive assay of limited value.

24.5.2   Proof-of-Concept Using Primary Rat Hepatocytes

Most published *in vitro* toxicogenomic studies have evaluated rat liver cells for several reasons. First, liver is a common target organ of toxicity. Second, rat liver cells are most commonly used for *in vitro* toxicologic studies. Third, the use of hepatocytes offers the opportunity to assess the toxicity associated with certain metabolites without prior metabolic activation. Finally, since most *in vivo* studies have focused on liver, liver-derived cells can be used to correlate *in vitro* and *in vivo* data. An *in vitro* system for hepatotoxicity could consist of isolated perfused livers, liver slices, isolated hepatocytes, or liver cell lines. Isolated perfused livers and liver slices maintain intact cellular interactions and spatial arrangements and allow for long-term studies [74, 77]. These models are also the most appropriate for studying toxic effects on the biliary system, because they contain phenotypically and functionally intact biliary epithelial cells. However, isolated livers and liver slices are resource intensive, low-throughput systems. Cell lines are readily available, cost effective, and generally yield reproducible results over time. However, liver cell lines are quite different from liver or primary hepatocytes in terms of function and phenotype. Gene expression profiles were compared for rat livers, rat liver slices, primary rat hepatocytes cultured on collagen monolayer or collagen sandwich, and two rat liver cell lines (BRL3A and NRL clone 9 cells) [20]. Liver slices were the most similar to intact rat livers, followed by primary hepatocytes in culture. In contrast, the two rat liver cell lines showed little correlation to intact rat livers. In particular, the cell lines expressed very low or undetectable levels of phase I metabolizing enzymes, both at the RNA and protein levels [20]. These results are consistent with data generated in our laboratory (Fig. 24.7).

Isolated hepatocytes are not identical but are sufficiently close to intact livers in terms of gene expression analysis (Fig. 24.8) [20, 78]. In addition, they maintain the enzyme architecture and metabolizing capabilities of intact liver in short-term cultures [79, 80]. However, isolated hepatocytes, especially of human origin, can be very difficult and expensive to obtain. Furthermore, in the case of human hepatocytes, lifestyle differences of the donors, such as smoking or drinking habits, medications, or general health, lead to substantial interindividual variability in gene expression profiles. However, this variability is overall not a major concern, since preliminary

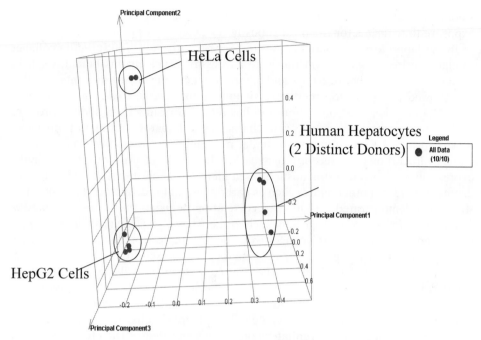

FIGURE 24.7 Principal component analysis of Affymetrix HG-U133A microarray-generated gene expression profiles from primary human hepatocytes, HeLa cells, and HepG2 cells. This analysis illustrates the major differences at the transcriptome level between primary human hepatocytes and liver cell lines, such as HepG2 cells, which are almost as dissimilar to human hepatocytes as HeLa cells, which are derived from a cervical carcinoma.

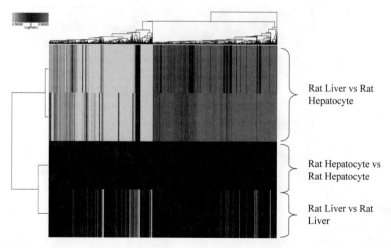

FIGURE 24.8 Heatmap illustrating the differences in gene expression profiles between rat liver and primary rat hepatocytes. Gene expression profiles were generated using Affymetrix rat RAE230A microarrays. Genes that are at least showing a two fold difference in expression levels with a p value less than 0.01 between the two systems are shown.

studies indicate a surprisingly low interindividual variability in response to high exposure to toxicants for the most robustly regulated genes [81].

In our laboratory, we routinely use primary rat hepatocytes cultured on collagen to characterize compounds at the gene expression level. In this model, we have profiled a large number of compounds, thereby generating an internal database that has allowed us to develop predictive signatures for several toxicologic endpoints (Fig. 24.9). For instance, our laboratory has reported results from a study profiling at the gene expression levels 15 well-characterized hepatotoxicants in primary rat hepatocytes [75]. Compounds with similar mechanisms of toxicity, such as the aromatic hydrocarbon (Ah) receptor ligands Aroclor 1254 and 3MC, resulted in similar expression profiles and, using unsupervised hierarchical clustering, could clearly be distinguished from other agents such as carbon tetrachloride and allyl alcohol. This study also demonstrated a significant correlation between the genes regulated *in vivo* and *in vitro* for some toxicants, such as the Ah receptor ligands. Similar results have been confirmed, reproduced, or expanded in studies conducted by others. For instance, in a study using primary rat hepatocytes exposed to 11 different hepatotoxicants and a low-density array platform containing only 59 genes, compounds could correctly be classified into different mechanistic hepatotoxic classes [82]. Other studies have also used liver-derived cell lines with some success. Three separate studies used a human hepatoma cell line (HepG2 cells) to demonstrate that transcriptional analysis differentiates compounds and that *in vitro* toxicogenomics can be used to further the understanding of toxic mechanisms [21, 83, 84].

24.5.3   Use of Gene Expression Profiling to Assess Genotoxicity

Toxicogenomics has also been applied in other cell systems. In particular, gene expression analysis has been evaluated as a potential tool to gain a better under-

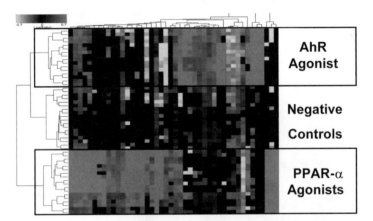

FIGURE 24.9 Heatmap of gene expression changes following treatment of primary rat hepatocytes with 16 aryl hydrocarbon receptor (AhR) agonists, 18 negative control compounds, and 18 peroxisome proliferator-activated receptor-α (PPAR-α) agonists for 48 hours. The genes shown were selected by linear discriminant analysis. Using a small internal database of *in vitro* gene expression profiles in primary rat hepatocytes, small gene sets can be identified using various statistical algorithms (in this case linear discriminant analysis) to classify compounds according to their toxic properties for specific toxicologic endpoints.

standing of genotoxic mechanisms. The current *in vitro* genotoxicity assays using mammalian cells (mammalian mutation and/or chromosomal damage assays) provide a limited insight into genotoxic mechanisms [22, 85]. Not surprisingly, the majority of positive genotoxicity findings for marketed drugs with negative carcinogenicity data have been observed in these *in vitro* mammalian assays, demonstrating their low specificity and the need to develop approaches enabling mechanism-based risk assessment [86]. More specifically, the differentiation of DNA-reactive versus DNA-nonreactive mechanisms of genotoxicity would facilitate risk assessment of positive findings in the *in vitro* mammalian cell-based assays. Several studies have addressed the question of whether gene expression profiling of *in vitro* systems would allow a better risk assessment of genotoxicants [85, 87]. Data from these studies demonstrated differences in gene expression profiles between DNA damaging and non-DNA-damaging compounds. In various cell types (p53-deficient mouse lymphoma cells L5178Y/TK$^{+/-}$, TK6 cells), DNA-damaging compounds regulated genes involved in cell cycle regulation, DNA repair, apoptosis, and cellular signaling that were distinct from those regulated by non-DNA-damaging agents [22]. This suggests that, although toxicogenomics will not replace the current standard genotoxicity assays for hazard identification, it can serve as a useful follow-up experimental approach to evaluate compounds with positive findings in these standard assays.

24.5.4 Current and Future Use of *In Vitro* Toxicogenomics

A tremendous amount of work remains to be done for *in vitro* toxicogenomics to become a routine tool for toxicologic characterization of compounds in discovery. However, this area is moving at an extremely rapid pace, and several companies are already using gene expression-based *in vitro* assays for compound characterization and prioritization. For instance, our laboratory has identified predictive signatures for specific toxicologic endpoints in the rat hepatocyte model. Some of these signatures, as well as the methods used to generate them, have already been published [18, 75, 88]. One can envision that efforts in this field will soon clarify the strengths and limitations of the *in vitro* toxicogenomic approach and thus establish the role of *in vitro* toxicogenomic assays in drug discovery.

24.6 TOXICOGENOMICS IN MECHANISTIC TOXICOLOGY

24.6.1 Objectives of Mechanistic Toxicology

The impact of gene expression profiling in drug discovery and development has so far been mostly evident when used to elucidate the mechanism of a specific toxicity. Toxic changes are commonly identified in preclinical studies and obviously not all toxic changes are worth investigating. The decision regarding whether a specific toxicologic change needs to be mechanistically understood is based on multiple factors. These factors include, for instance, the nature of the toxicologic change, the exposures at which the change occurs, the species affected, the availability of good backup compounds, or the stage of the program [18]. For instance, there is clear value in trying to understand the mechanism of tumorigenesis for test article-related tumors detected in a lifetime bioassay. At this stage of a program, clinical trials are well underway and an enormous amount of resources have already been invested. In contrast, in an early program, if several backup compounds with a different chemistry but similar physicochemical and pharmacological properties are available, it may not be worth investigating the mechanism of a specific toxicologic change occurring with a single lead compound. However, if backup compounds are not yet available, understanding the molecular basis of toxicologic changes may be useful to properly select backup compounds without this toxicologic liability through early structure–toxicity relationship studies during lead optimization. Indeed, when the mechanism of toxicity is understood, appropriate counterscreens can rationally be developed that allow for the selection of backup compounds unlikely to induce the same toxic change. Finally, there is a lack of sensitive and specific biomarkers for some toxic changes. Because gene expression profiling provides a global view of the transcriptional effects induced by a compound, it may identify biomarkers that can subsequently be used in preclinical and conceptually in clinical studies to monitor toxicity.

24.6.2   Case Examples of Mechanistic Toxicology

Hepatotoxicity   Early studies have shown that changes in expression of small gene sets can reliably discriminate compounds with distinct mechanism of toxicity in the liver. These gene sets can be used to mechanistically classify compounds and assign a compound with an unknown toxicologic mechanism into predefined classes based on mechanism [23, 70]. This allows one to identify toxicity using predictive gene expression signatures as discussed before and also to establish mechanistic hypotheses by comparing expression profiles with those present in a database. For instance, our laboratory has investigated the hepatic effects of A-277249, a thienopyridine inhibitor of NF-κB-mediated expression of cellular adhesion molecules [89]. This compound induced hepatic changes in rats in a repeat-dose toxicity study, including increased liver weights, changes in serum chemistry (elevations of serum transaminases, alkaline phosphatase, and gamma glutamyl transferase), and histopathologic changes (hypertrophy and hyperplasia of hepatocytes and biliary epithelial cells). To investigate the mechanism of this hepatotoxicity, a 3-day repeat-dose rat toxicity study was conducted. Livers were collected and gene expression profiles were generated using microarrays. The compound was observed to induce extensive changes in gene expression. Using a proprietary gene expression database of known hepatotoxicants, agglomerative hierarchical cluster analysis demonstrated that A-277249 had a gene expression profile similar to Aroclor 1254 and 3-methylcholanthrene (3MC), two well-characterized activators of the aryl hydrocarbon nuclear receptor (AhR), indicating that A-277249 hepatic changes were, at least in part, mediated by the AhR either directly or through effects on NF-κB [89]. The AhR is a nuclear receptor that mediates responses to various toxicants, such as the halogenated aromatic toxicants [90]. In this particular case, the chemical class was abandoned. But, in a case where backup compounds would have been available, one could have used these data to set up an appropriate counterscreen to rapidly evaluate the backup compounds for this toxic mechanism. In particular, one could have evaluated whether these compounds induce an upregulation of CYP1A1 in primary rat hepatocytes, since ligands of the AhR are known to induce CYP1A1.

Intestinal Toxicity and Notch Signaling   Gene expression profiling has rarely been applied to study toxicity of the gastrointestinal tract. The complexity and heterogeneity of this tissue makes it very difficult to investigate toxic changes at the level of the transcriptome. However, two recent studies demonstrated that toxicogenomics can be used to elucidate the toxic mechanisms and identify markers of toxicity for this tissue [26]. In the last few years, functional γ-secretase inhibitors (FGSIs) have been developed as potential therapeutic agents for Alzheimer disease [26, 91]. FGSIs can block the cleavage of several transmembrane proteins, including the cell fate regulator Notch-1, which plays an important role in the differentiation of the immune system and gastrointestinal tract. Rats treated with several FGSIs develop a unique gastrointestinal toxicity, characterized by an increase in gastrointestinal weight, distended stomach and small and large intestines, and a mucoid enteropathy related to goblet cell hyperplasia [26, 91]. Microarray analysis of the duodenum or ileum of FGSIs-treated rats identified changes in the expression of several genes, and these changes confirmed that perturbation in Notch signaling was the mechanism for this characteristic enteropathy. These gene expression studies went further and also identified that the gene encoding the serine protease adipsin was significantly upregulated following treatment with FGSIs. The investigators followed up on this interesting finding and demonstrated elevated levels of the adipsin protein in gastrointestinal contents and feces of FGSIs-treated rats, as well as increased numbers of ileal enterocytes expressing adipsin by immunohistochemistry. Based on these data, both laboratories concluded that adipsin may be potentially exploited as a specific, sensitive, and noninvasive biomarker of FGSIs-induced gastrointestinal toxicity.

Testicular Toxicity   Early toxicant-induced testicular changes are typically subtle in early stages without striking morphologic changes, which may easily be missed unless more sophisticated techniques, such as tubular staging, are used [92]. However, in longer term *in vivo* studies (4 weeks or longer), changes are typically more pronounced and advanced. Approaches that would allow for an earlier detection of testicular changes would be beneficial in preclinical safety assessment. Current well-established correlating biomarkers (such as serum FSH or semen analysis) are not sensitive enough to allow for an early detection of toxic changes both in preclinical studies and in clinical trials. Recently, a project sponsored by the ILSI Health and Environmental Sciences Institute (HESI) evaluated the suitability and limitations of additional biomarkers, such as Inhibin B, to detect modest testicular dysfunction in rats [93]. While the complete results of this study have not been communicated at this point, preliminary data have indicated that plasma inhibin B is not a useful marker. Finally, little is known in general about the mechanism of toxicity for testicular toxicants. This lack of understanding relates probably to a lower degree of interest by toxicologists in general in contrast to tissues like liver, but also to the complexity of the tissue. The testis is a tissue composed of several different cell types with striking differences in functions and morphology, which can all be targets for toxicants. Furthermore, these different cell types closely interact with each other, modulating their respective functions and status. Consequently, a toxicant targeting a specific cell type will ultimately affect, by a secondary mechanism, the status of another cell type. For instance, a toxicant that affects the function of Sertoli cells, the cell supporting the growth, differentiation, and release of germ cells, will ultimately lead to effects on germ cells, such as failure of sperm release or germ cell depletion. This complex cellular interdependence has limited the use of *in vitro* studies to investigate the mechanism of testicular toxicity.

Several elegant studies have demonstrated that gene expression profiling can elucidate the molecular basis of testicular toxicity [94–96]. For instance, gene expression changes in the testis were evaluated following exposure of mice to bromochloroacetic acid, a known testicular toxicant. Using a custom nylon DNA array, numerous changes in gene expression were detected in genes with known functions in fertility, such as Hsp70–2 and SP22, as well as genes encoding proteins involved in cell communication, adhesion, and signaling, supporting the hypothesis that the toxicologic effect was the result of disruption of cellular interactions between Sertoli cells and spermatids [94, 97]. Our laboratory has used DNA microarrays to investigate the testicular toxicity of another halogenated acetic acid, dibromoacetic acid (DBAA). Oral treatment of rats with DBAA at high doses (250 mg/kg/day) induces specific early morphologic changes in the testis, characterized by failed spermiation or failure of release by Sertoli cells of mature step 19 spermatids (Fig. 24.10). While this morphologic change strongly suggests that the Sertoli cell is the target cell for DBAA, our results using whole testes indicated that DBAA induced a small but consistent downregulation of cytochrome P450c17α (CYP17), an enzyme essential for the production of testosterone by gonads (Fig. 24.10). These results led us to hypothesize that DBAA may induce, at least in part, its toxicity through an effect on testicular testosterone production. In fact, we were able to show that following treatment of rats with DBAA for as little as 4 days, testicular testosterone contents were significantly decreased, indicating that the decrease in CYP17 expression likely has biological implications. This specific study illustrates two important points. First, because gene expression analysis represents a new and

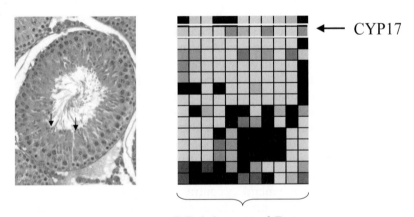

DBAA-treated Rats

FIGURE 24.10   Histologic and gene expression changes induced in rat testis by dibromoacetic acid (DBAA). Oral treatment of rats with DBAA at high doses (250 mg/kg/day for 4 days) leads to failed spermiation, characterized by the failure of release by Sertoli cells of mature step 19 spermatids (arrows). This histologic change correlates with a significant downregulation of cytochrome P450c17a (CYP17) mRNA in the 11 rats evaluated.

global approach to study the molecular mechanism of various pathologies, one should be extremely cautious not to focus exclusively on earlier hypotheses and not to rely on old dogma. In fact, microarray analysis offers the unique opportunity to generate global molecular data that should be used to generate new, unbiased hypotheses. Once generated, these hypotheses should be addressed using appropriately designed studies. Second, although laser-capture microdissection represents a useful technique to study gene expression in complex tissues by focusing on single cell populations, it should also be used with the understanding that critical cell–cell interactions may govern changes in gene expression. In the present case, should we have focused on Sertoli cells only, we probably would have been unable to implicate the decrease in testosterone production as a significant part of the DBAA-induced testicular toxicity.

24.7 TOXICOGENOMICS AND TARGET-RELATED TOXICITY

The recent advances in genomics have spurred a proliferation of novel potential therapeutic targets. The traditional target validation procedure is designed to demonstrate that modulation (inhibition or activation) of target activity in relevant disease models can lead to a therapeutic benefit. The target validation step frequently does not include an assessment of the effects of target modulation on normal cellular, organ, or body function. Yet, developing a good understanding of the potential safety liabilities associated with a target is clearly a critical phase of target drugability assessment. Most of the genomics-derived novel targets play major roles in normal cellular function, and consequently modulation of their activity can lead to toxic changes or what is often referred to as target-related toxicity, mechanism-based toxicity, or on-target toxicity.

Gene expression profiling can provide invaluable information about the biology of these novel targets and help proactively identify target-related safety liabilities. Ideally, this assessment should be conducted at the earliest stages of the discovery process, namely, the target identification/validation stage. With the proliferation of novel attractive targets and the limited resources of discovery units to focus on novel programs, this step becomes especially critical, as it allows a discovery organization to prioritize novel targets based not only on expected therapeutic benefits but also on potential safety liabilities. This ultimately leads to a greater focus on programs most likely to ultimately succeed.

Part of this step involves the evaluation of target expression in normal tissues from both preclinical species and human beings, with the development of quantitative expression tissue maps [54, 98–100]. These tissue maps allow one to proactively identify tissues more likely to be affected by toxic changes. The availability of complete tissue repositories or banks is necessary to generate these tissue maps. Target expression can be evaluated at the level of mRNA expression, protein expression, and enzymatic activity in the case of an enzyme or using assays such as receptor binding assays. Evaluation of mRNA levels is clearly the easiest way to generate expression data, but one should remember that, for a large proportion of proteins, mRNA levels do not necessarily correlate well with protein or activity levels. Therefore, it is usually recommended to confirm or complement mRNA data with appropriate secondary assays. Furthermore, total tissue expression may not always reflect the critical role played by some targets, especially in cases where a target is expressed in a small compartment of a complex tissue. These situations can be more effectively addressed with either *in situ* hybridization or immunohistochemistry.

The generation of expression tissue maps, albeit useful, is usually insufficient to evaluate potential safety liabilities associated with a target. In particular, these novel targets are frequently identified based on overexpression in diseased samples. Expression in normal tissues does not necessarily translate into nondrugability or on-target toxicity. The difference in expression levels may result in safety margins sufficient enough for development. Determination of a safety window, however, is not a trivial task early in a program. Ideally, it should be determined using appropriate tool compounds (i.e., compounds with adequate pharmacologic activity against and specificity for the target). These tool compounds do not need to have candidate properties as long as sufficient systemic exposure can be achieved for a short repeat-dose study. To control for toxicity related to a chemical class, one should use several tool compounds from different chemical classes and, if available, inactive compounds with close structural similarities (such as inactive enantiomers). In our laboratory, we typically use a 3-day repeat-dose study in male rats using carefully selected tool compounds for target assessment. Doses are selected to result in exposures sufficient to achieve efficacy (as determined by concurrent studies in relevant preclinical efficacy models), but also in higher exposures, so target-related safety margins can be determined. These high exposures are obviously dependent on the characteristics of the tool compounds available (pharmaceutical properties, ADME/PK, and toxicity) and are often limited early in a program. Tissues for gene expression profiling are then selected and prioritized based on the biology of the target (partly generated from the expression tissue maps, but also from the literature), as well as prior evaluation of clinical pathology and histopathology changes. Gene expression changes are evaluated in the context of available reference databases and of our battery of gene expression signatures.

Other approaches have been proposed to proactively evaluate on-target toxicity. These approaches use the same tools as for target validation, such as antibodies, genetically engineered mice, or technologies to modulate mRNA expression levels, such as antisense oligonucleotides, ribozymes, or siRNA [101–103]. In particular, siRNA has gained popularity in the last few years. We have explored the use of siRNA to understand on-target and off-target effects of compounds *in vitro* with mixed results. Clearly, issues such as potency and selectivity of siRNA need to be better understood for this approach to be useful in toxicogenomics. Furthermore, gene silencing approaches induce varying degrees of mRNA and protein downregulation, which may not mimic the pharmacologic inhibition necessary to achieve efficacy. Recent advances in viral and nonviral delivery methods have led to the use of RNA interference for *in vivo* functional genomic studies with successful gene downregulation [104, 105]. Because of the costs of siRNA, these *in vivo* studies are typically conducted in mice, a species for which robust toxicogenomic databases are not available. Furthermore, the required delivery techniques also induce mild adverse effects that complicate the interpretation of gene expression profiles. Our current experience with *in vivo* RNAi studies is too limited to provide a reliable assessment of the potential use of gene silencing to better predict target-related toxicity. However, conceptually, this approach appears promising.

24.8 TOXICOGENOMICS AND IDIOSYNCRATIC TOXICITY

24.8.1 Definition of Idiosyncratic Toxicity

Idiosyncratic toxicity refers to a toxicity not related to the pharmacology of the drug that occurs unexpectedly in a small proportion of treated patients, often in a non-dose-dependent manner [106]. This toxic effect is typically not detected in animals and consequently cannot be predicted during preclinical testing or the early phases of clinical trials. This could be due to host specificity of the toxic reaction or to the insufficient size of preclinical animal studies. Examples of drugs that result in idiosyncratic toxicity include troglitazone (withdrawn in 2000 due to liver toxicity), bromfenac (withdrawn in 1998 due to liver toxicity), fenfluramine (withdrawn in 1997 because of heart valve disease), and cerivastatin (withdrawn in 2001 due to rhabdomyolysis).

Several mechanisms have been proposed to explain the development of idiosyncratic drug toxicity. These include the formation of reactive metabolites in certain individuals due to the presence of polymorphisms in drug-metabolizing enzymes, the development of immune-mediated responses to the drug or one of its metabolites, a synergistic effect of concurrent low-level inflammatory reactions, and changes in mitochondrial function and integrity [107–111]. While substantial experimental evidence exists that these mechanisms occur for certain drugs, there is currently no reliable way to proactively identify compounds that may lead to idiosyncratic responses in a large patient population. Because gene expression profiling allows for a global view of responses occurring simultaneously in cells or tissues, it represents a new approach to study the mechanisms of idiosyncratic reactions and to potentially identify predictive signatures of idiosyncratic toxicity. We illustrate this concept using idiosyncratic hepatotoxicity.

24.8.2 Preclinical Models of Idiosyncratic Toxicity

Several models have been used to study the mechanism of idiosyncratic toxicity. Only a few models are covered here. The brown Norway rat has been commonly used as an animal model of idiosyncratic toxicity, especially for the study of suspected immune-mediated idiosyncratic reactions. For instance, following exposure to nevirapine or D-pencillamine, brown Norway rats develop toxic changes similar to those seen in humans [112, 113]. Another model is a two-hit model for idiosyncratic toxicity, where compounds with potential idiosyncratic liabilities require another underlying factor (such as alcohol intake or concurrent infection) to cause toxicity. This has led to the development of a lipopolysaccharide (LPS)-enhanced toxicity rat model, where rats are coadministered a single dose of compound and LPS. Using this model, several compounds (such as chlorpromazine, ranitidine, and trovafloxacin) known to cause idiosyncratic toxicity in humans have been shown to induce similar changes in rats [114–116]. This LPS-enhanced toxicity rat model has also been investigated at the gene expression level to generate novel hypotheses regarding the exact molecular cascade associated with the toxicity [116, 117].

Idiosyncratic toxicity has also been studied in *in vitro* models. In particular, an assumption is that these types of toxicity are host specific and that, consequently, only the use of human cells will lead to an accurate insight into the molecular and biochemical events occurring during toxicity. Using this approach, for instance, troglitazone was shown to lead to decreases in cellular ATP and mitochondrial membrane potential in HepG2 cells, and that, consequently, mitochondrial dysfunction may be, at least in part, the cause of the idiosyncratic toxicity induced by troglitazone [118]. Since the liver is often the target organ of idiosyncratic drug reactions, the latter are commonly studied using cultured human hepatocytes or liver-derived cell lines. Although cell lines such as HepG2 can be useful, recent advances in culturing of human hepatocytes have facilitated their use in toxicogenomic studies.

24.8.3 Case Example: Idiosyncratic Hepatotoxicity

As mentioned earlier, the liver is a common target organ of idiosyncratic toxicity and the focus of most research. In particular, the quinolone trovafloxacin has been a tool compound often used in our laboratory. Quinolones are antibacterial agents that act by inhibiting bacterial DNA gyrase and DNA topoisomerase IV [119]. As a class, they are generally well tolerated, except for trovafloxacin [120]. Before its regulatory approval in 1997, trovafloxacin had been tested in over 7000 patients and had not caused any hepatic failures or deaths. Over 2 million people have since received trovafloxacin and 150 cases of liver toxicity have been reported, including 14 cases of acute liver failure. Four patients required liver transplants and an additional five patients died [121]. Because of this hepatotoxicity, severe restrictions were placed on the use of trovafloxacin. The drug can now only be administered in life-threatening situations. The mechanism underlying this adverse effect has not yet been determined.

Our objective was, using human hepatocytes and gene expression profiling, to determine the molecular mechanism of the idiosyncratic toxicity induced by trovafloxacin. Human hepatocytes from four different donors were treated with six quinolone agents (trovafloxacin, levofloxacin, grepafloxacin, gatifloxacin, ciprofloxacin, and clinafloxacin). Using gene expression profiling, trovafloxacin could clearly be distinguished from the other quinolones; the treatment with trovafloxacin resulted in far more gene expression changes than the other compounds [81]. Many of these gene expression changes involved crucial biological pathways that may be involved in the mechanism underlying trovafloxacin-induced hepatotoxicity. In particular, trovafloxacin regulated a number of mitochondrial genes that were not regulated by the other quinolones [81]. In parallel, male Sprague–Dawley rats were treated with levofloxacin (600 mg/kg/day) and trovafloxacin (200 mg/kg/day) for 7 days. Consistent with other measures of toxicity (serum chemistry, histopathology), microarray analysis of the rat livers failed to identify unique gene expression changes induced by trovafloxacin.

Troglitazone is also commonly investigated as a reference compound for idiosyncratic hepatotoxicity. Troglitazone is a thiazolidinedione PPAR-γ agonist that was developed for the treatment of type II diabetes. Troglitazone induced idiosyncratic hepatotoxicity in a small percentage of patients and was removed from the market [106]. In a study similar to ours, human hepatocytes were treated with three thiazolidinedione compounds (troglitazone, rosiglitazone, and pioglitazone). Troglitazone also resulted in a large number of gene expression changes that were not observed with the two other thiazolidinedione compounds [122].

Albeit preliminary, these studies demonstrate two important points. First, the combined use of human hepatocytes and gene expression profiling allowed for the distinction of compounds associated with idiosyncratic hepatotoxicity (trovafloxacin, troglitazone) from compounds of the same chemical classes and not associated hepatotoxicity, suggesting that this *in vitro* system may be appropriate for studying idiosyncratic hepatotoxicity, and potentially for the early identification of safety liabilities. Second, rat repeat-dose studies did not differentiate trovafloxacin from another quinolone known not to induce liver failure in humans, indicating that, at least in the case of the quinolones, the traditional rat model may not be suited to detect potential idiosyncratic toxic liabilities even when coupled with a toxicogenomic evaluation.

24.9 TOXICOGENOMICS IN REGULATORY SUBMISSIONS

24.9.1 Overview of the FDA Pharmacogenomics Guidance

Because of the potential of gene expression profiling to improve the safety assessment of new chemical entities, the FDA issued a guidance in March 2005 for the regulatory submission of pharmacogenomic data (http://www.fda.gov/cder/guidance). This guidance reflects the effort of the FDA to promote the use of genomic technologies in drug development and is also designed to enhance the agency's knowledge of these emerging technologies. In finalizing these guidelines, the FDA has openly cooperated with the various stakeholders and has organized appropriate forums to focus on the major issues and principles that the document should cover. The pharmaceutical industry has welcomed this guidance, as it represents an important stepping stone toward the development of genomics-based drugs and the use of genomics-based safety data. In addition, this guidance provided reassurance to companies that early-stage toxicogenomic experiments would not bring negative regulatory consequences, an important aspect for the wider acceptance of this new technology in the relatively conservative environment of drug safety evaluation.

The guidance clarifies the FDA's policy on the use of pharmacogenomic data in the drug application review process and covers the application of genomics concepts and technologies to nonclinical, clinical pharmacology, and clinical studies. It provides guidelines to sponsors on pharmacogenomic data submission requirements, the format and procedure for data submission, and how the data will be used in regulatory decision making. In general terms, gene expression data for which submission is required include data used for decision making within a specific trial; data used to support scientific arguments about mechanism of action, dose selection, safety, or effectiveness; data that will support registration or labeling language; and data generated on previously validated biomarkers. This guidance demonstrates that the FDA is open to and expects the submission of gene expression profiling data that were generated to support scientific contentions related to toxicity.

The guidance defines pharmacogenomic tests as follows: "An assay intended to study interindividual variations in whole-genome or candidate gene, single-nucleotide polymorphism (SNP) maps, haplotype markers, or alterations in gene expression or inactivation that may be correlated with pharmacological and therapeutic response. In some cases, the pattern or profile of change is the relevant biomarker, rather than changes in individual markers." This implies that gene expression datasets could ultimately be recognized as validated biomarkers. The guidance also defines "valid biomarkers" and distinguishes between "known valid biomarkers" and "probable valid biomarkers." Valid biomarkers are measured in an analytical test system with well-established performance characteristics, and an established scientific framework or body of evidence exists to understand the significance of the test results. For a known valid biomarker, a widespread agreement exists in the medical or scientific community about the significance of the results. In contrast, for a probable valid biomarker, there is no widespread agreement, but only a scientific framework or body of evidence sufficient to elucidate the significance of the test results. An example would be a biomarker developed by a sponsor and not available for public scientific scrutiny or for independent verification. This distinction also reemphasizes the enormous amount of work and improvement that will be needed in the future to make gene expression data suitable for regulatory decision making. This includes obviously an improved scientific framework for data interpretation through the use of larger, more complete reference databases, but also improved quality control of laboratory procedures, a better understanding of the comparability of different platforms, and some better-defined processes to validate biomarkers.

The FDA recognizes that, currently, most gene expression profiling data are exploratory and would therefore not be required for submission. However, to be prepared to appropriately evaluate future submissions, FDA scientists need to develop an understanding of a variety of relevant scientific issues. The Voluntary Genomic Data Submission (VGDS) provides the material necessary to develop this understanding and is reviewed by a cross-center Interdisciplinary Pharmacogenomic Review Group (IPRG). For more information, the reader is referred to the FDA web site, which reviews the frequently asked questions regarding VGDS (http://www.fda.gov/cder/genomics/FAQ.htm). All VGDS data are protected from disclosure either outside the FDA or to review divisions, are routed directly to the IPRG, and stored on a secured, separate server. These data are not distributed outside the IPRG without the prior agreement of the sponsor and are not to be used for regulatory decision making. The concept of VGDS has in general been well received by the pharmaceutical industry. Voluntary submissions allow sponsors to familiarize FDA scientists with genomic data and their interpretation and, at the same time, to learn about the regulatory decision-making process and expectations involving genomic data. Ultimately, this could prevent delays in future submissions containing required genomic data. So far, many formal submissions have occurred.

24.9.2   Future Impact of Toxicogenomic Data in Regulatory Decision Making

The development of a guidance demonstrates that the FDA is expecting genomic data to become an integral part of the risk assessment of pharmaceuticals. It is, however, difficult at this point to objectively predict the role that a rapidly evolving technology will have in regulatory decision making. When the concept of toxicogenomics first emerged, expectations were high and to some extent unrealistic. While the technology and the development of appropriate analytical tools have considerably improved the ability to generate and interpret large sets of data, it still should not be considered a mature approach to evaluate toxicology. Furthermore, it is unlikely that toxicogenomics will replace most traditional toxicology studies that are currently part of a regulatory package. Rather, toxicogenomics will more likely complement and increase the value of these studies by providing an improved understanding of the relevance of preclinical toxicologic changes to humans. Toxicogenomics also represents a largely needed novel approach to identify additional biomarkers of safety that could potentially be used to improve monitoring of adverse events in the clinics, resulting in safer clinical trials and potentially earlier identification of outliers with increased sensitivity to particular adverse events. However, it is still unclear how genomics-based biomarkers will be validated to become an integral part of regulatory decision making. The validation of these biomarkers is complex and clearly context specific.

24.10   CONCLUSION

To address the high failure rate due to toxicity, the preclinical toxicologist in the pharmaceutical industry needs to more accurately identify a hazard earlier and provide an improved risk assessment of compounds in discovery and development. In contrast to what was available in the past, toxicogenomics requires a broader and slightly different expertise, often only achieved by multidisciplinary teams composed of toxicologists, molecular biologists, bioinformaticians, and biostatisticians, among others. The formation of productive teams composed of people with strikingly different scientific backgrounds, diverse expertise, and sometimes conflicting interest can be a significant challenge. Properly generated and curated reference databases are also needed to fully exploit the potential benefits of toxicogenomics. Furthermore, major improvements are needed for the microarray technology to become cost effective and meet performance characteristics amenable to its routine implementation in preclinical risk assessment. All these requirements can only be achieved through a substantial investment in human resources and hardware. Most major pharmaceutical companies have committed to significant investments, but so far toxicogenomics still has not been fully integrated in many organizations. This may reflect the current shortage of experts with a pragmatic vision of the future use of this technology, as well as the traditionally conservative nature of toxicology departments in the pharmaceutical industry. Nevertheless, if the trend seen in the last few years continues, it is realistic to predict that molecular toxicology and toxicogenomics will play a growing strategic role in the risk assessment of new chemical entities in the pharmaceutical industry.

REFERENCES

1. Service RF. Surviving the blockbuster syndrome. *Science* 2004;303:1796–1799.
2. Grabowski HG, Vernon JM. Returns to R&D on new drug introductions in the 1980s. *J Health Econ* 1994;13:383–406.
3. Rawlings MD. Cutting the cost of drug development? *Nat Rev Drug Discov* 2004;3:360–364.

4. Kola I, Landis J. Can the pharmaceutical industry reduce attrition rates? *Nat Rev Drug Discov* 2004;3:711–715.

5. Prentis RA, Lis Y, Walker SR. Pharmaceutical innovation by the seven UK-owned pharmaceutical companies (1964–1985). *Br J Clin Pharmacol* 1988;25:387–396.

6. Ulrich RG, Friend SH. Toxicogenomics and drug discovery: will new technologies help us produce better drugs? *Nat Rev* 2002;1:84–88.

7. MacNeil JS. Genomics goes downstream. *Genome Technol* 2005;54:24–30.

8. Segal E, Friedman N, Kaminski N, Regev A, Koller D. From signatures to models: understanding cancer using microarrays. *Nat Genet* 2005;37(Suppl):S38–S45.

9. Chu TM, Deng S, Wolfinger R, Paules RS, Hamadeh HK. Cross-site comparison of gene expression data reveals high similarity. *Environ Health Perspect* 2004;112:449–455.

10. Shi L, Tong W, Fang H, Scherf U, Han J, Puri RK, et al. Cross-platform comparability of microarray technology: intra-platform consistency and appropriate data analysis procedures are essential. *BMC Bioinformatics* 2005;6(Suppl 2):S12.

11. Yauk CL, Berndt ML, Williams A, Douglas GR. Comprehensive comparison of six microarray technologies. *Nucleic Acids Res* 2004;32:e124.

12. Chuaqui RF, Bonner RF, Best CJ, Gillespie JW, Flaig MJ, Hewitt SM, et al. Post-analysis follow-up and validation of microarray experiments. *Nat Genet* 2002;32(Suppl): 509–514.

13. Baker VA, Harries HM, Waring JF, Duggan CM, Ni HA, Jolly RA, et al. Clofibrate-induced gene expression changes in rat liver: a cross-laboratory analysis using membrane cDNA arrays. *Environ Health Perspect* 2004;112:428–438.

14. Waring JF, Ulrich RG, Flint N, Morfitt D, Kalkuhl A, Staedtler F, et al. Interlaboratory evaluation of rat hepatic gene expression changes induced by methapyrilene. *Environ Health Perspect* 2004;112:439–448.

15. Thomas RS, Rank DR, Penn SG, Zastrow GM, Hayes KR, Hu T, et al. Applications of genomics to toxicology research. *Environ Health Perspect* 2002;110:919–923.

16. Schena M, Shalon D, Davis RW, Brown PO. Quantitative monitoring of gene expression patterns with a complementary DNA microarray. *Science* 1995;270:467–470.

17. Nuwaysir EF, Bittner M, Trent J, Barrett JC, Afshari CA. Microarrays and toxicology: the advent of toxicogenomics. *Mol Carcinog* 1999;24:153–159.

18. Yang Y, Blomme EA, Waring JF. Toxicogenomics in drug discovery: from preclinical studies to clinical trials. *Chem Biol Interact* 2004;150:71–85.

19. *Innovation or Stagnation? Challenge and Opportunity on the Critical Path to New Medical Products*. Washington, DC: US Department of Health and Human Services, FDA; 2004.

20. Boess F, Kamber M, Romer S, Gasser R, Muller D, Albertini S, et al. Gene expression in two hepatic cell lines, cultured primary hepatocytes, and liver slices compared to the *in vivo* liver gene expression in rats: possible implications for toxicogenomics use of *in vitro* systems. *Toxicol Sci* 2003;73:386–402.

21. Hong Y, Muller UR, Lai F. Discriminating two classes of toxicants through expression analysis of HepG2 cells with DNA arrays. *Toxicol In Vitro* 2003;17:85–92.

22. Newton RK, Aardema M, Aubrecht J. The utility of DNA microarrays for characterizing genotoxicity. *Environ Health Perspect* 2004;112:420–422.

23. Hamadeh HK, Bushel PR, Jayadev S, Martin K, DiSorbo O, Sieber S, et al. Gene expression analysis reveals chemical-specific profiles. *Toxicol Sci* 2002;67:219–231.

24. Lee J, Richburg JH, Shipp EB, Meistrich ML, Boekelheide K. The Fas system, a regulator of testicular germ cell apoptosis, is differentially up-regulated in Sertoli cell versus germ cell injury of the testis. *Endocrinology* 1999;140:852–858.

25. Fielden MR, Eynon BP, Natsoulis G, Jarnagin K, Banas D, Kolaja KL. A gene expression signature that predicts the future onset of drug-induced renal tubular toxicity. *Toxicol Pathol* 2005;33:675–683.

26. Searfoss GH, Jordan WH, Calligaro DO, Galbreath EJ, Schirtzinger LM, Berridge BR, et al. Adipsin, a biomarker of gastrointestinal toxicity mediated by a functional gamma-secretase inhibitor. *J Biol Chem* 2003;278:46107–46116.

27. Shi L, Tong W, Goodsaid F, Frueh FW, Fang H, Han T, et al. QA/QC: challenges and pitfalls facing the microarray community and regulatory agencies. *Expert Rev Mol Diagn* 2004;4:761–777.

28. Mattes WB, Pettit SD, Sansone SA, Bushel PR, Waters MD. Database development in toxicogenomics: issues and efforts. *Environ Health Perspect* 2004;112:495–505.

29. Shi L, Tong W, Su Z, Han T, Han J, Puri RK, et al. Microarray scanner calibration curves: characteristics and implications. *BMC Bioinformatics* 2005;6(Suppl 2):S11.

30. Churchill GA. Fundamentals of experimental design for cDNA microarrays. *Nat Genet* 2002;32(Suppl):490–495.

31. Higgins MA, Berridge BR, Mills BJ, Schultze AE, Gao H, Searfoss GH, et al. Gene expression analysis of the acute phase response using a canine microarray. *Toxicol Sci* 2003;74:470–484.

32. Sugai T, Kawamura M, Iritani S, Araki K, Makifuchi T, Imai C, et al. Prefrontal abnormality of schizophrenia revealed by DNA microarray: impact on glial and neurotrophic gene expression. *Ann NY Acad Sci* 2004;1025:84–91.

33. Mirnics K, Pevsner J. Progress in the use of microarray technology to study the neurobiology of disease. *Nat Neurosci* 2004;7:434–439.

34. Galvin JE, Ginsberg SD. Expression profiling and pharmacotherapeutic development in the central nervous system. *Alzheimer Dis Assoc Disord* 2004;18:264–269.

35. Todd R, Lingen MW, Kuo WP. Gene expression profiling using laser capture microdissection. *Expert Rev Mol Diagn* 2002;2:497–507.

36. Irwin RD, Boorman GA, Cunningham ML, Heinloth AN, Malarkey DE, Paules RS. Application of toxicogenomics to toxicology: basic concepts in the analysis of microarray data. *Toxicol Pathol* 2004;32:72–83.

37. Hayes KR, Bradfield CA. Advances in toxicogenomics. *Chem Res Toxicol* 2005;18:403–414.

38. Vinciotti V, Khanin R, D'Alimonte D, Liu X, Cattini N, Hotchkiss G, et al. An experimental evaluation of a loop versus a reference design for two-channel microarrays. *Bioinformatics* 2005;21:492–501.

39. Kolaja K, Fielden M. The impact of toxicogenomics on preclinical development: from promises to realized value to regulatory implications. *Preclinica* 2004;2:122–129.

40. Fielden MR, Pearson C, Brennan R, Kolaja KL. Preclinical drug safety analysis by chemogenomic profiling in the liver. *Am J Pharmacogenomics* 2005;5:161–171.

41. Guerreiro N, Staedtler F, Grenet O, Kehren J, Chibout SD. Toxicogenomics in drug development. *Toxicol Pathol* 2003;31:471–479.

42. Ganter B, Tugendreich S, Pearson CI, Ayanoglu E, Baumhueter S, Bostian KA, et al. Development of a large-scale chemogenomics database to improve drug candidate selection and to understand mechanisms of chemical toxicity and action. *J Biotechnol* 2005;119:219–244.

43. Bushel PR, Hamadeh HK, Bennett L, Green J, Ableson A, Misener S, et al. Computational selection of distinct class- and subclass-specific gene expression signatures. *J Biomed Inform* 2002;35:160–170.

44. Ellinger-Ziegelbauer H, Stuart B, Wahle B, Bomann W, Ahr HJ. Characteristic expression profiles induced by genotoxic carcinogens in rat liver. *Toxicol Sci* 2004;77:19–34.

45. Thomas RS, Rank DR, Penn SG, Zastrow GM, Hayes KR, Pande K, et al. Identification of toxicologically predictive gene sets using cDNA microarrays. *Mol Pharmacol* 2001;60:1189–1194.

46. Waring JF, Jolly RA, Ciurlionis R, Lum PY, Praestgaard JT, Morfitt DC, et al. Clustering of hepatotoxins based on mechanism of toxicity using gene expression profiles. *Toxicol Appl Pharmacol* 2001;175:28–42.

47. Waring JF, Cavet G, Jolly RA, McDowell J, Dai H, Ciurlionis R, et al. Development of a DNA microarray for toxicology based on hepatotoxin-regulated sequences. *Environ Health Perspect* 2003;111:863–870.

48. Brazma A, Hingamp P, Quackenbush J, Sherlock G, Spellman P, Stoeckert C, et al. Minimum information about a microarray experiment (MIAME)—toward standards for microarray data. *Nat Genet* 2001;29:365–371.

49. Mattes WB. Annotation and cross-indexing of array elements on multiple platforms. *Environ Health Perspect* 2004;112:506–510.

50. Luhe A, Suter L, Ruepp S, Singer T, Weiser T, Albertini S. Toxicogenomics in the pharmaceutical industry: hollow promises or real benefit? *Mutat Res* 2005;575:102–115.

51. Tennant RW. The national center for toxicogenomics: using new technologies to inform mechanistic toxicology. *Environ Health Perspect* 2002;110:8–10.

52. Waters MD, Fostel JM. Toxicogenomics and systems toxicology: aims and prospects. *Nat Rev Genet* 2004;5:936–948.

53. Castle AL, Carver MP, Mendrick DL. Toxicogenomics: a new revolution in drug safety. *Drug Discov Today* 2002;7:728–736.

54. Searfoss GH, Ryan TP, Jolly RA. The role of transcriptome analysis in pre-clinical toxicology. *Curr Mol Med* 2005;5:53–64.

55. Suter L, Babiss LE, Wheeldon EB. Toxicogenomics in predictive toxicology in drug development. *Chem Biol* 2004;11:161–171.

56. Natsoulis G, El Ghaoui L, Lanckriet GR, Tolley AM, Leroy F, Dunlea S, et al. Classification of a large microarray data set: algorithm comparison and analysis of drug signatures. *Genome Res* 2005;15:724–736.

57. Golub TR, Slonim DK, Gaasenbeek JR, Caligiuri MA, et al. Molecular classification of cancer: class discovery and class prediction by gene expression monitoring. *Science* 1999;286:531–537.

58. Tusher VG, Tibshirani R, Chu G. Significance analysis of microarrays applied to the ionizing radiation response. *Proc Natl Acad Sci USA* 2001;98:5116–5121.

59. Khan J, Wei JS, Ringner M, Saal LH, Westermann F, et al. Classification and diagnostic prediction of cancers using gene expression profiling and artificial neural networks. *Nat Med* 2001;7:673–679.

60. Cristianini N, Shawe-Taylor J. *An Introduction to Support Vector Machines*. Cambridge UK: Cambridge University Press; 2000.

61. Furey TS, Cristianini N, Duffy N, Bednarski DW, Schummer M, Haussler D. Support vector machine classification and validation of cancer tissue samples using microarray expression data. *Bioinformatics* 2000;16:906–914.

62. Steiner G, Suter L, Boess F, Gasser R, de Vera MC, Albertini S, et al. Discriminating different classes of toxicants by transcript profiling. *Environ Health Perspect* 2004;112:1236–1248.

63. Thukral SK, Nordone PJ, Hu R, Sullivan L, Galambos E, Fitzpatrick VD, et al. Prediction of nephrotoxicant action and identification of candidate toxicity-related biomarkers. *Toxicol Pathol* 2005;33:343–355.

64. Greim H, Gelbke HP, Reuter U, Thielmann HW, Edler L. Evaluation of historical control data in carcinogenicity studies. *Hum Exp Toxicol* 2003;22:541–549.

65. Kramer JA, Curtiss SW, Kolaja KL, Alden CL, Blomme EA, Curtiss WC, et al. Acute molecular markers of rodent hepatic carcinogenesis identified by transcription profiling. *Chem Res Toxicol* 2004;17:463–470.

66. Ellinger-Ziegelbauer H, Stuart B, Wahle B, Bomann W, Ahr HJ. Comparison of the expression profiles induced by genotoxic and nongenotoxic carcinogens in rat liver. *Mutat Res* 2005;575:61–84.

67. Waring JF, Ulrich RG. The impact of genomics-based technologies on drug safety evaluation. *Annu Rev Pharmacol Toxicol* 2000;40:335–352.

68. Cattley RC. Peroxisome proliferators and receptor-mediated hepatic carcinogenesis. *Toxicol Pathol* 2004;32(Suppl 2):6–11.

69. Holden PR, Tugwood JD. Peroxisome proliferator-activated receptor alpha: role in rodent liver cancer and species differences. *J Mol Endocrinol* 1999;22:1–8.

70. Hamadeh HK, Bushel PR, Jayadev S, DiSorbo O, Bennett L, Li L, et al. Prediction of compound signature using high density gene expression profiling. *Toxicol Sci* 2002; 67:232–240.

71. Kramer JA, Blomme EA, Bunch RT, Davila JC, Jackson CJ, Jones PF, et al. Transcription profiling distinguishes dose-dependent effects in the livers of rats treated with clofibrate. *Toxicol Pathol* 2003;31:417–431.

72. Badr MZ, Belinsky SA, Kauffman FC, Thurman RG. Mechanism of hepatotoxicity to periportal regions of the liver lobule due to allyl alcohol: role of oxygen and lipid peroxidation. *J Pharmacol Exp Ther* 1986;238:1138–1142.

73. Butterworth KR, Carpanini FM, Dunnington D, Grasso P, Pelling D. The production of periportal necrosis by allyl alcohol in the rat. *Br J Pharmacol* 1978;63:353P–354P.

74. Amin K, Ip C, Jimenez L, Tyson C, Behrsing H. *In vitro* detection of differential and cell-specific hepatobiliary toxicity induced by geldanamycin and 17-allylaminogeldanamycin using dog liver slices. *Toxicol Sci* 2005;87:442–450.

75. Waring JF, Ciurlionis R, Jolly RA, Heindel M, Ulrich RG. Microarray analysis of hepatotoxins *in vitro* reveals a correlation between gene expression profiles and mechanisms of toxicity. *Toxicol Lett* 2001;120:359–368.

76. Burczynski ME, McMillian M, Cirvo J, Li L, Parker JB, Dunn RT, et al. Toxicogenomics-based discrimination of toxic mechanism in HepG2 human hepatoma cells. *Toxicol Sci* 2000;58:399–415.

77. Gomez-Lechon MJ, Ponsoda X, Bort R, Castell JV. The use of cultured hepatocytes to investigate the metabolism of drugs and mechanisms of drug hepatotoxicity. *Altern Lab Anim* 2001;29:225–231.

78. Waring JF, Ciurlionis R, Jolly RA, Heindel M, Gagne G, Fagerland JA, et al. Isolated human hepatocytes in culture display markedly different gene expression patterns depending on attachment status. *Toxicol In Vitro* 2003;17:693–701.

79. Li AP, Reith MK, Rasmussen A, Gorski JC, Hall SD, Xu L, et al. Primary human hepatocytes as a tool for the evaluation of structure–activity relationship in cytochrome P450 induction potential of xenobiotics: evaluation of rifampin, rifapentine and rifabutin. *Chem Biol Interact* 1997;107:17–30.

80. Ulrich RG, Bacon JA, Cramer CT, Peng GW, Petrella DK, Stryd RP, et al. Cultured hepatocytes as investigational models for hepatic toxicity: practical applications in drug discovery and development. *Toxicol Lett* 1995;82–83:107–115.

81. Liguori MJ, Anderson LM, Bukofzer S, McKim J, Pregenzer JF, Retief J, et al. Microarray analysis in human hepatocytes suggests a mechanism for hepatotoxicity induced by trovafloxacin. *Hepatology* 2005;41:177–186.

82. de Longueville F, Surry D, Meneses-Lorente G, Bertholet V, Talbot V, Evrard S, et al. Gene expression profiling of drug metabolism and toxicology markers using a low-density DNA microarray. *Biochem Pharmacol* 2002;64:137–149.

83. Harries HM, Fletcher ST, Duggan CM, Baker VA. The use of genomics technology to investigate gene expression changes in cultured human cells. *Toxicol In Vitro* 2001;15:399–405.

84. Morgan KT, Ni H, Brown HR, Yoon L, Crosby LM, et al. Application of cDNA microarray technology to *in vitro* toxicology and the selection of genes for a real-time RT-PCR-based screen for oxidative stress in Hep-G2 cells. *Toxicol Pathol* 2002;30:435–451.

85. Aubrecht J, Caba E. Gene expression profile analysis: an emerging approach to investigate mechanisms of genotoxicity. *Pharmacogenomics* 2005;6:419–428.

86. Snyder RD, Green JW. A review of the genotoxicity of marketed pharmaceuticals. *Mutat Res* 2001;488:151–169.

87. Dickinson DA, Warnes GR, Quievryn G, Messer J, Zhitkovich A, Rubitski E, et al. Differentiation of DNA reactive and non-reactive genotoxic mechanisms using gene expression profile analysis. *Mutat Res* 2004;549:29–41.

88. Yang Y, Abel S, Ciurlionis R, Waring JF. Development of gene expression-based *in vitro* assays for the efficient toxicity characterization of compounds. *Pharmacogenomics* 2006;7:177–186.

89. Waring JF, Gum R, Morfitt D, Jolly RA, Ciurlionis R, Heindel M, et al. Identifying toxic mechanisms using DNA microarrays: evidence that an experimental inhibitor of cell adhesion molecule expression signals through the aryl hydrocarbon nuclear receptor. *Toxicology* 2002;181–182:537–550.

90. Denison MS, Nagy SR. Activation of the aryl hydrocarbon receptor by structurally diverse exogenous and endogenous chemicals. *Annu Rev Pharmacol Toxicol* 2003;43:309–334.

91. Milano J, McKay J, Dagenais C, Foster-Brown L, Pognan F, Gadient R, et al. Modulation of notch processing by gamma-secretase inhibitors causes intestinal goblet cell metaplasia and induction of genes known to specify gut secretory lineage differentiation. *Toxicol Sci* 2004;82:341–358.

92. Creasy DM. Evaluation of testicular toxicity in safety evaluation studies: the appropriate use of spermatogenic staging. *Toxicol Pathol* 1997;25:119–131.

93. Stewart J. Inhibin B as a potential biomarker of testicular toxicity. *Toxicologist* 2005; 74:6.

94. Richburg JH, Johnson KJ, Schoenfeld HA, Meistrich ML, Dix DJ. Defining the cellular and molecular mechanisms of toxicant action in the testis. *Toxicol Lett* 2002; 135:167–183.

95. Adachi T, Ono Y, Koh KB, Takashima K, Tainaka H, Matsuno Y, et al. Long-term alteration of gene expression without morphological change in testis after neonatal exposure to genistein in mice: toxicogenomic analysis using cDNA microarray. *Food Chem Toxicol* 2004;42:445–452.

96. Adachi T, Koh KB, Tainaka H, Matsuno Y, Ono Y, Sakurai K, et al. Toxicogenomic difference between diethylstilbestrol and 17beta-estradiol in mouse testicular gene expression by neonatal exposure. *Mol Reprod Dev* 2004;67:19–25.

97. Rockett JC, Christopher LJ, Brian GJ, Krawetz SA, Hughes MR, Hee KK, et al. Development of a 950-gene DNA array for examining gene expression patterns in mouse testis. *Genome Biol* 2001;2:14.1–14.9.

98. Zappa F, Ward T, Pedrinis E, Butler J, McGown A. NAD(P)H: quinone oxidoreductase 1 expression in kidney podocytes. *J Histochem Cytochem* 2003;51:297–302.

99. Su AI, Wiltshire T, Batalov S, Lapp H, Ching KA, Block D, et al. A gene atlas of the mouse and human protein-encoding transcriptomes. *Proc Natl Acad Sci USA* 2004;101:6062–6067.

100. Su AI, Cooke MP, Ching KA, Hakak Y, Walker JR, Wiltshire T, et al. Large-scale analysis of the human and mouse transcriptomes. *Proc Natl Acad Sci USA* 2002;99:4465–4470.

101. Honore P, Kage K, Mikusa J, Watt AT, Johnston JF, Wyatt JR, et al. Analgesic profile of intrathecal P2X(3) antisense oligonucleotide treatment in chronic inflammatory and neuropathic pain states in rats. *Pain* 2002;99:11–19.

102. Semizarov D, Frost L, Sarthy A, Kroeger P, Halbert DN, Fesik SW. Specificity of short interfering RNA determined through gene expression signatures. *Proc Natl Acad Sci USA* 2003;100:6347–6352.

103. Zambrowicz BP, Turner CA, Sands AT. Predicting drug efficacy: knockouts model pipeline drugs of the pharmaceutical industry. *Curr Opin Pharmacol* 2003;3:563–570.

104. Lu PY, Xie F, Woodle MC. *In vivo* application of RNA interference: from functional genomics to therapeutics. *Adv Genet* 2005;54:117–142.

105. Li L, Lin X, Staver M, Shoemaker A, Semizarov D, Fesik SW, et al. Evaluating hypoxia-inducible factor-1alpha as a cancer therapeutic target via inducible RNA interference *in vivo. Cancer Res* 2005;65:7249–7258.

106. Waring JF, Anderson MG. Idiosyncratic toxicity: mechanistic insights gained from analysis of prior compounds. Curr *Opin Drug Discov Dev* 2005;8:59–65.

107. Williams DP, Park BK. Idiosyncratic toxicity: the role of toxicophores and bioactivation. *Drug Discov Today* 2003;8:1044–1050.

108. Knowles SR, Uetrecht J, Shear NH. Idiosyncratic drug reactions: the reactive metabolite syndrome. *Lancet* 2000;356:1587–1591.

109. Uetrecht J. Prediction of a new drug's potential to cause idiosyncratic reactions. *Curr Opin Drug Discov Dev* 2001;4:55–59.

110. Roth RA, Luyendyk JA, Maddox JF, Ganey PE. Inflammation and drug idiosyncrasy—is there a connection? *J Exp Ther* 2003;307:1–8.

111. Park BK, Kitteringham NR, Powell H, Pirmohamed M. Advances in molecular toxicology—towards understanding idiosyncratic drug toxicity. *Toxicology* 2000;153:39–60.

112. Shenton JM, Teranishi M, Abu-Asab MS, Yager JA, Uetrecht JP. Characterization of a potential animal model of an idiosyncratic drug reaction: nevirapine-induced skin rash in the rat. *Chem Res Toxicol* 2003;16:1078–1089.

113. Masson MJ, Uetrecht JP. Tolerance induced by low dose D-penicillamine in the brown Norway rat model of drug-induced autoimmunity is immune-mediated. *Chem Res Toxicol* 2004;17:82–94.

114. Luyendyk JP, Maddox JF, Cosma GN, Ganey PE, Cockerell GL, Roth RA. Ranitidine treatment during a modest inflammatory response precipitates idiosyncrasy-like liver injury in rats. *J Pharmacol Exp Ther* 2003;307:9–16.

115. Buchweitz JP, Ganey PE, Bursian SJ, Roth RA. Underlying endotoxemia augments toxic responses to chlorpromazine: is there a relationship to drug idiosyncrasy? *J Pharmacol Exp Ther* 2002;300:460–467.

116. Waring JF, Liguori MJ, Luyendyk JP, Maddox JF, Ganey PE, Stachlewitz RF, et al. Microarray analysis of LPS potentiation of trovafloxacin-induced liver injury in rats suggests a role for proinflammatory chemokines and neutrophils. *J Pharmacol Exp Ther* 2006;316:1080–1087.

117. Luyendyk JP, Mattes WB, Burgoon LD, Zacharewski TR, Maddox JF, Cosma GN, et al. Gene expression analysis points to hemostasis in livers of rats cotreated with lipopolysaccharide and ranitidine. *Toxicol Sci* 2004;80:203–213.

118. Tirmenstein MA, Hu CX, Gales TL, Maleeff BE, Narayanan PK, Kurali E, et al. Effects of troglitazone on HepG2 viability and mitochondrial function. *Toxicol Sci* 2002;69:131–138.

119. Drlica K, Zhao X. DNA gyrase, topoisomerase IV and the ;4-quinolones. *Microbiol Mol Biol Rev* 1997;61:377–392.

120. Ball P, Mandell L, Niki Y, Tillotson G. Comparative tolerability of the newer fluoroquinolone antibacterials. *Drug Safety* 1999;21:407–421.

121. Bertino J, Fish D. The safety profile of the fluoroquinolones. *Clin Ther* 2000;22:798–817.

122. Kier LD, Neft R, Tang L, Suizu R, Cook T, Onsurez K, et al. Applications of microarrays with toxicologically-relevant genes (tox genes) for the evaluation of chemical toxicants in Sprague Dawley rats *in vivo* and human hepatocytes *in vitro*. *Mutat Res* 2004;549: 101–113.

25

TOXICOPROTEOMICS: PRECLINICAL STUDIES

B. Alex Merrick and Maribel E. Bruno

National Center for Toxicogenomics, National Institute of Environmental Health Sciences, Research Triangle Park, North Carolina

Contents

25.1   INTRODUCTION

The primary purposes of this chapter are to define the field of toxicoproteomics, describe its development among "omics" technologies, and demonstrate its utility in experimental toxicological research, preclinical testing, and emerging applications to medicine. Subdisciplines within the field of proteomics deployed in preclinical research are described as Tier I and Tier II proteomic analysis. Tier I analysis involves global protein mapping and protein profiling for differential expression. Tier II proteomic analysis includes global methods for description of function, structure, interactions, and posttranslational modification of proteins. Preclinical toxicoproteomic studies with model liver and kidney toxicants are critically reviewed to assess their contributions toward understanding pathophysiology and in biomarker discovery. Toxicoproteomic studies in other organs and tissues are briefly discussed as well. A literature citation analysis matching proteomic and toxicity publications reveals that most toxicoproteomic research involves Tier I proteomic analysis and that biomarker development is a primary focus of many studies. The final section discusses five key developments in toxicoproteomics, encompassing new tools and research focus areas for the field.

25.2   THE FIELD OF TOXICOPROTEOMICS

Toxicoproteomics is the application of global protein measurement technologies to toxicology research. Chemical exposure frequently modifies proteins directly, produces changes in protein expression, and dysregulates critical biological pathways or processes leading to toxicity. Primary aims in toxicoproteomics are the discovery of key modified proteins, the determination of affected pathways, and the development of biomarkers for eventual prediction of toxicity. A growing base of pharmacogenomic knowledge should also strengthen the field of preclinical assessment and predictive toxicology [1–4].

    The wide application of proteomics has generated great interest and enthusiasm in many established scientific disciplines in basic biology and medicine, including the field of toxicology. There are well over 10,000 publications relating to some aspect or application of proteomics in the biosciences. However, the number of published proteomic studies is quite limited in reporting primary data for drug-mediated adverse reactions, biochemical toxicities, or undesirable phenotypes [5–7].

Compared to toxicogenomics or those technologies using DNA microarrays to study the effects of toxic substances, preclinical toxicoproteomics is indeed a smaller enterprise.

Fundamental reasons for the emerging state of preclinical toxicoproteomics compared to other omics fields relate to DNA technologies' ability to exploit the knowledge of whole genome sequence and apply it in mass parallel formats. DNA slides spotted with synthetic oligonucleotides can essentially hybridize and measure expression of every gene in human and many preclinical species. DNA microarrays are the most common transcriptomic format compared to other powerful gene expression methods like SAGE (serial analysis of gene expression) and MPSS (massively parallel signature sequencing). DNA microarray platforms provide high data output and rapid sample throughput in a way that proteomics cannot yet match in providing a "protein for every gene." Thus, as a hybrid "technofield" of proteomics and toxicology, toxicoproteomics is still becoming established as a specialized subject area. For the moment, toxicoproteomics has been placed under the aegis of toxicogenomics [8] or mass spectrometry [9].

The capabilities and critical issues for toxicogenomics and toxicoproteomics in pharmaceutical data submission for nonclinical safety testing to regulatory agencies have recently been reviewed [10]. Some of the unresolved issues raised for regulatory omic data submission include proper data quality standards, disparate platforms and data formats, meaningful data validation, relevance to traditional toxicological endpoints, potential added-value to established biochemical and molecular methods, animal-to-human extrapolation, mechanism of action, impact on the NOAEL, early versus adaptive, nonpharmacologic responses, limitations of bioinformatics algorithms, tools and available databases, and criteria for how genomic and proteomic data would influence regulatory decisions.

Some reviews in the field have closely scrutinized toxicoproteomics and metabonomics for their contributions in biomarker discovery beyond traditional clinical chemistry and histopathology indicators. A review of thirteen toxicoproteomic and metabonomic studies with various nephrotoxic agents examined various endpoints for their respective abilities to determine specificity and sensitivity of renal toxicity. The review concluded that proteomic (and metabonomic) data compared very poorly with traditional methods of blood and urine chemistries and histopathology without significant improvements [11]. However, it is the potential for discovery and new insights into pathobiology and therapeutics that fuels interest in omics technologies. The path to discovery is unfortunately seldom linear or formulaic. For example, progress in cystic kidney disorders leveraged prior proteomic mapping studies [12] to show MSK1 mutations underlie ciliary dysfunction in embryonic development [13]. Apparently, normal ciliary function is critical in renal tubule development and its dysfunction produces several forms of polycystic kidney disease. Clearly, the discovery potential of proteomics is a major driver in the push for better biomarkers of injury and disease.

Despite the discovery potential of toxicoproteomics, the strategies for conducting proteomic analysis and using such data in drug development, preclinical safety, and regulatory submission are far from standardized. The complexity of protein expression, multiple technology platforms, and emerging technical standards are major challenges for continued growth of the field. Researchers are also finding that no one platform is best suited for toxicoproteomic research.

One of the major goals for toxicoproteomics is to translate identified protein changes into new biomarkers and signatures of chemical toxicity that can provide much greater definition than current indicators [7]. The imprecise meaning of the term "biomarker" accounts for its wide variation in use (and misuse) in scientific and regulatory communities [14, 15]. At a biochemical and molecular level, biomarkers can be narrowed down to "singular biological measures with reproducible evidence of a clear association with health, disease, adverse effect or toxicity." This is a necessarily limited definition for quantitative biochemical or molecular measures. Historical and more current examples of biomarkers are the detection of a single *protein* such as C-reactive protein in cardiovascular disease [16], an *enzyme activity* like alanine aminotransferase activity in liver injury [17], *gene transcription* products such as Her2/neu [18] in breast malignancies, gene mutations/polymorphisms like slow acetylators that affect xenobiotic metabolism [19], or small molecules/metabolites such as serum glucose, insulin, and urinary ketone bodies in pathologic or drug-induced diabetes.

Many subcategories of biomarkers are in popular usage as well, including biologic, surrogate, prognostic, diagnostic, and bridging biomarkers [15, 20]. Importantly, a major development of the large datasets derived from omic technologies is the possibility of greater molecular topography compared to a singular biomarker. One of the major tenets of toxicoproteomics and other omic analyses is that specific patterns of protein changes can comprise a consistent "signature" of toxicity [21] or "combinatorial biomarker" [22] that is robust enough to be observed in spite of variations in biology, experimental design, or technology platforms. This is a critical assumption—first, because there is great potential for including nonspecific or indirect protein changes in such a signature, and second, because of the inherent challenges in establishing a causal linkage of multiple protein changes to a toxic or adverse phenotype. Discovery and definition of such toxicity signatures are at an early stage of progress in the field of toxicoproteomics [6, 21].

25.3 DISCIPLINES IN PROTEOMICS FOR TOXICOPROTEOMIC RESEARCH

Proteomics in a global protein analysis mode generally links separation and identification technologies to create a protein profile or differential protein display. Although the focus of proteomics has been grouped in various ways, Fig. 25.1 shows representative subdisciplines of proteomics that provide a means to categorize toxicoproteomic research.

Four factors often shape the manner in which researchers pursue their activities in toxicoproteomics that include (1) the complex nature of proteins, (2) that portion of the proteome targeted for study, (3) the integrative relationship of toxicoproteomic studies with other omic technologies, and (4) the driving forces behind specific toxicoproteomic projects.

Each of these four factors should be considered. First, a primary objective in proteomics is the isolation and identification of individual proteins from complex biological matrices. In toxicoproteomic analysis, the first tier of proteomic analysis is to determine individual *protein identities* (fingerprint, AA sequence), their relative (or absolute) *quantities*, and their *spatial location* within cell(s), tissues, and biofluids

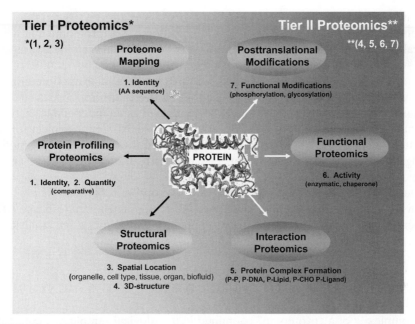

FIGURE 25.1 Disciplines of proteomics for application to preclinical drug assessment. Major areas of proteomics attempt to describe some portion of seven protein attributes (1–7) in a global manner. Tier I proteomic analysis (1–3) involves identification and quantitation of all proteins from a defined space for protein mapping or profiling. Tier II proteomic analysis (4–7) involves determination of three-dimensional structures, protein complexes, functions, or posttranslational modifications of proteins in a global manner.

of interest. The second tier of analysis globally screens for protein *functions, protein interactions*, three-dimensional *structure*, and specific *posttranslational modifications*. These first and second tiers of proteomic analysis encompass the seven intrinsic attributes of proteins that factor into toxicoproteomic analysis [23] as shown in Fig. 25.1. Proteomic platforms vary greatly in their respective abilities to deliver data on all protein attributes simultaneously during one analysis.

Proteome mapping is the most descriptive of proteomic inquiries and usually focuses on identifying all proteins in the sample or at a cellular location at hand. Profiling experiments necessarily require quantitation (relative to control, or absolute) to be comparative among samples. Implicit in protein mapping and profiling are considerations about the spatial "origin" of the sample. Often, sample origins are the same in profiling experiments for comparability; for example, serum samples are most comparable to serum, livers to livers, and so on. Structural proteomics is usually defined as high-throughput determination of protein structures in three-dimensional space and is often determined by X-ray crystallography and NMR spectroscopy. This definition has been expanded in Fig. 25.1 to include spatial location of proteins within the organism rather than continue to divide proteomic fields by specific levels of protein organization that might range from subcellular, cellular, organ, tissue, or organism to species proteomics.

A second factor to consider in toxicoproteomics is that the proteomes of most cells, tissues, and organs are so vast that, unlike whole genome queries, proteomes cannot be completely analyzed by existing proteomic platforms. By default, toxico-proteomic studies most often analyze only a portion of the proteome contained in typical biological samples. A frequent strategy to broaden protein coverage is to take steps prior to analysis to reduce sample complexity (analyze a portion of the proteome or "subproteome") by such procedures as subcellular fractionation, affinity or adsorptive chromatography, or electrophoretic separation.

Third, toxicoproteomic analysis may be conducted as an independent activity or alternately as a component of a large, formalized gene expression project for which the study design, type of experimental subjects, and the availability or amount of biological specimens may greatly impact sample preparation procedures and proteomic platform selection [24].

Fourth, the forces and individuals driving toxicoproteomic studies such as drug discovery, biophysical and chemical analyses, safety assessment, drug efficacy, ADME properties, and clinical trials will greatly influence the study design, analysis, and, importantly, biological interpretation of toxicoproteomic data.

25.4 PROTEOMIC PLATFORMS FOR TOXICOPROTEOMIC STUDIES

The complexity of a "proteome" contained in a biological sample presents numerous challenges for comprehensively describing the seven attributes of protein expression during any single proteomic analysis [7]. The primary aims of proteomic analysis are to (1) achieve maximal coverage of the proteome (i.e., Tier I analysis) in each sample, (2) complete analysis at high throughput, (3) produce an accurate quantitative protein measurement, (4) deliver data and interpretable results in a timely period, and (5) use discovery-oriented, open platforms.

All proteomic platforms typically share two common capabilities: a means of global *separation* and a technology for *identification* of proteins. Identification usually means assignment to international gene (i.e., NCBI) or protein (i.e., Uniprot or SwissProt) identification numbers. The following proteomic platforms represent a brief description of the principal technologies used for separating and identifying proteins during toxicoproteomic studies.

25.4.1 Two-Dimensional Gel Electrophoresis and Mass Spectrometry

Two-dimensional (2D) gel electrophoresis systems have been combined with mass spectrometry in an established and adaptable platform since 1975 and it is the most commonly used proteomic platform to separate and comparatively quantitate protein samples [25]. Current state-of-the-art 2D gels use immobilized pH gradient (IPG) gels first to separate proteins by charge and then subsequently to resolve by mass using SDS gel electrophoresis for effective separation of complex protein samples. Proteins are sufficiently separated to homogeneity by 2D gels to permit mass spectrometry (MS) identification. Typical IPG gels at 18–24 cm fitted with similarly sized SDS-PAGE gels can separate between 2000 and 3000 proteins. Each spot represents not a unique protein (i.e., gene product) but often posttranslationally modified forms of the same protein. Fluorescent staining is often the most sensitive means of protein detection (nanogram to microgram range). After electronic alignment (registration) of stained proteins in 2D gels by image analysis software, intensities of identical protein spots are compared among treatment groups and a ratio (fold change) is calculated for each protein using specialized software. In DIGE 2D-MS (*di*fferential *g*el *e*lectrophoresis two-dimensional gel mass spectrometry), protein samples to be compared are labeled with Cy2-, Cy3-, or Cy5-based linkers. Labeled samples are mixed together and electrophoresed on the same gel. This procedure minimizes image analysis errors from trying to electronically register different gels, since each dye (sample) is read at a different wavelength on the same gel [26]. Up to three or four samples can be run on the same 2D gel.

The combination of 2D gel separation of proteins with mass spectrometry provides a ready means of protein identification after protein excision, enzymatic digestion, and MS analysis. The 2D-MS platform forms a versatile and discovery-oriented standardized approach for use in toxicoproteomic studies [27]. A downside to this platform is the limited coverage of a proteome that can be realized on 2D gels by even the most sensitive fluorescent stains.

One-dimensional gel-based proteomic platforms—1D gel LC-MS/MS—may also be extremely effective for protein separation and identification using SDS-PAGE only (i.e., mass separation) with specially preprocessed samples such as immuno-depleted plasma [28] or cell secretomes [29]. Such preprocessing sufficiently reduces the original protein complexity to allow small amounts of sample protein (μg) or serum (μL) to be resolved to near protein homogeneity in stained protein bands. Bands are enzymatically digested to obtain diagnostic peptides for protein identification after amino acid sequencing by LC-MS/MS.

25.4.2 Multidimensional, Quantitative LC-MS/MS: MuDPIT, ICAT, iTRAQ, and SILAC

Multidimensional liquid chromatography (LC-LC) is used to separate protein digests (ng–μg peptides) by charge (strong anion exchange) and hydrophobicity (C18) immediately prior to entry into a tandem mass spectrometer (MS/MS) for protein identification [30]. A premier representative of LC-MS/MS proteomics is the multidimensional protein identification technology or "MuDPIT" platform. This approach has also been called "shotgun proteomics" since entire protein lysates are trypsin digested into thousands of peptide fragments without the need for any fractionation or processing prior to LC-LC separation and MS/MS identification. Advantages of this newer platform are the potential for detection and identification of low abundance proteins that may not be observed in gel-based protein separations. However, the MuDPIT platform is only semiquantitative. The platform is very effective in proteomic mapping and discovery studies and should find great utility in toxicoproteomics.

Other variations on the LC-MS/MS approach, closely linking LC separation to tandem MS instruments, have incorporated isotopic labeling strategies for protein quantitation and in-depth proteomic profiling of samples. Examples of such platforms are ICAT (isotope coded affinity tags), iTRAQ (isobaric tag for relative and absolute quantitation), and SILAC (stable isotope labeling with amino acids in cell culture). These methods use "light" and "heavy" forms of isotopes in linkers that bind to functional groups of proteins (i.e., cysteines or amino groups) in lysates. SILAC and iTRAQ are particularly effective for metabolic incorporation of "light" and "heavy" forms of amino acids (i.e., $^1H:^2H$, $^{12}C:^{13}C$, $^{14}N:^{15}N$) into cellular proteins during cell culture incubations. Although sample throughput is slow and analysis time is lengthy, the protein coverage has been greatly expanded with the development of these new multidimensional proteomic platforms. Careful sample, dose, and time selection to a few samples appears to be a successful strategy in achieving the most value from multidimensional, quantitative LC-MS/MS platforms.

25.4.3   Retentate Chromatography–Mass Spectrometry: SELDI

Retentate chromatography–mass spectrometry (RC-MS) is a high-throughput proteomic platform that creates a laser-based mass spectrum from a chemically absorptive surface. The principle of this approach is the adsorptive retention (pg–ng protein) of a subset of sample proteins on a thin, chromatographic support (i.e., hydrophobic, normal phase, weak cation exchange, strong anion exchange, or immobilized metal affinity supports). The adsorptive surfaces are placed on thin metal chips, which can be inserted into a specially modified MALDI-type mass spectrometer. The laser rapidly desorbs proteins from each sample on a metal chip to create a mass spectrum profile.

RC-MS can be performed on any protein sample but thus far this platform has found the greatest utility in the analysis of serum and plasma for disease biomarker discovery [6, 31]. The lead commercial platform of the RC-MS proteomic platform is the SELDI-TOF-MS instrument or, *s*urface-*e*nhanced *l*aser *d*esorption *i*onization *t*ime-*o*f-*f*light [32]. Analysis of samples is relatively rapid (100/day). Only a few microliters of biofluid sample are necessary and hundreds of samples can be screened in a few days. Downsides are that only a fraction of the proteome is analyzed (what adsorbs to the particular chemical surface), there are sample reproducibility issues, and protein identification of peaks is not readily achieved without additional analysis [33]. However, the RC-MS approach fits many problem areas as a proteomic discovery tool for defining drug or chemical exposure when rapid screening is needed for hundreds or thousands of preclinical or clinical samples.

25.4.4   Protein Capture Arrays: Antibody Arrays

Protein capture arrays (any mass parallel array of proteins, peptides, capture ligands, or adsorptive surfaces for protein analysis) represent a promising new proteomic tool that closely emulates the design for parallel analysis of DNA microarray technology [34]. Many different types of capture molecules can be arrayed (recombinant proteins, aptamers, peptides, drug libraries) but the most prevalent are antibody arrays that directly separate proteins from each other by affinity binding to specific protein targets. Generally, commercial antibody array platforms have widely varying sensitivities (pg–µg peptides) that fall into three classes based on targeted proteins: cytokine/chemokine arrays, cellular function protein arrays, and cell signaling arrays. However, antibody arrays are not presently available for any given cell type, biofluid, or species. This platform provides a rapid screen for limited sets of proteins that may fit some applications in toxicoproteomics.

25.5   TOXICOPROTEOMIC STUDIES IN LIVER INJURY

The liver is the primary site of xenobiotic metabolism and is a major organ for biotransformation and elimination of pharmaceuticals from the body [35]. Many of the initial studies in toxicoproteomics have been performed to gain insight into drug-induced liver injury and to test the capabilities of proteomic analysis with well studied drugs and chemicals in rodent models of toxicity. While rodent models of liver toxicity may predominantly show one phenotype such as necrosis, hepatitis, cholestasis, steatosis, fibrosis, cirrhosis, or malignancy, many different cellular and molecular processes are ongoing [36].

The removal from the marketplace of several widely prescribed drugs due to hepatotoxicity has attracted considerable attention and there are active efforts to better understand and identify hepatic risk prior to drug approval. Factors affecting susceptibility to drug-induced injury include age, sex, drug–drug interactions, and genetic polymorphism in metabolic pathways involved in activation or disposition of therapeutic drugs [37]. Reactive intermediates produced during metabolism can be toxic or some compounds may dysregulate critical biochemical pathways or functions of the liver [35].

Acute hepatic necrosis is a reproducible phenotype characteristic of many types of drugs and model compounds in preclinical species. The above considerations provide a rationale for exploring and testing the capabilities of emerging omics technologies like proteomics and transcriptomics upon acute hepatic injury. Which agents might be worthwhile for toxicoproteomic studies? A recent toxicogenomic study for classifying hepatotoxicants evaluated a representative list of 25 well-known model compounds or substances showing hepatotoxicity during testing [38]. The aim of this preclinical research report was to determine if biological samples from rats treated with various compounds could be classified based on gene expression profiles. Such model agents causing acute hepatonecrotic injury included acetaminophen, carbon tetrachloride, bromobenzene, hydrazine, and others. Hepatic gene expression profiles were analyzed using a supervised learning method (support vector machines—SVMs) to generate classification rules. The SVM method was combined with recursive feature elimination to improve classification performance. The goal was to identify a compact subset of probe sets (transcripts) with potential use as biomarkers. DNA microarray data have been generated for each substance in this study [38]. Their list of representative hepatotoxic agents for preclinical testing served as a basis for examining the literature for corresponding toxicoproteomic studies.

Table 25.1 summarizes available primary data from toxicoproteomic studies. Generally, these studies have been conducted on representative, model liver and kidney damaging agents relevant to preclinical assessment of toxicity. The agent, proteomic analysis platform, tissue or preparation, and brief results for each study are summarized in the table. Liver toxicants are addressed first.

25.5.1   Acetaminophen

Acetaminophen has been one of the most commonly tested agents for inducing hepatic injury in toxicoproteomic studies of the liver. It produces centrilobular hepatic necrosis in most preclinical species. Acute hepatocellular injury from acetaminophen (*N*-**a**cetyl-**p**ara-**a**mino**p**henol—APAP) exposure is primarily initiated by CYP2E1 bioactivation to form reactive intermediates such as *N*-acetyl-*p*-benzoquinone imine (NAPQI) that deplete glutathione and then bind to critical cellular

TABLE 25.1 Toxicoproteomic Analysis of Liver and Kidney Toxicants[a]

Reference	Chemical	Platform	Tissue	Results
46	APAP, AMAP	2D-MS	Mouse liver	35 proteins identified; altered proteins are known APAP adducts
47	APAP	2D DIGE MS	Mouse liver	Optimization study for 2D DIGE separation; several proteins altered with APAP
48	APAP	2D DIGE MS	Mouse liver	DNA array/proteomics; ↓ Hsps; protein changes in 15 min
49	APAP, others	NEPHGE 2D-MS	Rat liver, HepG2	113, 194 proteins identified in rat liver, HepG2 cells; catalase, carbamoylphosphate synthetase-1, aldo-keto-reductase, altered
53	APAP	ICAT	Mouse hepatocytes	Optimization study for ICAT analysis
50	APAP, CCl₄, amiodarone	2D-MS	Rat hepatocytes	31 proteins identified of 113 proteins altered by APAP
52	APAP	ICAT	Mouse liver	1632 proteins identified with 247 proteins differentially expressed; ↑ hepatoprotective proteins in SJL resistant strain; ↑ loss mitochondrial proteins from C57B1/6 susceptible strain
74	APAP, ANIT, Wy14643, Pb	2D DIGE MS	Rat liver, serum	Liver (124), serum (101) proteomics (proteins identified); five serum biomarkers for liver toxicity—PNP, MDH, GcBP PON1, RBP
51	APAP, TCN, amiodarone	2D-MS	Rat hepatocytes	For APAP, ↑15 and ↓25 proteins identified; ↓GPx; ↑PRx1,2
128	APAP	2D-MS	Rat liver, serum	Cluster analysis of transcriptomic, proteomic, and clinical chemistry data
129	CCl₄	2D-MS	Rat liver stellate cells	150 proteins identified; ↑ calcyclin, calgizzarin, galectin-1
55	CCl₄	2D-MS	Rat liver	30 proteins identified; proliferation and apoptosis proteins altered
57	BB	2D-MS	Rat liver	DNA array/proteomics; identified proteins infer degradation, oxidative stress from toxicity
29	Aflatoxin B1	1D gel LC-MS/MS	Rat hepatocyte	Rat secretome of 200 proteins identified; ↓α1-antitrypsin and 2-macroglobulin secretion with aflatoxin
60	Wy14643, rosiglitizone	2D-MS	ob/ob Mouse liver	↑ FA oxidation, lipogenesis in ob/ob with both PPAR activators; gluconeogenesis, glycolysis, AA metabolism affected with both
59	Wy14643, oxazepam	2D-MS	Mouse liver	DNA array/proteomics; subcellular fractions; protein identification unique to each chemical

130	Hydrazine	2D-MS	Liver mitochondria	Detection of carbonylated proteins after hypoxia
63	Hydrazine	2D DIGE MS	Rat liver	Lipid, Ca^{2+}, thyroid, stress pathways activated by toxicity
62	Hydrazine	2D DIGE MS	Rat liver	↑10, ↓10 proteins identified in lipid, Ca^{2+}, thyroid, stress pathways
67	Thioacetamide	2D-MS	Rat liver	STAP protein, stellate cells related to TAA-cirrhosis model
66	Thioacetamide	SELDI, MALDI-TOF/TOF	Rat liver	His-rich glycoprotein in serum related to TAA-cirrhosis model
65	Thioacetamide	2D-MS	Rat liver	Liver cirrhosis model found ↓ FA β-oxidation, branched chain AA, and methionine breakdown; ↑oxidative stress, lipid peroxidation pathways
78	Cyclosporin A	2D	Rat liver, kidney	Multiple 2D gel spots changed with cyclosporine in kidney (19 spots) and liver (29 spots)
79	Cyclosporin A	2D AA sequencing	Rat kidney	Specific ↓ of calbindin in kidney by cyclosporine; identified by AA sequencing; ELISA validation
82	Cyclosporin A	2D gel, 35S-labeling	Murine T cells	Cyclosporin A induces >100 proteins not found in resting or activated murine T-cells; proteins, like CSTAD, identified in later study [83]
90	Puromycin	2D-MS	Rat kidney	Proteomics/metabolomics to study renal glomerular toxicity
131	PbAc	2D-MS	Rat kidney, medulla, cortex	Subacute Pb altered 76 cortex proteins and 13 medullar proteins; ↓ calbindin, calcineurin, arginino-succinate synthetase; ↑ GSTM1
88	Gentamicin	2D-MS	Rat urine	20 proteins identified; mitochondrial dysfunction in renal cortex
95	4-Aminophenol, D-serine	2D-MS	Rat plasma	FAH identified as kidney damage biomarker
94	4-Aminophenol, D-serine, cis-Pt	2D-MS	Rat plasma	T-kininogen, inter-α-inhibitor H4P, complement c3 identified as kidney damage biomarkers
108	DCVC	2D DIGE MS	Porcine renal LLC-PK1 line	↑14, ↓9 proteins with DCVC; Hsp27 phosphorylation isoform found as marker of prosurvival by maintaining cell adhesion

ªSummaries of liver and kidney toxicoproteomic studies are intended to briefly overview study details and results. Only abbreviations that are helpful in interpreting the summary notes are included. For further explanation, please refer to the citation. Abbreviations are listed in order of appearance in the table. APAP, acetaminophen; AMAP, 3'-isomer of acetaminophen; 2D-MS, 2D gel mass spectrometry; 2D DIGE MS, 2D gel differential gel expression (Cy3,5 dyes) mass spectrometry; ↑, ↓, increase, decrease; Hsps, heat shock proteins; NEPHGE, nonequilibrium pH gel electrophoresis; ICAT, isotope coded affinity tags; CCl_4, carbon tetrachloride; ANIT, α-naphthylisothiocyanate; Wy14643, Wyeth 14643 compound; Pb, phenobarbital; PNP, purine nucleotide phosphorylase; MDH, malic dehydrogenase; GcBP, vitamin D binding protein; PON1, paraoxonase; RBP, retinol binding protein; TCN, tetracycline; GPx, glutathione peroxidase; PRx1,2, peroxiredoxin 1 and 2; BB, bromobenzene; LC-MS/MS, liquid chromatography tandem mass spectrometry; PPAR, peroxisome proliferator-activated receptor; Ca^{2+}, calcium; STAP, stellate cell activation associated protein; TAA, thioacetamide; SELDI, surface enhanced laser dissociated ionization; MALDI TOF/TOF, MALDI-based tandem MS; His, histidine; FA, fatty acid; AA, amino acid; CSTAD, cyclosporin A-conditional, T cell activation-dependent gene; PbAc, lead acetate; GSTM1, GSH transferase M1; FAH, fumaryl-acetoacetate hydrolase; cis-Pt, cisplatin; H4P, inter-α inhibitor H4P heavy chain; DCVC, dichlorovinyl-L-cysteine.

macromolecules [35]. Mitochondria are thought to be primary targets in acetamino-phen toxicity with particular attention on the mitochondrial permeability transition [39]. It is worth noting that mitochondrial dysfunction underlies the pathogenesis of several toxicities in preclinical species especially in liver, skeletal, and cardiac muscle, and the CNS [40]. Evidence has also been accumulating for the contribution of nonparenchymal cells such as Kupffer cells, NK cells, neutrophils, and endothelial cells that secrete cytokines and chemokines during acetaminophen-induced liver injury [41–45].

Some of the earliest toxicoproteomic studies using 2D-MS platforms were con-ducted using standard 2D-MS [46] analysis as well as the 2D DIGE MS platform alone [47] or in combination with DNA microarrays [48]. Proteomic analysis of livers from these studies in mice identified altered proteins that are known targets for adduct formation such as mitochondrial proteins, HSPs, and other structural and intermediary metabolism proteins. A different type of 2D gel separation using a nonequilibrium approach to charge separation of proteins (NEPHGE) found 100–200 differentially expressed proteins in rat liver and HepG2 cells, especially in enzymes involved in intermediary metabolism [49].

Studies using rat hepatocytes exposed to acetaminophen and analyzed by 2D-MS have found it helpful to concurrently evaluate other cytotoxic pharmaceutical agents such as tetracycline, amiodarone, and carbon tetrachloride [50, 51]. These studies found alterations in several metabolic enzymes and identified glutathione peroxi-dase and peroxiredoxins 1 and 2 (PRX1, PRX2), which serve as cellular responsive antioxidative enzymes during toxicant exposure.

One of the first LC-MS/MS studies using ICAT technology that involved acetaminophen toxicity in mouse liver was published in 2005 [52], which was preceded by an earlier optimization study for ICAT in mouse hepatocytes [53]. This study combined the more comprehensive ICAT analysis procedure with an adept choice of resistant (SJL) and susceptible (C57B1/6) mouse strains to investigate potential susceptibility factors (proteins and pathways) in acetamino-phen toxicity [52]. Inherent differences in liver homogenate protein expression levels between resistant SJL and susceptible C57B1/6 mice were found by com-parison of hepatic proteomics after vehicle (saline) treatment at 6h. Of the 1236 protein identified, 121 were differentially expressed between the two mouse strains. After 6h of 300mg/kg acetaminophen by intraperitoneal treatment, 1632 proteins were identified from which 247 were different between the two strains and 161 proteins were more abundant in the SJL strain. Some of these naturally more abundant proteins (in the absence of toxicant) may have protective roles against toxicity including two- to fourfold increases in lactoferrin, galectin-1, tripeptidyl-peptidase II, proteasomal subunit β-Type1, and DnaJ homolog A1. Upon administration of acetaminophen, comparative expression showed that SJL mice expressed from 3- to 10-fold higher levels of ubiquitin-like 2 (SUMO1) activating enzyme E1B, complement c5, COX1, peroxiredoxin 1, Grp170, Hsp70, GSTμ-2, and regucalcin. In addition to antioxidant enzyme functions, many of these upregulated proteins may have a reparative role in degrading denatured and damaged proteins, cell proliferation and regeneration, and cellular stress response. A selective loss of several mitochondrial proteins from susceptible C57B1/6 mice suggested this organelle is particularly vulnerable in acetaminophen-induced hepatic injury.

25.5.2 Carbon Tetrachloride

Carbon tetrachloride produces acute centrilobular hepatic necrosis but has frequently been used in a repeated exposure regimen over several weeks to produce an animal model of liver fibrosis [54]. Activation of hepatic stellate cells from a quiescent vitamin A-storing cell to a myofibroblast-like cell is a key event in excessive accumulation of fibril-forming extracellular matrix proteins and development of liver fibrosis. Proteomic analysis was performed on cellular and secreted proteins of normal and activated rat hepatic stellate cells either *in vitro* or *in vivo* after carbon tetrachloride for 8 weeks. Of the 43 altered proteins identified, 27 showed similar changes *in vivo* and *in vitro* including upregulation of calcyclin, calgizzarin, and galectin-1 as well as downregulation of liver carboxylesterase 10. These changes were confirmed in fibrotic liver tissues. A compendium of 150 stellate cellular and secreted proteins were identified.

Another carbon tetrachloride fibrosis study conducted a 2D-MS proteomic analysis on liver tissues from rats exposed to carbon tetrachloride for a period of 4–10 weeks [55]. During this exposure period, collagen deposition and hydroxyproline content of fibrotic livers increased continuously. Differentially expressed proteins from proteomic analysis were categorized as proliferation-related proteins/enzymes (proliferating cell nuclear antigen p120, p40, and cyclin F ubiquitin-conjugating enzyme 7—UBC7), and apoptosis-related proteins, mainly caspase-12, which was absent in the control rats. These researchers found that proliferation- and apoptosis-related proteins are dynamically expressed during different stages of rat liver fibrosis induced by carbon tetrachloride.

25.5.3 Bromobenzene

Bromobenzene is another well-characterized model liver toxicant whose metabolism, reactive intermediates, protein adducts, and liver toxicity phenotype (centrilobular necrosis) have been well characterized [56]. A transcriptomic and proteomic comparison of bromobenzene conducted after 24 h exposure to a single dose of bromobenzene showed alterations in transcripts and genes involved in drug metabolism, oxidative stress, sulfhydryl metabolism, and acute phase response [57]. Of the 1124 proteins resolved from liver homogenates, 24 proteins were differentially expressed and identified as intermediary or drug metabolism enzymes.

25.5.4 Wyeth 14643

The peroxisome proliferator-activated receptors (PPARs) are ligand-activated transcription factors that modulate lipid and glucose homeostasis [58]. Wyeth 14643 is a hepatic metabolic enzyme inducer and acts as a potent agonist of peroxisome proliferator-activated receptor alpha (PPAR-α), a member of the nuclear hormone receptor superfamily and a key transcriptional regulator of many genes involved in free fatty acid oxidation systems in liver. Global gene and protein expression changes were compared by cDNA microarray of mouse liver and 2D-MS of mouse liver subcellular fractions from B6C3F1 mice treated from 0.5 to 6 months with oxazepam and the peroxisome proliferator, Wyeth 14643 [59]. Each compound produces hepatocellular cancer after a 2 year bioassay of dietary exposure. The hypothesis was that each compound would produce cancer by different biochemical pathways and that transcript and protein changes measured prior to tumor formation (up to 6 months) would provide mechanistic insights into carcinogenesis. After 6 months, only 36 transcripts were altered after oxazepam compared to 220 transcripts with the Wyeth compound. Notable genes upregulated in the signature profile for oxazepam were Cyp2b20, Gadd45β, TNFα-induced protein 2, and Igfbp5. Upregulated genes with Wyeth compound were cyclin D1, PCNA, Igfbp5, Gadd45β, and CideA. Altered expression of over 100 proteins by proteomic analysis showed upregulation of the cancer biomarker α-fetoprotein in cytosol and cell cycle-controlled p38-2G4 protein in microsomes during both treatments. Both transcriptomic and proteomic analyses were deemed complementary in distinguishing between two chemical carcinogens that appear to proceed through different mechanisms and eventually lead to liver cancer as the common phenotype.

Insights into the therapeutic action of PPAR-α and PPAR-γ agonists, WY14643 and rosiglitazone, respectively, were reported in proteomic analysis of the ob/ob animal model of obesity disease [60]. Hepatic protein expression profiles were developed by 2D-MS analysis of lean and obese (ob/ob) mice, and obese mice treated with WY14643 or rosiglitazone. Livers from obese mice displayed higher levels of enzymes involved in fatty acid oxidation and lipogenesis compared to lean mice and these differences were further amplified by treatment with both PPAR activators. WY14643 normalized the expression levels of several enzymes involved in glycolysis, gluconeogenesis, and amino acid metabolism in the obese mice to the levels of lean mice. Rosiglitazone only partially normalized levels of enzymes involved in amino acid metabolism. This study used an established mouse model of obesity disease to map metabolic pathways and discriminate between PPAR-α and PPAR-γ agonist effects by proteomic analysis.

25.5.5   Hydrazine

Hydrazine is a model, cross-species hepatotoxicant used as an industrial reagent and found as a drug metabolite of the structurally related pharmaceutical isoniazid (antituberculosis drug) and the antihypertensive agent hydralazine. Hydrazine typically causes initial steatosis, macrovesicular degeneration, followed by marked hepatic necrosis. Transcriptomic studies suggest hydrazine initiates a process whereby the production and intracellular transport of hepatic lipids is favored over the removal of fatty acids and their metabolites [61].

Proteomic studies using 2D DIGE MS on the hepatotoxic effects of hydrazine were conducted in rats from 48 to 168 h [62, 63]. In one study, 2D gel patterns from liver were analyzed by principal component analysis (PCA) and partial least squares regression. PCA plots described the variation in protein expression related to dose and time. Regression analysis was used to select 10 upregulated proteins and 10 downregulated proteins that were identified by mass spectrometry. Hydrazine treatment altered proteins in lipid metabolism, Ca^{2+} homeostasis, thyroid hormone pathways, and stress response. In a second study, low density cDNA microarrays and 2D DIGE MS proteomics of liver tissue and metabonomic analysis of serum were performed from hydrazine-treated rats at 48–168 h [62]. Their findings supported known effects of hydrazine toxicity and provided potential biomarkers of hydrazine-induced toxicity.

25.5.6 Thioacetamide

Thioacetamide is metabolically activated in liver to produce thioacetamide-S,S-dioxide as a reactive intermediate that binds to liver macromolecules to initiate centrilobular necrosis [64]. Repeated administration of thioacetamide is an established technique for generating rat models of liver fibrosis and cirrhosis depending on dose and length of administration (weeks). A 2D-MS proteomic approach was used to profile liver protein changes in rats receiving thioacetamide for 3, 6, and 10 weeks to induce hepatic cirrhosis [65]. Expression of 59 protein spots altered by thioacetamide can be identified, including three novel, unannotated proteins. Down-regulation of enzymes was noted in pathways such as fatty acid β-oxidation, branched chain amino acids, and methionine breakdown, which may relate to succinyl-CoA depletion and affect heme and iron metabolism. Increased levels were found for enzymes responding to oxidative stress and lipid peroxidation such as GSH trans-ferases. Finally, these proteomic data were integrated into a proposed overview model for thioacetamide-induced liver cirrhosis affecting succinyl-CoA and cytochrome P450 production combined with iron release and hydrogen peroxide generation.

In another model of thioacetamide-induced liver cirrhosis in rats, researchers probed for potential serum biomarkers using the SELDI proteomic approach [66]. A weak cation exchange surface was used to analyze serum by SELDI MS from control (normal) rats, thioacetamide-induced liver cirrhosis rats, and rats with bile duct ligation-induced liver fibrosis. A consistently downregulated 3495 Da protein in cirrhosis samples was one of the selected significant biomarkers. This 3495 Da protein was purified on-chip and was trypsin digested on-chip for MS/MS identification of a histidine-rich glycoprotein. The new protein was proposed as a new preclinical biomarker for the rat cirrhosis model that might eventually prove useful for early clinical detection of liver cirrhosis and classification of liver diseases.

An innovative study involving stellate cell activation by 8 week treatment with thioacetamide utilized a proteomic approach that led to the discovery of a novel protein named STAP for "stellate cell activation-associated protein" [67]. Quiescent and thioacetamide-activated stellate cells were analyzed by 2D-MS (ESI-MS/MS) to identify 43 proteins altered during the activation process including upregulation of collagen-α_1 (I and III), γ-actin, neural cell adhesion molecule (N-CAM), calcyclin, calgizzarin, and galectin-1. In particular, STAP was highly increased both in activated stellate cells and in fibrotic liver tissues induced by thioacetamide treatment. These researchers cloned the STAP gene and found it was a cytoplasmic protein, expressed only in stellate cells, with molecular weight of 21,496 Da and a 40% amino acid sequence homology to myoglobin. Biochemical characterization showed STAP is a heme protein exhibiting peroxidase activity toward hydrogen peroxide and linoleic acid hydroperoxide. These results indicate that STAP is a novel endogenous peroxidase catabolizing hydrogen peroxide and lipid hydroperoxides, both of which have been reported to trigger stellate cell activation and consequently promote progression of liver fibrosis. STAP was postulated to play a role as an antifibrotic scavenger of peroxides in the liver.

25.6   NEW BLOOD BIOMARKERS IN LIVER INJURY

Blood is one of the most accessible and informative biofluids for specific organ pathology in preclinical studies. Biomarkers that can be assayed in biological fluids from preclinical species may hold relevance for human subjects [17]. A comprehensive mapping of soluble human blood elements of the plasma proteome is currently underway for improved understanding of disease and toxicity by the Human Proteome Oganization (HUPO) [68]. Results from an international survey of soluble human blood proteins by chromatographic and electrophoretic separation have revealed several thousand resolvable proteins for which mass spectrometry has provided evidence for over 1000 unique protein identifications [68, 69]. Researchers are also mapping the mouse [70] and rat [71] serum and plasma proteomes for use in preclinical and experimental studies. An excellent review has been published for 2D gel mapping of rat serum and rat tissue proteomic studies [71].

The sensitivity of 2D gel proteomic approaches to detect and measure alterations in the mouse or rat plasma proteomes has only recently been tested by various labs. Researchers examined changes in the mouse plasma proteome, focused upon inflammation after cutaneous burn injury with superimposed *Pseudomonas aeruginosa* infection [72]. Upregulations of inter α-trypsin inhibitor heavy chain 4 and hemopexin were detected along with other mouse acute-phase proteins, including haptoglobin and serum amyloid A. In another inflammation study, reference maps of the mouse serum proteome were generated by 2D-MS from control animals and from mice injected with lipopolysaccharide (LPS) to induce systemic inflammation, and from mice transgenic for human apolipoproteins A-I and A-II [73]. The greatest changes were noted for haptoglobin and hemopexin.

Finally, a comparative plasma proteome analysis has been reported in which investigators used 1D gel LC-MS/MS analysis upon a few microliters of plasma from lymphoma-bearing SJL mice experiencing systemic inflammation [28]. After removal of albumin and Igs from plasma, these researchers identified a total of 1079 nonredundant mouse plasma proteins; more than 480 in normal and 790 in RcsX tumor-bearing SJL mouse plasma. Of these, only 191 proteins were found in common. Many of the upregulated proteins were identified as acute-phase proteins but several unique proteins, including haptoglobin, proteosome subunits, fetuin-B, 14–3-3ζ, and MAGE-B4 antigen, were found only in the tumor-bearing mouse plasma due to secretion or shedding by membrane vesicles, or externalized due to cell death. These results are very encouraging for the effectiveness of a proteomic approach for protein identification from small sample amounts, and for comparative proteomics in animal models of drug-induced toxicity or disease.

The application of serum or plasma protein maps in toxicoproteomics such as serum profiling of liver injury has just begun to take shape. A recent study reported identification of serum proteins altered in rats treated with four liver-targeted compounds including acetaminophen, ANIT (1-naphthylisothiocyanate), phenobarbital, and Wyeth 14643 at early, fulminant, and recovery periods of effect [74]. Nineteen serum proteins were identified as significantly altered from the four studies and, among them, five serum proteins were of special interest as serum markers for early hepatic toxicity or functional alterations in rats, including vitamin D-binding protein (Gc binding protein), purine nucleotide phosphorylase (PNP), malic dehydrogenase (MDH), paraoxonase (PON1), and retinol-binding protein (RBP). Some of these proteins may serve as early predictive markers of hepatotoxicity for new drug candidates or may be more sensitive than other conventional methods.

The soluble portion of blood, serum or plasma, is regarded as a complex biofluid tissue. While many organs contribute various proteins as blood solutes, the liver is by far the most productive member of all organs and tissues. It has occurred to some researchers to study the secreted proteome of hepatocytes since liver parenchyma are often primary targets of drug-induced toxicity, and they also secrete many plasma proteins, which can be measured in preclinical species. Secreted proteins were separated and identified from primary rat hepatocytes using a collagen gel sandwich system. Proteomic analysis was conducted by a 1D gel LC-MS/MS procedure. More than 200 secreted proteins were identified that included more than 50 plasma proteins, several structural extracellular matrix proteins, and many proteins involved in liver regeneration. Secretion of two proteins, α_1-antitrypsin and α_2-macroglobulin, was greatly reduced in aflatoxin B1 exposed hepatocytes. This study provides evidence that proteomic analysis of medium from hepatocyte sandwich culture might represent a new *in vitro* model and general approach for future discoveries of secreted biomarkers in drug-induced chemical toxicity.

25.7   TOXICOPROTEOMIC STUDIES IN KIDNEY INJURY

Kidney is a primary organ for preclinical assessment in pharmaceutical development since its metabolic and excretory functions often render it susceptible to drug-induced toxicity [75]. The kidney is a major organ for filtration, reabsorption, and secretion to maintain homeostasis of water-soluble salts and small molecules. The organ also has a considerable capacity for biotransformation of drugs and xenobiotics. Specific physiological characteristics of the kidney are localized to specific cell types (i.e., vascular endothelial and smooth muscle cells, mesangial cells, interstitial cells, podocytes, proximal and distal tubular epithelial cells), with each demonstrating selective susceptibility to toxicity. Renal damage can be due to several different mechanisms affecting different segments of the nephron, renal microvasculature, or interstitium. The nature of renal injury may be acute and recoverable. However, other drugs with repeated exposure can produce chronic renal changes that may lead to end-stage renal failure. The abilities to perform kidney transplants and other organ replacements have saved many lives because of immunosuppressive drug treatment to prevent organ rejection. However, immunosuppressive drugs also run the risk of renal toxicity over time. New nephrotoxic markers amenable for multiple preclinical models and high throughput screening are major goals for toxicoproteomic and toxicogenomic technologies [75, 76].

25.7.1   Cyclosporin A

Some of the groundbreaking studies that initiated the field of toxicoproteomics took place in the mid-1990s and involved investigating the side effects of the immunosuppressant drug cyclosporin A. Cyclosporin A is a calcineurin inhibitor that has been a mainstay for immunosuppressive therapy following solid-organ transplantation. Cyclosporin A blocks immune responses by inhibiting the calcineurin-dependent dephosphorylation of the nuclear factor of activated T cells (NFAT). However, a dose-dependent nephrotoxicity occurs with high incidence that is characterized by nonhistologic functional deficits or functional decline, with calcium loss in urine (hypercalciuria), vascular-interstitial lesions, and calcification of renal tubules [77].

Initial 2D gel studies were conducted in rat liver and kidney samples that showed changes in 48 proteins in these tissues in rats treated with cyclosporin A in which an unidentified protein present only in the kidney was uniquely downregulated [78]. A subsequent 2D gel study of kidney homogenates identified a decrease in the 28 kDa kidney protein as calbindin-D using protein microsequencing. Importantly, this same study validated a time-dependent decrease in calbindin expression by ELISA for up to 28 days of cyclosporin A treatment [79]. These toxicoproteomic studies published a decade ago represented a significant advance in understanding an important part of cyclosporine-induced pathophysiology in kidney.

More recently, the contribution of calbindin-D28k has been clarified by the generation of genetically modified mice. Cyclosporin A-induced hypercalciuria represents two pathophysiological processes: a downregulation of calbindin-D28k with subsequent impaired renal calcium reabsorption and a cyclosporin A-induced high turnover bone disease [80]. In addition, there is evidence that one biochemical mechanism underlying cyclosporin A and other calcineurin inhibitors may be a drug-induced mitochondrial dysfunction [81].

The effects of cyclosporin A on gene upregulation were advanced by a 2D gel proteomic analysis of newly synthesized ^{35}S-methionine-labeled proteins in murine T cells activated in the absence or presence of cyclosporin A [82]. Remarkably, these investigators found more than 100 proteins not present in resting or activated T cells that could be induced by cyclosporin A exposure. It is important to emphasize that the discovery nature of this proteomic study was capitalized upon (same researchers) in identification of the corresponding genes under the same treatment conditions using a transcript enrichment technique called "representational difference analyses" [83]. Among the upregulated transcripts, a new gene was found, named *CSTAD*, for "CSA-conditional, T cell activation-dependent" gene. *CSTAD* encodes two proteins of 104 and 141 amino acids that are localized in mitochondria [83]. *CSTAD* upregulation is observed in mice after cyclosporin A treatment, suggesting that upregulation of *CSTAD* and perhaps many other genes may be newly implicated in cyclosporin A toxicity. Thus, toxicoproteomics has played an important role in furthering the understanding of the critical proteins and biological pathways in cyclosporin A toxicity that should lead to better biomarkers for this important class of pharmaceuticals.

25.7.2   Puromycin and Gentamicin

The regionally specific structure and function of the kidney renders specialized areas to be more susceptible to toxicity from exposure to certain pharmaceutical agents. For example, puromycin aminonucleoside is an antibiotic that causes glomerular podocyte necrosis, nephrosis, and proteinuria in rodent models [84]. Gentamicin is an aminoglycoside antibiotic that accumulates in proximal tubular epithelia and inhibits cell lysosomal function, producing phospholipidosis and tubular degeneration [85]. Some studies have begun to proteomically characterize specific regions such as the medulla and cortex [86] or subcellular structures of kidney cell types such as the nucleus [87]. In one study, the nephrotoxic effects of gentamicin upon protein expression were studied in rat kidney. Results revealed the identities of more than 20 proteins involved in the citric acid cycle, gluconeogenesis, fatty acid synthesis, and transport or cellular stress responses [88]. The authors believed that impairment of energy production and mitochondrial dysfunction were involved in gentamicin-induced nephrotoxicity.

Another approach to studying nephrotoxicity is by proteomic characterization of urine. Proteomic mapping of rat urine proteins studied by 2D-MS resolved 350 protein spots from which 111 protein components were identified including transporters, transport regulators, chaperones, enzymes, signaling proteins, cytoskeletal proteins, pheromone-binding proteins, receptors, and novel gene products [89]. One toxicoproteomic study examined urinary protein expression profiles to gain insight into puromycin-induced kidney toxicity [90]. Nephropathy and proteinuria caused by puromycin aminonucleoside in rats was studied by metabonomics and a 2D-MS proteomic analysis of urinary proteins from 8 to 672 h after dosing. Prior to exposure, major urinary protein (MUP), α_2-microglobulin, and glial fibrillary acid protein isoforms were the major urinary proteins found in addition to many other unidentified low mass urinary proteins. Following puromycin treatment, a gradual increase in higher mass proteins was observed on 2D gels, particularly albumin, at 32 h after dosing. By 120 h, albumin, transthyretin, and Gc-binding protein were identified as major urinary proteins from puromycin-induced kidney damage. After 672 h, the urinary protein profile in 2D gels had largely returned to normal. Many of these plasma-derived proteins appearing in the urine over 0–672 h following puromycin administration were consistent with loss of glomerular integrity and major leakage of plasma protein in urine. This study suggests that urinary proteomics, in conjunction with these other techniques, has the potential to provide significantly more mechanistic information than is readily provided by traditional clinical chemistries and may be a productive means for biomarker discovery of nephrotoxic agents in preclinical species.

25.7.3   4-Aminophenol, D-Serine, and Cisplatin

The nephrotoxin 4-aminophenol (4-AP) produces severe necrosis of the pars recta of the proximal tubule in the rat that is thought to occur through formation of the toxic metabolite 1,4-benzoquinoneimine [91]. D-Serine, an enantiomer of L-serine, is another model nephrotoxicant that selectively damages the pars recta of proximal tubules in the kidney, which may involve formation of toxic oxidative metabolites [92]. The chemotherapeutic agent cisplatin is also a model nephrotoxicant and targets different portions of the kidney. It is metabolized to cytotoxic intermediates in proximal tubular epithelial cells and induces necrosis in distal tubules and collecting ducts along with causing mild glomerular toxicity [93]. Proteomic profiling using 2D-MS was used to investigate plasma protein changes in rats treated with 4-aminophenol, D-serine, and cisplatin compared to saline controls [94]. Nontoxic isomers, L-serine, and transplatin were also studied. Many plasma proteins were found that displayed dose- and time-dependent response to toxicants. Several isoforms of T-kininogen protein were identified as increasing in plasma at early time points and returning to baseline levels after 3 weeks with each nephrotoxicant but not with nontoxic compounds. In addition, inter-α inhibitor H4P heavy chain was increased in the 4-AP and D-serine studies. A further set of proteins correlating with kidney damage was found to be a component of the complement cascade and other blood clotting factors, indicating a contribution of the immune system to the observed toxicity. It was proposed that T-kininogen may be required to counteract apoptosis in proximal tubular cells in order to minimize tissue damage following a toxic insult.

In a related study, plasma samples from 4-aminophenol and D-serine treated rats were profiled by 2D-MS showing dose- and time-dependent effects of various plasma proteins in response to these nephrotoxicants [95]. One toxicity-associated plasma protein was identified as the cellular enzyme fumarylacetoacetate hydrolase (FAH), a key component of the tyrosine metabolism pathway. FAH was elevated in the plasma of animals treated with 4-aminophenol and D-serine at early time points and returned to baseline levels after 3 weeks. The protein was not elevated in the plasma of control animals or those treated with the nontoxic isomer L-serine. The investigators raised the possibility that FAH might serve as a marker of kidney toxicity in preclinical species.

25.7.4   Dichlorovinyl-L-Cysteine

Dichlorovinyl-L-cysteine (DCVC) is a model nephrotoxicant taken up by renal proximal tubular epithelia, where it is bioactivated by renal cysteine conjugate (β-lyase) to form reactive, cytotoxic intermediates [96]. DCVC is a metabolite of trichloroethylene but can be chemically synthesized for use in experimental studies [97].

A proteomic study of DCVC toxicity was conducted in LLC-PK1 porcine renal epithelial cells by 2D DIGE MS to determine early changes in stress-response pathways preceding focal adhesion disorganization linked to the onset of apoptosis. DCVC treatment caused a greater than 1.5-fold up- and downregulation of 14 and 9 proteins, respectively, prior to apoptosis including aconitase and pyruvate dehydrogenase, and those related to stress responses and cytoskeletal reorganization, such as cofilin, Hsp27, and alpha-β-crystallin. Most noticeable was a pI shift in Hsp27 from phosphorylation at Ser-82. Only inhibition of p38 with SB203580 reduced Hsp27 phosphorylation, which was associated with accelerated reorganization of focal adhesions, cell detachment, and apoptosis. Inhibition of active JNK localization at focal adhesions did not prevent DCVC-induced phosphorylation of Hsp27. Overexpression of a phosphorylation-defective mutant Hsp27 acted as a dominant negative and accelerated DCVC-induced focal adhesion changes and the onset of apoptosis. Early p38 activation appears to rapidly phosphorylate Hsp27, to maintain cell adhesion, and to suppress renal epithelial cell apoptosis. This toxicoproteomic study combines both protein identification and posttranslational modification to elucidate critical proteins (Hsp27) and protein attributes (phosphorylation) in critical pathways (p38 stress pathway) to gain insight into mechanisms of renal epithelial cell death.

25.8   TOXICOPROTEOMICS OF ADVERSE EFFECTS AND TOXICANTS: CITATION ANALYSIS

The application of proteomics to toxicology is in its early stages. Published toxicoproteomic reports relevant to pharmaceutical research so far have focused on liver, kidney, and blood, as described in the previous sections of this chapter. However, it is of great interest to further stratify the areas of toxicoproteomic research. Citation analysis is one approach for further discriminating specific research areas in toxicoproteomics. A citation analysis was performed using SciFinder® software (CAS, Columbus, OH) to acquire an overview of how proteomics has been used in toxicology. A search of "proteomics" and "toxicity" terms retrieved a total of 895 documents from Medline and Chemical Abstract services that included primary literature, reviews, commentary, and chemical and patent oriented data. A subgroup of 323 citations of the total is shown in a two-dimensional bar graph in Fig. 25.2. The bar graph matches the SciFinder preset subcategories in "Toxicology"

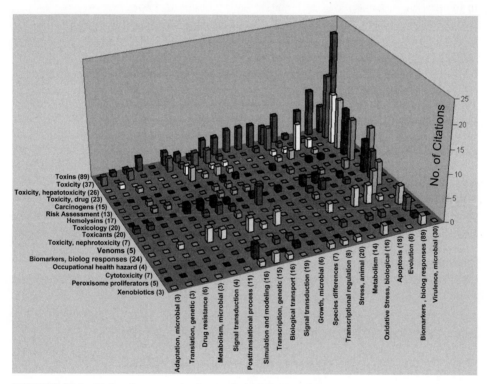

FIGURE 25.2   Role of proteomics in preclinical assessment and toxicology research. A 3D histogram displays the frequency and distribution of proteomic research citations in toxicology research as of March 2006. SciFinder® citation analysis matched the terms *proteomics* and *toxicity* and retrieved a total of 895 documents to comprise available toxicoproteomics references. The algorithm searches both Medline and Chemical Abstracts for published journal and conference literature and patents. A subgroup of 323 citations is shown in the bar chart to give more definition to citation analysis. The subgroup of 323 citations is the product of matching the category "Processes and Systems" (its selected subcategories on the *x*-axis) with the category "Toxicology" (its selected subcategory on the *y*-axis). Categories and subcategories are preset divisions of SciFinder software. The *z*-axis shows the number of citations (number in parentheses) for each bar, which represents the product of matching subcategories from the *x*- and *y*-axes. (SciFinder data display output from CAS, a division of the American Chemical Society.) In some subcategories, "biological" is abbreviated as "biolog."

with "Processes and Systems" categories to give more definition to the citation analysis.

The most cumulative citations occurred in the subcategory "Biomarkers, biolog responses," at 89 citations when matched with selected subcategories of toxicology. Similarly, the subcategory "Toxins" had 89 cumulative citations when matched with selected subcategories of "Processes and Systems." Other notable subcategories in "Processes and Systems" with high citations were "Virulence, microbial" (30), "Apoptosis" (18), "Stress, animal" (20), and "Signal transduction" (19). In "Toxicology," notable citations were in subcategories for "Toxicity" (37), "Toxicity, hepatotoxicity" (26), "Toxicity, drug" (23), and "Biomarkers, biolog responses" (24). Clearly, biomarker development is a primary focus in toxicoproteomic studies, particularly in liver.

The interest in preclinical development of biomarkers for drug toxicity may leave one to wonder why there are not more primary data reports in pharmaceutical toxicoproteomics. One reason is that linkages of mass spectrometry to separation technologies have only been available for 6–7 years and are just becoming more widely accessible in the last few years. A second reason is that some excellent toxicoproteomic research in the commercial sector may not be publicly accessible because of proprietary concerns unless compound structures can be coded [98] or only partially divulged [99]. A third reason is that meaningful differential protein expression is not easily achieved in many drug-exposed systems. Often drug targets are specific for receptors, signaling pathways, or portions of the cell that are at low levels of expression and not easily detectable (i.e., membrane receptor proteins). Alternately, there may be an overabundance of noninformative, interfering proteins (i.e., albumin removal from serum) that mask important low level proteins. Reduction of complexity or enrichment can be an extremely useful and necessary strategy for achieving differential protein expression prior to toxicoproteomic analysis. Undoubtedly, the range of citations in toxicoproteomics will widen, particularly as mass spectrometry becomes more pervasive and accessible.

25.9   FUTURE DEVELOPMENTS IN TOXICOPROTEOMICS

25.9.1   Toxicoproteomic Studies in Other Organs and Tissues

The brief historical development of toxicoproteomics has focused primarily on liver and kidney. However, protein profiling studies are being conducted in many other organs and tissues to profile adverse effects of therapeutics. Proteomic approaches are revealing new blood serum and tissue biomarkers in animal models of human neurodegenerative diseases like Parkinson disease, Alzheimer disease, and amyotrophic lateral sclerosis (ALS) [100, 101]. Proteomic studies are being conducted in cardiotoxicity models with doxorubicin [102] and renin–angiotensin models of hypertension [103]. Comparative protein expression studies are systematically examining testicular toxicity in rats with several reproductive toxicants such as cyclophosphamide, sulfasalazine, 2,5-hexanedione, and ethylene glycol monomethyl ether [104]. The effects of formaldehyde on rat lung [105] and protein adduct formation of 1-nitronapthalene metabolites in rat lung [106, 107] are being examined by proteomic techniques to provide insight into pulmonary pathology by these agents.

Thus, protein mapping and profiling studies are exploring a variety of preclinical assessment animal models of toxicity and disease.

25.9.2 Expectations and Reality

The expectations of omics technologies in pharmaceutical development are very high, but the breakthroughs in drug discovery and improvements over traditional measures in preclinical assessment have lagged behind. This situation is understandable since the platforms for proteomics continue to be in dynamic development. Furthermore, applications to toxicology settings are still being explored to match platform sensitivity for differential protein expression with preclinical biological samples. Many of the published toxicoproteomic reports reviewed herein have served as proof-of-principle studies using Tier I proteomic analysis as referred to in Fig. 25.1. The approach has been to examine a well-characterized toxicant(s) and compare proteomic data output with known toxicological endpoints (i.e., serum and urine chemistries, histopathology). These efforts might be described as the discovery phase of toxicoproteomics, where differential protein expressions are determined in response to compound exposure. However, many of these initial studies have often not been accompanied by any confirmation analysis using ELISA, Western blot, immunohistochemistry, or functional assay (i.e., enzymatic activity). Two other areas show a slow progress in toxicoproteomic research. One is in the follow-up *hypothesis-driven research* that further characterizes discovery findings and establishes causal linkage of toxicant exposure and effect. The other area is in *validation studies* of proposed biomarkers using independent and blinded study samples. However, the full cycle of discovery, focused confirmation analysis, and hypothesis-testing for causality is achievable [67, 82, 83, 108]. Validation studies to determine the general applicability of each biomarker represent a more long-term commitment.

Good study design in toxicoproteomic experiments (or any omic experiment) would be expected to include multiple doses, several time points, positive and negative control compounds, nontoxic chemical isomers, single and multiple dosing, confirmation of results, validation in blinded samples, and many other considerations that are standard practice in good science. Such design considerations have not been evenly applied in many of the reviewed toxicoproteomic studies. These shortcomings should be interpreted to determine where we are with state-of-the-art toxicoproteomics. Long data analysis times in interpreting mass spectra, large data volumes per experiment, statistical analyses, and bioinformatics challenges in deriving biological meaning from complex datasets have made toxicoproteomic studies cumbersome and time consuming. The inability organize, integrate, and communicate data within organizations and across many laboratories [109] underscores the continuing need for international proteomic data standards [110], accessible databases [8], and proteoinformatic tools [111] to most efficiently extract biological meaning from toxicoproteomic experiments [112, 113].

25.9.3 Future Trends and Tools in Toxicoproteomics

Future trends in toxicoproteomic studies will see developments in several areas where special attributes of proteins can be exploited by proteomics in preclinical assessment. First, further refinements of tandem mass spectrometry with intimately integrated multidimensional separation schemes will continue to dominate proteomic analysis. MS instruments will become more accessible. A driving force is the complementary nature of LC/MALDI and LC/ESI tandem mass spectrometry platforms that provide increased proteome coverage for almost any sample to be analyzed [114].

Second, reduction of sample complexity or any prepurification strategy prior to toxicoproteomic analysis will be the most useful when innovatively applied to appropriate biological samples (e.g., immunodepletion of albumin, Igs in plasma) or research problem areas (e.g., phosphoprotein enrichment in protein signaling).

Third, Tier II proteomics will begin to be applied to four toxicoproteomic problem areas: (1) global and targeted protein phosphorylation [115–117], (a) chemoproteomics [118] using pharmaceuticals or enzyme substrates like ATP [119] as mass capture ligands for proteins, (3) protein–protein interactions via pull-down approaches [120, 121], and (4) the introduction of innovative, functional proteomic screens such as those recently reported for Fas ligand [122].

Fourth, an enormous opportunity for toxicoproteomics lies in exploiting accessible biofluids (i.e., serum/plasma, urine, and cerebrospinal fluid) for biomarker development [123]. These activities in toxicoproteomics might be combined with transcriptomic analysis of blood leukocytes for a parallel approach in biomarker discovery [124]. Furthermore, serum/plasma may be screened for autoantibodies responsible for adverse drug reactions by incubation of serum with protein autoantigens. Autoantibodies to aldolase B have been reported that might be partially responsible for troglitazone-induced liver dysfunction [125].

Fifth, the insightful use of genetically altered animals and cell models will enhance discovery of protein targets and mechanistic insights into adverse drug reactions. The following studies might serve as examples. Proteomic analysis has been used to study important protein differences in leptin deficient ob/ob mice [60] or growth hormone receptor knock-out mice [126]. Molecularly altered cell systems (i.e., siRNA, RNAi, gene mutated) are highly adaptable to toxicoproteomic analysis and discovery such as ATM deficient cell models used to find hnRNP as a p53-coactivator in DNA damage and repair [127]. Use of genetically susceptible animal strains [52] can be highly informative tools in toxicoproteomics such as the use of SJL-resistant and C57B1/6-susceptible mice to acetaminophen toxicity [52].

Finally, continued efforts for integration of proteomics, transcriptomics, and toxicology data to derive mechanistic insight and biomarkers will be a continuing goal to maximize return on the investment in omics technologies [24, 113, 128].

25.10   CONCLUSION

Challenges for toxicoproteomics in preclinical risk assessment are for use as a discovery tool for specific proteins affected by drug and toxicant action, for better understanding of biochemistry and cell biology, and for biomarker development. The discipline of proteome mapping will be a different and more complex enterprise from the high throughput, linear sequencing activities that have been so useful in mapping the human genome. While the mapping and measuring of attributes in any one proteome is a large undertaking, biofluid proteomes such as serum/plasma, urine, and CSF hold the most immediate promise for preclinical assessment in terms of better biomarkers.

Strides in improving proteomic technologies to map and measure proteomes and subproteomes are being made. However, no one proteomic platform appears ideally suited to quantify the broad range of protein expression in a given tissue, to distinguish the multiple forms and posttranslational modifications of proteins, to address the inadequate annotation of proteomes, or to accomplish integration of proteomic data with transcriptomic and metabolomic data. More than one proteomic platform may likely be needed for complex experimental problem areas. While 2D gels will always be a flexible and adaptable tool in toxicoproteomics, the ascendancy of liquid chromatography-based tandem mass spectrometry (LC-MS/MS) in its many and varied platforms will eclipse most gel-based proteomic platforms. Additionally, toxicoproteomic researchers should make effective use of transcriptomic data that in many cases may likely precede any toxicoproteomic analysis of tissues or blood. In fact, such transcriptomic studies may prove an invaluable guide to inform and guide toxicoproteomic studies of the relevant subproteome for analysis by identifying pathways and subcellular structures affected by toxicity as inferred by changes in the transcriptome. The further challenge lies in conducting the follow-up, hypothesis-driven studies that bring biological meaning to the data contained in lists of altered proteins, transcripts, and metabolites.

Although there are many challenges for toxicoproteomics in preclinical assessment, the opportunities are also close at hand for a greater understanding of toxicant action, the linkage to accompanying dysfunction and pathology, and the development of predictive biomarkers and signatures of toxicity.

ACKNOWLEDGMENTS

This work was supported by the Intramural Research Program of the NIH, National Institute of Environmental Health Sciences.

REFERENCES

1. Chapal N, Molina L, Molina F, Laplanche M, Pau B, Petit P. Pharmacoproteomic approach to the study of drug mode of action, toxicity, and resistance: applications in diabetes and cancer. *Fundam Clin Pharmacol* 2004;18:413–422.

2. Leighton JK. Application of emerging technologies in toxicology and safety assessment: regulatory perspectives. *Int J Toxicol* 2005;24:153–155.

3. Ross JS, Symmans WF, Pusztai L, Hortobagyi GN. Pharmacogenomics and clinical biomarkers in drug discovery and development. *Am J Clin Pathol* 2005;124(Suppl): S29–S41.

4. Siest G, Marteau JB, Maumus S, Berrahmoune H, Jeannesson E, Samara A, Batt AM, Visvikis-Siest S. Pharmacogenomics and cardiovascular drugs: need for integrated biological system with phenotypes and proteomic markers. *Eur J Pharmacol* 2005;527:1–22.

5. Bandara LR, Kennedy S. Toxicoproteomics—a new preclinical tool. *Drug Discov Today* 2002;7:411–418.

6. Petricoin EF, Rajapaske V, Herman EH, Arekani AM, Ross S, Johann D, Knapton A, Zhang J, Hitt BA, Conrads TP, Veenstra TD, Liotta LA, Sistare FD. Toxicoproteomics: serum proteomic pattern diagnostics for early detection of drug induced cardiac toxicities and cardioprotection. *Toxicol Pathol* 2004;32(Suppl 1):122–130.

7. Wetmore BA, Merrick BA. Toxicoproteomics: proteomics applied to toxicology and pathology. *Toxicol Pathol* 2004;32:619–642.

8. Waters MD, Fostel JM. Toxicogenomics and systems toxicology: aims and prospects. *Nat Rev Genet* 2004;5:936–948.

9. Turner SM. Stable isotopes, mass spectrometry, and molecular fluxes: applications to toxicology. *J Pharmacol Toxicol Methods* 2006;53:75–85.

10. Kasper P, Oliver G, Lima BS, Singer T, Tweats D. Joint EFPIA/CHMP SWP workshop: the emerging use of omic technologies for regulatory non-clinical safety testing. *Pharmacogenomics* 2005;6:181–184.

11. Gibbs A. Comparison of the specificity and sensitivity of traditional methods for assessment of nephrotoxicity in the rat with metabonomic and proteomic methodologies. *J Appl Toxicol* 2005;25:277–295.

12. Keller LC, Romijn EP, Zamora I, Yates JR, 3rd, Marshall WF. Proteomic analysis of isolated chlamydomonas centrioles reveals orthologs of ciliary-disease genes. *Curr Biol* 2005;15:1090–1098.

13. Kyttala M, Tallila J, Salonen R, Kopra O, Kohlschmidt N, Paavola-Sakki P, Peltonen LKestila M. MKS1, encoding a component of the flagellar apparatus basal body proteome, is mutated in Meckel syndrome. *Nat Genet* 2006;38:155–157.

14. Hackett JL, Gutman SI. Introduction to the Food and Drug Administration (FDA) regulatory process. *J Proteome Res* 2005;4:1110–1113.

15. MacGregor JT. The future of regulatory toxicology: impact of the biotechnology revolution. *Toxicol Sci* 2003;75:236–248.

16. Yeh ET. High-sensitivity C-reactive protein as a risk assessment tool for cardiovascular disease. *Clin Cardiol* 2005;28:408–412.

17. Amacher DE. A toxicologist's guide to biomarkers of hepatic response. *Hum Exp Toxicol* 2002;21:253–262.

18. Ross JS, Fletcher JA, Linette GP, Stec J, Clark E, Ayers M, Symmans WF, Pusztai L, Bloom KJ. The Her-2/neu gene and protein in breast cancer 2003: biomarker and target of therapy. *Oncologist* 2003;8:307–325.

19. Thier R, Bruning T, Roos PH, Rihs HP, Golka K, Ko Y, Bolt HM. Markers of genetic susceptibility in human environmental hygiene and toxicology: the role of selected CYP, NAT and GST genes. *Int J Hyg Environ Health* 2003;206:149–171.

20. Bilello JA. The agony and ecstasy of "OMIC" technologies in drug development. *Curr Mol Med* 2005;5:39–52.

21. Merrick BA, Bruno ME. Genomic and proteomic profiling for biomarkers and signature profiles of toxicity. *Curr Opin Mol Ther* 2004;6:600–607.

22. Koop R. Combinatorial biomarkers: from early toxicology assays to patient population profiling. *Drug Discov Today* 2005;10:781–788.

23. Merrick BA. Introduction to high-throughput protein expression. In Hamadeh HK, Afshari CA, (Eds). *Toxicogenomics: Principles and Applications*. Hoboken, NJ: Wiley; 2004, pp 263–281.

24. Merrick BA, Madenspacher JH. Complementary gene and protein expression studies and integrative approaches in toxicogenomics. *Toxicol Appl Pharmacol* 2005; 207:189–194.

25. Righetti PG, Castagna A, Antonucci F, Piubelli C, Cecconi D, Campostrini N, Antonioli P, Astner H, Hamdan M. Critical survey of quantitative proteomics in two-dimensional electrophoretic approaches. *J Chromatogr A*, 2004;1051:3–17.

26. Freeman WM, Hemby SE. Proteomics for protein expression profiling in neuroscience. *Neurochem Res* 2004;29:1065–1081.

27. Yates JR. Mass spectral analysis in proteomics. *Annu Rev Biophys Biomol Struct* 2004;33:297–316.

28. Bhat VB, Choi MH, Wishnok JS, Tannenbaum SR. Comparative plasma proteome analysis of lymphoma-bearing SJL mice. *J Proteome Res* 2005;4:1814–1825.

29. Farkas D, Bhat VB, Mandapati S, Wishnok JS, Tannenbaum SR. Characterization of the secreted proteome of rat hepatocytes cultured in collagen sandwiches. *Chem Res Toxicol* 2005;18:1132–1139.

30. Macdonald N, Chevalier S, Tonge R, Davison M, Rowlinson R, Young J, Rayner S, Roberts R. Quantitative proteomic analysis of mouse liver response to the peroxisome proliferator diethylhexylphthalate (DEHP) *Arch Toxicol* 2001;75:415–424.

31. Petricoin E, Wulfkuhle J, Espina V, Liotta LA. Clinical proteomics: revolutionizing disease detection and patient tailoring therapy. *J Proteome Res* 2004;3:209–217.

32. Issaq HJ, Conrads TP, Prieto DA, Tirumalai R, Veenstra TD. SELDI-TOF MS for diagnostic proteomics. *Anal Chem* 2003;75:148A–155A.

33. Diamandis EP. Mass spectrometry as a diagnostic and a cancer biomarker discovery tool: opportunities and potential limitations. *Mol Cell Proteomics* 2004;3:367–378.

34. Cutler P. Protein arrays: the current state-of-the-art. *Proteomics* 2003;3:3–18.

35. Park BK, Kitteringham NR, Maggs JL, Pirmohamed M, Williams DP. The role of metabolic activation in drug-induced hepatotoxicity. *Annu Rev Pharmacol Toxicol* 2005;45:177–202.

36. Kaplowitz N. Drug-induced liver injury. *Clin Infect Dis* 2004;38(Suppl 2):S44–S48.

37. Maddrey WC. Drug-induced hepatotoxicity: 2005. *J Clin Gastroenterol* 2005;39:S83–S89.

38. Steiner G, Suter L, Boess F, Gasser R, de Vera MC, Albertini S, Ruepp S. Discriminating different classes of toxicants by transcript profiling. *Environ Health Perspect* 2004;112:1236–1248.

39. Kon K, Kim JS, Jaeschke H, Lemasters JJ. Mitochondrial permeability transition in acetaminophen-induced necrosis and apoptosis of cultured mouse hepatocytes. *Hepatology* 2004;40:1170–1179.

40. Amacher DE. Drug-associated mitochondrial toxicity and its detection. *Curr Med Chem* 2005;12:1829–1839.

41. Ishida Y, Kondo T, Tsuneyama K, Lu P, Takayasu T, Mukaida N. The pathogenic roles of tumor necrosis factor receptor p55 in acetaminophen-induced liver injury in mice. *J Leukoc Biol* 2004;75:59–67.

42. Ito Y, Bethea NW, Abril ER, McCuskey RS. Early hepatic microvascular injury in response to acetaminophen toxicity. *Microcirculation* 2003;10:391–400.

43. James LP, Simpson PM, Farrar HC, Kearns GL, Wasserman GS, Blumer JL, Reed MD, Sullivan JE, Hinson JA. Cytokines and toxicity in acetaminophen overdose. *J Clin Pharmacol* 2005;45:1165–1171.

44. Laskin DL, Laskin JD. Role of macrophages and inflammatory mediators in chemically induced toxicity. *Toxicology* 2001;160:111–118.

45. Liu ZX, Govindarajan S, Kaplowitz N. Innate immune system plays a critical role in determining the progression and severity of acetaminophen hepatotoxicity. *Gastroenterology* 2004;127:1760–1774.

46. Fountoulakis M, Berndt P, Boelsterli UA, Crameri F, Winter M, Albertini S, Suter L. Two-dimensional database of mouse liver proteins: changes in hepatic protein levels following treatment with acetaminophen or its nontoxic regioisomer 3-acetamidophenol. *Electrophoresis* 2000;21:2148–2161.

47. Tonge R, Shaw J, Middleton B, Rowlinson R, Rayner S, Young J, Pognan F, Hawkins E, Currie I, Davison M. Validation and development of fluorescence two-dimensional differential gel electrophoresis proteomics technology. *Proteomics* 2001;1:377–396.

48. Ruepp SU, Tonge RP, Shaw J, Wallis N, Pognan F. Genomics and proteomics analysis of acetaminophen toxicity in mouse liver. *Toxicol Sci* 2002;65:135–150.

49. Thome-Kromer B, Bonk I, Klatt M, Nebrich G, Taufmann M, Bryant S, Wacker U, Kopke A. Toward the identification of liver toxicity markers: a proteome study in human cell culture and rats. *Proteomics* 2003;3:1835–1862.

50. Kikkawa R, Yamamoto T, Fukushima T, Yamada H, Horii I. Investigation of a hepatotoxicity screening system in primary cell cultures—what biomarkers would need to be addressed to estimate toxicity in conventional and new approaches? *J Toxicol Sci* 2005;30:61–72.

51. Yamamoto T, Kikkawa R, Yamada H, Horii I. Identification of oxidative stress-related proteins for predictive screening of hepatotoxicity using a proteomic approach. *J Toxicol Sci* 2005;30:213–227.

52. Welch KD, Wen B, Goodlett DR, Yi EC, Lee H, Reilly TP, Nelson SD, Pohl LR. Proteomic identification of potential susceptibility factors in drug-induced liver disease. *Chem Res Toxicol* 2005;18:924–933.

53. Lee H, Yi EC, Wen B, Reily TP, Pohl L, Nelson S, Aebersold R, Goodlett DR. Optimization of reversed-phase microcapillary liquid chromatography for quantitative proteomics. *J Chromatogr B Analyt Technol Biomed Life Sci* 2004;803:101–110.

54. Weber LW, Boll M, Stampfl A. Hepatotoxicity and mechanism of action of haloalkanes: carbon tetrachloride as a toxicological model. *Crit Rev Toxicol* 2003;33:105–136.

55. Liu Y, Liu P, Liu CH, Hu YY, Xu LM, Mu YP, Du GL. [Proteomic analysis of proliferation and apoptosis in carbon tetrachloride induced rat liver fibrosis]. *Zhonghua Gan Zang Bing Za Zhi* 2005;13:563–566.

56. Nelson SD. Mechanisms of the formation and disposition of reactive metabolites that can cause acute liver injury. *Drug Metab Rev* 1995;27:147–177.

57. Heijne WH, Stierum RH, Slijper M, van Bladeren PJ, Van Ommen B. Toxicogenomics of bromobenzene hepatotoxicity: a combined transcriptomics and proteomics approach. *Biochem Pharmacol* 2003;65:857–875.

58. Staels B, Fruchart JC. Therapeutic roles of peroxisome proliferator-activated receptor agonists. *Diabetes* 2005;54:2460–2470.

59. Iida M, Anna CH, Hartis J, Bruno M, Wetmore B, Dubin JR, Sieber S, Bennett L, Cunningham ML, Paules RS, Tomer KB, Houle CD, Merrick AB, Sills RC, Devereux TR. Changes in global gene and protein expression during early mouse liver carcinogenesis induced by non-genotoxic model carcinogens oxazepam and Wyeth-14,643. *Carcinogenesis* 2003;24:757–770.

60. Edvardsson U, von Lowenhielm HB, Panfilov O, Nystrom AC, Nilsson F, Dahllof B. Hepatic protein expression of lean mice and obese diabetic mice treated with peroxisome proliferator-activated receptor activators. *Proteomics* 2003;3:468–478.

61. Richards VE, Chau B, White MR, McQueen CA. Hepatic gene expression and lipid homeostasis in C57BL/6 mice exposed to hydrazine or acetylhydrazine. *Toxicol Sci* 2004;82:318–332.

62. Kleno TG, Kiehr B, Baunsgaard D, Sidelmann UG. Combination of "omics" data to investigate the mechanism(s) of hydrazine-induced hepatotoxicity in rats and to identify potential biomarkers. *Biomarkers* 2004;9:116–138.

63. Kleno TG, Leonardsen LR, Kjeldal HO, Laursen SM, Jensen ON, Baunsgaard D. Mechanisms of hydrazine toxicity in rat liver investigated by proteomics and multivariate data analysis. *Proteomics* 2004;4:868–880.

64. Chilakapati J, Shankar K, Korrapati MC, Hill RA, Mehendale HM. Saturation toxicokinetics of thioacetamide: role in initiation of liver injury. *Drug Metab Dispos* 2005;33:1877–1885.

65. Low TY, Leow CK, Salto-Tellez M, Chung MC. A proteomic analysis of thioacetamide-induced hepatotoxicity and cirrhosis in rat livers. *Proteomics* 2004;4:3960–3974.

66. Xu XQ, Leow CK, Lu X, Zhang X, Liu JS, Wong WH, Asperger A, Deininger S, Eastwood Leung HC. Molecular classification of liver cirrhosis in a rat model by proteomics and bioinformatics. *Proteomics* 2004;4:3235–3245.

67. Kawada N, Kristensen DB, Asahina K, Nakatani K, Minamiyama Y, Seki S, Yoshizato K. Characterization of a stellate cell activation-associated protein (STAP) with peroxidase activity found in rat hepatic stellate cells. *J Biol Chem* 2001;276:25318–25323.

68. Omenn GS, States DJ, Adamski M, Blackwell TW, Menon R, Hermjakob H, Apweiler R, Haab BB, Simpson RJ, Eddes JS, Kapp EA, Moritz RL, Chan DW, Rai AJ, Admon A, Aebersold R, Eng J, Hancock WS, Hefta SA, Meyer H, Paik YK, Yoo JS, Ping P, Pounds J, Adkins J, Qian X, Wang R, Wasinger V, Wu CY, Zhao X, Zeng R, Archakov A, Tsugita A, Beer I, Pandey A, Pisano M, Andrews P, Tammen H, Speicher DW, Hanash SM. Overview of the HUPO Plasma Proteome Project: results from the pilot phase with 35 collaborating laboratories and multiple analytical groups, generating a core dataset of 3020 proteins and a publicly-available database. *Proteomics* 2005;5:3226–3245.

69. Ping P, Vondriska TM, Creighton CJ, Gandhi TK, Yang Z, Menon R, Kwon MS, Cho SY, Drwal G, Kellmann M, Peri S, Suresh S, Gronborg M, Molina H, Chaerkady R, Rekha B, Shet AS, Gerszten RE, Wu H, Raftery M, Wasinger V, Schulz-Knappe P, Hanash SM, Paik YK, Hancock WS, States DJ, Omenn GS, Pandey A. A functional annotation of subproteomes in human plasma. *Proteomics* 2005;5:3506–3519.

70. Duan X, Yarmush DM, Berthiaume F, Jayaraman A, Yarmush ML. A mouse serum two-dimensional gel map: application to profiling burn injury and infection. *Electrophoresis* 2004;25:3055–3065.

71. Gianazza E, Eberini I, Villa P, Fratelli M, Pinna C, Wait R, Gemeiner M, Miller I. Monitoring the effects of drug treatment in rat models of disease by serum protein analysis. *J Chromatogr B Analyt Technol Biomed Life Sci* 2002;771:107–130.

72. Duan X, Yarmush D, Berthiaume F, Jayaraman A, Yarmush ML. Immunodepletion of albumin for two-dimensional gel detection of new mouse acute-phase protein and other plasma proteins. *Proteomics* 2005;5:3991–4000.

73. Wait R, Chiesa G, Parolini C, Miller I, Begum S, Brambilla D, Galluccio L, Ballerio R, Eberini I, Gianazza E. Reference maps of mouse serum acute-phase proteins: changes with LPS-induced inflammation and apolipoprotein A-I and A-II transgenes. *Proteomics* 2005;5:4245–4253.

74. Amacher DE, Adler R, Herath A, Townsend RR. Use of proteomic methods to identify serum biomarkers associated with rat liver toxicity or hypertrophy. *Clin Chem* 2005;51:1796–1803.

75. Witzmann FA, Li J. Proteomics and nephrotoxicity. *Contrib Nephrol* 2004;141:104–123.

76. Davis JW, Kramer JA. Genomic-based biomarkers of drug-induced nephrotoxicity. *Expert Opin Drug Metab Toxicol* 2006;2:95–101.

77. Mihatsch MJ, Thiel G, Ryffel B. Cyclosporin A: action and side-effects. *Toxicol Lett* 1989;46:125–139.

78. Benito B, Wahl D, Steudel N, Cordier A, Steiner S. Effects of cyclosporine A on the rat liver and kidney protein pattern, and the influence of vitamin E and C coadministration. *Electrophoresis* 1995;16:1273–1283.

79. Steiner S, Aicher L, Raymackers J, Meheus L, Esquer-Blasco R, Anderson NL, Cordier A. Cyclosporine A decreases the protein level of the calcium-binding protein calbindin-D 28 kDa in rat kidney. *Biochem Pharmacol* 1996;51:253–258.

80. Lee CT, Huynh VM, Lai LW, Lien YH. Cyclosporine A-induced hypercalciuria in calbindin-D28k knockout and wild-type mice. *Kidney Int* 2002;62:2055–2061.

81. Serkova N, Christians U. Transplantation: toxicokinetics and mechanisms of toxicity of cyclosporine and macrolides. *Curr Opin Investig Drugs* 2003;4:1287–1296.

82. Mascarell L, Frey JR, Michel F, Lefkovits I, Truffa-Bachi P. Increased protein synthesis after T cell activation in presence of cyclosporin A. *Transplantation* 2000;70:340–348.

83. Mascarell L, Auger R, Alcover A, Ojcius DM, Jungas T, Cadet-Daniel V, Kanellopoulos JM, Truffa-Bachi P. Characterization of a gene encoding two isoforms of a mitochondrial protein up-regulated by cyclosporin A in activated T cells. *J Biol Chem* 2004;279:10556–10563.

84. Guan N, Ding J, Deng J, Zhang J, Yang J. Key molecular events in puromycin aminonucleoside nephrosis rats. *Pathol Int* 2004;54:703–711.

85. Sundin DP, Meyer C, Dahl R, Geerdes A, Sandoval R, Molitoris BA. Cellular mechanism of aminoglycoside tolerance in long-term gentamicin treatment. *Am J Physiol* 1997;272:C1309–C1318.

86. Witzmann FA, Fultz CD, Grant RA, Wright LS, Kornguth SE, Siegel FL. Differential expression of cytosolic proteins in the rat kidney cortex and medulla: preliminary proteomics. *Electrophoresis* 1998;19:2491–2497.

87. Shakib K, Norman JT, Fine LG, Brown LR, Godovac-Zimmermann J. Proteomics profiling of nuclear proteins for kidney fibroblasts suggests hypoxia, meiosis, and cancer may meet in the nucleus. *Proteomics* 2005;5:2819–2838.

88. Charlwood J, Skehel JM, King N, Camilleri P, Lord P, Bugelski P, Atif U. Proteomic analysis of rat kidney cortex following treatment with gentamicin. *J Proteome Res* 2002;1:73–82.

89. Thongboonkerd V, Klein JB, Arthur JM. Proteomic identification of a large complement of rat urinary proteins. *Nephron Exp Nephrol* 2003;95:e69–e78.

90. Cutler P, Bell DJ, Birrell HC, Connelly JC, Connor SC, Holmes E, Mitchell BC, Monte SY, Neville BA, Pickford R, Polley S, Schneider K, Skehel JM. An integrated proteomic approach to studying glomerular nephrotoxicity. *Electrophoresis* 1999;20:3647–3658.

91. Crowe CA, Yong AC, Calder IC, Ham KN, Tange JD. The nephrotoxicity of *p*-aminophenol. I. The effect on microsomal cytochromes, glutathione and covalent binding in kidney and liver. *Chem Biol Interact* 1979;27:235–243.

92. Kaltenbach JP, Carone FA, Ganote CE. Compounds protective against renal tubular necrosis induced by D-serine and D-2,3-diaminopropionic acid in the rat. *Exp Mol Pathol* 1982;37:225–234.

93. Kuhlmann MK, Horsch E, Burkhardt G, Wagner M, Kohler H. Reduction of cisplatin toxicity in cultured renal tubular cells by the bioflavonoid quercetin. *Arch Toxicol* 1998;72:536–540.

94. Bandara LR, Kelly MD, Lock EA, Kennedy S. A correlation between a proteomic evaluation and conventional measurements in the assessment of renal proximal tubular toxicity. *Toxicol Sci* 2003;73:195–206.

95. Bandara LR, Kelly MD, Lock EA, Kennedy S. A potential biomarker of kidney damage identified by proteomics: preliminary findings. *Biomarkers* 2003;8:272–286.

96. Chen JC, Stevens JL, Trifillis AL, Jones TW. Renal cysteine conjugate beta-lyase-mediated toxicity studied with primary cultures of human proximal tubular cells. *Toxicol Appl Pharmacol* 1990;103:463–473.

97. Lash LH, Qian W, Putt DA, Hueni SE, Elfarra AA, Krause RJ, Parker JC. Renal and hepatic toxicity of trichloroethylene and its glutathione-derived metabolites in rats and mice: sex-, species-, and tissue-dependent differences. *J Pharmacol Exp Ther* 2001;297:155–164.

98. Gao J, Ann Garulacan L, Storm SM, Hefta SA, Opiteck GJ, Lin JH, Moulin F, Dambach DM. Identification of *in vitro* protein biomarkers of idiosyncratic liver toxicity. *Toxicol In Vitro* 2004;18:533–541.

99. Meneses-Lorente G, Guest PC, Lawrence J, Muniappa N, Knowles MR, Skynner HA, Salim K, Cristea I, Mortishire-Smith R, Gaskell SJ, Watt A. A proteomic investigation of drug-induced steatosis in rat liver. *Chem Res Toxicol* 2004;17:605–612.

100. Sheta EA, Appel SH, Goldknopf IL. 2D gel blood serum biomarkers reveal differential clinical proteomics of the neurodegenerative diseases. *Expert Rev Proteomics* 2006;3:45–62.

101. Vercauteren FG, Bergeron JJ, Vandesande F, Arckens L, Quirion R. Proteomic approaches in brain research and neuropharmacology. *Eur J Pharmacol* 2004;500:385–398.

102. Merten KE, Feng W, Zhang L, Pierce W, Cai J, Klein JB, Kang YJ. Modulation of cytochrome C oxidase-va is possibly involved in metallothionein protection from doxorubicin cardiotoxicity. *J Pharmacol Exp Ther* 2005;315:1314–1319.

103. Elased KM, Cool DR, Morris M. Novel mass spectrometric methods for evaluation of plasma angiotensin converting enzyme 1 and renin activity. *Hypertension* 2005; 46:953–959.

104. Yamamoto T, Fukushima T, Kikkawa R, Yamada H, Horii I. Protein expression analysis of rat testes induced testicular toxicity with several reproductive toxicants. *J Toxicol Sci* 2005;30:111–126.

105. Yang YH, Xi ZG, Chao FH, Yang DF. Effects of formaldehyde inhalation on lung of rats. *Biomed Environ Sci* 2005;18:164–168.

106. Wheelock AM, Boland BC, Isbell M, Morin D, Wegesser TC, Plopper CG, Buckpitt AR. *In vivo* effects of ozone exposure on protein adduct formation by 1-nitronaphthalene in rat lung. *Am J Respir Cell Mol Biol* 2005;33:130–137.

107. Wheelock AM, Zhang L, Tran MU, Morin D, Penn S, Buckpitt AR, Plopper CG. Isolation of rodent airway epithelial cell proteins facilitates *in vivo* proteomics studies of lung toxicity. *Am J Physiol Lung Cell Mol Physiol* 2004;286:L399–L410.

108. de Graauw M, TijDens I, Cramer R, Corless S, Timms JF, van De Water B. Heat shock protein 27 is the major differentially phosphorylated protein involved in renal epithelial cellular stress response and controls focal adhesion organization and apoptosis. *J Biol Chem* 2005;280:29885–29898.

109. Rauch A, Bellew M, Eng J, Fitzgibbon M, Holzman T, Hussey P, Igra M, Maclean B, Lin CW, Detter A, Fang R, Faca V, Gafken P, Zhang H, Whitaker J, States D, Hanash S, Paulovich A, McIntosh MW. Computational Proteomics Analysis System (CPAS): an extensible, open-source analytic system for evaluating and publishing proteomic data and high throughput biological experiments. *J Proteome Res* 2006;5:112–121.

110. Orchard S, Hermjakob H, Julian RK Jr, Runte K, Sherman D, Wojcik J, Zhu W, Apweiler R. Common interchange standards for proteomics data: public availability of tools and schema. *Proteomics* 2004;4:490–491.

111. Hamady M, Cheung TH, Resing K, Cios KJ, Knight R. Key challenges in proteomics and proteoinformatics. Progress in proteins. *IEEE Eng Med Biol Mag* 2005;24:34–40.

112. Ekins S, Nikolsky Y, Nikolskaya T. Techniques: application of systems biology to absorption, distribution, metabolism, excretion and toxicity. *Trends Pharmacol Sci* 2005; 26:202–209.

113. Quackenbush J. Extracting meaning from functional genomics experiments. *Toxicol Appl Pharmacol* 2005;207:195–199.

114. Bodnar WM, Blackburn RK, Krise JM, Moseley MA. Exploiting the complementary nature of LC/MALDI/MS/MS and LC/ESI/MS/MS for increased proteome coverage. *J Am Soc Mass Spectrom* 2003;14:971–979.

115. Collins MO, Yu L, Husi H, Blackstock WP, Choudhary JS, Grant SG. Robust enrichment of phosphorylated species in complex mixtures by sequential protein and peptide metal-affinity chromatography and analysis by tandem mass spectrometry. *Sci STKE* 2005;16.

116. Kim SY, Chudapongse N, Lee SM, Levin MC, Oh JT, Park HJ, Ho IK. Proteomic analysis of phosphotyrosyl proteins in the rat brain: effect of butorphanol dependence. *J Neurosci Res* 2004;77:867–877.

117. Wang M, Xiao GG, Li N, Xie Y, Loo JA, Nel AE. Use of a fluorescent phosphoprotein dye to characterize oxidative stress-induced signaling pathway components in macrophage and epithelial cultures exposed to diesel exhaust particle chemicals. *Electrophoresis* 2005;26:2092–2108.

118. Gagna CE, Winokur D, Clark Lambert W. Cell biology, chemogenomics and chemoproteomics. *Cell Biol Int* 2004;28:755–764.

119. Beillard E, Witte ON. Unraveling kinase signaling pathways with chemical genetic and chemical proteomic approaches. *Cell Cycle* 2005;4:434–437.

120. Brandt M, Madsen JC, Bunkenborg J, Jensen ON, Gammeltoft S, Jensen KJ. On-bead chemical synthesis and display of phosphopeptides for affinity pull-down proteomics. *Chembiochem* 2006;7:623–630.

121. Uhlen M, Ponten F. Antibody-based proteomics for human tissue profiling. *Mol Cell Proteomics* 2005;4:384–393.

122. Hauptschein RS, Sloan KE, Torella C, Moezzifard R, Giel-Moloney M, Zehetmeier C, Unger C, Ilag LL, Jay DG. Functional proteomic screen identifies a modulating role for CD44 in death receptor-mediated apoptosis. *Cancer Res* 2005;65:1887–1896.

123. Gao J, Garulacan LA, Storm SM, Opiteck GJ, Dubaquie Y, Hefta SA, Dambach DM, Dongre AR. Biomarker discovery in biological fluids. *Methods* 2005;35:291–302.

124. Merrick BA, Tomer KB. Toxicoproteomics: a parallel approach to identifying biomarkers. *Environ Health Perspect* 2003;111:A578–A579.

125. Maniratanachote R, Shibata A, Kaneko S, Yamamori I, Wakasugi T, Sawazaki T, Katoh K, Tokudome S, Nakajima M, Yokoi T. Detection of autoantibody to aldolase B in sera from patients with troglitazone-induced liver dysfunction. *Toxicology* 2005;216:15–23.

126. Beyea JA, Sawicki G, Olson DM, List E, Kopchick JJ, Harvey S. Growth hormone (GH) receptor knockout mice reveal actions of GH in lung development. *Proteomics* 2006;6:341–348.

127. Moumen A, Masterson P, O'Connor MJ, Jackson SP. hnRNP K: an HDM2 target and transcriptional coactivator of p53 in response to DNA damage. *Cell* 2005; 123:1065–1078.

128. Fostel J, Choi D, Zwickl C, Morrison N, Rashid A, Hasan A, Bao W, Richard A, Tong W, Bushel PR, Brown R, Bruno M, Cunningham ML, Dix D, Eastin W, Frade C, Garcia A, Heinloth A, Irwin R, Madenspacher J, Merrick BA, Papoian T, Paules R, Rocca-Serra

P, Sansone AS, Stevens J, Tomer K, Yang C, Waters M. Chemical effects in biological systems—data dictionary (CEBS-DD): a compendium of terms for the capture and integration of biological study design description, conventional phenotypes, and omics data. *Toxicol Sci* 2005;88:585–601.

129. Kristensen DB, Kawada N, Imamura K, Miyamoto Y, Tateno C, Seki S, Kuroki T, Yoshizato K. Proteome analysis of rat hepatic stellate cells. *Hepatology* 2000;32:268–277.

130. Reinheckel T, Korn S, Mohring S, Augustin W, Halangk W, Schild L. Adaptation of protein carbonyl detection to the requirements of proteome analysis demonstrated for hypoxia/reoxygenation in isolated rat liver mitochondria. *Arch Biochem Biophys* 2000;376:59–65.

131. Witzmann FA, Fultz CD, Grant RA, Wright LS, Kornguth SE, Siegel FL. Regional protein alterations in rat kidneys induced by lead exposure. *Electrophoresis* 1999;20:943–951.

26

REGULATORY CONSIDERATIONS

Evan B. Siegel[1] and Duane B. Lakings[2]

[1]*Ground Zero Pharmaceuticals, Inc., Irvine, California*
[2]*Drug Safety Evaluation Consulting, Inc., Elgin, Texas*

Contents

Preclinical Development Handbook: Toxicology, edited by Shayne Cox Gad
Copyright © 2008 John Wiley & Sons, Inc.

26.1   THE STRATEGIC PRECLINICAL PLAN: AN INTEGRAL ELEMENT IN THE FDA PRE-IND CONSULTATION PROCESS

The advent of new approaches to small organic molecule (novel chemical entity or NCE) and macromolecule (biological) development, particularly in the biotechnological arena, has provided new opportunities for treatment and prevention of human disease, which has a major impact on patients, the healthcare system, and human productivity. The rapidly increasing cost (both in time and other resources) of new product development has led to unprecedented pressures on sponsors to move their programs from the discovery laboratory through preclinical testing and into human clinical trials.

Sponsors often find it difficult to incorporate formidable intellectual property into the realities of new product development, including the need to perform a logical, efficient, and targeted preclinical development program that effectively characterizes the drug-like attributes of drug candidates and may identify undesirable properties (i.e., demerits) that can prevent successful development. We see many new product failures in Phase III clinical trials, in some cases because poor planning and/or poorly designed preclinical work has been performed prior to the initiation of first-in-human or Phase I clinical trials. Since drug candidates that eventually fail during Phase II or Phase III clinical trials may have already cost sponsors $50–100 million (U.S.) or more, we need to ask ourselves whether a more intensive (not necessarily extensive) preclinical development testing plan could have resulted in early decisions to discontinue drug candidates in late discovery (i.e., discovery lead optimization or developability assessment), preclinical development, or early (Phase I) clinical phases, for which far smaller amounts of precious funding and other resources (personnel time and facilities) will have been spent. We suggest that sponsors, sponsor consultants, contract research organizations (CROs), and advisors undertake preclinical strategic planning for development programs before decisions are made (or not made) that might avoid these later clinical trial phase new product failures.

One approach is to enter into "pre-pre-IND" strategic preclinical discussions with the FDA, before beginning the formal pre-IND preclinical safety (toxicology and pharmacokinetic) studies that often lead to the officially sanctioned pre-IND and IND processes. Informal telephone conversations, submission of small amounts of summary pharmacology, pharmacokinetic, and toxicology data for FDA review, and skeletal proposals for strategic preclinical study plans can be accomplished by agreement with FDA Regulatory Project Managers and Reviewers. The FDA has launched its own initiatives to informally discuss new product development in the early preclinical stage, even before provisional products move into clinical trials via an IND. Sometimes a sponsor assumes that only limited animal pharmacology studies for "proof of principle" and perhaps one or two toxicology studies are needed prior to initiation of human clinical trials. In fact, the preclinical development program may require (usually does require) support from other study types, such as cross-reactivity, safety pharmacology, toxicokinetics, metabolism, genotoxicity and/or immunogenicity, and other development disciplines, such as manufacturing and clinical: in other words, a more sophisticated and detailed preclinical approach. In other situations, the sponsor may be under the misconception that he/she has to embark on a multimillion dollar preclinical development program, with the generation of reams of data and multiple publications, prior to planning a first-in-human clinical trial. By planning strategically, approaching the FDA early, receiving advice, and putting this advice into practice for a relatively modest expenditure of time and money, the overall development program for a drug candidate may well have a very smooth entry into preclinical development and/or early clinical development.

Since oncology NCEs and biologicals represent a significant percentage of those new products entering preclinical development and clinical trials and are projected to treat a life-threatening human disease (i.e., various types of cancer) for which safe and effective pharmaceutical products are not yet available, sponsors feel a great deal of urgency to move these novel drug candidates quickly into human clinical testing. This chapter uses oncology products as examples that can benefit from strategic preclinical development planning. The considerations included are generally applicable to all new product development programs and we cite regulatory guidances (FDA Guidance for Industry and International Conference on Harmonization (ICH) guidelines) that sponsors can (should) use for preparing a drug development plan and in the design of recommended preclinical studies for the effective characterization of drug candidates.

Several categories of preclinical issues and the associated studies to investigate these issues need to be considered for all NCE and biologicals development programs, including those involving biotechnologically derived active drug substances. A careful review of the specific "flags" for potential clinical safety that might be related to the particular chemical structure, mechanisms of action (if known), or other characteristics of the drug substance will allow the development team to focus on the preclinical development program that will best support a rapid movement of the NCE or biological into human trials. Key preclinical development considerations are discussed in the following sections, which are followed by short sections on preclinical development considerations for the manufacture of drug substance and proposed drug product and for the clinical aspects for submitting an IND for a first-in-human clinical trial.

26.2 PHARMACOLOGY

26.2.1 Primary and Secondary Pharmacodynamics

We recommend that sponsors consider the following when discovery and preclinical pharmacology development studies are designed and conducted to fully evaluate and characterize the pharmacological profiles of active antitumor agents:

- Antitumor animal models evaluated should explore the establishment of a disciplined dose–response relationship as well as the identification of a dose giving maximum biological activity, particularly if a safety margin for significant antitumor activity in animals cannot be established against the no observable adverse effect level (NOAEL) in the same animal species during toxicology studies (discussed later).
- A tissue specificity evaluation to determine if the active pharmaceutical ingredient (API) or drug candidate interacts with (i.e., binds to) specialized tissues such as vascular endothelium from various species, including humans. The

results from this research effort will assist in defining and confirming toxicology animal species that are relevant to humans as the development program unfolds.

- If the drug or biological candidate is expected to cause adverse effects in humans with inflammatory disorders and an appropriate animal model of inflammation is available, we recommend that the provisional product be evaluated in that model.

26.2.2 Safety Pharmacology

The ICH S7a guideline [1] recommends that a standard battery of safety pharmacology (SP) studies be conducted prior to the initiation of clinical trials on a new drug substance. This standard battery normally includes cardiovascular, central nervous system (CNS), and respiratory SP studies to investigate potential undesirable pharmacological effects of a drug substance on physiological functions in relation to exposure in the projected therapeutic range and above. The cardiovascular SP study should be designed to evaluate the potential to cause prolongation of the QT interval (as discussed in the ICH S7b guideline [2]), an area of concern for both the FDA and ICH primarily for NCEs but also for macromolecules.

For drug candidates intended to act in or be delivered via the gastrointestinal (GI) system (i.e., orally administered compounds), additional work should be performed exploring safety for the GI system, including effects on GI motility. Other SP studies that sponsors will need to consider (depending on the characteristics of the drug candidate) include effects on the renal/urinary system for drug candidates and/or their known metabolites cleared from the body by the kidney and on the autonomic nervous system for drug candidates that may have undesirable effects on the autonomic nerves. For drug candidates to be administered as part of a combination therapeutic regimen that contains an oncologic drug known to have adverse effects on the autonomic nervous system (i.e., platinum-containing compounds), SP studies should be designed to evaluate potential undesirable effects to the autonomic nervous system by the drug candidate alone and in combination with the agent known to produce adverse effects in this system.

26.3 PHARMACOKINETICS

We recommend that pharmacokinetic (PK) studies be conducted in the animal species to be evaluated in toxicology studies conducted in compliance with Good Laboratory Practice (GLP) regulations (as described in the Code of Federal Regulations, 21 CFR Part 58) and over the dose range proposed for these toxicology studies. These animal PK studies should be designed to evaluate the proposed clinical route of administration and, if possible, intravenous (IV) dosing to assess the absolute bioavailability (commonly referred to as F) of a drug candidate to be administered by a route other than IV. If appropriately designed, toxicokinetic (TK) evaluations during the subchronic and other toxicology studies may be sufficient to describe the PK profile of the NCE or biological in these animal species. This planning can save sponsors both time and funding. The ICH S3a guideline [3] on toxicokinetics can be referenced for further information on this topic. However, if a drug candidate has limited absorption into systemic circulation after a non-IV route of administration, we recommend that sponsors design and conduct animal PK studies to evaluate the rate and extent of delivery (i.e., the delivery profile) and to obtain information on the delivery characteristics of possible drug candidate formulations. These animal PK studies should be conducted prior to starting the toxicology studies needed for supporting human clinical trials so that drug candidate formulation that provides the desired delivery profile (and the one proposed for use in human trials) can be evaluated in the toxicology studies, thus allowing these animal safety studies to support the proposed first-in-human clinical trial.

26.3.1   Methods of Analysis: Bioanalytical Chemistry Method Development and Validation

Bioanalytical chemistry (BAC) methods for the pharmacologically active drug substance (i.e., parent compound and/or its metabolites, if known) in physiological fluids (e.g., serum/plasma and urine) from each toxicology species (e.g., rat, dog, nonhuman primate) will need to be developed and appropriately validated to provide TK support for toxicology studies and to analyze specimens collected during animal PK evaluations. The developed BAC method, after appropriate intermatrix and interspecies validation, can also be used to support human clinical trials. The *FDA Guidance to Industry: Bioanalytical Method Validation* [4] provides information on the various aspects and parameters (e.g., specificity, sensitivity, linearity, accuracy, precision, and stability) considered necessary to appropriately validate a BAC method.

26.3.2   ADME

In general, nonclinical ADME studies include protein binding, mass balance (including metabolite profiling, isolation, and identification, and metabolite pathway definition and comparison for various species, including humans), single- and possibly multiple-dose tissue distribution in a rodent (usually rats) species, special TK studies to support reproductive and developmental toxicology (reproductive toxicity) studies in a rodent (usually rats) and nonrodent (commonly rabbits) species, evaluation of the potential inhibition or induction of various drug metabolizing enzymes (particularly CYP450 isozymes such as CYP3A4, CYP2C9, CYP2D6), and possibly PK evaluations of metabolites (especially metabolites that have pharmacological or toxicological activity). Many of these ADME studies require an appropriately radiolabeled drug candidate. Where possible, the sponsor should prepare, or have prepared, a carbon-14 radiolabeled drug candidate in order to conduct these nonclinical ADME studies and also to be used in a possible mass balance study in humans (which is considered necessary in order to obtain the physiological samples for comparing the extent of metabolism and the metabolic profiles of a drug candidate in the toxicology animal species and in humans). However, not all these nonclinical ADME studies are necessary for the preclinical (e.g., prior to the first-in-human clinical trial) evaluation of a drug candidate. Sponsors normally conduct *in vitro* metabolism and protein binding studies in the projected toxicology animal species and in humans and mass balance assessments with metabolite profiling in the rodent toxicology animal species to support an IND submission for a first-in-human clinical trial and then conduct the other animal ADME studies on a drug candidate concurrently with clinical development.

Absorption   For small organic molecule and macromolecule drug candidates to be administered intravenously, absorption studies are not necessary. However, for NCEs with limited aqueous solubility and most macromolecules, studies to determine that the drug candidate is compatible with blood components are considered necessary, especially for a protein drug candidate to be administered intravenously.

If the proposed clinical route of administration for the provisional drug product is oral or another non-IV route (e.g., dermal, pulmonary, nasal, buccal), preclinical information on the rate and extent of absorption is usually necessary to show that the absorption profile is linear over the dose range to be evaluated in the toxicology studies, is not substantially different for each of the toxicology species, and is comparable to the absorption profile in humans (when human data are available). We recommend that the sponsor consider conducting an absolute bioavailability, dose proportionality study in each of the toxicology animal species (e.g., rat or other rodent and dog or nonhuman primate) and that the dose range evaluated include the projected pharmacological active dose for that species (if available) and the maximum projected dose level for toxicology assessments.

Distribution   Types of nonclinical distribution studies conducted on most drug candidates include protein binding and distribution in blood cells, single- and multiple-dose tissue distribution (TD), and feto-placental transfer and lacteal excretion studies. Preclinical distribution studies considered necessary to support an IND for a first-in-human clinical trial are protein binding and distribution into blood cells. Some sponsors also conduct single-dose TD studies with whole body autoradiography (WBA) prior to initiating first-in-human clinical trials but multiple-dose TD studies (if considered necessary as described in ICH S3b [5]) are conducted concurrently with human clinical studies. If the human disease to be evaluated during clinical trials is gender specific (females only) and/or pregnant or nursing women or women of child-bearing potential are to be studied in the first-in-human clinical trial, feto-placental transfer and lacteal excretion studies may be necessary prior to the initiation of clinical trials.

Metabolism   The similarity or difference in the extent of metabolism and possibly in the metabolites formed among the various toxicology animal species and humans should be explored to demonstrate the relevance of the animal model for human exposure. Thus, as part of the strategic preclinical development program planning, the sponsor should consider evaluating the extent of metabolism and *in vitro* metabolism profile of the active drug substance in animals and in humans. These *in vitro* metabolism studies can be conducted in microsomes, which express the various CYP450 isozymes, or hepatocytes, which express all the phase I (oxidation, reduction, hydrolysis) and phase II (conjugation) metabolism systems. If the drug candidate is extensively metabolized in *in vitro* systems from animals and humans, the sponsor may want to develop a metabolite profiling BAC method to determine if the metabolites formed are similar or different for the various species in order to select metabolically-relevant-to-human animal species for toxicology studies.

For a protein drug candidate, *in vitro* or *in vivo* metabolism studies are generally not considered necessary (as discussed in ICH S6 [6]) unless the biological contains not natural amino acids or other structural modifications. However, the potential of a macromolecule drug candidate to induce or inhibit drug metabolism enzymes (i.e., CYP450 isozymes) can be assessed from liver samples collected from the rodent and nonrodent animal species at necropsy during subchronic toxicology studies.

Excretion The rate and routes of excretion for the drug candidate and its metabolites in the toxicology animal species and later in humans are determined during mass balance (MB) studies (using the radiolabeled drug candidate). These animal mass balance studies, especially in the toxicology rodent animal species, are usually completed prior to the submission of an IND for a first-in-human clinical trial. Excreta (urine, bile, feces), and in some cases expired air, collected over various time intervals and blood/plasma at various time points after dosing are collected and counted for total radioactivity or total drug-related material (parent compound and any formed metabolites) to determine the routes of excretion and the extent of excretion by each route of elimination. As development continues, the collected samples from MB studies are profiled for drug candidate metabolites using a developed BAC profiling method (usually HPLC with a radiochemical detector). These collected physiological matrices (or from *in vitro* metabolism systems if the formed metabolites in MB studies and the earlier conducted *in vitro* metabolism evaluations are the same) can also be used for isolating sufficient quantities of each metabolite for identification, which is commonly conducted concurrently with clinical trials.

If urine samples collected and analyzed for total radioactivity during MB studies show little or no renal elimination of drug-related material, additional excretion studies may be necessary to evaluate how the drug candidate and its metabolites are cleared from the body and to obtain the necessary physiological matrices (i.e., bile) for metabolite profiling. If substantial radioactivity is eliminated in the urine, additional studies to evaluate the extent of renal elimination may be necessary and a safety pharmacology study on the renal/urinary system may be warranted.

26.3.3 Pharmacokinetic Drug–Drug and Drug–Food Interactions

Prior to the initiation of clinical trials on drug candidates to be administered concurrently with another active agent (e.g., a novel anticancer agent plus an approved cytotoxic agent), we recommend that animal drug–drug interaction studies be conducted to determine if the PK profiles of the drug candidate and the other anticancer agent are (or are not) changed by the combination regimen. Similarly, information on the optimal time (in relation to meals) for administration of a drug candidate can be evaluated with an appropriately designed drug–food interaction study.

If a particular species (e.g., the nonhuman primate) is a relevant animal model for evaluating the safety and metabolism of a drug candidate, this animal species is also relevant for evaluating potential drug–drug and drug–food interactions and the desired results can be obtained at a substantial reduction in time and cost (compared to that for human clinical trials). Thus, we recommend that the sponsor consider first conducting possibly needed human drug–drug or drug–food interaction studies in the key (i.e., relevant to humans) animal species. If no or only minimal interaction is found for a particular drug–drug combination or if food and the time of feeding do not adversely affect the extent of absorption or the absorption profile for the drug candidate, evaluations in humans would not be necessary. If substantial drug–drug or drug–food effects are noted in the nonhuman primate or other appropriate animal species, the results can be confirmed with relatively simple clinical trials.

26.4   TOXICOLOGY

In general, toxicology studies conducted prior to a first-in-human clinical trial are to establish a margin of safety for the first dose to be administered to humans and to identify potential tissues and organs of toxicity so that human clinical trials can be appropriately designed. Other animal safety aspects evaluated during preclinical development and recommended for completion prior to the first-in-human clinical trial include safety pharmacology (discussed earlier) and genotoxicity and local tolerance (see Sections 26.4.3 and 26.4.6). Preclinical approaches for evaluating the animal toxicology profile of NCEs and biologicals intended for monotherapy and combination/adjunctive therapy are considered next.

26.4.1   Single-Dose Toxicology

Lethal dose (LD_{50}) studies are no longer considered necessary (and are not recommended) and have been replaced by acute toxicology evaluations where dosing is continued until a dose level with marked toxicological effect is identified. Acute toxicology studies (as discussed in *FDA Guidance for Industry: Single Dose Acute Toxicity Testing for Pharmaceuticals* [7] and ICH M3 [8]) are conducted in two species, one of which is a nonrodent, and use both the proposed clinical route of administration and intravenous (if possible).

Monotherapy   For a drug candidate to be administered as a monotherapy, acute (single dose or the number of doses planned to be administered over a 24-hour period during clinical testing) toxicology studies in two species, one of which is a nonrodent, are generally considered necessary, unless there is ample evidence that a second species is inappropriate and would not be scientifically supportable. The acute studies should be designed to determine a no-observable-adverse-effect-level (NOAEL) and a dose that causes marked toxicity and to determine if the observed acute toxicity is reversible. The results of the acute studies should be available to assist the sponsor in the design and dose selection for subchronic toxicology studies, which should be conducted on the same animal species as completed acute toxicology studies.

Combination Therapy   Acute toxicology studies on the provisional experimental drug product administered concurrently with another anticancer therapy may be beneficial in showing that the toxicity profiles of the combination therapy are (or are not) substantially different from the profiles of either agent administered alone.

We recommend that combination therapy acute toxicology studies be conducted to assist in the design of the recommended subchronic combination therapy toxicology evaluations. Even when a drug candidate is to be part of a combination therapy, we recommend that the acute toxicology studies discussed previously for a monotherapy agent be conducted in order to establish the toxicological profile for the drug candidate.

26.4.2   Repeat-Dose Toxicology

Monotherapy   For an NCE or macromolecule as a monotherapy and to support single-dose administration to humans, subchronic toxicology studies in two species (one of which is a nonrodent) with a dosing duration of 14 days are recommended (as discussed in ICH M3 [8]). The duration of a proposed multiple-dose clinical trial should not be longer than that for the completed subchronic toxicology studies (i.e., a proposed clinical trial dosing duration of 30 days requires completed subchronic toxicology studies in two species with a duration of dosing of 30 days or longer). The high dose of the drug candidate for subchronic toxicology studies should be sufficient to produce toxic effects and to identify potential tissues and organs of toxicity while the low dose of the drug candidate should produce little or no toxic effect (i.e., NOAEL) in order to establish an acceptable safety margin for the dose levels to be evaluated in the first-in-human clinical trial.

Combination Therapy   Prior to initiating clinical trials on a provisional new product to be administered concurrently with another active agent, subchronic toxicology studies in two species (one of which is nonrodent) and using the proposed clinical route of administration, dosing frequency, and duration for each agent are generally necessary. Recommended dose groups for these combination therapy subchronic toxicology studies are vehicle control (no active pharmaceutical agent), active concomitant agent alone (at a dose above the planned clinical dose), and the experimental product at various dose levels with concurrent administration of the known therapy at the dose level evaluated for the active concomitant agent alone. The selection of dose levels should be based on previously conducted dose range-finding studies and/or an appropriately designed pilot study. An FDA (draft) Guidance to Industry [9] on the nonclinical safety evaluations for drug combinations is available. This guidance document provides information on the development recommendations when the combination includes (1) two or more previously marketed drugs, (2) one or more previously marketed drug plus one drug candidate, which could be either an NCE or a macromolecule, and (3) two or more drug candidates. We recommend that sponsors carefully review this draft FDA Guidance to Industry prior to beginning a preclinical development program wherein combination therapy will be studied in humans.

26.4.3   Genotoxicity

All small organic molecule drug substances (NCEs) need to be supported by the standard ICH battery of genotoxicity studies [10, 11], unless specific waiver is given by the FDA Reviewing Division. This standard battery of genotoxicity tests consists of the following:

1. A test for gene mutation in bacteria.
2. An *in vitro* assessment of chromosomal damage using mammalian cells or an *in vitro* mouse lymphoma tk$^{+/-}$ assay.
3. An *in vivo* test for chromosomal damage using rodent hematopoietic cells.

According to *FDA Guidance to Industry: Recommended Approaches to Integration of Genetic Toxicology Study Results* [12], the results from *in vitro* genetic toxicology studies should be available prior to the initiation of Phase I first-in-human clinical trials and the *in vivo* test can be conducted concurrently with clinical trials.

As discussed in ICH S6 [6], most biologicals (e.g., monoclonal antibodies or other proteins) do not require safety support from genotoxicity studies. However, if the macromolecule contains not natural amino acids or other structural modifications, the possible need for genotoxicity studies prior to first-in-human clinical trials should be addressed with the FDA during the pre-IND consultation.

26.4.4   Carcinogenicity

For most NCEs and then only under special circumstances, carcinogenicity studies are not initiated prior to the first-in-human clinical trial and thus are not considered as preclinical studies but are nonclinical studies. However, most small organic molecule development plans will need to include carcinogenicity studies in the rat and in the mouse, each of which are usually initiated after Phase II clinical trials have shown the drug candidate can mediate a human disease or disorder in patients without causing unacceptable toxicity in these patients. ICH S1a [13], S1b [14], and S1c [15, 16] provide guidance on the need for and dose selection for carcinogenicity studies. ICH S1b indicates that one rodent (usually the rat) carcinogenicity study plus one other study (commonly in a transgenic, p53$^{+/-}$ mouse model) that supplements the carcinogenicity study and provides additional information that is not readily available from the long-term assay can be used to support the development of a drug candidate. Thus, we recommend that careful thought be given in the strategic preclinical plan for negotiation with the FDA for conducting one carcinogenicity study plus one additional supportive study. These studies might be conducted during Phase III clinical development, thus deferring the significant cost until the provisional drug product shows enough promise in patients to justify the initiation of these long-term animal studies. A sponsor assumes some risk with this approach, particularly when the clinical development program is able to be truncated (i.e., substantial evidence of efficacy is observed during Phase II clinical trials, which is relatively common for many oncology drug candidates) and a marketing application can be submitted earlier than expected. In this case, a sponsor may be able to submit the completed carcinogenicity study(ies) during the formal NDA review, or as a postapproval, Phase IV commitment.

For macromolecule drug candidates, such as monoclonal antibodies or other proteins with no unusual structural characteristics [6], carcinogenicity studies are generally not necessary. We recommend that during the pre-IND consultation or another early meeting with the FDA, sponsors confirm that carcinogenicity studies for a biological will not be required.

26.4.5   Reproductive and Development Toxicity

Before pregnant or lactating women or women not practicing acceptable methods of birth control can be entered in clinical trials on a provisional drug product, completion of the recommended battery of reproductive and developmental toxicology studies, as delineated in the ICH S5a [17] and S5b [18] guidelines, will normally be necessary. These guidelines indicate that the rat, or other appropriate mammalian species, and a second mammalian species (most commonly the rabbit) should be used for embryotoxicity studies. The timing of inclusion of these studies is dependent on the particular characteristics of the experimental drug substance and any species-specific issues, as well as the speed with which the development program is moving. For most, but not all, NCE and biological drug candidates, these reproductive and developmental toxicology studies are not conducted during preclinical development but are initiated after Phase I clinical trial results are available and are frequently conducted concurrently with early Phase II clinical trials. As noted in Section 26.3 on pharmacokinetics, a question usually asked when reproductive toxicology studies show no apparent adverse effect to the fetus is whether the fetus was appropriately exposed to the test article and/or its metabolites. To obtain this information, sponsors usually conduct feto-placental transfer studies (using a radiolabeled drug candidate to demonstrate exposure of the fetus to drug-related material and not just the parent compound) in the rodent and nonrodent species used in reproductive toxicology studies. The results of these TK studies should also be available prior to the entry of women of childbearing potential and pregnant women into clinical trials on the provisional drug product.

26.4.6   Local Tolerability

Local tolerability assessments on a provisional experimental drug product can be, and frequently are, obtained during acute, subchronic, and chronic toxicology studies. Separate local tolerance studies in animals may not be necessary. However, sponsors need to ensure that the local tolerance evaluations are generated using the same provisional drug product that will be studied in clinical trials. For some formulation types, particularly for dermal, pulmonary, and nasal formulations, the extent of local exposure, and thus local tolerability, may be determined by the formulation type, the excipients in the formulation, and the rate of release of the drug substance from the formulation. In these cases, the sponsor will need to conduct formulation studies early (i.e., prior to the initiation of toxicology testing) so that the local tolerance or intolerance of provisional drug product can be established. For NCE and biological drug candidates to be administered by the IV, SC, or IM routes, local tolerance studies are important, particularly when the formulation is not similar to physiological conditions or when the drug candidate has limited aqueous solubility.

26.4.7   Immunogenicity

The potential for a biological, such as a chimeric monoclonal antibody, to cause an untoward immune response [6] in animals can be evaluated using samples collected during the subchronic toxicology studies and thus is commonly determined during preclinical development. Appropriate assays to determine the ability of the drug substance to cause the stimulation of antibody formation *in vivo* will be necessary.

26.4.8 Immunotoxicity

As noted in ICH S6 [6], the ability of the drug candidate to adversely affect the immune system (i.e., immunotoxicity) should be evaluated early in the drug development process, commonly during preclinical development. If appropriately designed, these results can be obtained during the subchronic toxicology studies in rodent and nonrodent animal species that are conducted prior to the first-in-human clinical trial.

26.4.9 Other Toxicology Studies

Other toxicology studies commonly conducted during drug development include determining the toxicological profile of drug candidate metabolites, drug substance impurities, and novel formulation excipients. Since the need for these study types cannot always be defined during preclinical development, the strategic drug development plan should be updated as necessary. For drug candidate metabolites that occur only in humans (i.e., novel human metabolites) or are at substantially higher levels in humans than in animals, the *FDA Guidance for Industry* (draft): *Safety Testing of Drug Metabolites* [19] is available to assist sponsors.

If a drug candidate has potential application for a human disease or disorder in elderly and/or pediatric patients, we recommend that sponsors conduct at least some toxicology studies in old or young animals, respectively, to ascertain if the observed toxicity profile is age related. If the toxicity profile is age-related, sponsors will need to carefully design clinical trials in elderly and/or pediatric patients to ensure that the patient population is not exposed to toxic levels of the drug candidate.

26.5   PRECLINICAL CONCLUSIONS

In this chapter, we have described and discussed the preclinical drug development studies considered necessary to effectively characterize the pharmacology, pharmacokinetic, and toxicology profiles of drug candidates, both NCEs and macromolecules. We have also provided references to FDA guidances and ICH guidelines that can be used by sponsors to assist in designing these preclinical studies and to determine when these studies need to be conducted in the overall strategic drug development plan. Table 26.1 provides a summary of the types of preclinical studies that are considered necessary prior to a first-in-human clinical trial on a drug candidate. Since each drug development program is unique, the preclinical studies listed may not be required for all drug candidates and/or additional studies may be necessary to appropriately evaluate whether or not a drug candidate has the necessary attributes, and does not have major demerits, to be a successful clinical drug candidate.

TABLE 26.1   Prxeclinical Drug Development Studies Commonly Conducted on NCE and Biological Drug Candidates

Study Type	Study Purpose and Goal	Reference
	Pharmacology	
Primary pharmacodynamics	*In vitro* and animal pharmacology studies on the mode of action and/or effects of a drug substance in relation to the therapeutic target.	
Safety pharmacology	Studies to evaluate the effects of a drug candidate on vital functions, such as the cardiovascular, central nervous, and respiratory systems (standard battery) and renal/urinary, autonomic nervous, gastrointestinal, and other organ systems (supplemental).	ICH S7a and S7b
	Pharmacokinetics	
Absorption	Studies to determine rate and extent of absorption of a drug candidate to be administered by a non-IV route. Studies may be *in vitro* and/or *in vivo* and results may be during toxicokinetic evaluations on a drug candidate.	ICH S3a
Distribution	*In vitro* studies to determine the extent of protein binding in animal species and in humans.	
Metabolism	*In vitro* studies to determine the extent of metabolism and possible drug metabolizing enzyme systems involved in the metabolism of a drug candidate in toxicology animal species and in humans.	
Excretion	Mass balance studies in the rodent and possibly the nonrodent toxicology animal species to determine the routes and extent of elimination. Profiling of drug candidate metabolites may be initiated.	
Drug–drug interaction	For drug candidates to be administered concurrently with other pharmaceuticals, animal interaction studies may be desirable to determine if the pharmacokinetic profiles of either agent are affected when coadministered.	

TABLE 26.1 *Continued*

Study Type	Study Purpose and Goal	Reference
	Toxicology	
Acute toxicology	Single-dose studies conducted in two species, one of which is a nonrodent, and using both the proposed clinical route of administration and intravenous (if possibly). Dosing should continue until evidence of marked toxic effect is observed.	ICH M3 and FDA Guidance to Industry
Repeat-dose toxicology	Repeat-dose studies in two species, one of which is not a rodent and using the proposed clinical route of administration and dosing frequency. Duration of dosing should be equal to or greater than that for the proposed clinical trails on the drug candidate.	ICH M3 and S4a
Genotoxicity	For NCEs, a standard battery of tests consisting of a test for gene mutation in bacteria, an *in vitro* assessment of chromosomal damage using mammalian cells or an *in vitro* mouse lymphoma tk$^{+/-}$ assay, and an *in vivo* test for chromosomal damage using rodent hematopoietic cells. For macromolecules, genotoxicity studies are usually not necessary.	ICH S2a, S2b, and S6
Carcinogenicity	Not required during preclinical development for NCEs. Not normally required for macromolecules.	ICH S1a, S1b, and S1c
Reproductive and developmental toxicology	Not usually required during preclinical development.	ICH S5a and S5b
Local tolerance	Tolerability at the site of dosing for both NCEs and biologicals should be conducted using the route of administration proposed for clinical trials and formulation to be evaluated in humans.	ICH M3 and S6
Immunogenicity and immunotoxicity	Studies recommended for macromolecules to evaluate the effects of the drug candidate on the immune system.	ICH S6
Other toxicology studies	Toxicology assessments on drug candidate metabolites and/or impurities and novel formulation excipients. Not usually conducted during preclinical development.	FDA Guidance to Industry

26.6 PRE-IND MANUFACTURING ISSUES

Prior to submitting an IND for a first-in-human clinical trial on a drug candidate, a sponsor will need to prepare the chemistry, manufacturing, and control (CMC) section (Item 7) of IND Form FDA-1571. This section consists of five subparts:

Subpart a: Manufacturing and controls information on the drug substance or active pharmaceutical ingredient (API)

Subpart b: Manufacturing and controls information on the proposed drug product

Subpart c: Manufacturing and controls information on the placebo to match the proposed drug product

Subpart d: Copies of labeling to be supplied for the clinical trials

Subpart e: Environmental impact analysis statement

CMC information on the API and proposed drug product in an IND should be of sufficient quality and detail to justify and support the use of the API during clinical development; should demonstrate that the sponsor utilized an API of similar quality during preclinical toxicology studies; and that the proposed drug product to be used in clinical trials was evaluated in animal safety studies. If the proposed drug product to be used in clinical trials was not evaluated in toxicology studies, sponsors will need to have conducted "bridging" studies to show that the rate and extent of absorption and the disposition profile for the proposed drug product are not significantly different from those for the formulated API used in the toxicology animal species and possibly in the pharmacology animal models, if the pharmacological response in animals was used in establishing the initial dose for the first-in-human clinical trial.

Information on the API should include the following:

1. The name and address of the facility where the API is manufactured.
2. The manufacturing procedure flowchart and a detailed description of production, including in-process controls.
3. Information regarding proof of structure, which can be obtained by elemental analysis, UV, IR, NMR spectra, and mass spectrum analysis.
4. Physical chemical properties, which include description and appearance, solubility profile, dissociation constant(s) (if any), optical rotation (if necessary), partition coefficient (such as octanol/water for log P determination), UV absorbance, melting point and thermal analysis, X-ray powder diffraction pattern, and qualitative tests.
5. Raw materials, including solvents and water, used in the manufacture of the API.
6. Copies of release specifications or manufacturer's certificates of analysis (COA) for raw materials.
7. Release specifications for the API.
8. Analytical chemistry (AC) methods for raw materials and API release testing.

9. Reference Standard information.
10. Packaging and labeling information.
11. Stability results including methods, procedures, and system suitability for the stability-indicating assay.

For the manufacture of the API, a flowchart of synthesis is recommended and should provide information on the starting materials (with structures) for each step, catalysts and other reagents for each step, reaction conditions for each step, and products (with structures) for each step. Information commonly provided for the description of each step of the API synthesis includes equipment required (including suppliers and specifications), reactions (including amounts and order of addition), solvents, conditions (temperature, pressure, pH, time), tests for completion of reaction, isolation procedure for synthesis product (intermediate or API), purification steps for synthesis product, and yield of synthesis product.

Commonly employed API structure elucidation techniques include elemental analysis, mass spectroscopy, nuclear magnetic resonance, ultraviolet spectrum, infrared spectrum, molecular weight, stereochemistry (if the API has one or more chiral centers), X-ray analysis, and chromatography (usually HPLC for an NCE and SDS-PAGE for a macromolecule).

Sponsors are requested to provide information on the API impurity profile, which requires the development and validation of an impurity profiling AC method. The AC methods should provide chromatographic separation of API from all impurities and/or degradation products and should allow for calculation of the amount of each impurity and/or degradant. At this stage of development, sponsors should initiate a program for the isolation and identification of each impurity and/or degradant in the API. The API used in animal safety studies should have an impurity profile that is similar to the profile for the material to be used in the first-in-human clinical trial. If the clinical trial API material contains a novel impurity or an impurity at higher levels than present in the API material used in toxicology studies, sponsors should consider conducting toxicology studies on the clinical trial API material to ensure that an API impurity or degradant does not cause toxicity that might lead to adverse events or even serious adverse events in humans.

For the proposed drug product or the formulated API that is to be evaluated during the first-in-human clinical trial, sponsors should consider providing the following information:

1. The name and address of the facility where the proposed drug product is manufactured.
2. A detailed description of the manufacturing and packaging procedures.
3. A list and description of all raw materials used in the manufacture of the proposed drug product.
4. Release specifications on all raw materials and/or a Certificate of Analysis (COA) from the manufacturer or producer of the raw materials.
5. Release specifications, including acceptance and rejection criteria for the quantity of API in the proposed drug product, for the final proposed drug product formulation. For solid dosage forms, content uniformity and rate of dissolution or release may also be required.

6. Description of all AC methods and tests employed in the testing and release of raw materials.

7. Details on container and closure systems for storage of the proposed drug product.

8. Proposed drug product stability results, including detailed descriptions of stability-indicating AC methods and procedures.

The description of the manufacturing process for the proposed drug product will most likely not be the same process that will be used for the drug product to be marketed. Sponsors need to include sufficient details on the proposed drug product manufacturing process to demonstrate that the process is under control and will produce similar material during the manufacture of separate batches.

If the first-in-human clinical trial on a drug candidate is to be a placebo-controlled trial, sponsors are requested to provide information on the placebo to match the proposed drug product. This placebo information is to include the following:

1. Name and address of facility where the placebo is manufactured.

2. Detailed description of the manufacturing and packaging procedures for the placebo.

3. List of all raw materials used in manufacturing the placebo.

4. Release specifications on all raw materials and/or a Certificate of Analysis (COA) from the manufacturer or producer of the raw materials used in the placebo.

5. Release specifications for the final placebo formulation, including method to demonstrate the absence of the API. Stability results are not routinely required for the placebo.

6. Description of all AC methods and tests employed in the testing and release of raw materials.

7. Details on container and closure systems.

Copies of the labeling for the proposed drug product and placebo formulations to be used in the clinical trial studies are to be included. The type of clinical trial study to be conducted will generally dictate the information to be included on the label for the clinical trial supplies. In all cases, the statement "Caution: New Drug Limited by US (Federal) Law to Investigation Use Only" has to be placed on all labels for an investigational new drug.

An environmental analysis statement is required to be included in an IND (21 CFR § 312.23 (a) (7) (e)). Most sponsors include a claim for categorical exclusion in an IND since the manufacturing processes for the API and proposed drug product have not yet been fully defined or characterized.

26.7 PRE-IND CLINICAL ISSUES

The clinical development of a drug candidate cannot be initiated until an IND has been submitted to the FDA. This IND contains three major aspects:

1. The results from preclinical animal pharmacology, pharmacokinetic, and toxicology studies conducted on the drug candidate that show the material has an acceptable margin of safety for dosing to humans.
2. The results from CMC efforts to demonstrate that the manufacturing processes for the API and proposed drug product can be controlled and produce material of a sufficient quality for administration to humans.
3. The proposed clinical development program for the drug candidate, including a complete protocol for the first-in-human clinical trial, an Investigator's Brochure to provide summary information on the drug candidate to clinical investigators, and a summary of the proposed clinical development program.

The sponsor, usually the clinical department or group, will need to generate the clinical trial protocol to be included in the IND. ICH E6 [20] provides sponsors with recommendations for conducting clinical trials on a drug candidate in the following areas:

- Institutional Review Board (IRB) and Independent Ethics Committee (IEC)
- Clinical trial investigator
- Sponsor
- Clinical trial protocol and protocol amendment(s)
- Investigator's Brochure (IB)
- Essential documents for the conduct of a clinical trial

In general, the clinical trial protocol is to contain sections that provide background information, objectives and purpose, design, subject selection and withdrawal, subject treatment, assessments of efficacy and safety, statistics, access to source data, quality assurance (QA) and quality control (QC) procedures, ethics, data handling and record keeping, financing and insurance, and publication policy.

The IB usually contains an introduction, general considerations, confidentiality statement, summary on the disease indication, physical and chemical properties of the API and formulation, summaries of completed preclinical pharmacology, pharmacokinetic, and toxicology studies, effects in humans (if any), and guidance for the investigator. For a first-in-human clinical trial, information on effects in humans is not usually available unless the drug candidate has been administered to humans in foreign clinical trials or in investigator-IND clinical studies.

The summary of the proposed clinical development program should contain sufficient detail to explain the clinical testing strategy to determine the safety, pharmacokinetics, and efficacy of the drug candidate in patients with the disease or disorder to be studied and to establish the dosage regimen for treating the disease or disorder without causing unacceptable toxicity.

REFERENCES

1. ICH S7a Guideline: *Safety Pharmacology Studies for Human Pharmaceuticals*, July 2001.

2. ICH S7b Guideline: *Safety Pharmacology Studies for Assessing the Potential for Delayed Ventricular Repolarization (QT Interval Prolongation) by Human Pharmaceuticals*, released for consultation at Step 2 of the ICH Process, February 2002.

3. ICH S3a Guideline: *Toxicokinetics: The Assessment of Systemic Exposure in Toxicity Studies*, March 1995.

4. *FDA Guidance to Industry: Bioanalytical Method Validation*, May 2001.

5. ICH S3b Guideline: *Pharmacokinetics: Guidance for Repeated Dose Tissue Distribution Studies*, March 1995.

6. ICH S6 Guideline: *Preclinical Safety Evaluation of Biotechnology-Derived Pharmaceuticals*, July 1997.

7. *FDA Guidance for Industry: Single Dose Acute Toxicity Testing for Pharmaceuticals*, August 1996.

8. ICH M3 Guideline: *Nonclinical Safety Studies for the Conduct of Human Clinical Trials for Pharmaceuticals*, July 1997.

9. *FDA Guidance to Industry (draft): Nonclinical Safety Evaluations for Drug Combinations*, January 2005.

10. ICH S2a Guideline: *Guidance on Specific Aspects of Regulatory Genotoxicity Tests for Pharmaceuticals*, July 1995.

11. ICH S2b Guideline: *A Standard Battery for Genotoxicity Testing of Pharmaceuticals*, July 1997.

12. *FDA Guidance to Industry: Recommended Approaches to Integration of Genetic Toxicology Study Results*, November 2004.

13. ICH S1a Guideline: *The Need for Long-Term Rodent Carcinogenicity Studies of Pharmaceuticals*, March 1996.

14. ICH S1b Guideline: *Testing for Carcinogenicity of Pharmaceuticals*, July 1997.

15. ICH S1c Guideline: *Dose Selection for Carcinogenicity Studies of Pharmaceuticals*, March 1995.

16. ICH S1c(R) Guideline: *Addendum to Dose Selection for Carcinogenicity Studies of Pharmaceuticals: Addition of a Limit Dose and Related Notes*, July 1997.

17. ICH S5a Guideline: *Detection of Toxicity to Reproduction for Medicinal Products*, September 1994.

18. ICH S5b Guideline: *Detection of Toxicity to Reproduction for Medicinal Products: Addendum on Toxicity to Male Fertility*, April 1996.

19. *FDA Guidance for Industry (draft): Safety Testing of Drug Metabolites*, June 2005.

20. ICH E6 Guideline: *Guideline for Good Clinical Practice*, May 1996.

27

REGULATORY ISSUES IN PRECLINICAL SAFETY STUDIES (U.S. FDA)

KENNETH L. HASTINGS[1] AND WILLIAM J. BROCK[2]

[1]*sanofi-aventis, Bethesda, Maryland*
[2]*Brock Scientific Consulting, LLC, Montgomery Village, Maryland*

Contents

27.1 INTRODUCTION

In drug development, it is important to know and understand the legislation and other "high level" documents (e.g., case law) establishing the regulatory authority of the FDA as well as the specific enabling documents that have been published (e.g., 21 CFR, ICH Guidances, FDA Guidances) and the supporting guidelines [1–10]. However, it is of practical importance to understand the scientific approach that ultimately drives decision making in the drug review divisions that constitute the real world of pharmaceutical development. The pivotal individual in applying pharmacology/toxicology principles and practice to drug development is the FDA reviewer. This individual has the task of interpreting data submitted by the sponsor and making the decisions critical to clinical drug development. Sometimes in trying

Preclinical Development Handbook: Toxicology, edited by Shayne Cox Gad
Copyright © 2008 John Wiley & Sons, Inc.

to understand the drug review process, it is easy to lose sight of the "big picture" and become lost in the minutia. A very useful approach to understanding the review and decision-making process is knowing the fundamental questions needed to be answered by the somewhat bewildering list of published documents. The following list of questions will form the framework for discussing regulatory issues that, when dealt with incorrectly, can derail a drug development program:

- Have sufficient preclinical (nonclinical) toxicology data been submitted?
- Are the doses proposed for clinical trials safe based on submitted data?
- Is the length of exposure proposed for clinical trials safe?

If sponsors keep these questions in mind when designing, conducting, and interpreting preclinical drug safety studies, they will be thinking along the same lines as the pharmacology/toxicology reviewer. Each of these questions is discussed in turn.

27.2   HAVE SUFFICIENT PRECLINICAL (NONCLINICAL) TOXICOLOGY DATA BEEN SUBMITTED?

When attempting to answer this question, two documents are absolutely pivotal: ICH M3 and ICH S6. These documents provide key information on what studies are needed to enable clinical trials. ICH M3 also contains a chart that lists the studies needed to be completed prior to conduct of specific clinical studies (Table 27.1).

There are several issues that should be considered when interpreting what appears to be a rather simple paradigm. The first is that the term "repeat-dose toxicity studies" is generally interpreted to mean daily oral doses. This is a relatively straightforward matter when considering a new molecular entity (NME) that will be administered in clinical trials by the oral route. However, when a drug will be administered by another route, interpretation becomes more complicated. There is no simple paradigm to which reference can be made, but rather a number of points to consider. The first is whether the drug is an NME or not. If the drug has been previously developed for use by oral administration, it may be sufficient to conduct what are generally referred to as "bridging studies." For example, if a drug was originally developed for oral administration and sufficient oral toxicology data are

TABLE 27.1   Duration of Toxicity Studies and Clinical Trials

| | Duration of Clinical Trials Toxicity Studies | |
Duration of Clinical Trials	Rodents	Nonrodents
Single dose	2 weeks	2 weeks
Up to 2 weeks	2 weeks	2 weeks
Up to 1 month	1 month	1 month
Up to 3 months	3 months	3 months
Up to 6 months	6 months	6 months
>6 months	6 months	Chronic: 9 months and longer

available, it may be possible to support clinical trials with repeat-dose toxicology studies by the new route of exposure (e.g., topical, inhalation) in one species (usually a nonrodent). Route-specific studies may need to be conducted (such as local irritation), and toxicokinetic studies should be incorporated into the nonclinical development program to establish comparative local and systemic exposure. However, the important point is that a complete replication of toxicology studies conducted by the original route of exposure may not be necessary.

An interesting issue that often arises in the nonclinical toxicology evaluation of drugs is the role of acute dose studies. As a general rule, the package of enabling studies should contain acute dose toxicology studies in both rodents and nonrodents. Several points should be considered. The first is the issue of what constitutes an acute dose study. Although occasionally a point of debate, it is generally accepted that an acute dose study is one in which the test article (drug) is administered as a single dose, or as more than one dose, in a single 24 hour period, followed by appropriate clinical and anatomical evaluation. The studies should be conducted over a dose range sufficient to demonstrate adverse effects and should be GLP compliant (21 CFR part 58). The second is that acute studies, as a general rule, are not usually sufficient to support clinical trials. They are essentially "discovery" or *hazard identification* studies intended to determine the toxic potential of the test article. In fact, several studies may need to be conducted (usually in rodents) to determine the doses necessary to produce toxicity. There are examples of drugs for which acute toxicity studies may be adequate to support clinical trials (basically, agents that will be administered as a single dose in very circumscribed clinical settings, such as radioimaging agents or inhalation anesthetics), and there are specific situations recognized in regulatory guidances discussed later, but in general these are not sufficient to initiate clinical trials. Finally, under most circumstances it is not necessary (in fact, it is discouraged) to determine lethal doses. Although acute dose toxicity studies may be useful in evaluating and managing overdose situations in clinical trials, and may eventually be used to write the overdose section of a product label, they are of limited practical use in the design and conduct of clinical trials. This leads to a consideration in designing toxicology studies to enable clinical trials: if appropriate repeat-dose toxicology studies have been conducted, GLP-compliant acute dose studies may not be needed, or even appropriate, especially in nonhuman primates.

As mentioned earlier, there are specific guidance documents that allow for the use of acute dose toxicity studies to enable clinical trials. For the development of imaging agents, for example, it is acceptable to conduct acute dose toxicity studies with significant caveats. First, the studies will need to be GLP compliant and conducted in both rodents and nonrodents, and animals should be monitored for the core battery of safety pharmacology parameters (cardiovascular, central nervous system, and pulmonary function) unless separate single-dose studies are conducted as described in ICH S7A. Second, complete clinical observations, clinical pathology (clinical chemistry and hematology), as well as necropsy and complete histological examinations must be conducted on day 2 (24 hours after test article administration). Third, a recovery group must be included for every dose group with complete clinical and necropsy/histology determinations.

The second example is the *screening IND*. In most respects, screening IND studies should be conducted in a manner identical to those needed to support clinical trials with imaging agents. There are several additional considerations, however. The screening IND is designed to allow a sponsor to submit safety data on several related compounds. Although not explicitly defined, the term "related compounds" is assumed to mean both structurally and pharmacologically related. If the drugs are to be administered by the oral route in clinical trials, acute toxicity studies should be conducted by the intravenous route as well, with complete safety pharmacology, clinical pathology, and pathology determinations. Toxicokinetic determinations also should be included with particular emphasis on oral bioavailability. An ICH-compliant battery of genotoxicity studies should be conducted with each compound. The specific purpose of the screening IND paradigm is to enable single-dose clinical studies in healthy volunteers in order to select the most promising candidate compound. For further discussion of the different types of INDs and the regulatory process, the reader is referred to Mathieu [11].

In 2006, the FDA published a comprehensive guidance entitled *Exploratory IND Studies* [8]. Although often referred to as a single approach, in fact the guidance describes several alternative approaches to first-in-human (FIH) clinical trials, and the types of nonclinical studies needed to support these trials. The general approach is discussed later, but one concept in particular utilizes acute toxicity studies—the *microdose* clinical trial. Essentially, the design of acute dose toxicity studies builds on the screening IND approach described earlier with the notable exception that the safety of a proposed single-dose clinical trial can be determined using one mammalian species. Selection of the species should be justified using comparative *in vitro* pharmacokinetic and pharmacodynamic data (essentially, using animal and human tissues/cells), and the dose selected for use in clinical trials should be no more than 1/100 of the no-observed-adverse-effect level (NOAEL) in the test species, based on relative body surface area and not a mg/kg dose. Safety pharmacology and genotoxicity studies are not needed. As a practical matter, the clinical trials are likely to be conducted using doses in the low microgram level (nanomole level for protein drugs), and the studies are designed primarily to determine (relative) oral bioavailability. Another possible clinical study endpoint is specific receptor binding (discovery pharmacodynamics).

In most instances, a battery of genotoxicity studies should be conducted and submitted for review prior to FIH clinical trials. These are hazard identification tests and should include bacterial mutagenicity (Ames test) and at least one *in vitro* mammalian genotoxicity study (the mouse lymphoma assay and/or a chromosomal aberration assay). Prior to Phase II clinical trials, a complete battery of ICH S2B genotoxicity tests should be completed, which as a practical issue means an *in vivo* rodent micronucleus assay in addition to previously completed studies.

Other studies that are needed according to ICH M3 include determination of local tolerance (if the drug is to be administered by a nonoral route), a battery of ICH S7A safety pharmacology studies, and, prior to Phase III clinical trials, the ICH equivalent of Segment II reproductive toxicology studies. Other studies may also be needed, such as an intravenous toxicology study to enable clinical studies to determine absolute oral bioavailability. Studies to determine potential drug effects on cardiac function (e.g., hERG assay, *in vivo* cardiac function studies), as described in ICH S7B, should be submitted although these are not required. ICH S8 immunotoxicity studies may be needed based on a weight-of-evidence analysis, primarily using results of repeat-dose toxicology studies. Some specific studies, such as assays to determine the ability of topical drugs to cause allergic contact dermatitis, may be needed.

Chronic nonrodent toxicology studies are likely to be needed if the drug is to be used for more than 3–6 months. As discussed later, there are considerations in deciding the need for chronic toxicology studies, but these apply to a minority of drugs. There are "regional differences" in the definition of chronic use. In the United States, "chronic toxicity studies" are defined as 3 months of repeated exposure to the drug, or intermittent exposure equivalent to 3 months. ICH specifies that a repeat-dose toxicology study in rodents of 6 months duration is adequate. For nonrodents, ICH defines the duration of a chronic repeat-dose toxicology study to be 9 months. However, for an NME that is the first molecule in a class of compounds, it is likely that a 12 month repeat-dose study will be needed. Another situation in which a 12 month study may be expected is "accelerated approval," where a fairly small clinical database is available for evaluation and, especially, where a surrogate marker is used as the efficacy endpoint. On the other hand, a 6 month repeat-dose toxicology study might be deemed sufficient if the drug belongs to a well-known class of drugs. Toxicities are sometimes observed that clearly limit the ability to conduct repeat-dose toxicity studies of greater than 6 months duration at clinically relevant doses. Lifetime rodent carcinogenicity bioassays (mouse and rat) will almost always be needed for drugs that will be used on a chronic basis. These studies are usually conducted late in the development of a drug and occasionally will be performed as part of postmarketing commitments. The FDA does not provide specific guidance on the conduct of most types of nonclinical toxicology studies (with the notable exception of food additives), but in the case of carcinogenicity bioassays, concurrence on the study design should be requested by the sponsor via the protocol assessment review process.

Finally, biologic therapeutics (basically, protein drugs) represent a unique class of therapeutics and nonclinical studies needed to enable clinical trials are considered in ICH S6. It is important to remember that ICH S6 and ICH M3 are complementary documents, and both apply to protein therapeutics. It is the exceptions to ICH M3 that should be noted when planning the development of protein drugs. For example, under most circumstances, rodents are not likely to be appropriate for evaluating the safety of protein drugs. In fact, it is the entire concept of "appropriate animal model" that leads to much of the misunderstanding in the design and interpretation of nonclinical toxicology studies with biologic products. Many of these drugs are immunogenic in animals other than nonhuman primates, and production of neutralizing antibodies in repeat-dose toxicology studies can render findings irrelevant to human safety. If a protein drug is pharmacologically inactive in a species, it is highly likely that safety information will also be uninformative in this model. Unlike small molecular weight drugs, most toxicity observed with protein drugs are likely to be essentially exaggerated pharmacodynamics. There are certainly exceptions, but even under most circumstances these apparently "off-target" adverse effects will be observed only in species fairly closely related to humans.

There are many ways of dealing with the issue of species specificity such as the use of homologous proteins that are pharmacologically active in a standard toxicology species (usually rodents) or the genetic manipulation of mice or rats such that they express the human receptor of interest (drug target) or lack the molecule (especially useful for evaluating protein antagonists or monoclonal antibodies to endogenous proteins). There are certain studies that are not needed to evaluate the safety of protein therapeutics. For example, genotoxicity studies and hERG assays are usually uninformative. In some cases, there may simply be no relevant animal model to evaluate the safety of a protein therapeutic, and consideration should be given to using *in vitro* data using human cells/tissues. This approach is discouraged by the FDA, but sometimes there will be no justifiable alternative. For example, consider a monoclonal antibody (mAb) directed at a human pathogenic virus. A standard method useful in evaluating potential safety concerns with the mAb is tissue cross-reactivity. Essentially, the mAb is tested with a bank of human (and animal) tissues to detect specific binding to expressed epitopes. If no binding is observed, it is highly likely that nonclincial toxicology studies will not be useful and that the safety of clinical studies cannot be evaluated using standard techniques. In the case of monoclonal antibodies to human epitopes, where no pharmacological effects are observed in nonhuman primates or other standard toxicology species, there are *in vitro* methods that utilize human cells and may be useful. For many (if not most) protein therapeutics, case-by-case study design should be the expected approach.

27.3   ARE THE DOSES PROPOSED FOR CLINICAL TRIALS SAFE BASED ON SUBMITTED DATA?

Extrapolation of doses from animals to humans is a critical issue in evaluating non-clinical toxicology studies. The key document to consult when converting animal doses to human equivalent doses is *FDA Guidance for Industry: Estimating the Maximum Safe Starting Dose in Initial Clinical Trials for Therapeutics in Adult Healthy Volunteers* [6]. The general method presented in this guidance is based on comparative body surface areas and utilizes the standard conversion formula:

$$\text{Human Equivalent Dose} = \text{Animal Dose (mg/kg)} \times (\text{Animal Weight/Human Weight})^{0.33}$$

This method is an inherently conservative approach and is intended to estimate systemic exposure to low molecular weight drugs. For example, if a dose of 30 mg/kg, when administered by the oral route to cynomolgus monkeys, produces an AUC of 50 μg·h/mL, using this formula, the human equivalent dose (HED) would be 10 mg/kg, and if this dose is administered to an adult human volunteer, the measured AUC should also be ~50 μg·h/mL. There are of course many assumptions made in this method and include similar oral bioavailability and metabolism, and the method assumes that the drug has never been administered to humans, so no comparative pharmacokinetic data exist to test the calculation. In addition, the method is meant to apply to FIH doses in healthy volunteers. Therefore, an additional safety factor should be applied to the calculated HED. The default safety factor advocated in the guidance is 10, so the dose calculated in the example given above would be 1 mg/kg. The guidance allows for several considerations in calculating HED, such as steepness of the dose–response curve and nature of adverse effects observed (reversible or not, monitorable or not, etc.), and provides the sponsor the opportunity to present data supporting an alternative method for estimating relative doses (such as body weight comparison). Although the default dose adjustment is referred to as a safety factor, it is in fact an uncertainty factor. Experience has demonstrated the method to be reliable for most classes of drugs. The exceptions include drugs delivered by routes of administration that do not result in appreciable systemic exposure, drugs that are extensively metabolized (where the object of the calculation is estimating comparative exposure to the parent drug), and protein drugs with a molecular weight $\geq 100,000$ where distribution is primarily confined to the vascular compartment.

An important consideration in calculating a safe starting dose for clinical trials in healthy volunteers based on animal data is that a NOAEL has been determined. The NOAEL is the animal dose that will be used to calculate the FIH dose. In most cases, the FDA will take a conservative approach in identifying a NOAEL. Since most Phase I studies will be conducted in healthy volunteers, essentially no adverse effects should be anticipated when administering FIH doses. An issue frequently debated with sponsors is the simple question of whether a finding in an enabling repeat-dose toxicology study is in fact "adverse." For example, should an increase in blood pressure of 10% compared to controls be considered adverse? Chances are the FDA would want to see a dose at which *no* increase in blood pressure was observed, but for certain drug classes this might be an unrealistic expectation. As discussed later, the pharmacologically active dose (PAD) is a consideration in calculating a safe starting dose. Depending on the intended use of the drug, blood pressure effects may be an important consideration, and if the HED at which the blood pressure effect is observed is higher than the anticipated PAD based on animal pharmacology studies, the PAD should be used to calculate the FIH dose. If the PAD is *greater* than the dose at which elevations in blood pressure are observed, it is likely that the FDA will consider the NOAEL to be the lower dose, and although pharmacokinetic data can be obtained in healthy volunteers, it is likely that pharmacologic activity studies will need to be conducted in patients rather than healthy volunteers.

The concept of NOAEL is important in one clinical trial design allowed under the *Exploratory IND Studies* guidance. The essential approach is that the sponsor would conduct a standard 2-week repeat-dose toxicity study in animals (usually rodents), and a NOAEL would be determined. The sponsor would include a determination of key pharmacokinetic (PK) parameters in this study, most importantly the AUC, C_{max}, and $t_{1/2}$. A 2-week repeat-dose oral toxicity study would then be conducted in a second animal species (usually dogs), using only one dose level, calculated to be the NOAEL equivalent based on the first species, and the same PK parameters determined. If the NOAEL in the first species is equivalent to the second species based on relative body surface area, and if PK parameters at the NOAEL are equivalent, then the HED can be calculated and used to establish the FIH dose. If one species appears to be more sensitive based on observed effects (essentially, this would mean that adverse effects were observed in the second species at the NOAEL equivalent in the first species), the sponsor would use the second species to determine the NOAEL in a 2-week repeat-dose study. In either case, the FIH dose would be no greater than 1/50 of the NOAEL in the more sensitive species based on the relative body surface area calculation. The *maximum* clinical dose would be the lowest of the following:

- One-fourth of the NOAEL determined in the first species (usually rodents)
- One-half of the AUC at the NOAEL in the first species, or the AUC in the second species (usually dogs) at the dose equivalent to the NOAEL in the first species (whichever is lower)
- The PAD in humans, or
- The dose at which an adverse clinical effect is observed

Although this seems a complicated scheme, it has the advantage of requiring less test article than would be needed for standard toxicity studies needed to enable FIH clinical trials, and the sponsor could conduct clinical trials of up to 7 days in duration in healthy volunteers to include the determination of PK parameters at steady-state blood levels. Other issues would also need to be addressed, such as genotoxicity and safety pharmacology, but the study design could support more rapid initiation of repeat-dose Phase I clinical trials.

One issue missing from this discussion has been studies to support traditional ascending-dose PK and maximum tolerated dose (MTD) Phase I clinical trials. These still have an important role in drug development. The body surface area dose calculation is relevant to dose setting in these studies. However, some classes of drugs continue to be evaluated in symptomatic patients rather than healthy volunteers, and determination of safe starting dose may follow a different paradigm. For example, when developing cytotoxic chemotherapeutic agents for the treatment of cancer, Phase I studies are typically conducted in patients who are suffering from end-stage disease. In this situation, it has been judged acceptable to use a much more aggressive strategy in determining acceptable clinical doses. A traditional approach is to determine the lethal dose in 10% of animals (LD_{10})—usually mice—and calculate the starting dose based on relative body surface area. Although rodents have been used to determine FIH doses, there is evidence that dogs may be more sensitive. However, there is an ongoing debate over whether increased sensitivity results in more effective dosing strategies. One issue to be considered in assessing the usefulness of a more sensitive species is that nonclinical toxicity studies in these animals may be limited with respect to discovering potential adverse effects. That is, it is at least worthy of consideration that use of a less sensitive species could allow for testing higher doses for longer durations, maximizing the possibility that important, clinically relevant toxicities may be revealed.

27.4   IS THE LENGTH OF EXPOSURE PROPOSED FOR CLINICAL TRIALS SAFE?

This is essentially a cumulative toxicity question. As presented earlier, ICH M3 explicitly states the length of nonclinical toxicity studies needed to support the safety of clinical trials. When designing a drug development program, it is important to consider the timing of nonclinical studies with respect to the duration of clinical trials. For example, the entire amount of time needed to conduct and evaluate findings can be underestimated, which can result in "delayed" clinical development. As a general rule, the importance of this issue is often overestimated. That is, it is much more important to design and conduct enabling toxicology studies correctly—even if this seems to take more time than might be judged necessary—than to rush studies and commit errors that compromise the reliability of study results. Recruitment of subjects into clinical trials often takes much more time than anticipated; the clinical investigator usually underestimates this time and the numbers of subjects that can be recruited. Carefully conducted nonclinical studies can be extremely valuable, especially with respect to discovering toxicities that require repeated exposure— and often repeated insult—to demonstrate. Although in-life determinations can be useful, clinical chemistry and hematology signs are usually not "leading indicators." When elevations in creatinine are observed, for example, it is likely that extensive kidney pathology has already been produced. Thus, reliance on in-life observations in nonclinical toxicology studies can be a risky clinical trial strategy.

One issue that has arisen repeatedly is the impact of positive findings in genotoxicity studies on the safety of clinical trials. When considering the significance of genotoxicity in length of exposure, a weight-of-evidence approach should be taken [9]. Experience has indicated that often positive genotoxicity findings can be related to product impurities, and it is important to make this determination as soon as possible. If positive genotoxicity findings are due to drug contaminants, this may be a fairly easy situation to address. Another typical situation is a positive finding in an *in vitro* chromosomal aberration assay. This argues for inclusion of *in vivo* micronucleus assays as early as possible in nonclinical development. Many times the situation that needs to be addressed is that the positive findings *in vitro* were produced at high drug concentrations, bacterial mutagenicity assays were negative, and the mouse micronucleus assay is needed to clarify the nature of the hazard.

Carcinogenicity studies are rarely needed to enable clinical trials, but there are exceptions [4]. Clinical development of peroxisome proliferator-activated receptors (PPARs) represents a significant departure from the norm. Current ad hoc policy in the FDA is to allow clinical trials with PPAR agonists for up to 6 months duration provided there are no other toxicities, especially genotoxicity or cardiotoxicity findings, in nonclinical studies. However, in order to proceed with studies of longer duration, it may be necessary to complete carcinogenicity bioassays, thus significantly affecting clinical trials. Although this has not been adopted as formal policy, it remains the practice within the FDA.

27.5   ADDITIONAL CONSIDERATIONS

In addition to the three issues just discussed, there are other questions that the pharmacology/toxicology reviewer will likely want to answer. These may include:

- Are there patient or condition of use restrictions?
- Do studies indicate the need for special monitoring or need for available antidotes?
- Are the demonstrated pharmacological effects relevant to the intended indication?
- Are adverse effects expected at effective doses?
- What is known about related drugs?
- What are the types and sites of toxic effects?

- Has the sponsor established a no observed adverse effect level (NOAEL)?
- What is the apparent therapeutic index?
- Are there irreversible or unmonitorable adverse effects?
- Are there differences in metabolism of the drug, especially between animals used in pivotal toxicology studies and humans?

These "supplemental" questions are no less important, but either apply to a subset of nonclinical studies or have been answered as part of the larger issues dealt with earlier. However, each deserves some comment.

Are There Patient or Condition of Use Restrictions?   This question usually can be taken as referring to special populations. For example, if a drug is to be studied in clinical trials to prevent transmission of infections from mother to infant (perinatal transmission, e.g., HIV), the sponsor should conduct Segment I and III reproductive toxicology studies earlier than is usually expected [3]. Although these studies are conducted prior to submission of the NDA, these studies would need to be conducted prior to Phase II clinical trials (assuming pregnancy would not be an issue in Phase I studies). Although a relatively simple timing issue for most drugs, this could be a complicated issue with biologics. In fact, the entire issue of reproductive toxicology studies becomes complex when evaluating protein drugs. This is the single case where these types of studies may need to be conducted in nonhuman primates (NHPs). Although great effort is made to avoid these studies (e.g., development of transgenic rodent models expressing the target of interest for use in reproductive toxicology studies), often cynomolgus monkeys or other NHPs may be the only practical choice. A somewhat related topic is studies to enable pediatric drug trials. The FDA has published guidance on the types of juvenile animal studies useful in supporting the safety of clinical trials in infants, children, and adolescents, but the most important point is that these may not always be needed, and consultation with the FDA is encouraged. Length of exposure, age of the clinical trial subjects, and what is already known concerning the adverse effects of the drug are all issues that should be considered in deciding the need for juvenile animal studies [10].

Another issue that should be dealt with under this question is the issue of phototoxicity and photoallergy [5]. The usefulness of nonclinical phototoxicity studies has been debated, and the FDA has published a guidance on this topic, but it is still somewhat unclear under what conditions nonclinical phototoxicity studies may be needed. Although generally considered in the development of topical drug products, this may also be an issue with drugs administered by other routes where systemic exposure results in significant skin deposition. In fact, some of the most important phototoxic drugs (e.g., fluoroquinolones) are given orally. The guidance relies on two parameters to determine the need for nonclinical phototoxicity studies: (1) significant molecular absorption in the UV-VIS spectrum and (2) concentration of the drug and/or metabolite(s) in the skin. Whether these are appropriate criteria can be questioned, however. Recently, the FDA has not requested photoallergy nonclinical studies since interpretation of the results continues to be debated.

Do Studies Indicate the Need for Special Monitoring or Need for Available Antidotes?   Although often overlooked, risk management is an important issue to be dealt with in toxicology studies. Unfortunately, nonclinical toxicology studies have not been utilized as well as possible in clinical trial design. There are examples of how these studies may be used. For example, if an association has been established in nonclinical studies between drug AUC and liver toxicity, this should be considered in the design and conduct of clinical trials. If a drug has been shown to cause anaphylactoid reactions, conditions associated with this adverse effect (such as rate of infusion for drugs given intravenously) should be used in the design of clinical trials, and appropriate antidotes (e.g., epinephrine) should be available during (and after) drug administration. There are a number of examples that could be cited, but the important point is to take into consideration toxicity findings when considering the issue of risk management. The effort to discover and apply biomarkers of toxicity is a major driver in the FDA's Critical Path Initiative.

Are the Demonstrated Pharmacological Effects Relevant to the Intended Indication?   The answer to this question is often put in the "nice to know" category, but the importance of the issue should not be underestimated. An important consideration is that the review team at the FDA develops a perception of how effective a drug is likely to be and will sometimes act accordingly. Consider, for example, a drug intended to prevent organ transplant rejection. Especially in renal transplantation, there are a number of effective drugs currently available. None are without adverse effect problems, but in general these have proved to be "miracle" drugs when used correctly. Thus, in developing a new drug for this indication, it is very important that proof-of-concept pharmacology studies provide compelling efficacy data. One consideration is that usually a candidate drug for an organ transplant indication will likely be added to an ongoing cyclosporine-based immunosuppressive regimen. Nonclinical pharmacology studies should take this into consideration, and studies should be designed to demonstrate whether the candidate drug in any way interferes with the efficacy of cyclosporine. The important consideration here is that sponsors ignore good proof-of-concept studies at their peril.

Are Adverse Effects Expected at Effective Doses?   This is another risk management question and should be considered as early as possible in the development of a drug. There are many effective drugs on the market that produce headache, nausea, diarrhea, and so on, in a significant portion of the patient population. Many of these adverse effects will only be discovered in clinical trials, but signs of toxicity should be carefully considered in the design and conduct of these trials. Among the signs that can be misinterpreted are neurological effects in animals. Many animals can demonstrate signs of neurotoxicity, such as aberrant behavior in a functional observation battery, that at first seem not predictive of human effects. It is important to remember that animal behavior in response to adverse neurological effects may not, in fact often does not, have a direct correlation in humans. It is entirely conceivable that convulsions in animals may not be associated with similar effects in clinical trials but may signal that the drug does have the potential to produce seemingly unrelated effects in humans, such as depression or anxiety. Once again, sponsors ignore such findings at their peril, especially where obvious adverse effects are observed in animals at target doses for development.

What Is Known About Related Drugs?   As was pointed out earlier, the FDA has experience with a vast array of drugs. Many have failed in development due to adverse effects, but findings were never made public in publications. As part of the drug development program, it is incumbent on the sponsor to determine as thoroughly as possible what is known in publicly available sources about possible drug class effects. It is also important that the sponsor address these potential class effects, often by design and conduct of specialized nonclinical studies or incorporation of additional observations in standard toxicology studies. Also, it is important to "listen to the reviewer." All too often suggestions are made to a sponsor that particular attention be given to a specific issue and the advice is ignored. A wise sponsor listens to what is essentially free advice and considers it carefully.

What Are the Types and Sites of Toxic Effects?   This is essentially a review issue, but as with so many questions in this list there are potentially important points to consider. One is related to the previous question. Simply put, if a drug belongs to a class with known toxicities, and these are not seen in submitted toxicology studies, several questions could be raised by the review team and include:

- Have they been conducted correctly?
- Has a true MTD been achieved?
- Were appropriate observations made and endpoints included?
- Do TK data support that sufficient systemic exposure was achieved?

As you can see, what is a seemingly straightforward issue that should be answered by the results of standard toxicology studies could become a very complicated problem. Another point to consider is whether the types of toxicities are "acceptable" given the intended indication. This can be a very complicated issue and should be addressed. For example, consider a drug that is intended to be administered by the topical route, and dermal toxicity studies have demonstrated relatively minor adverse effects at reasonable multiples of expected clinical doses. However, studies that maximize systemic exposure—that is, the studies were conducted by a parenteral route of administration—demonstrate significant toxicities associated with effective topical doses. These effects should not be ignored. It is frankly impossible to consider every scenario of use and discovery of a hazard should drive appropriate *risk assessment* studies. In this example, it may be adequate to demonstrate that, under conditions of use, significant systemic exposure is so unlikely as to render the toxicity findings irrelevant. A sponsor should never take such issues lightly—it is almost certain that the FDA will not.

Has the Sponsor Established a No Observed Adverse Effect Level (NOAEL)? Although discussed extensively earlier, it is included here for emphasis. The sponsor *must* establish a NOAEL in most cases in order to enable FIH clinical trials. There are the usual exceptions (such as chemotherapeutic agents), but these are relatively obvious. A classic mistake made by sponsors is to conduct a nonclinical toxicology study intended to support the safety of a clinical trial in which no adverse effects are observed at one dose and serious toxicities, including death on study, are observed at the next highest dose. Based on the results of the study, the sponsor will claim to have established a NOAEL. Although technically correct, the sponsor has ignored the obvious implications of the study results. That is, either the range of doses was too great to observe something equivalent to a lowest-observed-adverse-effect level (LOAEL) so that clinically appropriate toxicities were observed (i.e., adverse effects that may be monitored and when observed can be used to determine a reasonable stopping dose in a dose–escalation trial), or the dose–response curve is so steep with respect to serious toxicities that development of the drug is likely to be problematic. Issues such as this can seriously affect a drug development program and should not be taken lightly.

What Is the Apparent Therapeutic Index?   This question is related to the previous one. All too frequently, sponsors will fail to consider results of nonclinical pharmacology studies in the context of potential safety implications of findings. A common mistake is to conduct a proof-of-concept pharmacology study in an animal model, demonstrate promising effects, and ignore serious toxicities. Enabling nonclinical toxicology studies are conducted, a NOAEL is established, Phase I studies are conducted, and what is discovered is that although a safe dose can be administered to humans, it is nowhere near the projected efficacious dose based on pharmacology studies. This is actually a relatively easy issue to deal with as long as the sponsor conducts good studies and is willing to "live with" the results.

Are There Irreversible or Unmonitorable Adverse Effects?   This issue can be a "drug killer." There are a number of toxicities for which there are no adequate biomarkers of effect useful in clinical trials (especially prodromal markers). When observed, often the most important determination to make is the dose multiple at which the toxicity is observed. Although sometimes "irreversible or unmonitorable adverse effects" may be toxicologically insignificant, this is not the usual case. Thus, it is very important to establish the apparent therapeutic index. Other parameters that are important to establish include blood levels at which these adverse effects are observed (AUC, C_{max}); it is important to determine whether doses or systemic exposures needed to produce the adverse effects change with length of treatment (especially if the doses needed to produce the adverse effect are lower with longer exposures), and whether a clinically useful dose can be found where irreversible/unmonitorable adverse effects are not produced, with an appropriate safety margin. Although this is essentially the same as establishing an apparent therapeutic index, in fact, the toxicity used to determine this might occur at doses lower than those associated with the irreversible/unmonitorable effect and could provide an additional margin of safety.

Are There Differences in Metabolism of the Drug, Especially Between Animals Used in Pivotal Toxicology Studies and Humans?   This has emerged in recent years as a serious potential problem in drug development. Some authorities maintain that this is essentially an "artifact" of increased sensitivity of analytical methodology (tandem mass spectrometry, etc.). It is important that the sponsor determine as early as possible in the drug development program whether there is/are relatively unique drug metabolite(s) produced by humans that have not been assessed for safety in nonclinical toxicology studies. The FDA has published guidance on this topic [6]. Essentially, the guidance recommends that the sponsor determine, possibly using *in vitro* methods such as isolated human hepatocytes/liver slices/microsomes, whether unique (or disproportionately abundant) metabolites exist compared to species used in toxicology studies, and be prepared to deal with the issue proactively. This could mean that the sponsor might need to conduct essentially "bridging toxicology" studies with synthesized metabolite. There are other considerations, however, such as relative amount of metabolite. The FDA guidance has set (rather arbitrarily) 10% of administered dose or systemic exposure (both relative to parent drug) as the "concern level" for a unique or "overabundant" metabolite. It is recommended that the sponsor consult the FDA when such situations arise during drug development.

27.6   CONCLUSION

A wise man once said that every new drug requires a new development program. This is very close to the truth. Drug development should be approached as what it, in fact, is: a scientific experiment. There are few if any "givens" in drug development, which is why it is a risky proposition. Seek advice whenever needed, and consider it carefully when offered.

REFERENCES

1. FDA Guidance website: http://www.fda.gov/cder/guidance/index.htm.

2. ICH Guidance website: http://www.ich.org/cache/compo/276-254-1.html.

3. *Integration of Study Results to Assess Concerns about Human Reproductive and Developmental Toxicities.* Washington, DC: FDA; 2001.

4. *Carcinogenicity Study Protocol Submissions.* Washington, DC: FDA; 2002.

5. *Photosafety Testing.* Washington, DC: FDA; 2003.

6. *Guidance for Industry: Estimating the Maximum Safe Starting Dose in Initial Clinical Trials for Therapeutics in Adult Healthy Volunteers.* Washington, DC: FDA; 2005.

7. *Safety Testing of Drug Metabolites.* Washington, DC: FDA; 2005.

8. *Exploratory IND Studies.* Washington, DC: FDA; 2006.

9. *Recommended Approaches to Integration of Genetic Toxicology Study Results.* Washington, DC: FDA; 2006.

10. *Nonclinical Safety Evaluation of Pediatric Drug Products.* Washington, DC: FDA; 2006.

11. Mathieu M. *New Drug Development: A Regulatory Overview*, 7th ed. Waltham, MA: Parexel; 2005.

28

SELECTION AND UTILIZATION OF CROs FOR SAFETY ASSESSMENT

JOANNE R. KOPPLIN AND WARD R. RICHTER

Druquest International, Inc., Leeds, Alabama

Contents

28.1   INTRODUCTION

Outsourcing preclinical development and safety testing to Contract Research Organizations (CROs) has become common in the biopharmaceutical, chemical, medical device, and food additive industries. It is important to understand the culture of the

Preclinical Development Handbook: Toxicology, edited by Shayne Cox Gad
Copyright © 2008 John Wiley & Sons, Inc.

CRO industry and how to locate, evaluate, and work with individual CROs when outsourcing work. In this chapter, we discuss these processes based on personal experience working with and working for preclinical CROs. Our combined experience is derived from outsourcing preclinical work as employees of a major pharmaceutical company, a major chemical company, and a young biotechnology company and as consultants for these industries. We have also held senior management positions in three different CROs during the course of our careers.

28.2 HISTORICAL DEVELOPMENT OF THE PRECLINICAL CRO POST-WWII

Contract Research Organizations (CROs) conducting preclinical testing provide services in pharmacology, pharmacokinetics, analytical chemistry, toxicology, pathology, and associated disciplines. Most were established and/or grew after Word War II as a result of growth in the pharmaceutical industry and because of increasing government regulations. The preclinical contract industry has been concentrated in the United States and the United Kingdom. Smaller laboratories are found in Canada, France, Italy, Japan, and other countries.

Early growth of the preclinical contract industry was fueled by rapid growth of the pharmaceutical industry when construction of new toxicology laboratories and animal facilities did not keep up with the number of new drug candidates selected for development. Surplus work was outsourced but sponsors outsourced only work that was deemed less critical and simpler to conduct because contract laboratories did not have the same level of scientific expertise, facilities, or equipment as the sponsoring companies. The scientific capabilities of the contract laboratories grew in quality and depth over the years and by the 1990s they were generally perceived as the equivalent of that found in the largest pharmaceutical firms. For many specialized technologies they often were superior to the sponsoring companies because of extensive experience in technologies that were used only occasionally by a single company.

Rapid growth of toxicology contract laboratories occurred during the 1960s and the early 1970s. Industrial Biotest (IBT) was an industry leader and was utilized by many major pharmaceutical and chemical companies in the United States, Europe, and Japan. IBT was favored because it turned out studies and reports on time and at low cost and was perceived to provide quality work. By 1975, it was learned that Industrial Biotest fabricated some of the data in its reports and the laboratory was eventually closed with several members of the management team convicted of criminal activity. The criminal behavior of this laboratory was one of the motivators for the establishment of the Good Laboratory Practice Act of 1978. Because so many large companies had relied on this laboratory and because some of the work was invalidated, there was a significant backlash against outsourcing to contract laboratories. Pharmaceutical and chemical companies rapidly built new toxicology laboratories and established policies of conducting all preclinical testing in-house. The amount of outsourcing for preclinical safety testing leveled off or contracted in the 1980s, as a result.

Another unrelated event occurred in 1976 that was to have a major negative financial impact on the preclinical contract laboratory industry when the Toxic

Substances Control Act (TOSCA) was passed, regulating an estimated 75,000 chemicals. Most people in the industry and government expected that TOSCA would mandate extensive toxicology testing of thousands if not tens of thousands of chemicals in industrial use. The contract laboratory industry viewed this as an opportunity and a major new source of revenue and expansion. Many of the laboratories, including the industry leaders, built new facilities, increasing their animal capacity by as much as 30–40%. The work predicted by passage of the Toxic Substances Control Act never materialized due to the manner in which the law was interpreted by regulatory agencies and because of intense lobbying pressure by the chemical industry. By the early 1980s there was a serious surplus of animal rooms in the contract industry and most facilities were not filled. The industry became very competitive and companies cut prices to cost or even below cost to cover overhead. This oversupply of animal and laboratory facilities kept prices and margins depressed until the late 1990s when growth of the pharmaceutical industry caught up with capacity. Prices of studies remained at relatively flat level for 15 years in spite of inflation.

Starting in the 1990s, a series of factors dramatically improved the financial outlook for preclinical toxicology laboratories. (1) The biotechnology industry, considered as a subset of the pharmaceutical industry, matured and grew to spend significant amounts of money on development. (2) The contract laboratories achieved recognition that they were fully as capable as in-house laboratories of sponsors and they no longer carried the stigma of the Industrial Biotest incident. (3) Combinatorial chemistry and new automated early screening technologies increased the number of potential drug candidates in development. (4) Financial administrators in the large pharmaceutical and chemical companies put more and more pressure on the corporations to outsource for economic reasons, because of the lower operating costs in contract laboratories. Purchasing departments became involved and they pressed for preferred provider agreements with one or more CROs.

Today the involvement of CROs is recognized and supported by the FDA. In a speech to the Association of CROs (ACRO) in October 2002, the FDA Commissioner, Dr. Mark McClellan, stated that "CROs hold great potential" to help the process of reducing development time for new drug applications and getting safe, critical products to market more quickly.

28.3 ROLE OF THE CRO IN PRECLINICAL DEVELOPMENT TODAY

The trends just described have filled the empty animal rooms in the major preclinical CROs in the last several years. Pharmaceutical companies have their own laboratories but contract excess or specialized work to CROs. We estimate the annual value of outsourced work (preclinical and clinical) to be in excess of $8 billion (U.S.). Of this $8 billion, an estimated $600–750 million was outsourced for preclinical testing in 2002. It is unclear whether analysts developing these estimates have included the potential outsourcing from the smaller biotechnology companies. Small biotechnology companies without their own internal capabilities exclusively use CROs to conduct their safety testing. Even the largest biotechnology companies have limited animal facilities, usually limited to efficacy testing and pre-GLP safety testing.

Testing procedures conducted by preclinical CROs are standardized by government regulation and all competitors conduct the same process. All of the major players in the marketplace produce a quality report on time, conforming to government regulations with the process being driven by experienced managers and technical staff. Companies differentiate themselves by experience, unique technologies, automation, scientific expertise, and service. The product is the process rather than the end report.

Pharmaceutical companies generally do not feel comfortable with laboratories that appear to be too academic or culturally aligned with practices in government laboratories. These groups are perceived to pay less attention to timeliness and efficiency and to have less understanding of the drug development process. Pharmaceutical companies contract work to laboratories that have familiar facilities and familiar cultural behavior. They contract to laboratories with a known track record or those laboratories that employ experienced staff familiar with the pharmaceutical corporate culture. David Cavalla [1] in *Modern Strategy for Preclinical Pharmaceutical R&D* stated it in this way: "Enduring added value can only come from a strong knowledge base of the core business. In this case this is the technical and scientific complexity of the pharmaceutical development process. CROs who can capture this knowledge through employing professionally experienced leaders, who can then cultivate the scientific culture of pharmaceutical development into their organization, will be the winners of the fight to capture increased market share."

28.4   LOCATING CANDIDATE CROS

For new startup companies it is important to begin the identification and evaluation of CROs early to enroll one or more in assisting development of their business plan. "Before a company even has a drug candidate to test, when it is still devising its business plan and is concerned with matters such as financing, infrastructure, and early-stage discovery, it should begin researching the services available for outsourcing, the economics of pursuing an outsourcing strategy" [2]. For established companies, it is important to establish an ongoing relationship with several CROs to allow them to move rapidly in outsourcing new drug candidate testing.

Colleagues who have worked with several CROs can be the single most useful source of locating companies that are candidates for your outsourcing requirements. They can provide the benefit of their experience in working with specific companies and their positive as well as negative experiences. Frequently, they will have useful contacts on the staffs of the CROs they have worked with. An individual new to the preclinical development business may not have colleagues in the business. Attendance at local and regional biotechnology meetings is useful in making contact with new colleagues on an informal basis.

Consultants in preclinical development, safety assessment, or toxicology work with many CROs and they are usually in the business of assisting in evaluation of CROs and in outsourcing studies. While the major CROs all conduct a broad range of studies and have most technologies available, they are not all equally adept at conducting studies that are not part of the standard core of toxicology studies. Consultants can be very useful in assessing specific capabilities. Interviewing and getting the assistance of one or more consultants for suggestions on CROs helps develop a useful relationship with the consultant early on in the preclinical development process. If problems develop or unusual findings appear in safety studies, consultants can be invaluable in designing an approach to elucidate the problem and if necessary in working with the FDA to develop a strategy that will satisfy the agency's questions when the data are submitted in an IND. The consultant may not be needed for anything further in the preclinical development program but an established relationship is invaluable, should a consultant's assistance be needed.

Trade shows are a great place to review the capabilities of a large number of CROs, especially those with specialized technologies. The 2005 SOT meeting had 51 exhibitors who classified themselves as CROs. In addition, there were specialty laboratories with a single technology who didn't classify themselves as CROs. It is possible to meet scientists and scientific directors of the companies at shows such as the SOT Exhibition. It is possible to discuss a proposed development program and outsourcing requirements at the trade show and get a sense of the CRO's approach to a relationship with a new client. Develop a file of candidate laboratories for future reference and keep it up to date. We maintain a library of literature from at least 12 companies that we are interested in utilizing. In addition to literature, web sites are useful in getting an overview of a company's capabilities.

28.5 TELEPHONE INTERVIEWS FOR INITIAL SCREENING

Telephone interviews of candidate CROs save time and travel costs. They are useful in developing a short list of potential partners. The telephone will become one of the primary means of communication during the negotiating period and during study design, initiation, and conduct. The telephone interview will provide a sense of how easily the organization deals with you by phone. Determine if it easy to reach the scientific staff, whether you are routed only to marketing staff, and whether your calls are returned in a timely manner.

28.6 SITE VISIT: THE KEY TO EVALUATION

An actual site visit and inspection of the CRO's facilities and staff is the most important single activity in evaluating a new company. Mid-size and large companies considering outsourcing will conduct site visits by their in-house staff, while small virtual companies and new startups may conduct site visits through a consultant. Consultants often have working knowledge of the CRO under consideration and may not need to conduct a new inspection in the detail outlined here. For small companies relying on a consultant, it is still beneficial for a staff member to accompany the consultant on a site visit to meet the staff and begin to develop a working relationship. A site visit provides the opportunity to see work in progress and systems in action. It is the best way to evaluate security and the procedures to protect the confidentiality of data. Breaches of confidentiality can be very subtle and three examples follow. One of the authors (Richter) was alerted to a breach of security in his own CRO by a client. The client arrived at the laboratory early, 15 minutes before the front door was open for business. He walked behind some bushes adjacent to the front door to peer through the window. The desk of the director of pathology was next to the window and he saw the business cards of two of his colleagues who had visited the week before and he could read pages of a report for his compound. He was very unhappy. One of the authors (Kopplin) inspected a GLP compliant CRO that was affiliated with a university, but operated as an independent agency. They were self-contained except for the ability to print reports and they used the university central reproduction facility in another building. Confidential reports of safety studies were left on a table in the hallway for pickup after completion. They were accessible to the general public walking by. This laboratory was not placed on a list of acceptable CROs. One of the authors (Richter) inspected a large well established CRO and was getting a tour of the facility. They were visiting the test material storage room when the host was paged to a phone call. The author was left alone with access to the stock test material from dozens of companies. The laboratory was not placed on a list of acceptable CROs. These examples provide insight into the type of things that can only be determined by a site visit. A checklist (Table 28.1) is provided to outline the conduct of an inspection of a new CRO.

28.7   EVALUATION OF THE PROCESS: NOT THE FINAL REPORT

While the checklist covers very specific items, the overall evaluation of the candidate CRO should depend on an evaluation of its culture and an evaluation of the process involved in conducting the work. Unlike the manufacturer of a widget, the process of conducting the research, interpreting it, and summarizing it in a report is critical to its quality and elegance. The widget manufacturer can tolerate mistakes by having a good quality control system that eliminates defective products. That simplistic approach to quality is not applicable to a highly regulated knowledge-based industry. Evaluating the process is fundamental to finding a CRO that meets your needs. All of the major CROs can produce a report on time that is free from error. The quality of the process is what differentiates them. Thus, the culture of the CRO, its systems, and its staff are critical elements in success. When inspecting a CRO, look for signs that the process has broken down, such as piles of work on a study director's desk and floor or rooms full of materials that should have been archived or disposed of. One of the authors (Richter) discovered that a CRO's inability to validate an analytical procedure occurred when a reference standard for another compound that should have been archived was left in the analytical laboratory and used by mistake.

The reliability and quality of the process influence the time to completion of studies and reports. Pharmaceutical companies are under strong pressure to cut the time from drug discovery to market. It is important to determine the CRO's record for on-time reports. Late reports are an indication of failure in the processes or inadequate staffing.

28.8   SPECIAL CONSIDERATIONS IN SELECTING A SPECIALIZED OR UNIVERSITY LABORATORY

Working with university laboratories can require some extra effort. There are times when a specialized procedure performed only in a university setting is needed to

TABLE 28.1   Checklist for Site Visit Evaluation

Meet Key Personnel, Marketing, Management, Scientific and Technical

Marketing Representative
Senior Scientific Management
Study Director(s)
Director of Pathology
Director of Clinical Pathology
Directors of Analytical and Bioanalytical Chemistry
Director of Quality Assurance
Director of the Pharmacy
Managers and/or supervisors of other specialty services or laboratories

Staff Qualifications

Resumés of key scientific and technical staff
Certifications, scientists and technicians
Training records, evidence of ongoing training
Publication record and presentations at scientific meetings
Consultant's and part-time specialist's qualifications
Determine whether you would be comfortable working with this staff;
go to lunch and/or dinner with some of them;
ask to meet key people in their office, view their work environment

Special Things to Observe or Determine During Visit

Determine in-house capabilities. Are any key services outsourced?
Assess the morale of the staff
Observe how busy the facility is. Are animal rooms mostly full or mostly empty?
Find out their on-time record for delivery of reports
Establish who will be your primary contact during negotiations and during conduct of
    work
Develop an impression of whether the laboratory management appear to be interested in
    working with you or whether your visit is treated as a routine
Evaluate the degree of automation for data capture and reporting

Physical Plant Areas to Inspect

Reception
Conference room
Offices
Laboratories, chemistry, histology, clinical, specialty
Necropsy room(s)
Animal rooms
Technician work areas, desks and facilities for data review and organization
Pharmacy
Information Technology
Restrooms
Cage washing
Storage, clean and dirty cages, food, bedding, supplies

TABLE 28.1   *Continued*

What to Inspect Physical Physical Plant For

Organization of overall facility for efficient work flow; user friendly
HVAC, environmental monitoring system, review temperature records
Cleanliness of the facility
Cleanliness of uniforms
Maintenance
Organized work flow in laboratories
Work flow into and out of animal rooms, clean versus dirty corridors
Security and confidentiality. Can you see any data left in open view during a tour?
Availability of SOPs in work areas
Availability of MSDSs in work areas

Security

Reception and visitor entrance
Employee entrance
Deliveries and loading dock
Data security, hard copy and electronic
Computer backup, stored on site or off-site
Disaster recovery plan
Compound and formulation security
Background check on employees
Is work left unattended on desks?
Pathologists computers on or off while away from desk?
End of work day security for active paper files?
Backup generator
Emergency planning: snow, sleet, or other event

Standard Operating Procedures (SOPs)

Review table of contents for general overview
Review key SOPs and those for specialized procedures needed for proposed project(s)
Are the SOPs reviewed and updated on a specific schedule?
Are the SOPs accessible to the staff in the laboratories and animal rooms? Ask to see the
    SOPs for a specific procedure during a tour of the laboratories. Is it readily available and
    does it appear that the staff are following the SOPs?
Is the format of SOPs user friendly?
Is the process of SOP approval overly bureaucratic?
Do you find hand-written notes derived from SOPs in the laboratory—a GLP violation?
Evaluate employee health and emergency medical assistance
Review animal care program

Other Documentation

FDA and/or EPA inspections and audits, key findings
Maintenance records on equipment, view examples for critical equipment
Sample contracts and confidentiality agreements
Sample protocols
Statistical procedures
Examples of reports—final, interim, and periodic progress updates
Facility certifications, local
AAALAC accredited; date of last inspection, inspection report

evaluate the safety of a drug candidate. Unless the testing procedure has a widespread demand by the pharmaceutical industry, the laboratory is unlikely to be in compliance with the Good Laboratory Practices Act. The requirements of full compliance are of such a magnitude that it is not economically practical for the university laboratory to meet all of the specific details. The FDA and EPA will accept studies from these university laboratories, if the procedures are not available from a fully compliant GLP laboratory and if the laboratory meets the spirit of the GLP requirements. University laboratories generally do not have access to help in setting up the major requirements of GLP compliance. It will be necessary for the sponsoring organization to work with the laboratory to meet minimum standards. An inspection of the facilities and an evaluation of systems is the first step in outlining the deficits for the laboratory director and staff. We have found that the first and most glaring deficiency in many university laboratories is control of the test material and its security. Often the laboratories are used by graduate students who have unlimited access along with their visiting friends in the middle of the night. It is not difficult, but it is necessary, to develop locked and secure cabinets or rooms for the test material, related materials, data records, as well as the appropriate logs of the materials. The extent of installing GLP procedures depends on how critical the laboratory procedure is to determining the ultimate safety of the test article. The sponsor should be prepared to provide QA inspection of the work. At a minimum, the sponsor should be prepared to assist in any or all of the following:

Outlining the SOPs needed

Developing the protocols

Advising and/or assisting in the preparation of SOPs

Preparing forms for data recording, when not automated

Documenting staff performing individual procedures

Determining validation needs for instrumentation and processes

Maintaining CVs and training of staff

Defining raw data

Establishing data security procedures

We have also found that an hour of time spent in reviewing the background and need for GLP standards is productive with an inexperienced academic staff. Most individuals grasp the concept of documentation and chain of evidence for forensic purposes as an analogy and this goes a long way in achieving compliance with the general concept of Good Laboratory Practices.

28.9 SELECTING A SINGLE LABORATORY VERSUS SPREADING THE WORK AMONG MULTIPLE LABORATORIES

Early in the evolution of the CRO industry, many in the sponsor industry worried about the stability of an individual CRO and placed their studies in different laboratories because they felt it reduced the risk. If anything were to go wrong, financially, technically, or logistically in one lab and a study was compromised, the damage was limited. The rest of the development program would be safe.

With the maturation of the CRO industry, the individual companies have become financially stable, they have well established and reliable procedures, and they maintain a staff that is just as stable as that of the sponsoring organizations. With that change, it is usually wiser to place all of the development outsourcing with a single company once a working relationship has been established. The company will have experience with the compound, its formulation, and expected compound effects. Dose setting studies do not transfer well from one lab to another because of subtle differences in animal environment and care. A second lab will almost always insist on repeating dose-ranging studies before undertaking the next step in a development program even though dose ranging was done earlier at another laboratory. They will have learned from experience that they risk running a study that may not meet regulatory guidelines for establishing dose levels. It is critical to place major studies in the same laboratory that did the dose-ranging studies in the same species and strain of animals.

There are distinct financial advantages to placing all of a safety testing program at one laboratory in addition to eliminating the need for several dose-ranging studies. CROs will negotiate favorably on packages of all of the studies needed to reach an IND. Even those sponsors who only outsource one or two studies from a development program will get favorable treatment in pricing if they are repeat clients. However, it may be necessary to use several CROs because the laboratory of choice may not offer all types of studies or may be relatively inexperienced in a specialized study such as reproductive toxicology or genetic toxicology.

28.10 INITIAL SELECTION OF A CRO FOR A NEW PROGRAM OR SINGLE LARGE STUDY

For budget purposes, CROs will provide general prices for specific types of studies. The final price will depend on the specific protocol and variations of the protocol related to the type of compound, mechanism of action, and clinical indication being tested. CROs will also provide templates of protocols for sponsor review and modification or they will modify a protocol to meet the sponsor's specific requirements. Once the protocol is close to the final version, it is time to get specific prices for the work. This may involve submitting a single study for pricing or submitting a whole series of studies for pricing.

When outsourcing a new development package or a single large study such as a carcinogenicity study, it is useful to get prices from at least three different laboratories that have met your criteria during the screening process. The favored laboratory may not be able to start the projected studies on a realistic schedule because it is busy. Laboratories that are busy and fully booked usually do not negotiate on price. By letting the CRO know that you are getting three bids on the program, it will be sure to quote its best price for fear of being underbid by a competitor.

When getting bids from several laboratories and comparing prices, it is important to be certain that all are bidding on the exact same protocol. Rather than asking for the price of a 28 day rat gavage toxicity study, a specific and identical protocol should be submitted to each of the CROs. In that way, prices won't be affected by variations in the several laboratories standard protocols for that type of study. Inform the bidding companies that the protocol may be modified in final negotiations but that the initial protocol will be the basis for selection based on price. It helps to build future relationships, if you agree to share the pricing information after bids are returned. It is not necessary to disclose the bidding laboratory, only the range of prices from them.

Since the laboratories are competitive, bids usually are quite similar. If they are, the choice should be your favorite providing they all meet your time frame for completion of the work. Occasionally, there may be a laboratory that is especially high and out of range. The high price may indicate that the lab is booked and overworked or that it didn't review the protocol carefully, both bad signs. Bids that are significantly lower than the rest may indicate that the laboratory is having difficulty marketing or that it did not review the protocol carefully. If awarded the contract, the lab could be tempted to cut corners to keep costs down. When we were outsourcing studies for our respective employers, we never recommended accepting a price that was significantly below others or that was well below the expected range based on previous experience.

28.11 TACTICS FOR DEVELOPING A RELATIONSHIP WITH THE CRO STAFF AND ENLISTING THEM AS MEMBERS OF THE DEVELOPMENT TEAM

Nothing is more important to the success of outsourcing than developing an effective working relationship with the staff of the CRO. They should be considered part of the development team with just as much invested in the success of the project as the sponsor's staff. They should share the agony of failure and the elation of success. Decades ago, many sponsors felt it necessary to develop an adversarial relationship with a CRO to ensure due diligence in the conduct of the project. Nothing destroys a successful outcome more than a paranoid attitude over the conduct of a study. It is possible to exercise proper quality control over the outsourcing process without making it an adversarial relationship. The staff of the CRO expect that the sponsor will be looking over their shoulders and evaluating their work as it proceeds but this process does not need to be confrontational.

Developing a relationship that makes the technical staff as well as the scientific staff feel part of the team helps ensure success of the project. A good sponsor will present one or more seminars on the drug candidate and the development progress for the CRO staff. Progress reports on the development program keep enthusiasm high for the testing project and encourage careful work on the part of the technical staff. CRO management usually encourages such inclusion of the staff as part of your development team. It helps morale of the staff to have a stake in the outcome of the drug candidate's progress through the development process.

28.12 DEALING WITH UNEXPECTED COMPOUND-RELATED CHANGES OR TECHNICAL PROBLEMS

It is human to immediately assume that errors were made in the conduct of a study when there are unexpected adverse effects. It is in the best interest of the CRO to detect errors if they occur and the staff will assist in resolving the cause of unexpected results. One of the authors (Richter) worked with a sponsor on an intravenous infusion study that caused the death of all animals at the high dose level with severe damage to the veins. Studies on vein irritation had shown that the compound was not especially irritating. The sponsor immediately accused the laboratory of misdosing the animals, hired several consultants, and spent 3 months reviewing all of the records, interviewing technicians and scientific staff in an attempt to prove that the laboratory had made a serious error. The CRO staff had determined that the problem was related to the formulation within days of the deaths. The compound was only minimally soluble in the formulation and it precipitated out in the veins during infusion, actually obstructing them. It took the sponsor 3 months of lost time before the sponser accepted this interpretation and, working with another consultant, went back to the drawing board and reformulated.

28.13   MONITORING THE OUTSOURCED WORK

Monitoring of the work is a key to a successful outcome. Under GLP regulations, a study monitor is specified by the sponsor and this individual is the primary contact with the CRO's study director during the initiation, conduct, and reporting of the outsourced work. The study monitor should be in contact by email or phone at least weekly to review progress. The contract with the CRO should specify regular letter reports on a periodic basis, weekly or monthly, depending on the complexity of the study.

It is very helpful for the study monitor and/or additional sponsor representatives to visit the CRO laboratory site and review the work during the course of a study. The frequency and depth of these inspections depends on the complexity of the study. Short-term dose-ranging studies usually do not need a physical inspection unless the dosing procedure is unusually difficult. For definitive studies, such as 28 day, 90 day, or longer toxicology studies, it is desirable to have a sponsor representative on-site for at least the first day of dosing and the necropsies. Interim on-site inspections of the data on a monthly or quarterly schedule reduce the amount of time needed in reviewing the final report and in detecting problems. These visits are helpful in nurturing a sense of team work with the CRO staff and lets them know that they are part of the team. When unusual parameters are being measured or when a routine parameter is critical to the mechanism of action of the compound, the sponsor will want to be present for the event. Urinalysis is usually considered to be a very routine analysis in toxicological studies. We worked with a compound that was expected to cause changes in urinary parameters and this was so critical to the outcome of the study that sponsor representatives at the vice presidential level were on site to observe the urine collection and processing in the clinical pathology laboratory.

The best CROs occasionally make mistakes and sometimes these are not obvious to those who observe the work on a daily basis. A sponsor representative may look at the progress of the study with a different viewpoint. One of the authors (Richter) worked as a consultant for a carcinogenicity study at a CRO in which more than half of the female rats in all dose groups, including controls, developed uterine carcinomas. The spontaneous incidence of uterine carcinomas in rats of the strain used was less than 5%. The staff of the CRO were unable to determine the reason for the increased incidence after detailed review of all records. After the author found that there was light-induced damage to the retinas, he suggested that increased estrogen levels were responsible and that excessive exposure to light could increase estrogen. The CRO staff carefully checked the timers for the animal rooms and found that they were correctly set to go off and on at the protocol specified times. After the author insisted that the timers be checked again, the building engineers revealed that they had disconnected the timers from the lights and although the timers were running, they had no effect on the lights. The rats had been exposed to light 24 hours a day for 2 years! No one had checked to see if the lights actually went off every night. The book by Gralla [3] covers many issues in monitoring toxicology studies.

REFERENCES

1. Cavalla D. *Modern Strategy for Preclinical Pharmaceutical R&D* 1997;131.
2. Glaser V. *Outsourcing Drug Discov Dev* 2005;25(15):23–26.
3. Gralla EJ. *Scientific Considerations in Monitoring and Evaluating Toxicological Research.* Bristol, DA: Hemisphere Publishing Corporation; 1981.

29

AUDITING AND INSPECTING PRECLINICAL RESEARCH AND COMPLIANCE WITH GOOD LABORATORY PRACTICE (GLP)

N.J. DENT

Country Consultancy Ltd., Copper Beeches, Milton Malsor, United Kingdom

Contents

Preclinical Development Handbook: Toxicology, edited by Shayne Cox Gad
Copyright © 2008 John Wiley & Sons, Inc.

29.1   INTRODUCTION

The Good Laboratory Practice (GLP) Guidelines have been in existence for nonclinical safety studies since 1976 [1–8]. They have progressed through various transitional phases to become guidelines in some countries and regulatory/statutory instruments in others.

The current document is the Organisation for Economic Co-operation and Development (OECD) Principles of GLP [9] and is currently accepted as the industry standard. This was reviewed and published in January 1997 [10, 11] but must be used in conjunction with the appropriate Scientific Guidelines for the scientific side of the study, that is, the OECD Toxicology Guidelines and so on [12]. This sets out to cover all nonclinical safety studies and gives guidance as to how these studies should be conducted in conjunction with the appropriate regulatory toxicology guidelines and, on that basis, when encompassed in the various Directives of the European Union (EU) [13] or in other Memorandums of Understanding, allows data generated under this program to be mutually accepted by other OECD countries. One must not forget, however, the other equally important guidelines and regulations of other countries, such as those of the U.S. Food and Drug Administration (FDA) [14] and the U.S. Environmental Protection Agency (EPA) [15–20], and similar organizations in Japan [21]. All have basically similar rules and, being members of the OECD, data generated to the OECD principles will generally be accepted in the United States and Japan. The EPA regulations used to be quite different and were applied to agrochemical and pesticide products. However, having been revised recently, they have been brought in line with the documents of other agencies.

The guidelines themselves, with the exception of those in countries where they are featured as regulations, are, as stated, guidelines to the conduct of the study and aim to cover compliance with the GLP principles but in no way do they dictate how the science will be performed.

It must be remembered that compliance is monitored by adherence to GLP, whereas the regulatory authority and the receiving authority of the dossier when submitted for the application of a marketing permit or similar document review the science.

29.2   OBJECTIVE OF THE GUIDELINES

The general objective of the guidelines originates in the very early 1970s, when one pharmaceutical company in particular and a contract research organization (CRO) generated data that, when submitted to the FDA, gave them cause for concern in the accuracy of the data presented and, in certain instances, the honesty of the submission.

At that time, a full review of companies and institutions conducting nonclinical safety studies (toxicology) was undertaken by the FDA [22], and in general, the industry was found to be credible. One company (Industrial Biotest) was found to be generating extremely poor quality data—in many instances, in a fraudulent manner. Just prior to this, GD Searle had made a submission to the FDA where some data were apparently missing but subsequently sent, causing the FDA again to reconsider the total honesty of the pharmaceutical industry. The quote from the FDA was that it had "until that time assumed total honesty and integrity of the data supplied to the FDA for revision; however with recent events this has now given cause for concern."

Industrial Biotest basically set out with the prime objective to commit fraud, and many of the pesticide and agrochemical industries suffered through their lack of attention to detail, inventiveness, and basic dishonesty. Many of the test compounds sent for analysis and testing in animals for safety aspects remained unopened in the test substance store, although the client had received a report saying that the product had been tested and was extremely safe and able to be used. Around 200 studies were eventually rejected by the agencies, causing a great upheaval in the scientific research community and in the marketing of products. This caused the FDA to put together and implement the GLPs [23, 24].

Over the next 10 years, many countries introduced similar good practices guidelines. The EU [25] in general produced its guidelines, and eventually, despite the fact that the world was operating according to similar principles, a standard document was produced by the OECD in the early 1980s and became the industry standard. This was of benefit to the whole industry because it now precluded the fact that every submitting company would have to be inspected by each relevant monitoring authority and, when implemented into several directives and legal statutes [26, 27] within the OECD (particularly in the UK [28]), this allowed data generated by one company to be accepted by several receiving authorities without further inspection.

The objective of the GLPs is to ensure that a standard approach is undertaken, covering traceability and accountability and, while still allowing freedom for the scientists, to impose certain restrictions on the generation of data and the experimental work.

During the period of time when guidelines were being produced and inspections were taking place, several other instances of "dubious data" appeared. Notably, in the United States around the year 2000, a contract research company claimed full GLP compliance for its safety studies but in actual fact was cited by the FDA inspectors as having almost as many problems as Industrial Biotest. Later that year, an analytical contract research organization performing work for the EPA was found to operate a "two notebook system"—producing data as it was received from the machines and then manipulating that data to give better analytical results. Not only was this problem seen in the United States but similar instances were seen in laboratories in Scandinavia; in the United Kingdom a fraudulent submission was made to the regulatory authorities when a report was "doctored" to give better results on the product than had been seen in testing and, a product under license to a company was eventually found to have much of the data made up by the research technician.

The general aspect of nonclinical research could at this time be seen to be the ability to produce extremely poor quality data but in total compliance with GLP!

One cannot, however, use GLP to prevent any scientific person who is intent on committing fraud in its true sense from performing that act; it, however, has in the past and will in the future continue to enable this practice to be exposed more easily.

One should not consider that the whole scientific community is setting out to commit fraud or tempting to deceive the regulatory authorities; but, unfortunately, the whole concept of good laboratory practices was brought about and subsequently reinforced by those several issues and had brought the scientific community into disrepute with the regulatory agencies.

It must be remembered that GLP is merely common sense in a formal environment. The key phrases that are currently seen in a GLP environment include good documentation, good training, maintenance and calibration of all equipment, the archiving and storing of data in a formal and retrievable manner, and the use of high quality, validated equipment and accredited test systems (animals).

This in general is merely good science, and the GLPs have further enhanced this by the addition of an independent Quality Assurance Unit (QAU) and a study director/principal investigator who jointly controls and oversees the project and involves the management in putting together adequate resources and assuming overall responsibility for the study.

This can be seen as good science, with several slight enhancements. The details of these individual subjects are addressed later in this chapter.

29.3   WHO DOES IT AFFECT?

Any company or institution performing nonclinical safety studies for the submission of data for a new chemical entity; a new biological, immunological, pesticide, veterinary or agrochemical product; or, for that matter, a similar product that will eventually appear in the marketplace and be consumed by the general public must adhere to GLP in the conduct of their nonclinical safety study experimentation.

Although initially the GLPs were seen to be a bureaucratic restriction on research and development, over the thirty or so years since this practice has been established it is amazing the number of disciplines and companies that persistently apply to the regulatory authorities to enter into their GLP monitoring program while not performing any safety analysis or supporting safety analysis: the food industry, the analytical industry involved in assaying samples from human clinical trials, the microbiology laboratories, central laboratories in hospitals, and central laboratories performing safety analysis for human clinical trials. The list is endless but it merely demonstrates that good laboratory practices have been seen as a quality standard that is internationally accepted and therefore there is a definite bonus in having GLP as one if not the only quality standard within a company.

Within a company, every person from senior management to the junior technician is bound by these GLPs and must exhibit clear understanding and training in these practices.

To ensure that the practices are followed, a regulatory inspection takes place on a 2 year basis in most countries, and the objective of this is to review, as an independent group, how these good practices are being followed. Certification or a guarantee that the company is operating according to these standards is the benchmark standard. This is also addressed later in this chapter.

As we move into the 21st century, it is quite apparent that the industry will shrink as mergers and acquisitions [29–33] take place, and, with this, the emergence of the now familiar CRO will become ever more popular in the conduct of nonclinical safety studies. It is therefore very important that, in this area, the sponsor has the assurance that these facilities are operating not only to the highest standard of science but also in compliance with GLP and that, as a subcontractor, the data they generate will be equally accepted as if the data were generated by the company itself.

29.4   WHY HAVE IT?

In general terms, for companies conducting nonclinical safety studies [34], it is a regulatory requirement, and without this certificate or certification of compliance, data will generally not be accepted by the receiving/regulatory authorities.

However, one should not embark on the process of obtaining or working to GLP with this sole aim in mind. It should be used as an ongoing improving and quality standard for the laboratory. In fact, in my experience over the past five years, many companies have gone far beyond the requirements of GLP compliance [35], and the overall concept of good scientific design and good science has been superseded by the desire merely to obtain compliance. It is quite often seen that an extremely poor quality scientific study has been conducted in complete compliance with GLP. For example, on several occasions in a laboratory where the refrigerator was operated far from its permitted limits, but where the temperature was diligently recorded, signed, and dated as required by GLP, there was no attempt either to document the excursions outside the accepted range or to rectify the problem. The operative was merely under the impression that as long as temperature in the refrigerator is recorded, this is GLP despite the damage that excursions outside the temperature range may have caused to any investigational product stored in the refrigerator. Over the years, scientists who have worked according to the principles of GLP now readily admit without any prompting that they are unsure how they conducted scientific studies before the advent of these good practices: the ability to reconstruct studies, to work to a standard format across several differing laboratories or countries, and to be able to prove beyond reasonable doubt that these were the values obtained and the results submitted.

Certainly, data with a GLP compliance statement are being accepted more readily by the receiving authority, which has led to fewer repeated studies. This, in turn, is helping to achieve the aim of all scientists in reducing the use of animals.

From a company's point of view, working according to the principles of GLP shows that it has an attitude that is both ethical and moral to the production of scientific data with products that will eventually enter the human food chain or be of benefit to humankind.

29.5   HOW IS IT ENFORCED?

In the OECD countries, for at least 14 years, an Inspectorate has been set up, varying in inspector numbers from several hundred in the United States to one or two in countries not conducting a great deal of scientific nonclinical research. All countries, however, have a regulatory group that, in some instances, also acts as the receiving authority for the review of data and reports to the GLP Monitoring Authority (which visits on a 2 year basis or, in Germany, a 4 year basis, those companies who have claimed compliance and will then be on a rolling program of review [36]).

Unlike its role in many areas of regulatory compliance, it is still the responsibility of the sponsoring company to claim compliance from the Monitoring Authority. This claim is made for a particular company, laboratory, and/or series of tests. From the date of compliance when a letter is written to the Monitoring Authority, data generated from then on are assumed by that company to be in compliance with GLP. This claim in then verified in a visit from the regulatory inspector. The inspection may be performed by one or two persons for 1 to 5 days. At the end of the inspection, an exit meeting is held, and the company is usually given an indication of its performance. Noncompliance points are noted in writing and discussed, and a report is then prepared. In view of the findings, three levels of compliance can be obtained:

1. Sufficient deviations have been seen to question the integrity of the data and, therefore, a complete rejection of the claim of compliance is made, with a revisit necessary.

2. Minor points of compliance have been seen that can be handled in a specified period, in which case, the laboratory is placed under the category of pending compliance.

3. Very minor points of compliance have been seen, which, when addressed in writing by the management in a 1 month period with supportive paperwork and so on, lead to the company being given a Statement of Compliance, a Certificate of Compliance, or an indication that the laboratory is in compliance. It depends on the specific country whether a Certificate of Compliance is given. If a certificate is given, it generally states that on the particular day that the inspection took place, the laboratory was found to be in compliance with the OECD Principles of GLP. Also, the address of the facility is given as well as a listing of areas in which compliance has been confirmed. This could be stated as analytical support facilities, acute toxicology, mutagenicity, or similar designations.

Naturally, the benchmark standard is either the OECD Guidelines or similar standards in Japan or the United States. The Inspectorate carries out inspections against these documents. It could be said that often it is merely a review of the procedure and an opinion of compliance given by the inspector versus the interpretation of the individual conducting the experimental work. To try to overcome this criticism and to ensure that all inspectors work according to a standard format, over the past 4 years, the OECD has instituted a series of mutual joint visits (MJVs) [37]. The process of an MJV is that a company is inspected by its local inspector and that the inspector is accompanied by inspectors from two other countries as observers. At the conclusion of the inspection, the company is given the findings by its local inspector and, outside that meeting, a review of the performance of the inspector with positive and negative points is given by the two observing inspectors. To ensure continuity, one of these three inspectors would then be on the next MJV.

In the past, Memorandums of Understanding (MoUs) [38] have been instituted between certain major countries, such as Japan and the United Kingdom, the United States and Japan or Canada. However, these have generally fallen into nonuse for a variety of reasons, especially in Europe, where it is now, or has been for some time, not possible for a country to negotiate directly with another country. Brussels, however, being the center of the European Community, has to carry out that discussion with a proposed partner in another country. As such, at the time of this writing, very few MoUs are currently in force.

29.6   WHAT IS GLP?

As noted in Section 29.1, GLP is a series of guidelines that cover the conduct and data production for nonclinical safety studies.

The OECD covers a series of activities and personnel. Responsibilities, training, quality assurance (QA), Standard operating procedures (SOPs), study plans and study reports, data production and recording, equipment maintenance and calibration, computers and validation, test systems, test substances, and archiving are the primary areas covered by the GLPs. A very brief overview of each of these areas is given hereafter.

29.6.1   Responsibilities

The prime players in a GLP scenario would be the *management*, the *sponsor*, the *study director, the principal investigator*, and the *QA unit.*

In a hierarchical structure, management would be totally responsible for the conduct of the work and for the assurance that resources have been made available and that an active role is played by these people in overseeing the conduct of scientific research.

The sponsor is the company that places a contract with a CRO or requests from within a company that work in another department be undertaken. The sponsor supplies the money and the request for the work.

The study director is prime player and is ultimately responsible for the production of the study plan, the conduct of the study, and the overseeing or production of the final report. Naturally, a large amount of delegation may take place; however, this must always be in writing. The overall responsibility for the conduct of the study, the daily contact with the study staff, the prevention or recording of problems, and the assurance that the study has been conducted in line with the study plan, the GLP, and the scientific guidelines solely belongs to this individual.

The principal investigator is next in the line of responsibility after the study director and is generally the person seen in a field study situation where the crop spraying, for example, may be undertaken at a place remote from the GLP designated site where the study director works. The principal investigator is therefore the person responsible initially for that portion of the work, although the study in total is under the direct control of the study director. It may also be that, within a company, work is subcontracted to the Analytical Department, for example, for the analysis of formulated material. The person responsible for this particular aspect of the scientific work is the principal investigator, who is involved in the study plan and responsible to the study director. Another typical scenario is work conducted in a CRO under the control of the study director, where samples of plasma are taken for toxicokinetics, for example, and these samples are analyzed by the sponsor. The sponsor's analyst, therefore, may well be designated the principal investigator.

The quality assurance unit is an independent group that does not become involved in the conduct of the study but merely reviews the data, experimental work, and documents produced to ensure compliance with the SOPs, the study plans, and GLP. Other activities such as training and assistance in interpreting GLPs may be the responsibility of the QAU. (For more information, see Section 29.6.3 in this chapter or Section II, 1.4 pp. 17–19 of the OECD GLPs.)

29.6.2   Training and Recording: Confirmation of Suitability

It is the responsibility of management to ensure that training takes place and the responsibility of the study director to assure that the individuals conducting the work are adequately trained and have adequate records. At a minimum, there must be a CV, a training record, and a very clear job description. Specifically, with regard to a study director, there must be explicit details of how the study director position can be met and the responsibilities of that individual in carrying out the relevant duties.

There should be procedures detailing how the training will take place; recording of the training must be made on a regular basis, the records must be stored in archives and regularly updated, and a complete and historical review of a trainee's activities, previous training, and ability to conduct the work according to GLP must be documented. (See the OECD Principles, Section I 2a through 2d.)

29.6.3   Quality Assurance

This function, as already stated, is an independent review. The responsibilities here start with a review of the study plan and continue through the review of the study in the in-life phase, data audits, and the final study report audit.

In addition to these, *system audits* and *process audits* can be undertaken.

There is a total misconception within the industry, particularly in new companies applying good laboratory practice, about the concepts of quality assurance, which is frequently confused with quality control.

The easiest way of describing this would be: *quality control* is a system of regular checks made either 100% or as determined in standard operating procedures by all operatives on data, machines, standards, and so on; *quality assurance*, however, is an independent observation that the system of quality control has been operated.

Therefore, it should be quite clear that quality control is a system operated by all parties and can if necessary encompass elements seen in other accreditation systems; but the overall confirmation that quality control systems have been carried out is the independent review on a random or total basis carried out by the quality assurance unit.

The aim of QA is to assure management that compliance with GLP is maintained throughout the entire study, that the data integrity is maintained, and that compliance with the SOPs and the study plan is adhered to by all experimental study staff.

The study audit is a specific audit of the study in direct relation to the study plan.

A system audit, however, rather than proceeding in a vertical line, takes a horizontal line across all studies and would include such tasks as archiving, training,

SOPs, general computer validation, animal house operation, and management activities. These are but a few areas that would constitute a system audit but they give an idea of the type of activities across studies that would be audited.

Process audits, on the other hand, have specifically been addressed in the revised 1997 GLPs, and these are basically aimed at auditing short-term studies of a repetitive nature, generally undertaken by similar teams of people. A process audit assures that the system is working and that parts of the process are reviewed over a quoted period in the QA SOPs. The aim is to ensure that all critical aspects of this process are reviewed through different studies over a period of time. This does not necessitate QA review of all short-term studies on every occasion, nor does it require the review of such areas as analytical analysis on a batch-by-batch basis or the analysis of hematology or biochemistry samples each time these come up for analysis.

To enable the reader to understand quality assurance, examples of some checklists are included in Table 29.1. These should be classed as the minimum require-

TABLE 29.1   General Checklist For Audit/Inspection

- Introductory meeting to discuss studies (ongoing/completed).
- Review documentation produced for initial meeting.
- Review organizational structure, management awareness, study directors, support personnel, safety aspects relating to animal liberation and to protect the data and client identity.

Quality Assurance

Structure and status
Master schedule
Protocol review procedures
Study phase inspection procedures and frequency
Process based inspection
Facility inspection
Report auditing procedures
Reporting systems

Personnel

To cover training, policy for training, records, job descriptions, CVs.

Standard Operating Procedures (SOPs)

Their production, content, authorization, distribution, staff awareness, review procedure, and locations.

Animals

Source and supply
Receipt, acceptance, quarantine
Environmental design and control
Operational systems, clean/dirty regime and so on for stock, supplies, and staff
Cleaning regime
Identification and treatment allocation
Veterinary management
Dose administration

TABLE 29.1   *Continued*

Supplies
Collection of body fluids
Measurement, body weight, diet, consumption, clinical signs, and so on
Waste disposal and incinerator

Test Substance Control

Receipt, quarantine, characterization, formulation, accountability, dispatch to toxicology.

Laboratories

Clinical biochemistry, methods of analysis, QC, sample receipt, sample treatment
preanalysis, storage, raw data, reporting, authorization of results, equipment maintenance
and calibration.
Hematology, as for clinical chemistry.
Analytical chemistry, as for clinical chemistry.
ADME labs, for specific studies (e.g., WBA).

Computing Department

Validation, maintenance, backup, reporting, security, data handling, data manipulation,
programming and staff, CRF Part 11.

Histopathology

Autopsy procedures, dissection, preservation, labeling, processing.
Histology, tissue processing, slide production, slide QC, slide reading and recuts,
reporting.

Equipment

All areas other than those specifically addressed above, logs, service contract, non-
routine maintenance, and so on.

Archives

Design, security, operation, removal, return.

Documentation

To cover protocols, reports, amendments, their production, authorization, issue, review,
and distribution. Raw data: what is it and how is it approved?

Report Audit

Toxicology reports should be examined to produce an audit trail in the reverse direction
to the QA inspections carried out so far (i.e., report traced back through raw data to the
animal requisition records).

Management Briefing on Findings and Recommendations

ments: I am firmly convinced that the best tool given to a quality assurance auditor is the human body in terms of *eyes, ears*, and *nose*. While checklists can be a very useful memory aid, the best means of carrying out an audit is to look at the work being carried out, observe the operative in complying with the SOPs, and confirm adherence to the study plan or protocol. It must be of paramount importance to all staff and especially to the QA unit that the whole concept of quality assurance involves the study being in compliance with GLP, following the appropriate and up-to-date standard operating procedures, and being in strict adherence to the study plan or protocol. The scientific aspect is not the concern of quality assurance; this is solely the responsibility of the study director, the principal investigator, and the test facility management. Confirmation of satisfactory scientific study completion would be the basis of evaluation by the regulator.

Confirmation of quality assurance activities and compliance with GLP would eventually become the responsibility of the monitoring authority of the country concerned.

QA itself is required to produce SOPs that clearly detail operation, method of selection of critical phases, and studies, and to report its results to the management.

After every audit, a report is produced that is then discussed with the study director and circulated to the management with the overall agreement from the study director relating to the audit findings and their explanation of the resolution. (For in-depth review of QA, see Principles of GLP, Section II 2.1–2.2, p. 20.)

29.6.4 Standard Operating Procedures (SOPs)

These generally have been likened to a complete documented history of the entire aspect of conducting nonclinical safety studies. Any activity needs to be described in one of these documents. There may be a compilation of activities, or they may address single items such as the calibration and use of an electronic balance. They must be produced by the individual most familiar with the task, agreed on by management, and countersigned by a person senior to the author of the document.

Once produced, SOPs must be reviewed on a regular basis (approximately every 2 years), and any changes to these procedures must be made in writing, with the agreement of all parties, and circulated to each owner or user of the SOP. The SOP itself must be filed in the archive and additional copies produced. An SOP management system must be set up, whereby a responsible person knows the whereabouts of all SOPs and can retrieve and replace them with amended or superseded revisions and can make sure that they are reviewed regularly and disposed of when no longer required.

The SOP must appear immediately in the area adjacent to the workplace to be readily available to all persons. Frequently, SOPs are the basis of training, and most companies now have SOP-based training schemes. The content and receipt of the SOP should be acknowledged immediately upon receipt and a training program set up, whereby confirmation of the understanding and the ability to perform the duties stated in the SOP is documented in the appropriate training record.

SOPs should be adequately controlled to prevent unauthorized photocopying, which may lead to a superseded copy not being sent to the proper recipients. Someone making an illegal photocopy would not be on the distribution list and therefore would not always receive updated versions, with the possibility that an outdated method could be used.

The requirement for archiving historical copies is one of the key attributes of GLP in that traceability can be seen as originating at the archive. The dates and historical record of the SOPs can prove irrevocably that a particular action was the method in use at the time.

SOPs can be paper-based or electronic. The trend toward electronic record-keeping is becoming more common in laboratories. The only requirement made by the inspectorate is that accurate, controlled copies are available on the electronic media and that prevention of copying or unauthorized changing are built into the SOP system. (See GLP Principles Section II, 7 p. 24.)

29.6.5   Study Plans and Reports

Before any study can be undertaken satisfactorily, a study plan must be produced. The study plan is merely an indication of all of the activities that will take place, resources required, time frames, and objectives. The study plan can be likened to a road map that, when given to all the participants, will allow them to start at the beginning and to proceed through the various mazes to the final completion point indicated by the study report. The one golden rule in GLP is one study plan, one study director, and one report.

The study report itself is a mirror image of all the headings in the study plan and serves to confirm that the objectives of the study have been met and that the results and discussions of the data presented give an indication of the outcome of the particular experimental work.

Both the study plan and the report are audited by QA, and each study plan and report are generally determined by the company's format.

Typical headings must be given in both documents. (These can be found in Section II, 8.1–8.3, pp. 25–27 and 9.1–9.2, p. 28, of the OECD Principles of GLP.)

29.6.6   Data

Raw data, or source data, are generally considered the first records made, either electronically in computer-readable form or created the first time that the "pen hits the paper."

These should be original, signed and dated recordings that may be on any type of medium. When results are stored on media such as heat-sensitive paper, the results should be photocopied to insure against deterioration of the medium over time. Electronic data can be regarded as a disk, CD-ROM, or similar medium provided that this material, when reintroduced to the computer and the software, can generate the images stored on the disk or electronic medium in a 100% readable form.

There are many types of electronic media, machines, and source data or raw data within the toxicological environment. Ironically, the most common storage medium for raw data is paper. Paper and its storage partner microfilm have been around for many years, and their stability and reproducibility are well known. Other electronic media, however, do not have the same capability of reproduction known over a long period, and thus most industries and companies prefer paper.

The data should be recorded promptly, legibly, and signed and dated, and any corrections should be made in a format to allow the original record to be seen, the change should be described and justified where applicable, and the change should be signed and dated by the individual making the revision. This procedure, whether on paper or via computer, should have the same standards. With use of the computer, an audit trail is necessary to identify the change and the person making it, along with the reason.

29.6.7   Equipment

As can be imagined, equipment in a toxicological study may be varied, simple, or complex. As such, it is difficult to describe each individual type of equipment in this limited space.

GLP requires that equipment be maintained, calibrated, and generally demonstrated as fit for use.

Equipment such as can be seen in an analytical laboratory supporting toxicology studies, for example, high pressure liquid chromatography (HPLC) and other equally sophisticated equipment such as GC-MS/MS, should have checks of system suitability and installation, operation, and performance qualifications performed *at a minimum*.

Other equipment such as centrifuges and balances should be maintained and calibrated and, with regard to the latter, regular checks should be made with known, standardized, regularly calibrated weights. These should be placed on the balance with a frequency to guarantee that data from the machine are accurate. Even if the balance is an electronic calibrating balance, regular manual check weights should be applied.

Each piece of equipment should have a log book that gives a historical record of its use, breakdown, repair, and service. Generally, it is acceptable that these log books be placed by the equipment generating critical data to be presented in the final report.

All equipment should be clearly identified as to the time that it started producing raw data for experimental use and, when no longer required, the equipment should be removed from the laboratory or suitably labeled "not for GLP use."

The calibration and validation of equipment have been addressed extensively, but equipment that can be shown as "fit for purpose/use" within the GLP environment is generally acceptable to most regulatory inspectors. (For additional information on the GLP requirements for equipment, see Principles, Section II, 4, p. 22.)

29.6.8   Computers

Over the past few years, computers have played a very important role in many aspects of toxicology.

The general trend in the industry and particularly from the Inspectorate is to ensure that the computers are fully validated. Validation, however, means different things to different people. Some companies and their Information Technology Group (ITG) will dismantle the computer and its software components, reconfigure them, test them, and then reinstall them. Others will take a more realistic approach and work on the basis that the computer was brought in for a specific task and is considered validated provided that task is completed with the aid of the computer in a reproducible and acceptable manner.

However, in the most simplistic form, validation could be covered by *evidence that the computer will perform the task for which it was purchased and, more importantly, continue to perform that task for the foreseeable future.* In other words, as with other equipment, is the computer fit for the purpose?

Several documents have been written from a regulatory standpoint, the most useful being Monograph 10 of the OECD Principles, Application of GLP to Computer Systems [39]. Many books are available and vary in detail and content to cover everything that one would wish to know about computers but were afraid to ask, down to the simple documentation giving the essentials for validation and providing a disk with the SOPs to comply with GLP [40, 41].

The prime concern of the Inspectorate is that the user responsible for performing the validation and producing the report is in control of the equipment and can ensure and prove the integrity of the data when entered into the computer and regenerated in some other form.

It is generally accepted in the industry that acceptance testing is perfectly satisfactory for most computers and assures that the computer, when installed on company premises, will perform the function for which it was purchased. However, each computer must be viewed in the role it will play in the company, and suitable testing must be conducted to ensure that the data and integrity are of the highest quality and that total control over output is maintained.

As with all equipment, computer maintenance and calibration records are of paramount importance.

If in-house software programs are produced, they are tested and validated, and the source code is made available. One of the key elements required in the computer record-keeping is that of change control and password protection and training. (See GLP Principles Section II, 7(b), p. 25.) One very important rule is that the electronic signatures rule [42] must be observed when data are signed off electronically. This FDA requirement became effective 20 August 1997 and covers all data for which signatures are made electronically and requires that the FDA is officially notified.

However, in 2005 the FDA radically reviewed its requirements for electronic signatures and Part 11 compliance and basically required the industry to ensure that any use of computers in any form within a GLP study should follow the predicate rules, which were predominantly explained in the early good laboratory practices, and to confirm that the system is fit for use, adequately controlled, validated, password protected, and in essence completely controlled by the user and company. Much of what was seen to be bureaucratic and totally overenthusiastic approaches by the FDA and their guidance manuals were withdrawn at this time, but Part 11 is still alive and must be strictly adhered to in the situation where data are sent in whatever form to the FDA.

29.6.9   Test Systems

This really is a slightly complex name for what is generally considered the animal subject. Test system, however, has been utilized because, in many instances in toxicology, GLP now applies to such subjects as groundwater, soil, insects (such as earthworms and honey bees), and microorganisms (such as daphnia) and therefore the use of the word animal is not always applicable.

The main criteria are that the origin of the test system is known with its breeding history, where applicable, that these are purchased from well-known and, if possible, accredited suppliers, and that the quarantine period is observed to ensure that test systems are of high quality and fit for use.

Care, husbandry, intermediate sacrifice if the test system is found to be "in extremis," and humane sacrifice before necropsy are essentials for the test system. Separate housing among species and experimentation is critical, and all aspects of manipulation of the animal from clinical observations, dosing, and special tests such as electrocardiogram (ECG) need to be well documented and outlined in standard operating procedures.

Animal husbandry itself, the animal room, and the animal room diary giving an indication of exactly what occurred in the room and to the animal are essential items of documentation. Unique identification is also of paramount importance with the animals, cages, and the location of the cages.

The industry has very recently turned its attention to the use of individually ventilated cages (IVCs). The plus points for this are that the clean and dirty corridor situation, which has so frequently been vastly expensive in terms of HVAC, is no longer required and that a room with adequate ventilation and temperature control can house the IVC units, which are individually controlling the environment for the animal so that each cage can be considered as an individual animal room. Thus, for short-term toxicology studies, many more studies can be carried out in the same room, which was prohibited by earlier GLPs. Acute studies can therefore be conducted, and no longer is the volume of the room considered an issue by the toxicologist or regulator. New animal facilities can be constructed much quicker and at less cost than involved in the expensive clean and dirty corridor situation and ventilation. Existing animal units can readily be modified with a minimum of disruption to studies and with a minimum of expenditure in terms of reconstruction and HVAC. The animal itself is in a much more controlled environment, but the cautionary tale is that if an organization goes for IVCs, it is essential that the whole system be purchased: this includes not only the station controlling the temperature, humidity, and airflow within the cage, but cage cleaning stations and dosing and handling stations—all of which are filter air controlled to maintain the overall sterility and critical ambience of the experiment. Failure to do this and the purchase of only a partial system will doom the study to failure.

This system has been put into place where specific strains of mice, for example, are required to be used and their delicate nature would not allow for conventional animal housing; feeding studies particularly benefit here as the mass dust and contamination between study groups can be much more tightly controlled within the individual cage environment. The QA unit and regulator, however, must review these facilities in a totally different light with slightly more flexibility.

Compliance with GLP, however, brings particular problems and much of the QA audit and standard operating procedures need revising as do the formal GLP inspections of animal units comprised entirely of IVCs [43].

Full and documented histories of heating and ventilation are required, and, in barrier-maintained rooms, signed and dated records of positive to negative pressures are to be kept. These records should also reference any malfunction and its rectification. Furthermore, excursions outside the permitted range must be documented, and the effect on the study and data integrity must be identified and addressed by the study director in the final report. (Additional information is available in the GLP Principles, Section, II, 3.2, p. 21.)

29.6.10   Test Substance

In most instances, the test substance would be a new chemical entity (NCE) or an existing product; a comparator, pharmaceutical, veterinary, or agrochemical product; or even a device. Knowledge of the composition, characterization, stability, and other physiochemical properties is essential. Stability, however, may be determined as the short-term studies progress, with the proviso that the overall stability is known, along with full characterization by the time long-term toxicity studies are carried out. Stability testing may well be carried out in parallel as long as the stability of the active ingredient and formulated product is known sufficiently to allow for control of the dosing to be done within the period of stability known at that time.

One of the key elements of test substance control is accountability. A record of the amount received for toxicity testing should be accurately recorded, and 100% accountability of that product throughout the life of the testing is an essential element of GLP.

Again, formulation of the product is required to be covered in detail, and, in many companies, the elements of GLP are the benchmark standards when dealing with a test substance. Use of the test substance in the animal facility, the maintenance of homogeneity of suspensions, the mixing of the product in feed, and the testing of the product are all essential. This is one particular area in which, within the toxicology testing area, support functions such as analytical studies then come under GLP.

These functions will be required to test formulations and feedstuffs to ensure that the correct amount of the active ingredient is present as determined by the study plan for the various dosing groups. This requires that a validated method be available before any work is carried out, with the ability to analyze samples of the formulated product or plasma samples for toxicokinetics as the study progresses.

It is required that a reserve or retention sample of the active ingredient be retained. This should be retained for as long as it affords reasonable testing and within the expiry period determined by the analytical facility. It is also required that a retention sample be retained for studies that are not considered to be short term. This is one particular area in which revision of the GLPs is sometimes not well thought out. Originally, it had been stated that reserve samples should be taken for studies exceeding 4 weeks. This was subsequently revised to specify "studies that are not considered to be short-term." The glossary in the GLPs defines a short-term study as "a study of short duration with repetitive processes." This, one must admit, does not give a lot of guidance! (See additional information on systems in GLP Section II, 3.3, p. 21 and 6.1–6.2, p. 23.)

29.6.11   Archives

Having addressed all the various aspects of the study, one can see that much documentation, tissues, slides, and wax blocks could well be accumulating. The requirement is to store this material for "a period of time." Again, very little guidance is given in the GLP, and one is referred to the national guidelines for the storage of data. However, it is of great importance that this material be maintained in good condition in a retrievable format for at least 15 years or for 2 years past the availability of "the product," whichever is longer.

In 2006 the OECD Principles and GLP Compliance Monitoring Group produced a monograph detailing archiving in a GLP environment. This document gives valuable advice to the problematic subject of archiving [44].

Generally, companies themselves are maintaining that material for far longer, or for 2 years past the availability of the product.

All the material must be retained in a secure location for easy access, under the responsibility of a management-designated archivist and deputy. The security aspect of the archive should preclude damage from outside sources, fire, water, rodents, and so on.

Over the years, it has been seen that vast amounts of data must be retained. Most companies, bearing in mind the fifteen year retention period, tend to carry these documents in their archives for considerably longer periods of time. Many authorities still allow electronic archiving such as scanning to CD/DVD, but the FDA still requires the original paper document to be retained. This has led to a large explosion in contract archiving houses. While these are perfectly satisfactory, it is essential that the company QA unit inspect these for safety, security, long-term financial viability, and most importantly the general concepts that you would expect to see in your own archive. During 2006 the fragile nature of contract archiving was exposed when one major international company having a unit in London caught fire and at the same time a similar unit in The Netherlands also caught fire, both causing major loss of documentation. Either way, whether it is your own archive or the contract archive, this problem is always waiting around the corner.

The entire aspect of archiving is basically one of common sense, and guidance on how to archive these materials can be obtained from government agencies that store personnel records or from libraries. (Additional information on archiving is available in GLPs under Section II, 3.4, p. 22 and 10, p. 29.)

29.7 HOW CAN COMPLIANCE BE MAINTAINED WITHIN A FACILITY?

Compliance, having been granted after an inspection, should be monitored on a daily basis. However, it is my opinion that many companies' standards of compliance relax after the initial certificate has been granted only to find that, 2 years later, for example, an enormous rush 1 month before an announced inspection is required to generate the appropriate documentation and to update the system.

It is suggested that QC reviews be carried out on a regular basis to ensure that points likely to detract from the overall compliance are reviewed regularly and that project meetings be held where QA is invited to give a précis of the regular points seen during audits so that these can be addressed and rationalized.

Training and retraining, along with an awareness of the requirement to comply with GLP, are of immense importance. New equipment, major SOP revisions, and transfer of technicians or scientists among departments are always good signs that additional training should be carried out. It must be remembered that GLP is team-work. It is no good considering that there are the scientists and technicians on the one hand and QA on the other. There is no point in hoping that whatever happens and however little QC is carried out, QA will discover all the mistakes in the final report and review. Remember, it is not QA's problem; that department's role is to ensure that compliance has been maintained; QC and data checking are the responsibilities of every member of the staff team.

Improvement targets should be set in line with quality control manuals used in other accreditation systems. It is always a good point to review internally and on a regular basis (1) problems that have been encountered in experimentation, (2) audit findings, (3) ways to improve work by looking at new systems and reviewing SOPs to ensure that these are current, and (4) areas where improvements can be made.

An example can be taken from the accreditation systems [45], in which, in addition to QA audits, departments become involved in self-inspection. Each department can identify a QA representative whose daily responsibility is to review compliance issues, to look at the overall quality policy of the company, and to ensure that, between QA audits, self-inspection is performed and that a departmental review is made of these findings with action points and a time plan identified.

The primary impetus for the maintenance of compliance, however, is the regular external inspection by the Inspectorate. In addition, it is now becoming frequent for independent consultants to be brought in to do preregulatory inspections. Whichever way one views the system, whether through consultation or by assigning a department to perform inspections in one area and to conduct audits in another, the regular review of compliance should be maintained.

When using CROs, the whole aspect of auditing takes on a different light. Here, subcontracting is usually performed because of internal pressures, shortage of space, or lack of in-house expertise.

Dealing with CROs is no different from setting up an in-house GLP system. The CRO should be regarded as an extension of the facility in which the sponsor is conducting its own research.

29.8   PITFALLS AND BENEFITS

In conclusion, it is worthwhile to address the pitfalls and benefits of operating according to the principles of GLP.

A pitfall could be seen as a restriction on the scientist against performing free research. It could also be seen as an intrusion by an independent body looking at why problems occur and at the sorts of problems that occur and carrying out regular reviews with senior management about these problems. Costs will increase because of time pressures and the necessity of involving third-party reviews. The recording of data will now be subject to more QC, more required approvals, extra costs, and, generally, more data presented. Time must be taken to write and review SOPs. This in itself can be a very costly exercise; I know of one company that, having spent more than 6 months writing its SOPs, classed them as capital pieces of equipment and put a value of $20,000 on that volume.

Other companies and personnel may encounter similar pitfalls. The list is not intended to be exhaustive but merely to indicate areas in which additional time, money, and resources will be allocated. However, on the positive side, benefits can be seen immediately.

In talking to many people who have operated under the GLP system for the past 30 years, it is generally heard that the system allows for a better standard of research, less repeated work, the ability to have full accountability and traceability of everything within the experimental phase, and the knowledge that all documentation produced at the end of the study is now safe and secure in the archive and can readily be accessed for regulatory review or inspection.

Fewer studies are being repeated, and, therefore, the immediate benefit is the lowering of subject usage. The fact that data, when generated with a certificate or a compliance statement, will now be accepted by all OECD member countries means that once the study is completed and the regulatory submission made, the time for acceptance by several countries (if submissions are made in a multistate procedure) will be reduced dramatically.

Finally, the initial bureaucratic straitjacket of GLP thrust on the international research community in 1976 has rapidly turned full circle and now is seen as the quality standard to which all companies in all countries want to aspire. From that point of view, all nonclinical safety studies, when conducted according to the principles of GLP and adequately addressing science as well as compliance, can achieve a very high success rate both in the outcome of the science and in the acceptance of data for a regulatory submission.

REFERENCES

1. US Food and Drug Administration (FDA). Nonclinical Laboratory Studies. Proposed Regulations for Good Laboratory Practice Regulations. Proposed Rule. *Federal Register* 1976;41:51206–51228.

2. US Food and Drug Administration (FDA). Nonclinical Laboratory Studies. Good Laboratory Practice Regulations. Final Rule. *Federal Register* 1978;43:59986–60020.

3. US Food and Drug Administration (FDA). Good Laboratory Practice for Nonclinical Laboratory Studies: Amendment of Good Laboratory Practice Regulations. Amendment. *Federal Register* 1980;45:24865.

4. US Food and Drug Administration (FDA). Good Laboratory Practice Regulations. Proposed Rule. *Federal Register* 1984;49:43530–43537.

5. US Food and Drug Administration (FDA). Good Laboratory Practice Regulations. Final Rule. *Federal Register* 1987;52:33768–33782.

6. US Food and Drug Administration (FDA). Good Laboratory Practice Regulations. Minor Amendments. Final Rule. *Federal Register* 1989;54:15923–15924.

7. US Food and Drug Administration (FDA). Good Laboratory Practice Regulations. Removal of Examples of Methods of Animal Identification. Final Rule. *Federal Register* 1991;56:32088.

8. US Food and Drug Administration (FDA). Good Laboratory Practice Regulations. Technical Amendment. *Federal Register* 1994;59:13200.

9. OECD Series on Principles of Good Laboratory Practice and Compliance Monitoring. ENV/MC/CHEM/9817. As revised in 1997. http://www.oecd.org.ehs/ehsmono.

10. Dent NJ. Comparison between the principles of GLP 1992 as defined in Monograph 45 and the draft revision of the principles of GLP as published by OECD on 6th January 1997. *Qual Assurance J* 1997;2:7–12.

11. Dent NJ. European regulatory compliance issues: good research practices. *J Am Coll Toxicol* 1994;13 (1):79–85.

12. *OECD Guidelines for the Testing of Chemicals*. Paris: OECD; 1993.

13. Directives EEC/87/18, EEC/9, EEC/88/320. *Official J Eur Commun*, 1992.

14. US Food and Drug Administration. *Good Laboratory Practice for Nonclinical Laboratory Studies: Title 21, Part 58, Code of Federal Regulations*. FDA; 1993.

15. US Environmental Protection Agency (EPA). Pesticide Programs: Good Laboratory Practice Standards. Final Rule. *Federal Register* 1993;48:53946–53969.

16. US Environmental Protection Agency (EPA). Toxic Substance Control: Good Laboratory Practice Standards. Final Rule. *Federal Register* 1993;48:53922–53944.

17. US Environmental Protection Agency (EPA). Toxic Substance Control Act (TSCA): Good Laboratory Practice Standards. Final Rule. *Federal Register* 1989;54:34034–34050.

18. US Environmental Protection Agency (EPA). Federal Insecticide, Fungicide and Rodenticide Act (FIFRA): Good Laboratory Practice Standards. Final Rule. *Federal Register* 1989;54:34052–34074.

19. Good Laboratory Practice Standards (FIFRA), EPA. *Federal Register* 1993, Title 40, Part 160, Code of Federal Regulations, Final Rule revised as of July 1.

20. Good Laboratory Practice Standards (TSCA), EPA. *Federal Register* 1993, Title 40, Part 792, Code of Federal Regulations, Final Rule revised as of July 1.

21. Shillam KW. GLP Legislation. In Carson PA, Dent NJ, Eds. *Good Laboratory and Clinical Practices: Techniques for the QA Professional*. GLP Regulations Management Briefings—Post Conference Report. Rockville, MD: US Food and Drug Administration; 1979, pp 16–29.

22. Lepore PD. Overall responsibilities for GLP. In Carson PA, Dent NJ, Eds. *Good Laboratory and Clinical Practices: Techniques for the QA Professional*. Rockville, MD: US Food and Drug Administration; 1979, pp 29–39.

23. Lepore PD. Good Laboratory Practice Regulations: Questions and Answers, Subpart B. Available through FDA FOI, FDA, (HFI-35), Rockville, MD, 1979.

24. Lepore PD. Good Laboratory Practice Regulations: Questions and Answers, Subpart B. Available through FDA FOI, FDA, (HFI-35), Rockville, MD, 1981.

25. Broad RD, Dent NJ. An introduction to Good Laboratory Practice. In Carson PA, Dent NJ, Eds. *Good Laboratory and Clinical Practices: Techniques for the QA Professional*. Rockville, MD: US Food and Drug Administration; 1979, pp 3–16.

26. Commission Directive 1999/11/EC of 8 March 1999. *Official J Eur Commun* 1999; L77/8. 23.03.99.

27. Commission Directive 1999/12/EC of 8 March 1999. *Official J Eur Commun* 1999; L77/8. 23.03.99.

28. Good Laboratory Practice Regulations 1999. Statutory Instrument 1999 No. 3106. http://www.hmso.gov.uk/si/si1999/19993106.htm.

29. Dominated by the urge to merge. *Scrip Mag* 1999;Jan:46.

30. A strategic approach to R&D outsourcing. *Scrip Mag* 1999;July/Aug:29.

31. R&D trends give clues to future. *Scrip Mag* 1999;July/Aug:17.

32. How much of a threat is virtual pharma? *Scrip Mag* 1999;Nov:41.

33. The right treatment for the right patient. *Scrip Mag* 2000;Jan:11.

34. OECD Glossary. OECD Series on Principles of Good Laboratory Practice and Compliance Monitoring. ENV/MC/CHEM/9817. As revised in 1997. http://www.oecd.org.ehs/ehsmono.

35. Dent NJ. Forget compliance and concentrate on science. *Qual Assurance J* 1998;3:103–108.

36. Personal communication from OECD.

37. Personal communication from OECD.

38. Personal communication from OECD.

39. OECD GLP Consensus Document on The Application of the Principles of GLP to Computerised Systems, *Environ Monograph* 1997;10:116. OECD Series on Principles of Good Laboratory Practice and Compliance Monitoring. ENV/MC/CHEM/9817. As revised in 1997. http://www.oecd.org.ehs/ehsmono.

40. *The Red Apple II Symposium*, sponsored by DIA; (in press).

41. Chamberlain R. *Computer Systems Validation for Pharmaceutical and Medical Device Industries*. Buffalo Grove, IL: Interpharm Press; 1994.

42. US Food and Drug Administration. Electronic Records; Electronic Signatures; Final Rule. *Federal Register* 1997;62:13429–13466.

43. Dent NJ. Quality assurance and the use of individually ventilated cages (personal communication). Presentation to the British Association of Research Quality Insurance Symposium, Dublin.

44. Lawrence RG. Archives. In Carson PA, Dent NJ, Eds. *Good Laboratory and Clinical Practices: Techniques for the QA Professional*. Butterworth Heinemann; 1979, pp 155–171.

45. Piton A. Quality assurance: the present and future role of international standardization. In Dent NJ, Ed. *Implementing International Good Practices—GAPs, GCPs, GLPs, GMPs*. Interpharm Press; 1993, pp 251–256 (ISBN 0-935184-44-9).

Useful Websites and General References

Kracht WR. Implementing the ISO 9000 quality standards in a GMP or GLP environment. In Dent NJ, Ed. *Implementing International Good Practices—GAPs, GCPs, GLPs, GMPs*. Interpharm Press; 1993, pp. 267–277 (ISBN 0-935184-44-9).

Carson PA, Dent NJ. *Good Laboratory, Clinical and Manufacturing Practices*. London: Royal Society of Chemistry; 2007 (ISBN 978-0-85404-834-2).

Dent NJ, ED. *Implementing International Good Practices—GAPs, GCPs, GLPs, GMPs*.

Good Research Practices—A Practical Guide to the Implementation of the GXPs.

OECD homepage http://www.oecd.org.

European Quality http://www.euroqual.org.

US Federal Register—Environmental Issues http://www.epa.gov.fedrgstr.

GALPs http://www.epa.gov/doc/irm_galp.

EPA homepage http://www.epa.gov.

International Organization for Standardization http://www.iso.ch.

Good Laboratory Practice on Line http://www.glpguru.com.

Compliance Programme Manual http://www.fda.gov.ora.cpgm.default.htm.

Title 21 Code of Federal Regulations Part 58 http://www.access.gpo.gov/nara/cfr/index.html.

GLP Regulations Questions and Answers http://www.fda.gov/cder/guidance/index.htm.

Website for further information: www.countryconsultancyltd.co.uk.

30

DRUG IMPURITIES AND DEGRADANTS AND THEIR SAFETY QUALIFICATION

Robin C. Guy

Robin Guy Consulting, LLC, Lake Forest, Illinois

Contents

Preclinical Development Handbook: Toxicology, edited by Shayne Cox Gad
Copyright © 2008 John Wiley & Sons, Inc.

30.1   INTRODUCTION

In the United States, since very early times, traveling salespeople touted their latest miracle cures with enough publicity and fanfare to attract many to their circus-like shows. These cures were ointments, elixirs, and creams that would cure everything including obesity, diabetes, tuberculosis, and cancer [1]. Unfortunately, almost all of these products were either toxic or not efficacious. Even some vaccines were not safe, as evidenced in the deaths of thirteen children from St. Louis, Missouri after receiving an inoculation from a diphtheria antitoxin that was contaminated with tetanus [2]. This incident prompted Congress to enact the Biologics Control Act of 1902, a law that required inspections of the manufacturers and sellers of biological products, including testing of these products for purity and strength [3, 4].

In 1906, due to the outcry from the public after publication of Upton Sinclair's novel, *The Jungle*, the original Food and Drug Act was passed by Congress. The law prohibited adulteration and misbranding of food and drugs. Offending products could be seized and condemned and offending persons could be fined and jailed. Drugs had either to abide by standards of purity and quality set forth in the United States Pharmacopoeia (USP) and the National Formulary (composed of committees of physicians and pharmacists; these are now combined) or meet individual standards chosen by their manufacturers and stated on their labels. Adulteration was defined as the removal of valuable constituents, the substitution of ingredients so as to reduce quality, the addition of deleterious ingredients, and the use of spoiled animal and vegetable products. Misbranding was making false or misleading label statements regarding a food or a drug as well as the failure to provide required information in labeling.

Sulfanilamide, a drug used to treat streptococcal infections, had been used safely for years in tablet and powder form. For marketing to children, a company prepared the drug in liquid form after dissolving it in diethylene glycol and adding a raspberry flavor. Unfortunately, the 1906 law did not address testing products for toxicity. Diethylene glycol, a chemical normally used in antifreeze, is a deadly poison. Over 100 people died, most of whom were children. Another public outcry from this incident helped pass the Food, Drug, and Cosmetic Act in June 1938. This new law included cosmetics and medical devices and was instrumental in providing evidence of safety in pharmaceutical products prior to administration in humans. It also authorized factory inspections and gave the agency the ability to use injunctions to enforce the law.

Impurities in drug products have triggered numerous laws and amendments. In 1941 almost 300 people were killed or injured by ingestion of sulfathiazole tablets that were contaminated with phenobarbital. This caused the FDA to revise manufacturing and quality control requirements, leading to what would later be called Good Manufacturing Practices (GMPs) [5]. In 1945, batch certification by the FDA became a requirement for penicillin. The Penicillin Amendment requires FDA testing and certification of safety and effectiveness of all penicillin products; later amendments extended this requirement to all antibiotics. In 1983 FDA testing was found to be no longer necessary and was abolished [6].

Through the years, the U.S. Food and Drug Administration (FDA) and other international regulatory agencies, working alone or with industry representatives, have set regulations and guidelines for the handling of impurities in pharmaceuticals. As per the GMPs, it is essential that the purity of the pharmaceuticals is preserved from manufacturing through delivery to the consumer.

Most drugs are not administered as neat chemicals but are mixed with inactive ingredients to form the specific drug product. Many have impurities, due to manufacturing, leachables, or degradants. Impurities are chemicals contained in raw materials or formed during manufacture, storage, or use. Their properties may be different from the desired product with respect to activity, efficacy, and safety. These impurities may be either intentional or unintentional. Intentional impurities may be due to the raw material itself or excipients. Unintentional impurities may occur due to a few determinants, including interactions between the other materials in the drug product, leaching from containers, or degradation due to environmental conditions. Regulations and guidances exist for the safety assessment of impurities. Many focus on different levels of testing, based on the amount of impurity detected. There are many different methods and equipment available for the analysis of impurities. Safety or toxicology studies to test the impurity may be needed, and there are guidances for the selection and design of these studies.

30.2 TYPES AND SOURCES OF IMPURITIES

Impurities may come from a variety of sources. Manufacturing impurities, leachable impurities, and degradants are the most common.

30.2.1 Manufacturing Impurities

Manufacturing impurities can come from raw materials, active ingredients, excipients, process impurities and packaging impurities.

Raw Material Impurities Contamination from raw material sources is important to control. The highest quality starting material is essential to obtain a high quality product. Raw materials with impurities may be cleaned up, and it is important to do so before they have a chance to interact with other materials in the formulation that can lead to additional impurities. Cleaning up a raw material such as a chemical is usually easier than cleaning up natural materials. The latter may contain complex sample matrices that include similar chemical compounds. In addition, the pharmacologically active compounds are usually present in small amounts and therefore may be difficult to separate out from the impurities. Thus, highly sophisticated analytical methodologies must be developed to ensure that the natural drug is uniform and pure.

Compounds Related to Parent   Pharmaceuticals may contain impurities that are similar in structure to the parent material. These impurities may be more difficult to detect and isolate depending on how similar the structure is as compared to the parent material. A chromatogram may indicate a "shoulder" on the main peak or an eluting peak indicating such an impurity. An example is given in Fig. 30.1.

Spurious Compounds   Although each known degradation pathway is considered, and every attempt is made to decrease or obliterate the impurities, pharmaceutical chemistry can still be fickle. The additional unpredicted peak found on the chromatogram or the inexplicable tan flecks in a powder material could be an extractable–leachable, a residual solvent, or an unforeseen degradant. These must be investigated and, depending on the amount of the impurity, must be identified. The active pharmaceutical ingredient (API) from a natural material is an example of how complicated raw materials and impurities can become.

Active Ingredients   Impurities arise from the manipulation of an active ingredient in a pharmaceutical. These impurities may be formed due to process or storage conditions.

Excipients   An excipient is any inactive ingredient that is intentionally added to therapeutic or diagnostic product, but is not intended to exert a therapeutic effect at the intended dosage. Excipients may act to improve product delivery (e.g., enhance absorption or control release of the drug substance) or allow the product to be formulated (e.g., tablet). Examples of excipients include fillers, extenders, diluents, wetting agents, solvents, emulsifiers, preservatives, flavors, absorption enhancers, sustained-release matrices, and coloring agents [7]. Within the context of this guidance, the term excipient applies to macromolecular substances, such as albumin, or substances such as amino acids and sugars that are used in drug and biological products. It does not, however, apply to process- or product-related impurities (e.g., degradation products, leachates, residual solvents) or extraneous contaminants. Excipients may interact with the active ingredient or container to form impurities or they may be formed due to process or storage conditions.

Chromatogram of a sample with an impurity (A) vs. sample with the impurity removed (B)

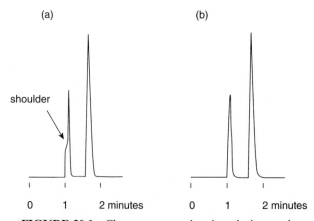

FIGURE 30.1   Chromatogram showing eluting peak.

Process Impurities   Process impurities, primarily residual solvents, are organic volatile impurities that remain in pharmaceuticals, even after processing, as well as oxygen left in lyophilized vials. Both the United States Pharmacopoeia (USP), the officially recognized drug standard-setting compendium [8], and the International Conference on Harmonisation of Technical Requirements for Registration of Pharmaceuticals for Human Use (ICH), Q3C [9], address commonly used chemical solvents, the latter of which has been adopted by the European and Japanese pharmacopoeias. Other process impurities may be due to by-products of synthetic reactions, chiral or stereoisomeric impurities, contamination, and residual process intermediates or reagents.

Biologics and biotechnology products have similar process impurity issues. The process needs to ensure that there are no residual cellular components in the biologic product. Biotechnology processing needs to avoid causing structural deformities to the protein. In all cases, the process must be scrutinized closely. Checking for impurities at various steps throughout the manufacturing phase may help to pinpoint where the impurities are produced.

Packaging Impurities   Packaging impurities can also be an issue in pharmaceuticals. These impurities can occur when chemicals from the packaging of the pharmaceutical are found in the product itself. These are discussed further in Section 30.2.3.

30.2.2   Degradants

Degradants are formed from the breakdown of the drug substance or product, possibly due to storage conditions, interaction of ingredients from the container, label or closing systems, or treatment of the material.

The ICH has published guidelines for the identification and qualification of degradant-related impurities. These guidelines take into account new and existing drugs and formulations. A forced degradation test is essential to assist in the determination of identifying any degradants and their degradation pathways. Forced degradation studies can be useful in the determination of the chemical and physical stability of crystal forms, the stereochemical stability of the drug substance alone and in the drug product, and for differentiating drug substance–related degradation products in formulations. Forced degradation tests are important to determine if extreme conditions will cause any impurities in the drug product. Forced degradation conditions can include storage under high temperatures, high humidity, extreme pH, freeze–thaw cycles, oxygen exposure, or UV light for specific time intervals. At certain timepoints, samples of the drug product are taken and analyzed for purity. One important consideration is that forced degradation experiments may only produce or release impurities into the drug product that would not generally be present during normal storage and handling conditions. A limitation of forced degradation testing is that a compound may not necessarily degrade under a given stress condition.

There are no specifics in the ICH guidelines for pH levels, temperature, conditions, or light intensity for forced degradation studies. However, for photodegradation, ICH Q1B [10] suggests that the light source should produce combined visible and ultraviolet (UV, 320–400 nm) outputs, and that exposure levels should be justified.

Degradation products if detected in significant amounts should be identified, tested for, and monitored against appropriately established acceptance criteria, according to ICH guidances [11, 12]. Investigation and identification of some specific degradation products may not be necessary if it has been proven that they are not produced under accelerated or long-term storage conditions [10, 13]. In addition, forced degradation may not be necessary when the routes of degradation and the suitability of the analytical procedures can be determined through use of data from stress testing of drug substance, reference materials for process impurities and degradants, data from accelerated and long-term studies on the drug substance, and data from accelerated and long-term studies on the drug product [14]. Additional corroborative information on the specificity of the analytical methods and on the degradation pathways of the drug substance may be available from literature sources.

Degradants will obviously vary for different drug products. Small chemicals may produce degradants that are similar to the parent compound. Biotechnological and biological products may encounter protein variants including truncated fragments, deamidated, oxidized, isomerized, aggregated forms, and mismatched disulfide links [15]. In these studies, there may also be difficulties in working with unstable degradation products.

As previously mentioned, many factors play a role in the formation of degradant products. Raw material handling is important to control early in the production phase. There should be no alteration of the material in any manner by chemicals or processing during manufacture. Changes in products can even lead to mutagenic degradants or degradants with increased immunogenicity, especially in biologics. The packaging used in various stages of the process may produce degradants. In addition, the choice of sterilization techniques may also play a role in producing degradation products, as different techniques may produce different degradants. Instability can lead to degradation over time. These factors would need to be taken into consideration prior to finalizing manufacturing, handling, and storage procedures.

30.2.3 Leachables and Extractables

Leachables and extractables are chemicals that may migrate from packaging or labeling, producing contamination in the drug product. These chemicals may be released throughout different stages of manufacturing, during storage or shipment of the drug components, during contact with processing materials in the plant, and even at the final stage while the drug product is in its primary storage container or in contact with labeling materials.

Extractables are compounds that can be extracted from the container, from the coatings of the container closure system, or from the label during forced degradation conditions including contact with an appropriate solvent or high temperature [16]. Forced degradation experiments may only release impurities into the pharmaceutical that would not generally be present during normal storage and handling conditions.

Leachables are compounds that migrate into the formulation from the label, container components, or coatings of the container and closure system as a result of direct contact with the formulation [17].These are impurities that have formed during normal storage and handling conditions. Certain types of storage or treat-ment conditions may also produce leachables more readily, including sterilization procedures.

Sources of leachable and extractable contamination from packaging may include accelerators, adhesives, antioxidants, coatings, components of the container or closure system, excipients, plastic or rubber components, plasticizers, processing aids, and vulcanizing agents. Plasticizers are used to make plastics more flexible. Plasticiz-ers such as bis(2-ethylhexyl)phthalate (BEHP) may be present throughout package manufacturing. Acrylonitrile is a leachable that may be present in manufactured products and is found in a number of pharmaceuticals [16]. Another potential source of leachable or extractable contamination is nitrosamines, which are found in prod-ucts made of rubber. Rubber and rubber products are used in packaging, in closure components, and in devices, primarily in O-rings. Inhalers are a medical device that is prepared with various plastic, rubber, and stainless steel components. The FDA has a draft guidance for inhalers, which basically states that the levels of degradation products and impurities should be determined by means of stability indicating methods, and that any impurities or degradation products appearing at levels 0.10% or greater should be specified [18]. Many drug products are distributed or adminis-tered in packages made of plastic and rubber components; therefore, phthalates and nitrosamines could come into contact with the drug product.

30.3   REGULATIONS

Both the U.S. Food and Drug Administration (FDA) and the ICH offer a plethora of information on dealing with impurities in pharmaceuticals. While the FDA is the regulatory authority in the United States, the ICH is an organization that brings together regulatory authorities and pharmaceutical associations of Europe, Japan, and the United States, in addition to experts from other non-ICH countries to discuss scientific and technical aspects of product registration. The purpose of the ICH is to make recommendations to achieve greater harmonization in technical guidelines and requirements for product registration in order to reduce or obviate the need to duplicate the testing carried out during the research and development of new pharmaceuticals.

It is essential that proper analyses be conducted for impurities. Knowledge gained from these analyses can be used to guide formulation development and improve manufacturing and packaging processes.

There are consequences when impurities are undetected or observed at higher levels than reported. For regulatory submissions for marketing applications, current FDA and ICH guidance recommends inclusion of the results, including chromato-grams of stressed samples, demonstration of the stability-indicating nature of the analytical procedures, and the degradation pathways of the drug substance in solu-tion, solid state, and drug product. The structures of significant degradation products and the associated procedures for their isolation and/or characterization also are expected to be included in the application. For the latest updates on these guidances and for more details, check the FDA or ICH websites (www.fda.gov, www.ich.org). The following discussions are summaries of the guidances and include authentic excerpts but are not intended to be all inclusive.

30.3.1   International Conference on Harmonisation (ICH) Guidance

Q3A   The ICH *Guidance for Industry, Q3A Impurities in New Drug Substances*, Revision 1, was published February 2003 [11]. It is intended to "provide guidance for registration applications on the content and qualification of impurities in new drug substances produced by chemical syntheses and not previously registered in a region or member state." A new drug substance is not the final marketed product, but the active ingredient used in the marketed product. An active ingredient is intended to furnish pharmacological activity or other direct effect in the diagnosis, cure, mitigation, treatment, or prevention of disease or to affect the structure or any function of the human body. The active ingredient does not include intermediates used in the synthesis of such ingredient. The term includes those components that may undergo chemical change in the manufacture of the drug product and be present in the drug product in a modified form intended to furnish the specified activity or effect (21 CFR 210.3(b)(7) and 21 CFR 314.3(b)). Impurities in new drug substances are addressed from both a chemistry and a safety perspective.

The guidance is not intended to apply to new drug substances used during the clinical research stage of development. Nor does it cover the following types of drug substances: biological/biotechnological, peptide, oligonucleotide, radiopharmaceutical, fermentation products and associated semisynthetic products, herbal products, or crude products of animal or plant origin. The guidance does not cover extraneous contaminants that should not occur in new drug substances and are more appropriately addressed as good manufacturing practice (GMP) issues, polymorphic forms, and enantiomeric impurities.

The guidance divides impurities into three categories: organic impurities (process– and drug-related), inorganic impurities, and residual solvents. These are defined in the guidance, along with their respective rationale for the reporting and control of impurities. The guidance further describes the circumstances in which impurities need to be reported, identified, and qualified.

The rationale for the reporting and control, identification, and qualification of impurities is discussed in the guidance. Organic impurities need to be summarized based on the actual and potential impurities most likely to arise during the synthesis, purification, and storage of a new drug substance. This discussion can be limited to those impurities that might reasonably be expected based on knowledge of the chemical reactions and conditions involved.

In addition, laboratory studies conducted to detect impurities in the new drug substance need to be summarized for the regulatory application. According to the guidance, "this summary should include test results of batches manufactured during the development process and batches from the proposed commercial process, as well as the results of stress testing used to identify potential impurities arising during storage. The impurity profile of the drug substance batches intended for marketing should be compared with those used in development, and any differences discussed" [13].

Studies conducted to characterize the structure of impurities present in a new drug substance at a level greater than the identification threshold (Table 30.1) should be described and any impurity from any batch or degradation product from stability studies should be identified. If identification of an impurity or degradant is not feasible, a summary of the laboratory studies demonstrating the unsuccessful effort should be included in the application. If an impurity is pharmacologically or

TABLE 30.1   Thresholds

Maximum Daily Dose[a]	Reporting Threshold[b,c]	Identification Threshold[c]	Qualification Threshold[c]
≤2 g/day	0.05%	0.10% or 1.0 mg/day intake (whichever is lower)	0.15% or 1.0 mg/day intake (whichever is lower)
>2 g/day	0.03%	0.05%	0.05%

[a]The amount of drug substance administered per day.
[b]Higher reporting thresholds should be scientifically justified.
[c]Lower thresholds can be appropriate if the impurity is unusually toxic.

toxicologically active, identification of the compound should be conducted even if the impurity level is below the identification threshold.

The guidance also states that "qualification is the process of acquiring and evaluating data that establishes the biological safety of an individual impurity or a given impurity profile at the level(s) specified. The applicant should provide a rationale for establishing impurity acceptance criteria that includes safety considerations. The level of any impurity that is present in a new drug substance that has been adequately tested in safety and/or clinical studies would be considered qualified. Impurities that are also significant metabolites present in animal and/or human studies are generally considered qualified. A level of a qualified impurity higher than that present in a new drug substance can also be justified based on an analysis of the actual amount of impurity administered in previous relevant safety studies. If data are unavailable to qualify the proposed acceptance criterion of an impurity, safety studies to obtain such data can be appropriate when the usual qualification thresholds are exceeded."

The "Decision Tree for Identification and Qualification," as revised for Q3B(R) (Fig. 30.2) describes considerations for the qualification of impurities when thresholds are exceeded. If the level of impurity cannot be decreased to below the threshold, or if adequate data is not available in the scientific literature to justify safety, then additional safety testing should be considered. The studies considered appropriate to qualify an impurity will depend on a number of factors, including the patient population, daily dose, and route and duration of administration. Toxicology studies are discussed briefly later in this chapter and in more detail in other chapters in this volume. Such studies can be conducted on the new drug substance containing the impurities to be controlled, although studies using isolated impurities can sometimes be appropriate.

ICH Q3A states that "safety assessment studies to qualify an impurity should compare the new drug substance containing a representative amount of the new impurity with previously qualified material. Safety assessment studies using a sample of the isolated impurity can also be considered." The latter is especially important to consider for genetic toxicology studies and the importance of testing the isolated impurity is discussed in more detail at the end of this chapter.

Therefore, according to the guidance, if the maximum daily dose of the drug is less than 2 grams per day and the impurity intake is more than 0.15% or 1.0 mg/day, the Qualification Threshold has been reached, meaning safety studies will need to be performed. Lower thresholds can be appropriate if the impurity is unusually toxic. In addition, the impurity will need to be reported and identified. These studies include general and genetic toxicology studies, and possibly other specific toxicology

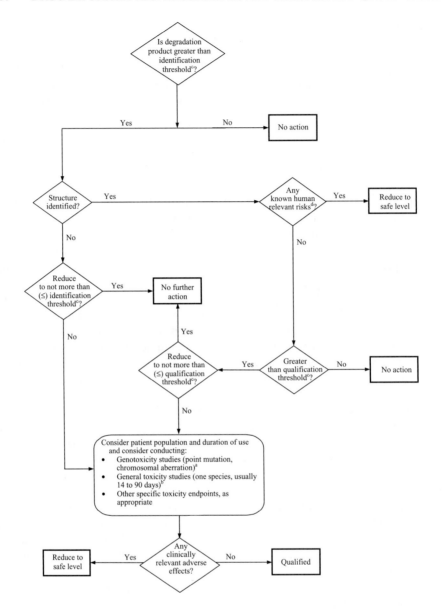

Notes

[a] If considered desirable, a minimum screen (e.g., genotoxic potential) should be conducted. A study to detect point mutations and one to detect chromosomal aberrations, both *in vitro*, are considered an appropriate minimum screen.

[b] If general toxicity studies are desirable, one or more studies should be designed to allow comparison of unqualified to qualified material. The study duration should be based on available relevant information and performed in the species most likely to maximize the potential to detect the toxicity of a degradation product. On a case-by-case basis, single-dose studies can be appropriate, especially for single-dose drugs. In general, a minimum duration of 14 days and a maximum duration of 90 days would be considered appropriate.

[c] Lower thresholds can be appropriate if the degradation product is unusually toxic.

[d] For example, do known safety data for this degradation product or its structural class preclude human exposure at the concentration present?

FIGURE 30.2 The "Decision Tree for Identification and Qualification," as revised for Q3B(R).

endpoints, as appropriate. It also recommended to have a discussion of specific toxicity testing with the appropriate FDA division.

The genetic toxicology studies can include a minimum screen (a study to detect point mutations and one to detect chromosome aberrations, both *in vitro*). The general toxicology studies should include one or more studies designed to allow comparison of unqualified to qualified material. The study duration should be based on available relevant information and performed in the species most likely to maximize the potential to detect the toxicity of an impurity. On a case-by-case basis, single-dose studies can be appropriate, especially for single-dose drugs. In general, a minimum duration of 14 days and a maximum duration of 90 days would be considered appropriate.

Inorganic impurities are normally detected and quantified using pharmacopoeial or other appropriate procedures. The need for inclusion or exclusion of inorganic impurities in a new drug substance specification should be discussed. Acceptance criteria should be based on pharmacopoeia standards or known safety data. The control of residues of the solvents used in the manufacturing process for a new drug substance should be discussed and presented according to ICH Q3C [9].

A registration application should include documented evidence that the analytical procedures are validated and suitable for the detection and quantification of impurities [19, 20]. Organic impurity levels can be measured by a variety of techniques, including those that compare an analytical response for an impurity to that of an appropriate reference standard or to the response of the new drug substance itself. Differences in the analytical procedures used during development and those proposed for the commercial product should be discussed in the registration application. Analytical results should be provided in an application for all batches of a new drug substance used for clinical, safety, and stability testing, as well as for batches representative of the proposed commercial process. The application should also contain a table that links the specific new drug substance batch to each safety study and each clinical study in which the new drug substance has been used. Any impurity at a level greater than the reporting threshold (Table 30.1) and total impurities observed in these batches of the new drug substance should be reported with the analytical procedures indicated. Table 30.2 is an illustration of reporting impurity results for identification and qualification in an application.

The guidance also states that when analytical procedures change, results provided in the application should be linked to the procedure used, with appropriate valida-

TABLE 30.2   Reporting Impurity Results in an Application

		Action	
Raw Result (%)	Reported Result (%)	Identification (Threshold 0.10%)	Qualification (Threshold 0.15%)
0.066	0.07	None	None
0.0963	0.10	None	None
0.12	0.12[a]	Yes	None[a]
0.1649	0.16[a]	Yes	Yes[a]

[a]After identification, if the response factor is determined to differ significantly from the original assumptions, it may be appropriate to remeasure the actual amount of the impurity present and reevaluate against the qualification threshold.

tion information provided, including representative chromatograms of representative batches. The applicant should ensure that complete impurity profiles (e.g., chromatograms) of individual batches are available, if requested.

The ICH Q3A guidance also states that the specification for a new drug substance should include a list of impurities. Individual impurities with specific acceptance criteria included in the specification for a new drug substance are referred to as specified impurities. Specified impurities can be identified or unidentified. A rationale for the inclusion or exclusion of impurities in a specification should be presented.

"Acceptance criteria should be set no higher than the level that can be justified by safety data and should be consistent with the level achievable by the manufacturing process and the analytical capability. Where there is no safety concern, impurity acceptance criteria should be based on data generated on batches of a new drug substance manufactured by the proposed commercial process, allowing sufficient latitude to deal with normal manufacturing and analytical variation and the stability characteristics of the new drug substance. Although normal manufacturing variations are expected, significant variation in batch-to-batch impurity levels can indicate that the manufacturing process of the new drug substance is not adequately controlled and validated" [21].

Q3B   ICH *Guidance for Industry, Q3B(R) Impurities in New Drug Products*, Revision 1, was published November 2003 [12]. It is intended to provide guidance for registration applications on the content and qualification of impurities in new drug products produced from chemically synthesized new drug substances not previously registered in a region or member state. A new drug product is a finished dosage form, for example, a tablet, capsule, or solution, that contains a drug substance, generally, but not necessarily, in association with one or more other ingredients [22]. The Q3B(R) complements the ICH guidance *Q3A guidance Impurities in New Drug Substances*, which should be consulted for basic principles along with ICH *Q3C Impurities: Residual Solvents*, when appropriate.

This guidance addresses only those impurities in new drug products classified as degradation products of the drug substance, or reaction products of the drug substance with an excipient and/or immediate container closure system (collectively referred to as *degradation products*). Generally, impurities present in a new drug substance need not be monitored or specified in new drug product unless they are also degradation products [21]. This guidance does not address impurities arising from excipients present in a new drug product or extracted or leached from the container closure system. This guidance also does not apply to new drug products used during the clinical research stages of development. It also does not cover the same types of products as in 3QA(R): biological/biotechnological, peptides, oligonucleotides, radiopharmaceuticals, fermentation products and associated semisynthetic products, herbal products, and crude products of animal or plant origin. Also excluded from this guidance are extraneous contaminants that should not occur in new drug products and are more appropriately addressed as GMP issues, polymorphic forms, and enantiomeric impurities.

The rationale for the reporting and identification of degradation products is similar to that in Q3A; however, identification thresholds are different (Table 30.3). The impurity profiles of the batches representative of the proposed commercial process should be compared with the profiles of batches used in development, and any differences should be discussed in the submission.

As expected, qualification of an impurity has similar concerns as Q3A. The main differences are the reporting, identification, and qualification thresholds (Table 30.3). The thresholds are basically higher than they were in Q3A; however, there are more categories for dosages. If the qualification thresholds given in Table 30.3 are exceeded and data are unavailable to qualify the proposed acceptance criterion of a degradation product, additional studies to obtain such data may be appropriate (Fig. 30.2).

The analytical procedures and reporting in 3QB(R) are similar to those in Q3A. Differences between the analytical procedures used during development and those proposed for the commercial product should also be discussed in the registration application. Reported results should be rounded using conventional rules (see Table 30.4). In Table 30.4, the doses have been divided into more categories than in 3QA, and, therefore, the action thresholds have changed.

The specification for a new drug product should include a list of degradation products expected to occur during manufacture of the commercial product and under recommended storage conditions. This section, again, is similar to Q3A, with the exception of the threshold levels being different. In addition, a final listing of impurities in the specifications should include the same items as in Q3A.

Q3C ICH *Guidance for Industry, Q3C Impurities: Residual Solvents* was published December 1997 [9]. It is intended to provide guidance for recommending acceptable amounts for residual solvents in pharmaceuticals for the safety of the patient. The guidance recommends use of less toxic solvents and describes levels considered to be toxicologically acceptable for some residual solvents. A complete list of the solvents included in this guidance is provided in a companion document entitled

TABLE 30.3 Thresholds for Degradation Products in New Drug Products

Maximum Daily Dose[a]	Threshold[b,c]
Reporting Thresholds	
≤1 g	0.1%
>1 g	0.05%
Identification Thresholds	
<1 mg	1.0% or 5 µg TDI, whichever is lower
1–10 mg	0.5% or 20 µg TDI, whichever is lower
>10 mg–2 g	0.2% or 2 mg TDI, whichever is lower
>2 g	0.10%
Qualification Thresholds	
<10 mg	1.0% or 50 µg TDI, whichever is lower
10–100 mg	0.5% or 200 µg TDI, whichever is lower
>100 mg–2 g	0.2% or 3 mg TDI, whichever is lower
>2 g	0.15%

[a]The amount of drug substance administered per day.

[b]Thresholds for degradation products are expressed either as a percentage of the drug substance or as total daily intake (TDI) of the degradation product. Lower thresholds can be appropriate if the degradation product is unusually toxic.

[c]Higher thresholds should be scientifically justified.

TABLE 30.4   Illustration of Reporting Degradation Product Results for Identification and Qualification in an Application

Raw Result (%)	Reported Result (%) (Reporting Threshold = 0.1%)	Total Daily Intake (TDI) of the Degradation Product (rounded result in μg)	Action	
			Identification Threshold 0.2%	Qualification Threshold 200 μg TDI (equivalent to 0.4%)
50 mg Maximum Daily Dose				
0.04	Not reported	20	None	None
0.2143	0.2	100	None	None
0.349	0.3[a]	150	Yes	None[a]
0.550	0.6[a]	300	Yes	Yes[a]

Raw Result (%)	Reported Result (%) (Reporting Threshold = 0.05%)	Total Daily Intake (TDI) of the Degradation Product (rounded result in mg)	Action	
			Identification Threshold 2 mg TDI (equivalent to 0.11%)	Qualification Threshold 3 mg TDI (equivalent to 0.16%)
1.9 g Maximum Daily Dose				
0.049	Not reported	1	None	None
0.079	0.08	2	None	None
0.183	0.18[a]	3	Yes	None[a,b]
0.192	0.19[a]	4	Yes	Yes[a]

[a]After identification, if the response factor is determined to differ significantly from the original assumptions, it can be appropriate to remeasure the actual amount of the degradation product present and reevaluate against the qualification threshold (see Attachment 1).

[b]Although the reported result of 0.18% exceeds the calculated threshold value of 0.16%, in this case the action is acceptable since the TDI (when rounded) does not exceed 3 mg. Chromatograms with peaks labeled (or equivalent data if other analytical procedures are used) from representative batches, including chromatograms from analytical procedure validation studies and from long-term and accelerated stability studies, should be provided. The applicant should ensure that complete degradation product profiles (e.g., chromatograms) of individual batches are available, if requested.

Q3C—Tables and List [23]. These tables are not included in this chapter but may be found in the ICH or FDA website. The list is not exhaustive, and other solvents may be used and later added to the list.

Residual solvents in pharmaceuticals are defined here as organic volatile chemicals that are used or produced in the manufacture of drug substances or excipients, or in the preparation of drug products. The solvents are not completely removed by practical manufacturing techniques. Appropriate selection of the solvent for the synthesis of drug substance may enhance the yield, or determine characteristics such as crystal form, purity, and solubility. Therefore, the solvent may sometimes be a critical parameter in the synthetic process. This guidance does not address solvents deliberately used as excipients nor does it address solvates. However, the content of solvents in such products should be evaluated and justified.

As there are no therapeutic benefits from residual solvents, all residual solvents should be removed to the extent possible to meet product specifications, good manufacturing practices, or other quality-based requirements. Drug products should contain no higher levels of residual solvents than can be supported by safety data. Some solvents that are known to cause unacceptable toxicities (carcinogens), such as benzene and carbon tetrachloride (Class 1, see Table 1 in Ref. 23), should be avoided in the production of drug substances, excipients, or drug products unless their use can be strongly justified in a risk–benefit assessment. Some solvents associated with less severe toxicity (nongenotoxic animal carcinogens or possible causative agents of other irreversible toxicity such as neurotoxicity or teratogenicity), such as acetonitrile and chlorobenzene (Class 2, see Table 2 in Ref. 23), should be limited in order to protect patients from potential adverse effects. Ideally, less toxic solvents, such as acetic acid and acetone (Class 3, see Table 3 in Ref. 23), should be used where practical.

Residual solvents in drug substances, excipients, and drug products are within the scope of this guidance. Therefore, testing should be performed for residual solvents when production or purification processes are known to result in the presence of such solvents. It is only necessary to test for solvents that are used or produced in the manufacture or purification of drug substances, excipients, or drug products. Although manufacturers may choose to test the drug product, a cumulative method may be used to calculate the residual solvent levels in the drug product from the levels in the ingredients used to produce the drug product. If the calculation results in a level equal to or below that recommended in this guidance, no testing of the drug product for residual solvents need be considered. If, however, the calculated level is above the recommended level, the drug product should be tested to ascertain whether the formulation process has reduced the relevant solvent level to within the acceptable amount. Drug product should also be tested if a solvent is used during its manufacture.

This guidance does not apply to potential new drug substances, excipients, or drug products used during the clinical research stages of development, nor does it apply to existing marketed drug products.

The guidance applies to all dosage forms and routes of administration. Higher levels of residual solvents may be acceptable in certain cases such as short-term (30 days or less) or topical application. Justification for these levels should be made on a case-by-case basis and discussed with the appropriate FDA division.

The methods for establishing exposure limits in compounds are discussed, as are reporting levels. Some analytical procedures for the determination of exposure typically include chromatographic techniques such as gas chromatography for solvents. Any harmonized procedures for determining levels of residual solvents as described in the pharmacopoeias should be used, if feasible. If only Class 3 solvents are present, a nonspecific method such as loss on drying may be used.

The limits of residual solvents may include a value for the Permitted Daily Exposure (PDE), which is the maximum acceptable intake per day of residual solvent in pharmaceutical products. These limits vary depending on the class.

For solvents to be avoided, solvents in Class 1 should not be employed in the manufacture of drug substances, excipients, and drug products because of their unacceptable toxicity or their deleterious environmental effect. However, if their use is unavoidable in order to produce a drug product with a significant therapeutic advance, then their levels should be restricted as shown in Table 1 of Ref. 23 of the companion document, unless otherwise justified. The solvent 1,1,1-trichloroethane is included (Table 1 in Ref. 23) because it is an environmental hazard. The stated limit of 1500 ppm is based on a review of the safety data.

For solvents to be limited, solvents in Class 2 (see Table 2 in Ref. 23) should be limited in pharmaceutical products because of their inherent toxicity. PDEs are given to the nearest 0.1 mg/day, and concentrations are given to the nearest 10 ppm. The stated values do not reflect the necessary analytical precision of determination. Precision should be determined as part of the validation of the method.

For solvents with low toxic potential, solvents in Class 3 (see Table 3 in Ref. 23) may be regarded as less toxic and of lower risk to human health. Class 3 includes no solvent known as a human health hazard at levels normally accepted in pharmaceuticals. However, there are no long-term toxicity or carcinogenicity studies for many of the solvents in Class 3. Available data indicate that they are less toxic in acute or short-term studies and negative in genotoxicity studies. It is considered that amounts of these residual solvents of 50 mg/day or less (corresponding to 5000 ppm or 0.5% under Option 1) would be acceptable without justification. Higher amounts may also be acceptable provided they are realistic in relation to manufacturing capability and GMPs.

For solvents for which no adequate toxicological data were found, the solvents listed (see Table 4 in Ref. 23) may also be of interest to manufacturers of excipients, drug substances, or drug products. However, no adequate toxicological data on which to base a PDE were found. Manufacturers should supply justification for residual levels of these solvents in pharmaceutical products.

30.3.2   U.S. FDA (CDER)

U.S. FDA (CDER) *Guidance for Industry, NDAs: Impurities in Drug Substances* was published February 2000 [24]. The guidance refers applicants to ICH *Q3A Impurities in New Drug Substances* when seeking guidance on identification, qualification, and reporting of impurities in drug substances that are not considered new drug substances. Q3A was developed by the ICH to provide guidance on the information that should be provided in a new drug application (NDA) in support of impurities in new drug substances that are produced by chemical syntheses. The FDA believes that the guidance provided there on identification, qualification, and reporting of impurities should also be considered when evaluating impurities in drug substances produced by chemical syntheses that are not considered new drug substances. ICH Q3A defines a new drug substance (also referred to as a new molecular entity or new chemical entity) as a designated therapeutic moiety that has not been previously registered in a region or member state. The definition also states that a new drug substance may be a complex, a simple ester, or a salt of a previously approved drug substance.

This recommendation applies to applicants planning to submit NDAs and supplements for changes in drug substance synthesis or process. It also applies to holders of Type II Drug Master Files (DMFs) that support such applications. Applicants should note that this recommendation would not apply to DMFs cited in an NDA or supplement if the DMF information has been deemed acceptable for that dosage form, route of administration, and daily intake prior to the publication of the final version of this guidance. Examples of NDAs affected by the recommendation include those submitted for new dosage forms of already approved drug products, or drug products containing two or more active moieties that are individually used in already approved drug products but have not previously been approved or marketed together in a drug product.

This guidance does not apply to applications for biological, biotechnological, peptide, oligonucleotide, radiopharmaceutical, fermentation, and semisynthetic products derived from herbal products or crude products of animal or plant origin, nor does it apply to Abbreviated New Drug Applications (ANDAs). Guidance on drug substances used for ANDA products is available [25].

In February 2005, the FDA published the *Guidance for Industry, ANDAs: Impurities in Drug Substances* [25]. This guidance provides revised recommendations on what chemistry, manufacturing, and controls (CMC) information to include regarding the reporting, identification, and qualification of impurities in drug substances produced by chemical synthesis when submitting original Abbreviated New Drug Applications (ANDAs), Drug Master Files (DMFs) including Type II DMFs, and ANDA supplements for changes in drug substance synthesis or process. The guidance also provides recommendations for establishing acceptance criteria for degradation products (specifically, degradation products of the active ingredient or reaction products of the active ingredient with an excipient(s) and/or immediate container/closure system) in generic drug products. The ANDA document refers to the ICH toxicology test scheme of up to 90 days in two species (rodent and nonrodent). The guidance does not apply to an ANDA or ANDA supplement that has been reviewed prior to the publication of the final guidance.

The submitter is referred to the ICH Q3B(R) guideline [12] that was developed to provide guidance on impurities in drug products for New Drug Applications (NDAs). However, the FDA believes that many of the recommendations provided on impurities in drug products also apply to ANDAs, including:

- Section I, Introduction
- Section II, Rationale for the Reporting and Control of Degradation Products
- Section III, Analytical Procedures
- Section IV, Reporting Degradation Products, Content of Batches
- Attachment 1, Thresholds for Degradation Products

The FDA recommends that the specification for a drug product include a list of degradation products and include in the submission a rationale for the inclusion or exclusion of degradation products in the drug product specification. It is important that the rationale include a discussion of the degradation profiles observed in stability studies and in the degradation profiles observed in the batch(es) under consideration together with a consideration of the degradation profile of the batch(es) manufactured by the proposed commercial process.

The FDA recommends the inclusion of general acceptance criteria of not more than the identification threshold (Fig. 30.2) for any unspecified degradation product and acceptance criteria for total degradation products. In addition, the drug product specification needs to include, where applicable, the following types of degradation products: each specified identified degradation product, each specified unidentified degradation product, any unspecified degradation product with an acceptance criterion of not more than the figure in the identification threshold in Q3B(R), and total degradation products.

The acceptance criterion for degradants should be set as in Q3B(R). In establishing degradation product acceptance criteria, the first critical consideration is whether a degradation product is specified in the United States Pharmacopoeia (USP). If there is a monograph in the USP that includes a limit for a specified identified degradation product, the FDA recommends that the acceptance criterion be set no higher than the official compendial limit. If the level of the degradation product is above the level specified in the USP, the FDA recommends qualification. Then, if appropriate qualification has been achieved, an applicant may wish to petition the USP for revision of the degradation product's acceptance criterion.

If the acceptance criterion for a specified degradation product does not exist in the USP and this degradation product can be qualified by comparison to an FDA-approved human drug product, the acceptance criterion should be consistent with the level observed in the approved human drug product. In other circumstances, the acceptance criterion may need to be set lower than the qualified level to ensure drug product quality. For example, if the level of the metabolite impurity is too high, other quality attributes, like potency, could be seriously affected. In this case, the FDA recommends that the degradation product acceptance criterion be set lower than the qualified level.

Recommended qualification thresholds for degradation products based on the maximum daily dose of the drug are provided in ICH Q3B(R). The decision tree (Fig. 30.2) describes considerations for the qualification of degradation products when the usual qualification threshold recommended in ICH Q3B(R) is exceeded.

30.4 TECHNIQUES

30.4.1 General

For safety and efficacy, it is important to know the purity of the drug substances and drug products. Useful information can often be obtained by carrying out a simple thin layer chromatographic analysis, and the ultraviolet spectrum can also be valuable. It is also possible to measure the absorbance of a solution of the drug and compare the result with tabulated specific absorbance values (the absorbance of a 1% (w/v) solution in a cell of 1 cm path length). For example, the specific absorbances for the drug colchicine in ethanol are 730 and 350 at 243 nm and 425 nm, respectively. Thus, a 10 mg/L solution in ethanol should give absorbance readings of 0.73 and 0.35 at 243 nm and 425 nm, respectively, in a cell of 1 cm path length. However, this procedure, along with other methods, does not take into account the presence of impurities with similar relative molecular masses and specific absorbance values or other impurities. Biologics have their own unique analytical challenges and may need both chemical assays and bioactivity assays (microbial, cellular, metabolic, enzymatic, gene expression). This section discusses chemical assays.

There are many different methods for the detection and quantitation of impurities in materials. Some of these are discussed next. Data on analytical methodology for specific chemicals is readily available on the Web. OSHA has an index of sampling and analytical methods for hundreds of chemicals at http://www.osha.gov/dts/sltc/methods/toc.html.

The National Institute of Standards and Technology (NIST) Chemistry WebBook provides access to data compiled and distributed by NIST under the Standard Reference Data Program and can be found at http://webbook.nist.gov/. The WebBook contains thermochemical data for over 7000 organic and small inorganic compounds, reaction thermochemistry data for over 8000 reactions, IR spectra for over 16,000 compounds, mass spectra for over 15,000 compounds, UV/Vis spectra for over 1600 compounds, gas chromatography data for over 27,000 compounds, electronic and vibrational spectra for over 5000 compounds, constants of diatomic molecules (spectroscopic data) for over 600 compounds, ion energetics data for over 16,000 compounds, and thermophysical property data for 74 fluids.

Method Validation   Method validation is an analytical procedure used to demonstrate that the analytical procedure in question is suitable for its intended purpose and is reproducible. A GMP requirement in 21 CFR 211.165(e) states that the accuracy, sensitivity, specificity, and reproducibility of test methods employed shall be established and documented [26]. The U.S. FDA (CDER) has a draft guidance that discusses analytical procedures and methods validation, chemistry, manufacturing, and controls documentation [27].

This draft guidance provides recommendations to applicants on submitting data for the validation study, including analytical procedures, validation data, and samples to support the documentation of the identity, strength, quality, purity, and potency of drug substances and drug products. The recommendations apply to drug substances and drug products covered in New Drug Applications (NDAs), ANDAs, Biologics License Applications (BLAs), Product License Applications (PLAs), and supplements to these applications. The principles also apply to drug substances and drug products covered in Type II Drug Master Files (DMFs). If a different approach is chosen, the applicant is encouraged to discuss the matter in advance with the center with product jurisdiction to prevent the expenditure of resources on preparing a submission that may later be determined to be unacceptable. Although this guidance does not specifically address the submission of analytical procedures and validation data for raw materials, intermediates, excipients, container closure components, and other materials used in the production of drug substances and drug products, validated analytical procedures should be used to analyze these materials.

The principles of methods validation presented apply to all types of analytical procedures. However, the specific recommendations in this guidance may not be applicable to certain unique analytical procedures for products such as biological, biotechnological, botanical, or radiopharmaceutical drugs. For example, many bioassays are based on animal challenge models, immunogenicity assessments, or other immunoassays that have unique features that should be considered when submitting analytical procedure and methods validation information. For questions on appropriate validation approaches for analytical procedures or submission of information not addressed in this guidance, applicants should consult with the appropriate chemistry review staff at the FDA.

FDA investigators inspect the analytical laboratory testing sites to ensure that the analytical procedures used for release and stability testing comply with GMPs (21 CFR part 211) [26] or good laboratory practices (GLPs; 21 CFR part 58) [28], as appropriate. These assure that proper guidelines and documentation are followed throughout the studies. All analytical procedures are of equal importance from a validation perspective. In general, validated analytical procedures should be used, irrespective of whether they are for in-process, release, acceptance, or stability testing. Each quantitative analytical procedure should be designed to minimize assay variation. Reference standards must be used. A list of information that should typically be included in a description of an analytical procedure is included in this guidance. Impurities and degradants are addressed in the method validation information and the following should be reported:

- Data to demonstrate the stability of all analytical sample preparations through the time required to complete the analysis.
- Representative calculations using submitted raw data, to show how the impurities in drug substance are calculated.
- Information from stress studies.
- Impurities labeled with their names and location identifiers (e.g., RRT for chromatographic data) for the impurity analytical procedure.
- For drug substances:

    A discussion of the possible formation and control of polymorphic and enantiomeric substances.

    Identification and characterization of each organic impurity, as appropriate. This information may not be needed for all products (e.g., botanicals). Other impurities (e.g., inorganics, residual solvents) should be addressed and quantitated.

    Recommendations on submitting information on impurities is provided in various FDA guidances such as the ICH guidance *Q3A Impurities in New Drug Substances* (January 1996).

    A list of known impurities, with structure if available, including process impurities, degradants, and possible isomers.

- For drug products:

    A degradation pathway for the drug substance in the dosage form, where possible.

    Data demonstrating recovery from the sample matrix as illustrated by the accuracy studies.

    Data demonstrating that neither the freshly prepared nor the degraded placebo interferes with the quantitation of the active ingredient.

The draft guideline lists examples of common problems that can delay successful validation.

- Failure to provide a sample of a critical impurity, degradation product, internal standard, or novel reagent.
- Failure to submit well-characterized reference standards for noncompendial drugs.
- Failure to provide sufficient detail or use of unacceptable analytical procedures. For example, use of arbitrary arithmetic corrections, failure to provide system suitability tests, and differing content uniformity and assay analytical procedures without showing equivalence factors for defining corrections as required by the current USP Chapter 905—Uniformity of Dosage Units.
- Failure to submit complete or legible data. For example, failure to label instrument output to indicate sample identity and failure to label the axes.

- Inappropriate shipping procedures. For example, failure to properly label samples, failure to package samples in accordance with product storage conditions, and inadequate shipping forms (e.g., missing customs form for samples from outside the United States).
- Failure to describe proper storage conditions on shipping containers.

Prior to the start of the validation study, conducting a feasibility study will help uncover issues early on so that the main study flows with ease. Feasibility studies address the setup method and system suitability, determine limits of detection (LOD) and quantitation (LOQ), perform forced degradation studies, check placebo for interferences, test related compounds, and check the label and specification claim.

The protocol needs to address specificity, linearity, accuracy, range, LOD/LOQ, precision, and robustness [29].

Specificity is the degree to which the measured response is due to the analyte of interest and not to other substances expected to be present in the sample matrix. For example, degradation products may be formed when the drug substance is exposed to environmental and/or chemical conditions, such as acid hydrolysis (HCl), base hydrolysis (NaOH), oxidation (peroxide), thermal degradation (heat), or photolysis (irradiation).

Linearity is the ability to obtain results that are directly proportional. Standards may be prepared at concentration levels ranging from 50% to 150% of the theoretical range of the analyte in a sample solution concentration prepared according to the method. The upper and lower limits of the linear range need to be reported. A graph of the standard curve and results of linear regression should also be determined. Low-level linearity for impurities needs to be determined, but sometimes impurity reference standards are unavailable. Since impurities are typically determined based on the active ingredient peak, demonstration of linearity at a low level is critical. A low-level linearity curve should include concentrations of 0.05%, 0.1%, 0.5%, 1.0%, 1.5%, and 2.0% of the active compound.

Accuracy is the measure of the total error of a method, including both systematic and random errors. For impurities assays, the accuracy should be assessed on samples (drug substance/drug product) spiked with known amounts of impurities. If impurities or degradation products are not available, it is acceptable to compare results obtained by a second, well-characterized method.

Range is the interval between the upper and lower concentration of analyte for which a suitable level of precision, accuracy, and linearity has been demonstrated.

Limit of Detection (LOD)   The LOD is the lowest concentration of analyte that can be detected, but not necessarily quantitated, by the analytical method. It is usually expressed as concentration of analyte generating an instrument response equivalent to three times the noise. The LOQ is the lowest concentration of analyte that can be determined with acceptable accuracy and precision by the analytical method. It is usually expressed as concentration of analyte generating an instrument response equivalent to ten times the noise.

Precision is the measure of how close the data values are to each other for a number of determinations under the same analytical conditions. ICH has defined precision to contain three components: repeatability (six replicate measurements of a single sample preparation), intermediate precision (ruggedness; second analyst repeats method precision on different instrument, column, day, etc.), and reproducibility (method precision, duplicate measurements of six sample preparations). Precision is expressed as the percent relative standard deviation (%RSD).

Robustness is similar to ruggedness. It is a measure of how the results are affected by variations of different factors internal to the method, as in the mobile phase pH, mobile phase composition, temperature, flow rate, injector/detector temperatures, and oven ramp rates. According to ICH Q2A, the robustness of an analytical procedure is a measure of its capacity to remain unaffected by small but deliberate variations in method parameters and provides an indication of its reliability during normal usage.

Metabolism of Impurities and Degradants   Although they are not true impurities in the drug substance or the drug product, metabolites might be produced *in vivo*. The drug substance or product is metabolized in a manner so that the animal becomes exposed to the new metabolite. These metabolites may be detected from bioanalysis samples (whole blood, plasma, serum, urine). Due to exposure *in vivo*, ICH Q3A states that impurities that are also significant metabolites present in animal and/or human studies are generally considered qualified.

30.4.2   Ultraviolet and Visible (UV/Vis) Spectroscopy

A number of the quantitative methods use ultraviolet (UV) (200–400 nm) or visible (400–800 nm) spectrophotometry. Quantitative analysis of solutions is commonly performed by ultraviolet spectroscopy [30]. The major problem encountered with this technique is interference, and some form of sample purification is needed, such as solvent extraction. The spectrophotometer may be of the single-beam or double-beam type. With a single-beam instrument, light passes from the source through a monochromator and then via a sample cell to the detector. With double-beam instruments, light from the monochromator passes through a beam-splitting device and then via separate sample and reference cells to the detector. Double-beam instruments with automated wavelength scanning and a variety of other features are also available.

30.4.3   Atomic Absorption Spectroscopy

Atoms can absorb energy of a specific wavelength that corresponds to the wavelength they would emit when eroded by a high energy source. In atomic absorption, the energy needed for the atomic emission is supplied by a source other than a flame. The flame is actually the cuvette that holds the sample. The decrease in the emission intensity of the source is proportional to the concentration of atoms in the sample. Atomic absorption spectroscopy is important for the analysis of trace metals in biological fluids [31].

30.4.4   Thin Layer Chromatography (TLC)

Thin layer chromatography (TLC) is a technique for determining the composition of a mixture. It involves the movement by capillary action of a liquid phase (usually an organic solvent) through a thin, uniform layer of stationary phase (usually silica gel, SiO_2) held on a rigid or semirigid support, normally a glass, aluminum, or plastic sheet or plate. Compounds are separated by partition between the mobile and stationary phases. It may be used to establish the extent of a reaction, the purity of a compound, or the presence or absence of materials in fractions from column chromatography. TLC is relatively inexpensive and simple to perform and can be a powerful qualitative technique when used together with some form of sample pretreatment, such as solvent extraction. However, some separations can be difficult to reproduce. The interpretation of results can also be very difficult, especially if a number of drugs or metabolites are present.

30.4.5 High Pressure Liquid Chromatography (HPLC)

In general, chromatography is used to separate mixtures of chemicals into individual components. Once separated, the components can be individually evaluated. With chromatography, separation occurs when the sample mixture is introduced (injected) into a mobile phase. In liquid chromatography (LC), the mobile phase is a solvent. The mobile phase transports the mixture through a stationary phase. The stationary phase is a chemical that can selectively draw components from a sample mixture. The stationary phase is usually contained in a tube (column). Columns can be glass or stainless steel of various dimensions.

The mixture of compounds in the mobile phase will interact with the stationary phase. Individual compounds in the mixture tend to interact at various rates. Those that interact the fastest will exit (elute from) the column first. Those that interact slowest will exit the column last. By changing characteristics of the mobile phase and the stationary phase, different mixtures of chemicals can be separated.

HPLC is commonly used for the separation, identification, purification, and quantification of chemical compounds (Fig. 30.3). Chemical separations can be accomplished since certain compounds have different migration rates given a particular column and mobile phase. Therefore, separation of compounds from each other can occur; the extent or degree of separation is mostly determined by the choice of the stationary phase and the mobile phase. The chromatographer may choose the conditions, such as the proper mobile phase, to allow adequate separation or purification in order to collect or extract the desired compound as it elutes from the stationary phase. Each compound should have a characteristic peak under certain chromatographic conditions. The migration of the compounds and contaminants through the column need to differ enough so that the pure desired compound can be collected or extracted without bringing on any other undesired compound.

Preparative HPLC is the process of isolation and purification of compounds. Analytical HPLC determines information about the sample compound, including identification, quantification, and resolution.

Identification of compounds by HPLC is a critical part of any HPLC assay and is accomplished by researching the literature and by trial and error. After a few steps, a separation assay must be developed. The parameters of this assay should be such that a clean, well-separated peak of the known sample is observed from the chromatograph.

Quantification of compounds by HPLC is the process of determining the unknown concentration of a compound in a known solution. It involves injecting a series of

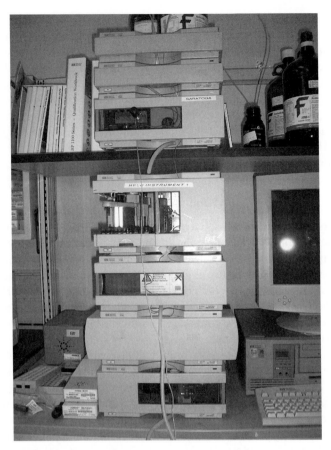

FIGURE 30.3   HPLC. Compliments of Midwest BioResearch, Evanston, IL.

known concentrations of the standard compound solution onto the HPLC for detection. The chromatograph of these known concentrations will give a series of peaks that correlate to the concentration of the compound injected.

30.4.6   Mass Spectrometry (MS)

Mass spectrometry is a powerful analytical tool because it can provide valuable structural information with a high degree of specificity. Compounds enter an electron ionization (mass spectrometer) detector and are bombarded with a stream of electrons causing them to break apart into fragments. These fragments can be large or small pieces of the original molecules and are charged ions with a certain mass. A group of four electromagnets (quadrupole) focuses each of the fragments through a slit and into the detector. The quadrupoles are programmed by the computer to direct only certain fragments through the slit. The rest bounce away. This happens repeatedly for a specific range of fragments. A graph, the mass spectrum, is then produced.

The production of a characteristic mass spectrum or fragmentation pattern acquired for each molecule makes it a definitive and effective tool for identifying unknown impurities or degradation products. This characteristic pattern is a "fingerprint." Comparing the MS "fingerprint" with large mass spectral databases further facilitates identification.

30.4.7 Gas Chromatography (GC) and Combination of GC and MS

As discussed previously, chromatography is used to separate mixtures of chemicals into individual components. The procedure for separation is similar for LC and GC with the exception of the mobile phase. In GC, the mobile phase is an inert gas such as helium.

With the combined GC/MS, the GC separates the components of a mixture. After the individual compounds elute from the GC column, they enter the electron ionization (mass spectrometer) detector. The fragments go through the same procedure as discussed for MS. MS characterizes each of the components individually. A 3D graph is produced, which provides qualitative and quantitative data. By combining the two techniques, an analytical chemist can take an organic solution, inject it into the instrument, separate the individual components, and identify each of them. Furthermore, the researcher can determine the quantities (concentrations) of each of the components.

ICH Q3C states that residual solvents are typically determined using chromatographic techniques such as gas chromatography. Any harmonized procedures for determining levels of residual solvents as described in the pharmacopoeias should be used, if feasible.

30.4.8 MS/MS

The tandem MS method has been used as an alternative to GC/MS. This method uses collision-activated dissociation on a triple quadruple mass spectrometer. This assists in the quick and direct qualitative and semiquantitative analysis. Other benefits of tandem MS include the elimination of most wet chemical and chromatographic separation steps, and the detection of both known and unknown compounds by molecular weight and functional group. A disadvantage is that tandem MS is somewhat less specific than GC/MS in the identification of some isomeric compounds.

30.4.9 HPLC/Mass Spectrometry (LC/MS or LC/MS/MS)

LC/MS data includes molecular weight and structural information that can help identify an impurity or a degradation product.

LC/MS/MS, also known as a triple-quad LC/MS, has become standard in the pharmaceutical analytical laboratory (Fig. 30.4). For the quantitative analysis of many analytes, LC/MS/MS is a fast, universal, selective, and sensitive tool. The quantitation is typically performed with high selectivity, which practically eliminates matrix components. LC/MS/MS is also a very important technique in the bioanalytical arena for characterizing large molecules such as botanicals, biologics, proteins, and peptides, which are typically present in challenging matrices.

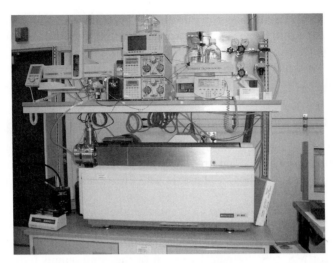

FIGURE 30.4   LC/MS/MS. Compliments of Midwest BioResearch, Evanston, IL.

30.4.10   Common Problems

Meeting GMP Standards for Maintenance and Recordkeeping   The FDA has promulgated 21CFR Part 211, *Current Good Manufacturing Practice for Finished Pharmaceuticals* [26]. There are other sections for the FDA-issued Good Manufacturing Practices (GMPs) and the manufacturer needs to look closely to ensure that the proper regulations are followed. The regulations in this part (21CFR Part 211) contain the minimum current GMP for preparation of drug products in general for administration to humans or animals: for drug products, in Parts 600 through 680, as they pertain to drugs that are also biological products for human use; and in Part 1271, as they are applicable to drugs that are also human cells, tissues, and cellular and tissue-based products (HCT/Ps) and that are drugs.

Maintenance and recordkeeping are addressed in many sections of 21CFR Part 211. Strict guidelines are in place, such as all equipment and utensils shall be cleaned, maintained, and sanitized at appropriate intervals to prevent malfunctions or contamination that would alter the safety, identity, strength, quality, or purity of the drug product beyond the official or other established requirements.

Virtually all actions need to be documented and stored. All records need to be maintained for specified periods, including any production, control, or distribution records; records for all components, drug product containers, closures, and labeling; records for maintenance; and use logs. Therefore, everything needs to be documented and explained so that the study can be reconstructed, if necessary.

For all impurities, approval of the drug product would be based on the applicant's ability to demonstrate that the product is manufactured to ensure both efficacy and safety for patients. This can only be achieved by paying detailed attention to identity, strength, quality, and purity of the products and their components during the entire manufacturing and distribution process.

Locating Suitable Standard and Reference Materials   Occasionally, there may be problems locating suitable standards and reference materials. Some of these may be purchases through a reputable dealer or the USP. Some may be custom made in a laboratory. But no matter which route is selected, documentation of all procedures and steps is critical to be in compliance with GMPs.

Difficulty of Separation of Chromatogram Background Noise If a chromatograph has a lot of peaks, there is a good possibility that all of the nonactive peaks are due to impurities. It is best to look for a method that puts your peak in a clear area. Depending on the type of equipment used for analyses, changes may be made to an existing method to place the peak in a clear area.

30.5   TOXICITY ASSESSMENT

Once it has been determined that an impurity needs to be qualified, research will need to be conducted to establish safety. The literature from peer-reviewed journals will need to be assessed. Toxicology and safety assessment studies may also need to be performed.

30.5.1   Literature-Based Approaches

Literature searches can be obtained in many different ways. There are many companies who offer subscriptions to their search programs, and Information Services professionals are also available to assist you in your search. For those who prefer to perform their own searches for no charge, many websites will provide you with results that include the citations and possibly abstracts. In many cases, there are fees for full text articles. Below is a brief introduction to some of the free databases on the Web. Links are current as of November 2007.

> The U.S. National Library of Medicine (www.nlm.nih.gov) has many links to other databases, including PubMed®, MEDLINE®, TOXNET®, LNM Gateway, LNM Catalog, the Hazardous Substance Data Bank (HSDB) and meeting abstracts. Other resources exist and it is worth a visit to the website.
>
> PubMed/MEDLINE (http://www.ncbi.nlm.nih.gov/entrez/query.fcgi to register) includes over 15 million citations from MEDLINE and other life science journals for biomedical articles back to the 1950s. PubMed includes links to full text articles and other related resources.
>
> TOXNET (http://toxnet.nlm.nih.gov/) contains databases on toxicology, hazardous chemicals, environmental health, and toxic releases. Databases include HSDB, IRIS, CCRIS, GENETOX, TOXLINE, EMIC, DART/ETIC, TRI, and ChemID/*plus*.
>
> LNM Gateway (http://gateway.nlm.nih.gov/gw/Cmd) can be used to search multiple NLM retrieval systems.
>
> LNM Catalog (http://www.ncbi.nlm.nih.gov/entrez/query.fcgi?db=nlmcatalog) provides access to NLM bibliographic data for journals, books, audiovisuals, computer software, electronic resources, and other materials. Links to the library's holdings in LocatorPlus, NLM's online public access catalog, are also provided.

Local, state, national, and international websites exist to provide information on impurities, chemicals, and regulations. For U.S. FDA information, including guidances and regulations, go to www.fda.gov.

30.5.2   Common Testing Requirements for New Impurities

New impurities, depending on the level present in the drug product, will need to be tested for safety. Studies to be performed are based on ICH and FDA guidances and will vary on a case-by-case basis. A few studies may be needed, or the entire list. Discussions with the appropriate division of the FDA for future study strategy may be prudent. Mammalian studies most likely are done in a rodent and a nonrodent species. Rat and dog, respectively, have previously been recommended, but recent tests have used the minipig in place of the dog. In certain specific cases, nonhuman primates may also be used.

The studies include but are not limited to:

- Pharmacodynamics
- Pharmacokinetics
- Safety pharmacology
- Genetic toxicology battery
- Acute dosing
- Repeated-dose studies
- Carcinogenicity
- Reproductive and teratology studies
- Multigeneration assessments
- Special testing as appropriate (i.e., phototoxicity, dermal, inhalation, sensitization, etc.)

If needed, a repeated-dose general toxicity study in rodents and nonrodents can range from a minimum duration of 14 days to 90 days. The clinical route of administration is recommended; however, other routes (i.e., intravenous, intraperitoneal) may be necessary if exposure is an issue. A minimal genetic toxicology battery, consisting of two *in vitro* assays to detect point mutations and chromosomal aberrations, should be conducted with the test article containing the contaminant, although more precision will be gained if the isolated impurity is tested. There may be a need for carcinogenicity studies if the drug product is administered daily for >3 months. Embryo-fetal development assessment may be necessary when the parent drug is used in a population that includes women of childbearing potential. Other reproductive toxicity studies may be requested on a case-by-case basis depending on results of the general toxicity and embryo-fetal developmental studies.

30.5.3   Study Design Based on Exposure, Route, Dosage, and Other Factors

Details of the studies may also need to be discussed with the FDA or other regulatory agencies. Details such as route, dosage, length of exposure, parameters measured, species, and age of animals are just a few considerations in the study design. Study protocols developed by the FDA or the Organisation of Economic Cooperation and Development (OECD) have been used.

30.5.4 Documentation Content and Format

Content of regulatory submissions will vary between regulatory bodies and types of submissions. Within the FDA, for example, there are differences between what is needed for approval of pharmaceuticals, biologics, and medical devices. In addition, each regulatory agency has a specific procedure for formatting. Many are moving toward the Common Technical Document (CTD). Virtually all agencies have guidelines posted on their websites to explain what is necessary for submission. More than one guideline for submissions may exist within an agency.

The FDA CDER Guidance page (http://www.fda.gov/cder/guidance/) has a few links to submission information, including information in Chemistry, Drug Safety, Electronic Submissions, ICH (final and draft), and IND (Investigational New Drug).

Providing the regulatory agency with the information that it needs for product approval is both a science and an art, and in many cases, expert assistance should be sought.

30.6 BRIDGING STUDIES

Changes are made many times during development of a drug substance or a drug product. When most of the preclinical safety testing has already been conducted, and changes are made, it may not be necessary to repeat all of the previous studies. However, a change in manufacturing techniques or a change in the impurity profile would necessitate testing to ensure that the materials before and after the change are comparable in terms of quality, safety, and efficacy. Comparability can often be deduced from available data alone but might sometimes need to be supported by comparability bridging studies.

Bridging studies may consist of toxicology studies in an appropriate species, either rodent and/or nonrodent. The nature of the bridging studies must be determined on a case-by-case basis. Examples of bridging studies are:

- An acute study.
- A repeated-dose study of 90 days' duration. Toxicokinetic samples should be analyzed and blood levels compared to levels observed in animals prior to the change.
- Pharmacodynamic studies would also need to be conducted to detect any possible changes.
- Teratology (Segment II) study in the most sensitive species (rat or rabbit, primarily).
- Pre- and postnatal development including maternal functions (Segment III).
- Other studies as needed.

Chapter 31, Bridging Studies in Pharmaceutical Safety Assessment, has more details of bridging studies.

30.7 DISCUSSION REGARDING TESTING THE DRUG WITH THE IMPURITY VERSUS ACTUAL IMPURITY

What exactly is tested for studies to determine the safety of impurities? As time goes on and the chemists have more experience with the drug substances, they find more efficient methods of producing the substance in hopes that the impurity profile will decrease. Most of the time, especially early on in development, the impurity is already present in the drug substance that is administered to the animals. If the impurity is present in a high enough concentration to provide a relevant dosage to the test systems in repeated-dose studies, the impurity may be considered adequately tested.

ICH Q3A states that the level of any impurity present in a new drug substance that has been adequately tested in safety and/or clinical studies would be considered qualified. ICH Q3B (R) describes considerations for the qualification of degradation products when thresholds are exceeded. If additional safety testing is needed, such studies can be conducted on the new drug product or substance containing the degradation products to be controlled, although studies using isolated degradation products can sometimes be appropriate.

Testing the actual impurity is important in some cases, and it would be prudent for the industry, FDA, and other agencies to hold discussions on this topic. Some impurities are present in rather small amounts. Toxicology tests may not be sensitive enough to characterize their individual toxicities if impurities are tested within a drug substance or product. Testing the toxicity of an impurity present in a drug substance or product in toxicology studies or bridging studies may very well be a waste of time, money, and animals if no toxicity from the impurity is observed due to low levels. However, using the predictive power of several structure–activity relationship (SAR) programs, specific toxicities identified for individual impurities could be assessed.

Testing the impurity at appropriate levels to produce appropriate safety factors for *in vivo* studies would elucidate specific toxicities from the impurity. But more crucial is testing the isolated impurity in genetic toxicology studies. If tested as a component of the drug substance, the exposure of the impurity to the target cells in these studies would be so low that only the most potent mutagens would be detected. To understand the toxicological implications of impurities, testing of the isolated impurity at appropriate concentrations is essential.

ACKNOWLEDGMENTS

I would like to thank Robert E. Osterberg, Office of New Drugs, Center for Drug Evaluation and Research, U.S. Food and Drug Administration, for his review of the draft manuscript for this chapter. I also thank Mike Schlosser, president of Midwest BioResearch, for allowing me to photograph the equipment.

REFERENCES

1. Janssen WF. The story of the laws behind the labels, Part I, 1906 Food and Drugs Act. *FDA Consumer*, June 1981. Available at http://vm.cfsan.fda.gov/~lrd/history1.html.

2. US FDA Center for Biologics Evaluation and Research. *Commemorating 100 Years of Biologics Regulation, Science and the Regulation of Biological Products From a Rich History to a Challenging Future*, 25 September 2002. Available at http://www.fda.gov/cber/inside/centscireg.htm.

3. US FDA Office of Women's Health. *FDA Milestones in Women's Health: Looking Back as We Move into the New Millennium*, 2000. Available at http://www.fda.gov/womens/milesbro.html.

4. Roberts R. *Safety Assessment in Pediatrics*. Center for Drug Evaluation and Research, US Food and Drug Administration; July 8, 1999. Available at www.fda.gov/cder/present/dia-699/sa-dia99/index.htm.

5. US FDA Center for Drug Evaluation and Research. *Time Line: Chronology of Drug Regulation in the United States*. Available at www.fda.gov/cder/about/history/time1.htm.

6. US FDA. *Milestones in U.S. Food and Drug Law History, FDA Backgrounder: Current and Useful Information from the Food and Drug Administration*, August 1995. Available at www.fda.gov/opacom/backgrounders/miles.html.

7. US Department of Health and Human Services, Food and Drug Administration, Center for Drug Evaluation and Research (CDER) and Center for Biologics Evaluation and Research (CBER). *Guidance for Industry, Nonclinical Studies for the Safety Evaluation of Pharmaceutical Excipients*, May 2005.

8. United States Pharmacopoeia (USP), 2005. Available at www.usp.org.

9. ICH. *Guidance for Industry, Q3C Impurities: Residual Solvents*, December 1997. Available at http://www.fda.gov/cder/guidance/index.htm.

10. ICH. *Guidance for Industry, Q1B Photostability Testing of New Drug Substances and Product*, November 1996. Available at http://www.fda.gov/cder/guidance/index.htm.

11. ICH. *Guidance for Industry, Q3A Impurities in New Drug Substances*, February 2003. Available at http://www.fda.gov/cder/guidance/index.htm.

12. ICH. *Guidance for Industry, Q3B(R) Impurities in New Drug Products*, November 2003. Available at http://www.fda.gov/cder/guidance/index.htm.

13. ICH. *Guidance for Industry, Q1A Stability Testing of New Drug Substances and Products*, August 2001. Available at http://www.fda.gov/cder/guidance/index.htm.

14. FDA website, 2005. Available at http://www.fda.gov/cder/guidance/cGMPs/packaging.htm.

15. ICH. *Guidance for Industry, Q6B Specifications: Test Procedures and Acceptance Criteria for Bio-technological/Biological Products*, August 1999. Available at http://www.fda.gov/cder/guidance/index.htm.

16. Osterberg RE. Extractables and leachables in drug products. *Am Coll Toxicol Newslett* 2005;25(1):1020.

17. Osterberg RE. Potential toxicity of extractables and leachables in drug products. *Am Pharm Rev* 2005;8(2):1020–1021.

18. US Department of Health and Human Services, Food and Drug Administration, Center for Drug Evaluation and Research (CDER). *Guidance for Industry, Metered Dose Inhaler (MDI) and Dry Powder Inhaler (DPI), Drug Products Chemistry, Manufacturing, and Controls Documentation*, October 1998. Available at http://www.fda.gov/cder/guidance/index.htm.

19. ICH. *Guideline for Industry, Q2A Text on Validation of Analytical Procedures*, March 1995. Available at http://www.fda.gov/cder/guidance/index.htm.

20. ICH. *Guidance for Industry, Q2B Validation of Analytical Procedures: Methodology*, November 1996. Available at http://www.fda.gov/cder/guidance/index.htm.

21. ICH. *Guidance for Industry, Q6A Specifications: Test Procedures and Acceptance Criteria for New Drug Substances and New Drug Products: Chemical Substances*, December 2000. Available at http://www.fda.gov/cder/guidance/index.htm.

22. Code of Federal Regulations; Title 21, Volume 5; Revised as of 1 April 2005. 21 CFR 314.3(b); Title 21—Food and Drugs, Chapter I—Food and Drug Administration Department of Health and Human Services, Subchapter D—Drugs for Human Use. Part 314, *Application for FDA Approval to Market a New Drug*, Subpart A—*General Provisions*, Sec. 314.3 *Definitions*. Revised as of 1 April 2005. Available at www.fda.gov.

23. ICH. *Guidance for Industry, Q3C—Tables and List*, November 2003, Revision 1. Available at http://www.fda.gov/cder/guidance/index.htm.

24. US Department of Health and Human Services, Food and Drug Administration, Center for Drug Evaluation and Research (CDER). *Guidance for Industry, NDAs: Impurities in Drug Substances*, February 2000. Available at http://www.fda.gov/cder/guidance/3622fnl.htm.

25. US Department of Health and Human Services, Food and Drug Administration, Center for Drug Evaluation and Research (CDER). *Guidance for Industry, ANDAs: Impurities in Drug Substances*, August 2005. Available at http://www.fda.gov/cder/guidance/index.htm.

26. US Department of Health and Human Services, Food and Drug Administration. 21CFR Part 211 *Current Good Manufacturing Practice for Finished Pharmaceuticals*. Revised 1 April 2005. Available at www.fda.gov.

27. US Department of Health and Human Services, Food and Drug Administration, Center for Drug Evaluation and Research (CDER). *Draft Guidance for Industry, Analytical Procedures and Methods Validation Chemistry, Manufacturing, and Controls Documentation*, August 2000. Available at http://www.fda.gov/cder/guidance/2396dft.htm.

28. US Department of Health and Human Services, Food and Drug Administration. 21CFR Part 58 *Good Laboratory Practice for Nonclinical Laboratory Studies*, Revised 1 April 2005. Available at www.fda.gov.

29. Thornton DJ, Thornton BL. Instrumentation systems: reliability and validity issues. In Ward KM, Lehmann CA, Leiken AM, Eds. *Clinical Laboratory Instrumentation and Automation—Principles, Applications and Selection*. Philadelphia: WB Saunders; 1994, Chap 15.

30. Bender JT. Ultraviolet absorption spectroscopy. In *Principles of Chemical Instrumentation*. Philadelphia: WB Saunders; 1987, Chap 6.

31. Narayanan S. Atomic absorption spectroscopy. In *Principles and Applications of Laboratory Instrumentation*. Chicago: American Society of Clinical Pathologists; 1989.

31

BRIDGING STUDIES IN PRECLINICAL PHARMACEUTICAL SAFETY ASSESSMENT

SHAYNE COX GAD

Gad Consulting Services, Cary, North Carolina

Contents

31.1 INTRODUCTION

Preclinical toxicology bridging studies are unique to the safety evaluation of pharmaceuticals [1–3]. While there have been analogues in clinical drug evaluation [4–6], only in the development of new drugs or new drug formulations are we faced with

---

TABLE 31.1   Reasons for Performance of Bridging Studies

Performed to Allow for Changes In:
  Formulations (most common)
  Manufacturing processes
  Optical isomer proportions
  Test species selection/issues
  Impurity or degradant issues
  Active metabolite issues

Performed to Accommodate:
  Correlation of effects between nonclinical species
  Correlation of surrogate markers with established effect on toxicity markers

the need to establish relative comparability between different formulations or dosing regimens of an active ingredient, or show the comparability of response of two different species of animals intended to predict toxicity and safety in humans. Such actions are usually attractive compared to having to repeat an entire nonclinical safety evaluation program. Rather, only one or two critical studies (most sensitive points/tests) are performed to establish relationships.

As technology (and the cost of drug development) has advanced, so has the need for carefully considered bridging studies.

Table 31.1 presents the primary reasons behind the conduct of preclinical bridging studies.

31.2   CAUSES AND SOLUTIONS

An excellent starting place is to consider the reasons for performing bridging studies, as listed in Table 31.1, as well as the issue behind each.

31.2.1   Formulation Changes

Frequently occurring after initial clinical trials, here bridging studies typically look at the change in pharmacokinetics, to assure that the new formulation components do not increase human tolerance issues.

Issue: Addition of new or alteration of combination of formulation components may either cause safety problems not previously seen or alter active ingredient pharmacokinetics in an unfavorable manner.

31.2.2   Changes in Manufacturing Processes or Site

Simple parallel comparative toxicity studies are commonly performed to establish that the active pharmaceutical ingredient (API) and/or clinical product are pharmacokinetically and toxicologically equivalent. These studies are also used if cell lines for producing biotechnology products are changed.

Issue: Changes in the process by which an API is manufactured or in the site where manufacture is performed may change the nature of the API in unforeseen ways; a bridging study serves to confirm equivalent biologic activity (both therapeutic and toxicological).

31.2.3   Alterations in Proportions of Optical Isomers

Assuming that they are not metabolically interconverted, a change in enantiomers in a racemic mixture of API generally calls for a comparative study.

Issue: As chemical development proceeds in parallel with other aspects of the development of a new drug, the proportion of optical isomers may change. As this can have widely different biologic effects, bridging studies seek to establish acceptability of any changes (which subquently can lead to changes in API specification).

31.2.4   Issues of Test Species Selection

First-in-Human (FIH) clinical trials reveal that one or both primary (rodent and nonrodent) species used to evaluate or predict safety to this point are not adequate—either in terms of pharmacokinetics or because a metabolite found in humans is not present (or present in inadequate amounts) in the test species. A bridge with another study must then be performed.

Issue: Nonclinical safety studies form the principal basis for providing confidence that the clinical development of a potential drug can be pursued with acceptable levels of risks. Change to a new process (rodent or more commonly nonrodent) requires adequate characterization of pharmacodynamics and toxicodynamics before longer term studies are conducted.

31.2.5   Impurity and Degradant Issues

These are perhaps becoming the most common types of bridging studies, although in this context the studies are sometimes called qualification studies. The needs arise either as extended stability studies disclose new or increased levels of a degradant formed as the result of a stability issue, or as impurities are discovered in newly produced lots of either API or clinical formulations.

Issue: The detection of an impurity or degradant in a pharmaceutical product presents a potential new and additional risk to patients exposed to the product. The magnitude (and acceptability) of potential risk must be established before use/evaluation clinically.

31.2.6   Active Metabolite Issues

Particularly in accordance with the new International Conference on Harmonization (ICH) and Center for Drug Evaluation and Research (CDER) guidelines, the need for these studies usually arises subsequent to the determination that there is an active metabolite present in humans at significant levels (the guidelines say 10% of the total area under the curve (AUC)), but lower levels have triggered FDA requests. The result may be a variation of the test species case. Selection of test species with the benefit of at least a metabolite profile in microsomes or hepatocytes will reduce but not exclude the possibility of this problem.

Issue: Active (or potentially active) metabolites that occur in human beings at levels not previously adequately evaluated in NCS studies may represent a significant risk to patients/subjects and must be evaluated for relevant potential clinical issues before further clinical development is pursued.

31.2.7 Correlation of Effects Between Nonclinical Species

It sometimes comes to pass that findings in one species are not readily apparent in another. This may be due to a wide variety of reasons but special studies "extending" evaluation in the species not showing the effect (such as achieving an equivalent level of systemic exposure) may serve to clarify relevance to humans.

Issue: As pointed out in Table 31.2, sometimes the identified potential toxicities in one of the species utilized in NCS evaluations are vastly different (usually to the worse) from the other species. In this case, unless there is a known basis for the difference that allows identification of which prediction is more relevant to potential clinical safety, such relevance (or basis for difference) needs to be established.

31.2.8 Correlation of Surrogate Markers with Established Effects on Toxicity Indicators

Subsequent to the performance of nonclinical systemic toxicity studies, it can occur that one wishes to demonstrate that surrogate markers may serve to identify an adverse effect in a less invasive manner, or to predict the early stages of effects before they become serious or irreversible. This particularly occurs when the actual toxic effect would be either unacceptable or highly undesirable in patients.

Issue: While Table 31.1 presents the major reasons for performing bridging studies, there are other potential reasons. There are a common set of inconsistencies or

TABLE 31.2 Troubleshooting in General Toxicology

Unexpected toxicity compared with prior tests	Change in formulation or batch of test chemical; poor predictivity of dose range-finder studies due to factors such as differences in animal age, supplier, or husbandry.
Variation in individual response	Metabolic polymorphism or other genetic factor; social factors in group housing (e.g., nutrition status)
Low systemic concentration or area under the curve (AUC)	Poor absorption or poor formulation; isotonicity is important in parenteral formulations; extensive first-pass effect; short half-life.
Low toxicity	Low availability; inappropriate route of administration or dose selection.
Interspecies differences	Different ADME; different mechanism of effect; species-specific mechanisms such as peroxisome proliferation; enterohepatic recirculation; different expression of or affinity for pharmacological receptors.
Different response in males and females	Especially in rodents; due to different activities of metabolism enzymes in liver particularly but also physiological differences such as α_2-microglobulin excretion in males.

problems that arise from many standard safety evaluation programs. Table 31.2 presents these, as well as the common genesis of their occurrence.

31.3 ISSUES OF BRIDGING STUDY DESIGN

31.3.1 Test Compound(s)

What test material is used in a bridging study is dictated by the issue to resolve because in most cases a portion of the question posed can be phrased as "Is the new drug material equivalent to that previously evaluated?" with equivalence potentially being pharmacokinetic, pharmacodynamic, or toxicodynamic. This being the case, there are two test materials/formulations to be included in a bridging study, with the first being the defined "standard" or material to date. This is often called the reference material.

The second (or "new" or "different") material will then generally be the "standard" with the extreme degree of changed nature (the most impurity or degradant or optical isomer) or isolated metabolite or new formulation.

31.3.2 Basic Bridging Study Design

The most common is the comparative study, in which at least two groups of test animals are given two different doses (low and high) of the reference material, two more are similarly given doses of the changed material (or metabolite), and a fifth group acts as a control, receiving only vehicle or formulations. The test animal species employed is determined by the issue to be resolved.

Test material administration is by the intended clinical route, with the intended frequency of administration (unless, of course, this is the issue to be addressed). Duration should be from 2 to 4 weeks.

31.3.3 Comparative (or Base) Species Data: Historical or Concurrent

While in bridging studies (unlike most other NCS studies), the direct comparison of concern is between the reference and new active material groups, this is not always or purely the case. Sometimes (such as with active metabolites), we are comparing responses or results between new material groups and a control group. While a concurrent control is almost always the most appropriate comparator, considerations of variability of the normal range in a historical population may be critical to understanding the relevance of a change or effect seen with a new material.

REFERENCES

1. Anderson C, et al. Bridging studies in Asia and the impact of the ICH E5 guideline. *Drug Information J* 2003;37:107(S)–116(S).
2. Arnold DL, Grice HC, Krewski DR. *Handbook of In Vivo Toxicity Testing.* San Diego: Academic Press; 1990.
3. Gad SC. *Drug Safety Evaluation.* Hoboken, NJ: Wiley-Interscience; 2002.

4. Liu JP, Chow SC. Bridging studies in clinical development. *J Biopharm Stat* 2002;12(3):359–367.

5. Naito C. Implementation of the bridging study strategy and extension of the "bridging" concept: current status. *Drug Information J* 2003;37:149(S)–154(S).

6. Naito C. Necessity and requirements of bridging studies and their present status in Japan. *Int J Clin Pharmacol Ther* 2000;38(2):80–86.

INDEX